KU-094-851

Principles

of Orthopaedic

Medicine

and Surgery

GWENT HEALTHCARE NHS TRUST
LIBRARY
ROYAL GWENT HOSPITAL
NEWPORT

2081744

617.3 WIE

Royal Gwent Hospital Library

GWR000006409

Principles
of Orthopaedic
Medicine
and Surgery

Sam W. Wiesel, M.D.

Executive Vice President for Health Sciences and
Executive Dean, Georgetown University Medical Center
Professor and Chairman, Department of Orthopaedic Surgery
Georgetown University School of Medicine
Washington, D.C.

John N. Delahay, M.D.

Peter Cyrus and Rose Dignan Rizzo Professor of Orthopaedic Surgery
Chief, Division of Pediatric Orthopaedics
Vice Chairman, Department of Orthopaedic Surgery
Georgetown University School of Medicine
Washington, D.C.

W.B. SAUNDERS COMPANY
A Harcourt Health Sciences Company
Philadelphia   London   New York   St. Louis   Sydney   Tokyo

W.B. SAUNDERS COMPANY
A Harcourt Health Sciences Company

The Curtis Center
Independence Square West
Philadelphia, Pennsylvania 19106

Library of Congress Cataloging-in-Publication Data

Principles of orthopaedic medicine and surgery / [edited by] Sam W. Wiesel, John N. Delahay.

p.   cm.

Includes bibliographical references and index.

ISBN 0–7216–8189–1

1. Orthopaedics.   2. Orthopaedic surgery.   I. Wiesel, Sam W.
II. Delahay, John N.   [DNLM: 1. Musculoskeletal Diseases—diagnosis.
2. Orthopaedic Procedures.   3. Orthopaedics—methods.
WE 140 P957 2001]

RD731. P9195 2001   616.7—dc21

DNLM/DLC   00–023913

Publisher Director, Surgery: Richard Lampert
Manuscript Editors: Thomas Stringer, Anne Ostroff
Production Manager: Natalie Ware
Illustration Specialist: Walter Verbitski
Book Designer: Gene Harris
Indexer: Dennis Dolan

PRINCIPLES OF ORTHOPAEDIC MEDICINE AND SURGERY   ISBN 0–7216–8189–1

Copyright © 2001 by W.B. Saunders Company.

All rights reserved. No part of this publication may be reproduced or transmitted in any form or by any means, electronic or mechanical, including photocopy, recording, or any information storage and retrieval system, without permission in writing from the publisher.

Printed in the United States of America.

Last digit is the print number: 9   8   7   6   5   4   3   2   1

This book is dedicated to Reverend Leo J. O'Donovan, S.J.,
President, Georgetown University,
with appreciation for his commitment to excellence
in medical education and for his friendship.

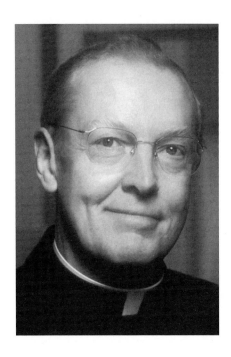

Contributors

Christopher E. Attinger, M.D.
Professor, Plastic Surgery, and Professor, Orthopaedic Surgery, Georgetown University School of Medicine; Director, Wound Healing Center, Georgetown University Hospital, Washington, D.C.
Wound Management in the Orthopaedic Patient

George P. Bogumill, Ph.D., M.D.
Distinguished Professor of Orthopaedic Surgery, Georgetown University School of Medicine, Washington, D.C.; Clinical Professor of Surgery, Uniformed Services University of the Health Sciences, Bethesda, Maryland; Consultant, Orthopaedic Surgery, Walter Reed Army Medical Center, Washington, D.C.
Tumors of the Musculoskeletal System

Daniel J. Clauw, M.D.
Associate Professor of Medicine and Chief, Division of Rheumatology, Georgetown University School of Medicine, Washington, D.C.
Rheumatic Disorders

Paul S. Cooper, M.D.
Associate Professor of Orthopaedic Surgery and Chief, Division of Foot and Ankle Surgery, Georgetown University School of Medicine, Washington, D.C.
Musculoskeletal Infections; The Foot and Ankle

John N. Delahay, M.D.
Peter Cyrus and Rose Dignan Rizzo Professor of Orthopaedic Surgery; Chief, Division of Pediatric Orthopaedics; and Vice Chairman, Department of Orthopaedic Surgery, Georgetown University School of Medicine, Washington, D.C.
The Development of the Musculoskeletal System and Growth Plate; Basic Science of Cartilage and Bone; Biomechanics and Biomaterials; Principles of Musculoskeletal Trauma; Musculoskeletal Infections; Metabolic Bone Disease; General and Regional Problems in Children; Musculoskeletal Trauma in Children

Brian G. Evans, M.D.
Associate Professor of Orthopaedic Surgery and Chief of Joint Reconstruction, Georgetown University School of Medicine, Washington, D.C.
Metabolic Bone Disease; The Hip and Femur

Maria Elmina D. Fernandez, M.D.
Fellow, Department of Neurology, Georgetown University School of Medicine, Washington, D.C.
Clinical Electrophysiology

Mustafa A. Haque, M.D.
Clinical Instructor in Orthopaedic Surgery and Chief of Hand Surgery, Georgetown University School of Medicine, Washington, D.C.
The Elbow and the Forearm; Hand and Wrist Surgery

William Harvey, M.D.
Radiology Resident, Georgetown University Medical Center, Washington, D.C.
Imaging in Orthopaedic Surgery

John J. Klimkiewicz, M.D.
Clinical Instructor in Orthopaedic Surgery and Chief of Sports Medicine, Georgetown University School of Medicine, Washington, D.C.
Physical Diagnosis

William C. Lauerman, M.D.
Associate Professor of Orthopaedic Surgery and Chief, Division of Spinal Surgery, Georgetown University School of Medicine, Washington, D.C.
Pediatric Spine; The Spine

Frank Petzke, M.D.
Fellow, Division of Rheumatology, Georgetown University Hospital, Washington, D.C.
Rheumatic Disorders

Steven C. Scherping, Jr., M.D.
Clinical Instructor in Orthopaedic Surgery, Georgetown University School of Medicine, Washington, D.C.
Physical Diagnosis

Benjamin Shaffer, M.D.
Clinical Associate Professor of Orthopaedic Surgery,
    Georgetown University School of Medicine,
    Washington, D.C.
*Principles of Sports Medicine; The Shoulder and Arm;
    The Knee and Leg*

Michael Sirdofsky, M.D.
Associate Professor and Interim Chairman, Department of
    Neurology, Georgetown University School of
    Medicine, Washington, D.C.
Clinical Electrophysiology

Sam W. Wiesel, M.D.
Executive Vice President for Health Sciences and
    Executive Dean, Georgetown University Medical
    Center; Professor and Chairman, Department of
    Orthopaedic Surgery, Georgetown University School of
    Medicine, Washington, D.C.
A Word About "Outcomes"; The Spine

Lawrence Yao, M.D.
Clinical Associate Professor of Radiology, Georgetown
    University School of Medicine, Washington, D.C.
Imaging in Orthopaedic Surgery

Preface

The purpose of this text is to give an overview of orthopaedic medicine and surgery. Although its intended audience is residents in orthopaedics and rheumatology, emergency and primary care physicians will also find it quite useful. *Principles of Orthopaedic Medicine and Surgery* is a practical guide to the diagnosis and management of musculoskeletal problems, as well as a reference for specific conditions.

Each pathologic entity is approached in a consistent manner: first, a clear definition of the condition is presented. Next, the history, physical findings, and laboratory/radiographic results are described. Third, a differential diagnosis is presented, to be considered before confirming or eliminating each disorder. The natural history is then reviewed, and finally the treatment options are discussed.

After the review of each condition in a specific anatomic area, an algorithm is provided. This device is helpful because patients present not with a specific pathologic problem but rather with a constellation of historical, physical, and radiographic findings. The task confronting the examining physician is to integrate these clinical variables into the formulation of a logical diagnosis and then to develop a treatment plan. The physician's ability to achieve this goal is determined by the accuracy of his or her thought process. An algorithm structures and teaches these processes.

During the preparation of this edition, it has been very exciting and stimulating to work with all the members of the Georgetown University Medical Center Department of Orthopaedics. Everyone has been enthusiastic and brings great expertise to his or her area of interest. We are most appreciative of each contribution, and we are very proud of the final text.

SAM W. WIESEL, M.D.
JOHN N. DELAHAY, M.D.

NOTICE

Medicine is an ever-changing field. Standard safety precautions must be followed, but as new research and clinical experience broaden our knowledge, changes in treatment and drug therapy may become necessary or appropriate. Readers are advised to check the most current product information provided by the manufacturer of each drug to be administered to verify the recommended dose, the method and duration of administration, and the contraindications. It is the responsibility of the treating physician, relying on experience and knowledge of the patient, to determine dosages and the best treatment for the patient. Neither the publisher nor the editor assumes any responsibility for any injury and/or damage to persons or property arising from this publication.

THE PUBLISHER

Contents

Section 1
Basic Science

Chapter 1

The Development of the Musculoskeletal System and Growth Plate

John N. Delahay, M.D.

A discussion of musculoskeletal anomalies must be based on a thorough understanding of the genetics, embryology, and postnatal development of the musculoskeletal system. Approximately 5% of babies are born with some type of congenital defect. Many of these defects have a genetic basis, and others do not. Conversely, a number of genetic diseases are not identified at birth and require a period of growth and development before they became apparent. Nevertheless, an appreciation of the normal development of the musculoskeletal system is integral to a more thorough understanding of these congenital defects.

GENETICS

In the era of molecular genetics, it is well documented that a number of biochemical abnormalities have a direct impact on subsequent structural and functional abnormalities of the musculoskeletal system. The Human Genome Project has given impetus to the identification of specific gene defects of heritable diseases. Great interest now exists in the development of gene therapy for some of these diseases, such as Huntington's disease and cystic fibrosis.

Advances in the techniques of gene mapping have permitted the identification of causative genes for many conditions, including many skeletal dysplasias, connective tissue disorders, muscular dystrophies, and peripheral neuropathies, as well as unusual syndromes with orthopaedic manifestations. It is striking to realize that such dramatic phenotypic anomalies can result from an isolated gene alteration.

In 1866 Gregor Mendel defined the classic patterns of inheritance. The rules governing the assortment of genetic information are as valid now as they were then. Most genetic diseases fall into one of three groups. In the first group are isolated gene defects, which are governed by the principles of mendelian inheritance. Abnormalities of the chromosomes, such as deletions and translocations, are in the second group. Third, the heterogeneous group of polygenic defects are somehow the result of the interplay between genetic and environmental factors.

Genetic diseases can present at any age. Specifically congenital diseases, such as clubfeet, developmental dys-

plasia of the hip (DDH), and various skeletal dysplasias, are present at birth. Some can present in childhood, such as Duchenne's muscular dystrophy and vitamin D–resistant rickets. Others, such as scoliosis, are more typically seen in the adolescent age group. The prevalence of various genetic diseases also varies widely. For example, DDH is seen in approximately 1 per 1000 live births, whereas achondroplasia is seen in approximately 1 in 50,000 live births.

It would seem obvious that a careful family history and subsequent development of a family pedigree would be an important step in the evaluation and subsequent management of a child with a genetic abnormality. There are legitimate reasons to develop an accurate pedigree. Genetic counseling, the determination of inheritance patterns, and an assessment of the likelihood that siblings will be affected all depend on this information.

Mendelian Inheritance

The common patterns that typify classic mendelian inheritance are specifically predicated upon the presence or absence of an abnormal gene on a chromosome. If the chromosome in question is unrelated to gender determination it is called an autosome. However if the gene is on one of the sex chromosomes, it is said to be X-linked. In addition, the pattern may be dominant, requiring only a single allele of the abnormal gene to express the trait, or it may be recessive, whereby two alleles are required to express the trait. Therefore, a heterozygous individual (with one allele of the abnormal gene) will express a dominant trait, whereas the homozygous state (with both alleles) is required to express a recessive trait. The four patterns typically seen are:

1. Autosomal dominant
2. Autosomal recessive
3. X-linked dominant
4. X-linked recessive

AUTOSOMAL DOMINANT CONDITIONS (Fig. 1–1)

This type of inheritance typically produces nonfatal structural abnormalities, such as tarsal coalition. As one would

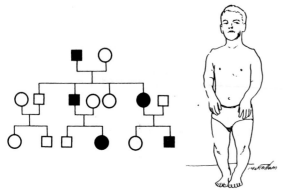

Figure 1–1. Pedigree chart—autosomal dominant inheritance pattern. (From Simon SR [ed]: Orthopaedic Basic Science. American Academy of Orthopaedic Surgeons.)

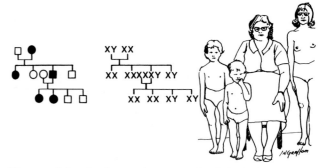

Figure 1–3. Pedigree chart—gender-linked dominant inheritance pattern. (From Simon SR [ed]: Orthopaedic Basic Science. American Academy of Orthopaedic Surgeons.)

expect, the heterozygote will express the condition. Expression of a genetic trait suggests a rather wide variation in the severity of the manifestation. Approximately half of the offspring will be affected, with no male/female preference. The unaffected individuals will not be able to transmit the trait. Achondroplasia is another example of this pattern. The fact that 50% of cases of achondroplasia result from spontaneous mutations is typical of this pattern of inheritance.

AUTOSOMAL RECESSIVE CONDITIONS (Fig. 1–2)

As a generalization, recessive conditions tend to be enzymatic defects, or as previously called, inborn errors of metabolism. Both alleles of a given gene must be abnormal for the condition to be expressed; therefore, only a homozygote will manifest the condition. It is possible for the parents to be unaffected but carriers of the abnormal gene. Approximately 25% of the offspring are affected, again with no male/female preference. Diastrophic dwarfism, the mucopolysaccharidoses, Ehlers-Danlos syndrome, and ochronosis are all autosomal recessive diseases.

X-LINKED DOMINANT CONDITIONS (Fig. 1–3)

The heterozygote manifests the condition, but it is the affected mother who transmits the X-linked gene to 50% of her daughters and 50% of her sons. An affected father will transmit the X-linked gene to 100% of his daughters and none of his sons. The fact that father-to-son transmission does not occur is a critical characteristic of this inheri-

tance pattern. Male children who inherit the trait are generally more severely involved than are females. The classic orthopaedic disease that is X-linked dominant is vitamin D–resistant rickets.

X-LINKED RECESSIVE CONDITIONS (Fig. 1–4)

Because two alleles carrying this trait are required in order to manifest the condition, those who will be affected are the homozygote female and the heterozygote male, because the male has only one X chromosome. The heterozygote female will be a carrier of the trait but will not manifest it. Therefore, the affected father will transmit the gene to all his daughters, who will become carriers, and to none of his sons. The carrier female transmits the gene to half of her daughters, who also will be carriers, and half of her sons, who will be affected. Two important diseases resulting from this form of inheritance are classic hemophilia and Duchenne's muscular dystrophy.

Polygenic Inheritance (Fig. 1–5)

It has been well recognized for years that many genetic diseases are the result of multiple genes that interact with environmental factors to produce a given trait. The typical gaussian curve (see Fig. 1–5) is frequently used to depict what has been referred to as the threshold of risk in a given population. If there is a first-degree relative who has a

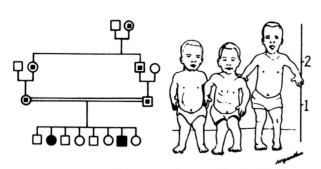

Figure 1–2. Pedigree chart—autosomal recessive inheritance pattern. (From Simon SR [ed]: Orthopaedic Basic Science. American Academy of Orthopaedic Surgeons.)

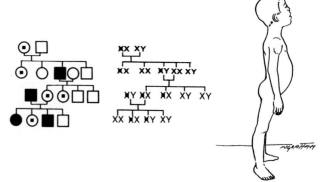

Figure 1–4. Pedigree chart—gender-linked recessive inheritance pattern. (From Simon SR [ed]: Orthopaedic Basic Science. American Academy of Orthopaedic Surgeons.)

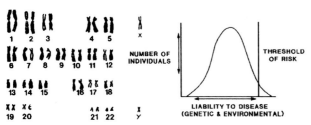

Figure 1–5. Composite diagram—polygenic inheritance. (From Simon SR [ed]: Orthopaedic Basic Science. American Academy of Orthopaedic Surgeons.)

given trait, such as scoliosis, there is clearly an increased risk for other relatives to manifest the trait. This can be represented by a shift of the curve or a lowering of the threshold. This threshold of risk is affected by race, sex, and to some degree by geography. Clubfoot is a good example of a polygenic trait. It is more common in males than females, with a ratio of 2:1. It is typically bilateral in about half of the patients. On the other hand, DDH, which has the same incidence as clubfoot, is a female dominant trait, with a ratio of 6:1. It is interesting to note that when clubfeet occur in the female or DDH in the male, these patients are generally more severely affected and more difficult to treat.

Chromosomal Abnormalities

This third category of genetic disease results from rearrangements within a given chromosome. These abnormalities can include extra chromosomes, referred to as a trisomy, or partial or complete loss of a chromosome, referred to as a deletion. In addition, mosaics and translocations of genetic material can also be grouped under this heading. Many of these chromosomal aberrations result in spontaneous abortions. It has been estimated that approximately 1% of live-born children have some type of chromosomal aberration. Trisomy 21 (Down syndrome) is certainly the most common disease in this category, with an incidence of 1 per 700 live births.

ORTHOPAEDIC EMBRYOLOGY

Following the introductory discussion on genetics, it appears appropriate to consider the prenatal development of the musculoskeletal system. All bone of the musculoskeletal system begins as mesenchymal condensations (Fig. 1–6) from a primary germ layer with multiple mechanical and chemotactic factors actively influencing the cellular differentiation. These condensations of cells typically form bone in one of two ways. Intramembranous bone formation occurs with the condensation of mesenchymal cells. They produce a mucoprotein matrix in which collagen becomes embedded. Subsequent mineralization converts the anlage to bone without an intermediate cartilage step. The second way is the more classic cartilage model bone (enchondral ossification).

Intramembranous Bone Formation

The skull is a good example of intramembranous bone formation. Initially, a small group of cells aggregate, divide, and form random cords of cells. These cells are high in alkaline phosphatase, and as one would expect, rapid calcification occurs and subsequent ossification forms primary trabecular bone. The calvarial portion of the skull forms in this manner. It is important to remember, however, that the basilar portions of the skull, such as the sphenoids, ethmoids, and petrous portions of the temporal bones, are formed enchondrally. The first fetal bone to ossify, the clavicle, is formed intramembranously.

Enchondral Ossification

The major components of the musculoskeletal system originate from the mesodermal layer of the trilaminar embryo.

Figure 1–6. Histologic study of fetus, at approximately 4 weeks' gestation, shows undifferentiated mesenchymal tissue within the limb bud, with early central condensation forming "anlage" of musculoskeletal structures. (From Bogumill GP, Schwamm HA: Orthopaedic Pathology: A Synopsis With Clinical and Radiographic Correlation. Philadelphia, WB Saunders, 1984.)

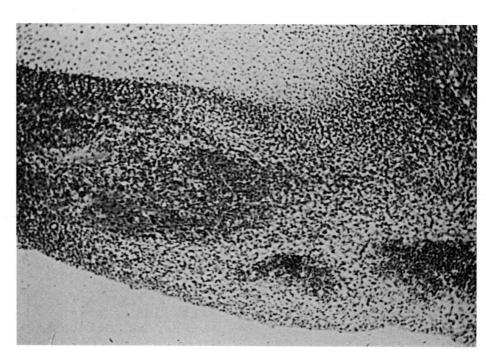

One can trace the development of the major long bones through the enchondral process. The primitive limb bud appears around the fifth week of embryonic life (Fig. 1–7). It is about that time that a tubular condensation of mesenchyme develops centrally in the limb bud. During the sixth week, the mesenchyme differentiates into cartilage through the process of chondrification. Both interstitial and apposi-

tional growth occur. In the seventh week, the cartilage model is penetrated by a vascular spindle, and subsequently, a sleeve of primitive bone is seen surrounding it (Fig. 1–8). Progressively, necrosis of the central cartilage occurs. Once this vascular spindle is established, the central portion of the model is populated by osteoblasts. As matrix is secreted, immature bone is formed. Once the central

A. Changes in Position of Limbs Before Birth

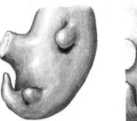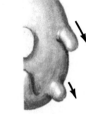

At 5 weeks. Upper and lower limbs have formed as finlike appendages pointing laterally and caudally

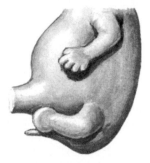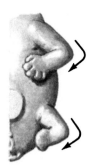

At 6 weeks. Limbs bend anteriorly, so that elbows and knees point laterally, palms and soles face trunk

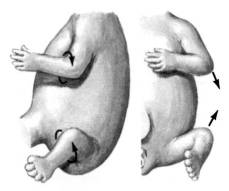

At 7 weeks. Upper and lower limbs have undergone 90° torsion about their long axes, but in opposite direction, so that elbows point caudally and knees cranially

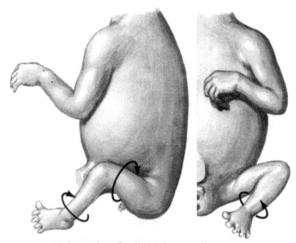

At 8 weeks. Torsion of lower limbs results in twisted, or "barber pole," arrangement of their cutaneous innervation

B. Precartilage Mesenchymal Cell Concentrations of Appendicular Skeleton at 6th Week

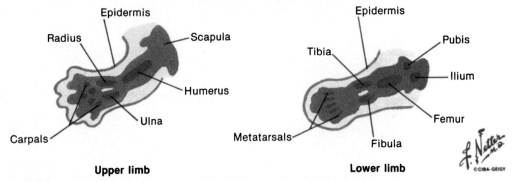

Upper limb

Lower limb

Figure 1–7. *A,* Changes in position of limbs before birth. *B,* Precartilage mesenchymal cell concentrations of appendicular skeleton at sixth week. (From Netter FH: The CIBA Collection of Medical Illustrations, Volume 8. Summit, NJ, CIBA-GEIGY Corporation.)

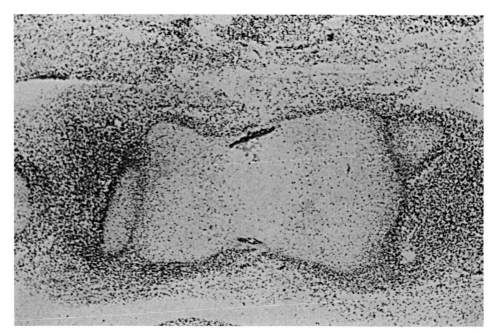

Figure 1–8. Histologic study of fetus, at approximately 8 weeks' gestation, shows earliest ossification. A sleeve, or collar, of bone is present on the outer surface of the cartilage model. (From Bogumill GP, Schwamm HA: Orthopaedic Pathology: A Synopsis With Clinical and Radiographic Correlation. Philadelphia, WB Saunders, 1984.)

portion of the model is ossified, it is referred to as a primary ossification center (Fig. 1–9). Further ossification of this primary ossification center can occur both enchondrally and intramembranously. Keep in mind that bone formed under the primitive periosteum does so intramembranously, whereas the bone formed at the ends is made enchondrally.

From the second through the sixth embryonic months, progressive changes occur in the tubular bones. First, the central (medullary) canal cavitates, leaving a hollow tube of bone with a large mass of cartilage persisting at each end. Within these masses of cartilage, the secondary ossification center, or epiphysis, will form (Fig. 1–10). A cartilage plate, the physis or growth plate, persists between the developing epiphysis and the metaphysis. This structure,

the physis, is responsible for longitudinal growth of the long bone. On the other hand, the periosteum is primarily responsible for latitudinal growth, thereby increasing the girth.

Neuromuscular Development

Recall that during the second week of embryonic life, the embryo itself is only bilaminar, that is, ectoderm and endoderm. At the caudal end of the bilaminar embryo is an area referred to as the primitive streak, a cluster of cells that invaginates between the two layers of the bilaminar embryo. This third layer subsequently formed is referred to as the mesoderm. This mesoderm is critical to the development of the bulk of the muscular and skeletal

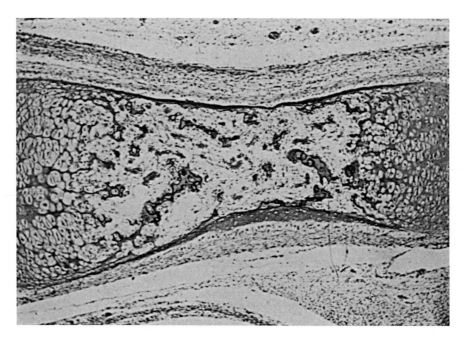

Figure 1–9. Primary ossification center of fetus, at approximately 14 weeks' gestation, shows that the cartilage cells have been removed almost entirely from the center, leaving remnants of acellular cartilage matrix. Bone deposits on the cartilage remnants will form primary trabeculae. Note that the primary sleeve, or collar, of bone has extended along both margins and is located adjacent to the hypertrophied cartilage at each epiphyseal end. (From Bogumill GP, Schwamm HA: Orthopaedic Pathology: A Synopsis With Clinical and Radiographic Correlation. Philadelphia, WB Saunders, 1984.)

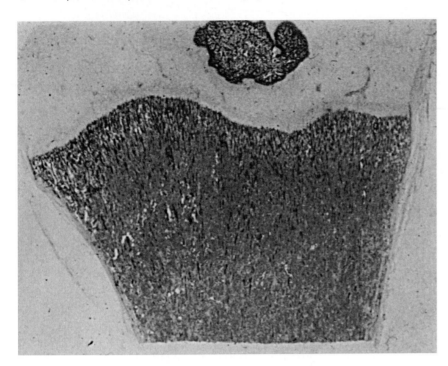

Figure 1–10. Early secondary ossification center of mature fetus. The formation of the secondary ossification centers in the lower tibia and upper femur coincide with fetal maturity. The secondary center does not begin in the center of the epiphysis, but nearer the growth plate. Expansion, therefore, is eccentric. (From Bogumill GP, Schwamm HA: Orthopaedic Pathology: A Synopsis With Clinical and Radiographic Correlation. Philadelphia, WB Saunders, 1984.)

systems. However, it should be remembered that the neural structures of the central nervous system are ultimately developed from cells originating from the ectoderm.

Around the third week, ectodermal induction results in the formation of a neural plate. The edges of this neural plate curl dorsally to form a neural tube (Fig. 1–11). Beginning in the center and continuing to each end, this neural tube will begin to close. Obviously, failure to close cranially results in anencephaly, and failure to close caudally results in spina bifida. A population of ectodermal cells parallel to the closed neural tube, referred to as neural crest cells, are the precursors of the dorsal root ganglia and much of the peripheral nervous system. Most of neural tube development is guided by notochordal induction. The notochord, which has been previously derived from the primitive knob, a cellular aggregate of the bilaminar embryo, has been cited by many to be the "pacemaker" of the neural tube. The mesodermal plate parallels the notochord in its development, thus elongating at the anterior end first, with more caudal elements being added later.

Mesodermal Differentiation

Two large masses of mesoderm are seen on each side of the neural tube and are thus referred to as paraxial mesoderm. Three distinct areas in this paraxial mesoderm have been identified: (1) medial mesoderm ultimately will form the axial musculature, (2) the intermediate portion of the paraxial mesoderm in large part develops into the genitourinary (GU) system, and (3) the lateral mesoderm will give rise to the musculature of the thoracic and abdominal cavities, as well as the rib cage. The intimate proximity of the medial and intermediate mesoderm clearly demonstrates why GU system anomalies are the most common associated defects in congenital musculoskeletal disease. Next in frequency are cardiac anomalies, owing to the fact that the heart is also of mesodermal origin.

At about 4 weeks of embryologic life, the paraxial mesoderm will segment into blocks of cells referred to as somites (Fig. 1–12). The somites will number between 42 and 44. Once the somites have segmented, beginning cranially and progressing caudally over a 10-day period, they will further differentiate into three cell masses—a dermatome, a myotome, and sclerotome, forming skin, muscle, and skeleton, respectively. The limb buds will develop from progressive differentiation of these somites. As mentioned earlier, the limb buds are identifiable around the fifth week of embryonic life.

Development of Joints (Fig. 1–13)

Condensations occur in the limb bud where mesenchyme aggregates. Ultimately these tubular condensations are separated by a discrete area referred to as the interzone. This interzone marks the primitive joint and typically has three layers of cells—two parallel chondrogenic layers and a third intermediate layer. The intermediate zone of cells will ultimately form the synovium and the intra-articular structures. Cavitation of this primitive joint usually awaits contouring of the joint surfaces. It has been suggested that cavitation is primarily an enzymatic process and is independent of fetal movement. The joint spaces are typically well established by the tenth week of embryonic life. Classically, the embryo becomes a fetus by the twelfth week. At that point all the embryonic organ systems and their respective organs have been formed. The remaining 6 months of fetal development is simply further growth and maturation of these previously formed embryologic structures.

Postnatal Development

As previously stated, the bones of the fetus are developing through the two mechanisms of intramembranous and en-

Differentiation of Somites Into Myotomes, Sclerotomes, and Dermatomes

Cross sections of human embryos

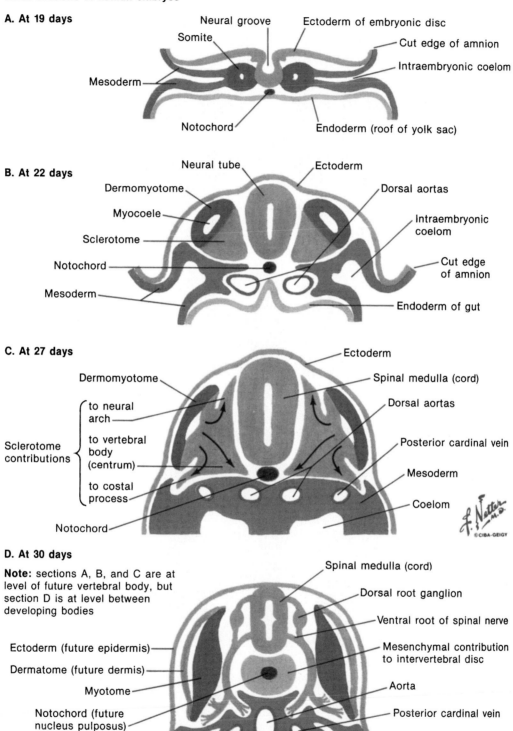

A. At 19 days

Neural groove — Ectoderm of embryonic disc
Somite — Cut edge of amnion
Mesoderm — Intraembryonic coelom
Notochord — Endoderm (roof of yolk sac)

B. At 22 days

Neural tube — Ectoderm
Dermomyotome — Dorsal aortas
Myocoele — Intraembryonic coelom
Sclerotome — Cut edge of amnion
Notochord — Endoderm of gut
Mesoderm

C. At 27 days

Ectoderm
Dermomyotome — Spinal medulla (cord)
Sclerotome contributions:
to neural arch — Dorsal aortas
to vertebral body (centrum) — Posterior cardinal vein
to costal process — Mesoderm
Notochord — Coelom

D. At 30 days

Note: sections A, B, and C are at level of future vertebral body, but section D is at level between developing bodies

Spinal medulla (cord)
Dorsal root ganglion
Ventral root of spinal nerve
Ectoderm (future epidermis) — Mesenchymal contribution to intervertebral disc
Dermatome (future dermis)
Myotome — Aorta
Notochord (future nucleus pulposus) — Posterior cardinal vein
Mesoderm — Coelom
Mesonephric kidney — Dorsal mesentery

Figure 1–11. Differentiation of somites into myotomes, sclerotomes, and dermatomes. (From Netter FH: The CIBA Collection of Medical Illustrations, Volume 8. Summit, NJ, CIBA-GEIGY Corporation.)

Progressive Stages in Formation of Vertebral Column, Dermatomes, and Myotomes

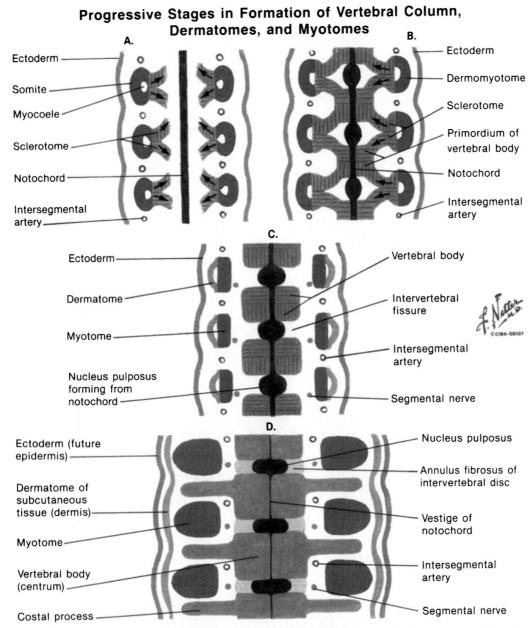

Figure 1–12. Progressive stages in formation of vertebral column *(A)*, dermatomes *(B)*, and myotomes *(C)*. Mesenchymal precartilage primordia of axial and appendicular skeletons at 5 weeks *(D)*. (From Netter FH: The CIBA Collection of Medical Illustrations, Volume 8. Summit, NJ, CIBA-GEIGY Corporation.)

Development of Three Types of Diarthrodial (Synovial) Joints

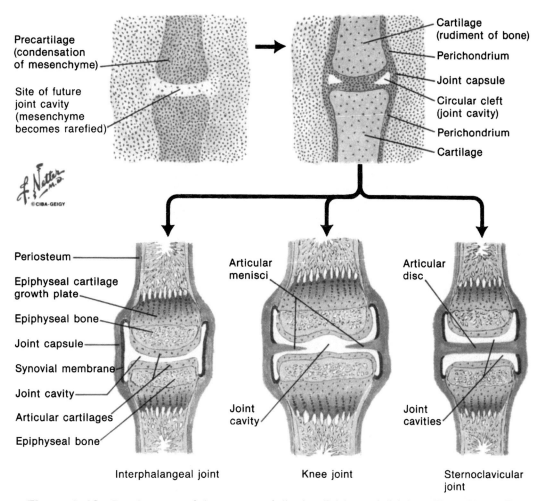

Precartilage (condensation of mesenchyme)

Site of future joint cavity (mesenchyme becomes rarefied)

Cartilage (rudiment of bone)

Perichondrium

Joint capsule

Circular cleft (joint cavity)

Perichondrium

Cartilage

Periosteum

Epiphyseal cartilage growth plate

Epiphyseal bone

Joint capsule

Synovial membrane

Joint cavity

Articular cartilages

Epiphyseal bone

Articular menisci

Joint cavity

Articular disc

Joint cavities

Interphalangeal joint   Knee joint   Sternoclavicular joint

Figure 1–13. Development of three types of diarthrodial (synovial) joints. (From Netter FH: The CIBA Collection of Medical Illustrations, Volume 8. Summit, NJ, CIBA-GEIGY Corporation.)

chondral bone formation. Following birth, these processes continue at an accelerated pace. The periosteal surfaces of all long bones, as well as large portions of the flat bones, continue to grow as a result of intramembranous bone formation. Bone is directly formed in a collagenized matrix by the activity of osteoblasts without the benefit of a cartilage model.

The most critical mechanism in postnatal bone maturation is the activity of the physis or growth plate. Significant knowledge currently exists as to the anatomy and physiology of the normal growth plate, as well as its biochemistry and its mechanical properties. This growth plate is a unique anatomic structure. It is the essential mechanism by which mammals are able to enlarge their endoskeleton. Whereas lesser animals must molt an exoskeleton in an effort to grow, the physis allows for longitudinal growth of the higher organism. It is clear, however, from the beginning that this unique anatomic structure has its own obsolescence built in. Not only does it stop producing bone, but it is in large measure consumed by its own product. During the time it exists, the physis, for all its unique and critical importance, creates a mechanical flaw in the bone. The

growth plate, therefore, is a critical entity in postnatal bone development and maturation.

THE PHYSIS (Fig. 1–14)

The characteristic cytoarchitectural pattern of the growth plate is typically present by the fourth month of fetal life. For most long bones, the discoid configuration is most typical. This is, of course, characterized by a planar area of rapidly differentiating cartilage, which blends into, but is nonetheless structurally distinct from, hyaline cartilage covering the chondroepiphysis. This discoid physis is located between the metaphysis and the epiphysis of a long bone.

The *epiphysis* is a secondary ossification center and typically ossifies from a central area, which then grows centrifugally. The epiphysis is normally subjected to compressive forces. Conversely, an *apophysis* is also a secondary ossification center, but one that ordinarily forms a point for muscle attachment and therefore is subjected to tensile forces. Both of these secondary ossification centers typically sit astride a discoid physis.

The growth plate histologically can be shown to have

Structure and Blood Supply of Growth Plate

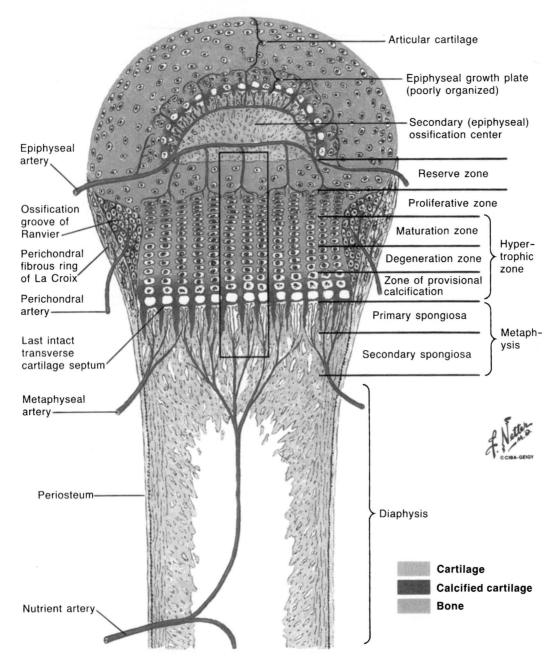

Articular cartilage

Epiphyseal growth plate (poorly organized)

Secondary (epiphyseal) ossification center

Epiphyseal artery

Ossification groove of Ranvier

Perichondral fibrous ring of La Croix

Perichondral artery

Last intact transverse cartilage septum

Metaphyseal artery

Periosteum

Nutrient artery

Reserve zone

Proliferative zone

Maturation zone

Degeneration zone

Zone of provisional calcification

Hyper-trophic zone

Primary spongiosa

Secondary spongiosa

Metaph-ysis

Diaphysis

Cartilage
Calcified cartilage
Bone

Figure 1–14. Structure and blood supply of growth plate. Branches of epiphyseal artery pass directly through reserve zone of cartilaginous growth plate without contributing capillaries to it, but on reaching proliferative zone, they arborize into capillaries that supply only top of cell columns. Metaphyseal and nutrient arteries subdivide into numerous small branches, which pass axially to bone-cartilage junction where they form loops or tufts but do not enter cartilage. Thus, metaphysis and bony portion of growth plate are well supplied with blood, but only uppermost portion of cell columns (proliferative zone of cartilage) is vascularized. Hypertrophic zone is avascular; cells are progressively poorly oxygenated and nourished from top downward, and lowermost cells degenerate and die. Peripherally located perichondral ring of La Croix and ossification groove of Ranvier have own distinct blood supply. These vascular phenomena have profound physiologic significance. (From Netter FH: The CIBA Collection of Medical Illustrations, Volume 8. Summit, NJ, CIBA-GEIGY Corporation.)

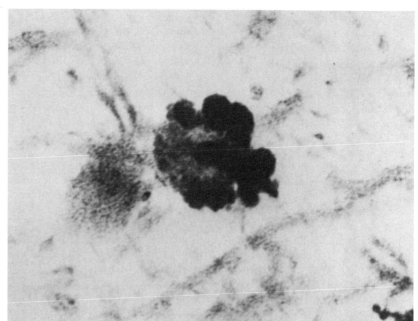

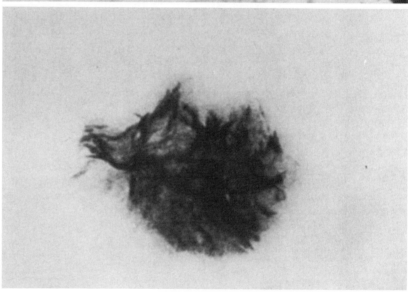

Figure 1-15. Electron micrographs of matrix vesicles from the middle and the bottom of the hypertrophic zone. The matrix vesicle in the top picture is from the middle of the hypertrophic zone and exhibits large clump-like calcium-stain complex either on or within the vesicle. The matrix vesicle in the bottom picture is from the bottom of the hypertrophic zone. Note that the typical crystal formation of hydroxyapatite is present within or upon the matrix vesicle (×240,000). (From Brighton CT: Orthop Clin North Am 15:586, 1984.)

four distinctly separate zones: (1) resting, (2) proliferating, (3) hypertrophic (degeneration), and (4) provisional calcification. Each zone has its own unique anatomy as well as its own unique function.

The Resting (Reserve) Zone. This histologic region is immediately subjacent to the bony epiphysis. The cells are roundish and occur in either singlets or doublets. The quantity of matrix is more than is seen in any other zone, and there is a high glycogen content stored in this region. Studies demonstrate a rather abundant endoplasmic reticulum, suggesting active synthetic activity. Although blood vessels have been identified, they tend to pass through this region and arborize lower. This feature may account for the relatively low oxygen tension in the resting zone. The location and histology of this region suggest that it has the capacity to produce cartilaginous matrix. However, additional physiologic studies show that the cells in this region remain relatively inert. Overall, the function of the resting zone remains somewhat cloudy.

The Proliferating Zone (Zone of Cell Columns). The cells in this region are typically flattened and arranged in longitudinal columns parallel to the long axis of the bone. Again, a significant amount of endoplasmic reticulum has been demonstrated in this region. The top cell in each of the columns is thought to be the germinal cell for longitudinal growth of the column below. Labeled thymidine studies have supported the germinal role of the top cell in each column. The extremely high content of proteoglycan identified in this zone suggests that it is synthesized there. Matrix vesicles (Fig. 1-15) are also present in high numbers, suggesting their role in matrix mineralization. Oxygen tension levels are highest in this zone, no doubt the result of the rich vascular supply seen here. Considering the anatomy and biochemistry of this region, the major functions of the proliferating zone are cell proliferation and matrix production, both of which are required for linear growth.

The Hypertrophic (Degeneration) Zone. The cells identified in this region are approximately five times the size of those in the zones above. Intracellular matrix gradually decreases in content as one goes deeper into this zone. The longitudinal septa of intercellular matrix persist into the deepest regions of the hypertrophic zone. However, thin transverse septa become progressively more sparse the deeper one goes into the plate. Similarly, glycogen, which is identified in the upper regions of the hypertrophic zone, is gradually lost in the lower half. The concentration of lysosomal enzymes is extremely high, and the concentration of proteoglycans and hydroxyproline is markedly low. Electron microscopy reveals the presence of an endoplasmic reticulum in the cells with increased vacuolation, cytoplasmic swelling, and increased numbers of mitochondria and lysosomes throughout this region. In addition, the previously noted matrix vesicles appear to be not only more prevalent but also more active in this region. It appears clear that the ultimate fate of cells in this region is necrosis. The process of cell necrosis is intimately entwined with the process of matrix calcification. The enzymatic interplay between the two processes, although suggested, is poorly elucidated. Similarly, the relatively low levels of oxygen tension indicate poor vascularity. All of these features: lysosomal enzymes, vacuolation, marginal blood supply, all support the idea that the role of the hypertrophic zone is the preparation of the matrix for calcification.

The Zone of Provisional Calcification. Some textbooks question the existence of this zone, saying that it actually consists of the bottom few cells in the hypertrophic zone and does not warrant its own designation as a zone. Others, however, prefer to identify this particular region as a specific zone. Nonetheless, this lowest region of the growth plate clearly is the area where calcification of the cartilaginous matrix occurs. It is here that the matrix vesicle concentration is highest, and it is here that these vesicles are most active. The mechanisms for the delivery and liberation of the calcium are still under active investigation. It is felt that the relative anoxia of this region plays a role in calcium release from the mitochondria (Fig. 1–16). Clearly, the function of this region is calcification. Typically, the mineral is deposited only in the longitudinal bars of matrix and not in the transverse septa.

THE METAPHYSIS

Any discussion of the growth plate would not be complete without a word about the subjacent metaphysis. Metaphyseal bone begins, by definition, just distal to the last intact transverse septum. One can identify a lacunar space that has been broken down and invaded by red blood cells. This specific region where the calcified cartilage becomes vascularized is referred to as primary spongiosa bone (see Fig. 1–14). Osteoblasts can be identified lining up on the longitudinal bars of calcified cartilage. Assuming this cartilage to be calcified, the process of ossification can begin spontaneously. In certain metabolic disease states, specifically rickets, in which calcification has not occurred, ossification cannot proceed normally. As one goes deeper in the metaphysis, the calcified cartilage cores of the trabeculae will be seen to disappear. At the point at which no calcified cartilage is present, the trabeculae are referred to as secondary spongiosa bone.

Clearly, the functions of the metaphysis are vascular invasion, bone formation, and bone remodeling. In regard to bone remodeling, resorption occurs on the external surface of the cortical bone, and formation occurs on the internal surface of the cortical bone. This mechanism is exactly the opposite of what one will see at the level of the diaphysis. The role of the metaphysis is to "cut back" or "funnelize" the trumpet-shaped end of a long bone.

Finally, two peripheral structures surrounding the growth plate are worthy of note. The first structure is the *ossification groove of Ranvier*, which is a wedge-shaped ring of cells surrounding the margins of the plate at the

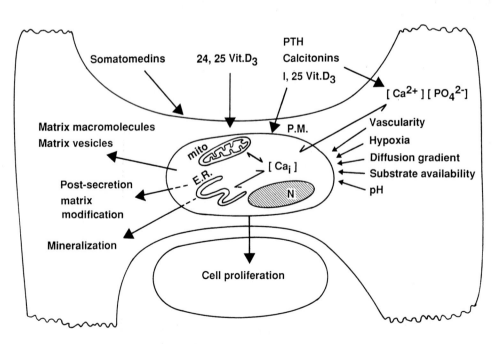

Figure 1–16. The factors influencing growth plate chondrocyte function and matrix mineralization. (From Iannoti JP: Orthop Clin North Am 1:6, 1990.)

level of the resting zone. Thymidine labeling has documented replication activity in these cells. The role of this structure is felt to be latitudinal growth of the plate.

The second peripheral structure is the *perichondrial ring of La Croix*. This is a fibrous sleeve, occasionally referred to as the "girdle of the growth plate." Some feel it acts as a limiting membrane and provides mechanical support for the plate.

BLOOD SUPPLY OF THE GROWTH PLATE

Essentially, the vasculature of the plate can be subdivided into three major groups: epiphyseal vessels, metaphyseal vessels, and a small group of perichondral vessels (see Fig. 1–14). The epiphyseal vessels enter the epiphysis or secondary ossification center. The terminal arborizations of these vessels pass through the resting zone of the physis and supply the upper portions of the proliferating zone. The entry point of this vessel depends on the amount of articular cartilage covering the bony epiphysis. In some bones, specifically the upper tibia, the course can be direct and nontortuous. However, in other bones, such as the proximal femur, the epiphyseal vessel has an extremely complex route to take in order to enter the bony epiphysis. Ordinarily, the vessel enters the bony epiphysis between the articular cartilage margin and the growth plate. In the case of the proximal femur, the vessel must travel beneath cartilage to the plate. During its very tortuous course, it is extremely vulnerable to shear injury. The metaphyseal vessels terminate in many straight branches, which penetrate the lowest regions of the growth plate. It is their presence that in some measure participates in the calcification of the matrix.

The perichondral vessels supply the peripheral cells and do not enter the depths of the epiphysis. As previously noted, the proliferating zone is the only area receiving a blood supply. The remainder of the plate is largely avascular.

PATTERNS OF GROWTH

Characteristically, long bone growth is generally considered to be a longitudinal phenomenon. The anatomy of the previously described physis clearly emphasizes its linear orientation and its predisposition to grow in this fashion. However, some latitudinal growth is essential for normal plate development. This growth is accomplished both by interstitial growth within the plate and appositional growth at the periphery in the region of the groove of Ranvier. Latitudinal expansion of the physis will obviously be precluded in areas that are juxtaposed to the subchondral plate once the subchondral plate has developed.

There are a number of regional variations in plate growth. Most of the time these variations result from mechanical limitation to interstitial expansion. As mentioned earlier, the subchondral plate is one of the major mechanical factors limiting plate growth. Differential growth of various ossification centers is also typical. The distal humerus is a good example of such differential growth. The trochlea and the capitellum initially are equal in size. However, the ossification center of the capitellum tends to develop earlier and more rapidly, and in doing so, it restricts its own interstitial expansion. The trochlea does not appear until later and therefore can ultimately achieve a larger size because it has a longer period of interstitial growth. Ultimately, when both of these centers fuse, latitudinal growth of the distal humerus becomes a peripheral function at the level of the epicondyles. A similar interplay of two epiphyseal nuclei is seen in the proximal femur, where initially the trochanteric apophysis and capital femoral epiphysis are of equal size but, due to differential and variational growth, ultimately end up with very different configurations.

CONTROL OF THE GROWTH PLATE

As one would expect, a number of factors affect normal plate growth and development. Both local and systemic factors have been clearly identified as manipulating the plate in the way in which growth is accomplished.

The Heuter-Volkmann law is an important local factor. It speaks to the subject of *mechanical load*, stating that there is a physiologic range of load within which the plate will grow successfully. Extremes of tension or compression, however, will tend to retard growth plate performance. The integrity of the periosteum acts as another mechanical restraint on the plate. Because it attaches directly to the groove of Ranvier, it will control the amount of latitudinal and longitudinal growth seen. Resection of portions of the periosteum will permit accelerated longitudinal growth. Obviously, pathologic mechanical loading, as seen in trauma, frequently has severe repercussions on the patterns of physeal growth. These effects will be discussed in the sections on pediatric trauma.

There is some preliminary information regarding *electrical effects* on the growth plate. Various experiments have been done subjecting plate cartilage to various electrical fields. Early indications suggest that under the proper circumstances of voltage gradients, accelerated growth of the plate can be seen. This growth response appears to be due to the voltage gradient and not to any current flow. It has been suggested that this is a direct response of the plate chondrocyte to the electrical field gradient.

Obviously the *vascular supply* to the plate is critical for growth integrity. Any disruption or damage to this supply of the plate will clearly impede its ability to function and grow normally.

A number of **systemic** factors have also been implicated in normal plate function. Genetic as well as nutritional factors certainly play a role in physeal manipulation. However, most indications are that hormonal control is the primary regulator of plate function.

The importance of *growth hormone* cannot be overemphasized. This is a peptide hormone produced by the pituitary gland that stimulates plate activity by affecting cellular proliferation. Growth hormone is felt to act through its mediators, the somatomedins and sulfation factor. Excessive levels of this hormone will cause an anticipated growth plate widening and ultimately gigantism. Should the plate be closed at the time of excessive growth hormone stimulation, acromegaly results. This condition is typified by increased appositional bone growth. On the other hand, deficiencies of this hormone typically slow plate growth. However, because the plate tends to remain open longer, ultimate height is variable. This finding suggests that growth hormone has no effect on plate closure, but rather a regulatory effect on rate of proliferation and osteogenesis.

Thyroid hormone is actually a sequence of peptide hormones produced by the thyroid gland. These hormones play a synergistic role with growth hormone. Thyroid hormone has primarily a trophic effect on cartilage growth and is essential to the normal health and growth of cartilage. Recently, a synergistic effect with insulin-like growth factor has been suggested. Excess levels of thyroid hormone have wide-ranging systemic effects but relatively few musculoskeletal manifestations. Low levels of thyroid hormone, however, result in growth retardation, erosion of the chondroepiphysis, and degradation of mucopolysaccharides.

Glucocorticoids are steroid hormones produced by the adrenal cortex and similarly seem to exert a trophic effect on cartilage. A physiologic level is required for normal physeal function. In the face of excessive levels, derived either endogenously or exogenously, there is a stunting effect on chondrocytes. This effect will be manifested by a decrease in mitotic activity, as well as synthetic activity. Inadequate levels of adrenal steroids can also cause stunting, but to a lesser degree.

Sex hormones, androgens and estrogens, are both steroid hormones. The androgens are felt to exert their effect in the hypertrophic zone. Testosterone seems to stimulate rapid cell division, calcification, and premature physeal closure. Conversely, deficiency states of androgenic hormones are characterized by a marked delay in physeal closure, resulting in the typical eunuchoid body habitus. Estrogen, on the other hand, apparently has a more complex effect on the plate. Some suppressive activity on plate function has been demonstrated with excessive levels of estrogen activity.

PLATE CLOSURE

Physiologic closure of the growth plate is a complex phenomenon. Clearly there are hormonal as well as local factors that manipulate this process. Once physeal growth has stopped, initial closure of the plate begins. The portion of the plate that closes first and the pattern of closure vary from bone to bone. Ultimately the growth plate, as we know it, disappears, and the metaphysis fuses to the secondary ossification center.

Females close their physes earlier than males, probably due to the estrogens, which accelerate cartilage replacement and osseous maturation. In any event, the process begins with the formation of an ossified bridge between the epiphysis and the metaphysis. It ends with complete disappearance of the cartilaginous physis. As mentioned previously, the location of the initial bridge in the transverse plane of the plate varies from bone to bone.

BIOMECHANICS OF THE GROWTH PLATE

The cartilaginous physis is clearly a mechanical defect at the end of a long bone. It is vulnerable not only to a number of chemical and toxic effects, but to mechanical disruption as well. As with all biologic tissues, injury to the plate can occur when the load exceeds the ultimate tensile strength. At that point, failure will occur. The result will be a function of the strength of the plate, as well as the magnitude of the load applied to it. The cross-sectional anatomy of a physis varies from bone to bone. Some plates are relatively planar with few metaphyseal interdigitations, such as the proximal tibia and the distal radius. Others are contoured to a significant degree, making failure patterns more complex.

In general, the growth plate is well adapted to absorb compressive stress. There is no question that failure in shear is the greatest risk that the plate must face. The undulations seen in the cross-sectional geometry of the plate are pegs that stabilize the plate relative to the metaphysis. These pegs are referred to as mammillary processes. These mammillary processes give the plate a certain resistance to the effect of shear forces. Unfortunately, the greater the constraint of the plate by these processes, the greater the risk of premature closure should the plate fail in shear, resulting in fracture of these pegs. Such is the case of the distal femoral physis; fractures typically fracture the mammillary processes, frequently resulting in premature physeal closure. As a generalization, it is fair to say that the plate is most vulnerable when it is actively growing. Therefore, in the prepubertal and pubertal individuals, one would anticipate the plate to be most susceptible to excessive mechanical load. Plate failure and its long-term complications can be relatively wide ranging. These issues will be discussed in the section on pediatric trauma elsewhere in the text.

Bibliography

Brighton C: Clinical problems in epiphyseal plate growth and development. *In* American Academy of Orthopedic Surgery Instructional Course Lectures XXIII. St. Louis, CV Mosby, 1974, pp 105–122.
This is the classic article on the subject. Dr. Brighton's work has provided the basis for most of the ongoing research on the physis.

Dietz F: Update on the genetic bases of disorders with orthopaedic manifestations. J Bone Joint Surg 1996;78A:1583–1595.
A current concepts review that is a "must" read for orthopaedic residents preparing for their board examinations. This article reviews the current information on the molecular genetic basis of several syndromes.

Iannotti J: Growth plate physiology and pathology. Orthop Clin North Am 1990;21:1–17.
A more up-to-date review of the subject provided by one of Dr. Brighton's collaborators.

Ogden J: The uniqueness of growing bones. *In* Rockwood CA (ed): Fractures in Children, 4th ed. Philadelphia, JB Lippincott, 1996, vol 3.
Excellent summary of the development of the musculoskeletal system by the leading authority on the subject.

Chapter 2

Basic Science of Cartilage and Bone

John N. Delahay, M.D.

CARTILAGE

Cartilage is a specialized, fibrous connective tissue. Its function varies, based on its histologic type. There are essentially three histologic types of cartilage. In addition, the growth apparatus of the skeleton includes physeal and epiphyseal cartilage, which are variants of these three basic types. Table 2–1 shows the composition of the types of cartilage.

Types of Cartilage

Hyaline Cartilage. This tissue covers the ends of long bones, forming their articular surfaces. Hyaline cartilage, therefore, is important for its ability to resist compressive forces and provide a relatively frictionless surface for smooth joint motion.

Fibrocartilage. The matrix of fibrocartilage is high in collagen fibers, as the name implies. These fibers tend to be visible by light microscopy. The menisci, the annulus fibrosis, and the symphysis pubis are largely fibrocartilage. Biomechanically, fibrocartilage is designed to resist tensile load.

Elastic Cartilage. As the name implies, elastic cartilage is composed primarily of elastic fibers. It is found in the external ear, the epiglottis, and the tip of the nose. Elastic cartilage has a moderate ability to resist tensile load, but it also allows for some controlled deformation. It is the least

common of the three types of cartilage and, in some respects, the most subject to damage.

Articular Cartilage

From an orthopaedic standpoint, the most important histologic type of cartilage is hyaline cartilage. The term "hyaline" was derived from the Greek word meaning "glass" and from the Latin word meaning "gristle." Hyaline cartilage is a very tough, resilient, firm material that, when applied to the bony endplates in diaphyseal joints, allows almost frictionless motion of those joints. The average thickness of the articular surface is between 2 and 4 mm, with some surfaces being as thick as 7 mm. Normal human adult articular cartilage is typically described as being divided into four histologic zones (Fig. 2–1).

HISTOLOGIC ZONES

Tangential (Gliding) Zone. The tangential zone is the most superficial zone of flattened cells. The axes of these cells are parallel to the articular surface.

Transitional (Intermediate) Zone. The cells in this zone are round or ovoid and are randomly distributed throughout the matrix in this region. These cells manifest small membrane processes, which are noted to extend into the matrix.

Radial Zone. The cells in this zone are arranged radially, that is, perpendicular to the articular surface. Membrane processes are similarly noted in this region and interconnect the cells. In addition, glycogen-containing storage granules can be found in these cells.

Calcified Zone. Small irregular cells with pyknotic nuclei are found in lacunae surrounded by huge amounts of hydroxyapatite crystal.

MORPHOLOGY AND PHYSIOLOGY

The tidemark is a wavy basophilic line described by some as a reverse epiphysis, meaning that this tidemark (Fig. 2–2) appears when the growth plate closes. This line is seen to be interposed between the radial zone and the calcified zone. Notably, no blood vessels can be seen to cross this line in normal articular cartilage.

Careful examination of the surface anatomy of articular

Table 2–1. Approximate composition of the various types of cartilage

| Cartilage | Water (%) | Solids (%) | | | |
		Collagen	GAG	Elastin	Other*
Articular	72	66	18	—	16
Epiphyseal	81	37	15	—	48
Fibrocartilage	74	78	2	0.6	19
Elastic	71	53	12	19	16

*Includes monocollagen proteins, calcium phosphorus, other ions, and macromolecules such as DNA and RNA.
From Gamble JG: The Musculoskeletal System: Physiological Basics. New York, Raven Press, 1988.

JOINT SPACE

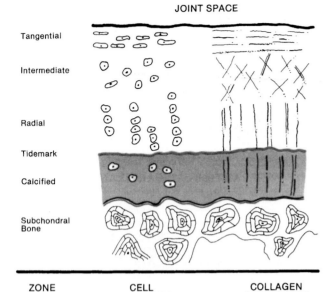

| ZONE NAME | CELL ORIENTATION | COLLAGEN ORIENTATION |

Tangential
Intermediate
Radial
Tidemark
Calcified
Subchondral Bone

Figure 2–1. Schematic representation of the cell orientation and collagen fibril orientation in the four histologic layers of articular cartilage. Chondrocytes are flattened, and collagen fibrils are mostly parallel to the surface in the tangential zone. Fibrils decussate in the intermediate zone and lie more perpendicular to the surface in the radial zone and in the calcified cartilage. (From Gamble JG: The Musculoskeletal System: Physiological Basics. New York, Raven Press, 1988.)

cartilage shows a zone of tightly packed collagen bundles tangential to the surface and slightly subjacent to it. This zone has often been referred to as the lamina splendens. At present, it is generally thought that this material causes the surface undulations seen on the articular surface and represents part of the complex lubricating system in a diarthrodial joint. It has been proposed that this surface

material in some way may trap synovial fluid and allow for appropriate gliding.

The cells that are integral to the articular surface are called chondrocytes. They account for only 0.1% of the volume of the tissue. As noted earlier, the shape of the chondrocytes varies slightly, depending on the zone in which they are found. Typically, the nucleus is eccentric and basophilically stained. It is not unusual to see more than one nucleus per cell. The cells are located in lacunae in the articular cartilage, and a halo of matrix surrounds the lacunae. Numerous organelles can be identified within these chondrocytes. Specifically, a Golgi complex, endoplasmic reticulum, mitochondria, and vacuoles have all been identified. As noted earlier, many of the cells possess cellular processes that are rudimentary when compared to those of the osteocyte.

Anatomically, articular cartilage is quite unique. Articular tissue is isolated in that it does not have a neural, lymphatic, or vascular supply. Also, the tissue is extremely hypocellular. Its hypocellularity led many to believe that it was metabolically inert, but this is simply not true. As will be seen, articular cartilage is an extremely active tissue.

The chemistry of articular cartilage is essentially the chemistry of its matrix (Table 2–2). As noted, the chondrocytes are distributed in the cartilage matrix. This matrix primarily is composed of water, accounting for 65 to 80% of the wet weight of cartilage. Approximately 10 to 20% of the wet weight of cartilage matrix is collagen, and approximately 5 to 7% is a unique proteoglycan commonly referred to as aggrecan. In addition, electrolytes are present in this fluid.

Looking at each constituent individually shows that the water molecules are loosely bound to the proteoglycan subunits. Heating is adequate to separate these molecules. In addition, the water content varies in different locations within the articular surface layer. In general, the more superficial the layer, the higher the water content.

Collagen constitutes 10 to 20% of the matrix when wet,

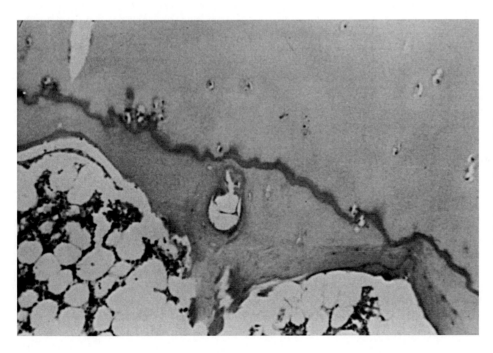

Figure 2–2. Higher magnification of tidemark, calcified cartilage, and bone. The tidemark delineates the forward limit of calcification. Calcified cartilage and bone are present beneath the tidemark. (From Bogumill GP, Schwamm HA: Orthopaedic Pathology: A Synopsis with Clinical and Radiographic Correlation. Philadelphia, WB Saunders, 1984.)

Table 2–2. Biochemical composition of articular cartilage

Component	% Wet Weight
Quantitatively Major Components	
Water	65 to 80
Collagen (type II)	10 to 20
Aggrecan	4 to 7
Quantitatively Minor Components	
(less than 5%)*	
Proteogycans	
Biglycan	
Decorin	
Fibromodulin	
Collagens	
Type V	
Type VI	
Type IX	
Type X	
Type XI	
Link protein	
Hyaluronate	
Fibronectin	
Lipids	

*Although these components are present in lower overall amounts, they may be present in similar molar amounts compared to type II collagen and aggrecan (for example, link protein), and may have major roles to play in the functionality of the matrix.

From Simon SR (ed): Orthopaedic Basic Science. American Academy of Orthopaedic Surgeons.

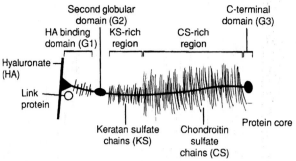

Figure 2–3. A schematic diagram of the aggrecan molecule and its binding to hyaluronate. The protein core has several globular domains (G1, G2, and G3), with other regions containing the keratan sulfate and chondroitin sulfate glycosaminoglycan chains. The amino-terminal G1 domain is able to bind specifically to hyaluronate. This binding is stabilized by link protein. (From Simon SR [ed]: Orthopaedic Basic Science. American Academy of Orthopaedic Surgeons, Chicago, 1992.)

and approximately 50 to 60% when dry. At present, the collagen is felt to be arranged in roughly three layers. The distribution of this protein is, however, not thought to be random. The surface layer of collagen is made up of fibers parallel to the articular surface. The central layer shows fibers that are spiral and oblique to the articular surface, and the deepest layer of articular cartilage, which is juxtaposed to the subchondral bony plate, demonstrates fibers that are perpendicular to that plate. This overall arrangement has been demonstrated by split pattern testing and is felt to be generally reliable despite the joint surface in question. The collagen present in cartilage is type II collagen. As can been seen in Table 2–3, each tropocollagen molecule is composed of three alpha-1 chains.

The third matrix constituent is a somewhat unique complex proteoglycan macromolecule, which has been referred to as aggrecan (Fig. 2–3). This molecule consists of a large,

lengthy, protein core to which are attached upwards of 100 chondroitin sulfate molecules and 40 to 50 keratan sulfate chains. These substances are polysaccharide molecules and are unique in articular cartilage. Relatively little is known about the protein core of the aggrecan molecule. It is known to be a complex protein with several distinct domains. The polysaccharide molecules, specifically the chondroitin and keratan sulfate, are attached roughly perpendicular to the protein core, which in turn is attached to a central filamentous core of hyaluronic acid. These large aggregate macromolecules may be noncovalently bonded to the collagen. The distribution of the aggrecan molecules is also not homogeneous. The highest concentrations can be found in the perilacunar areas, whereas the concentrations seem to be less in the superficial zones. Similarly, there is a variation in the amount of chondroitin-4-sulfate, chondroitin-6-sulfate, and keratan sulfate, based upon location, age, and disease state. The importance, however, of these macromolecules is unquestioned. They create huge electronegative fields about them. These large electrostatic domains bestow upon articular cartilage its biomechanical resiliency and resistance to deformity. The ability to hydrate the matrix is largely dependent on the concentrations of these large macromolecules.

Because cartilage is an avascular material, its nutrition depends upon diffusion. Although it was previously

Table 2–3. Types and properties of collagen

Type	Composition	Distinctive Features	Distribution
I	$[\alpha\,1(I)]_2\alpha\,2(I)$	Low hydroxylysine and carbohydrate; 90% of all collagen; forms thick fibrils	Bones, ligaments, tendons, skin
II	$[\alpha\,1(II)]_3$	High hydroxyproline and carbohydrate; forms thin fibrils	Hyaline and growth cartilage; nucleus pulposus
III	$[\alpha\,1(III)]_3$	High hydroxyproline; low carbohydrate; reticulin fibrils	Blood vessels, muscle, skin, internal organs
IV	$[\alpha\,1(IV)]_2\alpha\,2(IV)$	Very high hydroxylysine and carbohydrate	Basal lamina
V	$\alpha A\,(\alpha B)_2$	Unknown	Cell associated, widespread in small amounts

From Gamble JG: The Musculoskeletal System: Physiological Basics. New York, Raven Press, 1988.

thought that there were some small capillaries from the subchondral plate feeding the basilar layers of the articular surface, it has been relatively well documented that this is not the case. Adult articular cartilage essentially must depend on diffusion from synovial fluid through the surface layers to provide cartilage nutrition. Obviously, the rates of diffusion are a function of the size of the molecule and the concentration gradient. As one might expect, permeability is slower in the deeper layers because of the greater fixed charge. As this fixed charge decreases, as in the case of osteoarthritis and other disease states, permeability rates tend to increase.

As one would expect, the metabolism of articular cartilage is primarily anaerobic. This is consistent with its relative avascularity. Energy for metabolic activities is generally, therefore, derived from anaerobic pathways. Although there are a few aerobic pathways, they are far less developed and, therefore, of relatively little importance. Articular cartilage, which was once thought to be metabolically inert, has clearly been shown to be quite the opposite. It is capable of protein synthesis, as well as synthesis of polysaccharides, and the sulfonation of those polysaccharides. The chondrocytes are capable of synthesizing protein, specifically collagen, using standard pathways of DNA/RNA transcription. In addition, they can synthesize the glycosaminoglycan (aggrecan) component of the matrix. Currently, there is evidence to suggest that the entire proteoglycan molecule is synthesized simultaneously by the chondrocytes. Various labeling techniques have been used to measure the synthesis as well as the turnover of these matrix constituents. Specifically, glycine labeling has been used to follow protein synthesis, sulfate labeling has been used to plot glycosaminoglycan (GAG) synthesis, and thymidine labeling has been employed to measure DNA synthesis. Most studies have indicated that synthetic rates are linear with time. Although quite rapid in the immature animal, in the adult the rates are relatively constant, despite aging.

Turnover does exist in the articular surface. In the immature animal, mitotic figures can be seen and DNA synthesis measured. Once maturation is achieved and the tidemark develops, this type of activity ceases. It is safe to say that no mitotic activity is present in normal adult cartilage. All indications are, however, that the chondrocytes and their synthetic pathways are simply turned off rather than broken, and under certain situations, the chondrocytes can become active as chondroblasts, at least to a limited degree.

In addition to cellular turnover, there is also ongoing matrix turnover. An internal remodeling system has been proposed to modulate matrix degradation and formation. Cartilage enzymes are felt to be at the heart of this remodeling system. Proteolytic enzymes (proteinases) that are synthesized by the chondrocytes appear to be key in the degradation of articular cartilage. Two major groups of proteinases are currently receiving attention: metalloproteinases, such as collagenase and gelatinase, and the cathepsins. The metalloproteinases have garnered a significant amount of interest in the past several years. These compounds require the presence of zinc for their function, hence the name metalloproteinases. As the name implies, collagenase is key to the breakdown of the protein collagen. Cathepsins are critical for the degradation of aggrecan.

Cartilage as a tissue serves a favorable biomechanical role. It is an amazingly indentable tissue. This property is

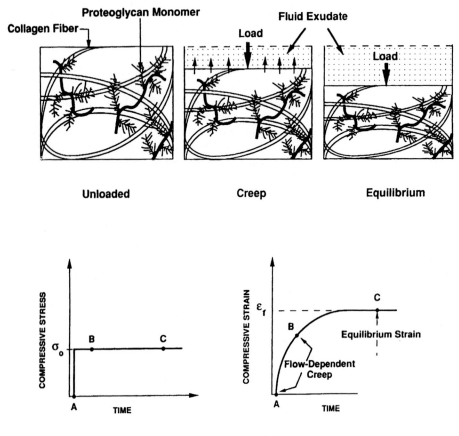

Figure 2–4. Biphasic creep behavior of a hydrated soft tissue such as articular cartilage during compression. Rate of creep is governed by the rate at which fluid may be forced out from the tissue, which, in turn, is governed by the permeability and stiffness of the porous-permeable, collagen-proteoglycan solid matrix. (From Simon SR [ed]: Orthopaedic Basic Science. American Academy of Orthopaedic Surgeons, Chicago, 1992.)

a function of its hyperhydrated state, which allows it to return to its original shape when indented (Fig. 2–4). Cartilage's ability to deform over time, or "creep," is a function of the thickness of the articular surface. Cartilage is also able to provide the diarthrodial joint with a certain level of shock absorption. This ability can occur passively, as a result of cartilage's deformation on impact, and actively, as a function of joint motion and muscle lengthening. Joint congruence, especially with loading, is dependent on the cartilage thickness and its pliability. There is an inverse relationship between cartilage thickness and joint congruence. Specifically, the thicker the articular surface, such as in the patellofemoral joint, the less congruent that joint will be. As the articular surface becomes damaged from various pathologic states, the ability of this cartilage to function normally in its biomechanical modes is markedly altered. This change simply compounds the rate of joint breakdown in a number of different pathologic situations.

PATHOLOGIC CHANGES

Aging. The chondrocytes in the aging articular surface tend to increase in size, achieving diameters two to three times greater than normal. In addition, there is an increase in lytic enzymes released by these cells, obviously causing increased rates of matrix degradation. As noted earlier, no mitotic figures, and therefore no DNA synthesis, is seen in the aging articular surface. With age, there is an overall decrease in the glycosaminoglycans and a relative increase in the protein content of the articular surface. As the aggrecan component of articular cartilage matrix decreases, the overall water content naturally decreases. With loss of water and proteoglycan, the mechanical well-being of the cartilage becomes slowly impaired. The cartilage simply becomes stiffer and less pliable.

Trauma to the Articular Surface. Mechanical as well as chemical injury can produce changes in the articular surface. Mechanical injury, such as superficial and deep laceration, is not uncommon. The healing of these chondral defects, however, varies depending on whether or not the subchondral plate is violated. Because cartilage is avascular, one would not expect significant healing and, indeed, that essentially is the case. Following superficial laceration, there is a local burst of mitotic activity with the generation of a small fibrous plaque. Lacking an inflammatory response and in the presence of early lysosome enzyme release, this plaque is very short lived. No significant healing is generally seen. However, in the presence of a deep laceration, that is, one that damages the subchondral bony plate, one will ordinarily see a vascular response. A fibrous plaque, which is adherent, initially forms. This plaque becomes populated with proliferating fibroblasts, and over a period of 2 to 6 months, healing occurs. Most feel that the cartilage filling this plaque is not normal hyaline cartilage. Rather, it is a variation of fibrocartilage that fills the void. This material is biomechanically less efficient than the normal hyaline surface. However, it does provide a continuity of the articular surface layer. Unfortunately, many of these new fibrocartilage plaques are quite vulnerable. Only half of the plaques, over 1 cm in diameter, survive for a protracted period of time.

Chemical injury to the articular surface is generally the result of a metabolic end product being deposited in the articular surface layer. Examples include ochronosis, gout, pseudogout, and hemachromatosis. Various chemical substances are deposited in the hyaline cartilage of the articular surface; hence, these are often referred to as deposition diseases. These materials alter the normal cartilage matrix and, therefore, the biomechanics of the articular layer. Usually this results in stiffening of the cartilage. As a result, shear injury and impact load injury are more likely to occur, thereby damaging this articular surface.

Osteoarthritis. Despite prior thinking, this pathologic state is not merely the wearing away of an inert material. Rather, it is in many ways a hypermetabolic state. Whether one believes the biomechanical or biochemical mechanism of osteoarthritis, clearly there are components of each in the progression toward the disease. Changes occur in the constituents of the entire articular surface. The cells tend to increase in number as well as demonstrate the phenomenon of cloning (Fig. 2–5). Specifically, this is the reason for the presence of more than one cell in the lacunae. In addition, some of these cells may demonstrate mitotic activity.

Matrix deterioration begins with an apparent healing phenomenon. Initially, there is an increase in the water content, and this water tends to be bound more tightly.

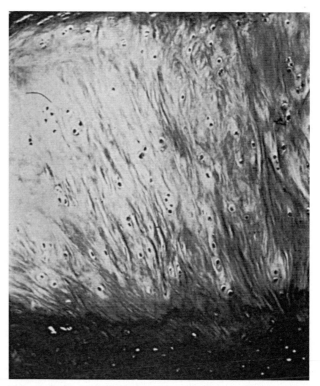

Figure 2–5. Osteoarthritis. Note fibrillation of the surface cartilage layers with unmasking of the fiber structure. Even though the fibers are identifiable and the arcade structure is unmasked, no fissures are present. The fibrillary pattern indicates dehydration, possible calcification, and brittle structure. Cloning extends through the full depth of cartilage instead of the normal limitation of a single stratum. (From Bogumil GP, Schwamm HA: Orthopaedic Pathology: A Synopsis with Clinical and Radiographic Correlation. Philadelphia, WB Saunders, 1984.)

Although there is also an initial burst of proteoglycan synthesis, there is overall a progressive loss in this important matrix constituent. The collagen content is the one thing that tends to remain relatively constant. There are generally some distribution changes of collagen between the various layers. Overall, cartilage metabolism varies proportionally with the severity of the disease. Early, there is an increased rate of DNA synthesis and cell replication. There is an increased rate of protein synthesis, and increased rate of glycosaminoglycan synthesis. Ultimately, the entire reparative effort fails, and at this point, water content, glycosaminoglycan content, and to a lesser degree collagen content gradually decrease. As these changes occur, the mechanical properties of the articular surface suffer and mechanical failure of the cartilage is imminent.

BONE

Bone, like cartilage, is a connective tissue. Because of its unique combination of an extracellular collagenous matrix impregnated with a mineral phase, bone is able to serve its major roles as a structural support for the musculoskeletal system in general, and as a dynamic reservoir for calcium. This latter function is essential in the maintenance of normal skeletal homeostasis as well as calcium and phosphorus metabolism. Bone is in a constant state of flux between continual bone formation and bone resorption; the processes are normally finely balanced. When the proper balance exists, skeletal mass is maintained and the properties of the skeletal system are optimized. In the face of pathologic states and the subsequent imbalance of bone formation and bone resorption, the maintenance of skeletal mass, calcium and phosphorus metabolism, and the biomechanical properties critical to the musculoskeletal system in general become dysfunctional.

The balance between resorption and formation is controlled by a number of local and systemic factors. The

Table 2–4. A classification of bone

Shape	Long, irregular
	Short, flat
Macroscopic	Cortical (compact)
	Cancellous (trabecular)
	Fine cancellous (embryonic)
Developmental	Membranous
	Endochondral
Microscopic	Woven
	Lamellar (haversian and nonhaversian)

From Gamble JG: The Musculoskeletal System: Physiological Basics. New York, Raven Press, 1988.

alteration in any of these systems will clearly affect the way in which the normal bone turnover is regulated.

Bone Morphology and Physiology

Bone is a connective tissue, as is cartilage, ligament, and tendon. It is unique, however, in that its extracellular matrix becomes impregnated with a mineral. On a macroscopic level, bone is typically described as being cortical or cancellous (Table 2–4). Cortical (compact) bone is the bone typically found in the diaphysis of long bones as well as subchondral plates, the outer and inner table of the skull, and the outer and inner tables of the pelvis. Cancellous (trabecular) bone is more typically seen in areas such as the metaphysis of a long bone and the diploic space of the skull. Cancellous bone is extremely responsive to mechanically applied stress and is primarily affected by Wolfe's law. Simply stated, this law emphasizes the observed fact that bone will be formed in areas where it is needed and will be resorbed in areas where it is not needed.

Microscopically, there are two levels of organization. The differentiation is determined based on the distribution of the collagen fibers in the matrix as well as the orientation

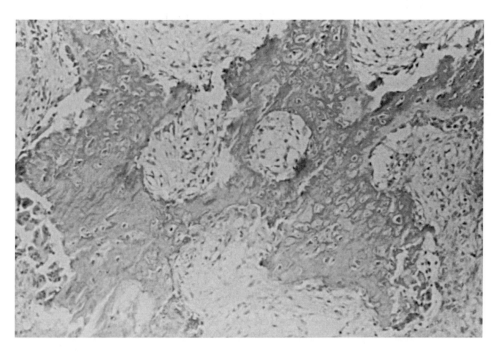

Figure 2–6. Immature bone (early callus). Note the large number of osteoblasts and osteocytes. (From Bogumill GP, Schwamm HA: Orthopaedic Pathology: A Synopsis with Clinical and Radiographic Correlation. Philadelphia, WB Saunders, 1984.)

of the cells. The most primitive type of bone is frequently referred to as woven bone (Fig. 2–6). Here the collagen fibers are randomly and loosely arranged. The cells are large and irregular and are located in very rudimentary lacunae. In the fetus, as well as in the child prior to puberty, it is not uncommon to see immature or woven bone in the cortex, as well as in the metaphysis. After growth completion, woven or immature bone is not seen except in the presence of pathologic states. In these situations, the presence of woven bone indicates high rates of bone turnover.

The second type of bone described at microscopic level is lamellar bone (Fig. 2–7). Lamellar bone is a highly ordered arrangement of collagen and cells that is critical to the normal biomechanical function of the skeleton. The woven bone present in the skeleton is slowly and methodically replaced by lamellar bone. By 1 year of age, only lamellar bone is forming, and as previously mentioned, this type of bone will ultimately replace all the woven bone present in the skeleton.

In the adult skeleton, all the bone present is lamellar bone. The implication is that both cancellous and cortical types of bone are lamellar at a microscopic level. The difference, however, is the three-dimensional structure of this lamellar bone (Fig. 2–8). In cancellous bone, the lamellar bone is configured in a very loose honeycomb with few, if any, blood vessels entering the bone surface itself. Resorption and formation take place at the surface of the trabeculae, and this type of structural organization is far more metabolically active than that in cortical bone.

The cortical bone (haversian bone), on the other hand, is a very highly ordered, geometrically arranged structure. The basic unit of cortical bone is the osteon, which refers to the osteonal or haversian system built around a capillary in a central canal. This canal is surrounded by layers and layers of mineralized bone matrix. The matrix collagen in each successive layer has a different orientation (Fig. 2–9), thereby giving the bone "ply strength," not unlike the arrangement of layers in plywood. The cells (osteocytes)

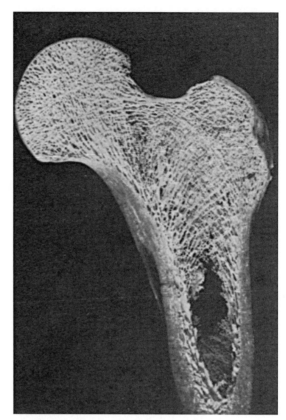

Figure 2–8. Although all the bone in the adult proximal femur is lamellar, the three dimensional structure is very different. The cortex is dense compact bone whereas the honeycomb of cancellous bone has responded to superimposed mechanical stress. (From Bogumill GP, Schwamm HA: Orthopaedic Pathology: A Synopsis with Clinical and Radiographic Correlation. Philadelphia, WB Saunders, 1984.)

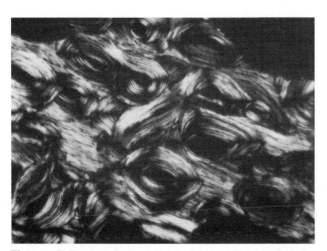

Figure 2–7. A polarized light picture of secondary haversian bone showing the circular arrangement of the lamellae around haversian canals and some longitudinally arranged lamellae in the interstitial bone (×100). (From Jowsey J: Metabolic Diseases of Bone. Philadelphia, WB Saunders, 1977.)

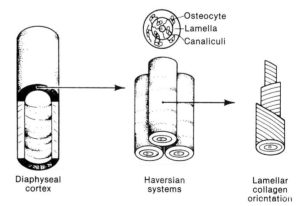

Figure 2–9. The diaphyseal cortex of a long bone is composed of haversian systems built around a central canal. The osteocytes lie within lacunae and communicate with the central canal via cytoplasmic processes running in canaliculi. Collagen fibrils have a different orientation in each lamella, adding to the composite strength. (From Gamble JG: The Musculoskeletal System: Physiological Basics. New York, Raven Press, 1988.)

Structure of Cortical (Compact) Bone

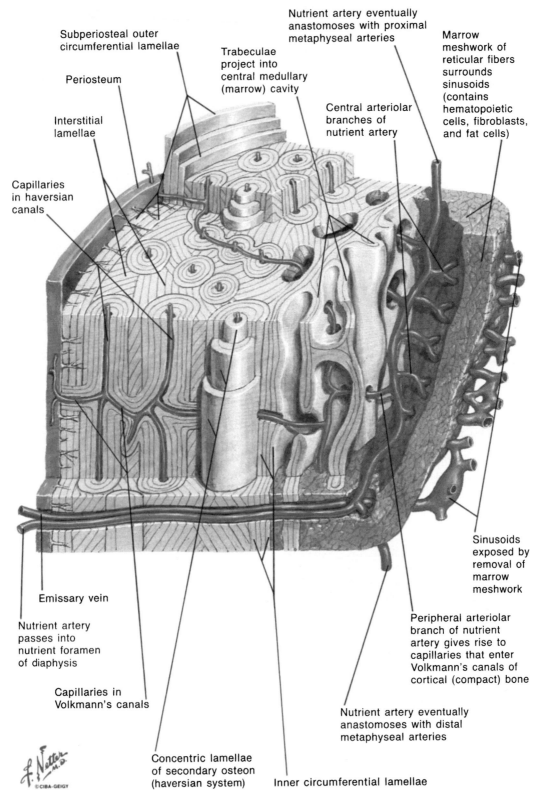

Subperiosteal outer circumferential lamellae

Periosteum

Interstitial lamellae

Capillaries in haversian canals

Trabeculae project into central medullary (marrow) cavity

Nutrient artery eventually anastomoses with proximal metaphyseal arteries

Central arteriolar branches of nutrient artery

Marrow meshwork of reticular fibers surrounds sinusoids (contains hematopoietic cells, fibroblasts, and fat cells)

Sinusoids exposed by removal of marrow meshwork

Emissary vein

Nutrient artery passes into nutrient foramen of diaphysis

Capillaries in Volkmann's canals

Concentric lamellae of secondary osteon (haversian system)

Inner circumferential lamellae

Peripheral arteriolar branch of nutrient artery gives rise to capillaries that enter Volkmann's canals of cortical (compact) bone

Nutrient artery eventually anastomoses with distal metaphyseal arteries

Figure 2–10. Structure of cortical (compact) bone. (From Netter FH: The CIBA Collection of Medical Illustrations, Volume 8. Summit, NJ, CIBA-GEIGY Corporation.)

are located in lacunae, and the cellular processes radiate from the lacunae in small channels called canaliculi (Fig. 2–10).

In any given section of haversian bone there are multiple osteonal systems. Between osteonal systems, there is additional lamellar bone filling the void. These lamellae are referred to as interstitial lamellae. In addition, surrounding the whole cortex itself is a layer of lamellar bone, referred to as the outer circumferential lamellae.

VESSELS AND NERVES

Bone, like most tissues, requires a vascular bed. Cartilage, as mentioned, is a notable exception. Bone has a vascular flow accounting for 8% of the cardiac output in the normal resting state. Most of the cells in adult bone are within 0.1 mm of a small blood vessel. In general, the blood flow to bone is between 5 and 20 mL/min per gram of wet bone. On a macroscopic level, the blood vessel enters the bone typically through a nutrient foramen. Many bones have more than one nutrient foramen. Once interiorized, the blood vessels arborize extensively through the medullary canal and peripherally to the periosteum. In addition, the blood vessels supplying the periosteum arborize over the surface of the bone. It is traditionally taught that the periosteal blood supply is adequate to feed the outer third of the cortex, whereas the interosseous or medullary supply carries the inner two thirds of the cortex. These small vessels continue to arborize, ultimately forming the artery and vein found in the haversian canal.

The nerves identified in the haversian canal are mixed in nature; specifically, some are myelinated and others are unmyelinated. They range in diameter up to about 130 μm. Some of these nerves are found closely approximated with the vessels, and others seem to be in a separate sheath. For many years, there has been a general debate as to the exact function of these nerves. Pain, proprioception, and trophic effects have all been attributed to the nervous system of bone. Whether or not these nerves play any significant role in the regulation of growth and repair remains to be elucidated.

BONE CELLS

Bone cells, like other cells in the body, have the usual cellular structure and cellular organelles. Physiologically, they perform the three fundamental cellular functions: cell replication, protein synthesis, and energy transformation. In bone, there are several different cell lines. First is a rudimentary population of progenitor cells. One line of progenitor cells is capable of differentiating into an osteoblastic line, and the other is capable of differentiating into an osteoclastic line. Although there has been some enthusiasm in the past to suggest that osteoblasts and osteoclasts are derived from a single preosteoblast, current information suggests that these are indeed separate cell lines. The basic bone-forming cell or osteoblast (Fig. 2–11) measures approximately 20 to 30 μm in diameter. The cell has a single nucleus and basophilic cytoplasm and is usually polyhedral in shape. Typically these cells are found in layers lined up on the surface of bony trabeculae. Tight junctions are typically found between the osteoblasts.

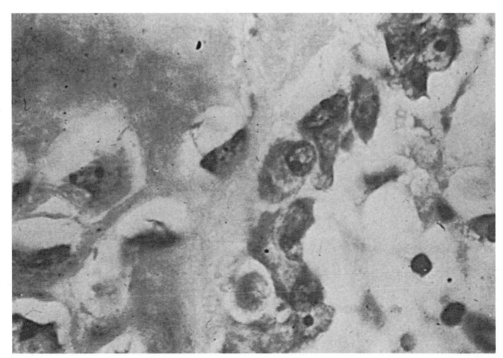

Figure 2–11. Osteoblasts secreting osteoid matrix. The light-staining matrix is deposited on the surface of existing bone. Some of the osteoblasts become encased in the osteoid matrix and modulate to become osteocytes (evident on the left). New relays of osteoblasts appear on the right. The large nucleus with prominent nucleolus, bluish-staining cytoplasm due to numerous ribosomes, and large demilune (Golgi apparatus) are characteristic of cells actively producing protein (osteoid). (From Bogumill GP, Schwamm HA: Orthopaedic Pathology: A Synopsis with Clinical and Radiographic Correlation. Philadelphia, WB Saunders, 1984.)

These junctional areas may be related to the bone-forming activity. The major function of these cells is the production of collagen matrix. Therefore, they typically contain abundant rough endoplasmic reticulum. In general, these cells can produce three to four times their own volume of matrix in a 3- to 4-day period. Initially, the organic matrix that they lay down, referred to as osteoid, is unmineralized. It remains so for about 15 days in the human. Because matrix is made at the rate of 1 μm per day, the normal width of osteoid on the surface of any given trabecula remaining unmineralized is about 15 μm. As the osteoid is formed by the osteoblast, the cells become incorporated into the matrix at regular intervals. The area of incorporation is referred to as a lacuna, and the osteoblast having buried itself in a lacuna becomes known as an osteocyte.

The osteocytes (Fig. 2–12) vary in shape and size based on their age. The young ones, which have just recently graduated from osteoblast status, still have a relatively abundant rough endoplasmic reticulum. As one would expect, this cellular organelle will decrease with age. In addition, as the cell ages, numerous cellular processes will be put out into the canalicular system of the surrounding mineralized bone. These cell processes do not completely fill the canalicular space, allowing room for an extracellular fluid component. These cellular processes of the aggregate number of osteocytes are exposed to a huge surface area, critical for mineral exchange and the maintenance of calcium homeostasis. The canalicular system ultimately links the cellular processes of the osteocyte with the vascular channel in the central canal of the osteonal system. In addition to their role in the maintenance of skeletal homeostasis and calcium metabolism, the osteocytes have been shown to be capable of a limited amount of bone resorption. This phenomenon is referred to as osteocytic osteolysis. Clearly, the osteocyte is not capable of bone resorption to the degree seen by the osteoclast. However, this limited amount of resorption is felt to be important in the physiologic maintenance of skeletal mass.

The fourth bone cell of significance is the osteoclast (Fig. 2–13). The osteoclast is a large, multinucleated cell containing numerous mitochondria and very dense granules. The paucity of rough endoplasmic reticulum indicates the absence of significant synthetic activity by these cells. The cytoplasm of the osteoclast appears to be acidophilic. Of significance is the presence of an unusual ruffled border at the active surface of these cells. This ruffled border appears to be the "active end" of the osteoclast. In this area numerous channels and vesicles are present, thereby increasing the active surface area of the cell critical for bone resorption. In this area, vesicles containing mineral and collagen fragments can be identified (Fig. 2–14).

The osteoclast is not a macrophage. It cannot devour multiple substances. The osteoclast is very restricted in its diet. It is able only to resorb bone. Based on its size, the osteoclast is far more efficient than the osteoblast. It is capable of undoing the work of 20 osteoblasts. The nuclear ratio alone (osteoclast to osteoblast ratio) is 6 to 1. This fact merely emphasizes the relative efficiency of this particular cell in fulfilling its physiologic role.

The osteoblast and the osteoclast, however, work in tandem. There is always a population of both cell lines active in the skeleton. Measurable levels of bone resorption and bone formation are ongoing. These processes, as noted earlier, are dramatically altered by pathologic states and changes in the secretion of critical hormones, such as parathormone. When bone resorption ceases and bone formation begins, this event is marked by the formation of a "cement line." Also called a reversal line, this histologic mark emphasizes the continuously reciprocating bone-forming and bone-resorbing activity essential for normal skeletal homeostasis. The average cement line is approximately 1 μm in width. It is easily stained with the usual

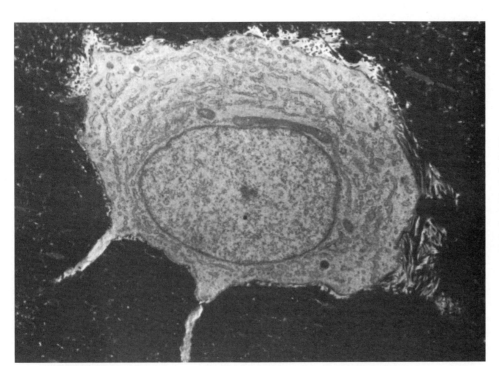

Figure 2–12. Electron microscopic appearance of an osteocyte with two canaliculi projecting from the cell cytoplasm (×10,000). (Courtesy of Dr. B. Boothroyd.) (From Jowsey J: Metabolic Diseases of Bone. Philadelphia, WB Saunders, 1977.)

Figure 2–13. Osteoclasts removing bone. The multinucleated osteoclast contains many mitochondria and proteolytic enzymes. The pale area adjacent to the bone is due to large numbers of villi and infolding of cell membrane typical of resorption surfaces. Digestive vacuoles are evident in the cytoplasm. Action by the osteoclast is rapid. Occasionally the osteoclast will have disappeared, leaving the empty space behind. These spaces are called Howship's lacunae. (From Bogumill GP, Schwamm HA: Orthopaedic Pathology: A Synopsis with Clinical and Radiographic Correlation. Philadelphia, WB Saunders, 1984.)

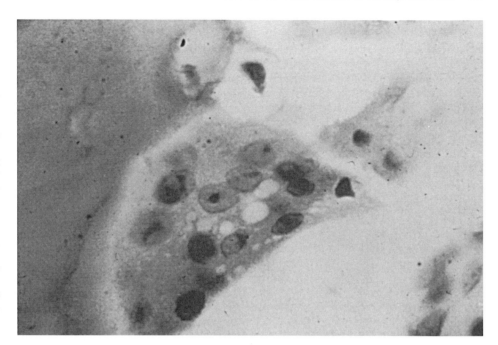

techniques because of its biochemical differences with the surrounding matrix. Some have suggested that these cement lines also represent an area of mechanical weakness and, as such, are at greater risk for shear failure than are other areas in the osteonal system.

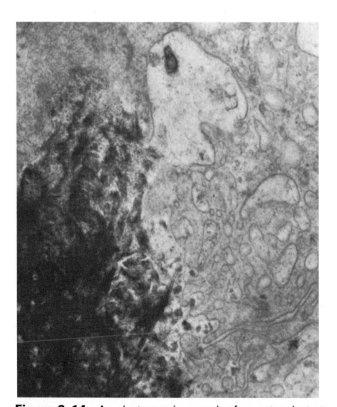

Figure 2–14. An electron micrograph of an osteoclast at high power. Both hydroxyapatite crystals and collagen can be seen in the vesicles that have formed in the cytoplasm (×60,000). (Courtesy of Dr. B. Boothroyd.) (From Jowsey J: Metabolic Diseases of Bone. Philadelphia, WB Saunders, 1977.)

Bone Matrix and Formation

Bone is a unique material in that it is biphasic. It is a composite structure, combining a blend of mineral in matrix. The mineral phase, accounting for 70% of bone by weight, is primarily the inorganic solid, calcium hydroxyapatite. The organic phase, or matrix, constitutes approximately 30% of bone by weight. This organic matrix is composed primarily of collagen, accounting for 95% of its weight. Therefore, like cartilage, collagen is an important component of the tissue matrix. In addition to collagen, small amounts of mucoprotein, phospholipid, and sialoproteins are present. Along with these chemical components, 2% by weight is water and the cells account for an additional 2% (Table 2–5).

Bone matrix is, for all intents and purposes, collagen. Therefore, the discussion of collagen is critical to the understanding of the organic matrix of bone. Collagen is essentially a protein, and as such, its basic component is an amino acid chain. Three of these chains are coiled

Table 2–5. The general composition of bone

Component	Percentage
Solids	92%
Water	8%
Solid composition	
Mineral phase	65%
Organic phase	35%
Mineral phase composition	
Calcium	60%
Phosphorus, Mg, Na, other ions	40%
Organic phase composition	
Collagen	95%
Cells	3%
Lipids, glycosaminoglycans, noncollagen proteins, etc.	2%

From Gamble JG: The Musculoskeletal System: Physiological Basics. New York, Raven Press, 1988.

together to form the basic molecular unit of collagen, referred to as tropocollagen (Fig. 2–15). The molecular weight of this basic unit is approximately 300,000. The sequence of the amino acids in the chain, as well as the tertiary and quaternary structure of these chains, determines the specific type of collagen, which varies with the specific tissue in question.

The synthesis of this important protein occurs in two stages (Fig. 2–16). The first stage is an intracellular phase that begins with amino acid activation. The amino acids are delivered to the ribosomes in the standard fashion, where they are linked together to form a protocollagen molecule. This chain is hydroxylated at the lysine and proline radicals. The hydroxylated proline radicals are subsequently glycosylated. At the point at which the glycosylation occurs, the chain is referred to as the procollagen monomer, or alpha chain. This procollagen monomer is intracellular at this point, and its molecular weight is approximately 120,000. Each of these chains has an amino terminal group and a carboxy terminal group. These terminal radicals are thought to play a role in cell wall transport and in the inhibition of fiber formation while intracellular. While still within the cell, three of these alpha chains aggregate to form the triple helix. The helix of procollagen (alpha chain) is a left-handed coil. Three of these coils are polymerized into a triple right-handed coil, which is now ready for cell extrusion.

Once the triple helical molecule is extruded from the cell, there occurs a limited proteolytic event that splits the amino terminal radical and the carboxy terminal radical from each procollagen molecule in the helix. Once this cleavage occurs, the basic unit, tropocollagen, remains. Fibrillogenesis can now proceed. The individual tropocolla-

gen molecules become bundled into submicroscopic microfibrils, which further bundle to form fibrils. Within the fibrils, specific side chain reactions occur. These reactions are responsible for the formation of cross-links within a given molecule (tertiary structure) as well as between adjacent molecules (quaternary structure). The development of this quaternary structure is critical to the normal biomechanical role of collagen, specifically to resist tensile load.

As the molecules of tropocollagen are bundled, there is a very specific pattern to this process (Fig. 2–17). The molecules create within the collagen fibrils so-called "hole zones." These zones are essentially voids within the collagen fibrils resulting from the quarter stagger arrangement of the individual collagen molecules. Specifically, each tropocollagen molecule overlaps the adjacent molecule about 25% of its length—hence quarter stagger. In addition, there are small "pores," which exist between the sides of these adjacent parallel molecules. The net effect of the "hole zones" and the unique quarter stagger array is to create, within the collagen fibril, spaces for the subsequent deposition of the inorganic phase. Electron microscopic examination of bone collagen reveals a typical and unique banding of the collagen, which reflects these voids within the collagen fibril. This banding is frequently referred to as the periodicity of collagen.

Bone collagen behaves differently from collagen in soft tissue. It is only sparingly soluble. It has a lower shrinkage temperature, and it does not denature. In addition, the intermolecular spacing is greater, as just mentioned, to make it more accessible for the deposition of mineral. These properties are the result of the unique cross-linking. The intramolecular and intermolecular interactions previously mentioned tend to stiffen the molecule and rein-

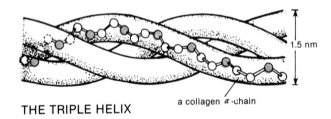

THE TRIPLE HELIX

a collagen α-chain

1.5 nm

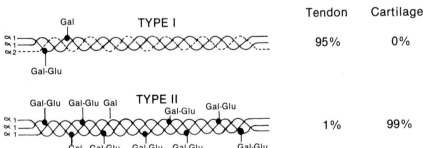

	Tendon	Cartilage
TYPE I	95%	0%
TYPE II	1%	99%
TYPE III	5%	1%

Figure 2–15. Structure of the triple helix and schematic of the three interstitial types of collagen, showing the distribution in tendon and cartilage. There are differences in alpha-chain amino acid compositions, collagen hydroxylation, and glycosylation among the types. Type III is the only one containing internal disulfide cross-links. (From Gamble JG: The Musculoskeletal System: Physiological Basics. New York, Raven Press, 1988.)

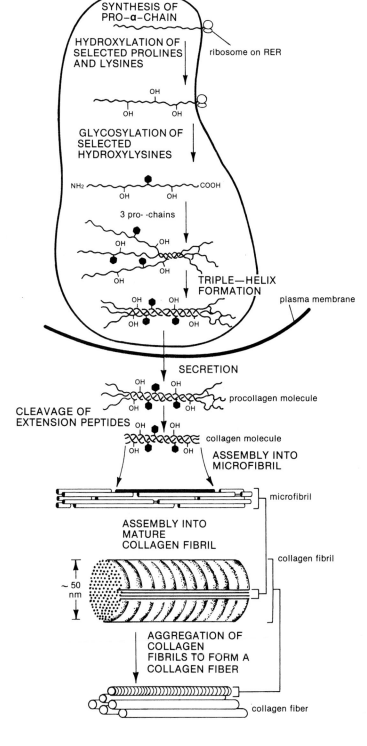

Figure 2–16. Intracellular and extracellular events of collagen synthesis and fibrillogenesis. Procollagen is secreted into the endoplasmic reticulum (ER) cisternae as it is synthesized and then packaged for secretion in the Golgi apparatus. Removal of propeptides permits fibril formation, aggregation, and cross-linking into fibers of ligaments, tendons, etc. Adapted with permission from Albers, et al. (1983). (From Gamble JG: The Musculoskeletal System: Physiological Basics. New York, Raven Press, 1988.)

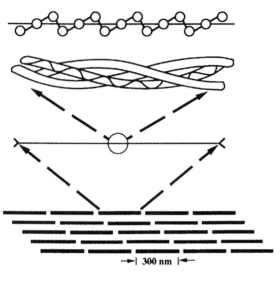

Alpha chain

Triple helix

Tropocollagen molecule

Collagen fibril with quarter stagger array

→| 300 nm |←

Figure 2–17. Schematic representation and photomicrograph of the collagen fibril structure. (From Mow VC, Hayes WC: Basic Orthopaedic Mechanics. New York, Raven Press, 1991.)

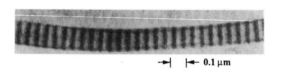

Fibril with repeated banding pattern seen under electron microscope

→| |← 0.1 μm

force its biomechanical function. There appears to be some increase in the amount of cross-linking with age. Aberrations in the extent of cross-linking are typical in certain pathologic states. Marfan's syndrome is characterized by a decrease in the usual number of cross-links, whereas scleroderma typically shows an increase in the amount of highly cross-linked collagen.

There are numerous different types of collagen. At the present time, it is estimated that there are at least 15 distinct variations with about 30 genetically distinct chains. All are members of the collagen family, and the triple helical structure is preserved. The differences are largely based on variations in amino acid sequencing as well as variations in chain combinations. Those most important to the musculoskeletal system are type I collagen, which is seen in bone, skin, tendon, and blood vessel wall, and type II collagen, which is seen in articular cartilage and the nucleus pulposus. A summary of the collagen types is included in Table 2–3. Investigations into collagen polymorphism and the molecular bases are actively ongoing. Numerous collagen dysplastic diseases, as well as their genetic defects, continue to be elucidated (Table 2–6).

Mineral Phase of Bone

Approximately two thirds of bone matrix by weight and approximately one half by volume are mineral. The most common form is calcium hydroxyapatite crystal. These crystals are 580 Å by 50 Å and are described as tubular hexagons. As is well known, chloride and fluoride ions can be substituted for hydroxyl radicals within the crystal lattice. Therefore, fluoride and chloride have been described as bone-seeking ions. Although hydroxyapatite is the most common form of the mineral present, there is also a small amount of amorphous calcium phosphate. Debate still exists as to whether this form of mineral is merely a finely divided apatite crystal.

As noted earlier, the unique feature of the bone mineral is its ordered association with bone collagen. The mineral is arranged along the long axis of the collagen fibril with an interval of 600 to 700 Å. This periodicity is identical to the normal periodicity of the unmineralized collagen fibril. Studies have clearly indicated that the mineral is found in the "hole zones" of the quarter stagger arrangement of the collagen molecules. Approximately 50% of the total mineral in bone is contained in these hole zones. Similarly, noncovalent "interactions" have been identified between the collagen and the apatite. This "bonding" bestows on this two-phase material properties that are greater

Table 2–6. Molecular defects in heritable diseases of collagen

Syndrome	Defect
Ehlers-Danlos syndrome	
Types I–III	Fibrillogenesis defects
Type IV	Decreased type III collagen
Type VI	Lysyl hydroxylase deficiency
Type VII	Persistence of N-propeptide
Type IX	Defective cross linking
Marfan syndrome	Abnormal pro-α 2(I) affecting structure of type I collagen
Osteogenesis imperfecta	
Type I	Probable deletion of d(1) gene
Type II	Defective secretion of α chains
Type III	Decreased pro-α 2(I) chains
Menkes syndrome	Cu metabolism abnormality causing defective cross linking

From Gamble JG: The Musculoskeletal System: Physiological Basics. New York, Raven Press, 1988.

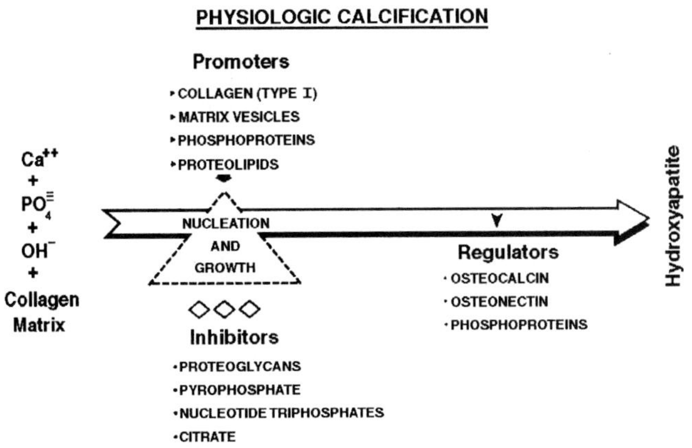

PHYSIOLOGIC CALCIFICATION

Promoters
- COLLAGEN (TYPE I)
- MATRIX VESICLES
- PHOSPHOPROTEINS
- PROTEOLIPIDS

Ca⁺⁺ + PO₄³⁻ + OH⁻ + Collagen Matrix → NUCLEATION AND GROWTH → Hydroxyapatite

Regulators
- OSTEOCALCIN
- OSTEONECTIN
- PHOSPHOPROTEINS

Inhibitors
- PROTEOGLYCANS
- PYROPHOSPHATE
- NUCLEOTIDE TRIPHOSPHATES
- CITRATE

Figure 2–18. Scheme for initial calcification. (From Simon SR [ed]: Orthopaedic Basic Science. American Academy of Orthopaedic Surgeons, Chicago, 1992.)

than the sum of the parts. The remaining bone mineral is postulated to be contained in the central core of the collagen fibril.

MINERALIZATION

Having reviewed the two components of this biphasic material, it is important to consider the process whereby they are put together in their unique relationship. The process of mineralization occurs in two distinct phases. The first is referred to as initiation, and the second is referred to as proliferation or accretion.

The process of *initiation* requires a combination of events (Fig. 2–18). Specifically, increase in the local concentration of precipitating ions, followed by exposure of those ions to mineral nucleators, begins the propagation process. Inhibitors and regulators modulate the formation of apatite. The process of initiation requires more energy

than does the addition of mineral to already existing crystals. Because sufficient energy is not always readily available, some have proposed that the initial mineral deposited is a metastable precursor of apatite, and as more energy becomes available, this unstable precursor is converted to the more stable forms of apatite crystal.

Within the extracellular environment are small structures referred to as matrix vesicles. These structures have been credited with the ability to facilitate calcification by concentrating calcium ions, by providing a microenvironment free of inhibitors, and by providing the needed enzymes for matrix modification.

Once the initial process of deposition occurs, the second phase of *proliferation* or *accretion* can begin (Fig. 2–19). At this time additional mineral is added to that which is already present. As previously discussed, this mineral is inserted into the "hole zones" of the collagen fibers. Obviously, the further deposition of mineral will serve to improve rigidity of the overall matrix.

Recently, the importance of calcium-binding proteins within the bone matrix has been emphasized. These noncollagenous proteins are felt to be critical in the facilitation of mineralization within the collagen. Specifically, phosphoproteins, osteonectin, and some of the GLA proteins have been cited. Osteocalcin, one of the recently isolated GLA proteins, is said to account for 10 to 20% of all of the noncollagenous proteins in bone. The role of these GLA proteins is still actively being investigated.

BONE RESORPTION

The process of bone formation clearly appears to be more complex than that of bone resorption. However, resorption is no less important. Bone resorption involves the hydrolysis of collagen and the dissolution of bone mineral. It is well documented that the osteoclast must simultaneously do both. There is no mechanism in place for the simple

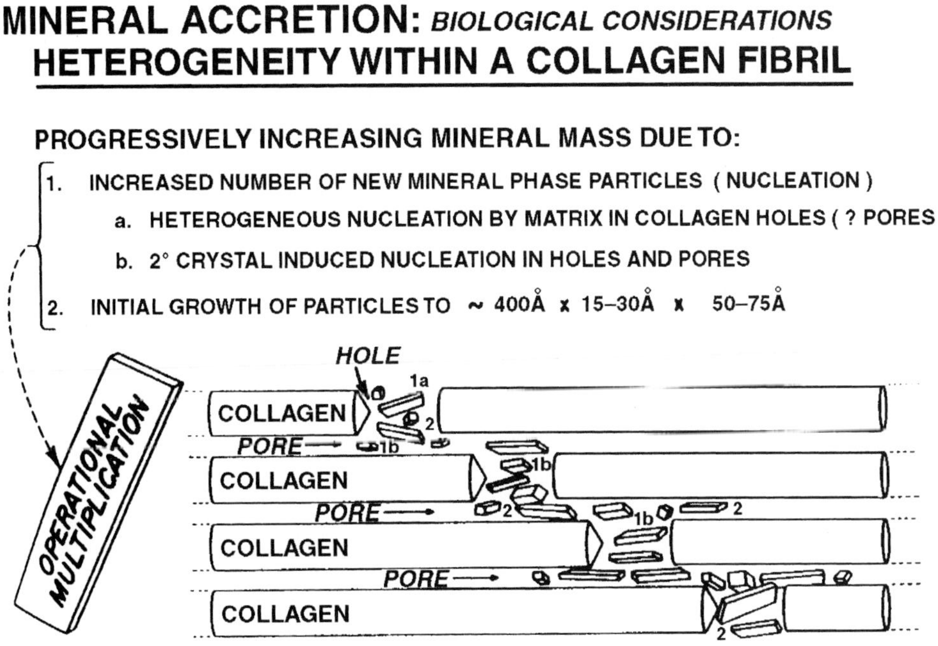

MINERAL ACCRETION: *BIOLOGICAL CONSIDERATIONS* HETEROGENEITY WITHIN A COLLAGEN FIBRIL

PROGRESSIVELY INCREASING MINERAL MASS DUE TO:

1. INCREASED NUMBER OF NEW MINERAL PHASE PARTICLES (NUCLEATION)
   a. HETEROGENEOUS NUCLEATION BY MATRIX IN COLLAGEN HOLES (? PORES)
   b. 2° CRYSTAL INDUCED NUCLEATION IN HOLES AND PORES
2. INITIAL GROWTH OF PARTICLES TO ~ 400Å x 15–30Å x 50–75Å

OPERATIONAL MULTIPLICATION

HOLE

COLLAGEN
PORE →
COLLAGEN
PORE →
COLLAGEN
PORE →
COLLAGEN

Figure 2–19. Diagram showing mineral accretion. (From Simon SR [ed]: Orthopaedic Basic Science. American Academy of Orthopaedic Surgeons, Chicago, 1992.)

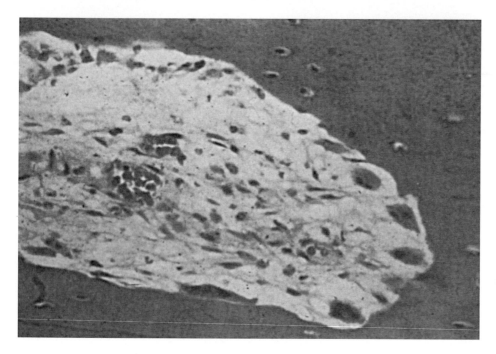

Figure 2–20. "Cutting cone." Successive relays of osteoclasts on the right resorb a tunnel of bone, making it longer and wider with each relay. Behind the cutting cone is a "filling cone" of successive relays of osteoblasts secreting osteoid. Resorption is facilitated by high-speed flow of well-oxygenated blood in small vessels, whereas refill is accompanied by dilated sinusoidal vessels with sluggish flow and low oxygen content. (From Bogumill GP, Schwamm HA: Orthopaedic Pathology: A Synopsis with Clinical and Radiographic Correlation. Philadelphia, WB Saunders, 1984.)

dissolution of bone mineral, leaving unmineralized osteoid. As described earlier, the osteoclast is the critical cell for the resorption of bone. The brush border of this multinuclear cell is always in contact with the bone that is actively being resorbed. Electron micrographs of these cells demonstrate an increased number of mitochondria adjacent to the brush border, suggesting their function in the transcellular transport of calcium ion. In addition, numerous lysosomes are identified in this area, which seems appropriate, considering the fact that these organelles contain numerous hydrolytic enzymes.

The process is thought to be initiated by the lysosomal degradation of bone collagen. Once the initial degradation begins, fragments of the disrupted collagen are taken up by the cell and further hydrolyzed. Collagenase cleaves tropocollagen into two major fragments. Parathormone seems to directly increase the local concentration of collagenase enzyme. Considering the role of parathormone in calcium release, this effect seems appropriate. Coincident with the degradation of the collagen is the solubilization of the hydroxyapatite crystal.

BONE REMODELING

The removal of bone and its subsequent redeposition is an ongoing process. The process is somewhat age-dependent. Approximately 80% of total skeletal mass is cortical bone, and approximately 20% of skeletal mass is cancellous bone. In the young skeleton, turnover rates can be as high as 50% per year in certain diaphyseal bones. With aging

this number decreases to 2 to 3% per year in the older individual. The process of resorption begins with a wave of osteoclastic activity in the form of "cutting cones" (Fig. 2–20). These osteoclastic cutting heads remove old bone, and in their wake, new osteoblastic activity can be seen. The process of bone remodeling and the rates of this process are under the control of numerous local and systemic factors. The control of bone turnover and the pathologic states resulting from aberrations of the process will be further discussed in Chapter 11, Metabolic Bone Disease.

Bibliography

Boden S: Calcium homeostasis. Orthop Clin North Am 1990;21:97–107.
Current reference on the management of mineral by the skeleton.

Boskey A: Mineral-matrix interactions in bone and cartilage. Clin Orthop 1992;281:244–274.
Well-written, easy-to-understand classic reference on the intricate relationships that exist between organic and inorganic phases.

Gamble J: The Musculoskeletal System: Physiologic Basics. New York, Raven Press, 1988.
Excellent compact text that is easy to read and yet adequately summarizes the orthopaedic sciences. Good section on neuromuscular physiology is included.

Mankin H: Current concepts review: The response of articular cartilage to injury. J Bone Joint Surg 1982;64A:460–466.
Although dated, this article explains the basis for much of the work on this subject.

Simon S (ed): Orthopaedic Basic Science. Chicago, Illinois, American Academy of Orthopedic Surgery, 1994.
This book has become the standard text for orthopaedic residents preparing for their boards. It has extensive information regarding the orthopaedic basic sciences and is well referenced.

C h a p t e r   3

Biomechanics and Biomaterials

John N. Delahay, M.D.

The purpose of this chapter is to assist the reader in understanding the basic principles of biomechanics and biomaterials. The study of mechanics is critical to an understanding of the principles of orthopaedic surgery, both in terms of the normal functioning of the musculoskeletal system, as well as aberrant behavior in this mechanical environment. The study of biomaterials is also an integral part of the field of orthopaedic surgery in as much as many implants are used in the management of musculoskeletal afflictions. An understanding of these implants and the properties of the material from which they are made is critical to an appreciation of their use.

BIOMECHANICAL FORCES

Because most of the bones of the extremities function as levers upon which muscles act, and because these muscles are essentially forces in a mechanical sense, it seems appropriate to begin with a discussion of forces. A force is simply defined as a push or pull and technically is one of three types:

1. Tensile force tends to pull objects apart.
2. Compressive force tends to push objects together.
3. Shearing force tends to make one part of an object slide over an immediately adjacent part.

Forces can act separately or in combination with one another. It is important to understand that forces are essentially vector quantities (Fig. 3–1). That is, they have a magnitude, a line of application, a direction or sense, and a point of application. Unlike scalar quantities, which are

described by a single number such as time, weight, and temperature, the manipulation of a vector quantity involves different rules. Specifically, if any one of the four characteristics of the force vector is changed, the entire vector itself is altered. For example, should the direction or point of application be altered, the entire vector quantity, the force acting on the system, is similarly altered.

When multiple forces act on a structure, it is possible to resolve these forces into a single vector. This resultant vector then represents these multiple forces and demonstrates their combined effect as a single force. Most loading situations feel the effect of forces. Therefore, the techniques of vector analysis permit the summation of these forces and a graphic demonstration of their combination (Fig. 3–2). Joints are no exception. Multiple muscle forces tend to pull structures with varying magnitudes, points of attachment, and directions. These forces require resolution in order to be able to evaluate the loading environment. By resolving these multiple forces into a single vector, their net effect can be anticipated (Fig. 3–3).

Forces that act at different points on a body tend to result in moments. Moments cause bending or rotation of the body in question. A *moment*, because it results from a force, can be expressed as the product of that force and the perpendicular distance from the line of action of the force to the axis of rotation (Fig. 3–4). It is important to keep in mind that the distance (d) in the standard formula for moment ($M = F \times d$) is the *perpendicular distance* from the line of application to the axis of rotation. In the seesaw example, each child creates a bending moment on the board. This moment tends to bend the board at the fulcrum (A). In Figure 3–4 these two moments are represented by Ba and Cb. For the system to be in equilibrium, these moments must be equal.

There are numerous examples in the musculoskeletal system of the effects of a moment. The classic example frequently used is that of the bending moment felt by a dynamic hip compression screw used to fix an intertrochanteric fracture. As shown in Figure 3–5, a moment is created by the vertical force (Wy), which is tending to bend the plate. With a higher angle plate, d will decrease; hence, the bending moment will decrease.

The term *torque* is occasionally used to indicate a moment that produces rotational motion about an axis. Essentially, a moment and a torque can be considered to be the

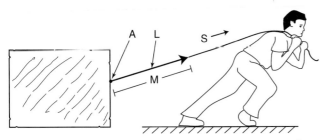

Figure 3–1. Forces are vector quantities. They have four characteristics: magnitude (M), line of application (L), sense (S), and point of application (A).

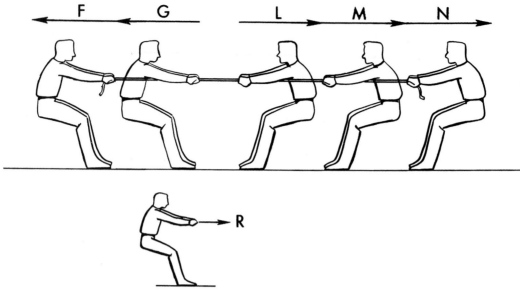

Figure 3–2. Forces F, G, and L, M, N are tension forces acting on the rope; R is the equal and opposite force of the rope pulling on the man. (From Le Veau B: Williams and Lissner: Biomechanics of Human Motion. Philadelphia, WB Saunders, 1977.)

same. Despite the fact that the formulas for calculating these force effects are different, they produce similar results—bending or rotation about an axis. A special example of torsional moments is the force couple (Fig. 3–6). This force system is created by two equal, parallel forces that are not colinear. Their resultant effect is additive and is represented by F × d.

For an object to be in equilibrium, all of the forces must equal zero *and* all of the moments must equal zero. The concept of equilibrium is important, if one is to use mathematical models to determine the loading of various joints and the effect of load on various implants.

The formula for force is F = ma (mass × acceleration), which allows one to define force in terms of any unit desired. The standard force unit is the newton, which is defined as the force needed to accelerate 1 kg of mass 1 m/s². Inertia is the resisting force that tends to keep the 1 kg of mass in its existing state of motion. The term *weight* represents a special form of force, specifically that which results from gravity. The force with which a given mass is attracted toward the center of a gravitational body is represented by its weight. Unfortunately, the term kilogram is widely used to indicate weight and mass. Therefore, the use of that term creates confusion as to the force. The term newton is the preferred term to indicate force (Table 3–1).

ELASTICITY, STRESS, AND STRAIN

The orthopaedic surgeon deals with many solid structures, some biologic, such as bone and cartilage, and others

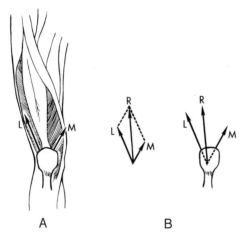

Figure 3–3. *A* and *B,* In locating the single resultant vector, R, of the combined vastus lateralis, L, and medialis, M, muscle forces on the patella, their action lines are extended to the point of intersection. (From Le Veau B: Williams and Lissner: Biomechanics of Human Motion. Philadelphia, WB Saunders, 1977.)

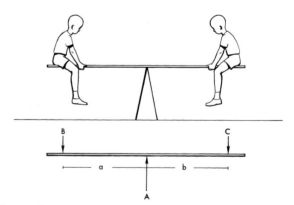

Figure 3–4. Here the forces are on opposite sides of the axis; B tends to turn the board in a counterclockwise direction, and C to turn it clockwise. In equilibrium, B + C (downward forces) = A (upward force). (From Le Veau B: Williams and Lissner: Biomechanics of Human Motion. Philadelphia, WB Saunders, 1977.)

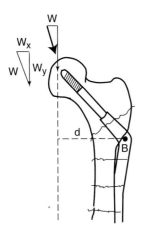

Figure 3–5. Bending moment (M) on a compression hip screw is calculated as follows:

$$M = W_y \times d$$

where d = distance from line of application to axis of rotation (B) and W_y = component of force W (body weight) acting along y axis (tending to bend the screw).

Table 3–1. Comparison of force units

System of Units	Force*	Mass	Acceleration
SI (uses meter-kilogram-second units, MKS)	Newton (N)	Kilogram (kg)	1.0 m/s²
Modified metric	Kilopond (kp, kg-f)	Kilogram (kg)	9.8 m/s²
centimeter-gram-second (cgs) units	Dyne	Gram (g)	1.0 cm/s²
foot-pound (mass) second (f-lb[m]sec)	Poundal	Pound (lb-m)	1.0 ft/s²
foot-pound (force) second (f-lb[f]sec)†	Pound	Slug	1.0 ft/s²

*Force = mass × acceleration.
†In this system, a gravitational type force is considered a fundamental quantity, defined arbitrarily as the pound, just as the meter is considered a fundamental quantity in the metric system. It is this difference that leads to some of the confusion over mass and force. Maintaining the use of the -m and -f nomenclature is a great aid to keeping things straight when kg and lb are used. An excellent discussion of the new SI System is given by Carter in Frankel and Nordin (1980). From Cochran GVB: A Primer of Orthopaedic Biomechanics. New York, Churchill Livingstone, 1982.

nonbiologic, such as metals and plastics. In the pure science of mechanics, one assumes that the objects or bodies analyzed are rigid. In biologic systems, this is not a valid assumption. It is important to be able to consider the change in shape or volume of an object as external forces

are applied. The elasticity of matter is demonstrated simply by a diving board that bends under load and returns to its original shape when the load is removed. For many materials, this ability to return to its original configuration is nearly perfect; these materials are said to be elastic (Fig. 3–7). This, of course, assumes that the deforming force does not exceed the elastic limit of the material. Some materials, such as dough or putty, have exceedingly low elastic limits and are said to be inelastic. The behavior of elastic materials is governed by Hooke's law, which states that the deformation of an elastic body is directly proportional to the magnitude of the applied force provided that the elastic limit is not exceeded. This law tends to be valid for most metals and other structural materials. However, it is not valid for plastic materials.

The analysis of the behavior of a material hinges on the principles of stress and strain. *Stress* is defined as a force per unit area of material and is a measurement of the intensity of the force. Stress essentially represents the intermolecular resistance within an object to the action of an

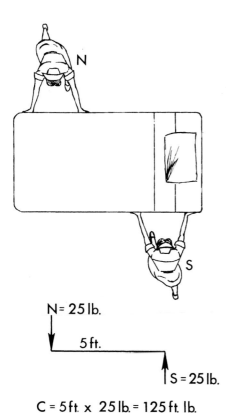

N= 25 lb.

5 ft.

S = 25 lb.

C = 5 ft. x 25 lb. = 125 ft. lb.

Figure 3–6. Example of a couple, C, in which equal and opposite forces are applied to either end of a bed to turn it around. C = the product of one of the forces and the distance between them. (From Le Veau B: Williams and Lissner: Biomechanics of Human Motion. Philadelphia, WB Saunders, 1977.)

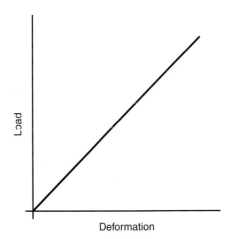

Figure 3–7. Load deformation curve for a perfectly elastic material. This is the graphic representation of Hooke's law: load is proportional to deformation.

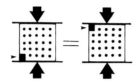

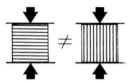

Figure 3–8. The material depicted at the top is isotropic; that is it is homogeneous. The properties, therefore, are the same throughout the material despite the direction of loading. The lower material is anisotropic or heterogeneous and therefore the properties and behavior will vary with the direction of loading. (From Cochran GVB: A Primer of Orthopaedic Biomechanics. New York, Churchill Livingstone, 1982.)

outside force that has been applied. Stress cannot be measured directly; however, its magnitude can be calculated by various formulas. The use of these formulas to determine a material's stress-related properties is predicated upon the fact that the material is isotropic. This description implies a homogeneity of the material such that the physical properties are the same regardless of the direction of testing. Conversely, in an anisotropic material, the physical properties vary with the direction of testing (Fig. 3–8). Obviously, the stress-related behavior in an anisotropic material would be more difficult to evaluate.

There are two basic types of stress (Fig. 3–9):

Normal stress is perpendicular to the plane of any cross section of material. Therefore, compressive forces and tensile forces will generate a normal stress in the structure.

Shear stress is defined as the intensity of force parallel to the surface on which it acts. The classic example used to demonstrate shear stress most dramatically is a pair of scissors.

When forces create stress within a structure they typi-

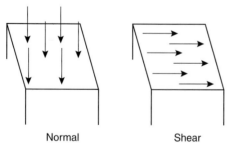

Normal   Shear

Figure 3–9. Stress is force per unit area acting in a given plane within a material. Normal stress: perpendicular to the plane. Shear stress: parallel to the plane.

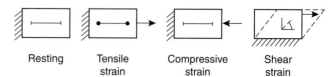

Resting   Tensile   Compressive   Shear
          strain   strain   strain

Figure 3–10. Strain is a deformation or dimensional change, representing the internal effect of a force on a body. Normal stress produces linear strain. Shear stress produces angular deformation.

cally produce strain. *Strain* is defined as the deformation within a structure (Fig. 3–10). Before a structure or a material breaks, it usually stretches or bends. This stretching or bending prior to failure is called strain, and it is defined as the change in unit length or angular deformation of a material subjected to load. Similar to stress, there are two types of strain:

Normal strain is caused by either stretching, which results from tensile force, or shortening, which results from compressive force.

Shear strain is defined as the angular deformation suffered by an object subjected to a shearing force.

At this point it is necessary to clarify the terms force, deformation, stress, and strain. Force and deformation are said to be *structural properties*. Thus, when a force is applied to a given structure, some degree of deformation is produced. The force obviously can vary from situation to situation, and the degree of deformation similarly will be a function of the material that composes the structure. Stress and strain, on the other hand, are said to be *material properties*; that is, they are the same for a given material no matter what structure is made from that material. Essentially, stress is force normalized per unit area. By this normalization one can compare the behavior of one material to another without reference to a specific structure. In other words, a steel hip screw and a steel suspension bridge will have the same material properties (assuming the steel to be the same).

STRESS-STRAIN CURVE

When an elastic material is subjected to an increasing tensile stress that carries the material beyond the elastic limit, a stress-strain curve can be plotted, as seen in Figure 3–11. In considering this curve, the line between zero and B is straight, showing that stress is proportional to strain for small strains in accordance with Hooke's law. The elastic limit is reached at point B; beyond that point stress is no longer proportional to strain, and the deforming object is no longer capable of regaining its original length when the disturbing force is removed. If the force is removed at point C, the strain retraces the broken line back to the base line and the object is left with permanent deformation (permanent set). The important features of this curve are as follows:

• *Yield point* is the stress at which marked increase in deformation occurs without an increase in load (point B).
• *Ultimate tensile strength* (UTS) is the highest point

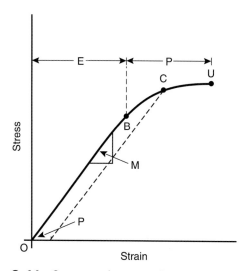

Figure 3–11. Stress-strain curve. B = elastic limit; P = permanent set; U = ultimate tensile strength; E = elastic portion of the curve; P = plastic portion of the curve; M = modulus of elasticity (Young's modulus) = slope of the curve.

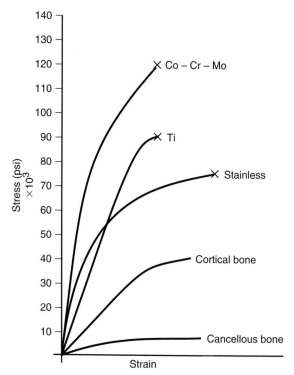

Figure 3–12. Stress-strain curve for orthopaedic materials.

on the curve. This is the maximum apparent stress that the material can withstand. UTS is frequently referred to as the strength of the material.

- *Elastic region* is the portion of the curve from zero to B. This portion of the curve is typically linear. It is within this portion that stress is proportional to strain and Hooke's law is valid.
- *Plastic region* is the portion beyond point B where the deforming strain is not proportional to the applied stress.
- *Modulus of elasticity* is represented by the slope of the line in the elastic portion. The modulus is also a material property. The higher the number, the greater the hardness of the material. Essentially this modulus indicates the pounds per square inch (psi) of stress that must develop to gain a certain amount of strain. For stainless steel the modulus is approximately 20 × 10⁶ psi.

These curves can be used to compare the behavior of various materials. Specifically in orthopaedics, one can compare the material properties of the commonly used metals—chrome-cobalt, titanium alloys, and stainless steel—as they relate to cortical and cancellous bone. The curves showing these relationships are shown in Figure 3–12.

LOADING

Forces can load an object in a number of ways. The object frequently used to model loading mechanisms is a solid bar of material or a beam. This bar of material can be used to compare the changes that are seen as various loads are applied and as the direction of those loads is altered. *Tensile loading* results from a force applied along the long axis of the bar, stretching the bar and causing any given cross-sectional area to decrease in size. *Compressive loading* conversely will tend to shorten the bar and, in doing

so, will tend to increase any given cross-sectional area. The specific dimensions of the change can be determined using Poisson's ratio.

Bending is actually a form of composite loading. Using the model of a cantilever beam (Fig. 3–13) in which material is fixed at one end and loaded at the other, isolated loading patterns can be appreciated as the beam is bent. On the convex side of bending, tensile stresses are generated and tensile strain is observed. On the opposite, or

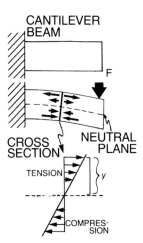

Figure 3–13. Bending of a beam. Application of load F causes tensile stresses to be generated on the convex side of the bend and compressive stresses to be generated on the concave side of the bend. (From Cochran GVB: A Primer of Orthopaedic Biomechanics. New York, Churchill Livingstone, 1982.)

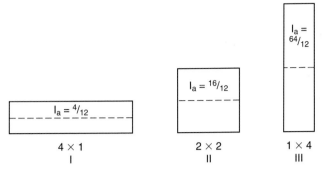

Figure 3–14. Area moment of inertia. The three beams have the same cross-sectional area; however, the material is distributed differently about the neutral plane. Formula for area moment of inertia is:

$$\frac{BH^3}{12}$$

The behavior of these three beams in bending will vary greatly despite the fact that the cross-sectional area of the three is the same. Based on this, beam III clearly is the most rigid and therefore has the greatest resistance to bending.

concave, side of the bend, compressive strain is noted, resulting from compressive stresses generated. Located in the center of the beam is a neutral plane, where the stresses are zero. These principles are applicable to the failure of long bones. When subjected to bending loads, the bones behave much like a cantilever beam, i.e., tensile stress on the convex side and compressive stress on the concave side.

The way in which the material is distributed over the cross section in any beam of material will alter the loading pattern. An important property, the *area moment of inertia*, defines this material distribution and therefore is needed to determine the resistance to bending of a structure under static loading (Fig. 3–14).

Torsional loading results when a torque is applied to a cylinder of material. In doing so, stresses are created within this cylinder. The *polar moment of inertia* is that property of the cross-sectional area of a cylindrical structure that is a measure of the distribution of the material about an axis perpendicular to the cross section. For example, the distribution of the material at greater distances from this central axis tends to improve the torsional rigidity of the cylinder in question. The polar moment of inertia can dramatically affect torsional loading and, as such, plays an important role in the fracture patterns seen in long bones. For example, the polar moment in the proximal tibia is greater than that in the distal tibia. Therefore, torsional failure is predictably more likely to occur distally, and clinically, that is the case (Fig. 3–15).

Combined loading occurs in most structures, biologic as well as nonbiologic. The loading patterns in these situations tend to be significantly more complex. Most fractures, when they occur, are not the result of a single isolated form of loading, but rather a combination of mechanisms: compression, tension and shear, bending, and torsion.

STRESS CONCENTRATION EFFECTS

Stress in a smooth bar of an isotropic material is rather easy to calculate. However, if the material is anisotropic,

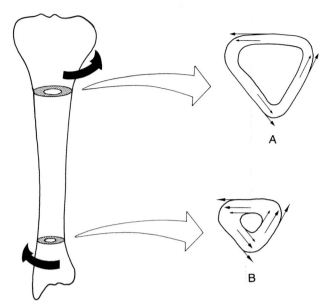

Figure 3–15. Distribution of shear stresses in two cross sections of a tibia subjected to torsional loading. The proximal section *(A)* has a higher moment of inertia than the distal section *(B)*, because more bony material is distributed away from the neutral axis. (Adapted from Frankel and Burstein, 1970; from Frankel VH, Nordin M: Basic Biomechanics of the Skeletal System. Philadelphia, Lea & Febiger, 1980.)

or if there is a missing section, the calculation becomes far more complex. The principle of stress concentrators (stress raisers) has broad clinical significance. Albert Burstein and others demonstrated that the presence of a screw or drill hole in the femur of a rabbit was able to decrease by 70% the ability of that bone to store energy when stressed torsionally. Further, it was shown that upon removal of a screw from a long bone, it took between 8 and 10 weeks for the stress concentration effect to be negated (Fig. 3–16). In essence, a hole in a long bone significantly weakens that

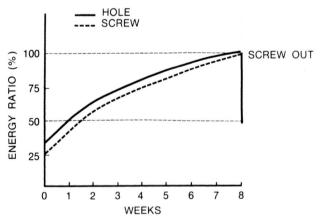

Figure 3–16. Effect of screws and screw holes on the energy storage capacity of rabbit femora. The energy storage for experimental animals is expressed as a percentage of the total energy storage capacity for control animals. (Adapted from Burstein et al., 1972; from Frankel VH, Nordin M: Basic Biomechanics of the Skeletal System. Philadelphia, Lea & Febiger, 1980.)

bone in the presence of torsional load. Similarly, an open section effect is created when a larger segment of bone is removed from the circumference of a long tubular bone. The cortical discontinuity functions as a large stress raiser, and in torsional testing of the human tibia, such an open defect can reduce the load to failure and the ability to store energy by up to 90%.

ENERGY CONSIDERATIONS

The term energy has been used on several previous occasions, specifically as it relates to the ability of a bone to store energy. In its purest sense, *energy* is a measure of the capacity or the ability to do work. It, like work, is a scalar quantity and is expressed in the same units, that is, foot-pounds or joules. The amusement park roller coaster provides the best and most vivid model for energy considerations. As the train is moved to the top of the track, it acquires potential energy. Work must be put into the system to take the train to the top of the track. Once there, it has the maximum potential energy that it can acquire. Work has been done on the object against the force of gravity. In this position, the train is now capable of transferring its energy into a kinetic form. That is, as it starts down the track it gives up its potential energy in exchange for kinetic energy, or the energy of motion. Therefore, kinetic energy is the ability of a moving object to produce work. Work, in physics, is the product of a force multiplied by the displacement of that force (W = F × s). Unlike moment, the distance (s) is the distance traveled by the object. Once the train reaches the bottom of the track the energy transfer is complete, and if it were an idealized frictionless environment, the coaster would just keep going in the same direction at constant velocity.

The principle of this roller coaster can be applied to human gait (Fig. 3–17). The vertical oscillation of the center of gravity during the normal gait cycle is essentially no different from the coaster going up and down on its track. As the center of gravity rises, energy is being put into the system, and as the center of gravity falls, that energy is being recovered in the form of kinetic energy.

These energy concepts are perhaps more important when considering the use of implants and their significance in fractures. The behavior of a metallic implant and that of a long bone both depend on their ability to store energy. The

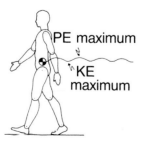

Figure 3–17. Energy exchange occurs during normal gait. To elevate the center of gravity work must be done by the organism and potential energy is stored. This is subsequently recovered as kinetic energy as the center of gravity falls. (From Cochran GVB: A Primer of Orthopaedic Biomechanics. New York, Churchill Livingstone, 1982.)

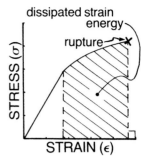

Figure 3–18. Energy storage can be graphically represented as the area under the stress-strain curve (strain energy). The energy represented by the white triangle is recoverable whereas that identified in the shaded area is dissipated—all is strain energy. (From Cochran GVB: A Primer of Orthopaedic Biomechanics. New York, Churchill Livingstone, 1982.)

energy that a body is capable of absorbing, by changing its shape under the application of external loads, is referred to as *strain energy*. Bone is such a material. It is capable of absorbing energy under the application of external loads. As a bone or implant deforms with the application of load, a certain amount of potential energy is placed into the structure. As the structure returns to its original shape, that energy is recovered in a kinetic form. Stated another way, the potential energy stored in the structure at the time of deformation is referred to as strain energy. The strain energy in a deformed structure would best be represented as the area under the stress-strain curve. Further, that area graphically shown under the elastic portion of the curve represents the stored strain energy that is completely recoverable. However, the area under the plastic portion of the stress-strain curve is the absorbed strain energy, which is dissipated (Fig. 3–18). This dissipation results in the process of producing permanent deformation. Dissipation of energy is used frequently to protect both structures as well as human beings. The bumper of a car is frequently designed to deform, thereby dissipating energy and decreasing the risk of further damage to the rest of the vehicle or to its inhabitants.

In the case of fractures, the energy stored within the bone is completely released. It stands to reason that the more energy stored prior to bony failure, the greater will be the risk of collateral soft-tissue damage. Again, only the energy stored under the elastic portion of the curve is recovered at the time of fracture. Therefore, one can argue that the ability of a bone or an implant device to deform plastically somehow protects the adjacent soft tissues from damage. It is important to note that in biologic systems, the ability of bone to absorb energy is rate-dependent. Specifically, this means that the speed at which the bone is loaded determines the ability of that bone to store energy (Fig. 3–19).

These principles are best exemplified by considering the result of applying a torsional load to the tibia. The higher the speed of loading, the more energy the bone stores prior to failure. Conversely, if the load is applied slowly, the energy stored tends to be less. The implications of this are significant. With low-velocity failure, the energy released at the time of fracture is approximately half of that released

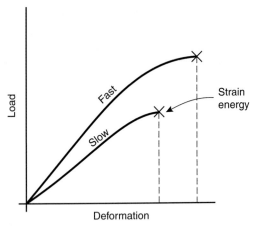

Figure 3–19. Strain energy stored is shown relative to the rate of loading. As seen the more rapid the rate of load application, the greater the amount of stored energy (strain energy).

if the bone had been loaded more rapidly. Hence, the natural conclusion is that soft-tissue damage is far more likely with high-velocity trauma.

VISCOELASTICITY

As discussed previously, many nonbiologic materials behave in a purely elastic manner. That is, the stress and strain are linearly proportional and constant. Most of the metals and ceramics that are used in orthopaedics behave in a classically elastic fashion. Polymers, on the other hand, behave differently. Polymers, much like bone, show a degree of rate dependence. That is, the stress developed depends not only on the strain, but also on the time taken to reach that strain. This behavior of rate dependence is referred to as *viscoelasticity.*

For a viscoelastic material the stress developed depends on the strain and the time. For a viscoelastic material, the stress-strain curve can be altered by changing the strain rate. The model frequently used to demonstrate biologic viscoelastic behavior is the ear lobe (Fig. 3–20). In reviewing Figure 3–20, with application of a weight to the ear lobe, there will be an initial instantaneous deformation, with further deformation occurring over time. This deformation over time will reach a limiting or steady state value. Upon removal of the load, there will be an immediate recoil toward the baseline with a slow return to the original state.

Using this curve as a reference one can identify three phenomena that are typical of a viscoelastic material:

Damping. This phenomenon is exemplified by the syringe, in which the resistance or force required to move the plunger into the syringe increases as the rate of movement of the plunger increases. This action is analogous to the shock absorbers of a car, which moderate the sharp vibrations imparted to the wheels. This property of a material, offering greater resistance as the speed is increased, is called damping.

Creep. Following the sudden application of a given load, there is an initial deformation, followed by a subsequent additional deformation, which occurs as a function of time under the same initial load. For example, we lose some height during the course of the day. This loss of height is due to creep of the intervertebral disks. Slowly over time, they thin down; the net effect when summated is loss of height.

Relaxation. Relaxation describes a decrease in stress within a deformed structure over time, when the deformation is held constant. When a Harrington rod is used on the concave side of a scoliotic curve to straighten the spine, there is an immediate tightening of the ligamentous structures on the concavity of the curve. However, the stresses within those ligamentous structures lessen with time. In addition, the stresses within the rods themselves can be noted to decrease.

MECHANICAL PROPERTIES OF TISSUES

Bone

Despite the fact that both cancellous and cortical types of bone are fabricated from the same material, their structural properties vary enormously.

CANCELLOUS BONE

Cancellous bone is an organized, load-bearing material. Mechanically, its presence seems to be associated with the need to provide a transition of direction of forces, such as between the femoral neck and the femoral cortices. In addition, there may be a role to play in the absorption of impulse loading. Cancellous bone, by its very nature, is anisotropic; therefore, its behavior varies with the direction of loading. It tends to be stiffer in tension than in compression. It also fails at lower strain in the direction parallel to the axis of the spicule. For example, in the proximal femur it is well known that the calcar is a condensation of cancellous bony trabeculae that is stress-generated. This region is capable of absorbing high compressive stresses. In addition, it has been theorized that once a microfracture

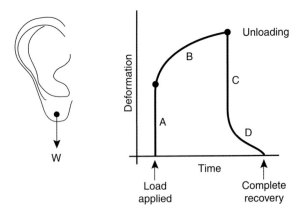

Figure 3–20. Principles of viscoelastic behavior. As load is applied to a viscoelastic material, immediate deformation *(A)* occurs. With the load held constant, slow progressive additional deformation (creep) continues to occur with time *(B).* When unloading occurs, there is immediate recoil *(C),* followed by a prolonged period of stress relaxation *(D).*

occurs in a bony trabeculum, the site will become stiffer upon healing, most likely as a result of the effect of the microcallus in increasing the polar moment of inertia. In turn, the subchondral trabeculae stiffen. Whether this change in turn leads to stiffening of the subchondral plate with subsequent development of osteoarthritis remains an open question.

The obvious major difference between cancellous and cortical bone is the degree of porosity. Because of its far greater porosity, cancellous bone behaves very poorly during compression. Despite its ability to absorb energy upon impact, the application of significant loads will cause failure at strain rates of 0.5. At that point, crushing of the trabeculae has already begun to occur. As is the case in a vertebral body compression fracture, once a certain amount of compression and failure has occurred, the overall construct does become somewhat stiffer. This ability to become "stronger" with the application of compressive load is in contrast to the application of tensile load. Once yielding of cancellous bone occurs in tension, rapid fracture is likely to follow. The ability to absorb energy in tensile loading is markedly less than in compressive loading.

CORTICAL BONE

Cortical bone is a unique tissue. In light of its organized, mineralized structure, it is clearly designed to carry load. The classic lamellae (parallel sheets of bone) are 3 to 4 μm thick. The haversian systems are suited and designed to withstand bending about their long axis. Cortical bone, although viscoelastic by nature, is characterized by its elastic properties, especially at low strain rates. The ability of bone to deform plastically is a function of its hydration. In the fully hydrated state, cortical bone exhibits elastic behavior up to 0.3% strain. When it is dry, bone exhibits a higher modulus in both tension and compression, but it is more brittle. Therefore, in vivo, in its normal hydrated state, bone has a far greater ability to absorb strain energy. The fact that bone is viscoelastic only enhances its behavior in the mechanical environment within which it must function. This ability to behave differently at different strain rates protects the structure from failure within a wide range. The mechanical properties of bone are intimately related with its chemistry.

For example, aging causes an anticipated effect mechanically. The decrease in water, collagen, and glycosaminoglycan content causes the bone to be stiffer. As a result, the tensile and compressive moduli are greater. Unfortunately, the strain energy to failure and ultimate tensile strength tend to decrease, making fracture more likely. Although the bone is stiffer, this does not mean that it is stronger, as some might think. In fact, the stiffer bone is more brittle and absorbs less energy prior to failure.

Articular Cartilage

The biomechanical behavior of cartilage can best be understood by appreciating the fact that it is a biphasic tissue: matrix and water. Cartilage, as noted previously, is a fluid-filled porous medium. The chemical constituents of the organic matrix (collagen and proteoglycan) and the interstitial water interact with each other to create a unique tissue capable of impact load absorption and near frictionless

interfaces. Articular cartilage is viscoelastic, as is bone. Therefore, it is capable of creep. The ability of cartilage to creep is important in the normal lubricating mechanics of diarthrodial joints. As the cartilage is loaded, fluid is expressed, creating what has been referred to as an elastohydrodynamic mechanism of joint lubrication. This subject will be further discussed in the section on joint mechanics later in this chapter.

Collagenous Tissues

Ligament and tendon are essentially passive structures and inherently are not responsible for active motion. Histologically, they are composed of three fiber types: (1) collagen, which gives them strength and stiffness, (2) elastic fibers, needed for extensibility under load, and (3) reticular fibers, essentially present for bulk. Both ligament and tendon function primarily in tension. Their mechanical properties are a function of the orientation of the fibers, the material properties of the fibers, and the relative proportion of collagen to elastin.

Structurally, the direction of the fibers varies between tendon and ligament. In tendon, the collagen bundles are parallel, as one would expect, making them the ideal tissue to withstand high tensile load. Ligament, on the other hand, must function throughout the full range of a given joint. In order to meet this demand, the fiber orientation must be far more diverse and therefore somewhat random. Typically, nonparallel arrays of collagen fibers are seen.

The properties of the two fibers are also somewhat different. Collagen is a ductile material, showing a stress-strain curve similar to that of bone. The elastic fibers, on the other hand, behave much like a rubber band. That is, they show significant deformation or strain with relatively minimally applied load, but once failure occurs, it occurs quickly.

The proportion of the fibers in different tissues varies as well. Tendon, as a tissue, is composed almost entirely of collagen fibers. This makeup gives it its ability to translate force directly from muscle to bone. Ligaments, on the other hand, primarily function to stabilize joints during motion. They must allow a certain amount of "play" as the joint moves. Although composed primarily of collagen, they have a much larger proportion of elastic fibers. Indeed, up to two thirds of some ligaments, such as the ligamentum nuchae and the ligamentum flavum, are elastic fibers.

Noyes and coworkers demonstrated a load elongation curve for collagenous tissues (Fig. 3–21). Specifically, Noyes' work employed the Rhesus monkey knee as a model. These knees were tested in tension to failure of the anterior cruciate ligament (ACL). The force/elongation curve shown graphically represents the behavior of these ligaments and, by inference, those in the human. In Figure 3–21, region 1 represents "toeing in" of the collagen. The initial application of load serves only to straighten the wavy collagen fibers. Once they are straight, the curve becomes linear, confirming primarily elastic behavior. At point 2, which can be compared to the yield point on a stress-strain curve, microfailure of collagen fibers begins. This process continues out to region 3, at which point the tissue has sustained 6 to 8% strain. Although appearing grossly normal up to this point, the anterior cruciate liga-

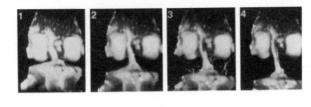

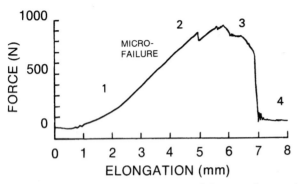

Figure 3–21. Progressive failure of the anterior cruciate ligament from a cadaver knee tested in tension to failure at a physiologic strain rate (Noyes, 1977). Almost 8 mm of joint displacement took place before the ligament reached complete failure. The force-elongation curve generated during this experiment is correlated with various degrees of joint displacement. (Courtesy of Frank R. Noyes, M.D., and Edward S. Grood, Ph.D; from Frankel VH, Nordin M: Basic Biomechanics of the Skeletal System. Philadelphia, Lea & Febiger, 1980.)

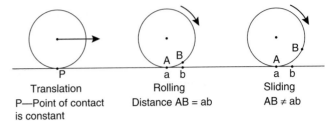

Figure 3–22. Types of joint motion.

ment has undergone significant in-substance failure. From this point forward, major failure of the tissue develops, with disruption occurring at 50% strain.

Further studies have elaborated on this important basic work. Clearly, other factors determine the strength of a given ligament under loading. The size and shape of a ligament are critical issues in its behavior. As one would expect, the larger the cross-sectional area, the stronger the ligament. The speed of loading, as is the case with other viscoelastic biologic tissues, also plays a role in ligament failure. The ACL has been shown to function much like bone in that, as the loading rate increases, the ligament is able to store more energy prior to failure. Unfortunately, when the ligament does fail at these high rates, it tends to be within the substance of the ligament with disastrous consequences. At lower loading rates, the bony insertion of the ligament is more vulnerable and therefore tibial spine avulsion is more likely. This data suggests that with an increase in loading rate, the strength of the bone increases more than the strength of the ligament. Hence, ligament failure occurs at higher loading rates.

JOINT MECHANICS

In order to evaluate the way in which a given diarthrodial joint functions, it is important to look at two specific aspects of that joint. First is the evaluation of its *kinematics*, which is the study of the relative motion of the two articulating surfaces in relation to each other. The other is to evaluate the *kinetics* of joint motion, which refers to the

forces that are creating the motion as well as the loads that are created across the articular surface.

The kinematics of any given joint will clearly be a function of the geometry of the juxtaposed bony surfaces. In general, three types of motion occur between surfaces of joints: translational, rolling, and sliding motions (Fig. 3–22). Translational motion is the movement of one surface past another with no rotational component. This movement can be seen to some degree in the spine and in the shoulder. Rolling and sliding motions imply a degree of rotational motion, which is an extremely complex subject. Suffice it to say that pure rolling motion between two surfaces occurs when the instant center of rotation is always at the point of contact between the two surfaces. On the other hand, a sliding motion implies that the instant center is not at the point of contact of the two surfaces. This motion results when the moving segment is rotating without moving an equivalent distance along the surface beneath.

In point of fact, most diarthrodial joints demonstrate a degree of sliding motion and translational motion. Pure rolling is more theoretical than real when applied to a biologic system. The implication, however, is that in hinged joints, such as the knee and the elbow, there is no fixed, single axis of rotation. Rather, this axis of rotation changes throughout the arc of motion. Therefore, rather than a

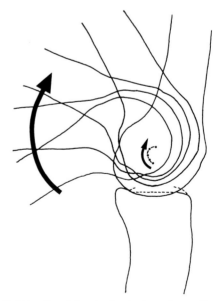

Figure 3–23. Semicircular instant center pathway for the tibiofemoral joint in a 19-year-old man with a normal knee. (From Frankel VH, Nordin M: Basic Biomechanics of the Skeletal System. Philadelphia, Lea & Febiger, 1980.)

single axis of rotation, one can calculate what is called an "instant center pathway," which is a line representing the summation of individual instant centers throughout the full arc of motion. The knee is a classic example. The instant center path has been carefully worked out and is represented by a small semicircle in the femoral condyle (Fig. 3–23). Pathologic intra-articular defects alter this normal path, thereby causing jamming of the joint surfaces and subsequent damage.

The kinetic analysis of joint function is even more complex because joints are in motion, and any change of position alters the forces as they are applied to the joint. Specifically, the forces acting on a given joint (Fig. 3–24) during activity are those due to the muscle forces pulling across it, the superimposed body weight, the force of the floor pushing back against the joint in question, and the infamous J-force. The J-force, or joint reaction force, is intrinsic to a given joint and is the force felt by the articular cartilage in any given load-bearing situation. For example, the J-force on the undersurface of the patella performing certain exercise protocols has been calculated relatively carefully. Similarly, the J-force across the hip in various models with and without external aids has been reviewed.

The final consideration regarding joint mechanics is *lubrication*. From an engineering standpoint, there are only two fundamental types of lubrication: (1) boundary lubrication and (2) fluid film lubrication. In point of fact, both forms are operational in the lubricating mechanism of a diarthrodial joint.

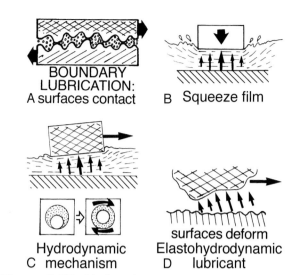

Figure 3–25. Modes of lubrication. *A*, Boundary lubrication. *B*, Squeeze film. *C*, Hydrodynamic. *D*, Elastohydrodynamic (a combination of *B* and *C* mechanisms). (From Cochran GVB: A Primer of Orthopaedic Biomechanics. New York, Churchill Livingstone, 1982.)

Boundary lubrication (Fig. 3–25*A*) depends on the chemical absorption of a monolayer of lubricant molecules to the surface of the contacting solids. During relative motion of the surfaces, the bearing components are protected by these lubricant molecules, which slide over each other. This lubrication prevents adhesion and abrasion of the naturally occurring surface asperities. Boundary lubrication is essentially independent of the physical properties of either the lubricant or the contacting bodies. In general, it is believed that hyaluronate is the key boundary lubricant in diarthrodial joints. Its role is primarily to decrease the friction between soft tissue and bone, therefore acting as a boundary lubricant. It has been suggested, although not proved, that under severe loading conditions synovial fluid and hyaluronate can act as a boundary lubricant for articular cartilage. However, under normal loading a fluid film mechanism is proposed for articular cartilage (Fig. 3–25*D*).

These fluid film mechanisms involve the generation of a fluid wedge between the bearing surfaces to keep them apart. A number of different fluid film models have been proposed by several authors. The term elastohydrodynamic lubrication seems to be the biologic model that most authors accept. In this model it is proposed that the porous articular cartilage surface retains water molecules. With superimposed pressure, water is squeezed (Fig. 3–25*B*) from the articular surface and is interposed between the bearing surfaces. With motion, a wedge of fluid is created that is wide on the advancing edge and resorbed on the trailing edge of motion (Fig. 3–25*C*). In other words, fluid is squeezed from the cartilage into the articular space as the bearing surfaces approximate each other, and resorbed as the load decreases on the backside of motion.

This model of joint lubrication is generally accepted, although some authors argue over details. In general, it is safe to say that the lubrication of soft tissue on bone is primarily a boundary phenomenon with hyaluronate as the lubricant. The articular cartilage on articular cartilage

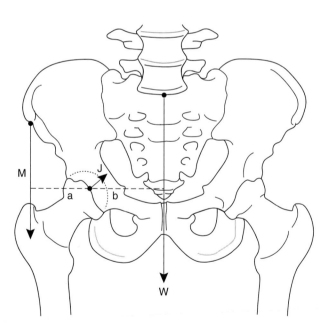

M—Abductor muscles
W—Body weight
J—Joint reaction force

Figure 3–24. Forces acting on the hip (one-leg stance) are the force of abductor muscles (M) and body weight (W) and the joint reaction force (J). Force M (acting over distance a) and force W (acting over distance b) create moments. For equilibrium to exist, these two moments must be equal. The J-force acts through the center of rotation and therefore does not create a moment.

bearing is a squeeze film elastohydrodynamic mechanism with water and glycoprotein functioning as the lubricants.

It has been well documented that articular cartilage injury or disease will clearly alter the normal lubricating mechanisms of the joint. For example, loss of the glycosaminoglycan content of the articular cartilage, as seen in aging and osteoarthritis, will markedly decrease the ability of the articular surface to retain water. Therefore, its ability to function in the squeeze film mechanism is severely impaired. This change would likely increase the rate of degenerative breakdown of the articular surface.

BIOMATERIALS AND IMPLANTS

In this section the principles of biomaterials will be reviewed as they relate specifically to orthopaedic implants. The orthopaedic surgeon is the major user of foreign materials, whether they be from the simplest and most commonly used implant, the screw, to highly complex diversified implants of multiple materials, such as in joint replacement arthroplasties.

There are reports of metallic implants being used as far back as the 1500s. Gold plates were used for the correction of cleft palate deformities, bronze suture materials were popular, and silver wire was employed as an internal fixation device in the 1800s. It was not until the Listerian era that the use of foreign bodies proliferated. Prior to that time, infection, drainage, and skin necrosis complicated the use of virtually all metallic devices. At the turn of the century, Sherman, Hausmann, and others were employing plates and screws made from such metals as brass, silver, and nickel-plated alloys. As the use of these metallic implants proliferated through the early 1900s, the problem of wear and corrosion became progressively apparent. These factors presented complicated treatment decisions in the management of fractures and nonunions. In 1936, Venable and Stuck reported on their extensive use of metals, specifically chrome-cobalt alloy, which then became popular. It was in the 1950s that titanium and the titanium-based alloys were introduced as potential metallic implant materials.

Obviously, any foreign implant needs to survive in the environment in which it is placed. Biocompatibility became one of the major concerns in implant development. The problems related to strength of the implant were carefully studied, and at the present time, it is probably fair to say that most implants currently available are able to adequately withstand the loads placed upon them.

Metallurgy

Metals are essentially aggregates of metallic ions. The metallic bond between these atoms is unique in the world of matter. Pure metals are similar to crystals in that they have a crystalline surface, an ionic core, and to some degree, some free electron gas. As a result, lattices are created and are a function of the specific metal, the type of bonding present, and the way in which the metals were fabricated (Fig. 3–26). Alloys are formed by mixing various elemental metals. These alloys are substances with metallic properties due to the presence of at least one

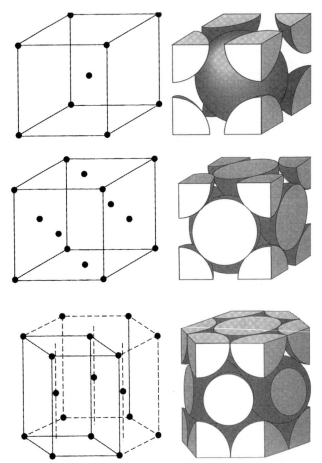

Figure 3–26. Unit cell structure for body-centered cubic *(top)*, face-centered cubic *(center)*, and hexagonal close packed *(bottom)* crystal structures. (Adapted with permission from Ralls KM, Courtney TH, Wulff J: Introduction to Materials Science and Engineering. New York, John Wiley & Sons, 1976.)

elemental metal, which has been mixed with either other metals or nonmetallic chemical elements.

The manipulation of metallic alloys is critical in the determination of their mechanical properties. Typically, molten metals are mixed and allowed to cool. During this cooling phase, the alloys nucleate into a crystalline structure. These crystals slowly grow together, and as one crystalline group encounters another, a boundary is formed and becomes known as the grain boundary. The size of these crystals is determined by the rate at which the molten metal is cooled. This cooling process is referred to as *quenching*. It has been demonstrated that the smaller the grain size, the harder, stronger, and tougher will be the alloy. Therefore, one can appreciate the importance of grain size manipulation. In addition to the quenching rate, impurities such as holes, bubbles, inclusions, surface scratches, and other imperfections will alter the mechanical properties. Finally, the mechanical manipulation of the alloy, once it is cooled, also plays a role in the manipulation of its properties. This mechanical manipulation such as rolling sheets of the metal between heavy rollers, is referred to as *cold working*. Specifically, cold working of a metal can make it less ductile and harder, should that be required for its application.

The process of *annealing*, which is the process of reheating an alloy to manipulate its properties, is frequently used to create a more desirable metal for implant use. For example, annealing of chrome-cobalt allows the metallurgist to make a more corrosion-resistant alloy. In addition, the fatigue properties can also be altered, using the techniques of cold working and annealing.

In orthopaedic surgery, essentially three metallic alloys are employed for implant fabrication (see Fig. 3–12): (1) stainless steel, (2) chrome-cobalt alloy, and (3) titanium.

Stainless steel is a mixture of primarily iron and nickel and has the longest history of use. The early stainless implants were problematic because of a high incidence of corrosion and fatigue failure. The more recent fabrication techniques have dramatically improved the alloy's behavior. Stainless steel has the lowest yield strength of the three alloys. However, its benefit is a long plastic region of the curve, making it the most ductile of the three materials; therefore, it is able to absorb large amounts of strain energy prior to failure. Most fracture fixation implants are fabricated from stainless steel.

Chrome-cobalt alloy has the highest ultimate tensile strength (UTS), and is therefore the strongest. It also has the highest modulus of elasticity, making it the stiffest of the three materials. Some would argue that its modulus is the most disparate from that of cortical bone, and therefore, it is not optimal for implant use. However, joint replacement implants on the market today are fabricated from this alloy.

Titanium-based alloys include aluminum and vanadium to harden the material. These alloys have excellent corrosion resistance and good fatigue properties; however, wear has been a significant problem. The modulus is the lowest of the three alloys. Therefore, many suggest that this is the best for implant applications, because its modulus is closest to that of bone. However, it is important to realize that none of the three are even close to the modulus of bone, making this argument somewhat specious. In addition, the UTS is below that of chrome-cobalt, despite the fact that the yield strength is somewhat higher. In addition, its ability to deform plastically is limited.

The choice of a metal for a given application has historically been somewhat idiosyncratic. Depending on the application, the cost, the surgeon's prejudice, and other factors, different metals have been chosen over the years. As one can see, reviewing Table 3–2, the properties of metals when compared to bone, polymethyl methacrylate, and ultra high molecular weight polyethylene are dramatically different. Even within the class of chrome-cobalt alloys, one notices significant differences in properties based upon preparation techniques (cast versus forged).

Polymers

Polymers have found increasing use since World War II. Their early failures were primarily due to fracture of the implant itself. A number of different polymers have been used over the years including acrylics, Teflon, and other materials. At the present time the polymer of choice in the fabrication of implant components is ultra high molecular weight polyethylene (UHMWPE), which is essentially a long-chain threadlike molecule of very high molecular weight, which tends to vary because of the chain lengths (Fig. 3–27). These chains are mesomorphic, in that they have regular atomic arrangements in some directions but not in others. As one would expect, the polymers are stronger as the chain length increases. Strength can be improved by the addition of a chemical that increases the cross-linking. Unlike metals, polymers are difficult to characterize with any degree of accuracy because they vary somewhat from batch to batch of new materials. The manufacture of polymers involves the use of a number of chemical additives, such as catalysts, inhibitors, accelerators, and chain transfer agents. These are all essential in the preparation of these materials. Polyethylene itself is a whole class of compounds, which differ by molecular weight, branching, density, and capacity for crystallization. In general, the higher the molecular weight, the higher the crystallinity and the harder the product. The mechanical properties depend on the molecular weight, the density, and the crystallinity (Fig. 3–28). Ultra high molecular weight polyethylene is a thermoplastic resin. This means that the polymer softens with increasing temperature, making molding and manufacture feasible, and allowing a superior finish to be achieved. This process is reversible with reheating of the material. This property explains the reason that implant components cannot be heat sterilized. They will distort and their properties will be altered.

Table 3–2. Properties of implant materials and bone

Material	Elastic Modulus (GPa)	Yield Stress (MPa)	Ultimate Stress (MPa)	Fatigue Endurance (MPa)
Ti-6Al-4V	110	800	965	414
316L SS	200	700	965	345
Co-Cr-Mo (cast)	210	450	655	310
Co-Cr-Mo (forged)	210	896	1207	414
Bone	17	130	150	34
PMMA	3	—	35	10
UHMWPE	1	12	14	—

*At 10^6 loading cycles.
Note: 1 GPa = 1000 MPa = 1000 MN/m^2 = 1 × 10^9 N/m^2. "Cast" refers to the manufacturing method whereby molten alloy is poured into a preformed mold. "Forged" refers to the process of cold working.
Key: SS, stainless steel; PMMA, polymethyl methacrylate; UHMWPE, ultra high molecular weight polyethylene.

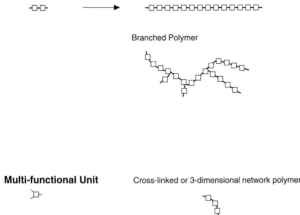

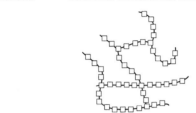

Figure 3–27. Linear, branched, and cross-linked polymer backbones. (From Simon SR: Orthopaedic Basic Science. American Academy of Orthopaedic Surgeons, Chicago, 1993.)

POLYMETHYL METHACRYLATE

Polymethyl methacrylate (PMM) has frequently been referred to as "cement." It is essentially a luting agent, which creates a mechanical interlocking bond between adjacent surfaces. A "glue" or adhesive, on the other hand, creates a chemical bond between the surfaces. PMM is supplied in the form of a white powder, which consists of small balls of polymethyl methacrylate polymer and a vial of monomer (liquid form). The monomer vial contains a stabilizer to prevent polymerization until after mixing. When the mono-

mer is mixed with the polymer, benzol peroxide catalyzes the process of polymerization. This particular polymeric material is a thermosetting resin. The polymerization occurs in the presence of heat. However, once the material has set, no amount of heating can reverse its configuration. The single most important factor in the setting time of polymethyl methacrylate is the ambient temperature of the room (Fig. 3–29). The cooler the room, the longer the setting time. In addition, the type of mixing, the rate of mixing, and the patient's body temperature all will alter the rate of setting.

Implant Failure

A number of mechanisms can cause the failure of a given implant. Metal, plastics, and cement are all vulnerable to various types of failure. Mechanical as well as chemical breakdown of the implant can occur.

FATIGUE

Most implants are made to tolerate the loads encountered below their yield point. Although designed to function in a mechanical environment, some implants will fail under extreme cyclic loading conditions due to the process of fatigue. Fatigue is the result of repetitive or fluctuating application of load. Each measured load application is below the yield point, but when applied cyclically, fatigue failure with crack propagation can occur. The endurance limit is that critical load below which no amount of cyclic loading will produce failure. Implants should be designed to function below the endurance limit. As loads exceed the endurance limit or are applied cyclically, fatigue of the implant may occur. Ductility does not in and of itself preclude fatigue, because only a moderate amount of plastic deformation of an implant can be tolerated before failure is seen. Imperfections in design or fabrication such as cracks, notches, impurities, and sharp angles predispose the implant to fatigue failure.

WEAR

Wear is the mechanical removal of material from surfaces in relative motion to each other. For example, the sliding of one object over another produces wear. It is key to

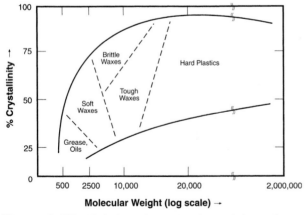

Figure 3–28. Variations in molecular weight and crystallinity have a profound effect on the material properties of polymers, as shown here for polyethylene. (Adapted with permission from Ralls KM, Courtney TH, Wulff J: Introduction to Materials Science and Engineering. New York, John Wiley & Sons, 1976; from Simon SR: Orthopaedic Basic Science. American Academy of Orthopaedic Surgeons, Chicago, 1993.)

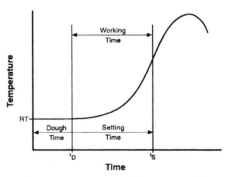

Figure 3–29. Curing curve of polymethylmethacrylate bone cement. (Adapted with permission from Black J: Orthopaedic Biomaterials in Research and Practice. New York, Churchill Livingstone, 1988; from Simon SR: Orthopaedic Basic Science. American Academy of Orthopaedic Surgeons, Chicago, 1993.)

remember that wear is a mechanical process. When two surfaces are loaded together in intimate contact, the surface roughness or asperities create points of frictional contact. It has been demonstrated that fragments from one surface may adhere to the opposite surface. Typically this adherence results from intermolecular actions. As the surfaces continue to rub against one another, further disruption of surface smoothness can occur. This process is referred to as adhesive wear (Fig. 3–30).

Abrasive wear occurs when a hard rough surface slides on a softer material, such as metal on polyethylene. The harder material tends to cut grooves (troughing) in the softer material. In addition, the presence of particulate debris between the surfaces that may have arisen from the process of adhesive wear accentuates the process of abrasive wear. When fragments are present between the bearing surfaces, the process is referred to as "three-body wear." As the distance over which the bearing surfaces slide will increase over time, there tends to be a volumetric increase in the number of wear particles.

CORROSION

Corrosion is essentially the electrochemical breakdown of a metallic surface. The ionic transfer, from one metal to a more base level, produces the surface breakdown of the metallic implant. Stainless steel is the best example of the corrosion problem. If the surface coating of a metallic implant were to be disrupted, the underlying base metal is exposed to the surrounding milieu. Depending on the base metal, corrosion may then proceed. In the case of stainless steel, exposure of the base metal (iron) usually stimulates an obvious corrosive response. If extensive, blackening of the adjacent soft tissues can be seen. The surface protective layer of an implant is referred to as the *passivation layer*. The coating is designed to protect the implant from corrosive attack and is applied at the time of manufacture.

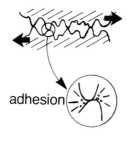

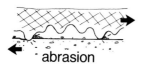

Figure 3–30. Adhesive wear and abrasive wear. (From Cochran GVB: A Primer of Orthopaedic Biomechanics. New York, Churchill Livingstone, 1982.)

Biologic Response to Implants

In general, the host organism will respond to the presence of a foreign material. This response can be local in the region surrounding the implant, systemic, or a combination. Tissue reaction to the presence of an implant is time-related. Its severity is related to the size and the shape of the implant, the movement between the implant and the tissues, the amount of corrosion and degradation of the implant, and the biologic activity of the corrosive and degradative by-products. In large part, these factors determine the local tissue reaction. The systemic reaction on the other hand can be far-reaching and variable but fortunately, for the most part, is really quite benign. Hypersensitivity reactions to metallic particles and metallic ions have been reported. The metal reported to have the worst record is nickel. If there is a question about nickel allergy, patients should be skin-tested prior to the use of stainless steel implants.

Metallic particles resulting from implant wear are typically taken up by cells of the reticuloendothelial system, which phagocytose these particles. Cells containing these particles can be identified in distant organs such as the lung and the spleen. In addition, cobalt levels in hair and nails have been noted to be elevated by a factor of 15 in patients with metal on metal implants. It was primarily for this reason that the use of these types of implants has been discontinued.

Finally, speculation regarding carcinogenesis due to presence of metallic ions or metallic particles in vivo arose because of concerns about industrial exposure to agents such as nickel and quaternary chromium compounds. Despite intensive investigation in a number of animal models, there has been no adequate documentation that metallic implants place their host at any risk for carcinogenesis. Most metallic implants become surrounded by a benign fibrous barrier, which separates them from the host tissues. This relatively avascular membrane remains inert throughout the life of the implant.

Polymers, on the other hand, tend to be a bit more reactive in the tissues, especially in the finely divided, particulate form. In the case of polyethylene, the particle size is critical. It has now been relatively well accepted that what was once known as "cement disease" is in fact the result of particulate ultra high molecular weight polyethylene in the tissues. The presence of these minute plastic particles permits them to be taken up by RE cells and histiocytes. This response promotes the release of a number of substances detrimental to bone. Specifically, interleukins, prostaglandins, and tumor necrosing factor are seen in elevated levels adjacent to this material. The net result of these intermediaries is the production of bony osteolysis. Osteolysis adjacent to polyethylene implants can be the harbinger of loosening and ultimate failure of the implant itself.

Polymethyl methacrylate, once thought to be the culprit in the osteolytic cycle, has now been somewhat pardoned. The particle size is absolutely critical in the determination of soft-tissue reaction. Polymethyl methacrylate remains relatively inert within the phagocytes. Occasionally, small granulomas can be seen adjacent to areas of cement breakdown. Probably of greater significance is the systemic effect of "monomer toxicity." At the time of cement insertion into the femoral canal, cases of hypotension and vascular collapse advancing to cardiac arrest have been reported. This phenomenon is felt to be related to the effect of methyl methacrylate monomer as a powerful vasoactive substance.

Other Implant Materials

SILICONE

This material is uncommonly used in orthopaedic applications. Other than joint arthroplasties in the hand and occasional use of freehand carved blocks used as spacers, there are few applications for silicone. In block form, it is an extremely stable and relatively inert material. Unfortunately, it is mechanically weak, and as a result, it tends to fail and fatigue, with fractures, cracks, and release of particles. The "silicone synovitis" that results adjacent to these implants can be intense, to the point of chronic drainage, mandating removal of the implant.

CERAMICS

This very heterogeneous class of materials is difficult to characterize. Essentially, these are materials consisting of mechanical mixtures of two or more compounds, usually including oxides, sulfides, phosphates, or sulfates of metals. They are extremely resistant to wear and corrosion. They have a very high UTS with virtually no ability to deform plastically. Therefore, they are brittle. Glasses and sand are two compounds that are considered ceramics. Currently in orthopaedic surgery, ceramics are used for several applications: implants, bone graft substitute, and implant coating.

Implants. Ceramic femoral heads, fabricated from aluminum hydroxide compounds (alumina) and a newer compound referred to as zirconia, are currently available. Their theoretical benefits are marked wear resistance resulting in minimal particulate debris, an excellent frictionless environment when paired with a polyethylene cup, and an extremely high UTS. Unfortunately, their brittleness and, even more important, their high expense tend to mitigate against general use.

Bone Graft Substitute. Various ceramic materials are currently on the market for use in filling bone defects and in promoting bone healing. Both naturally occurring and synthetic ceramics have been demonstrated to have an osteoconductive effect. Therefore, they are achieving popularity as a bone graft substitute. Newer information suggests that their efficacy may be improved by the addition of an osteoinductive material such as bone marrow.

Implant Coatings. Hydroxyapatite is a ceramic material. Synthetic hydroxyapatite crystals are currently being plasma-sprayed onto the surface of the metallic femoral stem. Titanium alloys are currently favored as the substrate metal. The hope is that biologic ingrowth will be stimulated by the material, thereby improving implant fixation. The exact role for ceramic coating and the long-term results of these ingrowth layers have yet to be documented.

SUMMARY

Materials and design both play a major role in implant selection. The use of any given implant for a particular clinical application still hinges on a balance struck between the characteristics of the ideal orthopaedic implant. One needs to weigh the features of biologic compatibility, adequate strength, the mirroring of physical and mechanical properties of the part to be replaced, the biologic environment into which the implant will be placed, the potential interference with normal anatomy, and most unfortunately, the cost of fabrication when determining the choice of an implant for a specific use. In addition, the experience and prejudices of the surgeon cannot be underestimated. Needless to say, the specific indications for an implant, as well as the technical considerations for its use, are beyond the scope of this chapter and will be discussed elsewhere in the text.

Bibliography

Burstein A: Fundamentals of Orthopaedic Biomechanics. Baltimore, Williams & Wilkins, 1994.
    This text is updated and readable, although slightly technical. Good sections on joint mechanics related to arthroplasty.
Cochrane G: A Primer of Orthopaedic Biomechanics. New York, Churchill Livingstone, 1982.
    Most readable text for the nonengineer. It clearly elucidates the principles of biomechanics, using excellent marginal illustrations. Excellent for board review.
Dumbleton J: An Introduction to Orthopaedic Biomaterials. Springfield, IL, Charles C Thomas, 1975.
    Excellent sequentially developed review of biomaterials with tests available at the end of each section. These are particularly helpful study guides. Unfortunately, a bit out of date.
Frankel V: Basic Biomechanics of the Musculoskeletal System. Philadelphia, Lea & Febiger, 1980.
    Places emphasis on specific joint mechanics.
Frankel V, Burstein A: Orthopaedic Biomechanics. Philadelphia, Lea & Febiger, 1971.
    The original, classic work. Relatively unsophisticated.
Gozna E: Biomechanics of Musculoskeletal Injury. Baltimore, Williams & Wilkins, 1982.
    Excellent, well-illustrated text. Discusses mechanics in terms of trauma, and the resulting injury to the skeleton.
Noyes F: The strength of the anterior cruciate ligament in humans and rhesus monkeys: Age related and species related changes. J Bone Joint Surg 1976;58A:1074–1082.
    Classic article that is the basis for most of the current knowledge on the subject of ACL strength. Implications for the reconstruction of this ligament are based on the work.

Section II
Evaluation of the Patient

GWENT HEALTHCARE NHS TRUST
LIBRARY
ROYAL GWENT HOSPITAL
NEWPORT

C h a p t e r   4
Physical Diagnosis

John J. Klimkiewicz, M.D.
Steven C. Scherping, Jr., M.D.

GENERAL PRINCIPLES

Physical examination of the patient with a suspected disorder of the musculoskeletal system is driven, in large part, by the history given by the patient. The maxim "listen to the patient" certainly holds true in orthopaedic history taking and physical diagnosis. However, it is also essential, when evaluating the musculoskeletal system, to be aware of the very real possibility that the underlying source of a patient's symptoms may be well removed from the focus of the patient's complaints. Referred pain, such as hip disease or injury causing pain on the medial aspect of the knee, or a cervical spine disorder causing pain in the area of the scapula and shoulder, is common. Both must be considered when the patient describes his or her symptoms. With the exception of the hand or foot, examination of the musculoskeletal system cannot be adequately accomplished without having the extremity completely exposed. Establishing a routine practice of having the patient change into an examining gown facilitates thorough physical examination and is encouraged.

With an understanding that distal symptoms in an extremity may be related to pathology more proximally, or even in the spine, it is essential that an examination of any part of an extremity include examination of the entire limb. Furthermore, many musculoskeletal conditions are best diagnosed by comparing the affected extremity to its unaffected counterpart. One should routinely examine the opposite extremity to determine the significance and the degree of abnormal findings such as instability, weakness, or atrophy. Examination of the cervical spine, in the case of upper extremity disorders, and the lumbar spine, for disorders of the lower extremity, is frequently necessary to ensure that there is no central nervous system component to the patient's problem.

A final general principle in the approach to physical diagnosis of the musculoskeletal system is the benefit of observing the function of the affected body part. The musculoskeletal examination should routinely begin with observation of the patient's gait, and it can be quite helpful to observe upper extremity function when evaluating a shoulder, elbow, or hand problem.

This chapter will be devoted to reviewing some of the basic principles of physical diagnosis as they pertain to specific areas of the musculoskeletal system. Further details, as well as correlation of history and physical findings, are discussed in those individual chapters.

PHYSICAL EXAMINATION OF THE UPPER EXTREMITIES

Cervical Spine

Physical findings in both the cervical and lumbar spine are obtained through careful observation and inspection, palpation of the bony and soft tissue structures, determination of the range of motion, and the performance of a detailed neurologic examination, along with other special tests. The findings from these examinations fall into two broad categories: (1) nonspecific findings that are present in most patients with a problem in their neck or lower back and that provide little clue as to the location or source of the problem; and (2) specific findings that are most useful in localizing the exact site of pathology.

Examination of the spine cannot proceed until the patient is changed into an examining gown. This is particularly important because any examination of the patient with a suspected cervical spine disorder should also include an examination of the shoulders and upper thoracic spine to search for other sources of referred pain to the neck. The examination begins by observing the patient ambulate. The examiner's attention is directed at the patient's station, gait, and attitude and posture of the head. Tandem walking, whereby the patient walks heel to toe, is also assessed in an effort to elicit more subtle signs of imbalance or a lack of coordination. Particular difficulty with tandem walking may be an early sign of myelopathy.

The examination proceeds with palpation of the bony and soft tissue structures of the neck. Tenderness to deep palpation in the muscles around the neck, such as the trapezius, rhomboids, and the cervical paraspinal muscles, is ubiquitous in individuals with neck pain but is nonspecific. Midline tenderness is less common and can be helpful in localizing the site of pathology to a particular level, or to levels if there are specific sites of midline tenderness. Particularly in assessing acute injuries, and in the emergency department setting, careful palpation from the occiput to the upper thoracic spine is a mandatory component of the physical examination. The C7 and T1 spinous processes, as opposed to the other posterior cervical elements, are usually palpable and can help to serve as anatomic landmarks. The C2 spinous process may occasionally be palpable, and notable prominence should arouse suspicion of atlantoaxial instability.

Range of motion testing should include an objective

assessment of cervical flexion-extension, axial rotation, and lateral bending. Range of motion testing of the cervical spine will routinely demonstrate diminished motion in patients with neck pain. Although this decrease generally provides little useful information regarding the etiology of the problem, range of motion testing can be a very helpful way of monitoring the patient's response to treatment. In general, limited cervical extension is characteristic of cervical spondylosis, and restricted and painful flexion is characteristic of a muscular or ligamentous injury, or a myofascial syndrome.

Careful neurologic examination of the upper extremities is an essential part of the physical examination of the cervical spine patient. Characteristic sensory, motor, and reflex changes can be seen in the patient with compression of various cervical nerve roots; although some overlap may occur, it is usually possible to identify a specific nerve root that is compressed or inflamed and to determine the disk level involved. Reflex testing at the biceps, brachioradialis, and triceps tendons is graded. The sensory component of the examination involves perceived sensation to pinprick and light touch in the upper extremity dermatomes (Fig. 4–1). Manual motor testing is used to grade the strength of each muscle group, and a score from 0 to 5 is given. In this scoring system: 0 indicates no evidence of contractility, 1 is slight contractility but no joint motion, 2 is complete range of motion with gravity eliminated, 3 is complete range of motion against gravity, 4 is complete range of motion against gravity with some resistance, and 5 is normal strength. A deficit in a particular reflex, sensory level, or muscle group can often be traced back to the exact level of cervical root involvement (Table 4–1).

Another important part of the neurologic examination is the search for evidence of spinal cord compression and a resultant myelopathy. A broad-based, shuffling gait is characteristic of the individual with cervical spondylotic myelopathy. Upper motor neuron findings such as hyperreflexia, Hoffman's sign (reflex contraction of the thumb interphalangeal [IP] joint with flicking of the distal phalanx of the middle finger), ankle clonus, or Babinski's sign are all important findings that suggest spinal cord dysfunction. Weakness, wasting, and evidence of hand clumsiness, such as the loss of mirror movement (dysdiadochokinesia), are also suggestive of myelopathy.

There are other special tests that may be useful in the assessment of patients with cervical spine pathology. Reproduction of shoulder and arm pain with extension and rotation of the neck toward the painful extremity (Spurling's sign) is a specific test indicative of cervical radiculopathy. The distraction and compression tests are other maneuvers sometimes useful in the patient with a presumed cervical radiculopathy (Fig. 4–2). In the distraction test, manual traction is applied to the cranium in an effort to lessen the pain associated with a compressive radiculopathy. In the compression test, force applied to the apex of the cranium often increases the radicular pain of a patient with a compressed cervical root. Adson's test is performed by palpating the patient's radial pulse first with him or her in the resting position and then by having the patient hunch the shoulders forward, turn the head toward the affected extremity, and extend the arm backward; diminution of the pulse represents a positive test and may be indicative of thoracic outlet syndrome (Fig. 4–3).

Shoulder

Evaluation of the shoulder begins with inspection and palpation of the entire shoulder girdle, followed by the testing of active and passive ranges of motion, motor and sensory testing, and finally, special tests. The frequent overlap of neck and shoulder pathology, as well as their propensity to coexist in a given patient, make it essential that, as in all other upper extremity complaints, evaluation of the cervical spine be performed.

Inspection and observation are helpful in evaluating patients with shoulder pathology. Viewing patients as they take off their shirt can provide clues as to the function of shoulder girdle mechanics. Inspection for evidence of bony prominences, such as a prominent distal clavicle in patients with a history of acromioclavicular dislocation, or asymmetric deltoid or rotator cuff atrophy is important. Palpation of the areas surrounding the shoulder is frequently a direct way to determine the site of pathology. Localized tenderness over the acromioclavicular (AC) joint, the bicipital tendon, the coracoacromial ligament, or the greater tuberosity may point to such corresponding disorders as AC arthritis, bicipital tendinitis, impingement syndrome, and rotator cuff tendinitis, respectively. Finally, prior surgi-

Table 4–1. Physical findings in cervical and thoracic radiculopathies

Dermatome	Sensory Testing	Motor Testing	Reflex Testing
C4	Lateral neck		
C5	Area over the middle deltoid	Deltoid Biceps brachii (secondary)	Biceps reflex
C6	Dorsum of the first web space and thumb	Biceps brachii Wrist extensors	Brachioradialis reflex Biceps reflex (secondary)
C7	Long finger	Wrist flexors Long finger extensors Triceps brachii	Triceps reflex
C8	Little finger and ulnar side of hand	Long digital flexors (grip)	
T1	Medial arm at the elbow	Finger abduction and adduction (interossei)	
T2	Medial upper arm and adjacent chest		
T4	Nipple line		
T10	Umbilicus	Trunk flexion (Beevor's sign)	Abdominal muscle reflex

From Reider B: The Orthopaedic Physical Examination. Philadelphia, W.B. Saunders, 1999, p 319.

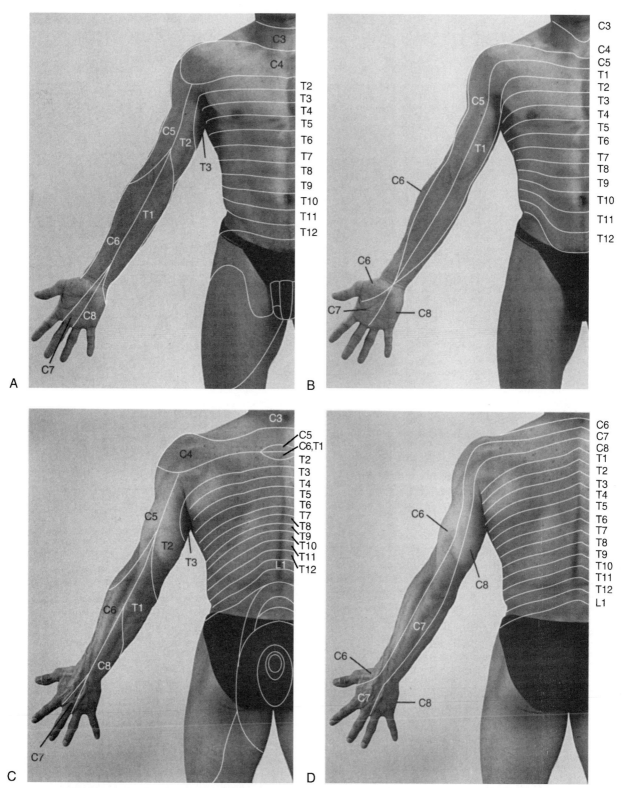

Figure 4–1. Cervical and thoracic dermatomes. *A and C*, After Foerster. *B and D*, After Reegan and Garrett. (From Reider, B: The Orthopaedic Physical Examination. WB Saunders, Philadelphia, 1999, p 322.)

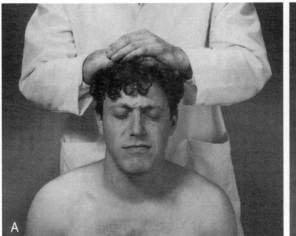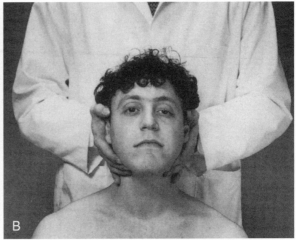

Figure 4–2. *A*, Axial compression test. *B*, Distraction test. (From Reider, B: The Orthopaedic Physical Examination. WB Saunders, Philadelphia, 1999, p 388.)

cal incisions are important to recognize because previous procedures often complicate a patient's presentation. The competence of the deltoid in patients who have undergone prior procedures is important, and any palpable defects localized to its insertion suggesting dehiscence should be recognized.

Active and passive ranges of motion are then tested. Normal motion at the shoulder includes elevation (combined abduction and forward flexion) of 180 degrees, internal rotation of 55 degrees, external rotation of 45 degrees, and extension of 45 degrees. Internal rotation can be better quantified by asking the patient to reach behind the back, noting the vertebral level or posterior anatomic structure reached with an extended "hitch-hiker's thumb" (Fig. 4–4). Additionally, external rotation should be measured with the arm at the side, and at 90 degrees of abduction, as

these positions have been found to selectively tighten the anterosuperior and anteroinferior aspects of the shoulder capsule, respectively, in these positions. Comparison with the opposite side is necessary when evaluating a patient's motion because these values are extremely variable between patients. Markedly limited and painful motion in all planes with both active and passive testing suggests adhesive capsulitis, and active motion that falls short of passive motion may be indicative of a rotator cuff tear. By palpating the scapula, one can differentiate glenohumeral from scapulothoracic motion. Patients often substitute their scapulothoracic musculature for weakness in the rotator cuff. Palpation of crepitus with motion may be suggestive of degenerative arthritis in the shoulder joint, and a rotator cuff tear may result in palpable grinding of the greater tuberosity under the acromion on shoulder elevation. Dis-

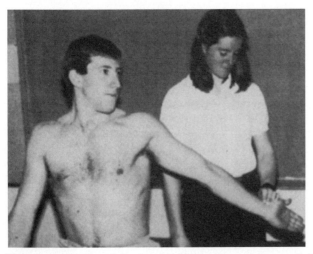

Figure 4–3. The Adson test. Diminution of the radial pulse when the patient turns the head, with the arm extended, abducted, and externally rotated, suggests compression of the subclavian artery, which may be a cause of thoracic outlet syndrome. (From Magee DJ: Orthopaedic Physical Assessment, 2nd ed. Philadelphia, WB Saunders, 1992, p 122.)

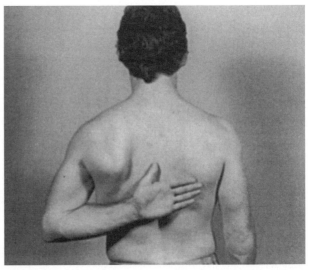

Figure 4–4. Internal rotation. Internal rotation is recorded by noting the position of the "hitch-hiker's thumb" referenced to the posterior anatomy. Here, the subject has internal rotation to T7. (From Rockwood C: The Shoulder, 2nd ed. Philadelphia, WB Saunders, 1998, p 181.)

tinction between glenohumeral and subacromial crepitation can respectively distinguish between these conditions.

Shoulder injuries may result in injuries to the brachial plexus. Motor and sensory testing of the affected upper extremity should routinely be carried out. Atrophy of the deltoid or the supraspinatus and infraspinatus muscles is an important physical finding and is suggestive of long-standing axillary or suprascapular nerve injuries, respectively. In the acute setting, sensory loss in the autonomous zone of the axillary nerve, on the lateral aspect of the shoulder over the deltoid, is evidence of axillary nerve dysfunction. However, deltoid motor weakness is a more reliable indicator of injury to this nerve. Strength testing in general should be performed for both the deltoid and the rotator cuff and the results compared to the opposite side. Isolation of the supraspinatus, infraspinatus, serratus anterior, and subscapularis muscles can be performed. Subscapularis strength is best tested with either the "lift-off sign" or "belly press test" (Fig. 4–5). The lift-off test is performed by asking the patient to internally rotate and extend the shoulder to a posterior spinous process and to actively lift the hand off from the spine, isolating the subscapularis muscle. Patients unable to maintain this position have a nonfunctioning subscapularis muscle. Similarly, the "belly press test" can be used in patients who are unable to reach backward. In this case the patient places the palm flat against the anterior abdomen and is asked to maintain the elbow in a plane anterior to the abdomen. Inability to obtain or hold this position suggest weakness in the subscapularis muscle. Supraspinatus strength is best tested with the extremity abducted 90 degrees and forward flexed 30 degrees with the thumb of the hand facing downward against resistance placed on the upper arm region. Finally, the long thoracic nerve supplying the serratus anterior

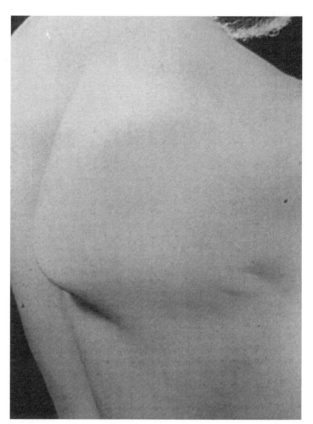

Figure 4–6. Winging of the right scapula. Palsy of the right serratus anterior muscle leads to migration of the scapula superiorly, with the inferior angle moving medially and protruding. (From Rockwood C: The Shoulder, 2nd ed. Philadelphia, WB Saunders, 1998, p 172.)

should be evaluated. Nerve palsy can lead to "winging" of the scapula (Fig. 4–6).

Patients with rotator cuff injury normally present with pain and limitation of function in the form of weakness and limitation of active motion. Functional impairment is suggestive of a more severe problem involving the rotator cuff, and pain is normally present throughout the spectrum of impingement syndrome/rotator cuff pathology. Pain with overhead activities is commonly present with either inflammation or tearing of the rotator cuff, but the presence of night pain is highly suggestive of more severe damage to these structures. Several special tests are extremely useful in evaluating patients with rotator cuff disease, and include the impingement sign, the impingement reinforcement sign, the drop-arm test, and the impingement test. Neer's impingement sign is elicited by passively flexing the shoulder to 90 degrees with the examiner's opposite hand stabilizing the acromion. Reproduction of pain with this maneuver is evidence of rotator cuff tendinitis, or impingement syndrome and the sensitivity of this test can be enhanced by internally rotating the shoulder once it has been elevated to 90 degrees (Hawkin's impingement re-enforcement sign) (Fig. 4–7). The impingement test is done by sterilely injecting a local anesthetic into the subacromial space and to repeat these tests several minutes later. The elimination of pain is highly suggestive of an impingement process occurring in the rotator cuff causing the associated

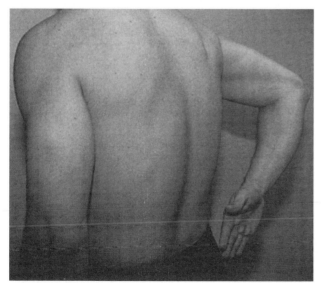

Figure 4–5. The lift-off test is performed by having the patient lift the palm of the hand backward, away from the small of the back. The patient must have sufficient internal rotation to allow this test to be performed. It is suggestive of a subscapularis rupture if the patient cannot lift off. (From Rockwood C: The Shoulder, 2nd ed. Philadelphia, WB Saunders, 1998, p 192.)

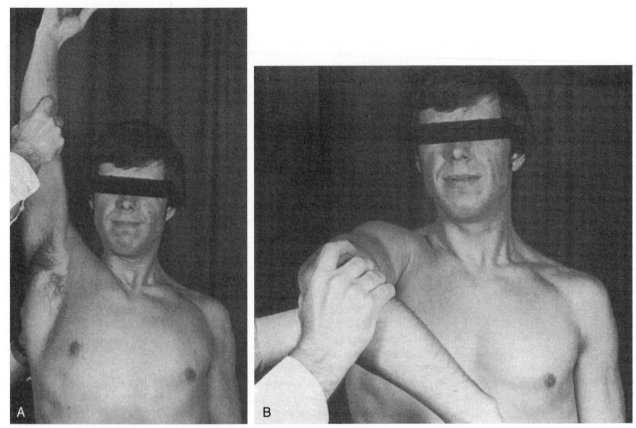

Figure 4–7. The impingement sign is elicited by forward elevation of the shoulder (A), compressing the greater tuberosity against the anterior acromion. Further internal rotation (B) brings the greater tuberosity under the coracoacromial ligament, increasing the sensitivity of this test. (Modified from Hawkins RJ, Kennedy JC: The impingement syndrome in athletes. Am J Sports Med 1980;8:57.)

pain. Finally, the drop-arm test evaluates rotator cuff strength and is performed by abducting the arm to 90 degrees, and asking the patient to slowly lower it to the side. Failure to control the arm as it "drops" to the side is suggestive of a large tear in the rotator cuff.

Patients presenting with instability may complain of either pain or instability as their presenting problem. Important when evaluating these patients is a thorough history that can provide valuable insight as to the nature of this process. The mechanism of injury, along with arm position, and number of prior dislocations can help classify the nature of the instability. Similar complaints in the opposite shoulder are also significant in this respect. It is important to distinguish an atraumatic versus traumatic etiology, as well as the directional component of this process. Traumatic mechanisms are often unidirectional, but more subtle atraumatic cases often demonstrate a multidirectional element. On physical examination, the presence of generalized ligamentous laxity is important. Recurvatum of the elbows as well as the ability to hyperextend the first metacarpophalangeal joint often suggests more generalized ligamentous laxity often seen in patients with multidirectional instability. The presence of a sulcus sign is also an important finding in these patients. Traction on the elbow flexed 90 degrees often produces a sulcus beneath the acromion in ligamentously lax individuals with multidirectional instability (Fig. 4–8). It represents an inferior component as part

of the multidirectional nature of their problem. Function of the rotator interval capsular structures in patients with a demonstrable sulcus sign can be tested for by externally rotating the shoulder. Patients with a functioning rotator interval capsule should demonstrate a decrease in their sulcus sign with this maneuver. Anterior and posterior drawer testing should then be performed and the results compared to the opposite shoulder to detect pathologic laxity with anterior and posterior stress maneuvers. With the patient relaxed in a supine position, the arm is placed in approximately 90 degrees of abduction, the humeral head is loaded with an axial stress to center it on the glenoid, and then anterior and posterior vectors are applied to test for translation. Normal posterior translation usually exceeds that of its anterior counterpart, and comparison to the opposite side is necessary. Grading of translation is displayed in Figure 4–9. Next provocative testing maneuvers for instability should be performed. The anterior apprehension test is performed in individuals in whom anterior shoulder instability is suspected. Standing behind the patient, the examiner slowly abducts, extends, and externally rotates the shoulder. Patients with an anterior component to their instability will experience, at a certain point, sense recurrence of their instability and resist this maneuver (Fig. 4–10). Pain in this position is less predictive for this phenomenon. The posterior apprehension can be performed similarly. In this test, the shoulder is forward flexed to 90

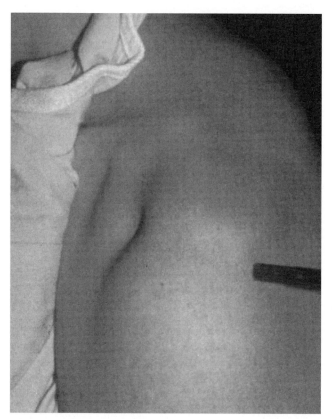

Figure 4–8. Patient with multidirectional instability with a sulcus sign demonstrating the inferior component to her instability pattern.

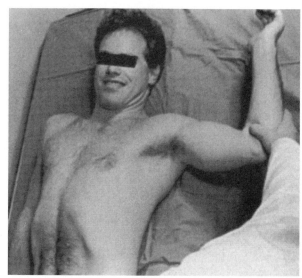

Figure 4–10. Apprehension test—supine (fulcrum test). The patient is positioned with the scapula supported by the edge of the examining table. The arm is positioned in abduction and external rotation, which produces a feeling of impending anterior instability, accompanied by apprehension on the part of the patient. (From Rockwood C: The Shoulder, 2nd ed. Philadelphia, WB Saunders, 1998, p 187.)

firms the predominant direction of instability. In this test, the examiner places the patient supine. A posteriorly directed stress on the proximal humerus is then applied that often relieves the sensation of apprehension with the arm in an abducted and externally rotated position in patients with anterior instability.

Elbow

Examination of the elbow is facilitated by observation of its use during function of the upper extremity. Inspection of the elbow at rest includes evaluation of the carrying

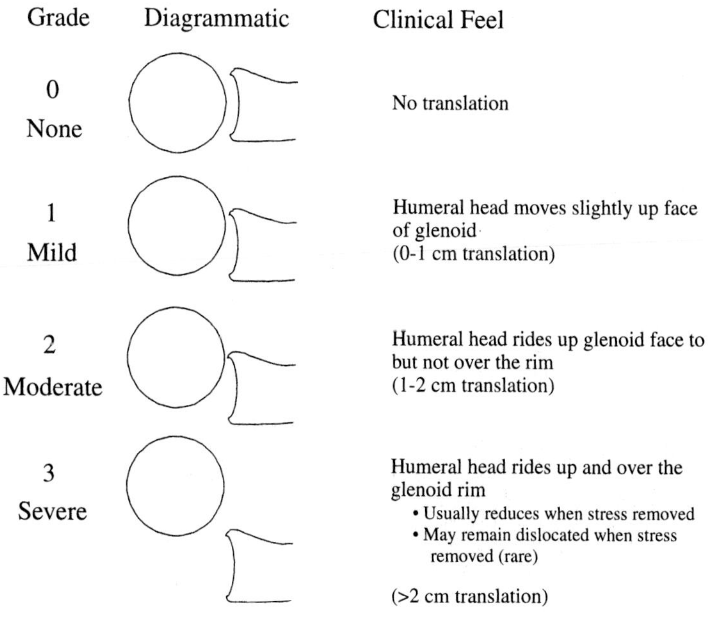

degrees and internally rotated with a posterior force vector applied at the elbow. A sensation of instability in this position is more suggestive of a posterior component to the instability pattern. Again, pain is a less suggestive sign. The anterior relocation test can then be performed with the arm in the anterior apprehensive position, and often con-

Figure 4–9. Clinical evaluation of a translation of the humeral head within the glenoid fossa, utilizing the load and shift test. (From Rockwood C: The Shoulder, 2nd ed. Philadelphia, WB Saunders, 1998, p 185.)

Grade	Diagrammatic	Clinical Feel
0 None		No translation
1 Mild		Humeral head moves slightly up face of glenoid (0-1 cm translation)
2 Moderate		Humeral head rides up glenoid face to but not over the rim (1-2 cm translation)
3 Severe		Humeral head rides up and over the glenoid rim • Usually reduces when stress removed • May remain dislocated when stress removed (rare) (>2 cm translation)

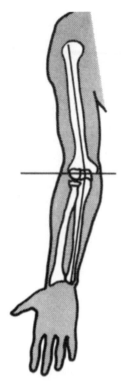

Figure 4–11. The carrying angle, measured clinically as the angle formed by the arm and the forearm, with the elbow extended. (Modified from Morrey BF: The Elbow and Its Disorders, 2nd ed. Philadelphia, WB Saunders, 1993, p 74.)

angle, which is the angle subtended by the arm and forearm with the elbow in full extension (Fig. 4–11). This angle is usually 5 degrees of valgus (the apex or elbow pointing toward the midline) in males and 10 to 15 degrees in females. An abnormal carrying angle can be the result of malunion of a fracture of the distal humerus or a growth injury following a pediatric fracture, and it can result in

delayed ulnar nerve symptoms as well as a cosmetically displeasing appearance.

Palpation of the elbow is extremely helpful in determining the source of pathology. Palpable bony landmarks include the medial and lateral epicondyles, the olecranon process, and the radial head. The ulnar nerve, the medial and lateral collateral ligaments, the annular ligament, and the origin of the extensor and flexor muscle groups are soft tissue structures that can be palpated directly and identified as sources of the patient's complaints. The distal tendons of the biceps and triceps should be palpated, and evidence of tendinitis or tendon rupture should be appreciated. In addition, palpation of the olecranon bursa, and observation of an enlarged, fluctuant, or erythematous mass can be made in individuals with olecranon bursitis (Fig. 4–12).

The elbow is a highly mobile joint, and stiffness or loss of motion is a frequent complaint of individuals with disorders in this region. Normal flexion and extension of the elbow is in excess of 135 degrees of flexion and 0 degrees of extension, respectively. Hyperextension may be present in females, although it is not uncommon for heavily muscled males to lack several degrees of full extension. Normal pronation and supination are 90 degrees each. This assessment is most easily made by comparing one side with the other and asking the patient to hold a pen or pencil while rotating the forearm. It can be quite helpful, when examining the elbow, to palpate for crepitus or irregular motion as the extremity is passively taken through a full range of flexion, extension, pronation, and supination. Manual motor testing of the flexors, extensors, pronators, and supinators of the elbow is carried out. Of note, the biceps functions as both a flexor and supinator of the elbow. Sensory testing in the dermatomal and peripheral nerve distributions is also carried out (see Fig. 4–1).

Special tests about the elbow include the tennis elbow test, Tinel's test, and tests for ligamentous stability. Individuals with tennis elbow (lateral epicondylitis) have reproduction of their lateral elbow pain with resisted active extension of the wrist (Mill's sign) (Fig. 4–13). Lateral

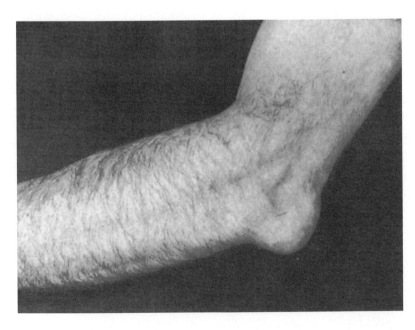

Figure 4–12. Olecranon bursitis in a patient with tophaceous gout. (Modified from Polley HF, Hunder GG: Rheumatologic Interviewing and Physical Examination of the Joints, 2nd ed. Philadelphia, WB Saunders 1978, p 83.)

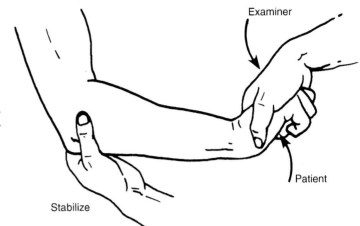

Figure 4–13. Mill's test for tennis elbow syndrome. (From Magee DJ: Orthopaedic Physical Assessment, 2nd ed. Philadelphia, WB Saunders, 1992, p 153.)

tenderness when resisting active extension of the third metacarpophalangeal joint further isolates the extensor carpi radialis brevis as the pathologic structure. Tinel's sign refers to the production of pain and radiating paresthesias when tapping over an injured nerve or neuroma. The ulnar nerve, as it passes within the cubital tunnel, is a frequent site of pathology, with pain on the medial aspect of the elbow and pain and parethesias down the medial forearm into the ulnar aspect of the hand.

The medial and lateral collateral ligaments of the elbow can be tested with the elbow slightly flexed 30 to 45 degrees and a varus or valgus force is applied. Testing for medial laxity of the ulnar collateral ligament should be done with the forearm in pronation as this isolates this structure. The examiner's hand can stabilize the elbow, act as a fulcrum, and palpate for gapping on the involved side, and the results should be compared to the uninvolved elbow as the instability is often subtle. Pain with these maneuvers is often more apparent than valgus laxity with

ulnar collateral injuries. The history is extremely important when evaluating these patients. Injuries to the medial side are often in repetitive throwers. Although there can be a single event with a "pop" felt upon throwing an object, often the complaints with this injury center on pain with throwing maneuvers, or the loss of control or velocity. In contrast, injuries to the lateral collateral structures most commonly follow trauma to the elbow region.

Chronically, subtle posterolateral instability is more often a problem. This pattern of instability is isolated by the lateral pivot shift test (Fig. 4–14). In this test a valgus and axial load is applied to the supinated forearm while the patient is in the supine position. Often a palpable "clunk" and pain can be appreciated as the arm is brought from 30 to 45 degrees of flexion to full extension as the radius is subluxed or dislocated from a reduced position. Apprehension is also significant and common in patients with this complex pattern of injury when frank instability cannot be demonstrated on physical examination.

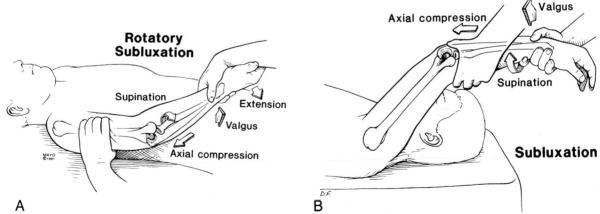

Figure 4–14. *A,* The posterolateral rotatory subluxation or lateral pivot-shift test of the elbow. The elbow is supinated and a valgus moment is applied with axial compression while extending it from a flexed position. This causes the ulna to subluxate off the humerus, permitting the radial head to move with the ulna. *B,* The test is performed much more easily with the arm over the patient's head (we now use this method exclusively). Full external rotation of the shoulder provides a counterforce for the supination of the forearm and leaves one hand of the examiner free to control valgus moments. (*A* from Morrey BF: The Elbow and its Disorders, 2nd ed. Philadelphia, WB Saunders, 1993, pp 566–580; *B* from O'Driscoll SW, Bell DF, Morrey BF: Posterolateral rotary instability of the elbow. J. Bone Joint Surg 73A:111, 1991.)

Wrist and Hand

Because of the complexity of the involved anatomy, the high functional demand, and the significance of the disability related to any loss of function, physical examination of the wrist and hand is the most complex area in physical diagnosis of the musculoskeletal system. Thorough documentation of a physical examination, including region by region testing for tenderness, swelling, range of motion, and neurologic function is essential. Because injuries to the hand are frequently associated with medicolegal or workers' compensation claims, a detailed and well-documented examination is crucial.

Inspection of the hand includes inspection of the patient's hands during function. Inspection of both the palmar and dorsal surfaces of the hand and wrist includes identifying changes in the general condition and color of the skin and fingernails. Identifying scars can be very helpful in determining potential disruption of tendons deep to the skin, as well as possible sources of contracture or neuroma formation. The intrinsic musculature of the hand should be carefully evaluated, and wasting of the intrinsic muscles, including the muscles of the thenar or hypothenar eminences, is suggestive of significant dysfunction of either the ulnar nerve or the anterior horn cells of the spinal cord. In addition, clubbing of the fingertips is an important sign of significant pulmonary disease and should not be overlooked.

Palpation of the skin, particularly on the palmar surface, can reveal pathology. Thickening of the palmar fascia, with associated contracture of the digits (Dupuytren's disease), is common, especially on the ulnar side of the hand in men. Bony palpation, including palpation of the radial styloid and the bones of the carpus, yields specific information regarding disorders of the wrist. In particular, palpation of the scaphoid in the anatomic "snuffbox" is an important sign of potential injury, particularly a nondisplaced fracture (Fig. 4–15). Careful palpation of the hook of the hamate, on the ulnar border of the palmar surface of the hand, may suggest injury to this structure. Other important sites of pathology, which may be tender on palpation, include the carpometacarpal joint of the thumb, the ulnar styloid process, the flexor carpi radialis tendon, and the tendons of the extensor pollicis brevis and abductor pollicis longus.

Range of motion of the wrist in flexion, extension, and radial and ulnar deviation should be measured and recorded. Range of motion of the fingers at the metacarpophalangeal as well as the distal and proximal interphalangeal joints is also checked. Normal range of motion is best evaluated by a side-to-side comparison. Differences between active and passive ranges of motion may be found and may serve as clues to tendon injuries. In addition, differences in the range of motion of the proximal interphalangeal (PIP) joint, with flexion and extension of the metacarpophalangeal (MP) joint (Bunnell-Littler test), can result from intrinsic contracture.

Other special tests for the hand and wrist include Phalen's test, Tinel's test, Allen's test, and tests for competence of the long finger flexors. Phalen's sign is elicited by having the patient flex the wrist to 45 degrees and wrist is left in this position for about 60 seconds. Reproduction of paresthesias into the thumb, index, and long fingers is a sensitive but relatively nonspecific sign of carpal tunnel syndrome. Tinel's sign is elicited at the wrist by tapping over the median nerve as it enters the carpal tunnel, just proximal to the wrist crease. Radiating pain and paresthesias along the distribution of the median nerve constitutes a positive test. Allen's test is performed by having the patient hold the hand above the level of the heart. The examiner manually exsanguinates the hand or asks the patient to open and close the fist tightly several times, and then manually occludes the ulnar and radial arteries. First one artery and then the other is released and the opposite hand checked for comparison. Delayed or incomplete reperfusion of the hand represents partial obstruction of flow in the involved artery. This test should always be checked before drawing an arterial blood gas from the radial artery. A similar version of Allen's test can also be performed on individual digits.

The status of the flexor digitorum superficialis and the flexor digitorum profundus tendons can be determined for each digit. The flexor digitorum superficialis tendon can be isolated and tested by holding the other fingers in full extension at the distal interphalangeal (DIP) joints. This blocks excursion of the flexor digitorum profundus for the involved digit and leaves only the superficialis to perform flexion of the PIP joint. Only by blocking profundus function can one be certain that the superficialis is functioning; isolated lacerations or ruptures of this tendon are relatively common. The flexor digitorum profundus is tested by holding the PIP joint of the involved digit in full extension. Active flexion of the DIP joint signifies a functioning profundus tendon in that finger (Fig. 4–16).

Careful neurologic examination of the hand involves motor and sensory testing. Sensory testing in the autonomous zones of the median (radial aspect of the volar distal phalanx of the index finger), ulnar (ulnar aspect of the volar distal phalanx of the little finger), and radial (dorsal aspect of the web space between the thumb and index finger) nerves is carried out. Two-point discrimination should also be tested whenever a digital nerve injury is suspected. Motor strength testing of the intrinsic muscles of the hand, including the lumbricals, interossei, thenar,

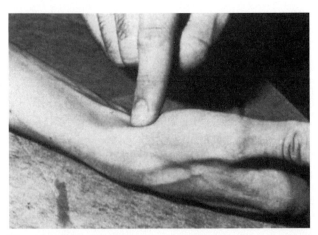

Figure 4–15. Tenderness to palpation over the anatomic snuff box may indicate injury to the scaphoid. (From Tubiana R [ed]: The Hand, vol 3. Philadelphia, WB Saunders, 1984.)

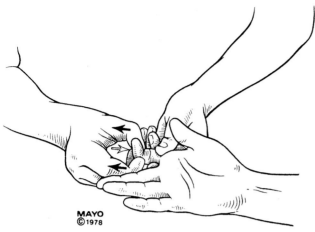

Figure 4–16. The integrity of the flexor digitorum profundus is tested by active flexion of the distal interphalangeal joint with the proximal interphalangeal joint held in extension by the examiner. (Modified from Polley HF, Hunder GG: Rheumatologic Interviewing and Physical Examination of the Joints, 2nd ed. Philadelphia, WB Saunders, 1978, p 142.)

and hypothenar groups, as well as the extrinsic wrist and finger flexors and extensors is carried out and recorded.

PHYSICAL EXAMINATION OF THE LOWER EXTREMITIES

LUMBAR SPINE

The examination of the lumbar spine replicates, in form, the steps used in examining the cervical spine. First the patient is carefully observed and attention directed at body position and freedom of movement through the lumbar spine. Palpation of the spine and adjacent structures is followed by an objective assessment of the lumbar range of motion and the performance of a thorough neurologic examination as well as other specialized tests. Examination of the low back, as in the neck, elicits findings that are either nonspecific but quite common or very specific for certain conditions or levels of nerve root involvement. Palpation of the lumbar spine commonly reveals areas of tenderness along the lumbar paraspinal muscles or over the posterior superior iliac spine, but does not point to a specific diagnosis. Tenderness directly over the spinous processes, in the trauma patient, may be evidence of a bony fracture. Tenderness to percussion, along the midline, is sometimes indicative of an infection of the spine. Tenderness over the buttocks or in the sciatic notch is a relatively common finding in patients with nerve root compression and sciatica. Finally, the trochanteric bursa should be palpated because trochanteric bursitis can sometime coexist with, or mimic, lumbar radiculopathy.

Decrease in the range of motion of the lumbar spine is most easy to elicit in flexion and extension and is a relatively nonspecific finding. Patients with lumbar spinal stenosis frequently have loss of lordosis and have pain on extension of the low back, but often a normal range of forward flexion. Isthmic spondylolisthesis often causes a painful limitation of extension as well. Segmental instability of the lumbar spine may be characterized by a "tortur-ous return from forward flexion," wherein patients have full forward flexion but have difficulty returning from the flexed position and may use their hands on their thighs to aid their return to neutral.

A thorough neurologic examination of the lower extremities is essential in evaluating the patient with lumbar spine pathology. Prior to this, however, it is important to evaluate the hip and consider this as a possible source of the patient's complaints. Patients with isolated groin pain more typically have primary hip joint rather than lumbar spine pathology. In addition, careful palpation of the distal pulses and evaluation of the quality of the skin for dysvascular changes should be undertaken in the patient with a history of leg pain. Both vascular and neurologic disease can be a source of leg pain, and differentiating the two is an essential component of any examination. Because intra-abdominal and pelvic pathology can cause back pain, the examiner should also be considering diagnoses such as pancreatitis, abdominal aortic aneurysm, colorectal disease, or peptic ulcer as the source of pain. The genitourinary system is also a frequent source of back pain.

Neurologic examination of the lower extremities begins with evaluation of the patient's gait, and asking the patient to walk on the toes and heels can help elicit subtle weakness in the gastrocnemius-soleus complex and ankle dorsiflexors, respectively. Light touch and pinprick testing for dermatomal sensory loss is carried out (Fig. 4–17). Proprioception in the great toe as well as vibratory sensation are evaluated to detect evidence of posterior column dysfunction, or more commonly a peripheral neuropathy. Manual motor testing and testing of the deep tendon reflexes is also performed (Table 4–2). Because the presence of a neurologic abnormality is such an important part of the diagnosis of neural compression, it is important to perform and document a complete neurologic examination and to be careful to pick up subtle abnormalities, particularly in motor strength. In the author's experience, mild weakness of the extensor hallucis longus is the most common neurologic abnormality seen, followed by asymmetry of the ankle jerks.

Nerve root compression caused by disk herniation frequently results in a positive "tension sign." The relevant tension signs are the straight-leg raising test and the femoral nerve stretch test. The straight leg raising test is performed with the patient in either the seated or supine position: with the knee extended, the leg is elevated by the examiner. The sciatic nerve does not realize tension until 30 to 35 degrees of elevation of the leg, but between 35 and 70 degrees there is an increasing stretch of the nerve, with increasing hip flexion. The reproduction of leg pain or paresthesias, radiating distal to the knee, represents a positive straight-leg raising sign and is an important component in the clinical diagnosis of a herniated disk at L4–L5 or L5–S1 (Fig. 4–18). The sensitivity of the test can be augmented by dorsiflexing the ankle at the point at which the patient has difficulty with further leg elevation. Also, a positive contralateral straight-leg raising test, whereby the performance of the straight-leg raising test on the unaffected limb produces characteristic pain in the affected extremity, is an even more specific sign of nerve root compression. The femoral nerve stretch test is performed by simultaneously extending the hip and flexing

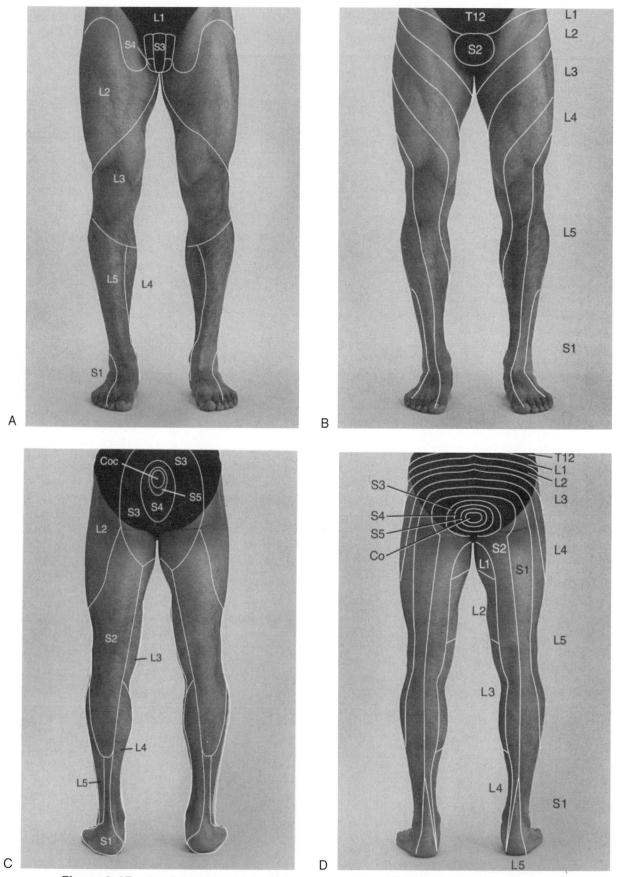

Figure 4–17. *A to D,* Lumbar and sacral dermatomes. (*A and C,* After Foerster. *B and D,* After Keegan and Garrett.) (From Reider B: The Orthopaedic Physical Examination. Philadelphia, WB Saunders, 1999, p 355.)

Table 4–2. Physical findings in lumbosacral radiculopathies

Dermatome	Sensory Testing	Motor Testing	Reflex Testing
L1	Anterior proximal thigh near inguinal ligament	Iliopsoas (seated hip flexion)	
L2	Mid anteromedial thigh	Iliopsoas (seated hip flexion)	
L3	Just proximal or medial to patella	Quadriceps	Patellar tendon reflex (secondary)
L4	Medial lower leg and ankle	Tibialis anterior	Patellar tendon reflex
L5	Lateral and anterolateral leg and dorsal foot	Extensor hallucis longus	Tibialis posterior reflex
		Extensor digitorum brevis	Medial hamstring reflex
		Gluteus medius	
S1	Posterior calf, plantar foot, and lateral toes	Gastrocsoleus	Achilles tendon reflex
		Peronei	
		Gluteus maximus	
S2	Posterior thigh and proximal calf	Rectal examination	
S3, S4, S5	Perianal area	Rectal examination	

From Reider B: The Orthopaedic Physical Examination. Philadelphia, WB Saunders, 1999, p 356.

the knee. Reproduction of the patient's pain down the anterior thigh is seen in patients with radiculopathy secondary to a herniated disk at L2–L3 or L3–L4. It is important to note that production of back pain with straight-leg raising is universal in patients with lumbar spine disorders, is nonspecific, and does not constitute a positive tension sign.

The Hip

Physical examination of the hip begins with observation of the patient's gait. Two common abnormalities of gait seen with hip pathology are an antalgic gait and a Trendelenburg (or gluteal) lurch. In single stance phase the hip abductors maintain the pelvis level, against the force of gravity. If the patient places the hands against a wall and stands on one leg, a normal hip will be able to prevent the pelvis

from drooping. Abnormal function of the hip abductors, which may be secondary to mechanical or neurologic causes, will result in drooping of the contralateral pelvis; this is a positive Trendelenburg sign. Because normal contraction of the hip abductors on single-leg stance results in an increase in the joint reactive force across the hip, the resulting pain can be another reason for a positive Trendelenburg sign. When a patient with a positive Trendelenburg sign walks, the tendency for the contralateral pelvis to droop is countered by swaying the torso over the involved (ipsilateral) hip to prevent contralateral pelvic drooping. This gait pattern is referred to as a "Trendelenburg gait" (Fig. 4–19). "Antalgic gait" refers to the patient's unconscious attempt to shorten the stance phase in order to reduce pain and is nonspecific for hip pathology. Trendelenburg and antalgic gait patterns can coexist.

The most specific finding on palpation of the hip is tenderness directly over the greater trochanter. Between the greater trochanter and the fascia lata is the trochanteric bursa, which is a common source of lateral hip pain.

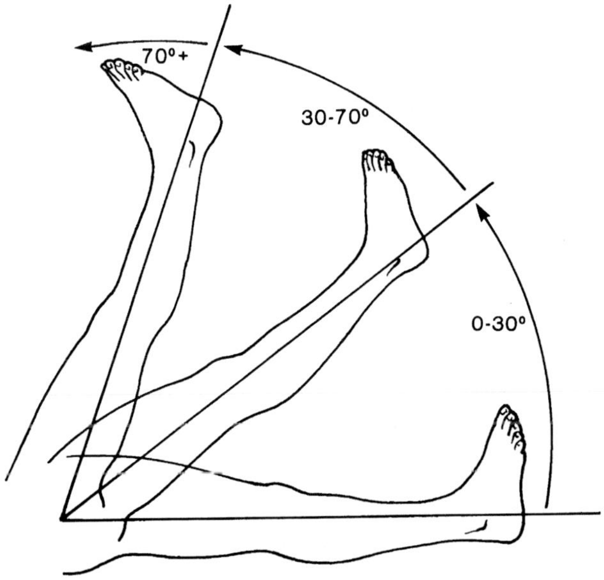

Figure 4–18. Dynamics of the straight-leg raising test. Maximal tension is applied between 30 to 70 degrees of hip flexion, with the knee extended. (Modified from Borenstein DG, Wiesel SW: Low Back Pain: Medical Diagnosis and Comprehensive Management. Philadelphia, WB Saunders, 1989, p 71.)

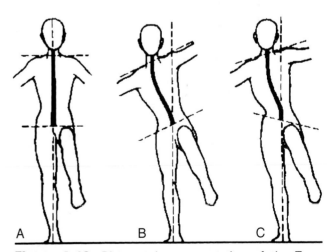

Figure 4–19. Diagramatic representation of the Trendelenburg sign and Trendelenburg lurch. A, negative Trendelenburg sign, normal gait. B, Trendelenburg lurch, but negative Trendelenburg sign. C, positive Trendelenburg sign and lurch. (Modified from Johnston RC, Fitzgerald RH Jr, Harris WH, et al: Clinical and radiographic evaluation of total hip replacement. J Bone Joint Surg 72A:165, 1990.)

Trochanteric bursitis is usually easily diagnosed by identifying tenderness about the greater trochanter. Range of motion of the hip is best tested in the supine position. Normal ranges of motion of the hip include at least 120 degrees of flexion, 10 to 20 degrees of extension, 40 to 45 degrees of abduction, 10 to 30 degrees of internal rotation, and 30 to 40 degrees of external rotation. Loss of internal rotation, particularly when accompanied by pain, is a very sensitive indicator of hip pathology, usually degenerative arthritis of the hip. Flexion contracture of the hip, or loss of full extension, often cannot be appreciated unless the lumbar lordosis is eliminated. The Thomas test involves flexion of the contralateral hip and knee to flatten the lordosis, followed by attempting to fully extend the hip. If this test is not performed, a flexion contracture of the hip can be masked by an increase in compensatory lumbar lordosis, thereby allowing the patient to appear to fully extend both hips when supine (Fig. 4–20).

Sensory and manual motor testing of the lower extremity is carried out, and it is essential to remember, in the patient with a complaint of hip pain, that the lumbar spine can be the source of referred or radicular pain. This is particularly true in patients with buttock and posterior thigh complaints, which they frequently describe as "hip" pain.

Knee

Evaluation of the knee begins with observation of gait and gross inspection of alignment. Gait observation is best performed with both the lower extremities exposed. Joint alignment should be simultaneously observed during gait and in double-leg stance. Varus (bowlegged) and valgus

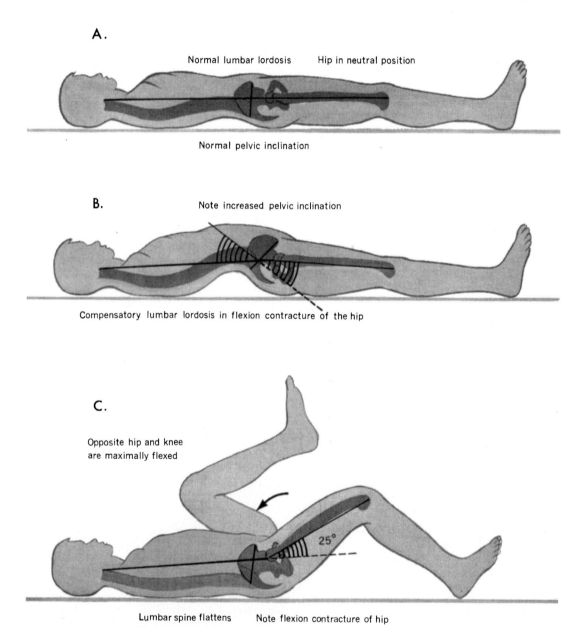

A.

Normal lumbar lordosis   Hip in neutral position

Normal pelvic inclination

B.

Note increased pelvic inclination

Compensatory lumbar lordosis in flexion contracture of the hip

C.

Opposite hip and knee
are maximally flexed

25°

Lumbar spine flattens   Note flexion contracture of hip

Figure 4–20. The Thomas test for hip flexion contracture, demonstrating how increased lumbar lordosis can mask a flexion contracture of the hip. (Modified from Tachdjian MO: Pediatric Orthopedics, 2nd ed. Philadelphia, WB Saunders, 1990, p 28.)

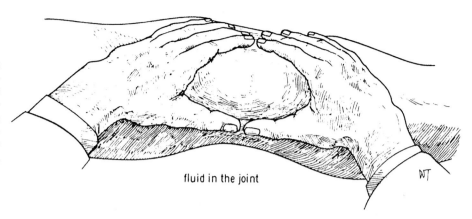

Figure 4–21. Palpation of a fluid thrill by alternately compressing medial and lateral to the patella, to demonstrate a joint effusion in the knee. (Modified from Insall JN, Windsor RE, et al: Surgery of the Knee, 2nd ed. New York, Churchill Livingstone, 1993, p 67.)

fluid in the joint

(knock-kneed) malalignment should be identified as well as any tendency toward hyperextension (recurvatum), giving way, or lateral thrusting on stance phase. Any side to side differences should be noted. Palpation of the knee should be performed in both the flexed and extended position, and the knee should be palpated as it is taken through a range of active motion. The presence of an effusion should then be documented. This is best performed with the knee extended. In this position the suprapatellar pouch is "milked" down to increase the volume of any fluid in the main joint space. A transmissible fluid wave between the medial and lateral parapatellar spaces is usually the most sensitive sign of a joint effusion (Fig. 4–21). A ballotable patella is usually not present unless there is a large joint effusion.

Examination of the patellofemoral joint should begin by flexing and extending the knee in search of retropatellar crepitus. Again side-to-side differences should be noted. The presence of any patellar facet tenderness should be noted on either the medial or lateral sides. Patellar mobility in both the medial and lateral direction, termed patella glide, should then be assessed. This is best quantified by subdividing the patella into quadrants in a medial to lateral direction to assess the excursion in this plane (Fig. 4–22). Often patients with generalized ligamentous laxity will demonstrate increased patellar glides often associated with patellar maltracking or instability. The presence of apprehension especially with a laterally directed force should be documented. Passive patellar tilt should then be quantitated in degrees to assess any tightness that may exist in the lateral retinacular structures. Additionally, measurement of the Q angle should be performed in cases in which patellar instability or maltracking is of concern. Normal values differ between the sexes but range from 5 to 10 degrees. Finally, quadriceps tone and the presence of atrophy or asymmetry should be noted.

Palpation of the medial and lateral joint lines with the knee extended and flexed is performed, and tenderness suggests injury to the menisci. Ecchymosis or tenderness to palpation along the medial or lateral collateral ligaments suggests injury to these structures. Tenderness along the quadriceps or patellar tendon is found in patients with tendinitis or disruption in these regions. The ability to perform a straight-leg raise is crucial when one suspects a violation of the extensor mechanism about the knee. Palpation about the knee should also include the subcutaneous bursae which are common sources of inflammation and pain.

The collateral and cruciate ligaments are then tested for stability. The results are best compared to those of the opposite knee, as a modest amount of laxity is frequently seen and may not have significance unless it is clearly different from the findings on the opposite side. The medial and lateral collateral ligaments are tested by applying a valgus or varus stress, with the knee flexed to 30 degrees, respectively. The most specific test for an anterior cruciate ligament (ACL) injury is the Lachman test. With the knee flexed to 30 degrees the examiner holds the distal thigh in one hand and applies an anterior stress to the proximal leg with the other. Anterior translation, exceeding that of the other knee, particularly if there is no discrete endpoint, suggests insufficiency to the ACL (Fig. 4–23). The anterior drawer sign, performed by applying an anterior stress to the knee when flexed to 90 degrees, is less sensitive because of the stabilizing effect of the posterior horns of the menisci. The pivot shift test is a more specific, but less sensitive maneuver for ACL insufficiency. With the leg internally rotated and a mild valgus force applied, the knee is flexed and extended between 0 and 45 degrees. Subluxation of

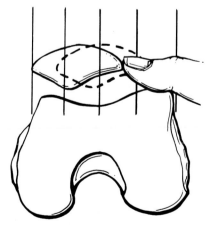

Figure 4–22. Assessment of patellar mobility medially and laterally. The patellofemoral joint can be mentally divided into quadrants and patellar mobility assessed in both directions. (From DeLee JC: Orthopaedic Sports Medicine: Principles and Practice. Philadelphia, WB Saunders, 1994, p 1179.)

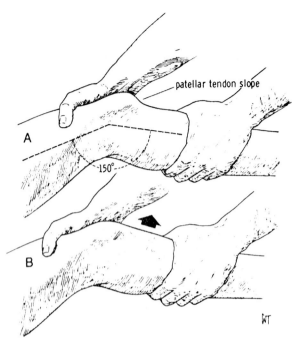

Figure 4–23. The Lachman test, performed with the knee in 20 to 30 degrees of flexion. (Modified from Insall JN, Windsor RE, et al: Surgery of the Knee, 2nd ed. New York, Churchill Livingstone, 1993, p 75.)

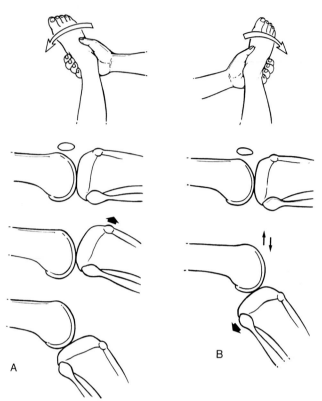

Figure 4–24. *A,* In the true pivot shift test, the lateral tibial plateau shifts from a reduced position in extension into anterior subluxation in slight flexion and reduces again at 30 degrees of flexion. In the reversed pivot shift test *(B),* the lateral tibial plateau falls from a position reduced in extension into posterior subluxation and flexion. (From Jakob RP, Hassler H, Stäubli HU; Observations on rotatory instability of the lateral compartment of the knee. Acta Orthop Scand 1981;191:6–27.)

the lateral compartment of the tibia in full extension, which reduces with flexion beyond 20 to 30 degrees and recurs with return to full extension, is diagnostic of anterolateral rotatory instability caused by insufficiency of the ACL (Fig. 4–24). It is essential to have the patient fully relaxed prior to attempting this maneuver as muscular guarding with the quadriceps can mask what would otherwise be a positive test.

Posterior cruciate ligament (PCL) insufficiency is characterized by a posterior drawer sign or by a positive "sag sign." The posterior drawer test is performed with the patient supine and the knee bent to 90 degrees. Application of a posterior force resulting in posterior translation of the tibia suggests injury to the PCL. A positive sag sign is elicited by flexing the hip and knee to 90 degrees with the patient supine. By holding the foot and allowing gravity to act on the leg, subluxation of the tibial tubercle beyond that seen on the opposite side is a very specific sign for PCL injury. This posterior subluxation is also evident on flexing the knees to 90 degrees and stabilizing the foot. Comparison with the opposite side is helpful when feeling for the normal "stepoff" present on the medial tibial plateau (Fig. 4–25). Both the degree of posterior sag and presence of an endpoint on posterior drawer testing are crucial in grading these injuries. The quadriceps active test is also often positive in PCL-deficient knees. In this test the patient lies supine with the knee flexed to 90 degrees and foot stabilized by the examiner. The patient is then asked to contract the quadriceps muscle, which acts to reduce a posterior subluxed knee in those who are PCL deficient (Fig. 4–26).

Important to assessing knee ligamentous injuries is to

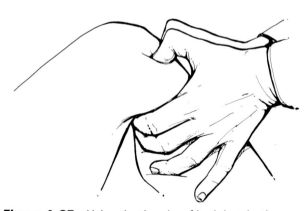

Figure 4–25. Using the thumbs of both hands, the examiner palpates the femoral condyles and then slides his thumbs down to rest on the tibial plateaus. Normally, there is a step-off between the femoral condyles and the tibial plateaus, allowing the thumbs to rest on the plateau. In the patient with PCL laxity, the tibia is subluxed posteriorly, resulting in absence of this step-off. (From DeLee JC: Orthopaedic Sports Medicine: Principles and Practice. Philadelphia, WB Saunders, 1994, p 1382.)

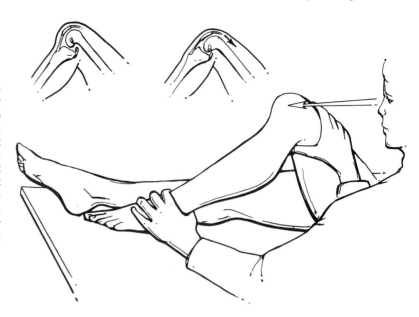

Figure 4–26. The quadriceps active drawer test. The examiner rests his elbow on the table. He uses the ipsilateral hand to support the subject's thigh *and* to confirm that the thigh muscles are relaxed. The foot is stabilized by the examiner's other hand, and the subject is asked to slide the foot gently down the table. Tibial displacement anteriorly resulting from quadriceps contraction confirms the presence of a PCL injury. (From DeLee JC: Orthopaedic Sports Medicine. Principles and Practice. Philadelphia, WB Saunders, 1994, p 1383.)

rule out the presence of an isolated or combined rotatory instability. Posterolateral instability is often present in the multiple-ligament injured knee. This is best tested in either the prone or supine position. External rotation of the foot with the knee in a neutral starting point is consistent with a posterolateral component to the instability pattern (Fig. 4–27). The external rotation recurvatum test and reverse pivot shift test are also positive with this condition. The external rotation recurvatum test is performed by straightening the leg in full extension by grasping the great toe distally. Those patients with posterolateral instability will demonstrate increased varus and recurvatum in comparison to the opposite side as a result of a deficient posterolateral corner. The reverse pivot shift is done by placing a external rotation and valgus stress to the knee and bringing an extended knee into a flexed position. Those patients with posterolateral instability will reduce from a posteriorly subluxed starting point at approximately 20 to 30 degrees of flexion (Fig. 4–28).

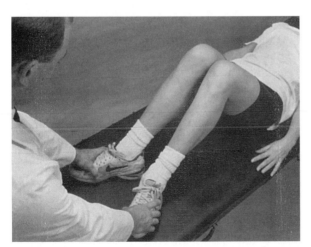

Figure 4–27. External rotation test. (From Reider B: The Orthopaedic Physical Examination. Philadelphia, WB Saunders, 1999, p 238.)

Measurement of any muscle atrophy and testing of active and passive range of motion is then carried out. Normal individuals have full extension with a very distinct "bounce home" at the extreme of extension, and they have flexion to at least 135 degrees. Loss of a distinct end point on full extension suggests an intra-articular block, commonly a displaced bucket-handle tear of the medial meniscus. Flexion contracture of the knee is common and can be due to many causes. The presence of a flexion contracture should be distinctly sought and recorded. Often patients having a flexion contracture will present with anterior knee pain. Hamstring tightness can also be similarly observed in those complaining of patellofemoral symptoms. Pain on hyperflexion of the knee, particularly in the area of the posterior medial or posterior lateral joint lines, suggests injury to the meniscus, particularly when associated with tenderness to palpation.

Several special tests about the knee are then performed to further identify sources of pathology. McMurray's test is performed by hyperflexing the knee and applying a valgus stress and external rotation. A palpable or audible click over the medial joint line suggests injury to the medial meniscus, most commonly in its posterior half. Other helpful tests include the Apley compression and distraction test. The compression test also aids in the diagnosis of a torn meniscus. With the patient prone on the examining table the knee is flexed to 90 degrees. Downward compression on the heel with internal and external rotation increases the force on the meniscus; if pain is reproduced, this finding suggests a meniscal injury. This test can be simulated by asking the patient to "duck walk," which, when painful, also suggests a meniscal injury (Fig. 4–29). The distraction test is also performed with the patient prone and the knee flexed to 90 degrees. Stabilizing the thigh with the examiner's knee, the foot is distracted and the leg internally and externally rotated. Pain with this maneuver over the medial or lateral joint line suggests injury to the respective collateral ligament. These two tests, performed in sequence, are designed to help differentiate meniscal from ligamentous pathology. Finally, Ober's test

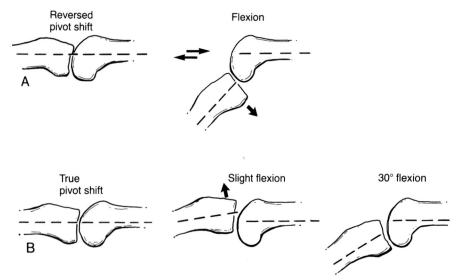

Reversed pivot shift

Flexion

A

True pivot shift

Slight flexion

30° flexion

B

Figure 4–28. *A,* Reversed pivot shift test. The knee is reduced in extension. The knee is flexed, the posterolateral tibial plateau subluxes posteriorly on the femur. This produces a shifting sensation similar to the classic pivot shift noted in patients with ACL laxity. *B,* In the true pivot shift the tibia is subluxed anteriorly in extension and reduced in flexion. (From DeLee JC: Orthopaedic Sports Medicine. Principles and Practice. Philadelphia, WB Saunders, 1994, p 1386.)

can be helpful in those complaining of lateral knee pain. The patient is asked to lie on the unaffected side with the contralateral hip flexed. The affected hip is then extended and adducted; this operation will demonstrate pain and tightness of the iliotibial band in those with iliotibial band friction syndrome (Fig. 4–30).

Foot and Ankle

No other structure in the musculoskeletal system is subjected to the repetitive forces experienced by the foot. These forces are applied and can create pathology in every component of the foot, including the skin, subcutaneous tissue, muscles, tendons ligaments, and bones. Disorders

of the foot and ankle are common sequelae of many general medical conditions, the most notorious being diabetes mellitus, and are experienced by individuals of all ages.

Examination of the foot begins with evaluation of the patient's gait. Inspection includes inspection not only of the foot itself, but of the patient's shoes. Patterns of shoe wear offer very useful information about abnormal wear patterns and pathology in the foot or leg. Any orthoses routinely worn by the patient should also be evaluated. Palpation, careful neurologic examination, testing for stability, and testing for range of motion are also important parts of the examination. Like any other extremity the normal side should be utilized for comparison. Evaluation of gait should be performed with the patient barefoot. Abnormal gait patterns, deformities of the foot that change through the gait cycle, as well as changes in gait with shoeing should be noted.

Inspection of the foot is perhaps the most important part of the entire examination. Many deformities can be appreciated with inspection alone, including hallux valgus (bunions), bunionette deformities, hammer toes, claw toes, and excessive inversion or eversion of the foot (Fig. 4–31). The foot should be inspected in both the non–weight-bearing and weight-bearing posture, and differences, specifically in inversion of the heel should be noted. Careful

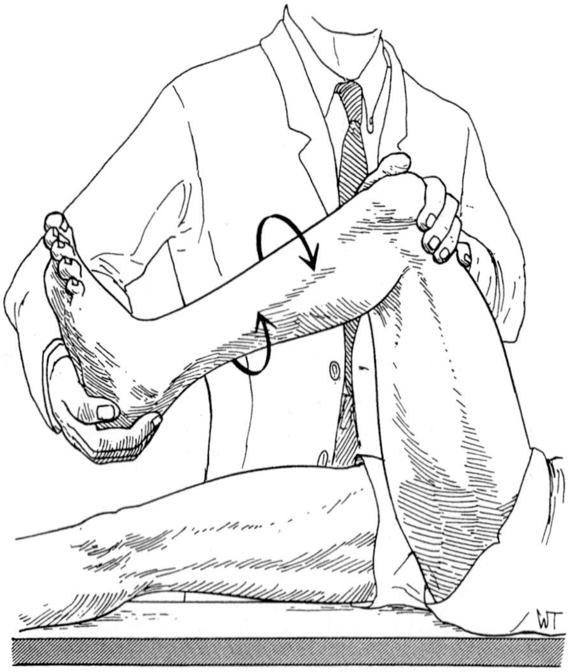

Figure 4–29. McMurray's test. (From Insall JN: Surgery of the knee. New York, Churchill Livingstone, 1984.)

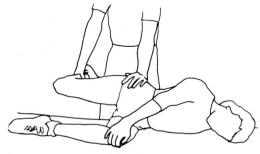

Figure 4–30. Clinical evaluation of flexibility in the iliotibial band (Ober's test). (From DeLee JC: Orthopaedic Sports Medicine. Principles and Practice. Philadelphia, WB Saunders, 1994, p 263.)

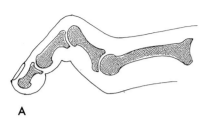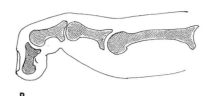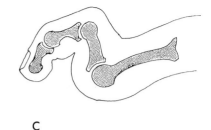

A   B   C

Figure 4–31. Lesser toe deformities. *A,* Hammer toe. *B,* Mallet toe. *C,* Claw toe. (From Tachdjian MD: Congenital deformities. *In* Jahss MH [ed]: Disorders of the Foot, Philadelphia, WB Saunders, 1982, p 212.)

inspection of the skin, particularly in middle-aged and older adults, is essential. Peripheral vascular insufficiency and diabetic neuropathy are common causes of foot complaints and may be misinterpreted by the patient as causing foot pain of a mechanical nature. The dorsalis pedis and posterior tibial pulses should be carefully palpated and recorded. Equally important are inspection and palpation of the skin; color, temperature, and the presence of hair on the dorsum of the foot and toes should all be assessed. It is helpful at the time of inspection of the foot and skin to proceed to sensory testing. Pinprick and light touch sensation are routinely tested, but it is important to realize that the first sensory modality lost in many patients with diabetes mellitus and peripheral neuropathy is position sense. It is important, therefore, to note that retention of light touch sensation does not by itself constitute a normal sensory examination in the patient with diabetes.

Evaluation of the longitudinal arches is especially important and should be carried out in the weight-bearing and non–weight-bearing positions. A supple flatfoot is characterized by contact of the medial border of the foot with the floor on weight bearing, with restitution of a normal longitudinal arch in the non–weight-bearing position. This supple flatfoot is a common developmental condition and is usually bilateral. New onset or acquired flatfoot in the middle-aged or older adult, particularly with a history of posterior and medial ankle pain in the area of the medial malleolus and posterior tibial tendon, may be evidence of posterior tibial tendon rapture and is important to diagnose as early as possible. Other findings consistent with this diagnosis include loss of active heel inversion when the patient stands on tiptoes (Fig. 4–32) and asymmetric splaying of the affected foot ("too many toes sign") when viewed from behind, compared to the opposite foot.

Bony and soft tissue palpation is carried out. Careful bony palpation allows the examiner to localize the source of pain, which may be quite vague based solely on the patient's history. Knowledge of the underlying anatomy and careful inspection and palpation of the foot frequently allows one to very accurately arrive at a clinical diagnosis without further testing. Palpation of the malleoli, the head of the talus, the base of the fifth metatarsal, the shafts of each of each of the metatarsals, and the area of the heel pad and plantar fascia is carried out. Fixed deformities, particularly of the forefoot, are assessed, and the presence of skin changes such as corns and calluses or crowding or overlapping of the toes is identified.

Range of motion testing of the foot and ankle can be

readily carried out, and the results should be compared to the opposite side. Normal ankle dorsiflexion extends to 20 degrees beyond neutral and plantar flexion to 50 degrees. Inversion and eversion occur at the subtalar joint and extend 5 to 10 degrees in each direction. The normal forefoot can adduct 20 degrees and abduct 10 degrees. Motion of the great and lesser toes should also be noted, and fixed deformities such as hammer toes identified. It is important to be aware of the mobility present in the normal great toe metatarsophalangeal (MTP) joint, because loss of this motion is a common source of pain and gait alteration. The first MTP joint has a normal range of flexion of 45 degrees and can dorsiflex from 70 to 90 degrees. The IP joint of the great toe, on the other hand, cannot dorsiflex beyond neutral but is routinely capable of 80 to 90 degrees of plantarflexion. The lesser toes have slightly less motion at the MTP and PIP joints, and loss of motion of the lesser toes is tolerated somewhat better than loss of motion of the great toe.

The final part of the examination is testing for ankle joint stability and joint line pain. The anterior drawer test is designed to test the competence of the anterior talofibular ligament. It is performed by stabilizing the patient's leg, just above the malleoli, with the examiner's hand and applying an anterior stress with the opposite hand, cupping the patient's heel (Fig. 4–33). Any significant anterior translation is usually an abnormal finding, although as

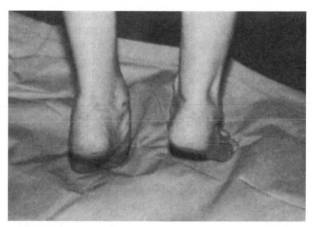

Figure 4–32. Loss of active heel inversion, with the patient standing on tiptoes, suggests a rupture of the posterior tibial tendon. (Modified from Mann RA: Surgery of the Foot, 5th ed. St. Louis, CV Mosby, 1986, p 477.)

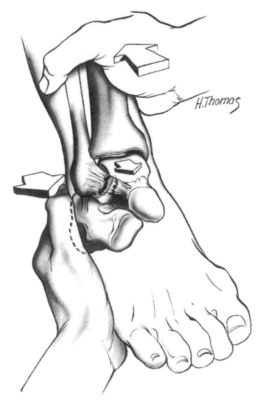

Figure 4–33. The anterior draw test for ankle instability. (Modified from Jahss MH: Disorders of the Foot. Philadelphia, WB Saunders, 1982, p 108.)

with all stress testing, comparison to the opposite side is mandatory. Straight inversion of the foot and ankle can be performed, with the examiner's thumb placed over the calcaneofibular ligament to test the combined integrity of the anterior talofibular and calcaneofibular ligaments. Finally, deltoid ligament instability can be determined, on occasion, by the presence of excessive motion over the deltoid with the application of an eversion stress. Assessment of joint line tenderness with the presence of an effusion is often helpful in defining an intra-articular source of generalized ankle pain.

CONCLUSION

Several principles have been stressed in the examination of the patient with a musculoskeletal injury or complaint. The interplay between the patient's history and the physical examination is common to all areas of physical diagnosis, but the musculoskeletal system is unique in the ability of the examiner, in many cases, to look directly at, and palpate, the affected body part. The need to expose the area in question and its contralateral control cannot be overemphasized, as is true for the benefit of observing function of the extremity, particularly gait. Finally, the examiner must be reminded of the possibility that pain in a given area (e.g., shoulder, knee) may be related to pathology in a more proximal region. The remainder of this text will deal with a variety of conditions, a careful approach to physical examination adhering to the foregoing principles will facilitate accurate diagnosis and appropriate treatment.

Bibliography

Boyes JH: Bunnell's Surgery of the Hand. Examination of the Hand. Philadelphia, JB Lippincott, 1970, pp 108–129.

DeLee JC, Drez D: Orthopaedic Sports Medicine: Principles and Practice. Philadelphia, WB Saunders, 1994, pp 1275–1400.

Fu FH, Harner CD, Vince KG: History and Physical Examinations in Knee Surgery. Baltimore, Williams & Wilkins, 1996, pp 253–274.

Hoppenfeld S: Physical Examination of the Spine and Extremities. New York, Appleton-Century-Crofts, 1976.

Hoppenfeld S: Orthopaedic Neurology. A Diagnostic Guide to Neurologic Levels. Philadelphia, JB Lippincott, 1997.

Jahss MH: Examinations in Disorders of the Foot. Philadelphia, WB Saunders, 1982, pp 81–102.

Morrey BF: The Elbow and Its Disorders, 2nd ed. Philadelphia, WB Saunders, 1993, pp 566–580.

Reider B: The Orthopaedic Physical Examination. Philadelphia, WB Saunders, 1999.

Rockwood CA, Matsen FA: The Shoulder, 2nd ed. Philadelphia, WB Saunders, 1998, pp 149–177.

Tachdjian MO: Pediatric Orthopaedics. The Orthopaedic Examination. Philadelphia, WB Saunders, 1990, pp 4–58.

Chapter 5

Imaging in Orthopaedic Surgery

Lawrence Yao, M.D.
William Harvey, M.D.

This chapter offers a brief introduction to the major imaging modalities used in orthopaedic practice. Plain film radiography still plays the biggest role in the orthopaedic imaging evaluation, despite the ever-growing repertoire of high-technology imaging tests. Attention will be given to the often overlooked but important technical aspects of imaging, particularly when relevant to the best clinical application of these tests. Sections will be organized around imaging modalities. Finally, a general approach to the imaging workup of broad categories of disease will be provided, as an algorithmic approach to disease workup is increasingly emphasized in our cost-conscious practice environment.

RADIOGRAPHY

Technique

For the radiographic evaluation of the extremities, dedicated extremity cassettes employing a single emulsion film are considered the gold standard, because they provide extremely high spatial resolution, approaching 14 line pairs (lp) per millimeter, albeit at the cost of a slightly higher radiation dose. There is an increasing use of computed or digital radiography in many practice settings, and some departments are striving to become "all digital." Most popular, commercial digital or computed radiographic (CR) systems utilize a light-sensitive phosphor plate. This plate is digitally read with a laser scanner after the phosphor cassette is exposed by an x-ray tube in the conventional manner.

The real advantage of CR systems is that they facilitate the integration of radiography into picture archiving and communication systems (PACS). A digital imaging system and associated infrastructure may permit the transfer of images to distant and multiple sites using ever-improving network and teleradiology technology. A PACS overcomes the pitfalls of lost films and facilitates simultaneous physician access to imaging from various locations (clinic, office, operating suite, intensive care unit). Currently, CR is most often still printed on film and viewed in the conventional manner. The small size of the hard copy film format generated by CR systems may discourage practitioners who are accustomed to viewing and measuring from life-size radiographic images on conventional film.

The primary disadvantage of CR for skeletal imaging is the limited spatial resolution of phosphor cassette systems, which is usually on the order of 3 to 4 lp/mm. High-resolution CR cassette systems improve the resolution to 5 to 6 lp/mm, but these cassettes are currently available only in smaller size formats. Newer "direct to digital" technology is emerging, which does not depend on a phosphor screen and a laser scanning procedure for image acquisition and digitization. These direct to digital radiographic systems utilize charge-coupled device (CCD) array technology, or flat panel designs (selenium plates) and enable faster patient throughput than phosphor CR systems. Current direct to digital systems offer a spatial resolution that is no better than that of CR systems. From an image quality perspective, the possible advantages of CR technology include improved contrast resolution for lower spatial frequencies, and wider receptor latitude.

The Radiographic Workup

Plain film radiography is the most common imaging test used in evaluating trauma and musculoskeletal pain. It gives excellent, high-resolution visualization of the osseous structures and some indirect information about the surrounding soft tissues. Plain radiographs are almost always the initial step in the imaging workup, and diagnostic errors can result when they are omitted. It is important to tailor the radiographic view to the clinical problem, and to know when special views may be necessary. This chapter cannot present recommended protocols for every clinical indication but will review some common radiographic examinations that are of regular relevance and utility for orthopaedics. Readers are referred to other references for more detailed descriptions of radiographic positioning and technique.

SHOULDER

The radiographic assessment of the shoulder usually includes an anteroposterior (AP) view obtained with the humerus in external rotation. This depicts the major bony structures and is useful in evaluating for calcification of

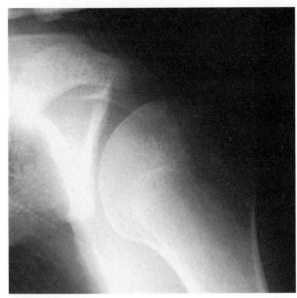

Figure 5–1. Grashey view. This posterior oblique view of the shoulder demonstrates the glenohumeral joint space, which cannot be visualized on a routine anteroposterior (AP) view. This view is sometimes called a true AP view of the shoulder.

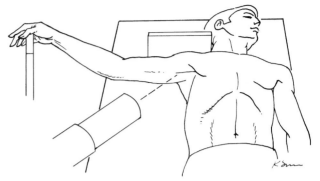

Figure 5–2. Axillary view of the shoulder. If the hand is supported as shown, this view can be performed in even severely traumatized shoulders. (From Resnick D: Bone and Joint Imaging, 2nd ed. Philadelphia, WB Saunders, 1996, p 25.)

the supraspinatus tendon. AP views in internal rotation of the humerus superimposes the greater tuberosity over the humeral head, permitting better visualization of calcification in the infraspinatus and teres minor, which will project laterally, and in the subscapularis, which will project medially. AP views will not show the glenohumeral joint space, which is shown on a true AP or Grashey view, which is obtained by placing the patient at an oblique angle of approximately 40 degrees to the side of interest (Fig. 5–1).

The axillary view is orthogonal to the frontal radiograph and evaluates the glenohumeral joint and the relative positions of the humeral head and glenoid fossa. This is usually performed with a horizontal x-ray beam aimed at the axilla, with the arm fully abducted and the film placed above the acromioclavicular (AC) joint. This view is particularly important to evaluate fracture displacements and can be performed in almost all cases of proximal humeral fractures if the patient's arm is supported adequately (Figs. 5–2 and 5–3).

A modification of the axillary view is the Westpoint view, which improves detection of an anteroinferior glenoid rim fracture after dislocation. The patient is positioned prone with the arm abducted 90 degrees and the central ray angled 20 to 30 degrees cephalad and 25 to 30 degrees medially. The Stryker or "notch" view can be used to visualize Hill-Sachs defects in the humeral head and is obtained with the patient supine, the arm flexed, and the palm placed on top of the head. The central ray is directed 10 degrees cephalad.

A trans-scapular or so-called "scapular Y view" can assess glenohumeral dislocation without the attendant discomforts of arm abduction, but it gives less information about fracture displacement. The humeral head should normally be superimposed over the glenoid fossa between the coracoid process anteriorly and scapular spine posteriorly.

Anterior and posterior dislocations can usually be confirmed on this view.

The outlet view demonstrates the bony margins of the supraspinatus outlet and profiles the leading, anterior edge of the acromion where enthesophytes may form and contribute to impingement syndrome. The patient is obliqued as for a trans-scapular view, but the x-ray tube is angled 10 to 30 degrees to parallel the axis of the scapular spine (Fig. 5–4).

Evaluation of the clavicle and AC joint requires a frontal view with the beam angled 10 to 15 degrees cephalad. In cases of suspected AC joint instability or sprain, bilateral views are helpful (Fig. 5–5). Obtaining upright images with

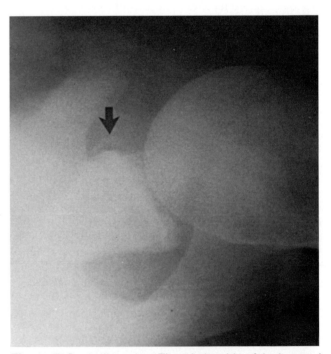

Figure 5–3. Axillary view. The relationship of the humeral head to the glenoid fossa is clearly demonstrated on this axillary projection. The *arrow* indicates a small avulsion fracture from the anterior rim of the glenoid, or so-called Bankart fracture.

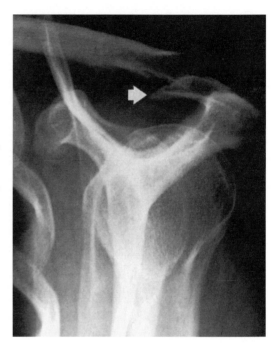

Figure 5–4. Supraspinatus outlet view. This view, taken along the axis of the supraspinatus muscle belly, depicts the bony margins of the supraspinatus outlet. Anterior acromial spurs *(arrow)* are readily identified, and the type of acromion can be determined according to the classification of Bigliani and Morrison. (From Bergman AG: Rotator cuff impingement: Pathogenesis, MR imaging characteristics, and early dynamic MR results. Magn Reson Imaging Clin North Am 1997;5:709).

and without weights suspended from the wrists is helpful in distinguishing type 2 from type 3 injuries.

PELVIS AND HIP

The standard AP view of the pelvis is obtained with the patient supine and the feet internally rotated approximately 15 degrees so that the long axis of the femoral neck is parallel to the film. Judet views are 45-degree oblique views of the pelvis. These views better assess the posterior acetabular rims, the pubic rami, and the degree of congruency across the acetabular dome in cases of intra-articular fracture. Major pelvic ring disruptions my be further assessed with inlet (beam angled 20 degrees caudally) and outlet (beam angled 20 degrees cephalad) views. The inlet view depicts the degree of AP displacement across the pelvic ring, while the outlet view depicts superoinferior displacement. Outlet views also nicely depict pubic rami fractures that can be missed on the routine AP radiograph.

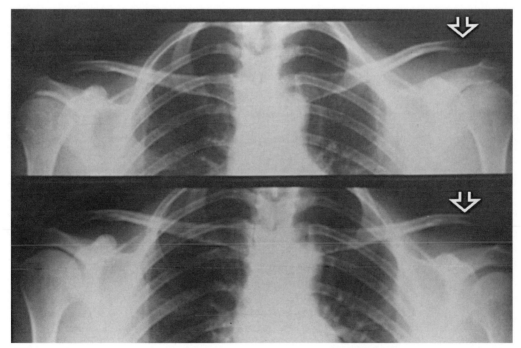

Figure 5–5. AC joint evaluation. Frontal views are performed without *(above)* and with *(below)* 5-pound weights suspended from the wrists. Dislocation of the distal clavicle is evident *(arrow)*, as well as widening of the coracoclavicular interval on the radiograph with weights, indicating a type 3 injury.

Pelvic instability can be assessed by acquiring standing AP views while the patient bears weight on one foot and then the other. Pelvic instability is confirmed when there is greater than 2 mm of movement across the symphysis. Instability in major pelvic fractures, however, can usually be inferred from computed tomographic (CT) findings.

The sacroiliac joints are best assessed using coned AP views with a cephalad beam angulation of 30 degrees, also known as the Ferguson view, or prone views with a similar caudal beam angulation (Fig. 5–6). Oblique projections may be of some value, but are difficult to optimize.

Routine evaluation of the hip includes a coned-down AP view with internal rotation and a "frog leg" lateral view with the hip abducted and externally rotated. In this way two orthogonal views of the proximal femur are achieved without turning the patient. For trauma patients, an axiolateral or groin lateral view of the hip can be obtained with an angled, horizontal beam aimed at the groin, with the contralateral thigh flexed out of the beam (Fig. 5–7). This view affords a lateral view of the femoral neck without moving the hip, and permits assessment of the version angle of the acetabular component after hip arthroplasty.

The von Rosen view is an AP view of the pelvis obtained with the femurs maximally abducted and internally rotated. This view is used in newborns and infants to assess for hip subluxation. A line bisecting the femoral neck on this view should pass through the acetabular fossa. This view is more sensitive for subluxation than other inferences made on the routine AP view of the pelvis—such as disruptions in Shenton's line—but is more difficult to obtain.

KNEE

The full knee series includes the AP view, lateral view (knee flexed 20 to 35 degrees), and internal and external 45-degree oblique views. Weight-bearing AP views of the knee (usually in full knee extension) should be performed when assessing for joint space loss in osteoarthritis. AP weight-bearing views of the knees in 30 degrees of flexion are even more sensitive for early joint space loss but are more difficult to perform (Fig. 5–8).

In trauma patients, a cross table lateral view is obtained and may depict a fat-fluid level in the suprapatellar recess. This demarcation represents the sharp interface between marrow fat and blood, and indicates a lipohemarthrosis from

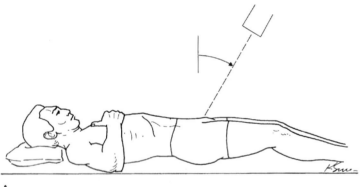

A

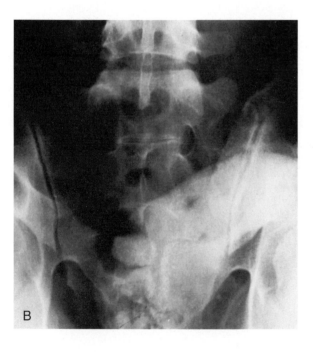

B

Figure 5–6. Ferguson view. This angled-beam AP radiograph improves depiction of the sacroiliac joints. The pubic symphysis projects over the midsacrum. (From Resnick D: Bone and Joint Imaging, 2nd ed. Philadelphia, WB Saunders, 1996, p 32.)

Figure 5-7. Groin or axiolateral view of the hip. This angled-beam cross table view of the hip facilitates a lateral projection while avoiding the need to move the affected hip. This can be useful in assessing trauma as well as the version angle of acetabular prostheses. (From Resnick D: Diagnosis of Bone and Joint Disorders, 3rd ed. Philadelphia, WB Saunders, 1995, p 29.)

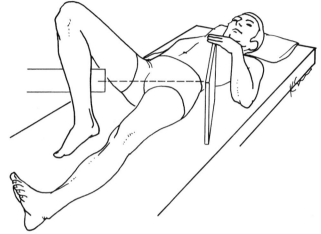

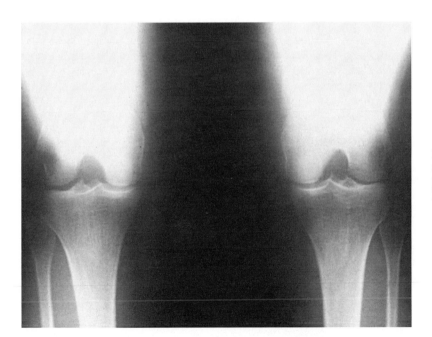

Figure 5-8. Bent knee weight-bearing AP view. This radiograph of the knees detects joint space narrowing earlier than weight-bearing studies done in full extension.

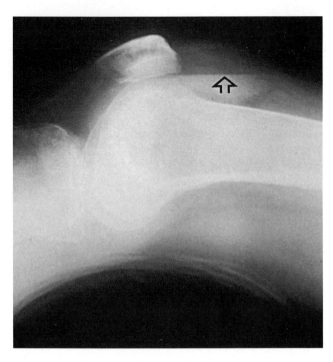

Figure 5–9. Cross table lateral views. These lateral views in severe trauma cases should be analyzed with attention to fluid-fluid levels in the suprapatellar bursa. A fat-fluid level *(arrow)* indicates an intra-articular fracture.

intra-articular fracture (Fig. 5–9). If AP and lateral views are normal, CT may be helpful for further evaluation.

The "sunrise" or "skyline" view of the patella is acquired with the knee in greater than 90 degrees of flexion, and provides an axial view of the patella (Fig. 5–10). It does not depict patellar malalignment or subluxation, which must be assessed at lesser degrees of knee flexion. One popular technique for assessing patellar position is the Merchant view, which is obtained with the patient supine and the knee flexed at a 45-degree angle (Fig. 5–11). The congruence angle can be measured on this view and is formed by line segments bisecting the femoral trochlea and connecting the patellar apex and the trough of the trochlea. A congruence angle greater than 12 degrees is an indicator of patellar subluxation. The Hughston view is similar to

the Merchant view, but does not require a special film holder (Fig. 5–12). The interpretation of patellar tilt optimally should be made on axial views performed in 30 degrees (Laurin view) or less of flexion.

A "tunnel" view or intercondylar notch view is obtained with the knee flexed 45 degrees and the beam angled along the axis of the tibial plateau (Fig. 5–13). This view is particularly useful in the assessment of possible loose bodies, osteochondritis dissecans, and tibial plateau fractures.

WRIST

The routine wrist series consists of posteroanterior (PA), oblique, and lateral views. In cases of trauma, a scaphoid view should also be done. This view is done in the PA projection, with ulnar deviation of the wrist and slight

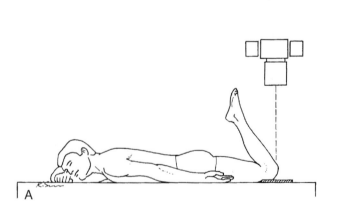

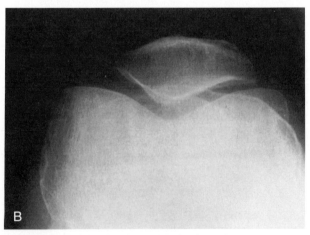

Figure 5–10. Sunrise view. This axial or skyline view of the patella is taken with the knee in greater than 90 degrees of flexion. Hence, this view does not convey information about patellar subluxation. (From Resnick D: Diagnosis of Bone and Joint Disorders, 3rd ed. Philadelphia, WB Saunders, 1995, p 32.)

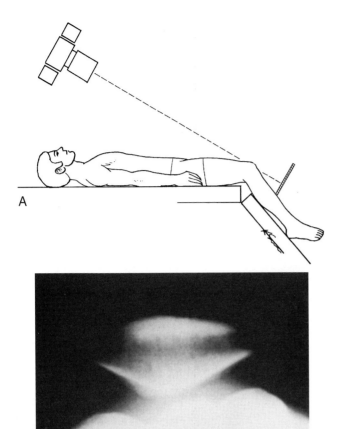

Figure 5–11. Merchant view. This view is performed at 45 degrees of knee flexion and requires beam angulation and a special film holder. The congruence angle is measured on this view to quantify patellar subluxation. (From Resnick D: Diagnosis of Bone and Joint Disorders, 3rd ed. Philadelphia, WB Saunders, 1995, p 33.)

cephalad angulation of the x-ray beam, thereby elongating the projection of the waist of the scaphoid (Fig. 5–14). The perinavicular fat plane should be seen on the PA and scaphoid views, and if not, a scaphoid fracture should be suspected. In cases of suspected arthritis, the Norgaard or "ball-catchers" view is useful to detect early erosions about the metacarpal heads and at the pisiform triquetral articulation.

The lateral view is used to exclude dislocations, mal-alignments, and intercalated segment instabilities of the carpal bones. On the lateral view, the pronator quadratus fat plane should always be assessed; if present, it is a helpful supporting sign that the distal radius is not fractured.

A carpal tunnel view evaluates the hook of the hamate and spine of the trapezium in cases of palmar pain after trauma; these sites cannot be assessed on the routine views. This view is obtained by hyperextending the hand and directing the central beam 25 to 30 degrees above the horizontal axis (Fig. 5–15). The hook of the hamate can also be evaluated nicely on a slightly off lateral view (semisupinated) with the wrist radially deviated.

ANKLE AND FOOT

Routine radiographic evaluation of the ankle includes AP, lateral, and mortise views. In the AP view the distal fibula obscures the lateral gutter of the ankle joint. The mortise view is performed with the foot internally rotated 15 to 20 degrees and should demonstrate both the lateral and medial gutters of the mortise joint. The mortise view depicts talar shift, secondary to ligamentous instability, and traumatic widening of the syndesmosis (normally less than 5 mm). The mortise view also best depicts the malleoli without overlap, and loose bodies in either gutter. If a posterior malleolar fracture is suspected, a 45-degree external oblique view may visualize this injury even when a lateral view is normal.

The Harris-Beath view is an axial view of the calcaneus, which assesses the calcaneal tuberosity, and also visualizes the middle and posterior facets of the subtalar joint, particularly useful after trauma (Fig. 5–16). The Broden view is obtained in the frontal plane with internal rotation of the ankle and a cephalad angled beam directed parallel to the posterior articular facet of the subtalar joint. The Broden view can help determine if there is joint involvement or incongruency in cases of calcaneal fracture (see Fig. 5–16).

Standard evaluations of the foot include the AP, lateral, and internal oblique views. The oblique view is obtained by elevating the lateral side of the foot by 30 degrees and aiming the central ray at the base of the fifth metatarsal; this view better depicts the mid- and forefoot. The AP and lateral views should be performed as weight-bearing films if there are concerns about foot alignment. The Cobey view is done PA with the patient standing on a platform, with the beam caudally angulated 20 degrees. This view nicely depicts heel position and axis relative to the main tibial weight-bearing axis, and is helpful in staging pes planus.

CERVICAL SPINE

The routine trauma series of the cervical spine includes a lateral view, an AP view, and an open mouth odontoid view (Fig. 5–17). The lateral view is improved by pulling down on the patient's arms; traction should never be placed on the head. A swimmer's view may be necessary if the entire cervical spine, and in particular, the alignment at C7–T1, is not clearly visualized on the lateral view. This view is obtained with one of the patient's arms raised and the other down at the side.

The utility of trauma oblique views, performed with the patient supine, is arguable, and they are not routinely obtained to "clear" the cervical spine. They may be effective in high-risk settings, in which a better evaluation of the articular pillars and the C2 segment can be made. Oblique views are most useful if a trauma table with an articulated C-arm is available, or if they are done upright, which is possible only in low-risk cases.

Lateral views of the cervical spine in flexion and extension are of very limited utility in trauma. They may provide added confidence in clearing low-risk cases, particularly when equivocal findings are noted on preliminary evaluation (degenerative subluxations, prevertebral soft-tissue prominence) or when patients report pain that is out of proportion with normal x-ray findings. Flexion and extension views are contraindicated when the patient's level of consciousness is altered. In cases in which the clinical

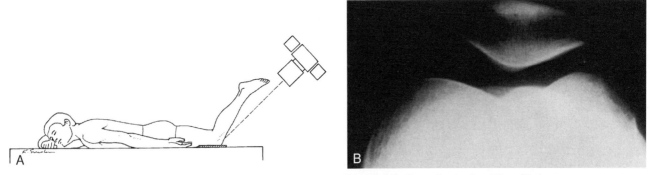

Figure 5–12. Hughston view. This skyline view of the patella is performed at 50 to 60 degrees of knee flexion and does not require a special film holder. (From Resnick D: Diagnosis of Bone and Joint Disorders, 3rd ed. Philadelphia, WB Saunders, 1995, p 32.)

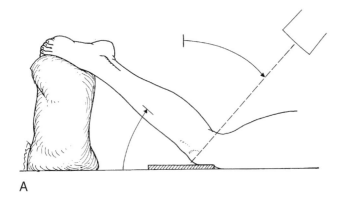

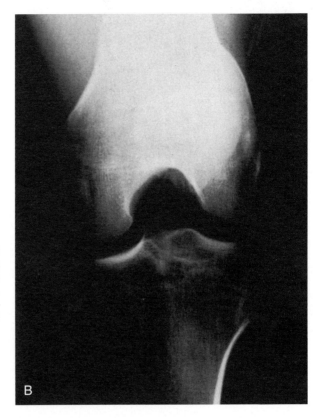

Figure 5–13. Tunnel view. In this view the knee is flexed and the beam is angled to roughly parallel the tibial plateau. This view may be difficult to achieve in the severely traumatized patient. (A from Resnick D: Bone and Joint Imaging, 2nd ed. Philadelphia, WB Saunders, 1996, p 35. B from Resnick D: Diagnosis of Bone and Joint Disorders, 2nd ed. Philadelphia, WB Saunders, 1988, p 43.)

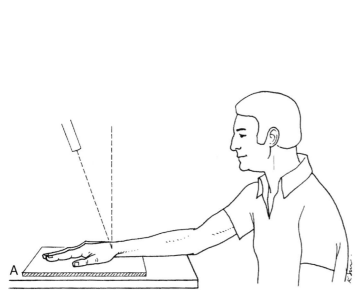
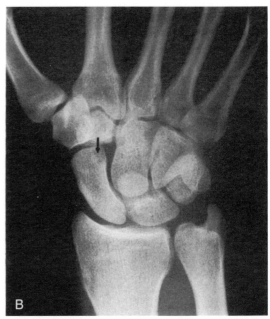

Figure 5–14. Scaphoid view. This angled-beam film in ulnar deviation of the wrist straightens out the waist portion of the scaphoid, which can be difficult to see on the straight PA view of the wrist. PA and oblique views are also necessary to fully evaluate the scaphoid. (*A* from Resnick D: Diagnosis of Bone and Joint Disorders, 3rd ed. Philadelphia, WB Saunders, 1995, p 10. *B* from Resnick D: Diagnosis of Bone and Joint Disorders, 2nd ed. Philadelphia, WB Saunders, 1988, p 10.)

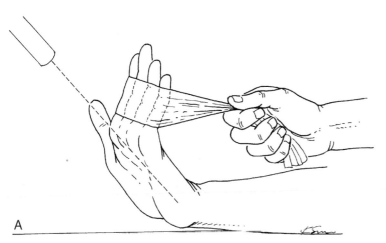
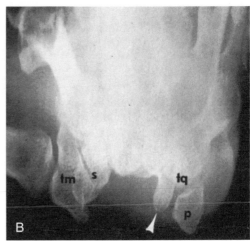

Figure 5–15. Carpal tunnel view. This view is important if a fracture of the hook of the hamate *(arrowhead)* or spine of the trapezium is suspected. Key: tm = trapezium, s = scaphoid, tq = triquetrum, p = pisiform. (From Resnick D: Diagnosis of Bone and Joint Disorders, 3rd ed. Philadelphia, WB Saunders, 1995, p 10.)

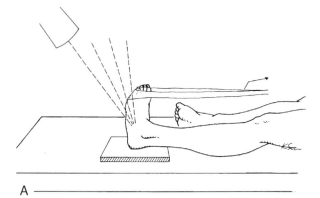

A

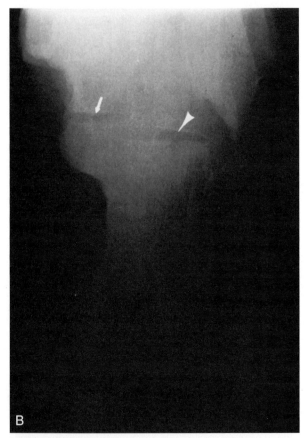

B

Figure 5–16. Hindfoot views. The Harris view of the calcaneus is performed with 45 degrees of beam angulation. Lesser degrees of beam angulation in combination with internal rotation of the ankle will improve visualization of the posterior subtalar facet joint; such views are known as Broden views. (From Resnick D: Diagnosis of Bone and Joint Disorders, 3rd ed. Philadelphia, WB Saunders, 1995, p 37.)

suspicion of instability or ligamentous injury is high, magnetic resonance imaging (MRI) is a better and safer test than flexion and extension radiographs.

The pillar view is an AP projection taken with the x-ray tube angled approximately 25 degrees in a caudal direction (Fig. 5–18). This view better visualizes the articular pillars and lamina of the lower cervical spine, which are at particular risk in hyperextension/compression injuries. A pillar view may be useful when the standard AP view suggests possible malalignment of the pillars.

With the increasing availability, speed, and utility of CT evaluation in traumatized patients, the threshold to perform CT should be low in high-risk patients, particularly if routine radiographs are suboptimal or suspicious, and the patient is already going to CT for evaluation of the head or body.

TOMOGRAPHY

Tomography or planigraphy, and especially complex motion tomography, can be useful for generation of cross-sectional radiographs. These images may be useful in resolving overlap of bony structures in areas of complex anatomy. The odontoid process of the cervical spine is an example of an area where plain tomography can been helpful. However, thin-section CT, particularly when combined with multiplanar image reformation, has largely replaced tomography in most clinical settings. Tomography is still useful in the evaluation of potential fracture nonunions where internal fixation hardware creates artifact, thereby greatly limiting CT. Tomography is a time-consuming modality, however, and delivers a very high radiation dose to the patient. Most clinical centers no longer support multidirectional tomography at this time. One enduring form of linear tomography is so-called panoramic tomography of the mandible and maxilla. These examinations are performed on a dedicated unit, which uses an x-ray source and curved film receptacle, which both rotate on separate axes about the patient (Fig. 5–19).

CONVENTIONAL ARTHROGRAPHY

Intra-articular needle placement under fluoroscopic guidance can be performed for purposes of contrast injection,

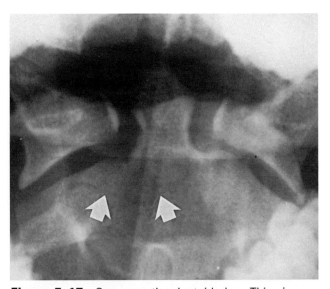

Figure 5–17. Open mouth odontoid view. This view assesses the dens and the C1–C2 alignment, but it may be challenging to project the teeth and skull base off the odontoid process and upper aspect of C2. In this case, a linear lucency is seen extending from the base of the odontoid into the body of C2, indicating a type 3 dens fracture *(arrows).*

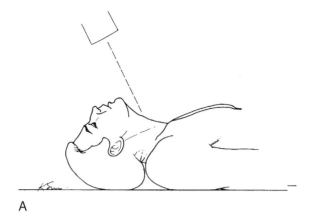

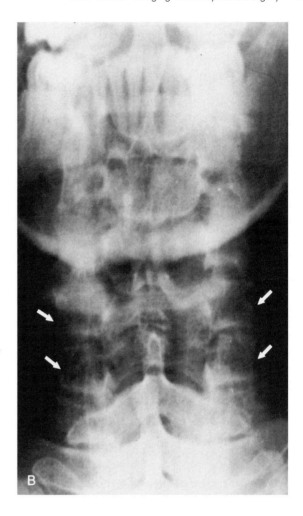

Figure 5–18. Pillar view. This AP angled-beam film is easy to perform, and evaluates the alignment of the lower cervical pillars and also assesses the lower lamina better than the standard AP view. (*A* from Resnick D: Diagnosis of Bone and Joint Disorders, 3rd ed. Philadelphia, WB Saunders, 1995, p 21. *B* from Resnick D: Diagnosis of Bone and Joint Disorders, 2nd ed. Philadelphia, WB Saunders, 1988, p 28.)

fluid aspiration, or instillation of steroid or analgesic medication. Injection of iodinated contrast medium or air followed by radiography is known as arthrography. Conventional arthrography has been largely replaced by MRI, but is still a useful tool for diagnosing full-thickness rotator cuff tears of the shoulder, and for evaluating the interosseous ligaments and triangular fibrocartilage of the wrist. Contrast arthrography is likely neither very sensitive nor specific for diagnosing loosening of arthroplasty components, but fluoroscopic needle placement and aspiration are still important for excluding deep infection in painful joint replacements.

C-arm fluoroscopy is an important tool for guiding needle injections of the disk and facet joints in an effort to determine specific pain sources in problematic and failed, postoperative backs. Epidural injections and nerve blocks using long-acting steroids can also be performed under fluoroscopy as therapeutic procedures.

Figure 5–19. Pantomographic radiograph: This specialized, linear tomography technique generates a single comprehensive view of the mandible, although the condyles and perisymphyseal regions are occasionally difficult to image with this technique.

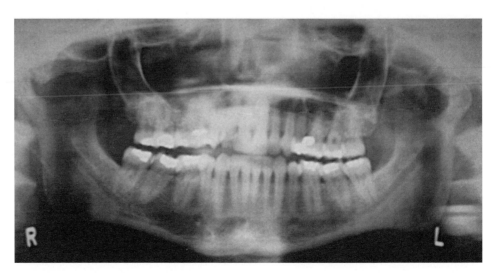

ULTRASONOGRAPHY

Ultrasound has the advantage of being semiportable, easily tolerated, and relatively inexpensive. With new transducer technology, ultrasound can easily surpass MRI and CT in spatial resolution, and can be used effectively in the imaging of small or superficial body parts. Common examples of the clinical application of high-resolution ultrasound include the diagnosis of Morton's neuromas and ganglion cysts.

Ultrasound is well suited to the evaluation of tendonopathy and reliably detects ruptures of tendons. Common clinical applications include evaluation of the Achilles tendon and the rotator cuff of the shoulder (Fig. 5–20). Whether ultrasound is as effective as MRI in grading the severity of tendonopathy is controversial at this time. Certainly, however, ultrasound is a more operator-dependent modality and requires a good deal of user experience to be effective. Ultrasound does visualize ligamentous structures as well, although a thorough working knowledge of anatomy is required of the user. For example, a targeted ultrasound examination can be used to assess for a Stenner lesion after ulnar collateral ligament injury of the metacarpophalangeal joint of the thumb, or the so-called gamekeeper's thumb injury.

Ultrasound perhaps has been underutilized in the evaluation of soft tissue mass lesions. It is particularly effective at determining the vascularity of lesions, particularly with the advent of real-time color Doppler imaging technology. Color Doppler maps the Doppler frequency shift, which is related to flow velocity, onto a gray scale ultrasound image. Power Doppler presents an integration of the power spectral density function, which is independent of flow velocity and direction. Thus, what power Doppler displays is analogous to the circulating blood volume, and it is highly sensitive to low-velocity flow. With these enhancements, ultrasound conveniently assesses the vascularity of lesions, and can identify hyperemia around inflammatory masses.

As a real-time imaging modality, ultrasound is also ideally suited to the safe performance of imaging guided biopsies. Ultrasound can be used to detect foreign bodies in the soft tissues that may not be evident on radiographs. Ultrasound can be used to guide foreign body retrieval under direct real-time visualization. Finally, relief from calcific peritendonitis or hydroxyapatite deposition disease (HADD), most commonly encountered in the region of the rotator cuff, can be facilitated by needle aspiration. In these patients who are refractory to conservative treatment, large-gauge needle aspiration of these deposits under direct ultrasound guidance can be curative. Ultrasound may facilitate joint aspiration in cases of suspected septic arthritis. In the pediatric patient, a short ultrasound evaluation may be useful in excluding the presence of joint effusion and possibly obviating needle aspiration in suspected cases of septic arthritis.

Because ultrasound is a real-time examination, it has the potential to evaluate dynamic, mechanical joint, and tendon problems. In the newborn and young infant with suspected hip dysplasia, ultrasound is the most sensitive means to diagnose both the subluxability of the hip and the degree of acetabular dysplasia. Ultrasound can be used to follow the maturation of the hip as well, at least until mineralization of the capital epiphysis begins to limit the examination. Another situation in which the real-time capability of ultrasound can be valuable is the assessment of the long head biceps tendon. Subluxation of the tendon can be diagnosed during provocative internal and external rotation of the shoulder.

COMPUTED TOMOGRAPHY

Technique

Computed tomography (CT) is a technique that generates cross-sectional images that are reconstructed from multiple digital radiographic projections or views. These views are combined through the method of "back-projection" to generate the cross-sectional image. Recent advances in CT include the development of helical or spiral scanners, in which "slip-ring" technology allows continuous unidirectional tube motion. Combined with improved tube heat capacities, the helical technique permits more rapid scan acquisition, and correspondingly, the coverage of large body areas in a relatively short period of time. This speed has been particularly valuable in imaging the chest and abdomen during suspended respiration. However, the increased speed has also facilitated the use of CT for the evaluation of the traumatized patient.

The helical CT also generates a three-dimensional projectional data set, which facilitates retrospective reconstruction of cross-sectional images at arbitrary intervals or locations throughout the data set. As a result, cross-sectional images can be reconstructed arbitrarily close to each other, in an overlapping fashion, without the penalty of an increased radiation dose to the patient. Such overlapping reconstructions improve the ability to subsequently re-

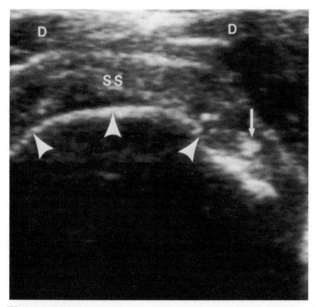

Figure 5–20. Shoulder ultrasound. Transverse view of the supraspinatus tendon demonstrates the moderately echogenic tendon (SS) between the dense shadow of the humeral head cortex *(arrowheads)* and the overlying deltoid muscle (D). The long head biceps tendon is seen as an echogenic focus *(small arrow)*. (From Resnick D: Diagnosis of Bone and Joint Disorders, 3rd ed. Philadelphia, WB Saunders, 1995, p 228.)

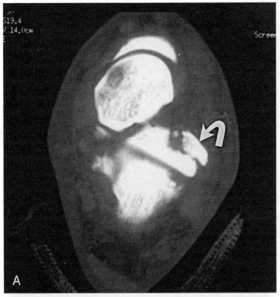

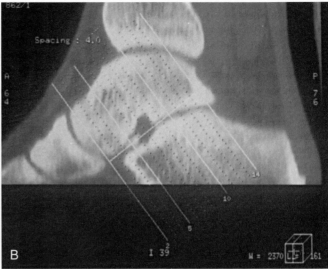

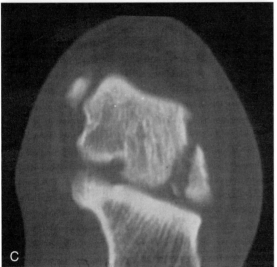

Figure 5–21. Helical CT of the hindfoot. Axial images *(A)* were acquired helically and reformatted into the sagittal *(B)* and oblique coronal planes *(C).* The optimal oblique coronal plane is prescribed from the sagittal reformatted image to best depict this lateral process fracture of the talus *(arrow)* and its relationship to the posterior facet of the subtalar joint. These versatile presentations of the axial scan data are facilitated by multiplanar reconstruction of the helical scan data.

format the axial source images into other imaging planes (multiplanar re-formation), such as coronal or sagittal planes. This improved multiplanar capability compensates for one of the traditional limitations of CT, that is, restriction to the axial imaging plane (Fig. 5–21).

Most recently, the emergence of multidetector-array CT will also allow retrospective reconstruction of images at variable scan collimation while dramatically increasing scan acquisition speed. Thinner scan sections (approaching 0.5 mm) can be achieved at reduced radiation dose. Implications for improved multiplanar resolution and 3D imaging are compelling, and the applications for CT will correspondingly continue to grow.

Clinical Applications

TRAUMA

CT is extremely helpful in clarifying the pattern and severity of traumatic bony injures and hence may be very helpful in preoperative planning. Compared to radiography, CT more accurately depicts the relationship and degree of comminution of fracture fragments. CT is particularly help-

ful in pelvic and complex acetabular fractures, as well as fractures of the calcaneus. Multiplanar re-formation of CT images is particularly useful in these areas, where for example, sagittal re-formations of the acetabulum and oblique coronal re-formations of the calcaneus can present the information from an axial data set in a more clinically useful and intuitive manner. Similarly, coronal re-formations of CT scans through the knee can be very helpful for pre-operative planning of tibial plateau fractures. The magnitude of joint surface depression and step-off can be accurately gauged on reformatted images, without resorting to the slow and antiquated technique of plain tomography.

CT data, if acquired using thin section collimation, and particularly if acquired helically, can be presented as shaded surface displays (Fig. 5–22). Although these surface renditions of axial image data do not contribute to fracture detection, they do improve visualization of the three-dimensional relationship of fracture fragments to each other and may aid in preoperative planning, particularly for acetabular fractures.

Although CT is chiefly used for problem solving and preoperative planning in cases of skeletal trauma, it can be

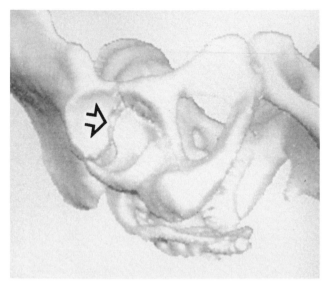

Figure 5–22. 3-D surface rendering. CT studies can be presented as shaded surface displays, which can improve appreciation of the relationships of fracture fragments to each other in the case of complex injuries. In this example, a T-shaped acetabular fracture is displayed as though the patient is supine. Helical scan acquisition was used.

or equivocal. This is a cost-effective strategy particularly if trauma patients require undergoing CT evaluation of other body parts. Again, helical CT is particularly well suited to evaluation of the cervical spine, where multiplanar re-formations may be helpful in visualizing fracture displacements and depicting the pillars or facet joints. Helical CT of the entire cervical spine may have utility as a primary screening method in very high risk trauma cases. More commonly, however, CT is only used to assess specific vertebral levels that are either suspicious or inadequately evaluated on the routine radiographs. The C7–T1 levels, and the odontoid process of C2, are typical problematic areas.

CT can be done after intra-articular administration of dilute iodinated contrast medium or air. The utility of so-called CT arthrography may be enhanced with improved, helical CT technology. CT arthrography is particularly useful in the shoulder in defining instability lesions of the labrocapsular ligamentous complex (Fig. 5–24). CT arthrography is ideally suited to the evaluation of joints for loose bodies, and also evaluates the joint surface for chondral defects and tears, although less accurately than MR arthrography. Finally, CT arthrography may provide information about the stability of chronic osteochondral lesions.

TUMORS

CT is often helpful in characterizing bony lesions and associated cortical bone destruction, periosteal reaction, and mineralization. By depicting lesion mineralization and patterns of bone destruction, CT may narrow differential diagnosis. However, CT is less effective than MRI in defining the extent of marrow involvement. In the case of bone lesions, CT is also useful in defining the extraskeletal extent of a bone lesion that extends through the cortex or arises on the surface of the bone. Similarly, CT is also

used as a primary modality for diagnosis in skeletal areas that are difficult to image with routine radiography, such as the spine and calcaneus (Fig. 5–23). Instabilities or subluxations of the distal radioulnar or sternoclavicular joints are very difficult to diagnose by radiography, but can be accurately assessed with a fast, very limited CT protocol. CT is now widely used in most trauma settings for clearing the cervical spine when radiographs are inadequate

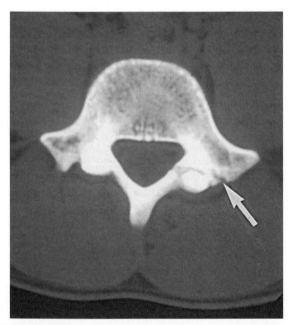

Figure 5–23. Spondylolysis. Axial CT scan demonstrates sclerosis surrounding an irregular lucency traversing the pars interarticularis on the left side *(arrow)*. These areas are easily identified on routine, 3-mm axial CT images.

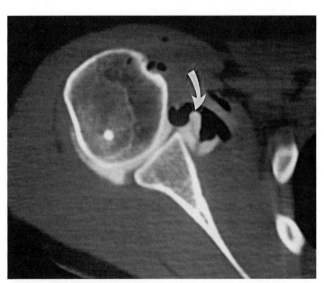

Figure 5–24. CT arthrogram. Air and dilute iodinated contrast medium have been injected into the right shoulder, outlining the labrocapsular structures. Elevation of a stripped labrum *(arrow)* is nicely demonstrated in this chronic Bankart lesion. The abnormal anterior labrum imbibes contrast material and therefore appears dense.

helpful in defining the involvement of neurovascular structures.

In the case of extraskeletal disease, the use of intravenous contrast material is usually helpful. In evaluation of intrinsic bony disease, the use of contrast material is not generally helpful. Soft tissue masses are generally better delineated and more sensitively detected with MRI than with CT. However, CT enhanced with intravenous contrast material is still a useful method for evaluating soft tissue masses. Specific findings can be seen on CT in the case of fat-containing lesions or lesions of vascular origin, and like MRI, CT can also distinguish cystic and necrotic components of soft tissue masses. CT is also well suited to the fast and accurate guidance of needle biopsy procedures.

MAGNETIC RESONANCE IMAGING

Magnetic resonance imaging has emerged as the most versatile and powerful means of imaging diagnosis. Clinical MRI is based on the detection of radiofrequency signals emanating from hydrogen nuclei as they resonate within a strong, static magnetic field. These signals, similar in frequency to FM radio signals, are generated by hydrogen nuclei after their selective and carefully timed radio frequency excitation. Radiofrequency signal strength is determined chiefly by the number of resonating protons per tissue voxel, or proton density, and by two relaxation constants, T_1 and T_2. So called T_1-weighted images favor proton species with short T_1 relaxation constants, such as the aliphatic hydrogen nuclei in fat. Intravenous paramagnetic contrast medium works chiefly by shortening the T_1 relaxation of neighboring protons. T_2-weighted images favor proton species with a long T_2 relaxation constants, such as the hydrogen nuclei in free water.

MRI innovation continues at a rapid pace, and newer MRI techniques are both faster and higher in resolution. For orthopaedic imaging, the resolution requirements are currently most important, but MRI can now generate information about tissue physiology, such as the diffusibility of water molecules, the relative perfusion of organs, and the circulating blood volume within tissues. Spectroscopic information from MRI can also measure and map biochemical markers of tissue structure and function. The utility of these functional MR tools for orthopaedic applications remains to be explored.

Technical Considerations

Resonating proton signals are larger, and correspondingly, image fidelity and resolution are improved at higher magnetic fields. One and 1.5 tesla scanners are considered "high field" units, and are typically of a closed-bore, tunnel-like design. These high field designs are more likely to result in claustrophobia for the patient, and their 55- to 60-cm bore diameter is commonly unable to accommodate very obese or broad patients. Open MRI designs usually employ a sandwich arrangement of permanent or resistive magnets and are usually of 0.3 tesla or lower field strength. These units are less claustrophobia inducing and can accommodate larger and broader patients. The "open" feature usually confers the additional advantage that patients

can be positioned such that the imaging area of interest is at "isocenter," or the most homogeneous portion of the magnetic field. The lower field strength of open magnet designs can be compensated for by longer scan times, but these units are still limited in their ability to image small parts at high resolution.

Also important to image fidelity and resolution are dedicated surface coils or volume coils used for signal detection. These are custom designed for different body parts. There is an intrinsic trade-off between the volume of coverage and signal to noise, such that the best images are acquired with the smallest receiver coils. Hence, a targeted MRI examination is always the most diagnostic. However, this approach to MRI requires a clear knowledge of the area of clinical concern, so that the appropriate receiver coil and the appropriate volume of interest are selected. These practical limitations of MRI are overcome to some degree with so-called phased-array technology in which multiple small receiver coils are applied and signals are acquired and processed simultaneously from each by different receiver circuits. This costly design innovation is available on most current state-of-the-art scanners.

Intravenous, paramagnetic contrast agents are chelates of gadolinium and are routinely administered for MRI of the central nervous system. The indications for intravenous MRI contrast material for musculoskeletal imaging are more limited. An intravascular agent does provide information about blood flow and capillary permeability or leakage within specific tissues of interest. This is occasionally helpful in characterizing mass lesions with MRI. Contrast enhancement may also be beneficial in outlining reactive or inflammatory tissues surrounding abscesses. Finally, contrast material enhancement may be of value in surveillance for recurrence of tumor after surgery or radiotherapy.

Direct intra-articular injection of either saline or a dilute solution of saline and a paramagnetic MRI contrast agent is known as MRI arthrography. This technique optimizes the delineation of synovial joints and their supporting structures. MRI arthrography is most widely used in the evaluation of instability lesions of the shoulder. It may also be of use in the evaluation of the knee after meniscal repair and optimizes the evaluation of the acetabular labrum of the hip.

Clinical Applications

The high-contrast resolution of MRI confers a considerable advantage over CT for evaluation of soft tissues. However, MRI is also extremely useful for evaluation of the marrow space, because the fat content of the marrow generates a high MRI signal, at least on T_1-weighted imaging. Pulse sequences that suppress fat signal are often useful in evaluation of the marrow, given that pathologic changes will show up as an area of high signal against the dark, fat-suppressed, normal marrow signal. Fat-suppressed imaging, particularly the STIR technique (short tau inversion recovery) are particularly sensitive to edema or inflammation whether in bone or soft tissue (Fig. 5–25), and are also quite effective at delineating disease extent in the case of neoplasia. MRI evaluation of supporting connective tissue structures requires high spatial resolution and an appropri-

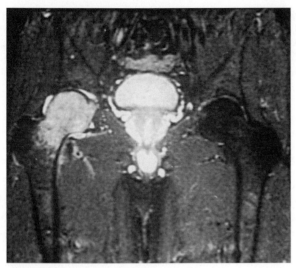

Figure 5–25. Marrow edema pattern. Coronal STIR MR image of the hips is highly sensitive to edema, as shown in the right proximal femur involving the head and neck. In this case of transient osteoporosis there is no demarcated necrotic zone.

ately tailored MRI examination that targets the specific structures of interest.

MRI is the best noninvasive test for evaluation of the joint surface. Traumatic chondral tears as well as advanced degenerative chondral loss are easily imaged, typically with some form of T_2-weighted imaging. Low-grade chondromalacia (grade 2) is also diagnosed accurately with high resolution techniques. Grade 1 chondromalacia is less reliably detected with current MRI techniques. High-resolution and particularly 3D MRI techniques can be used to measure the total cartilage volume within a joint, an index that may be of value in longitudinal studies designed to assess the efficacies of new treatments for arthritis. MRI, particularly when done with intravenous contrast material enhancement, is also much more sensitive than radiography for the detection of early bone erosion in the case of inflammatory arthritis. This increased sensitivity may have implications for evaluating new therapies for rheumatoid arthritis.

Unlike hyaline cartilage, the fibrocartilaginous meniscus of the knee is low in signal intensity on most MRI sequences. Fortunately, meniscal derangement appears as zones of increased signal against the normal, low signal fibrocartilage of the meniscus. Assessment of the knee for meniscal derangement is one of the most common indications for musculoskeletal MRI. On modern high field scanners, the sensitivity and specificity of MRI for meniscal tears are each approximately 90%. State of the art MRI scans also give information about the size and orientation of meniscal tears, and the presence of displaced flaps or bucket handle fragments. The postoperative meniscus continues to be a challenge for MRI, particularly if prior, postprocedural scans are not available for comparison. In these cases, intra-articular contrast medium injection may be of added value.

Fibrocartilaginous supporting structures in other joints, including the labrum of the shoulder and hip, can also be evaluated by MRI. Given their smaller size and more variable signal characteristics, they are less easily evaluated than the meniscus of the knee. MR arthrography is superior to conventional MR for the evaluation of the labra of the shoulder—particularly if SLAP lesions are suspected (superior labrum, anterior to posterior tears) (Fig. 5–26). MR arthrography is primarily indicated in the evaluation of suspected instability lesions of the shoulder. Images obtained after intra-articular injection better define Bankart and Bankart variants such as the anterior labroperiosteal sleeve avulsion (ALPSA), Perthes lesion, and glenoid labral articular disruption lesions (GLAD) (Fig. 5–27).

MRI is effective at diagnosing acute ligamentous injuries. Early experience in the MR evaluation of the knee revealed that MRI diagnoses ACL ruptures with high accuracy (sensitivity and specificity over 95%). MRI is similarly useful for evaluating acute ligamentous injuries in other locations. However, MRI is generally less good at assessing the severity or completeness of ligament insufficiency. This is particularly true in the subacute or chronic clinical setting.

The multiplanar imaging capability and high soft tissue contrast of MRI makes it ideally suited to the evaluation of the spine. Spinal canal and foraminal stenosis can be accurately assessed, as well as alterations in spinal alignment. The intervertebral disk is clearly depicted, with the nucleus being higher in signal than the annulus and posterior longitudinal ligament. Disk protrusions, extrusions, and sequestrations can be differentiated in the thoracic and lumbar spine (Fig. 5–28). Far-lateral disks are better visualized with MRI than with CT. CT still depicts osteophyte formation and annular ossification better than MRI, and may more accurately depict foraminal stenosis and spondylosis than MRI. The role for CT myelography evaluation of the spine continues to diminish as MRI techniques improve. In cases of major trauma and suspected instability, MRI may prove to be a safer and more effective test for ligamentous spinal derangement and potential instability than traditional, flexion, and extension radiographs.

MRI is quite sensitive for tendon disruptions if studies

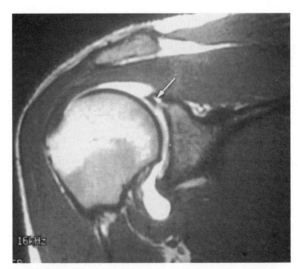

Figure 5–26. MR arthrography for SLAP lesion: A T_1-weighted image in the coronal oblique plane demonstrates contrast material extending into the superior labrum *(arrow)*.

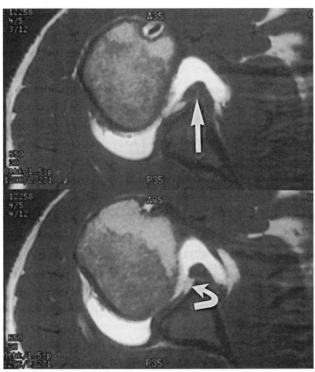

Figure 5–27. MRI arthrogram for shoulder instability. The joint has been distended after direct intra-articular injection of a dilute gadolinium chelate. Contrast medium outlines a partially detached anterior labral tear *(straight arrow)*, which is associated with an adjacent chondral tear *(curved arrow)*, the so-called GLAD lesion.

are performed with sufficient spatial resolution. This application has been particularly useful in staging impingement syndrome of the shoulder, in which MRI is accurate in identifying full-thickness rotator cuff tendon ruptures as well as gauging the size and severity of these lesions (Fig.

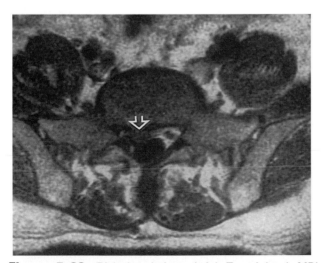

Figure 5–28. Disk herniation. Axial T_1-weighted MRI through the L5–S1 disk space demonstrates an anterior epidural mass *(arrow)* that displaces the right S1 nerve root and indents the thecal sac, consistent with a large right paramedian disk herniation.

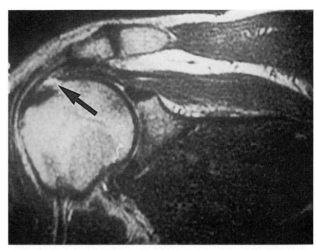

Figure 5–29. Rotator cuff tear. Oblique coronal T_2-weighted image is acquired along the axis of the supraspinatus tendon and muscle. A small full-thickness tear is well demonstrated as an area of focal hyperintensity *(arrow)*.

5–29). Degenerative and attritional changes in tendons, or tendinosis, is also detected on MRI scans, particularly when imaging is performed at short echo times. The imaging findings of tendinosis, however, may be difficult to distinguish from interstitial or partial thickness tendon ruptures. Signal characteristics do seem to be useful in making this distinction in the rotator cuff and Achilles tendon, in which macroscopic sites of rupture appear as areas of increased signal on T_2-weighted or longer echo time MR images. The ability of MRI to detect tendon changes in mild cases of clinically suspected "tendonitis" is still poorly documented.

MRI is sensitive in detecting muscle sprains and tears. In suspected cases of hamstring injury, for example, MR evaluation may be of some prognostic value, particularly in elite athletes, in whom the size of injuries, the extent of intramuscular fluid collections, and particularly the presence of hemorrhage can be delineated (Fig. 5–30). MRI is also sensitive to other physiologic and pathologic changes in muscle. Delayed onset muscle soreness (DOMS) is clearly depicted on T_2-weighted MRI images or STIR images. Transient changes in muscle signal are seen on MRI immediately after exercise, likely related to shifts in muscle water compartmentalization. These MR signal changes do bear a relation to muscle work, and therefore have implications for biomechanical research applications. For reasons that are not well understood, MRI and particularly STIR sequences are very sensitive to muscle alterations that occur very early in denervation states and neuropraxia, and thus may serve as a useful adjunct to electrodiagnostic studies. These MRI signal changes occur very early and do precede changes on electromyography. Finally, MRI effectively maps the often heterogeneous changes seen in inflammatory myopathies. This capability may contribute to more effective, image-guided muscle biopsy for diagnosis of these often complex and confusing disease entities.

Although cortical bone itself does not produce an MRI signal, the cellular and fatty elements in bone marrow do, and hence, MRI has become a powerful tool in diagnosing infiltrative, inflammatory, and traumatic conditions of bone.

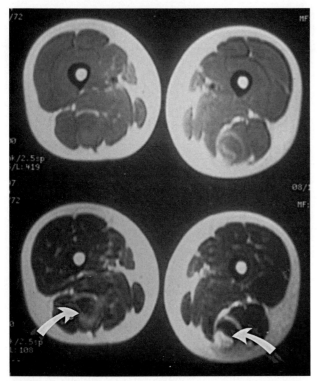

Figure 5–30. Muscle injury. Axial T$_2$-weighted MRI *(lower images)* demonstrates high signal involving the semitendinosus muscles bilaterally *(arrows)*, with greater severity on the left side. The presence of high signal on the T$_1$-weighted images *(upper left image)* indicates hemorrhage, a sign of greater injury severity.

Fairly specific MRI changes are seen in avascular necrosis of bone, in which zones of necrotic marrow become demarcated by reactive tissue and edema that exhibit abnormal MRI signals relative to normal marrow (Fig. 5–31). These changes are evident within weeks of the ischemic event, and the MRI findings are more specific and seen with greater resolution than they are with bone scan.

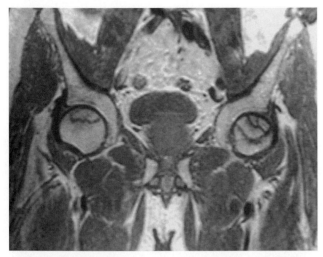

Figure 5–31. MRI of avascular necrosis. Coronal T$_2$-weighted MRI shows the well-defined serpentine-like interfaces that surround areas of marrow necrosis. The necrotic regions are occasionally surrounded by abundant marrow edema or reaction.

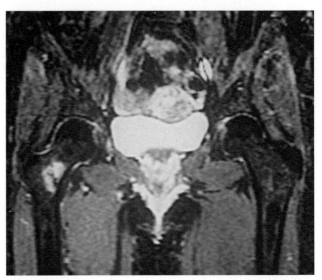

Figure 5–32. Stress fracture. Fat-suppressed MRI of the hips and the coronal plane demonstrates the conspicuity of marrow edema about a femoral neck stress fracture. The fracture is also visualized as a low signal fatigue or fracture line.

Similarly, the narrow reactions to both stress and trauma create alterations in the bone marrow signal that make MRI a very sensitive means to diagnose fractures, both of the fatigue and traumatic varieties (Fig. 5–32). In many cases, MRI will actually visualize the fracture or fatigue zone as a low signal line, which again confers greater specificity in diagnosis compared to bone scan (Fig. 5–33). MR, like bone scan, is highly sensitive for minor bone injury that

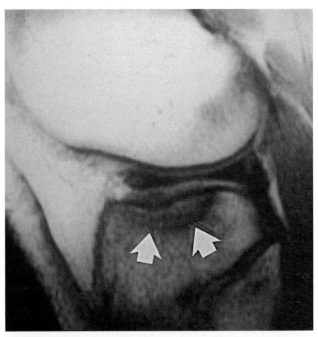

Figure 5–33. Nondisplaced fracture. Sagittal T$_1$-weighted MRI illustrates the sensitivity of MRI for subtle bony fractures. A slight deformity in the subchondral cortex of the lateral tibial plateau is easily seen as well as the zone of trabecular failure deep to the joint surface *(arrows)*.

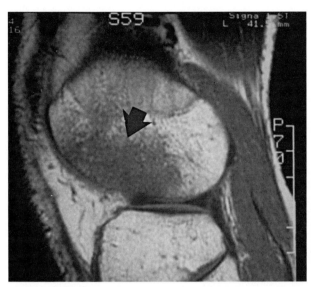

Figure 5–34. Occult bony injury. Sagittal intermediate MRI through the lateral femoral condyle demonstrates an ill-defined area of diminished signal intensity *(arrow)* within the subchondral bone. There was no discrete area of cortical interruption or deformity, consistent with a so-called "bone bruise" or occult trabecular injury. This marrow edema pattern is highly sensitive for bone injury.

occurs short of frank fracture, and these lesions are often referred to as bone bruises or occult trabecular injuries (Fig. 5–34). The multiplanar capabilities and relatively high resolution of the MRI scan constitute general advantages over bone scintigraphy in the diagnosis of stress or occult traumatic fracture.

The sensitivity of MRI to marrow edema and soft tissue inflammation make MRI an effective test for osteomyelitis (Fig. 5–35). The use of intravenous contrast material is not essential but may aid in identifying areas of necrosis or

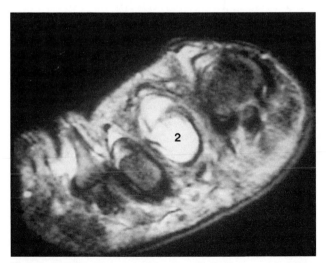

Figure 5–35. Osteomyelitis. T_2-weighted coronal oblique MRI through the forefoot demonstrates markedly increased marrow signal consistent with osteomyelitis involving the second metatarsal head (2). Corresponding radiographs were normal.

abscess formation. Again, the high resolution of MRI may make it more specific and also more useful for presurgical planning than bone scan. An important requirement for the effective use of MRI is prior knowledge of the anatomic region of concern, such that an appropriate, high-resolution study can be executed. Hence, a pertinent and accurate history is essential. Bone scan has the advantage of surveying larger areas than MRI and is less limited in this way. The utility of MRI and bone scan are both considerably diminished if there has been prior recent trauma or surgery that might impart alterations in bone marrow physiology, independent of those caused by infection.

MRI is very sensitive for detecting marrow replacement that occurs in metastatic and primary tumors of bone (Fig. 5–36). MRI is more sensitive and specific for metastatic disease to bone than either CT or bone scan. In the case of primary tumors of bone, MRI is indispensable for surgical planning, particularly in cases in which limb salvage procedures are anticipated. MRI accurately defines the extent of disease in the marrow space, and delineates extraosseous extension of tumor. Although the signal characteristics of tumors are usually not specific, MRI is quite effective in distinguishing cystic from solid masses, and also identifies the presence of aneurysmal bone cyst components and tumor necrosis. Problems may arise in using MRI to delineate tumors that are associated with reactive inflammation, such as histiocytosis or osteoid osteoma (Fig. 5–37). In these cases, it may be difficult to distinguish perilesional edema from the lesion or disease nidus itself.

MRI is not usually used to diagnose diffuse marrow diseases such as leukemia and myeloma. Actually, these infiltrative diseases are occasionally difficult to detect by MRI. MRI signal characteristics on routine imaging sequences may not reliably distinguish these marrow infiltrates from normal hematopoietic or red marrow. Often, the pattern or extent of marrow cellularity—that is, the replacement of normal yellow marrow—is more telling than the signal characteristics of the infiltrates themselves. More sophisticated imaging techniques including the use of contrast enhancement are likely to be of some value in both detecting pathologic marrow infiltration and gauging the efficacy of therapy in these diseases.

MRI is the modality of choice for the imaging evaluation of suspected soft tissue tumors. The utility of MRI is primarily in lesion detection and delineation, which aids management and surgical or biopsy planning. MRI has a higher sensitivity for soft tissue masses than CT, and although the MRI features are not usually specific for one histologic diagnosis, MR does often contribute information that may significantly narrow the differential diagnosis. Occasionally, specific diagnoses can be made with confidence based on MRI (Fig. 5–38), particularly in the case of vascular origin or fat-containing tumors. The use of intravenous contrast material may aid the identification of tumor necrosis, and the confirmation of the cystic nature of certain lesions, but it is not essential to the MRI evaluation of mass lesions.

NUCLEAR SCINTIGRAPHY

The specificity of nuclear medicine studies is determined by the radiopharmaceutical agent that is administered. Se-

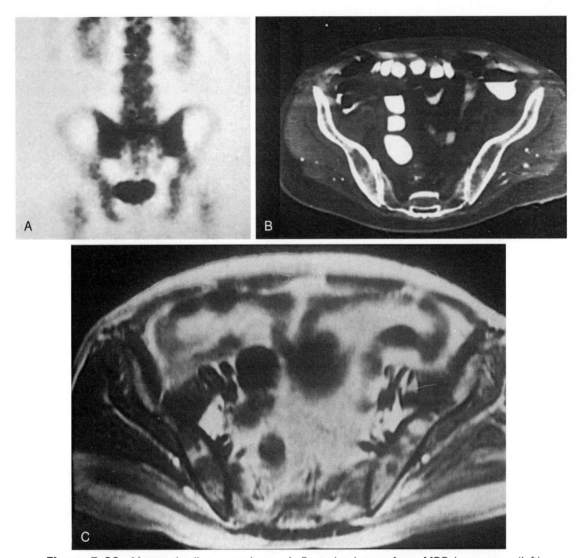

Figure 5–36. Metastatic disease to bone. *A,* Posterior image from MDP bone scan *(left)* shows no focal abnormalities. *B,* Axial CT *(right)* also shows no definite focal abnormalities or sites of bone destruction. *C,* Axial T_1-weighted MRI shows multiple, focal areas of discrete marrow hypointensity consistent with widespread metastatic disease to both iliac bones as well as portions of the sacrum.

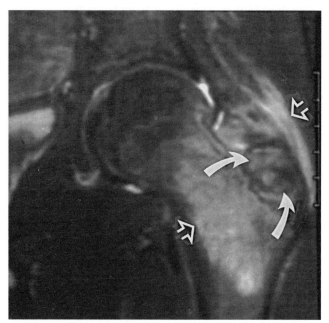

Figure 5–37. Lesion characterization on MRI. Coronal fat-saturated MRI after contrast administration demonstrates ill-defined enhancement *(open arrows)* in soft tissues and the surrounding marrow secondary to chondroblastoma in the greater trochanter *(solid arrows)*. The contrast enhancement is related to perilesional inflammation characteristic of this tumor. Contrast administration, in general, does little to aid lesion characterization on MRI.

lective uptake of radiopharmaceutical agents occurs in tissues in a temporally predictable fashion. The radiotracer portion of the radiopharmaceutical is typically a gamma-emitting isotope, and the distribution of radiopharmaceutical is imaged by a gamma (scintillation) camera. These

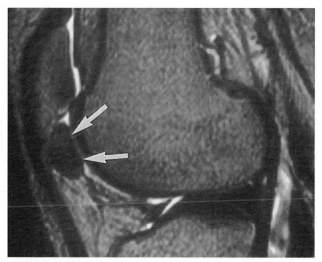

Figure 5–38. Soft tissue mass characterization. Sagittal T_2-weighted MRI through the extensor mechanism of the knee shows a well-defined mass inferior to the patella and deep to the tendon *(arrows)*. This demonstrates characteristic diminished signal intensity, due to hemosiderin deposition, which supports a diagnosis of focal pigmented villonodular synovitis.

cameras have large faces and can scan large areas of the body quickly to produce so-called planar images. Gamma cameras can also be designed to rotate around the patient to collect multiple views, which can then be reconstructed into tomographic or cross-sectional images in various planes. This application is referred to as SPECT imaging (single photon emission computed tomography) (Fig. 5–39). Technetium-99m (^{99m}Tc) is the radioisotope used most commonly for clinical scintigraphy because of its inexpensive production from portable generators, convenient half-life of 6 hours, and a principal photon energy of 140 keV, which is well suited to detection by gamma cameras.

Skeletal scintigraphy, or bone scan, is the nuclear medicine examination most commonly performed for the evaluation of orthopaedic problems. Imaging commences approximately 2 to 4 hours after the intravenous administration of the radiopharmaceutical, which is usually ^{99m}TC-methylene diphosphonate (MDP). The MDP bone scan is highly sensitive for a diversity of bony abnormalities, images the entire skeletal system, and is well tolerated by patients. Image acquisition requires 30 to 40 minutes. The uptake of ^{99m}Tc-MDP is determined by both the osteoblastic activity of bone as well as blood flow to the bone. MDP uptake is diminished in osteoporosis and in patients who are on bisphosphonate therapy.

The most common application of skeletal scintigraphy is in detecting metastatic disease, for which the sensitivity approaches 95%. Metastatic disease causes altered bone metabolism that causes focal increased uptake of MDP. Metastatic disease is detected much earlier on bone scans than on radiography. Bone density has to change by 30 to 50% before a plain radiograph will depict infiltrative disease. Certain aggressive and purely osteolytic tumors, however, such as multiple myeloma, renal cell carcinoma, and early Langerhans cell histiocytosis, may not produce increased uptake on bone scan, or may present as photon-deficient or "cold" areas that can be overlooked. For this reason multiple myeloma is conventionally staged with the radiographic skeletal survey.

Occasionally, after effective chemotherapy, metastatic bone lesions may exhibit increased osteoblastic activity that manifests as increased activity on follow-up bone scans and is known as the "flare" phenomenon. Hence, increased avidity for tracer should not be interpreted as a sign that metastatic bony disease has progressed. With advanced and diffuse metastatic disease (typically secondary to prostate or breast carcinoma) the bone scan may show such diffusely increased bone activity that it assumes a pseudonormal appearance, known as a superscan. This pitfall may be avoided by recognizing the diminished or absent renal tracer activity that also characterizes most of these cases.

Bone scintigraphy is of limited value in imaging primary bone neoplasms. The area of uptake may not reflect the true tumor margins, and soft tissue involvement will not be appreciated. Bone scintigraphy is not reliable in distinguishing malignant from benign lesions, although the pattern of uptake may reflect the aggressiveness of the lesion. In evaluating what is presumed to be a solitary bony lesion, bone scintigraphy is mainly useful in excluding multifocal disease or unsuspected metastatic disease.

Clinical history is important in interpreting bone scans, because tracer uptake is highly nonspecific. Sites of bony

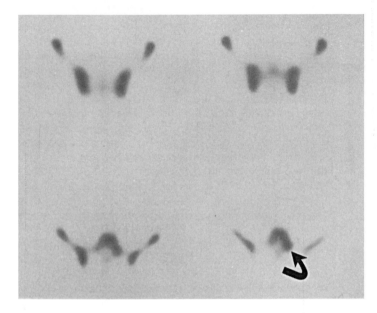

Figure 5–39. SPECT bone scan. Axial images are reconstructed from a ^{99m}Tc-MDP bone scan of the lumbar spine. Asymmetrical increased uptake in the posterior elements on the left *(arrow)* indicates the site of a pars interarticularis fracture.

trauma and of degenerative joint disease will regularly appear as incidental, focal areas of increased radiotracer uptake on bone scan. Bone scintigraphy is therefore a useful technique for detecting occult fractures or stress fractures. About 80% of traumatic fractures are seen at 24 hours and 95% by 3 days. The greatest tracer uptake is usually seen approximately 7 days after fracture. Bone scans will revert back to normal approximately 1 year after fracture, with 95% normalizing by 3 years. Stress fractures typically appear as focal areas of increased uptake, often eccentrically situated within a long bone. So-called stress reactions that occur from bone fatigue prior to actual fracture, and the related entity of shin splints, appear as more diffuse, cortical areas of increased tracer localization.

Avascular necrosis, whether related to trauma, sickle cell disease, steroid use, or alcoholism can be readily identified with bone scintigraphy, although the appearance will depend on the time course of the process. Because of decreased blood flow to the site, recently infarcted bone may appear photopenic. Detection of the photopenic, infarcted bony foci, however, requires adequate spatial resolution, which may require SPECT imaging or pinhole collimators. Later, healing and new bone formation will manifest as increased activity about the area of infarction. This presentation may be difficult to distinguish from that caused by arthrosis.

Osteomyelitis, particularly in its acute form, can be diagnosed by bone scanning with a sensitivity that far exceeds that of radiography. Radiotracer uptake will generally be increased at sites of osteomyelitis within the first 24 hours of the infection. Dynamic multiphase imaging heightens the specificity of bone scan by better differentiating osteomyelitis from cellulitis or septic arthritis. The first phase (the flow phase) consists of dynamic, acquisition of images over the area of interest every 2 to 5 seconds for the first 1 to 3 minutes after injection and reflects regional blood flow. In the second phase static images are obtained during the first 10 to 20 minutes after injection after adequate recirculation of tracer; this phase is known as the blood pool or tissue phase and reflects circulating blood volume. For the third, or delayed, phase, images are obtained 2 to 4 hours after injection, when substantial clearance of soft tissue and blood pool activity has occurred. Increased activity on all three phases of bone scan imaging is seen in osteomyelitis, but cellulitis is abnormal on only the first two phases. However, a positive three-phase bone scan is not entirely specific for osteomyelitis, and can be seen in inflammatory arthritis, gout, acute fracture, reflex sympathetic dystrophy, and neuropathic joint disease. The sensitivity of the three-phase bone scan may also be diminished in cases of severe peripheral vascular disease, and perhaps for similar reasons, in the diabetic foot.

In the 1970s, gallium-67 citrate was commonly used in conjunction with ^{99m}Tc-MDP bone scanning to increase the specificity of diagnosis for osteomyelitis. By the mid-1980s, however, scanning with labeled leukocytes largely supplanted gallium scanning in the scintigraphic evaluation of osteomyelitis and potential soft tissue abscesses. Gallium-67 is still of some value in the evaluation of potential disk space and vertebral infections. Gallium scans can also be helpful in the pediatric population in which uptake of ^{99m}Tc-MDP in the growth plates may mask adjacent uptake from infection. Gallium, which also localizes in tumors, is still routinely used for staging and assessing disease progression in patients with lymphoma.

Leukocyte scintigraphy has largely replaced gallium scanning for the assessment of complicated osteomyelitis. To perform leukocyte scintigraphy, white blood cells from the patient are separated from approximately 50 mL of whole blood, and are labeled with either indium-111 oxine, or ^{99m}Tc hexamethyl-propyleneamine oxime (HMPAO). The labeled cells are then reintroduced into the patient. Scanning is usually performed at approximately 6 and 12 hours after injection. The technetium-labeled white blood cell study is preferable to indium for most orthopaedic applications, because the shorter half-life of technetium permits a larger injected dose to be used. This more favorable dosimetry means that images have higher count rates and higher resolution, which is particularly important in evaluating the extremities. The utility of white blood cell scanning should greatly improve with the emergence of a new, in vivo white blood cell labeling technique using an antigranulocyte antibody tagged with [99m]Tc.

Scintigraphy with labeled white blood cells has proved to be useful in diagnosing infection about total joint arthroplasties or internal fixation hardware. Skeletal scintigraphy is of limited value in this setting, although it may confer some information about prosthetic loosening. Localization of white blood cells about orthopaedic implants, although far more specific than MDP, can still be seen to some degree around noninfected implants, and also about sites of neuropathic joint disease. This physiologic uptake is usually low in intensity, and generally decreases farther out from the time of surgery. However, when periprosthetic white blood cell localization occurs, diagnostic accuracy is greatly improved if the findings are correlated with a ^{99m}Tc sulfur colloid marrow scan. If the pattern of white blood cell localization parallels the marrow uptake of sulfur colloid in a congruent fashion, infection can be excluded and white blood cell localization can be regarded as physiologic (Fig. 5–40). However, areas of white blood cell localization that are incongruent with the uptake of sulfur colloid are diagnostic of osteomyelitis. The accuracy of white blood cell scanning for osteomyelitis is lower in the spine, and it may also be diminished after antibiotic therapy and in cases of chronic osteomyelitis.

The availability of whole-body positron emission tomography (PET) imaging is increasing. In particular, fluorine-18-fluorodeoxyglucose PET (FDG-PET) imaging has gained acceptance for its ability to effectively stage tumors and evaluate for recurrent neoplasia. This imaging technique, which identifies sites of increased glucose utilization, is also an alternative method to diagnose osteomyelitis in complicated clinical settings (Fig. 5–41).

BONE DENSITOMETRY

Osteoporosis is increasingly recognized as a major public health problem, with huge attendant health care costs and morbidity rates. Bone densitometry studies are increasingly used to assess fracture risk, and to guide treatment decision making in cases of suspected osteoporosis. Guidelines for the use of densitometry continue to evolve.

Quantitative CT (QCT) is an older technique for measuring bone density and is used to analyze the lumbar spine. For routine QCT evaluations, axial images of T12–L4 are analyzed using conventional, single energy CT equipment. With the aid of phantoms of known density that are scanned with the patient, bone mineral content can be calculated with reasonable precision (coefficient of variation is less than 3%). Quantitative CT is considerably less precise when used at the hip. The major advantage of QCT is that it allows a quantitative measure of true trabecular bone mineral content. Because trabecular bone is metabolically far more active than cortical bone, QCT may permit earlier and more sensitive detection of changes in bone mass resulting from treatment or disease. Special software may also permit separate quantification of cortical bone mass. The disadvantages of QCT include a relatively high radiation dose (0.5 to 1.0 rad), poor precision in comparison with dual-energy x-ray absorptiometry (DEXA), and a systematic error caused by variances in marrow fat content. An increase in the fat content of the marrow space will lower the measured attenuation values used to calculate bone mineral density, when using standard, single energy CT equipment.

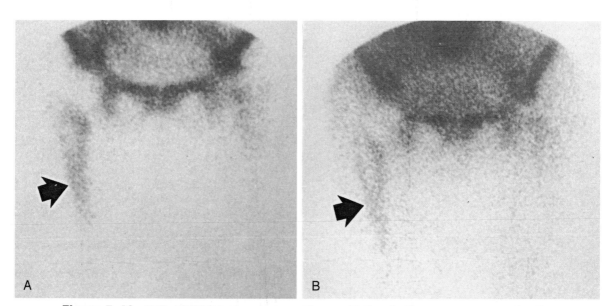

Figure 5–40. ^{99m}Tc-HMPAO leukocyte scan. Nonspecific localization can occur around orthopaedic implants *(arrow)* as in this case of a right total hip replacement *(A)*. Correlation with a ^{99m}Tc-sulfur colloid scan *(B)* is important to ascertain an incongruent pattern of white blood cell localization. In this case, a similar or congruent pattern of tracer localization is seen on sulfur colloid scan, indicating that this is physiologic or reactive white blood cell localization and not osteomyelitis.

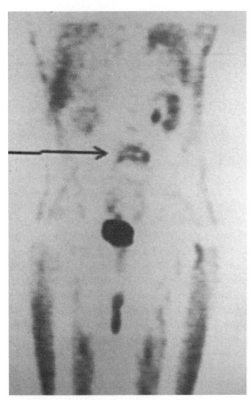

Figure 5–41. FDG PET. This coronal reformation from a whole-body FDG PET scan demonstrates increased uptake about a lower lumbar disk space *(arrow)* in this case of spondylodiskitis. Note normal tracer clearance in the urinary system and normal glucose utilization in the skeletal musculature of the thighs.

The technique used most widely for osteoporosis screening is DEXA. Routine DEXA screening is performed on the lumbar spine and hip, in the frontal projection. The dual energy feature of this examination permits separate calculation of x-ray attenuation from bone and from soft tissue. In this way, the bone mineral content can be derived from a two-dimensional, projectional (non–cross-sectional) technique. Modern DEXA scanners utilize a fan-beam x-ray source, and hence are quite fast (less than 5 minutes for image acquisition), and lateral DEXA is also possible for evaluating the vertebral bodies of the spine.

The advantages of DEXA are the extremely low radiation dose (less than 5 mrad), high precision (coefficients of variation less than 1% for the spine) and relatively low cost. For clinical purposes, measured bone mineral density from DEXA examinations are most commonly expressed as a standard deviation from the mean bone density of healthy young control subjects (T score), or less important, as a standard deviation from the mean for age- and sex-matched control subjects (Z score). Various regions of interest are reported for the hip region, but the bone mineral content of the femoral neck is probably the most useful and precise measurement.

Quantitative ultrasound techniques using small, dedicated units for analysis of the calcaneus are also gaining popularity, given their low cost. These units measure broadband ultrasound attenuation and speed of sound to calculate bone stiffness. These parameters also appear to effectively assess fracture risk. However, the precision of quantitative ultrasound is currently still significantly poorer than that of DEXA, and only peripheral sites can be assessed.

RADIATION EXPOSURE CONSIDERATIONS

X-rays and gamma rays are used in medical imaging and are part of the electromagnetic spectrum, which includes visible light, radio waves, and radiant heat. X-rays differ from gamma rays only in their origin—the former from electron and the latter from nuclear transitions. All ionizing radiation can damage biologic tissues. This damage can be immediate and result in cell death or it may take the form of DNA alteration and carcinogenesis. Alternatively, gonadal exposure may have deleterious affects on progeny.

The units used to measure radiation exposure can be confusing. The standard unit of measurement for radiation exposure is the roentgen, which is defined by the ionizing potential of radiation in air (expressed as $2.58 \times$ E-4 coulombs/kg of air). The roentgen is less biologically relevant than a measure of the amount of radiation that is absorbed in tissue. Absorbed radiation is measured in units of rads (the SI unit is a gray, which equals 100 rads). A dose of 1 rad is defined as 100 erg of energy absorbed by 1 g of tissue. A second unit closely related to the rad is the rem (roentgen equivalent in man), which relates the absorbed dose to biologic risk through a multiplicative quality factor. This adjustment accounts for the differing biologic impacts of different radiation type on tissue. For gamma and x-rays, however, the rad and rem are equal (quality factor = 1).

The easiest exposure to measure and compare is the skin or entry dose, but this may be a poor indicator of the dose delivered to the most biologically sensitive tissue, which is often deeper glandular or gonadal tissue. For example, an AP view of the foot will differ in the amount of radiation to sensitive organs compared to that given by a mammogram, even though the skin exposures may be similar. Effective whole-body or organ dose equivalents can be calculated that reflect the comparative biologic risk from different tests, but these calculations require a complex modeling process called dosimetry.

The typical entry doses for common tests include 10 to 30 mrem for a PA chest x-ray, 500 to 750 mrem for an AP lumbar spine, 2000 to 6000 mrem for a head CT, and 2000 to 5000 rem/minute for fluoroscopy. Natural background sources of radiation contribute up to 300 mrem a year, much of it in the form of cosmic gamma radiation and radon. Children are more susceptible than adults to the deleterious effects of radiation. Exposures during pregnancy are most damaging at the second to sixth weeks.

To put exposures in perspective, the minimum dose that causes skin erythema is approximately 200 to 300 rad. Death occurs in 10 to 24 hours after exposures of 600 to 1000 rad, and immediate death occurs at doses greater than 1000 rad. Of greater practical concern are the risks associated with low-level radiation exposures, and these are estimated from mathematical and statistical models. The incremental lifetime risk for cancer (usually leukemia or lymphoma) is estimated to be approximately 0.1% per rad. Expressed differently, if 100,000 people each received a dose of 1 rad, approximately two new cases of cancer would be anticipated per year, based on a life expectancy of approximately 75 years.

The National Council on Radiation Protection and Management (NCRP) has recommended that the lifetime exposure in rems should not exceed one's age in years. The maximum permissible whole-body dose for radiation workers is 5 rem per year (75 rem per year for the hands), and 0.1 rem per year for the general public. The use of protective barriers, such as lead aprons, and maximizing one's distance from the x-ray source are the two most effective measures that limit the dose to health care workers.

ALGORITHMS FOR IMAGING WORKUP OF MAJOR DISEASE CATEGORIES

Flow sheets are provided that describe the decision-making process that should guide the imaging evaluation of four important clinical problems. These guidelines continue to evolve as technology evolves, and the decisions about utilization may also vary as perspectives on cost efficacy change.

Osteomyelitis (Fig. 5–42)

Radiography is the first line imaging test for suspected osteomyelitis, and occasionally radiography alone is adequate. Hematogenous osteomyelitis can be effectively diagnosed by three-phase bone scan, but complex cases involving prior trauma, fracture, surgery, or neuropathic joint disease may require leukocyte scintigraphy. MRI may still

be effective if the surgery or trauma is subacute (i.e., more remote than 3 months). MRI is usually the test of choice in assessing for osteomyelitis secondary to spread from a contiguous soft tissue infection or ulcer, and may provide useful information on extent of bone involvement if surgery is planned. Prior surgery can be a difficult, confounding factor, however, in evaluation of persistent or recurrent infections.

Skeletal Tumors (Fig. 5–43)

Radiography is the most important test for narrowing differential diagnosis in the case of bony lesions. Cross-sectional imaging may help to elucidate potentially aggressive features of bony lesions, and plan or guide biopsy. Compared with radiography, CT or MRI can be a more sensitive means to follow equivocal lesions that do not quite warrant biopsy. The roles of CT and MRI are complementary, and both may be necessary for preoperative planning in the case of primary bone tumors. The bone scan is primarily useful for staging and for confirming that a solitary bony lesion is indeed solitary.

Cervical Spine Injury (Fig. 5–44)

CT plays an increasingly important role in the evaluation of acute cervical spine trauma, particularly if patients fall into high-risk categories. Risk of injury can be gauged by simple criteria, such as the mechanism and severity of injury, associated craniofacial injuries, neurologic signs, and advanced patient age. With improvements in helical CT, the entire cervical spine can be cleared primarily with CT in selected high-risk patients. There is little utility for

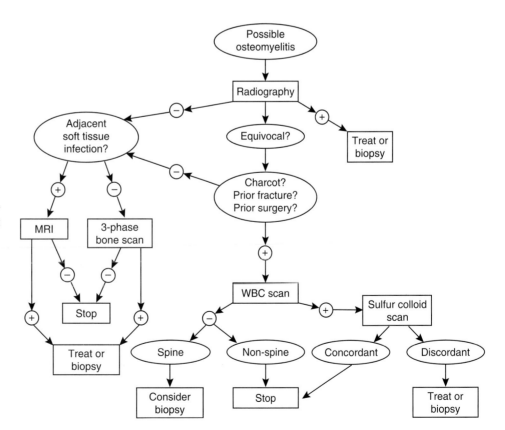

Figure 5–42. Algorithm for evaluation and management of possible osteomyelitis.

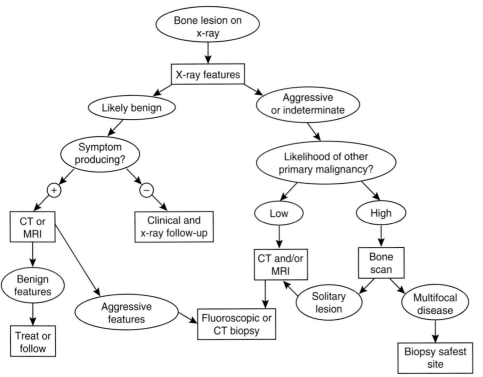

Figure 5–43. Algorithm for evaluation and management of a bone lesion found on x-ray.

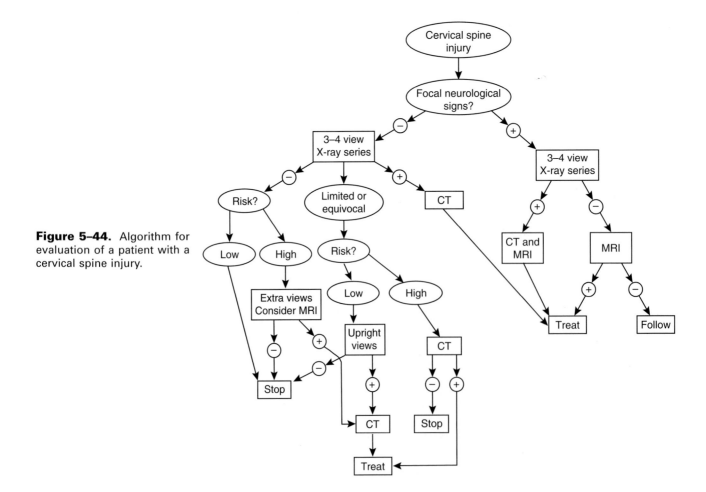

Figure 5–44. Algorithm for evaluation of a patient with a cervical spine injury.

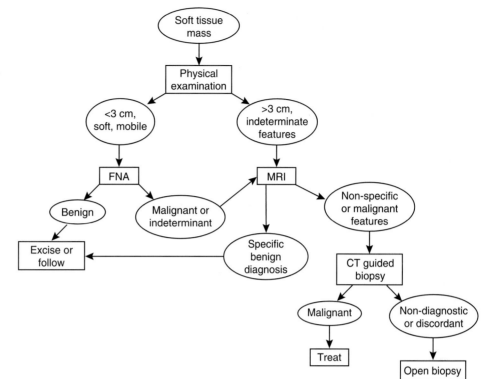

Figure 5–45. Algorithm for evaluation of a soft tissue mass.

flexion or extension views of the spine, although they may add diagnostic confidence of normality in low-risk patients with significant symptoms. A higher suspicion of ligamentous injury likely warrants an MR evaluation, as does the presence of neurologic signs.

Soft Tissue Masses (Fig. 5–45)

The decision to pursue an imaging workup is based on the size, chronicity, and physical characteristics of the mass. MRI is the imaging test of choice in cases of soft tissue masses. MR provides some degree of tissue characterization and, more important, accurately defines lesion extent. Alternatively, imaging may helpful to confirm or exclude the presence of a suspected mass lesion. CT is ideally suited to guide the core biopsy of deep or heterogeneous lesions.

Bibliography

Alazraki NP, Mishkin FS: Fundamentals of Nuclear Medicine, 2nd ed. New York, The Society of Nuclear Medicine, 1988.

Anderson JF, Reed JW, Steinweg J: Atlas of Imaging in Sports Medicine. Sydney, Australia, McGraw-Hill, 1998.

Ballinger PW: Merrill's Atlas of Radiographic Positions and Radiologic Procedures, 6th ed. St. Louis, CV Mosby, 1986.

Bergman AG: Rotator cuff impingement: Pathogenesis, MR imaging characteristics, and early dynamic MR results. Magn Reson Imaging Clin North Am 1997;5:709.

Berquist TH: Imaging of Orthopedic Trauma, 2nd ed. New York, Raven Press, 1992.

Berquist TH: MRI of the Musculoskeletal System, 3rd ed. Philadelphia, Lippincott-Raven, 1996.

Blackmore CC, Emerson SS, Mann FA, Koepsell TD: Cervical spine imaging in patients with trauma: Determination of fracture risk to optimize use. Radiology 1999;211:759–765.

Boutin RD, Brossmann J, Sartoris DJ, et al: Update on imaging of orthopedic infections. Orthop Clin North Am 1998;29(1):41–66.

Bushberg JT, Seibert AJ, Leidholdt EM, Boone JM: The Essential Physics of Medical Imaging. Baltimore, Williams & Wilkins, 1994.

Curry TS, Dowdey JE, Murry RC: Christensen's Physics of Diagnostic Radiology, 4th ed. Philadelphia, Lea & Febiger, 1990.

Graf R: Guide to Sonography of the Infant Hip. New York, Thieme, 1987.

Resnick D: Diagnosis of Bone and Joint Disorders, 3rd ed. Philadelphia, WB Saunders, 1995.

Stoller D: Magnetic Resonance Imaging in Orthopedics and Sports Medicine. Philadelphia, JB Lippincott, 1993.

Thrall JH, Ziessman HA: Nuclear Medicine: The Requisites. St. Louis, Mosby–Year Book, 1995.

Van Holsbeeck M, Introcaso JH: Musculoskeletal Ultrasound. St. Louis, Mosby–Year Book, 1991.

Chapter 6

Clinical Electrophysiology

Michael Sirdofsky, M.D.
Maria Elmina D. Fernandez, M.D.

Electromyography (EMG) and nerve conduction studies should be regarded as an extension of the clinical examination. A brief history and neurologic examination should be performed prior to the actual study itself. Once the differential diagnosis is made, the EMG should be tailored to prove or disprove the different diagnostic possibilities. This approach should take into account the referring physician's concerns but should be flexible enough to explore alternative etiologies and to change the scope of the testing as unexpected abnormalities are found. This open approach will take full advantage of the clinical and electrodiagnostic expertise of the neurophysiologist. Any other approach will not consistently yield clinically meaningful or even correct results. Although this practice sounds so intuitive that it need not be included for discussion, it is often not done consistently enough. For instance, EMG signs of denervation are common to most neurogenic conditions. A patient referred for radiculopathy because of painless atrophy and wasting in his right arm may on close clinical inspection be found to have a milder degree of similar changes in the left arm. A limited EMG restricted in scope to the right upper limb may have suggested the diagnosis of a C6 and C7 radiculopathy. A more widespread study would have revealed a generalized picture of denervation consistent with a systemic disorder such as amyotrophic lateral sclerosis. A patient referred to rule out thoracic outlet syndrome is found to have carpal tunnel syndrome and a patient with carpal tunnel syndrome is found on more widespread study to have this entrapment superimposed on a background polyneuropathy. Thus, the EMG is not a test that can be performed in a vacuum or by an unsupervised technician if reliable interpretive data are to be obtained. (Technicians often perform nerve conduction studies; however, the scope of their work is overseen by the neurophysiologist.)

BASIC ELECTROPHYSIOLOGIC PRINCIPLES

Nerve Conductions

When a cathode is applied to a nerve there is an accumulation of negative charges under this pole and an accumulation of positive charges under the anode. The inside of the axon underneath the cathode then becomes relatively positive, resulting in local current flow and depolarization. The resting mammalian transmembrane potential is around -90 mv. If the degree of depolarization drops the resting potential to approximately -70 mv, an all or none action potential will develop as a result of an energy-dependent morphologic change in sodium channels that will open, rendering them permeable to sodium ions. Unlike the unidirectional spread of current in the normal physiologic situation, in which the signal is initiated at the anterior horn cell or sensory nerve endings, when a cathode is used, current propagates in a bidirectional fashion from the point of depolarization. Because of heavy myelin insulation around the internodal segments, current created by the action potential can only pass to the bare axon in a saltatory fashion at the node of Ranvier. Any process that interrupts the myelin sheath will result in slowing of nerve propagation or dispersion of the recorded signal from the muscle or nerve. Dispersion occurs as a result of differential slowing of the population of nerve fibers that make up a nerve. The resultant waveform may possess many phases or may be of long duration. In pathologic situations there may also be conduction block at adjacent nodes secondary to current leakage. If there is enough current leakage secondary to disruption of the myelin insulation, adjacent nodes of Ranvier will not be depolarized, resulting in block of the propagating impulse. Thus, the hallmark of acquired demyelination is conduction slowing, waveform dispersion, and conduction failure or block.[1] Genetic demyelinating conditions usually result in uniform slowing of all the fibers of the nerve. It is therefore uncommon to see waveform dispersion with inherited conditions.[2]

Axonal neuropathies are associated with a dropout of sensory and motor axons. The resultant amplitude of the signal recorded from the muscle (compound muscle axon potential, or CMAP) or nerve (sensory nerve action potential, or SNAP), which is a measure of the number of viable axons, is subsequently reduced. The axon maintains a trophic influence over muscle. Axonal loss will lead to muscle atrophy with resultant diminution of the size of the CMAP. Thus, the hallmark of axonal neuropathies is drop in amplitude. Velocities may also slow in axonal neuropathies secondary to the loss of the fastest conducting axons. However, this is generally never below 70 percent of the lower limit of normal.[3]

The benefit of obtaining conductions in those felt to possess a clinical neuropathy are many. The clinical impression and severity can be documented. In addition, the type of neuropathy such as demyelinating, axonal, predominantly sensory, motor, or motor neuronopathy, often possesses distinctive differential diagnoses. Finally, in some cases the results can be followed sequentially to view for improvement with therapy or in therapeutic clinical trials.

Techniques

MOTOR CONDUCTIONS

The active or pickup electrode (G1) is placed over the motor point of the recording muscle of interest. An indifferent electrode (G2) is placed over the tendon of that muscle. A cathode is then placed over the nerve innervating the muscle of interest. The nerve is then depolarized and the response is displayed on a monitor. The stimulation is gradually intensified until the CMAP appears maximal. The intensity is then increased by 20 percent to a supramaximal stimulus that ensures that all the nerve fibers are depolarized. This procedure is then repeated at a proximal site or sites. Distances between cathodal sites of stimulation are measured and nerve velocities are calculated according to the following formula:

$$\frac{\text{Distance (mm)}}{T_p - T_d \text{ (msec)}}$$

Distance in millimeters is measured between the points of cathodal stimulation. T represents the time to the onset of a response in milliseconds between proximal site of stimulation (T_p) and the distal site of stimulation (T_d). This calculation will yield a result in meters/second over the desired nerve segment. The typical measurements would include median and ulnar forearm as well as peroneal and tibial leg velocities. The peroneal nerve segment across the fibula head and the ulnar nerve segment across the elbow are also frequently obtained when clinically required. Other measurements obtained include the distal motor latency, CMAP amplitude and duration (Fig. 6–1). The distal motor latency is a time measurement in milliseconds that represents the time to the onset of the CMAP from the most distal point of stimulation. This takes into account the delay at the neuromuscular junction and along the muscle fiber itself, which conducts only at 5 m/sec. Either standard distances or anatomic landmarks are used so that distal motor latency norms can be established. Distal motor latency is often delayed in focal compressive lesions such as carpal tunnel syndrome or early in the course of demyelinating neuropathies.[4]

SENSORY CONDUCTIONS

Sensory nerve action potentials (SNAPs) can be recorded in an orthodromic or antidromic fashion. Normal physiologic signaling is orthodromic. That is, the direction of impulse flow is from the end organ, in this case the sensory nerves, toward the spinal cord. In the upper limb, ring electrodes are placed around the distal interphalangeal DIP and proximal interphalangeal PIP joints of the fingers while recording over the nerve more proximally at the wrist or forearm. An antidromic sensory recording would involve stimulation of the nerve in the forearm or wrist while recording distally from the digits. This arrangement is the opposite of the normal physiologic direction of impulse propagation for a sensory nerve and represents an antidromic recording. Latency values are virtually identical for either method. Amplitude measurements tend to be greater in antidromic recordings as the pickup electrodes, particularly in the upper limbs, lie closer to the nerves they record from. Either method is acceptable (Fig. 6–2).

Sensory potentials often show abnormality earlier than

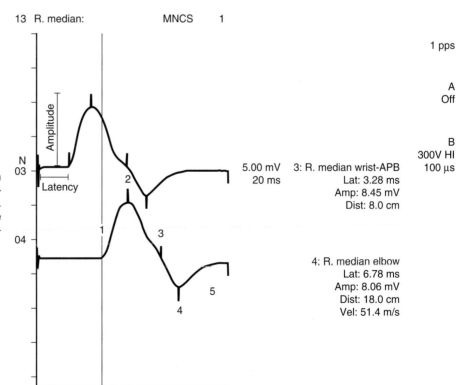

Figure 6–1. A normal median motor conduction. Latency is measured to the onset of the potential. Amplitude is measured from the baseline to the peak of the potential.

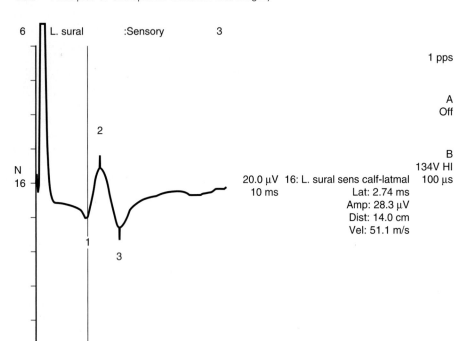

6 L. sural   :Sensory   3

1 pps

A
Off

B
134V HI
100 μs

N
16

20.0 μV 16: L. sural sens calf-latmal
10 ms   Lat: 2.74 ms
                         Amp: 28.3 μV
                         Dist: 14.0 cm
                         Vel: 51.1 m/s

2

1

3

Figure 6–2. A normal sural sensory nerve action potential (SNAP).

motor potentials in neuropathies and nerve compression injuries for reasons that are as yet unclear. For instance, it would be extremely unusual to find a distal motor latency delay in a carpal tunnel syndrome if the sensory potential were normal. In addition, because of the anatomic location of the dorsal root ganglion, central lesions involving the spinal cord or sensory nerve root will spare the sensory potential because the dorsal root ganglion sits outside the spinal cord at the level of the intervertebral foramina. Therefore, someone with a root avulsion injury and an anesthetic arm may have completely normal sensory nerve action potentials. Preservation of the dorsal root ganglion, the cell body of origin for the sensory nerve, will maintain the integrity of its distal nerve process. The corollary to this is that any lesion at or distal to the dorsal root ganglion will affect the sensory nerve action potential recorded distally. The anterior horn cell, by contrast, sits centrally in the ventral gray of the spinal cord. Therefore, a neurogenic lesion responsible for a reduced amplitude CMAP can lie anywhere between the anterior horn cell and muscle. This dichotomy between the anatomic origins for the motor and sensory nerves often proves useful for localization of disease, as already discussed in root avulsion injuries. Another example would be with primary motor disorders such as ALS, which involves degeneration of anterior horn cells. Conductions may reveal low amplitude CMAPs with completely preserved SNAPs as the dorsal root ganglion is not affected in this disorder. Selective motor involvement is not often seen in peripheral nerve lesions and should suggest the possibility of a central motor disorder.

F WAVES

F waves, so named because they were first discovered in foot muscles, are backfired responses from anterior horn cells recorded from the muscle in a similar fashion as that described for motor conductions. As previously described, stimulation of a nerve with a cathode results in a bidirectional wave of depolarization. An impulse then travels back toward the spinal cord in an antidromic fashion for a motor nerve. The anterior horn cell responds and depolarizes, sending a signal orthodromically back to the muscle. This response is purely motor as it can be obtained in deafferentiated limbs.[5–7] Approximately 5 percent of the anterior horn cell population responds and a different population of motor neurons responds to each impulse. This renders the response small in amplitude (5 to 10 percent of the CMAP) and variable in waveform morphology from stimulus to stimulus. The F wave should be obtainable from any nerve and its corresponding recording muscle. The latency to the onset of the shortest F wave out of 10 to 20 stimulations is generally accepted when establishing normal values. The spread between the shortest and longest F waves has also been used when establishing normative data. F wave latency is dependent on height, and nomograms have been established to determine normal values corrected for height. F waves may prove useful in trying to establish a proximal abnormality of the motor nerve. Because the impulse must traverse the proximal nerve segment twice, proximal lesions may delay the F wave or cause it to be absent. F wave abnormalities may be the only way to establish the early diagnosis of Guillain-Barré syndrome. This demyelinating disorder involves the proximal motor roots and nerves, yielding a high likelihood of F wave abnormalities.[8] Unfortunately, F wave abnormalities are nonspecific. They may indicate that there is a proximal abnormality, but that could lie anywhere along the course of the nerve, including the plexus, root, and spinal cord.

H REFLEXES

The H reflex, named so for Dr. Hoffman who discovered it, is the physiologic equivalent of the ankle jerk.[9] Instead of tapping the Achilles tendon, the reflex is usually obtained by selective electrical activation of the sensory Ia afferents of the tibial nerve at the popliteal fossa. A cathode is used to stimulate the nerve while recording from the gastrocnemius or soleus muscles in the leg. Low level stimulation is used to selectively activate the sensory fibers. This level will cause a monosynaptic return volley to the muscle. Because the same group of motor neurons is activated each time, the latency is virtually identical for each trial. Descending central inhibition of motor neuron excitability may cause variation in the amplitude of the response from trial to trial. Unlike the F wave, which can be found in any nerve muscle pair, the H reflex can be obtained only in adults from the flexor carpi radialis stimulating the median nerve and from the calf stimulating the tibial nerve.[10] Nomograms have been established for normal values taking into account leg length and the age of the patient. In addition to measuring the latency, interside latency differences are very sensitive in picking up a unilateral abnormality. There should be no greater than a 1.8 msec difference between sides.[11]

The H reflex, like the F wave, provides an indication of a proximal abnormality. Once again, the localization can be anywhere in the proximal portion of the nerve, plexus, root, or spinal cord. Unlike the F wave, which looks only at the motor portion of the nerve, the H reflex looks at the entire length of the nerve, including the sensory division. This measurement may be advantageous in disorders in which sensory involvement occurs early or may be the only area of involvement, as in radiculopathy. The H reflex is most often used as a test of the integrity of the S1 nerve root during tibial nerve stimulation. In the proper clinical setting, unilateral H reflex asymmetry or absence with tibial stimulation is supportive of S1 root involvement and may be of help in distinguishing L5 from S1 radiculopathy when the sole abnormality on EMG needle examination is lower lumbar paraspinal denervation.

The H reflex may be absent in normal elderly individuals as well as early in neuropathy. In addition, once abnormal, the H reflex usually remains abnormal and thus cannot be used to follow as a sign of improvement.

Physiologic Variables

AGE

Because nerves are not fully myelinated at birth, conduction velocities at birth are approximately one half of adult values and do not reach adult norms until approximately 3 to 5 years. Premature infants have even slower initial velocities.[12] Conductions slow with advancing age, possibly slowing by as much as 10 percent by the age of 60.[13] Sural sensory, plantar sensory, and long latency H reflexes may be absent in normal healthy elderly individuals over the age of 65.

NERVES AND NERVE SEGMENTS

Lower limb conduction velocities are slower than upper limb velocities, and proximal nerve segments tend to conduct faster than distal segments.[14] Possible reasons include shorter internodal segments and reduced axonal diameter in longer nerves. Proximal nerves may be better insulated with warmer temperatures resulting in faster velocities.

TEMPERATURE

Cold temperatures result in prolonged latencies, delayed velocities, and enlarged amplitudes.[15] Normal or enlarged amplitudes associated with conduction delay should be a warning to the physiologist that the patient may have cold extremities. Skin temperature should be at least 34°C.[16] A thermistor should be available to measure skin temperature, and the patient should be warmed if needed with infrared lamps, hair dryers, or warm water immersion. Correction formulas are available but are not necessarily reliable. Many patients are anxious, and this anxiety causes a sympathetic vasoconstrictive response. Skin temperatures which were normal at the beginning of the evaluation may not remain so as the testing proceeds. Failure to pay strict attention to skin temperature could, for instance, result in mislabeling patients as having carpal tunnel delay or diffuse polyneuropathy.

NERVE INJURIES

Neurapraxia

Experimental tourniquet-induced nerve compression with subsequent histopathologic evaluation has revealed invagination of myelin segments at the edges of the compressing tourniquet.[17] This type of nerve injury is known as neurapraxia and is associated with conduction block at the level of the compression. The physiologic correlate of this is the inability to pass a nerve impulse from above the site of block. Conduction distal to the site of block is normal. A clinical example of this would be a Saturday night palsy in which the radial nerve is compressed in the upper arm. Recovery from such an injury may occur within hours to months. If the degree of compression was mild, there will not be interruption of axons and the functional recovery will be excellent.

Axonotmesis

A more severe degree of nerve injury with interruption of axons but sparing their connective tissue sheaths and basal lamina is called axonotmesis. The interruption of axons causes wallerian degeneration distal to the site of injury. This dissolution of the distal stump will become unexcitable within 4 to 5 days from the time of injury.[18] Loss of the trophic influence of the axon will cause muscle weakness and atrophy below the level of the injury in a proximal-to-distal gradient. Axonal sprouting will eventually occur, along with reinnervation in a proximal to distal direction. Recovery may be incomplete and protracted, often taking 3 to 6 months or more as the axonal growth cone slowly expands at a rate of 1 mm/day.[19] A distal nerve injury has a better prognosis as there is less distance for the regenerating axons to grow. Causalgic pain may be an accompaniment of this type of injury.

Neurotmesis

Neurotmesis is the most severe type of nerve injury, implying complete nerve transection, including connective tissue sheaths and basal lamina. Wallerian degeneration occurs, as with axonotmesis. However, in the absence of the connective tissue sheaths, regenerating nerve fibers will have little chance to find their end organs and neuroma growth is frequent. Without surgical intervention, there is little chance for functional recovery.

Nerve Injury and Conduction Studies

When should nerve conduction studies be performed following an injury, and how can they predict the degree of injury? Because it takes 5 days for the distal segment of a nerve to become unexcitable following axonal interruption, studies performed approximately 1 week after injury can begin to clarify the type of and degree of injury. Conductions performed at the time of injury stimulating from above the level of the lesion may be absent with either conduction block or neurotmesis. Stimulation at this time below the site of injury will be normal for velocity and amplitude measurements given the continued presence of a functional distal segment. However, 1 week later a conduction block injury will continue to show a normal amplitude response below the site of injury, but a neurotmesis will show no response at all, given the complete wallerian degeneration that has taken place distal to the site of injury. With axonotmesis, the amplitude of the response will be reduced above and below the site of injury because of the incomplete loss of axons.

Medical legal issues may play a role in determining the timing of electrical studies. An obstetrician who delivers a baby who has a weak arm may want to obtain testing on day 1. If the baby has suffered in utero nerve compression, establishing a baseline conduction with follow-up over the next 5 to 7 days can help to determine chronicity versus evolving changes, which would suggest a new and acquired lesion. The presence of fibrillation potentials on initial needle EMG (to be discussed next) also provides very strong evidence of an in utero problem, as these discharges take 2 to 3 weeks to develop.

ELECTROMYOGRAPHY

The EMG needle examination is complementary to nerve conduction studies. The distribution of changes found on needle examination often establishes or confirms the diagnosis. For instance, bilateral abnormalities consistent with denervation in a distal to proximal gradient are suggestive of a length dependent, stocking, axonal neuropathy. Denervation restricted to a myotome in muscles innervated by a common root is suggestive of radiculopathy.

Insertional Activity

The patient is instructed to relax as much as possible while a recording needle is inserted into the desired muscle. An audio and video signal is obtained. The needle is moved in short steps and in multiple directions. This causes a discharge potential whose duration is slightly longer than the needle movement itself.[20] Reduction in insertional activity is often first noted as a loss of the audio signal during needle movement. This suggests that the muscle under study has been replaced by connective tissue, as in many dystrophic muscle diseases, or that there is neurogenic atrophy of muscle as seen with axonal interruption. Prolonged insertional activity may be associated with early denervation or inflammatory muscle diseases and is typically seen 10 to 14 days after nerve injury.

Spontaneous Activity

FIBRILLATIONS AND POSITIVE WAVES

A denervated muscle fiber deprived of its axon will begin to spontaneously discharge. These discharges are known as fibrillation potentials and are the most reliable signs of denervation, suggesting an acute or ongoing problem. They have small potentials, usually less than 200 μV in amplitude, with a regular discharge pattern. When abundant they sound like "rain on the roof." A form of fibrillation probably recorded from an injured part of the muscle fiber is called a positive sharp wave. These waves have a large positivity, fire rhythmically, and make a characteristic dull popping sound. Both fibrillations and positive sharp waves have the same significance, but for as yet unknown reasons, positive waves appear earlier than fibrillations after injury. Positive waves appear around 2 weeks and fibrillations up to 3 weeks after nerve injury. The timing is dependent on the proximity of the muscle to the site of nerve injury. Muscles closer to the site of injury will show the earliest signs of spontaneous activity than those more distal. Paraspinal muscle may reveal positive waves 5 to 7 days following root injury.[21]

Fibrillations and positive waves may be found in myopathies, particularly the inflammatory myopathies such as polymyositis or dermatomyositis (Fig. 6–3). Damage to end plate regions may account for the presence of fibrillations in these disorders.

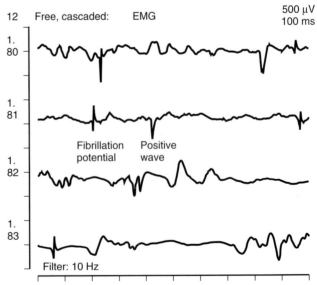

Figure 6–3. Positive waves and fibrillation potentials from paraspinal muscles in polymyositis.

FASCICULATIONS

A fasciculation represents a spontaneous discharge of a motor unit that is not under voluntary control. They may be seen as a small twitch on the skin surface or may be found on needle examination deeper within the muscle while the needle is at rest. When restricted in scope, they may be associated with local nerve injury. Widespread fasciculations associated with fibrillation potentials are commonly seen in ALS. Healthy individuals may have "benign" fasciculations and occasionally cramps in the absence of widespread denervation on needle study.

COMPLEX REPETITIVE DISCHARGES

These discharges are secondary to a group of muscle fibers firing repetitively at a rate of 5 to 100 impulses per second. They make a sound akin to a machine gun. They are commonly seen in chronic neurogenic or myopathic conditions and may be seen from the iliopsoas muscle in normal subjects.

Motor Unit Potentials

AMPLITUDE, DURATION, PHASES, AND RECRUITMENT PATTERNS

A motor unit consists of the anterior horn cell and all the muscle fibers supplied by that anterior horn cell. When a patient makes a slight contraction, motor units become activated and are described according to their amplitude, duration, number of phases, and how they are recruited. In general, enlarged motor units are a sign of a neurogenic lesion. They are enlarged because of an increased muscle fiber density in the region of the recording needle which may be secondary to collateral sprouting of surviving axons as they attempt to reinnervate the muscle. As the motor unit territory increases with reinnervation, there is an associated increase in axon terminals, causing the duration of the motor unit to increase. Increased amplitudes and durations are present within months of axonal interruption. Motor units consisting of more than four phases are called polyphasic. This level tends to appear within weeks to months after axonal disruption, although polyphasics have been reported as early as 7 days from the time of denervation.[22] In general, greater than 15 percent of analyzed motor units should be polyphasic before the muscle is termed abnormal. Occasionally, defining an abnormality solely on the basis of increased polyphasia will result in falsely positive studies. Other objective measures such as prolonged duration motor units are also generally present to support the contention of abnormality based on increased polyphasia.

Disorders of muscle tend to cause random dropout of muscle fibers, resulting in low amplitude and shortened duration motor units, which may be polyphasic. The acronym BSAAP (brief, small amplitude, abundant polyphasic) has been given to this type of motor unit. There are exceptions whereby neurogenic lesions are "myopathic" in appearance, and vice versa. However, the motor unit changes described here are generally useful in distinguishing between neurogenic and myopathic conditions.

The pattern of motor unit firing with slowly increasing force is called recruitment. This pattern is often of great use in distinguishing between a neurogenic and myopathic lesion. It may also be of use in detecting malingerers. The smallest motor units tend to be recruited first and generally fire up to 5 to 20 Hz before the next unit is recruited.[23] In neurogenic conditions there may be a reduction in the number of functional motor units. Thus, reduced numbers of motor units are firing more quickly in an effort to keep up the muscle strength. Myopathic recruitment patterns consist of an early or full level of motor activity filling the video display for the level of effort. Myopathy results in a random loss of muscle fibers from each motor unit. In order to keep up the muscle strength, more motor units are recruited early. Malingerers or those suffering from pain or upper motor neuron weakness may be unwilling or unable to recruit many motor units. However, the motor units they do recruit fire in a normal and often slow or tremulous fashion.

RADICULOPATHIES

The referral to an EMG facility for the evaluation of radiculopathy exceeds all other requests. Lumbar radiculopathy accounts for 62 to 90 percent[24] of all radiculopathies, whereas cervical radiculopathy accounts for 5 to 36 percent.[25] Thoracic radiculopathy is uncommon. Pain is the most characteristic symptom, followed by pain and weakness. Isolated weakness in the absence of pain is unusual. L5 followed by S1 are the most common roots affected in the lumbar region. C7, C6, and C8 are, respectively, the most commonly affected cervical root levels.[26] An isolated disk herniation is the most common cause of acute radiculopathy in young patients. Older patients may have a combination of bony and ligamentous abnormalities in addition to disk degeneration as the cause of their root compromise. The distribution of the sensory root is called a dermatome. The segmental motor root distribution to the muscle is a myotome. Most muscles are innervated by two and occasionally three myotomes. The clinical diagnosis is made on the basis of the sensory, motor, and reflex changes. The diagnostic impression is often supplemented by computed tomography (CT), CT myelography, and EMG. Of these tests, EMG is the only physiologic measure of function, whereas all the others assess anatomy or structure. Although other physiologic tests are available, such as somatosensory evoked potential (SEP) and root stimulation techniques, their diagnostic yields are low and still unproved. The EMG needle examination complemented by appropriate conduction studies remains the gold standard for physiologic evaluation of radiculopathy. The EMG result was positive in 73 to 94 percent of cases of radiculopathy versus 75 to 84 percent for myelography and CT.[27] Studies reveal that lumbar MRI may reveal up to 64 percent anatomic abnormalities in asymptomatic subjects.[28, 29] EMG can, therefore, play a very important role in trying to determine whether the anatomic abnormalities are of any functional significance. In addition, a patient with clinical radiculopathy with a completely normal imaging examination may prove to have a noncompressive etiology such as Lyme disease, diabetes, or carcinomatous meningitis. Only the EMG could have confirmed the diagnosis of radiculopathy suggesting the need for further diagnostic testing.

Needle Examination in Radiculopathy

The most characteristic change in radiculopathy is the presence of positive sharp waves or fibrillation potentials in a myotomal distribution consistent with acute or ongoing denervation. Paraspinal muscles may yield the sole abnormality in 5 to 40 percent of cases. The yield is dependent on the timing of the study.

Paraspinal muscles may reveal acute denervation with fibrillations and positive waves within 5 to 7 days of injury (Fig. 6–4). Limb muscles may take up to 3 weeks to reveal changes. If the EMG is performed after a 3-week period, the chance of finding both paraspinal and limb muscle denervation increases. The corollary of this is that delayed EMG study may show the absence of paraspinal changes with persistent and predominantly distal limb muscle changes because the first muscles to denervate are the first to reinnervate. In the cervical region false negative studies may occur after 6 months[30] and after 12 to 18 months in the lumbar region. Because distal limb muscles are the ones to most likely reveal ongoing denervation, it may be difficult to distinguish between a length dependent axonal neuropathy and radiculopathy. This distinction is especially confounding in elderly patients, in whom the absence of sensory potentials and H reflexes cannot be used to help distinguish between neuropathy and radiculopathy. As stated previously, these potentials may be absent in normal elderly patients above the age of 60.

Although paraspinal muscle denervation brings the level of the lesion up to the root or anterior horn cell, exact localization based only on paraspinal changes is not possible because paraspinal muscles are innervated by several overlapping segments. Previous laminectomy may injure the posterior ramus and render future paraspinal evaluation unreliable.[31] Other limitations with regard to paraspinal muscles are that they may reveal fibrillations in apparently normal individuals over the age of 40, in diabetics, and in muscle diseases, particularly myositis.

Enlarged and long duration motor units in a myotomal

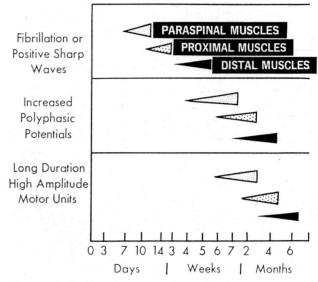

Figure 6–5. Development of needle electromyographic changes with time in different muscle groups in radiculopathies. (From Aminoff MJ: Symposium on electrodiagnosis. Neurol Clin 3[3]:505, 1985.)

distribution are evidence of chronic denervation and in the absence of associated fibrillations suggest a static situation (Fig. 6–5).

Cervical Radiculopathy

From 56 to 70 percent[32] of all cervical radiculopathies involve C7. Abnormalities are found frequently in the triceps, pronator teres, and flexor carpi radialis. There is occasional confusion with carpal tunnel syndrome, which is easily identified with appropriate conduction studies.

Radiculopathies involving C5 and C6 are often difficult to distinguish given their overlapping myotomes. The dorsal scapula nerve to the rhomboids is a direct extension of the C5 root, which is usually the sole innervation of the rhomboids. Denervation in this muscle is therefore helpful in distinguishing C5 involvement. The pronator teres with C6 and C7 innervation is more suggestive of C6 radiculopathy when other C5 and C6 muscles are involved. If the paraspinals are not denervated, an upper trunk brachial plexopathy cannot be ruled out (Fig. 6–6).

C8 radiculopathy may commonly involve intrinsic hand muscles, the flexor pollicis longus, and the extensor indicia proprius. Confusion with a lower trunk brachial plexopathy and an ulnar nerve compression is possible and usually can be ruled out by the appropriate conduction studies, including conduction across the elbow and ulnar sensory potentials, which should be normal in root lesions.

Lumbar Radiculopathy

In lumbar radiculopathy L5 is the most commonly affected lumbar root. The anterior and posterior tibialis muscles as well as the peroneus longus, tensor fascia lata, and gluteus medius muscles are useful muscles to survey when this root level is suspected. L5 radiculopathy with foot drop should be distinguished from a peroneal nerve entrapment

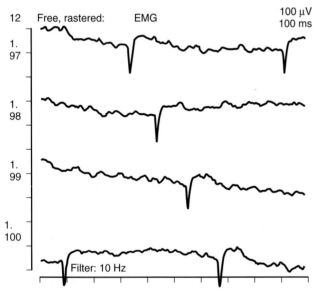

Figure 6–4. An example of positive waves seen in a patient with radiculopathy.

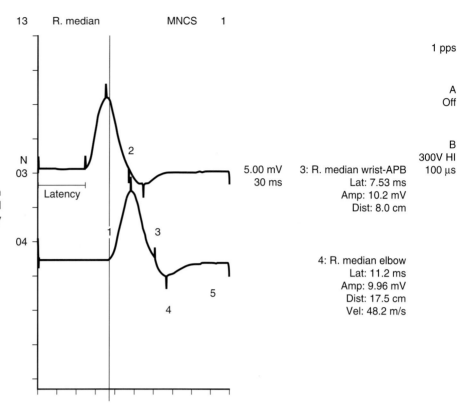

Figure 6–6. An abnormal median motor conduction with prolonged distal latency. Normal distal latency is less than 4.3 ms.

at the fibula head by the absence of slowing or conduction block across the fibula head and by the preserved peroneal sensory potential, which should not be affected by root level lesions.

S1 radiculopathies commonly affect the gastrocnemius, soleus, tibial intrinsic foot muscles, and the gluteus maximus. Because most of these muscles are innervated by the tibial division of the sciatic nerve, consideration should be given to the possibility of a sciatic neuropathy. Intact sural sensory potentials and involvement of the gluteus maximus would be evidence against a sciatic neuropathy. H reflexes are commonly abnormal in S1 radiculopathies (see Fig. 6–6).

L2, L3, and L4 are usually considered together because there is no way to isolate between these overlapping root levels. The adductors, quadriceps, and iliopsoas muscles may be involved. Confusion can exist when the paraspinal muscles are normal between a lumbar plexopathy and a femoral neuropathy. There is no good sensory potential, other than the saphenous, which is difficult to obtain in normal subjects, which can help distinguish between a peripheral and a root level lesion.

Lumbar stenosis is characterized by claudication-like symptoms that appear during walking and are relieved by sitting. Bilateral EMG abnormalities are common. These findings can be suggestive of bilateral symmetric or asymmetric S1 or L5 radiculopathies. Chronic motor unit changes are not uncommon. The H reflexes are often absent. Occasionally, the study is completely normal.

In lumbar radiculopathy, the anatomic level of abnormality may not correlate with the root level of abnormality found on EMG. This is because of the arrangement of the cauda equina which begins at L2. The distal lumbar and sacral roots must descend multiple segments intraspinally before exiting at their appropriate neuroforamina. Therefore, a lesion such as a neuroma attached to the L5 root at the L2 anatomic level may reveal discordant physiologic and anatomic data. In addition, because multiple roots descend together, a central disk could account for multiple root involvement or cauda equina syndrome. Imaging studies should be performed at least to the T12–L1 levels to ensure that a proximal lesion is not missed.

Finally, dependent on the degree or severity of either a cervical or lumbar radiculopathy, the predominance of sensory versus motor involvement, the ability of reinnervation to keep up with denervation, and the scope and timing of the EMG will determine whether or not the study is abnormal. For these reasons, a normal EMG never rules out the possibility of radiculopathy in the proper clinical setting.

ENTRAPMENT NEUROPATHIES

Entrapment neuropathies are compression syndromes that may produce numbness, tingling, pain, or weakness in an extremity. Clinical history and examination are very important in developing differential diagnoses and distinguishing these syndromes. Tinel's sign may be present on tapping the nerve at suspected site of entrapment. For example, tapping the median nerve at the wrist will reproduce the numbness in carpal tunnel syndrome, and tapping the ulnar nerve as it winds around the medial epicondyle will reproduce the tingling that runs down the little finger in ulnar entrapment at the elbow. Tarsal tunnel syndrome may also have a positive Tinel's sign. Because asymptomatic patients may have a Tinel's sign, to be meaningful it is important that the feeling elicited by the tap reproduces symptoms.

The other entrapment syndromes may have a diffuse, nonlocalizing pain, numbness, tingling, or loss of dexterity. Examples of these syndromes are the thoracic outlet syndrome with brachial plexopathy, resistant tennis elbow, piriformis syndrome, and pronator teres syndrome.

Entrapment neuropathies usually show conduction abnormalities on electrophysiologic studies secondary to focal demyelination. However, with severe compression causing axonal loss, EMG findings may also be seen.

Treatment for entrapment neuropathies may vary depending on the etiology, the severity of clinical symptoms, and electrophysiologic changes. Surgical entrapment release for carpal tunnel syndrome may relieve symptoms and prevent thenar atrophy. Compression secondary to tumors such as ganglion cysts may need to be surgically resected. Physical therapy and use of orthotics are also a significant part of management. Avoidance of repetitive activities that may precipitate symptoms may be sufficient treatment.

Median Neuropathy

CARPAL TUNNEL SYNDROME

Carpal tunnel syndrome (CTS) involves entrapment of the median nerve across the wrist as it traverses through the carpal tunnel under the transverse carpal ligament together with nine flexor tendons. Any bony deformity, inflammation, tenosynovitis which is frequently secondary to rheumatoid arthritis, or tumor may increase intracarpal pressure causing median nerve compression. Patients typically complain of numbness, tingling, and pain involving the lateral 3 1/2 digits, which are the thumb, index finger, middle finger, and lateral half of the ring finger. However, symptoms may include all five digits, the wrist, and even the forearm. Numbness and pain usually awaken the patient at night, and shaking the hands may relieve symptoms. Patient may also complain of thenar atrophy and loss of dexterity associated with difficulty in opening jars or dropping objects. Exacerbation of CTS may be precipitated by repetitive hand movement such kneading, knitting, typing, and use of a computer mouse, to name only a few. Driving may also exacerbate CTS.

Neurophysiologic testing for CTS involves nerve conduction studies (NCV) of the median nerve and ulnar nerve. The ulnar nerve is done for comparison and for detection of polyneuropathy if present. In our laboratory, we usually start with the orthodromic palmar stimulation. The median and ulnar nerves are stimulated at midpalm, 8 cm distal to the recording electrode at the wrist. The upper limit of both the median and ulnar mixed nerve peak latencies is 2.2 msec, and a significant difference between the two is greater than 0.3 msec.[34] This is a very sensitive test for detection of mild CTS. Kimura has shown that the palm to wrist sensory latency was delayed in 21 percent of hands in which conventional latencies were normal.[8] Another useful method for diagnosis of CTS is the median-ulnar sensory latency difference to the ring finger because

the ring finger has both median and ulnar innervation. Antidromic[35] or orthodromic[36] stimulation may be used. Significant difference between the median and ulnar peak latencies would be above 0.4 msec.[37] Potential error would be if the fourth digit is fully innervated by the ulnar nerve. When the median sensory peak latencies are prolonged, the median motor conduction recorded from the abductor pollicis brevis (APB) is done to evaluate latency and amplitude. Significant latency delay that we use in our laboratory is above 4.3 msec (Table 6–1). Amplitude should be greater than 3 μV. CTS is bilateral in 58 percent of patients. Prolonged median motor distal latencies recorded from the APB in other series of CTS vary from 29 to 81 percent.[33] Grading the severity of the CTS usually depends on median sensory peak latency and median motor distal latency delays, loss of amplitude of median sensory or motor potentials, presence of thenar atrophy, and severity of clinical symptoms. Mild CTS usually has only median sensory peak latency delays +/− sensory nerve action potential (SNAP) amplitude below the lower limit of normal associated with the symptoms. Moderate CTS shows median sensory latency delays and relative or absolute prolongation of median motor distal latency.[38] Severe CTS involves both median sensory and motor latency changes that may be associated with loss or reduction of sensory amplitude and reduction of median motor potential. Acute denervation changes in the form of fibrillations and positive waves are more likely to be seen in EMG of the APB or opponens pollicis when the median motor potential shows delayed latency and reduced amplitude signifying severe CTS.

Table 6–1. Muscles usefully examined by needle EMG when delineating which myotomes are involved

Upper Extremities	Lower Extremities
C5	L2, 3 4
Rhomboids	Vastus lateralis
C5, 6	Vastus medialis
Supraspinatus	Adductor longus
Infraspinatus	Gracilis
Deltoid	L4, 5–S1
Biceps brachii	Anterior tibial
C5–7	L5–S1
Serratus anterior	Biceps femoris
C6, 7	Peroneus longus
Pronator teres	Extensor digitorum longus
Extensor carpi radialis longus	Flexor digitorum longus
C6–8	Extensor hallucis longus
Latissimus dorsi	L5–S1, 2
C7, 8	Gastrocnemius
Triceps brachii	S1, 2
Extensor carpi radialis brevis	Soleus
Other wrist and digit extensors	Abductor hallucis
Flexor carpi radialis	Abductor digiti quinti
Flexors of the digits	First dorsal interosseous
C8–T1	
Abductor pollicis brevis	
First dorsal interosseous	
Abductor digiti minimi	

From Aminoff MJ: Symposium on electrodiagnosis. Neurol Clin 3(3):507, 1985.

Surgical evaluation for entrapment release is commonly recommended when the CTS is severe to prevent thenar atrophy and weakness. Resection of the carpal ligament is usually a simple outpatient procedure causing significant relief of symptoms. Nerve conduction studies usually have the greatest improvement during the first 6 weeks after surgery.[39] Some conductions may return to baseline. However, some studies remain abnormal even when symptoms have significantly improved.[40, 41] Conservative management with use of wrist splints especially worn at night is recommended for mild to less severe CTS. A trial of several months is advised before surgery is contemplated.

PRONATOR TERES SYNDROME

The median nerve may be compressed as it passes between the two heads of the pronator teres muscle at the elbow and then under the edge of the flexor digitorum sublimis. Symptoms may be similar to CTS. Symptoms may be aggravated by forearm pronation, elbow flexion, and flexion of the distal interphalangeal joint of the index finger. Tinel's sign may be elicited at the site of entrapment at the elbow. Denervation changes on EMG of the median innervated muscles above the wrist with sparing of the pronator teres would be characteristic of this syndrome. The pronator teres is usually innervated by a branch of the median nerve before it passes between the heads of the pronator teres and is therefore not usually affected in this syndrome.

ANTERIOR INTEROSSEUS SYNDROME

The median nerve usually gives off its anterior interosseus branch, which is a purely motor nerve, after passing through the pronator teres. The anterior interosseus division could be compressed by direct trauma to the forearm, forearm fractures, fibrous bands related to the flexor digitorum sublimis or the flexor digitorum profundus, blood drawing from the cubital vein.[42] The nerve could be partially compressed causing either weakness of the flexor pollicis longus or flexor digitorum profundus to index or middle finger. When the anterior interosseus division is completely compressed there would be paralysis of the flexor pollicis longus, flexor digitorum profundus to the second and third digits, and pronator quadratus muscles. The person with the syndrome would not be able to pinch using the flexion of the thumb and the distal interphalangeal joint of the index finger because the muscles responsible for this movement are weak. To check for pronator quadratus weakness, pronation has to be done with the elbow flexed to eliminate pronator teres effect. Ulnar innervated hand muscles may also be involved if a portion of the ulnar nerve is carried with the anterior interosseus nerve in the Martin Gruber anastomosis before it joins the ulnar nerve distally.[43] Sensory symptoms are not expected because the nerve is purely motor. However, diffuse aching pain may sometimes be felt at the elbow region.

Denervation changes on EMG of the flexor pollicis longus, flexor digitorum profundus to second and third digits, and pronator quadratus would confirm the diagnosis. The median nerve latency to pronator quadratus may show delays in some cases.

Ulnar Neuropathy

ULNAR NERVE INVOLVEMENT AT ELBOW

The ulnar neuropathies are commonly caused by compression of the nerve at the elbow as it winds around the medial humeral epicondyle. Symptoms usually involve numbness of the volar aspect of the fifth and medial half of the fourth digits and the dorsal tips of these fingers. The dorsal ulnar cutaneous branch may be involved causing numbness of the dorsum of the hand up to the wrist. There may be weakness of the dorsal interossei, deep head of the flexor pollicis brevis, the hypothenar muscles, the adductor pollicis, and occasionally the flexor digitorum profundus to the fourth and fifth digits and the flexor carpi ulnaris. Sensory symptoms typically are numbness or tingling radiating down fifth and medial half of fourth digit and could be precipitated by elbow flexion and leaning on the elbows. Recurrent trauma and recurrent subluxation of the nerve anterior to the epicondyle are the most common causes of ulnar neuropathy. Lesions could also be due to posttraumatic changes such as calcifications related to old fractures, gouty tophi, and tumors. Tardy ulnar palsy is the development of ulnar neuropathy years after an elbow fracture or dislocation.[44] Change in the carrying angle of the elbow and limited elbow extension are factors thought to cause traction of the ulnar nerve around the elbow region. Cubital tunnel syndrome may be due to compression of the nerve as it passes through the aponeurotic origin of the flexor carpi ulnaris.[45] This is the more likely cause if there is no history of trauma or bony deformity noted clinically.

Electrodiagnostic findings may depend on the severity of ulnar entrapment. The ulnar sensory potentials may be reduced or absent. The ulnar motor conduction is usually taken below and above the elbow and the significant ulnar motor velocity decrement across the elbow would be above 11 m/sec.[46] The ulnar motor amplitude is also noted below the elbow and above the elbow and the significant difference is more than 10 percent decrement in the above-elbow response compared with the below-elbow ulnar motor amplitude or above 25 percent decrement for the above-elbow compared with the ulnar response recorded from the wrist.[47] EMG of ulnar innervated muscles below the elbow may reveal denervation changes.

Treatment for ulnar neuropathy is mostly conservative with avoidance of repetitive elbow flexion activities or leaning on elbows, or wearing elbow splints. However, for more severe cases showing clinical deterioration surgery may be required. This may involve anterior transplantation of the ulnar nerve subcutaneously or into the flexor pronator mass, medial epicondylectomy, or simple release of the flexor carpi ulnaris aponeurosis.

ULNAR NERVE ENTRAPMENT AT THE WRIST

The ulnar nerve may be entrapped at different levels below the elbow. It may be compressed at the wrist as it passes through the Guyon's canal or distal to the canal on the palm itself, or at the forearm involving the dorsal ulnar cutaneous branch. The symptoms may be mixed motor and sensory when the ulnar nerve is compressed at the base of the palm as it enters into Guyon's canal or pure motor when compression is distal to the canal involving the deep palmar branch sometimes sparing the hypothenar muscles, or pure sensory if compression involves the dorsal ulnar sensory branch. Guyon's canal is formed by the pisiform and the hook of the hamate and bounded by the volar carpal ligament and transverse carpal ligament. The ulnar nerve travels with the ulnar artery and vein, and it divides into its motor and sensory branches within the ulnar tunnel. Any arteritis or thrombophlebitis involving these vessels may cause ulnar entrapment. Common etiologies for ulnar neuropathy at the wrist involve chronic trauma from occupational activities, such as polishing gold, chronic pressure from holding pliers or screwdrivers, or putting hubcaps on tires, or chronic pressure on handlebars in professional cyclists.[48] Fractures of the wrist, ganglion, tumor, osteoarthritis, and bursitis are other reported causes.[48]

Earliest electrodiagnostic findings may be abnormalities in the ulnar sensory latencies and amplitude reduction or loss. Latency delays in the ulnar motor conductions recorded from the abductor digiti quinti are commonly seen. In some cases with sparing of the hypothenar branch, the ulnar motor conduction has to be recorded from the first dorsal interosseus muscle to demonstrate the latency abnormality. Depending on the degree of compression, the ulnar motor potentials may be reduced signifying axonal loss. Proximal nerve conductions are usually normal. EMG may reveal denervation changes in the intrinsic ulnar innervated hand muscles and normal findings in ulnar innervated muscles proximal to the lesion.

Treatment may involve surgery for severe ulnar entrapment with release of the volar carpal ligament to decompress Guyon's canal and neurolysis with exploration as clinically warranted. Conservative management with splints may be sufficient for milder cases. For the dorsal sensory branch, which is usually injured by blunt trauma or laceration, treatment may vary from conservative for the former and exploration of the ulnar nerve with neurolysis or nerve release from scarring for the latter.

Radial Nerve Entrapment

The radial nerve may be injured anywhere from the axilla, above the elbow, around the elbow region, or at the forearm near the wrist involving the superficial radial nerve. Most of the radial nerve lesions are secondary to trauma,[49] but there have been a few reported cases of spontaneous entrapment following strenuous muscular effort.[50] Common radial nerve compression just below the axilla may be seen with Saturday night palsy, which is found among alcoholics who wake up with wrist drop after prolonged sleep with arm flung over a bench or with hyperabduction during sleep. This compression usually spares the triceps. Chronic pressure in the axilla from crutches used to be a common cause but has been corrected with proper guidance. The triceps may be involved if the lesion occurs before the branch to the triceps has been given off by the main radial nerve at the axilla. The radial nerve is commonly injured as it winds around the spiral groove by blunt trauma or more frequently fractures of the humerus in this region. There would be weakness of the radial innervated muscles including the brachioradialis, the wrist extensors, and the finger extensors. The triceps is spared. Elbow flexion may be preserved because of the intact biceps, brachialis, and coracobrachialis which are innervated by the musculocutaneous

nerve. A high radial nerve injury always involves weakness of the brachioradialis.

Electrodiagnostic studies involving segments of the radial nerve may demonstrate the site of injury or entrapment. Conduction block or temporal dispersion with less severe compression may be seen at the site of the lesion. The extensor indicis proprius is commonly used for attachment of the recording electrode, and stimulation may be applied at Erb's point, the posterolateral aspect of the upper arm below the insertion of the deltoid, on the lateral aspect of the arm halfway down, at the elbow between the biceps tendon and brachioradialis, and at the midforearm between the extensor digiti minimi and the extensor carpi ulnaris.[51] The motor and sensory conductions are usually preserved below the level of the lesion if there is no axonotmesis involved. If there is complete injury of the radial nerve, the motor and sensory potentials may be completely absent. EMG may reveal denervation in the radial innervated muscles below the lesion.

Treatment for radial nerve palsy depends on the etiology. For Saturday night palsy, treatment is usually conservative, and function may return after several weeks to months, depending on the degree of injury. For radial injuries secondary to trauma such as fractures, treatment may be conservative, waiting for return of function for 2 to 3 months before surgical exploration.[49] However, for comminuted fractures, the risk of nerve entrapment is higher, and surgical exploration may be necessary more emergently.[49, 50]

Posterior Interosseus Nerve Entrapment

The radial nerve splits into the posterior interosseus division, which is purely motor, and the superficial radial nerve, which is purely sensory distal to the elbow region. The posterior interosseus nerve may be entrapped as it enters the supinator through the arcade of Frohse. Compression may also be due to tumors, ganglion, or tenosynovitis within this region. Occasionally, entrapment may be secondary to fractures such as "Monteggia's fracture," which involves dislocation of the radial head with fracture of the ulna.[51, 52] Symptoms include weakness of wrist extensors and finger extensors. The extensor carpi radialis longus and brevis may be spared so that weakness of wrist extensors is only partial. Brachioradialis and triceps are also spared. The patient characteristically can extend the wrist with radial deviation. Paralysis of finger extensors at the metacarpophalangeal joint may be demonstrated by dorsiflexing the wrist, eliminating the tenodesis effect when the wrist is flexed. The distal phalangeal extension of the digits is preserved because it is attributed to the ulnar and median innervated lumbricals.

Nerve conduction studies would be able to localize the lesion at the region of the arcade of Frohse. EMG may show denervation of the muscles innervated by the posterior interosseus nerve, such as the extensor carpi ulnaris, extensor digitorum communis, extensor indicis proprius, abductor pollicis longus, and extensor pollicis longus. The extensor carpi radialis and supinator, which are innervated proximally by the radial nerve, are normal. The superficial radial sensory conduction would also be normal.

Treatment commonly involves surgery with removal of

cysts, ganglion, or tumors or release of the arcade of Frohse if entrapment is at this site.

RESISTANT TENNIS ELBOW

Tennis elbow pain is characterized by sharp pain secondary to lateral epicondylitis. Resistant tennis elbow pain may be mistaken for this. However, for the resistant tennis elbow, diffuse aching pain is maximal a few centimeters away from the lateral epicondyle within the extensor muscle mass and is due to compression of the posterior interosseus nerve by the radial head,[53, 54] by fibrous bands in the extensor carpi radialis, or by the arcade of Frohse.[55] Resistant tennis elbow pain will not respond to treatment for lateral epicondylitis. Instead, treatment requires decompression of the posterior interosseus nerve with resection of the bands entrapping it.

SUPERFICIAL RADIAL NERVE

The superficial radial nerve is more commonly injured by trauma such as lacerations at the wrist or distal forearm. However, there have been reported cases of compression secondary to tight watch bands, casts, handcuffs, or any tight band around the wrist.[56] Numbness and loss of sensation in the radial innervated portion of the dorsum of the hand is seen. Neurodiagnostically, there may be absence of the superficial radial sensory potential or reduction in the size of the potential. Treatment is usually conservative.

THORACIC OUTLET SYNDROME

Brachial plexopathy with compression of the medial cord or lower trunk is characteristic of thoracic outlet syndrome. True neurogenic thoracic outlet syndrome is rare,[57] and more common cervical or peripheral lesions should be ruled out before it is considered. Entrapment may be due to the presence of a cervical rib, constricting bands, or the anterior and medial scalene muscle, or Sibson's fascia.[58] Symptoms may include numbness, tingling, or pain in the hand or diffuse aching pain in the arm. Paresthesias could be precipitated by prolonged hyperabduction. Weakness with clumsiness could also be seen in some cases. CTS has been mistaken for thoracic outlet syndrome in the past and scalenectomy and rib resection have been done with no relief of symptoms.[59]

Characteristic neurodiagnostic findings would be abnormality in the ulnar sensory nerve potential, low amplitude median and ulnar CMAPs,[60, 61] and abnormal EMG of muscles with C8 and T1[62] innervation. CTS and ulnar entrapment across the elbow have to be ruled out. Since carpal tunnel syndrome was defined in the early 1950s, thoracic outlet syndrome surgery has dramatically decreased.[63]

Treatment for thoracic outlet syndrome may be conservative such as strengthening exercises for the shoulder to prevent slumping posture or use of devices such as corsets or belts that will prevent abduction of upper limb with placing of the hand behind the head during sleep. Surgical treatment may involve removal of the first rib, the scalene muscles, or any constricting bands via transaxillary approach or via supraclavicular approach.

In contrast to true neurogenic thoracic outlet syndrome, vascular thoracic outlet syndrome is due to compression of the subclavian or the axillary artery. Symptoms may range from a sense of coldness and aching pain during exercise in mild cases to painful emboli and digital gangrene in severe cases. There have also been rare episodes of arterial thrombus with extension of the clot, causing carotid occlusion or cerebral infarction secondary to embolic phenomenon.[64, 65] Workup for vascular thoracic outlet syndrome requires arteriography, and if this syndrome is found, surgical repair should follow soon because arterial damage will only worsen.

Digital Nerve Entrapment in the Hand

The digital nerves may be compressed by tumors, cysts, tenosynovitis, or osteophytes encroaching on the lateral and medial aspect of the digits. The digital nerves are also commonly injured by trauma. Symptoms may include numbness, pain, swelling, tenderness, and limited range of motion of the digits. Treatment depends on the etiology of the neuropathy. Surgery with resection of tumors or cysts could be the treatment of choice. For blunt trauma or chronic repetitive occupational trauma, treatment may be conservative.

Sciatic Nerve Entrapment

Sciatic nerve entrapment is uncommon. However, the sciatic nerve may be entrapped as it passes between the tendinous origin of the piriformis muscle.[66] Diffuse deep aching may be felt. The sciatic nerve may also be compressed by thick fascia between the biceps femoris and the adductor magnus.[67] The peroneal division is more commonly involved than the tibial division of the sciatic nerve. Compression of the peroneal and tibial nerves may also occur secondary to Baker's cysts[68] or any tumor at the popliteal fossa. History of hip fractures and dislocations and complications of hip joint replacement surgery may be other predisposing factors causing sciatic nerve entrapment. A less common etiology is due to anticoagulants with resultant retroperitoneal or pelvic bleeding.[69]

EMG is the useful modality in evaluation of sciatic nerve entrapment. Differentiation between radiculopathy and sciatic entrapment is the aim. The paraspinals should be spared. Muscles innervated by the inferior and superior gluteal nerves should be normal in sciatic involvement unless it is part of a more widespread sacral plexopathy.

Peroneal Entrapment

Injury to the peroneal nerve commonly occurs across the fibular head where it divides into the deep and superficial peroneal nerves. Peroneal palsy typically involves foot drop secondary to a weak or paralyzed anterior tibialis. All the toe extensors are weak with deep peroneal nerve palsy. Foot eversion may also be weak when the superficial peroneal nerve is involved. Foot inversion is spared because it is innervated by the tibial nerve. The extent of sensory loss depends on the involvement of deep peroneal nerve alone, or superficial peroneal nerve alone, or both. Peroneal palsy may be due to chronic compression secondary to tumors, cysts, or acute trauma such as fracture of the fibular head,[70] or hyperinversion of the ankle causing stretching of the peroneal nerve with resultant injury across the fibular head,[71] or chronic pressure across the fibular head by improperly molded casts, bandages, tight stockings, or during surgery, sleep, or stupor with prolonged pressure along the nerve causing ischemia and demyelination.[72] It can also be due to entrapment of the peroneal nerve as it passes through the fibular tunnel formed by the tendinous edge of the peroneus longus muscle and the fibula.[58] Diffuse aching pain is common in this form of peroneal entrapment. Otherwise, the foot drop is typically painless.

Peroneal nerve conduction study with demonstration of velocity slowing and conduction block across the fibular head due to demyelination is characteristically seen. The extensor digitorum brevis is used for the recording electrode and the peroneal nerve is stimulated proximal to the extensor digitorum brevis at the ankle, then below the fibular head and at the lateral popliteal fossa. The superficial peroneal sensory potential may also be absent. If the peroneal motor potential is absent on recording from the EDB because of marked atrophy, the peroneal motor response may be taken with the recording electrode over the anterior tibialis and stimulation done below the fibular head and at the lateral border of the popliteal fossa. EMG is helpful in differentiating peroneal nerve palsy from L5 radiculopathy, sciatic entrapment with peroneal involvement, or central lesions. Denervation changes may be seen only in the peroneal innervated muscles below the fibular head for peroneal palsy. Denervation in the short head of the biceps femoris indicates higher peroneal lesion, as this muscle is innervated by the peroneal division of the sciatic nerve. L5 radiculopathy may involve denervation in the paraspinals, the gluteal muscles, and the tibial innervated posterior tibial muscle. However, in some cases only the peroneal muscles below the fibula will show changes in sciatic or L5 lesions. Mononeuritis multiplex which commonly presents as foot drop will not show segmental slowing across the fibular head on nerve conduction study because the lesion is not demyelinating. Pyramidal lesion presenting as "peroneal palsy" will reveal normal motor and sensory conductions and normal EMG with poor activation of the muscle secondary to loss of voluntary control.

ANTERIOR TARSAL TUNNEL SYNDROME

The distal deep peroneal nerve may be entrapped as it passes under the dense superficial fascia of the ankle. Symptoms may involve paresthesias over the dorsum of the foot if the superficial peroneal branch is involved or sensory loss at the web between the first and second digits if the deep peroneal nerve is compressed. Occasionally, if the lateral peroneal branch, which is chiefly motor, is the only one entrapped, symptoms may simply be a diffuse aching over the dorsum of the foot associated with weakness of the extensor digitorum brevis.

Peroneal motor conduction with recording electrode over the extensor digitorum brevis and stimulation at the ankle and below the fibular head will reveal prolonged distal latencies in both. Denervation changes in the extensor digitorum brevis is not so helpful because this muscle is commonly injured by local trauma, such as by wearing tight shoes. People with this syndrome usually find a comfortable position that will lessen the symptoms. Treatment is often conservative, such as use of a foot orthosis to change the foot position, although there have been reported cases who only had relief of symptoms after the thick fascia or fibrous band compressing the nerve was resected.[73]

TARSAL TUNNEL SYNDROME

Tarsal tunnel syndrome usually refers to posterior tarsal tunnel syndrome caused by entrapment of the posterior tibial nerve within the tarsal tunnel. The tarsal tunnel is located behind the medial malleolus and is formed by the ankle bones, the flexor retinaculum, and the laciniate ligament. The posterior tibial nerve traverses this tunnel with the posterior tibial artery, the tendons of the tibialis posterior, the flexor digitorum longus, and the flexor hallucis longus. The posterior tibial nerve divides into the medial plantar, lateral plantar, and calcaneal branches as it passes or after it passes through the tibial tunnel. Symptoms typically include burning pain similar to that of CTS, and Tinel's sign may be elicited on tapping the tibial tunnel. Radiating pain along the sole of the foot may be felt. Location of sensory loss and pain may depend on involvement of one, two, or all three branches of the posterior tibial nerve. Weakness of the intrinsic foot muscles may also be seen because the distal posterior tibial nerve innervates these muscles. There should sparing of proximal tibial muscles in the lower legs.

Sensory nerve conduction of the medial plantar[74] and lateral plantar nerves are found to be sensitive indicators of tarsal tunnel syndrome. Comparison with the asymptomatic foot is indicated to evaluate for neuropathy, although there have been cases of bilateral tarsal tunnel syndrome.[75] Unfortunately, these potentials may be absent in normal individuals over the age of 50.

Treatment of tarsal tunnel syndrome may be conservative with use of medial arch supports and bracing the foot to avoid trauma.[76] Nonsteroidal anti-inflammatory agents are also helpful in treatment of bursitis or tenosynovitis, which may cause flare-up of the tarsal tunnel syndrome. The use of local steroid injection or short course oral cortisone may prove beneficial. Surgery with tarsal tunnel release relieving posterior tibial nerve compression is another mode of treatment if the conservative approach fails.[77]

References

1. Waxman SG: Conduction in myelinated, unmyelinated, and demyelinated fibers. Arch Neurol 1977;34:585.
2. Donofrio PD, Albers JW: Polyneuropathy, classification by nerve conduction studies and electromyography. AAEM Minimonograph No. 34. Muscle Nerve, 1990, p 6.
3. Kimura J: Clinical electrophysiology of peripheral nervous system axons. *In* Waxman S, Kocsis J, Stys P (eds): The Axon. New York, Oxford University Press, 1995, p 616.
4. Buchtal F, Guld C, Rosenflack P: Propagation velocity in electrically activated fibers in man. Acta Physiol Scand 1955;34:75.
5. Mayer RF, Feldman RG: Observations on the nature of the F wave in the baboon. J Neurol Neurosurg Psychiatry 1966;29:196.
6. Fisher MA: H reflexes and F waves: Physiology and clinical indications. Muscle Nerve 1992;15:1223–1233.
7. Kimura J: Clinical electrophysiology of peripheral nervous system axons. *In* Waxman S, Kocsis J, Stys P (eds): The Axon. New York, Oxford University Press, 1995, p 616.
8. Kimura J: Proximal versus distal slowing in motor nerve conduction velocity in the Guillain-Barré syndrome. Ann Neurol 1978;3:344.
9. Eisen A: Electrodiagnosis of radiculopathies. Neurol Clin 1985;3:495–510.

10. Jabre JF: Surface recording of the H reflex of the flexor carpi radialis. Muscle Nerve 1981;4:435–438.
11. Wilbourn AJ, Aminoff MJ: The electrodiagnostic examination in patients with radiculopathies. AAEM Minimonograph No. 72. Muscle Nerve 1998;12:1614.
12. Bougle D, Denise P, Yaseen H, et al: Maturation of peripheral nerves in preterm infants. Motor and proprioceptive nerve conduction. Electroencephalogr Clin Neurophysiol 1990;75:118–121.
13. Mayer RF, Feldman RG: Nerve conduction studies in man. Neurol 1963;13:1021–1030.
14. Kimura J, Yamada T, Steveland NP: Distal slowing of motor nerve conduction velocity in diabetic polyneuropathy. J Neurol Sci 1979;42:291–302.
15. Louis AA, Hotson JR: Regional cooling of human nerve and delayed sodium inactivation. Electroencephalogr Clin Neurophysiol 1986;634:371–375.
16. Todnem K, Knudsen G, Riise T, et al: The nonlinear relationship between nerve conduction velocity and skin temperature. J Neurol Neurosurg Psychiatr 1989;52:497–501.
17. Ochoa J: Nerve fiber pathology in acute and chronic compression. *In* Omer GE, Spinner M (eds): Management of Peripheral Nerve Problems. Philadelphia, WB Saunders, 1980, pp 487–501.
18. Gilliatt RW, Taylor JC: Electrical changes following section of the facial nerve. Proc R Soc Med 1959;52:1080.
19. Berger AR, Schaumberg H: Human peripheral nerve disease (peripheral neuropathies). *In* Waxman S, Kocsis J, Stys P (eds): The Axon. New York, Oxford University Press, 1995, pp 648–650.
20. Wiechers DO: Mechanically provoked insertional activity before and after nerve section in rats. Arch Phys Med Rehabil 1977;58:407.
21. Lambert E: Electromyography. *In* Youmans J (ed): Neurological Surgery. Philadelphia, WB Saunders, 1973, Vol 1, pp 358–367.
22. Colochis SC, Pease WS, Johnson EW: Motor unit action potentials in early radiculopathy. Their presence and ephaptic transmission as a hypothesis. Electromyogr Clin Neurophysiol 1992;32:27–33.
23. Clamann HP: Activity of single motor units during isometric tension. Neurology 1970;20:254.
24. Wilbourn AJ, Aminoff MJ: Radiculopathies. *In* Brown WF, Bolton CF (eds): Clinical Electromyography, 2nd ed. Boston, Butterworth-Heinemann, 1993, pp 177–209.
25. Love JG, Walsh MN: Protruded intervertebral discs: A report of one hundred cases in which operation was performed. JAMA 1938;111:396–400.
26. Marinacci AA: A correlation between operative findings in cervical herniated disc with the electromyograms and opaque myelograms. Electromyography 1966;6:5–20.
27. Wilbourn AJ: The value and limitations of electromyographic examination in the diagnosis of lumbosacral radiculopathy. *In* Hardy RW (ed): Lumbar Disc Disease. New York, Raven Press, 1982, pp 65–109.
28. Boden SA, Davis DO, Dina TS, et al: Abnormal magnetic resonance scans of the lumbar spine in asymptomatic subjects. J Bone Joint Surg Am 1990;72:403–408.
29. Jensen MC, Brant-Zawadski MN, Obuchowski N, et al: Magnetic resonance imaging of the lumbar spine in people without back pain. N Engl J Med 1994;331:69–73.
30. Waylonis GW: Electromyographic findings in chronic cervical radicular syndromes. Arch Phys Med Rehabil 1968;49:407–412.
31. See D, Kraft G: Electromyography in paraspinal muscles following surgery for root compression. Arch Phys Med Rehabil 1975;56:80–83.
32. Yoss RE, Corbin KB, MacCarthy CS, Love JG: Significance of signs and symptoms in localization of involved roots in cervical disc protrusion. Neurology 1957;7:673–683.
33. Jablecki CK, Andary MT, So YT, et al: Literature review of the usefulness of nerve conduction studies and electromyography for the evaluation of patients with carpal tunnel syndrome. AAEM Quality Assurance Committee. Muscle Nerve 1993;16:1392–1414.
34. Jackson DA, Clifford JC: Electrodiagnosis of mild carpal tunnel syndrome. Arch Phys Med Rehabil 1989;70:199–204.
35. Johnson EW, Kukla RD, Wongsam PE, Piedmont A: Sensory latencies to the ring finger: Normal values and relation to carpal tunnel syndrome. Arch Phys Med Rehabil 1981;62:140–141.
36. Valls J, LLanas JM: Orthodromic study of the sensory fibers innervating the fourth finger. Muscle Nerve 1988;11:546–552.
37. Charles N, Vial C, Chauplannaz G, Bady B: Clinical validation of antidromic stimulation of the ring finger in early electrodiagnosis of mild carpal tunnel syndrome. Electroencephalogr Clin Neurophysiol 1990;76:142–147.
38. Stevens JC: The electrodiagnosis of carpal tunnel syndrome. AAEM Minimonograph No. 26. Muscle Nerve 1997;20:1477–1486.
39. Pascoe MK, Pascoe RD, Tarrant E, Boyle R: Changes in palmar sensory latencies in response to carpal tunnel release. Muscle Nerve 1994;14:1475–1476.
40. Melvin JL, Johnson EW, Duran R: Electrodiagnosis after surgery for carpal tunnel syndrome. Arch Phys Med Rehabil 1968;49:502–507.
41. Goodwill CJ: The carpal tunnel syndrome: Long-term follow up showing relation of latency measurements to response to treatment. Ann Phys Med 1965;8:12–21.
42. Dawson DM, Hallett M, Millender LH: Median Nerve Entrapment at the Elbow. Entrapment Neuropathies. Boston, Little, Brown, 1983, pp 76–86.
43. Spinner M: The anterior interosseus nerve syndrome. J Bone Joint Surg 1970;52A:84.
44. Paine KW: Tardy ulnar palsy. Can J Surg 1970;13:255–261.
45. Feindel W, Stratford V: Role of cubital tunnel in tardy ulnar palsy. Can J Surg 1957;1:287.
46. Kincaid JC: The electrodiagnosis of ulnar neuropathy at the elbow. AAEE Minimonograph No. 31. Muscle Nerve 1988;11:1005–1015.
47. Olney RK, Miller RG: Conduction block in compression neuropathies: Recognition and quantification. Muscle Nerve 1984;7:662–667.
48. Dawson DM, Hallett M, Millender LH: Ulnar nerve entrapment at wrist. Entrapment Neuropathies. Boston, Little, Brown, 1983, pp 123–140.
49. Packer JW, Foster RR, Garcia A, Granthan SA: The humeral fracture with radial nerve palsy: Is exploration warranted? Clin Orthop 1972;88:34.
50. Lotem M, Fried A, Levy M, et al: Radial palsy following muscular effort. J Bone Joint Surg 1971;53B:500.
51. Jebsen RH: Motor conduction velocity in proximal and distal segments of the radial nerve. Arch Phys Med Rehabil 1966;47:597.
52. Morris AH: Irreducible Monteggia lesion with radial nerve entrapment. J Bone Joint Surg 1974;56A:1744.
53. Haggert CG: Entrapment of the posterior interosseus nerve causing forearm pain. Proceedings of the Scandinavian Society for Surgery of the Hand. J Hand Surg 1977;2:486.
54. Werner CO: Lateral elbow pain and posterior interosseus nerve entrapment. Acta Orthop Scand Suppl 1979;174:1.
55. Spinner M: The arcade of Frohse and its relationship to posterior interosseus nerve paralysis. J Bone Joint Surg 1968;50B:809.
56. Dawson DM, Hallett M, Millender LH: Radial nerve entrapment. *In* Entrapment Neuropathies. Boston, Little, Brown, 1983, pp 164–167.
57. Drake CG: Diagnosis and treatment of lesions of the brachial plexus and adjacent structures. Clin Neurosurg 1964;11:110.
58. Sunderland S: Nerves and Nerve Injuries, 2nd ed. London, Churchill Livingstone, 1978.
59. Gilliatt RW, LeQuesne PM, Logue V, et al: Wasting of the hand associated with a cervical rib or band. J Neurol Neurosurg Psychiatry 1970;33:615.
60. Gilliatt RW, LeQuesne PM, Logue V, et al: Peripheral nerve conduction in patients with a cervical rib and band. Ann Neurol 1978;4:124.
61. Gilliatt RW: Thoracic outlet compression syndrome. Br Med J 1976;1:1274.
62. Eisen AA: Radiculopathies and plexopathies. *In* Brown WF, Bolton CF (eds): Clinical Electromyography. Boston, Butterworth & Co, 1987.
63. Dawson DM, Hallett M, Millender LH: Thoracic outlet syndromes. *In* Entrapment Neuropathies. Boston, Little, Brown, 1983, pp 169–183.
64. Simon H, Gryska PF, Carlson DH: The thoracic outlet syndrome as a cause of aneurysm formation, thrombosis, and embolization. South Med J 1977;70:1282.
65. Banis JC Jr, Rich N, Whelan TJ Jr: Ischemia of the upper extremity due to non-cardiac emboli. Am J Surg 1977;134:31.
66. Pezina M: Contribution to the etiological explanation of the piriformis syndrome. Acta Anat 1979;105:181.
67. Banerjee T, Hall CD: Sciatic entrapment neuropathy. J Neurosurg 1976;45:216.
68. Nakano KK: Entrapment neuropathy from Baker's cyst. JAMA 1978;239:239.
69. Wallach HW, Orea ME: Sciatic nerve compression during anticoagu-

lant therapy: Computerized tomography aids in diagnosis. Arch Neurol 1979;36:448.

70. Storell DA, Hinterbuchner C, Green RF, Kalisky Z: Traumatic common peroneal nerve palsy: A retrospective study. Arch Phys Med Rehabil 1976;57:361.

71. Meals RA: Peroneal nerve palsy complicating ankle sprain. J Bone Joint Surg 1977;59A:966.

72. Dawson DM, Hallett M, Millender LH: Peroneal nerve entrapment. *In* Entrapment Neuropathies. Boston, Little, Brown, 1983, pp 201–210.

73. Borges LF, Hallett M, Selkoe DJ, Welch K: The anterior tarsal tunnel syndrome: Report of two cases. J Neurosurg 1981;54:89.

74. Guiloff RJ, Sherratt RM: Sensory conduction in medial plantar nerve. J Neurol Neurosurg Psychiatry 1977;40:1168.

75. Oh SJ, Sarala PK, Kuba T, Elmore RS: Tarsal tunnel syndrome: Electrophysiological study. Ann Neurol 1979;5:327.

76. Dawson DM, Hallett M, Millender LH: Tarsal tunnel syndromes. *In* Entrapment Neuropathies. Boston, Little, Brown, 1983, pp 211–218.

77. Kaplan PE, Kernahan WT: Tarsal tunnel syndrome: An electrodiagnostic and surgical correlation. J Bone Joint Surg 1981;63A:96.

C h a p t e r   7

A Word About "Outcomes"

Sam W. Wiesel, M.D.

Every clinician's goal is to make the patient better. Historically, the measure of what "better" meant was based on hard (objective) data. In musculoskeletal medicine, this could take the form of bone healing on x-ray or the resultant angle of an osteotomy. The old saying that "the operation was a success but the patient died" was not far from the truth of measuring the outcome of a particular procedure. Today, hard data are not sufficient when judging a patient's outcome for treatment efficacy. Physicians must take into account "soft" data.

Soft data are the patient's self-report on the assessment of the clinical outcome and should be considered in establishing a patient's health status. It is not based on an objective scale but rather on items such as pain magnitude and psychologic factors such as depression or anxiety. There are no physical measurements for these types of variables.

Over the past several years, a number of patient-based outcome assessment instruments have been developed. They include pain, function, and psychosocial measurements, as well as composite measurements of all three. Each involves a self-administered examination that assesses health in terms of the variable being evaluated. The reliability and validity of these examinations are not consistent from patient to patient nor for that matter in many instances for the same patient taking the same test several weeks apart. However, for a specific point in time, it does give the physician an evaluation of how the patient perceives the success of the treatment.

Physicians need to be cognizant of a patient's "soft" data as well as the "hard" data. Both are important in judging a patient's well-being. The future will bring a sophistication in measuring these soft variables with increased accuracy. The point of this "word about outcomes" is to encourage physicians not to lose sight of the complete picture when assessing a patient's health.

Section III
General
Orthopaedics

Chapter 8
Principles of Musculoskeletal Trauma

John N. Delahay, M.D.

It is probably safe to say that injury to the musculoskeletal system is a ubiquitous international problem. The management of trauma to bone and soft tissue was primarily responsible for the development of orthopaedic surgery as a specialty. Indeed, the specialty was founded and organized by individuals who had an expressed interest in guaranteeing quality care for patients with such injuries. The treatment of fractures and dislocations is historically an ancient art. Hippocrates (Fig. 8–1) and others wrote on their treatment methods hundreds of years ago. Fractures of the femur, dislocations of the shoulder, and infections in the extremity were all the subject of historical writings (Fig. 8–2). Physicians learned much from wartime experiences. The development of management techniques took a quantum leap forward in each postwar era. The development of improved anesthesia techniques (Fig. 8–3), the antibiotic era, and the progressing sophistication of internal fixation devices have all contributed to the rapidly expanding techniques used in the management of musculoskeletal trauma. This chapter is meant to serve as an introduction to the language of fractures and dislocations as well as to the general approaches in their management. Specific injuries as well as the principles guiding the management of musculoskeletal injury in children are discussed in more detail in the specific chapters related to those subjects.

TERMINOLOGY

Injuries to the musculoskeletal system are generally discussed in three major groups. First, are *fractures,* which by definition are a disruption in the continuity of cortical and/or cancellous bone. Second, are *dislocations,* which are disruptions of the normal articulating anatomy of a joint. Dislocations may be either complete, where the anatomy is grossly disturbed or partial, the latter referred to as a joint *subluxation.* Third, a combination of a fracture in proximity to a joint resulting in subsequent joint dislocation or subluxation is referred to as a *fracture dislocation.* It is important to recognize this is an entirely different injury than either of the other two.

Numerous words have become popular in the lexicon of skeletal trauma. These terms provide a common ground for communication amongst professionals discussing these injuries. First, fractures are either *open* or *closed.* Identifying whether or not the skin overlying the injury is intact is critical, if treatment is to be appropriate. The old term, "compound," is no longer used; the currently preferred term is "open." Fractures may also be *simple,* in that they have two major fragments; or they be *comminuted,* meaning the presence multiple fragments of bone present. Fractures may be *complete,* when the fracture line extends completely across the bone; or they may be *incomplete,* when the fracture line crosses only one cortex. Incomplete fractures are typically seen in the pediatric age group.

In addition to these terms, a number of words are used to describe the deformities seen in association with a given fracture. As one can surmise, fractures can deform in both the AP and sagittal plane as well as in a transverse plane. First, *displacement* (Fig. 8–4) of a fracture is noted. This specifically refers to any translatory deformity between the major fragments; by convention, the distal segment is described in relation to the proximal. For example, should the distal fragment be anterior to the proximal, the displacement is described as anterior. In this same vein, it is possible for the fracture ends to be *overriding,* in which case the two fragments are shortened in relation to one another; or conversely *distracted,* should the two bone ends be pulled apart. The latter situation, from the standpoint of healing, is far more problematic. Typically, soft tissue interposition delays fracture in the face of distraction; whereas overriding (bayonet apposition) may cause shortening, it does not seem to retard union.

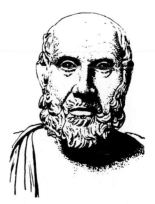

Figure 8–1. Hippocrates. (From Rang M: Anthology of Orthopaedics. Edinburgh, Churchill Livingstone, 1966, p 6.)

117

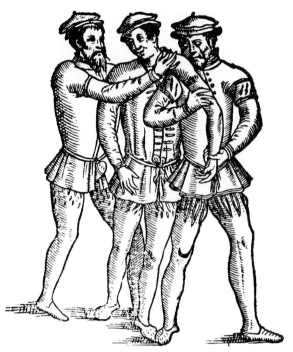

Figure 8–2. The technique of reducing a complete dislocation of the left shoulder, as illustrated in the *Ten Books of Surgery* by Ambroise Paré. New York Academy of Medicine. (From Lyons AS, Petrucelli RJ: Medicine: An Illustrated History. New York, Harry N Abrams, 1978, p 384.)

Angular deformity also can occur in both planes. The musculoskeletal system requires joint alignment for normal anatomic function. Should angular deformity exist, thereby creating malalignment of two joints, long-term dysfunction and disability can be anticipated. *Angulation* is typically described based on the apical direction of the two frag-ments. Specifically, should the apex point anteriorly, the fracture is said to be anteriorly angulated, etc. Again, this terminology is simply based on convention.

Thirdly, *rotational deformity* is important to recognize. Axial rotation of a long bone at a fracture site clearly causes rotational malalignment of the joint above and below. As mentioned previously, this will create an abnormal situation for joint function. Frequently, rotational malalignment can be obvious, such as in the midshaft of the tibia, when the foot and the knee do not line up. It can also be far more subtle, such as seen in the hand, where fractures in phalanges and metacarpals can frequently cause rotational deformity. This deformity can be missed if the examiner fails to have patients close the hand as part of the normal physical examination.

A number of descriptive terms have been used to define the *fracture pattern* (Table 8–1) itself. They include such terms as transverse, spiral, oblique, impacted, avulsed, and complex. In reviewing the adjacent figure in Table 8–1, one can see that a simple transverse fracture is one where the fracture line crosses the bone perpendicular to its long axis. A spiral fracture is one in which the fracture line twists around the bone, being oblique in both the AP and sagittal planes. In contradistinction, an oblique fracture is one that crosses the bone obliquely in one plane only. The oblique fracture (unlike the spiral fracture) shows the fracture line to be oblique in one plane and transverse in the other.

The significance of these terms is that they allow the examiner to more accurately analyze the *mechanism* by which the injury occurred. For example, had the bone been loaded in torsion, one would expect a spiral fracture. Axial loading on the hand tends to cause an impacted or compressed fracture. Conversely, the application of tensile load can be expected to produce an avulsion type injury. The common transverse fracture of a long bone results from

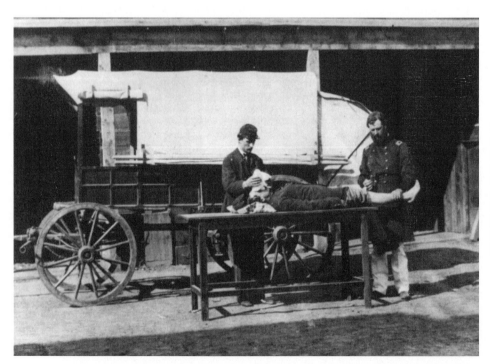

Figure 8–3. Contrary to popular belief, anesthesia was more the rule than the exception during the Civil War. A Union soldier receives anesthesia in this image. (From Kuz JE, Bengtson BP: Orthopaedic Injuries of the Civil War. Kennesaw Mountain Press, 1997, p 13.)

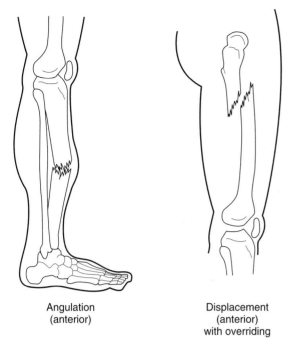

Angulation
(anterior)

Displacement
(anterior)
with overriding

Figure 8–4. Fracture deformities.

the application of bending load. In the latter case, the fracture line initiates on the convex side of bending (tensile side) and propagates across the bone to the concave side (compression side).

Obviously, many fractures result from the application of combined loading patterns. The best example is a pure oblique fracture. In order to create this injury, the bone

needs to be bent while axial load is being applied. This example of complex loading is one of the more common in the musculoskeletal system. The significance of the mechanical analysis of fracture patterns is of more than just academic interest. The interpretation of loading pattern will allow the examiner to gain insight into the amount force required to produce the injury, thereby suggesting the energy level of the injury itself. Complex loading patterns clearly require greater force (Fig. 8–5), and therefore more energy storage (strain energy) occurs. At the time of fracture, this energy is released; the greater the strain energy, the more collateral soft tissue damage is anticipated. In keeping with this concept, one would expect more soft tissue damage with a comminuted oblique fracture of the tibia than one would anticipate with a simple low-velocity spiral fracture.

SOFT TISSUES

Having just mentioned damage to the soft tissues in the extremity, it is appropriate to discuss these structures at this time.

Periosteum

The outer membrane covering a long bone is believed by most to be important for its healing. Although in a child, this outer layer is of great significance, it clearly has a role to play in the adult as well. The adult has a single layered fibrous periosteum, which provides a modicum of mechanical support as well as a site for osteogenic activity. In addition, the periosteal blood supply has been shown to feed the outer third of the bony cortex. Therefore, disrup-

Table 8–1. Summary of long bone fracture biomechanics

Fracture Pattern	Appearance	Mechanism of Injury	Location Soft Tissue Hinge	Energy
Transverse		Bending	Concavity	Low
Spiral		Torsion	Vertical segment	Low
Oblique-transverse or butterfly		Compression + Bending	Concavity or side of butterfly	Mod
Oblique		Compression + Bending + Torsion	Concavity (often destroyed)	Mod
Comminuted		Variable	Destroyed	High
Metaphyseal compression		Compression	Variable	Variable

From Gozna ER, Harrington IJ: Biomechanics of Musculoskeletal Injury. Baltimore, Williams & Wilkins, 1982.

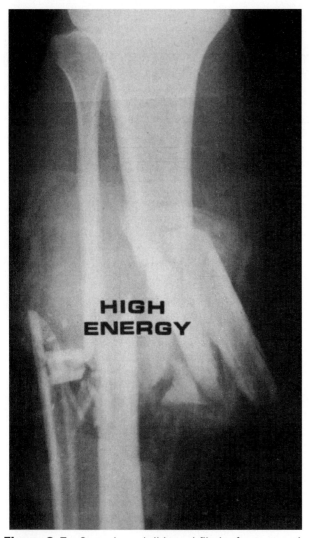

Figure 8–5. Comminuted tibia and fibular fracture as the result of a motorcycle accident. This high-energy fracture with its associated soft tissue injuries eventually required amputation. (From Gozna ER, Harrington IJ: Biomechanics of Musculoskeletal Injury. Baltimore, Williams & Wilkins, 1982.)

tion of this membrane has a deleterious effect, both on mechanical stability of the fracture and the biologic vascularization of the callus. Severe soft tissue stripping and periosteal disruption will clearly create a very unstable situation for fracture reduction as well as seriously disrupting the normal healing sequence due to vascular damage. Its ultimate effect will be a retardation of osteogenesis. In addition, the periosteum is frequently helpful in achieving a satisfactory closed reduction. It can be used not only to guide the reduction of a given fracture but also to maintain a fracture once reduced.

Vascular Structures

Injury to the circulatory system in association with fractures and dislocations is a relatively uncommon event. When it does occur, however, it is always an emergent situation. It is safe to say that in the extremities, the most

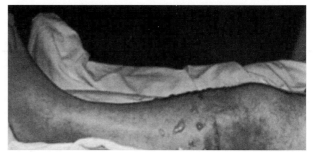

Figure 8–6. Acute compartment syndrome of the leg. (From Browner BD, Jupiter JB, Levine AM, Trafton PG: Skeletal Trauma, 2nd ed, Vol 1. Philadelphia, WB Saunders, 1998.)

common vascular lesion requiring immediate attention is an impending *compartment syndrome* (Fig. 8–6). Trauma to the musculature in a compartment typically results in bleeding within that compartment. As the intracompartmental pressure increases, collapse of small venous structures occurs. This only accentuates the increased pressure within the compartment by decreasing outflow of fluids from the compartment itself. Ultimately, intracompartmental pressures exceed the systolic pressure head, resulting in arterial collapse. This further amplifies the relative paucity of blood flow to the muscles and nerves within a given compartment. It is important to recognize that compartment syndrome is a progressive phenomenon and not a single isolated event. Ultimately, the process leads to myonecrosis. Necrosis of muscle tissue with further inflammation and liquefaction only antagonizes the entire process. Neural structures similarly suffer as a result of both pressure and circulatory deprivation. Left untreated, a compartment syndrome can result in a gangrenous extremity (Fig. 8–7).

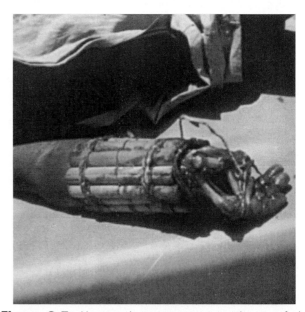

Figure 8–7. Untreated compartment syndrome of the forearm, secondary to excessive tightness of an occlusive dressing. (From Browner BD, Jupiter JB, Levine AM, Trafton PG: Skeletal Trauma, 2nd ed, Vol 1. Philadelphia, WB Saunders, 1998.)

All compartments are at risk for this injury; however, the anterior compartment of the leg and volar compartment of the forearm appear to be uniquely predisposed. It has only been in recent years that Myerson and others have called our attention to the significance of compartment syndrome in the foot itself.

With the disastrous consequences that can result from failure to diagnose an impending compartment syndrome in a timely fashion, it is critical for those who care for the trauma patient to recognize the early manifestations of this syndrome. It is key that one not wait for the appearance of the five "Ps" (pain, pallor, pulselessness, paresthesias, and paralysis) of arterial injury before making the diagnosis of an impending compartment syndrome. If one is lulled into a false sense of security by the presence of a pulse, myonecrosis may already be well underway. The characteristic findings in the patient with an impending compartment syndrome are as follows: tenderness of the compartment, palpatory firmness of the compartment, pain far out of proportion to what one would anticipate for the injury in question, and, what many believe to be the most important, pain with passive stretch of muscles contained within the compartment. In years past, when compartmental monitoring techniques were quite rudimentary, it was routine to surgically decompress a compartment based on clinical evaluation and judgment. Currently, with the benefit of newer monitoring devices (Fig. 8–8), one has the added advantage of direct measurement of compartmental pressures. These monitoring devices are effective and generally readily available. Normal tissue pressure within a compartment is 1 to 2 mmHg. Fasciotomy is generally recommended whenever the intracompartmental pressure exceeds 30 mmHg. In the polytrauma patient or patients with head injury, the tolerance is generally lowered and fasciotomy is performed when pressures exceed 20 mmHg. It is important to keep in mind that if the measuring device does not seem to be consistent with the clinical evaluation of the patient, it is far safer to proceed with compartmental decompression. Failure to do so is frequently disastrous for the patient.

At the time of surgical decompression, all soft tissue layers causing constriction need to be opened. The skin itself can frequently act as a constricting membrane and as such should be opened the entire length of the compartment. Although subcutaneous fasciotomy has been used in

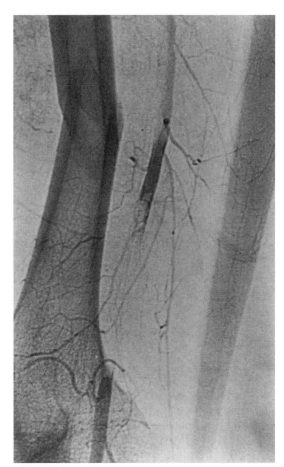

Figure 8–9. Occlusion of the superficial femoral artery is located below the site of the oblique fracture of the femur. (From Browner BD, Jupiter JB, Levine AM, Trafton PG: Skeletal Trauma, 2nd ed, Vol 1. Philadelphia, WB Saunders, 1998.)

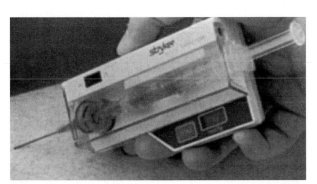

Figure 8–8. The Stic catheter. (Courtesy of Stryker Mississauga, Ontario, Canada.) (From Browner BD, Jupiter JB, Levine AM, Trafton PG: Skeletal Trauma, 2nd ed, Vol 1. Philadelphia, WB Saunders, 1998.)

the past and may still be used appropriately in certain situations, it is critical that adequate decompression be accomplished. The once popular fibulectomy for decompression of all four compartments in the leg has fallen into disrepute. Late deformity and ankle instability have made this a relatively poor choice for compartmental decompression. There should be no shame in the need for plastic surgical procedures to close a skin defect should it be required, rather than prematurely closing the skin and recreating inordinate amounts of pressure.

Direct arterial injury (Fig. 8–9) is less common a concern than compartment syndrome. Arteries in the extremities tend to be somewhat elastic as a function of their media. Their overall elasticity generally allows them to "get out of the way" of the oncoming bone at the time of fracture. From this, one can surmise that damage to major arteries can be anticipated, if for whatever reason they are inelastic or are fixed by adjacent soft tissues and therefore unable to "get out of the way." One can see crushing injuries as well as partial lacerations of arterial structures. The more common scenario, following a crushing injury, is the development of an intramural hematoma. Subsequent bleeding within the wall of the vessel will obviously occlude the vessel. Similarly, it makes clot removal impossible and the techniques for reestablishing flow usually involve either the use of a vein graft or a prosthetic segment to bypass the damaged segment of vessel. Partial vessel laceration, as one may see in association with pelvic fractures, creates the added problem of bleeding into either the retroperitoneal space or in an extremity. Hypovolemic shock or compartment syndrome is likely to follow these events.

Classically, arterial injury has been described in association with several specific injuries. Textbooks frequently cite clavicular fracture as potentially causing injury to the subclavian vessels. Most would agree that concerns regarding this injury are probably inflated. However, injuries about the elbow, especially in children, are of significant concern for damage to the brachial artery. The artery tends to be fixed anteriorly by the lacertus fibrosus, making trauma to this vessel a significant concern. The other injuries, specifically fractures in the distal third of the femur, fractures in the proximal tibia, and dislocations of the knee joint, all emphasize the unique vascular anatomy about the knee. The popliteal artery is fixed posteriorly at the knee as a result of its trifurcation. Therefore, with these specific injuries it is vulnerable. It is probably safe to say that most arterial injuries occur around the knee joint.

Neural Structures

Damage to nerves and branches of nerves in association with fractures has also been reported (Fig. 8–10). As with injuries to the arterial tree, these structures similarly can withstand only a certain amount of stretch or pressure. Typically, the nerve is compressed, contused, or stretched as a result of fracture in the vicinity. Seddon has classified peripheral nerve injury into the following three classic groups.

NEURAPRAXIA

Neurapraxia is defined as a physiologic disruption of neural function without anatomic abnormality of the nerve. The

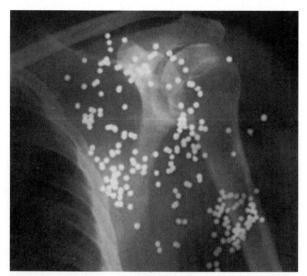

Figure 8–10. A close-range shotgun blast to the shoulder injured the brachial plexus. (From Browner BD, Jupiter JB, Levine AM, Trafton PG: Skeletal Trauma, 2nd ed, Vol 1. Philadelphia, WB Saunders, 1998.)

prognosis is best for this group with anticipated return of function in 4 to 6 months in many cases.

AXONOTMESIS

This is an anatomic disruption of the axonal sheath. The epineurial sheath of the nerve remains intact. As one might expect, this is a more severe grade of injury. For recovery to occur, wallerian degeneration and subsequent regeneration will be required. Frequently, recovery is incomplete at best, and depending on the nerve in question, it may be completely absent. The formation of intraneural neuromas may complicate this injury.

NEUROTMESIS

Neurotmesis represents a complete anatomic disruption of the entire nerve. This grade of injury is rare in closed fractures and is more typical in severe open injuries resulting from gunshot wounds, penetrating trauma, and the like. Obviously, this group has the poorest prognosis and mandates neural repair or graft if any hope of regeneration is to be anticipated.

PROGNOSIS

The prognosis for any given nerve depends not only on the grade of the injury but also on its location as well as its function. Nerves with more discrete motor control, such as the ulnar nerve, will clearly have a poorer prognosis than will a nerve supplying bulk muscle groups such as the axillary nerve. It is key that the examiner carefully evaluate and document the extent of neural injury should one be present. All too frequently, a cursory evaluation of the peripheral nerves leads to long-term medical and legal ramifications. It is important to carefully evaluate the sensory as well as the motor distribution for the nerves in the traumatized extremity. Often an injury is overlooked because the examiner feels secure finding a normal sensory distribution. One such example is the posterior interosseus nerve. This is purely a motor nerve. Therefore, if the physician is satisfied after finding the sensory distribution of the radial nerve to be intact, this injury will be missed.

Specific fractures mandate careful neural evaluation. Examples include the legendary humeral fracture with radial nerve palsy, the supracondylar fracture in the child with anterior interosseous nerve palsy, and posterior dislocation of the hip with sciatic nerve palsy.

Muscle-Tendon Unit Injuries

It goes without saying that bony injury in the extremity will likely produce trauma to the adjacent muscle-tendon units. The vast majority of these injuries are relatively benign and heal uneventfully. Tendon laceration itself is a rare phenomenon in association with fractures. Muscle contusion and laceration similarly will usually resolve uneventfully. However, a specific concern related to muscle trauma is the ultimate formation of *heterotopic ossification.* Trauma to major muscle groups can lead to the formation of bone within these muscles. The process of myositis ossificans traumatica is poorly understood. It also seems to be somewhat unique to specific anatomic sites. The brachialis muscle in the anterior arm, the quadriceps muscle in the anterior thigh, and the abductor muscles of the hip are uniquely predisposed to manifest this complication.

Ligaments

The strength of ligaments is a relative constant throughout life. As noted previously, ligaments essentially are pure collagen with some elastic fibers arrayed in a somewhat random pattern. Physiologically, they serve as check reins throughout the range of joint motion. Aging takes minimal toll on ligamentous structures. A slight increase in cross-linking of the collagen fibers in aging ligaments has been identified. This implies that the ligament may become slightly stiffer with age.

As is the case with any extremity injury, one must consider both bony trauma and the possibility of ligamentous disruption. In most cases, the "weak link" will be the tissue that fails first. Frequently, once the first failure occurs, the other adjacent tissues will be spared. A good example of this concept can be appreciated if one considers a "clipping injury" or valgus stress injury (Fig. 8–11) to the lower extremity. In the middle age group, with all tissues being normal, one can anticipate a ligamentous disruption of the knee joint. Failure of the medial collateral ligament or anterior cruciate ligament can be expected. The bony structures adjacent to these ligaments mechanically are stronger and, therefore, more likely to resist the abnormal load. In an elderly female with osteoporosis, however, the bony tissue is likely to be weaker and less able to resist load than the ligamentous structures. Therefore, in this age group, one should anticipate a plateau fracture of the proximal tibia instead of ligamentous disruption of the knee. As will be seen later, a child has open growth plates about the knee, and in that case one can anticipate physeal fractures of either the distal femur or proximal tibia. The physis is weaker than either bone or ligament in the pediatric age group. Therefore, age as well as mechanism of injury is a significant factor in the type of musculoskeletal injury that occurs.

SPECIAL TYPES OF FRACTURES

Generally, fractures of the musculoskeletal system involve normal tissues. Should the loading pattern be unusual or the host be abnormal, complex and atypical injuries should be suspected. There are several specific injuries that are unusual and therefore worthy of mention.

Pathologic Fractures (Fig. 8–12)

These result from an abnormality of the host bone. Should the bone be weakened by tumor, metabolic disease, or infection, it is more prone to fracture. Fractures through this abnormal bone are referred to as pathologic fractures. The management of these injuries will require individual-

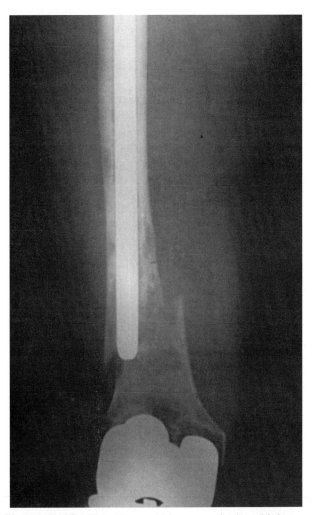

Figure 8–12. This 78-year-old woman had multiple myeloma and carcinoma of the breast and had undergone a previous total arthroplasty for degenerative disease of the knee. At 1½ years before admission, she also underwent a Zickel nail fixation for a subtrochanteric fracture. The patient had subsequent disease below the tip of the Zickel nail and above the total-knee arthroplasty and sustained a fracture at the tip of the Zickel nail. This required removal of the Zickel nail and fixation with an interlocking nail system to protect the entire femur. (From Browner BD, Jupiter JB, Levine AM, Trafton PG: Skeletal Trauma, 2nd ed, Vol 1. Philadelphia, WB Saunders, 1998.)

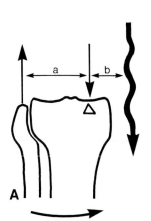
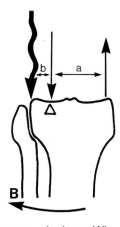

Figure 8–11. A first-class lever system at the knee. When the tibia is subjected to a bending moment that adducts the shank *(A)*, a tension force occurs in the lateral ligament and a compression force occurs over the medial tibial condyle. The reverse occurs when the knee is abducted *(B)*. (From Gozna ER, Harrington IJ: Biomechanics of Musculoskeletal Injury. Baltimore, Williams & Wilkins, 1982.)

ization based on the underlying disease. Standard treatment protocols are usually inadequate to manage these unique injuries.

Stress Fractures

These injuries typically result from cyclic loading of an extremity. Even though each single application of load may be below the yield point, repetition produces a summation of force and bony failure. Stress fractures are typically seen in the proximal medial tibia and the femoral neck in long distance runners and the neck of the second metatarsal in military recruits, hence the name "march fracture."

Intra-articular Fractures

Fractures, which occur adjacent to or entering a joint, cause disruption of the articular surface. Unlike long bone fractures, these injuries predispose the joint to late stiffness and osteoarthritic change. For this reason, the management of these complex injuries requires special protocols. The principles of managing intra-articular fractures have been well enunciated. They include the following:

A. Anatomic restoration of the articular surface
B. Rigid fixation of the bony structures
C. Early motion of the affected joint
D. Delayed weightbearing on the extremity

Pediatric Injuries

A section on pediatric trauma is found in Chapter 17. Several specific points are appropriate at this time related to injuries unique in children.

INCOMPLETE FRACTURES

As mentioned earlier, the bone of a child is able to deform plastically (Fig. 8–13), thereby bending without breaking. That being the case, children have the unique ability to sustain incomplete fractures. Although these injuries have been occasionally reported in adults, one needs to be very suspicious of this diagnosis. Adult bone tends to be stiffer than that of the child, making the possibility of incomplete fracture remote. The child's bone, because of its ability to deform plastically, typically will demonstrate one of two patterns:

1. *Greenstick fractures* occur in cortical bone and therefore are seen in the diaphysis. Typically the application of bending load initiates the crack on the convex (tensile) side of the bend.
2. *Torus (buckle) fractures* are seen in cancellous bone, hence occur in the metaphysis. Failure is seen on the concave (compression) side of the bend.

In general, incomplete fractures are benign injuries, requiring short-term immobilization and enjoying an excellent prognosis. Special concern exists in cases in which both bones in the same forearm are fractured. If the radial fracture is complete but the ulnar fracture is greenstick, it will usually be necessary to complete the fracture of the ulna. Otherwise, it will act as a spring and redeform the radial fracture.

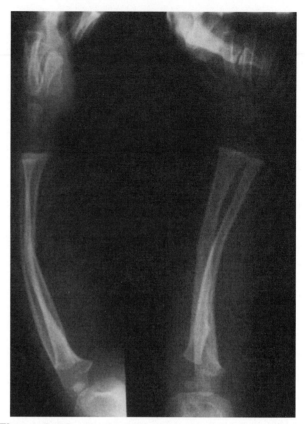

Figure 8–13. Plastic deformation in the radius and ulna of a 2-year-old following a fall. The bones are plastically deformed at midshaft, with volar compression and dorsal tension failure but without fracture propagation. (From Green NE, Swiontkowski MF: Skeletal Trauma in Children, Vol 3. Philadelphia, WB Saunders, 1998.)

PHYSEAL FRACTURES (Fig. 8–14)

The long bone of a child has a built-in mechanical flaw. This structure, the *physis,* is critical for normal bone growth. However, the physeal cartilage is a labile tissue and one subject to mechanical failure. This structure will fail with the application of excessive load. Physeal fractures are grouped using the classic Salter-Harris scheme. This classification not only allows the physician to anatomically describe the fracture line but also offers some general guidelines for treatment and expectations for prognosis.

The *type I* injury is a simple fracture across the entire physis. The physis is not a perfectly flat surface, making these injuries more common in the younger age group where the physis tends to more planar. Prognosis is good with adequate reduction.

The *type II* injury is a failure through the plate with the line exiting through the metaphysis. This results in a small metaphyseal fragment remaining with the physeal segment. On x-ray the finding of the metaphyseal fragment is called Holland's sign. Frequently this is the only radiographic finding and should alert the physician that failure has occurred through the plate itself.

The *type III* injury involves failure vertically through the epiphysis with the fracture line exiting horizontally through the plate. This injury can be complicated by prema-

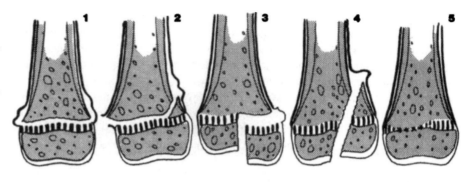

Figure 8–14. Illustration of Salter and Harris classification of epiphyseal injuries (see text). (From Salter RB, Harris WR: Injuries involving the epiphyseal plate. J Bone Joint Surg 45A: 587, 1963.)

ture physeal arrest of a portion of the growth plate. The juvenile Tillaux fracture is such an injury.

The *type IV* injury is characterized by a fracture line propagating vertically across the epiphysis, the physis, and the metaphysis. This injury is notorious for the late formation of a bony bar and the resultant tethering of the growth plate. Should this occur, angular deformity will result. The lateral condylar fracture of the humerus is such an injury.

The *type V* injury is the most subtle and yet the most dangerous. It has been described as a compression or crushing injury to the plate and is almost always complicated by partial or complete physeal arrest. The problem clinically with a type V injury is the initial negative radiograph. Only after physeal arrest has occurred is this injury diagnosed retrospectively.

There has been an addendum to the classification with the inclusion of thermal injuries to the plate. Some refer to these as type VI injuries.

In addition to the type of physeal fracture, other factors that impact on prognosis are the age of the patient at the time of the injury, the specific bone involved, the magnitude of displacement, and the appropriateness of treatment.

LONG BONE FRACTURES

Children have the unique ability to undergo extensive remodeling following long bone fractures. This is a function primarily of their periosteal anatomy and physiology. The periosteum of a child is richly vascular, significantly thick, and innately more osteogenic than that of the adult. As such, it bestows not only a degree of mechanical stability, but also a degree of active biologic potential. This potential is manifested by very early and frequently complete remodeling of the fracture. Not only do the fractures remodel significantly, but also their healing time is often shortened, because of this very active periosteum. By inference, it is uncommon to see a nonunion of a pediatric long bone fracture.

FRACTURE HEALING (Fig. 8–15)

The biology of fracture healing is not particularly complex. It parallels that of the healing of any other nonossified connective tissue. Essentially, fractures heal in three phases: a vascular phase, a metabolic phase, and a mechanical phase. These same three phases can be seen in skin, fascia, ligament, and other tissues of the human organism. What is unique about bone is not the phases of healing, but rather the end result of the ossification process, which results in this hard connective tissue.

The initial or *vascular phase* of healing begins at the time of insult and lasts for approximately 4 weeks, through the formation of a primary cellular (soft) callus. *Callus* by definition is a space-filling, space-bridging granulation tissue with the potential to form bone. At the time of fracture, a fracture hematoma is formed. There has been a great deal of research surrounding the role of this fracture hematoma. For many years, it was believed that the hematoma was actually a retardant to fracture healing and efforts were frequently made to aspirate this hematoma. Currently, it is safe to say that the hematoma is viewed as a favorable or trophic factor, needed for satisfactory fracture union. The microenvironmental changes that occur within this fracture hematoma appear to be important in the steps that follow. Initially, there is the synthesis of collagen in and around the hematoma, which results in the formation of a so-called organized hematoma. The primitive fibroblastic precursors appear to be responsible for the synthesis of this protein. Once the hematoma has become organized or collagenized, one can demonstrate small vascular twigs invading the margins of this hematoma. With the vascularization will subsequently be seen the differentiation of osteoblastic precursors. Ultimately, these osteoblastic cells begin to proliferate a very primitive form (woven) of bone. Once initial bone formation has begun, this mass of tissue can be viewed as the primary cellular (soft) callus.

The second or *metabolic phase* of fracture healing is initiated with the formation of the primary cellular callus and the subsequent differentiation and sophistication of this callus into a firmer, more mechanically sound hard callus. During this time, there are a number of chemical and electrical changes, which can be demonstrated within the callus. These not only stimulate osteoblastic proliferation and activity, but also modulate the areas within which bone is formed. The net result of this progressive, metabolically active phase is the formation of a hard mass of bony callus, which typically is defined in four regions about the fracture site. These four regions (Fig. 8–16) are referred to as bridging callus, buttressing callus, sealing callus, and uniting callus. The latter is the last completed and in most respects is the most important. For many long bone fractures, but certainly not for all, the metabolic phase is complete between 8 and 10 weeks after fracture.

The third or *mechanical phase* of fracture healing is initiated once the hard callus is formed. The duration of this phase is the longest, and terminates once the remodeling process has been completed. The age of the patient, the specific bone, and the overall health of the host are all factors that affect the rate of the mechanical phase of

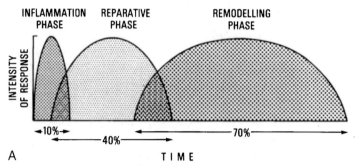

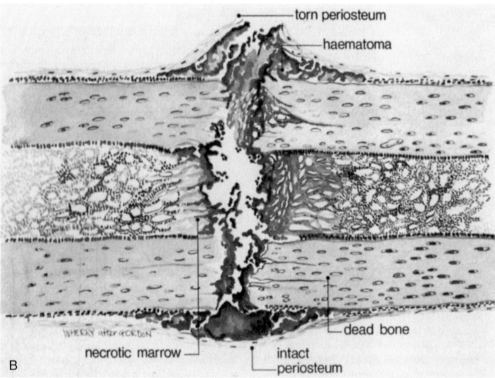

Figure 8–15. Phases of fracture healing. *A,* An approximation of the relative amounts of time devoted to inflammation, reparative, and remodeling phases in fracture healing. *B,* The initial events involved in fracture healing of long bone. The periosteum is torn opposite the point of impact and, in many instances, is intact on the other side. There is an accumulation of hematoma beneath the periosteum and between the fracture ends. There is necrotic marrow and dead bone close to the fracture line. (From Cruess RL: Healing of bone, tendon, and ligament. *In* Rockwood CA Jr, Green DP [eds]: Fractures in Adults, 2nd ed, Vol 1. Philadelphia, JB Lippincott, 1984, pp 148–150; reprinted by permission.)

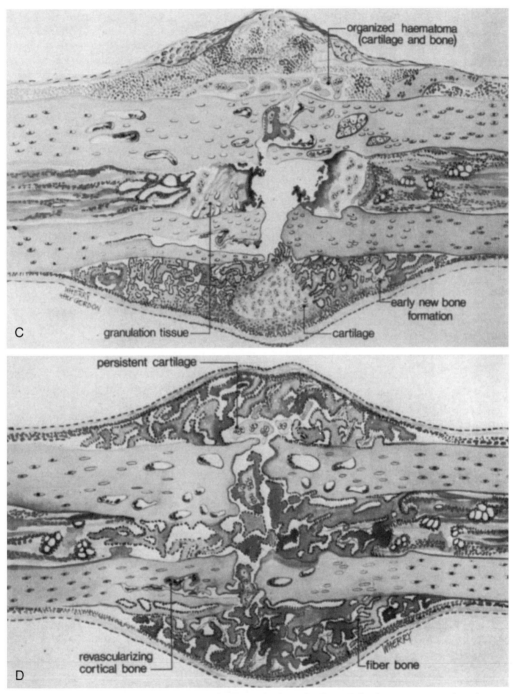

Figure 8–15 *Continued. C,* Early repair. There is organization of the hematoma, early primary new bone formation in subperiosteal regions, and cartilage formation in other areas. *D,* At a later stage in the repair, early immature fiber bone is bridging the fracture gap. Persistent cartilage is seen at points most distant from ingrowing capillary buds.

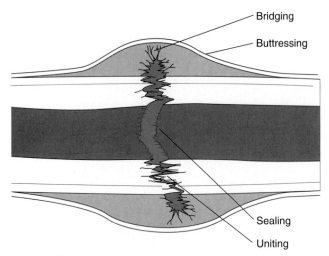

Figure 8–16. Regions of fracture callus.

healing. It is during this phase that Wolff's law is believed to be the primary factor. Wolff's law states that bone will be formed in the areas of need and will be resorbed where it is not required for mechanical demands. As with most of the "form follows function" rules, there are various signals that manipulate the hard callus. Extensive research has indicated that electrical signals are important in the callus to modulate the activity of various cell populations. Andrew Bassett, Carl Brighton, and others have been successful, not only in identifying the voltage gradients in the microenvironment, but also in using them clinically in an effort to manipulate the rate of fracture healing. It has been shown that in the areas of active fracture remodeling, both negative and positive potentials can be measured. Further, in the area of the negative pole, the aggregation of osteoblastic precursors has been demonstrated. Conversely, about the electropositive pole, osteoclastic cells can be seen. The external application of electrical currents has been demonstrated to be capable of manipulating these cell populations. Thus one is able to stimulate osteoblastic activity with the application of an electronegative field.

Once the mechanical phase of fracture healing has been completed, one can assume that the given bone is now mechanically sound and essentially restored to its pre-fracture integrity.

EVALUATION OF THE PATIENT WITH SKELETAL TRAUMA

Obviously, textbooks have been written on the subject of physical diagnosis and the surgical patient. There are, however, several specific points relative to the orthopaedic patient that are appropriate to highlight.

History of the Injury

As mentioned earlier, the mechanism of injury is extremely important in anticipating not the only the skeletal injury but also the associated soft tissue damage. The mode of application of force is frequently associated with a given type of injury. Frequently with a careful history, one can elicit whether the mechanism was bending, torsion, axial load, etc. This type of information can be invaluable in anticipating additional injury, as well as in planning treatment.

Occupation of the Patient

Frequently physicians tend to overlook the patient's occupation. For patients who have sustained skeletal trauma, this is particularly important. Restoring the patient to an active work status is frequently critical to the individual and his or her family. Therefore, it should be of great significance to the treating physician. It is important to know and to understand specifically what is required of the patient in the work place. The rigors of certain jobs may make it impossible to rapidly restore this patient to his or her previous occupation. On the other hand, aggressive rehabilitative and recuperative efforts may make return at the earliest time a reasonable goal.

Activity Level Prior to Injury

Many times, it becomes significant to be aware of the patient's activity level before a given injury is sustained. This is particularly important as it relates to the elderly patient who has sustained a significant musculoskeletal injury. The elderly woman who sustains a hip fracture and was marginally ambulatory in an assisted living facility prior to her injury is unlikely to achieve an activity level greater than this after her injury. Indeed, the injury may markedly decompensate an elderly individual who had been living "on the edge."

Documentation of Physical Findings

All too often in the heat of the trauma venue, important facts regarding the initial evaluation are not documented or not documented completely. Specifically, one needs to carefully document the presence and extent of any skin disruption in the involved extremity. Scrapes, abrasions, partial-thickness injuries, burns, and blisters, in addition to frank open wounds, should be recorded. Any partial or questionable abnormality in neural function must be recorded as well. The circulatory evaluation, as has been discussed previously, is critical if one is to avoid disastrous complications in this patient population. Failure to carefully examine and document these facts leaves the patient at greater risk for long-term disability and the physician at greater risk for legal liability.

PRINCIPLES OF FRACTURE MANAGEMENT

The goal in treating fractures and dislocations can be simply stated: first, *reduce* the fracture or dislocation; second, *maintain* that reduction until union has occurred. Despite these very simple and straightforward goals, there are many complex issues that complicate what might seem to be straightforward treatment algorithms.

In order to achieve a reduction of a fracture or a dislocation, one needs to correct the deformities that are present. These may be as simple as single plane displacement or as complex as multiplane rotational and angular deformities with associated joint subluxation. Careful radiographic evaluation, not only of the fracture, but also of the joint above and below, will allow the physician to carefully evaluate the injury and plan treatment. Special imaging studies may be required to completely assess the extent of the injury. It is imperative to emphasize the need for careful evaluation of the joint above and below a diaphyseal fracture. All too often, it is taken for granted that the obvious injury is isolated; diagnosis of associated articular injuries is therefore delayed. Should there be any question regarding position of the fracture or articulating anatomy, one should not hesitate to proceed with more advanced studies such CT and/or MRI scans.

Essentially, there are three ways in which a fracture can be reduced (Fig. 8–17). The first is closed manipulation, the second is surgical open reduction of the fracture and third is the application of traction. *Closed manipulative techniques* are as the name implies—the use of manually applied pressure to guide the bone ends into their pre-fracture position. Usually, this will necessitate increasing the deformity in an effort to unlock the fracture or disengage the fragments from a periosteal rent. Then reduction can frequently be completed. The techniques for reducing a joint dislocation are similarly based on the principles of disengagement of locked fragments and careful manual reduction of the articulating segments. It is generally uncommon that further damage is done at the time of closed reduction. Here again, it is important to carefully examine the patient, including the neurovascular status, before attempting any manipulation to reduce a fracture or dislocation.

Surgical open reduction is for the most part, in principle, straightforward. An incision over a fracture site allows the surgeon to access the injury and to reduce it under direct vision. Several fractures are amenable to an interim approach—that is, the closed manipulation of the fracture under fluoroscopic guidance and fixation of that fracture in a percutaneous mode. It goes without saying that surgical techniques should aim at reducing the fracture with the minimum of additional damage to the periosteum, bone, and other soft tissues.

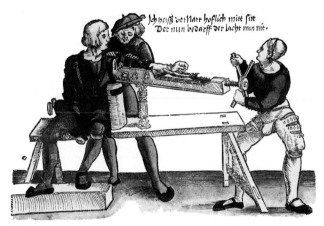

Figure 8–17.   Device used to reduce a dislocated shoulder in the Middle Ages. (From Lyons AS, Petrucelli RJ: Medicine: An Illustrated History. New York, Harry N Abrams, 1978, p 384.)

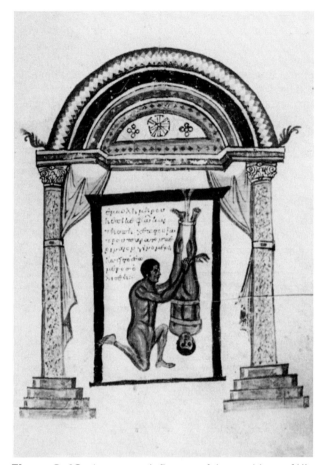

Figure 8–18.   Long-term influence of the teachings of Hippocrates (in this case, reducing a dislocation of the knee), seen in an 11th-century Byzantine copy of a century codex, Commentaries of Apollonios on the Peri arthron of Hippocrates. Medicea-Laurenziana, Florence. (From Lyons AS, Petrucelli RJ: Medicine: An Illustrated History. New York, Harry N Abrams, 1978, p 384.)

Lastly, the application of *traction,* whether skin or skeletal, is an age-old mechanism for the reduction of fractures and dislocations. Historically, many "unique" devices have been used in this effort. Longitudinal traction has been used for centuries in an effort to line up long bone fractures and "pull into place" dislocated joints (Fig. 8–18). Currently there are still traction protocols, which are more than appropriate for certain injuries. Traction can be applied through the skin using various adhesive bandages, as a point of attachment to the limb. Obviously, one is limited in the amount of weight that can be applied. Therefore, skeletal traction is far more efficient in the definitive management of fractures. The use of a K-wire (with a tensioning bow) or a Steinmann pin will allow fixation to the skeleton providing a point of attachment for the traction weight. In the current managed care environment, the use of traction with the requisite hospital stay has been disappearing from the armamentarium of treatment protocols. This, however, does not make these techniques any less appropriate or effective in fracture management.

Once the fracture has been reduced, it is essential that the reduction be maintained. Reduction without maintenance is only half of the battle fought. *Maintenance* of fracture reduction is clearly an important step in the management of any injury. Techniques for fracture maintenance include the application of external devices such as casts, splints, braces, and external fixators. The use of internal fixation devices continues to increase in popularity. Lastly, continuation of traction permits maintenance of a reduction previously achieved. The choice of immobilization devices frequently is quite obvious. For example, once one achieves the reduction of a distal radial fracture by closed manipulation, the use of a cast or external fixator usually follows. If one were to perform an open reduction of both bones of the forearm, typically one would fix these fractures with an internal fixation device. If traction had been used to achieve the reduction, continuation of the traction is often considered to maintain it.

The application of casts is an age-old technique for the maintenance of fracture reduction. Despite increasing sophistication of the materials used, the principles of cast application remain largely unchanged. The immobilization of the joint below and the joint above the fracture has been taught for years. Molding the cast in the area of the fracture site to achieve three-point fixation typically ensures one of a decreased risk of fracture displacement. The importance of recognizing the dangers of a cast cannot be overemphasized. Casts that are too tight, that are poorly molded, that have creases or that have been inappropriately wedged can create more problems than they solve. They can intensify an impending compartment syndrome. They can cause neural damage and skin damage as well. The risk of developing deep vein phlebitis should not be underestimated. Despite the increasing use of internal fixation devices, appropriate casting technique is an art that cannot be sacrificed.

The external fixator is a technique that has been employed for many years. Originally, these devices were popular tools of veterinary medicine. Their success in animals led to their use in humans. The use of pins, above and below the fracture site as fixation points for the externally applied frame, has been an important advance in the armamentarium of the trauma surgeon. Despite controversy surrounding the rigidity of these frames and its significance to fracture healing, the principles governing their use have been a constant. The problem of pin track sepsis has discouraged some from using these devices. Should the pin track become infected, it is usually due to skin sealing around the pin. This results in shear damage to the skin with subsequent sepsis. Frequently this is simply treated by merely opening the skin around the pin and applying local care. Should the drainage persist, removal and exchange of the pin would be necessary. The duration of fixator use and the post-fixator management of a given fracture are largely functions of the specific fracture and the practice of the individual surgeon.

Internal fixation devices continue to grow in popularity. This has been driven by numerous factors. First are improved anesthetic techniques; second, the improved use of prophylactic and therapeutic antibiotics; third, the sophisticated maketing of these implants over 20 to 30 years; and lastly, and sadly, the need to rapidly treat patients in an effort to decrease hospital time and thereby decrease cost. It is probably fair to say that the use of internal devices

has indeed shortened hospital stays; in addition, it has improved patient mobility in the post-fracture period and has allowed easier rehabilitation of the overall extremity. However, they are not without their complications; specifically, infection and implant failure are two of the most notable. The internal fixation devices in general use are for the most part fabricated from stainless steel. This not only moderates the cost of the device but also usually allows for some level of plastic deformation prior to failure. In general, ductility (ability to deform plastically) is desirable in a fracture fixation implant. Therefore, titanium is a less desirable choice in many surgeons' minds. Titanium alloys, despite high yielding strengths, have poor ductility.

BIOMECHANICS OF INTERNAL FIXATION DEVICES

The Screw (Fig. 8–19)

The screw certainly is the most common implant in current use. Mechanically, this device converts a torsional load into an axial compressive load. As the screw is tightened, the head advances to the bony cortex; once in contact, further tightening tends to create compression between bony fragments. Despite multiple different head designs and thread designs, it is the root diameter (the narrowest diameter of the threaded portion) and the root area of the tapped thread that determine the ultimate strength of the screw. Most screws tend to fail owing to pull-out, although occasionally breakage can cause failure. As stated, the single most important determinant of the pull-out resistance is the root area of the tapped hole. Essentially, this represents the area of bony contact with the threads, and as one would naturally expect, the greater the area of contact, the greater the resistance to pull-out.

Screws have been used in many different applications. The most rudimentary of these is as an interfragmentary screw fixing two bony fragments together. The other common application is for fixation of a plate to the bone.

Plates

The use of bone plates similarly has a long history in the management of fractures. The use of various metallic devices, which one could loosely call plates, were used as early as the mid-1800s. Because of the primitive metals and poor surgical techniques, most of these were abysmal failures. As techniques became more sophisticated, the use of plates became more widespread and at the present time these implants are very popular in fracture fixation. The role of this device is to transmit the force from one end of the bone to the other, thereby bypassing the fracture site. Thus, the fracture is protected from load application. The more basic role of the plate is to maintain proper alignment of the fragments throughout the healing process. From a mechanical standpoint, plates are of four basic types:

1. *Neutralization plates.* Essentially, these plates act as a bridge, transmitting forces from one bone fragment to the other and bypassing the fracture site, thus "neutralizing" the load.

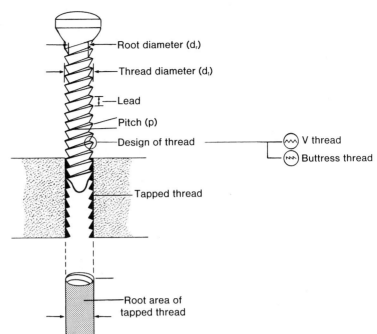

Figure 8–19. Design parameters of the orthopedic bone screw. (From Gozna ER, Harrington IJ: Biomechanics of Musculoskeletal Injury. Baltimore, Williams & Wilkins, 1982.)

2. *Compression plates* (Fig. 8–20). Through the use of several devices, both external and internal to the plate itself, these plates can be used to achieve compression of the fracture site. As previously noted, compression is believed to have a positive osteogenic effect as a result of the electrical stimulation of osteogenic precursors. Therefore, this technique itself can act as a stimulus to bone healing.

3. *Buttress plates* (Fig. 8–21). This plating technique is designed primarily for the management of metaphyseal fractures. They "shore up" (buttress) a metaphyseal segment from collapsing due to superimposed shear load.

4. *Condylar plates.* These plates are particularly appropriate for use in the treatment of intra-articular fractures, especially about the knee joint.

It is important to appreciate that plates, by their nature, are *load-bearing* devices. That means, by their design, they transmit the forces past the fracture site and carry the load within the plate itself. This spares the fracture site from "feeling the load." As a natural sequela of this fact, the fracture itself will not undergo complete mechanical remodeling until the plate has been removed. This phenomenon is referred to as *stress shielding.* This disadvantage of plates has frequently encouraged surgeons to opt for another choice when one is available for internal fixation.

Intramedullary Rods

A number of intramedullary rods have been designed over the years to fix fractures by creating an interference fit in the medullary canal. Both flexible and rigid rods are currently available for these applications. In general, the flexible rods achieve fixation by "stuffing the canal" with multiple implants. The older Rush rod and newer Enders rods are examples of this type of design. As noted, they achieve fixation by filling the canal and to a lesser degree creating an element of three-point fixation.

More popular are the solitary rigid rods that fix the fracture in two ways. First, they create an interference fit in the canal, especially at the narrowest region (isthmus).

Figure 8–20. Three methods of producing compression plate fixation. (Reprinted with permission from M. E. Müller, M. Allgöwer, H. Willeneger: Manual of Internal Fixation. Berlin, Springer-Verlag, 1970.)

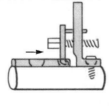

TENSIONING DEVICE

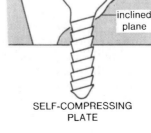

SELF-COMPRESSING PLATE

ECCENTRIC SCREW PLACEMENT

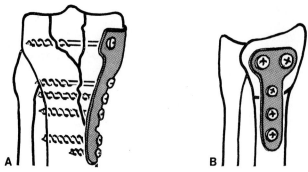

Figure 8–21. Buttress or "T" plates for tibial plateau fractures *(A)* or distal radius fractures *(B)*. (From Gozna ER, Harrington IJ: Biomechanics of Musculoskeletal Injury. Baltimore, Williams & Wilkins, 1982.)

Second, the use of proximal and distal locking screws adds to the fixation (Fig. 8–22). The sophistication of current intramedullary devices allows them to be used in a multiplicity of applications. Previously, certain fractures were not appropriate for rod fixation. The presence of severe comminution, segmental fractures, long bone fractures in the meta-diaphyseal region, and fractures with significant bone loss were all poor candidates for rod use. At the present time with improved metallurgy and improved design, as well as improved proximal and distal fixation, virtually all of these are amenable to rod management. The great benefit of the intramedullary rod is that it can usually be placed in a "closed" fashion. This has markedly decreased the risk of postoperative sepsis. The other perceived advantage is the fact that intramedullary rods for the most part are said to be *load-sharing* devices. Unlike the plate, which completely unloads the bone, the rod allows the bone to "feel" some of the applied loads. In doing so, the bone can progress well into the third stage of fracture healing, without the negative effect of stress shielding. Obviously, like all internal fixation devices, rods are not without their complications. "Technical misadven-

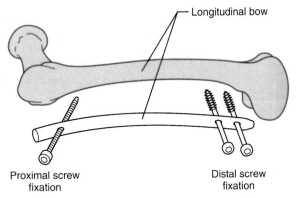

Longitudinal bow

Proximal screw
fixation

Distal screw
fixation

Figure 8–22. Basic anatomy of an intramedullary nail. The proximal end has an internally threaded opening for adaptation of driver/extractor instrumentation. It has a longitudinal bow that approximates that of the femur. Proximal and distal screw holes are placed in the nail for interlocking fixation. (From Browner BD, Jupiter JB, Levine AM, Trafton PG: Skeletal Trauma, 2nd ed, Vol 1. Philadelphia, WB Saunders, 1998.)

tures," such as further comminution of the fracture, incarceration of the rod and increase in the fracture deformity, are all issues to be considered. Late complications such as infections and rod breakage also can occur.

In summary, the use of internal fixation devices has clearly revolutionized the practice of orthopaedic trauma surgery. They have shortened the hospital stay, improved the overall rehabilitation of the limb, and decreased the disability time for the patient.

ORTHOPAEDIC EMERGENCIES

There are relatively few orthopaedic problems that mandate immediate intervention. However, those that do exist truly represent emergent situations. Specifically, these injuries are fractures and dislocations associated with vascular injury, dislocations of major joints, and open fractures.

Injuries associated with *vascular trauma* have been discussed earlier in this section. Clearly, it goes without saying that interruption of the blood supply in a limb, resulting from either a compartment syndrome or direct arterial trauma, mandates urgent intervention. Consultation with vascular surgeons and other professionals skilled in the area of managing vascular injury is appropriate in these situations. Noninvasive and invasive studies are usually mandatory to clearly define the specific injury in question and subsequently guide treatment.

Dislocations of major joints usually mandate early treatment for several specific reasons. First and perhaps foremost is the pain associated with these injuries. The traumatic alteration in the articulating anatomy of a major joint produces severe levels of pain. This is in part due to bleeding within the capsule; the resulting stretching of the capsular ligaments causes stimulation of the pain and pressure endings in these structures. In joints, such as the hip and shoulder, there is the added risk of avascular necrosis of the femoral and humeral head, respectively. Owing to bleeding within the joint and subsequent tamponade of retinacular vessels, it is easy to appreciate the paucity of blood flow to these bony structures. It is probably fair to say that hip dislocations left untreated for over 12 hours are complicated by avascular necrosis of the femoral head in numbers approaching 100%. Although it is true that perhaps the avascular necrosis may be spotty in the femoral head, it is also reasonable to assume that even without full head involvement, significant late degenerative disease can usually be anticipated. Similarly, dislocations of major joints can cause traction injuries to adjacent nerves. The reversibility of those injuries may well be a function of the duration of the dislocation. Specifically, stretch palsy of the ulnar nerve associated with elbow dislocations may be irreversible if the dislocation is not reduced promptly.

Open fractures are the third orthopaedic emergency. By definition, any fracture or dislocation, associated with an overlying disruption of the skin and soft tissue envelope, constitutes an open fracture or dislocation. It is imperative to recognize that this need not be a large gaping wound. A small puncture wound, suggesting penetration of the skin from a bony spicule, is more than adequate to signal an open fracture. Indeed, many of these small, relatively unassuming wounds are far more dangerous than large ones. This is of course because they are frequently underdiagnosed, underestimated, and/or undertreated. One must keep in mind that approximately a third of the patients who have sustained an open fracture are polytrauma victims. Therefore, multisystem injury must be considered. Despite the orthopaedic surgeon's desire to treat the open fracture in a timely fashion, it is far more important to be cognizant of other injuries and deal with them appropriately before the patient is taken to the operating room.

Open fractures have been classified by a number of different authors. Far and away the most commonly used classification scheme for open fractures is that of Ramon Gustilo. Although no classification can truly describe the extent of the skin and associated soft tissue injury, this one most closely approximates the need to do just that. Gustilo's three major categories are as follows:

Type 1 open fracture is typified by a puncture wound of 1 cm or less. It is also assumed that this wound is relatively clean and most likely was the result of a bony spike causing the wound "from within, out."

Type 2 open fracture is characterized by a wound greater than 1 cm in length. Also, minimal soft tissue damage adjacent to that wound is assumed.

Type 3 open fracture is a complex group (Fig. 8–23). Owing to the need to more carefully assess the associated soft tissue damage, this group has been further subdivided. These subtypes permit more exact analysis of these usually extensive injuries.

- *Subgroup 3A*: Fracture with extensive soft tissue damage without soft tissue loss or degloving.
- *Subgroup 3B*: Fracture with extensive soft tissue loss and degloving. Massive periosteal stripping and bone exposure is characteristic.
- *Subgroup 3C*: Fracture with associated arterial injury requiring repair. The amount of soft tissue damage is irrelevant in this group.

This classification is the frame of reference for many current articles on open fractures and has become essentially the standard in the reporting of such injuries. It is also worthy of note that some specific types of injuries, owing to their very nature and the magnitude of energy required to create them, are immediately classified as type 3. Some examples of this are open segmental fractures, such as those resulting from high-speed vehicular trauma, gunshot wounds as well as high-velocity missile wounds such as war wounds, and injuries that occur in a hostile environment, such as those occurring in contaminated water and those occurring in the barnyard. Despite the magnitude of the open wound, these should all be considered as type 3 injuries and treated appropriately.

Obviously, the concern with open fractures is the contamination of the wound resulting from the injury. At the time of injury, all of these wounds are contaminated by local bacteria. It is exactly this fact that mandates emergent management of these injuries. The goal of this management is to adequately cleanse and debride the wound in a effort to prevent the conversion of this contaminated wound into an infected wound. This difference, although subtle, is absolutely critical in the successful management of these injuries. Once the wound has become infected (that is,

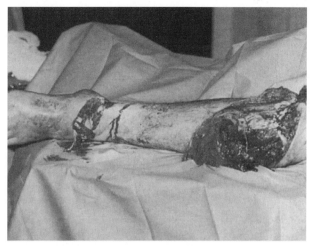

Figure 8–23. Type III B open fracture. Note massive soft tissue loss and evidence of degloving. (From Browner BD, Jupiter JB, Levine AM, Trafton PG: Skeletal Trauma, 2nd ed, Vol 1. Philadelphia, WB Saunders, 1998.)

once there is the presence of replicating bacteria), it is far more difficult to ultimately eradicate those organisms from the host.

Principles of Open Fracture Management

First, to restate the obvious, it is critical to recognize an open fracture and recognize that an open fracture is a surgical emergency. Second, complete evaluation for other life-threatening injuries is mandatory. Once this has been accomplished, the patient can safely be taken to the operating room for aggressive *irrigation and debridement* of the wound (Fig. 8–24). The importance of thorough wound cleansing cannot be overemphasized. All too often, the naive surgeon errs in the belief that an inadequately debrided wound can be compensated for by aggressive antibiotic administration. This is a blunder of monumental proportions and one that must be avoided at all costs.

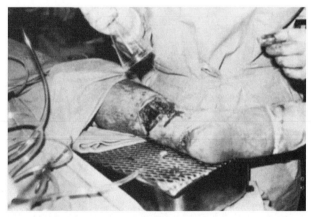

Figure 8–24. Adequate debridement of devitalized tissues, removal of foreign bodies, and copious irrigation are done with the aid of jet lavage, particularly in type II and type III open fractures. (From Gustilo RB, Gruninger RP, Tsukayama RT: Orthopaedic Infection: Diagnosis and Treatment. Philadelphia, WB Saunders, 1989, p 96.)

Aggressive and meticulous wound care is the sine qua non in the management of open fractures. Removal of all dead and devitalized tissue including muscle, fascia, skin, and bone fragments is required to remove all potential substrate for bacterial growth. If, after the initial debridement, there is uncertainty as to tissue viability, there is certainly no shame in returning the patient to the operating room for subsequent repeated debridements. Once the surgeon is convinced that the wound is meticulously clean, coverage should be the next priority. Obviously, the extent of soft tissue loss will dictate the type of coverage required. Whether this be delayed primary closure, healing by secondary intention, or the need for flaps, the ultimate goal is to achieve wound coverage. Chapter 14 more specifically addresses these issues.

The timing of *wound culture* has become somewhat controversial. Previously, Michael Patzakis indicated a high correlation (60%) between initial emergency room cultures and subsequent organisms retrieved. At the present time, these numbers are not believed to be valid. The use of prophylactic antibiotics as well as newer techniques of wound and bone management has altered the correlative relationship, making initial wound culture often misleading. Therefore, initial cultures are generally taken either just prior to debridement or, as recommended by many trauma surgeons, following complete debridement of the wound. It is probably fair to say that it is the post-debridement cultures that are the most critical in the management of these traumatized extremities.

Once adequate wound control has been achieved and appropriate antibiotics selected and delivered, stabilization of the fracture site itself is the next priority. Frequently this can be done at the time of wound management. However, depending on the type of open fracture, it may be necessary to either delay fracture management or alter the type of immobilization technique employed. In type 1 and type 2 open fractures, current recommendations are to employ the same techniques for fixation and immobilization that one would employ had that fracture been closed. However, in the presence of extensive soft tissue injury or complex fracture patterns, which constitute the type 3 group, it is usually necessary to alter the type of fixation and immobilization one chooses to employ. One such example of this principle is the use of intramedullary rods. It is a well-known fact that the cortex of a long bone receives its blood supply both from the periosteal arterial bed and the endosteal arterial bed. Rhinelander has shown that the outer third of the cortex receives its supply from the periosteum, whereas the inner two thirds of the cortex receives its supply from the endosteal or medullary bed. With extensive soft tissue stripping, it is typical for the periosteal supply to be ripped from the outer cortex. In that event, the current trend is to use an unreamed intramedullary rod for long bone fractures. The thought is that use of a reamed rod would further devascularize the cortex by reaming out the medullary blood supply, thereby markedly stunting any attempt of the fracture to heal. The decision to use an unreamed rod in a type 3 open fracture is predicated on a biologic mandate. The tradeoff in this situation is the sacrifice of device strength. The use of a reamed rod would ordinarily allow for the insertion of a larger device, thereby improving its torsional rigidity. In addition to intramedullary rods, the use of external fixators (Fig. 8–25) has a special place in the management of severe open fractures. Frequently, they can be employed to achieve adequate fixation in the face of severe soft tissue loss.

The use of prophylactic antibiotics is now the norm in the presence of open fractures. Since the most likely organism to complicate these injuries is *Staphylococcus aureus* as well as other gram-positive cocci, it is imperative that the agent chosen provide adequate coverage for these organisms. In general a semisynthetic penicillin or first-generation cephalosporin is chosen as the prophylactic agent for type 1 open fractures. With an extension of the soft tissue damage and the increased risk of other bacterial contaminants, additional agents may be added. For example, many recommend the use of two agents—one to cover gram-positive cocci and the other to cover gram-negative rods when dealing with a type 2 open fracture. Logically,

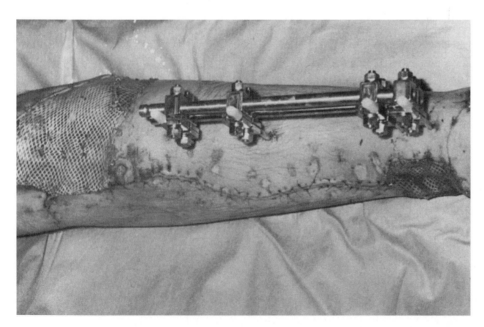

Figure 8–25. A rigid double-bar anterior external fixator maintains fixation of an open tibial fracture. (From Browner BD, Jupiter JB, Levine AM, Trafton PG: Skeletal Trauma, 2nd ed, Vol 1. Philadelphia, WB Saunders, 1998.)

many then choose a third antibiotic to cover anaerobes in the face of a type III open fracture.

The aggressive and appropriate management of open fractures has dramatically decreased the morbidity that used to be seen in the face of these injuries. The use of meticulous wound toilet, fracture stabilization, appropriate wound coverage, and prophylactic antibiotics has dramatically improved the prognosis for open fracture.

COMPLICATIONS OF FRACTURES

As with any other disease of the musculoskeletal system, trauma can be complicated by a number of different events. Some of these are the result of the injury itself; others are unfortunately the result of the treatment. In any event, it is critical to be cognizant of these complications, to anticipate their potential occurrence, and to be comfortable with their management.

Problems of Union

Perhaps the most basic issue surrounding fracture management is the primary goal: to get the fracture to heal. Problems related to healing of a fracture are therefore the most basic to be considered.

MALUNION

In malunion, the fracture has healed but the position is unacceptable. Most authors define unacceptable position as one that is inappropriate for normal limb function; however, there are some who more rigorously define it as any position other than anatomic. Clearly, there are many fractures allowed to heal in other than anatomic position. The best example is the clavicle, where overriding, frequently allowed to remain, does not compromise normal function. Therefore, most would not define this as a malunion. Conversely, a tibial fracture allowed to heal with 90 degrees of rotation is clearly a functional deficit for the patient, hence a malunion.

DELAYED UNION

Fractures heal at a specific rate. This is largely determined by the specific bone in question. Associated soft tissue damage will play a role. The use of the terms "delayed union" implies that a fracture has failed to heal in this statistically acceptable time frame. Many delayed unions will usually heal if more time is allowed to pass. It is important to mention the terms *clinical union* and *radiographic union*. Most fractures are treated on the basis of clinical union. This implies no tenderness and no false motion at the fracture site. Radiographs should show adequate bridging and uniting callus to suggest progress toward union. Radiographic union, on the other hand, implies that the fracture has completed the mechanical stage of healing. The radiographic changes are mature and no further changes are expected. Obviously, this takes significantly longer to achieve than clinical union.

NONUNION

Fractures that have not healed and additionally have lost their biologic potential to do so are referred to as non-unions. The use of the term not only indicates that the fracture remains un-united, but also more importantly, connotes a fracture that is unable to do so. The implications of the term are far reaching. Once the decision has been made that a given fracture has reached the point of nonunion, one is essentially indicating that the microenvironment around the fracture is "impotent." If that is the case, biologic stimulation of this microenvironment will be required to reinitiate the healing process.

Over the years, many factors have been implicated in the causation of a nonunion. These include excessive motion due to poor immobilization, infection, steroid administration, ionizing radiation, malnutrition, and local devascularization as a result of soft tissue stripping.

Typically, two types of nonunions are described:

- *Atrophic* nonunion is characterized by the interposition of fibrous tissue between the bone ends.
- *Hypertrophic* nonunion (Fig. 8–26) is typified by the presence of overexuberant callus, dominated by cartilage, with poor progression to union. A specific type of hypertrophic nonunion is the synovial pseudoarthrosis. In this extreme case, not only is there abundant cartilaginous callus, but also there is a cleft between the bone ends. This space is filled with fluid, giving the nonunion the appearance of a "false joint" (pseudoarthrosis).

The *diagnosis of a nonunion* is not always easy. The most objective criterion used by the majority of observers is the failure to see radiographic progression on three sequential x-rays, taken 1 month apart. Occasionally, equivocal changes may make longer follow-up necessary. Few generalizations are possible regarding specific times required for the development of a nonunion.

Once it has been clinically and radiographically determined that a nonunion exists, the treatment is specific to the anatomic site. Some generalizations regarding management are possible. First, an effort should be made to determine the cause of the nonunion: infection, extensive strip-

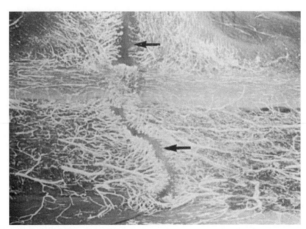

Figure 8–26. Microangiogram of a 6-week-old canine radial fracture. There is tremendous increase in vascularity, and the capillaries are unable to penetrate the interposed fibrocartilage *(arrows)* of this hypertrophic delayed union. (From Rhinelander FW: J Bone Joint Surg 50A:78, 1968.)

ping, etc. Stabilization of the fragments is usually required; this most often indicates the use of internal fixation devices. Anatomic site dictates the type of device used. Some do well with a plate, such as the humerus, whereas others show better results with rod fixation. Biologic stimulation of the microenvironment is required to promote healing. The indolent milieu that exists should not be expected to respond merely to the application of an internal fixation device.

Various techniques are available for biologic stimulation. The use of autogenous bone graft is by far the classic (Table 8–2). The success of autogenous graft is the standard to which other methods are compared. Success rates using this material are usually quoted to be in the 80% range. Autogenous bone graft is both osteoinductive and osteoconductive. Inductive phenomena are largely the result of bioactive substances transferred in the graft material, such as bone morphogenic protein (BMP). Few living osteogenic cells survive the transplant, again emphasizing the significance of these inductive substances. The osteoconductive role implies the ability of the grafted bone to function as a template or lattice upon which new bone can form (creeping substitution).

In the late 1970s, the use of electrical current in various forms was popular to stimulate bone healing. The creation of an electronegative field favors the differentiation of bone formative cells. The practical way in which these fields have been created has not always been overwhelmingly successful. Commercial devices such as transcutaneous electrodes (with battery pack) or implantable electrodes were used with varying results. At the present time, electromagnetic induction coils applied externally are the only technique that seems to have survived into the 1990s and beyond.

Currently, there is a huge interest in the development of *alternatives to bone graft.* Many centers are working furiously to develop options for the stimulation of this microenvironment. Because of the relative paucity of available autogenous material, especially in children, there is clearly a need for bone inductive substances. It must be remembered that cancellous (as opposed to cortical) autograft will remain the standard. Cortical autograft, although conductive, is not nearly as effective as an inductive material.

Perhaps the most obvious substitute is fresh-frozen or freeze-dried *allograft* material. Obviously, the former is problematic from the standpoint of disease transmission. The freeze-drying techniques do decrease this risk but do not alter the antigenicity of the material.

Table 8–2. Properties of autologous bone grafts

Property	Cancellous	Nonvascularized Cortical	Vascularized Cortical
Osteoconduction	+ + + +	+	+
Osteoinduction	+ +	?	?
Osteoprogenitor cells	+ + +	—	+
Immediate strength	—	+ + +	+ + +
Strength at 6 months	+ +	+ +	+ + +
Strength at 1 year	+ + +	+ + +	+ + + +

Source: © 1995 American Academy of Orthopaedic Surgeons. Reprinted from the Journal of the American Academy of Orthopaedic Surgeons: A Comprehensive Review, Volume 3 (1), p. 2, with permission.

Ceramic materials, both naturally occurring and synthetic, are commercially available as a bone substitute. These are calcium phosphate compounds similar in structure to calcium hydroxyapatite. They are available as granular particles as well as in block form. Currently, they are popular as bone substitutes in nonunion surgery as well as replacements for bone defects. Unfortunately, their mechanical weakness tends to be a factor limiting their use. The resorption of these materials and the replacement with host bone is the hoped-for end result.

Demineralized bone matrix has come on the market as a bone substitute. This material is a combination of noncollagenous proteins, bone growth factors, and collagen, which has been extracted from bone. The currently available material is packaged in a syringe, making it possible to apply the material much like a caulk. Again, indications include bone defects and nonunion surgery.

Bone marrow is an extremely rich source of osteoprogenitor cells. The aspiration of marrow is easily accomplished at the time of surgery without violating the iliac crest. It can be used alone or in combination with other material, such as ceramics, to fill defects or stimulate a nonunion site. Currently, the use of marrow is receiving a great deal of attention, since there is little morbidity encountered in its harvest or use. Combined with a ceramic, it becomes a composite graft, i.e., a combination designed to achieve both inductive and conductive effects.

Lastly, the purification and commercial use of *bone morphogenic protein (BMP)* is now in the investigational stages. The protein itself has been characterized for many years, largely the result of the work of Marshall Urist. Its ready availability and generalized use have yet to be realized. Early data are very encouraging.

Nonunions are frequently one of the most challenging problems in orthopaedic surgery. The failure of a fracture to heal will frequently require multiple trips to the operating room, challenging patient and surgeon alike.

Stiffness and Loss of Motion

These complications are unfortunately are all too common following fracture treatment. Limited joint motion may have many causes. Perhaps the most common is the formation of intra-articular scar tissue. This can result from the fracture itself, if intra-articular, or simply from the immobilization. This scarring is referred to as arthrofibrosis.

Intra-articular bone fragments can also block motion. Loose bodies can result from a displaced osteochondritis dissecans, a fragment of meniscus, or fractured osteophyte. Poorly reduced intra-articular fractures and resultant post-traumatic osteoarthritis clearly will restrict motion. It is critical for successful management of extremity trauma that restricted joint motion be avoided.

Infection

Through the mid-1950s, infection following open fracture was the most common cause of nonunions. With the advent of generalized antibiotic use, this is no longer the case. Nonetheless, infection can still complicate open fractures. Perhaps more important are the infections that complicate the operative treatment of closed fractures. The widespread use of internal fixation devices has clearly increased the incidence of postoperative infection. Obviously, the implant itself is not the cause of the infection. Rather, the implant acts as any other foreign substrate, providing a surface for adhesion of microorganisms (Fig. 8–27). These microorganisms, to a variable degree, are capable of excreting a protein polysaccharide coat around their microcolonies. This is referred to as the *glycocalyx*. This membrane is key to the discussion of implant sepsis. It not only makes it difficult to eradicate the infection from the surface of the implant by restricting antibiotic penetration, but it also makes retrieval and identification of the causative organism difficult. In addition, the presence of variable amounts of necrotic bone provide additional substrate for microbial growth.

Myositis Ossificans

The development of heterotopic ossification following fractures and soft tissue injuries is well known. Several specific sites are predisposed: the quadriceps muscle, the brachialis muscle, and the abductors of the hip. The bone formation is hamartomatous in nature. Criteria for removal are based on the determination of the maturity of heterotopic bone. Generally, it is best to wait at least 1 year from onset. In addition, a cold bone scan and mature x-ray are best awaited prior to excision. Premature excision is usually complicated by massive recurrence.

Implant Failure

Obviously, the ever-increasing popularity of fracture fixation devices accounts for the increasing incidence of implant failure. All too often, one makes the mistake of believing that an implant can substitute for an ununited fracture. Nothing could be further from the truth. Clearly, there is a race between fracture healing and implant failure. The fracture fixation device is only an internal splint. It is not designed to replace the bone. Implants fail primarily as a result of fatigue. Should one attribute too significant a role to the device, one is likely to be faced with the challenge of salvaging a failed implant.

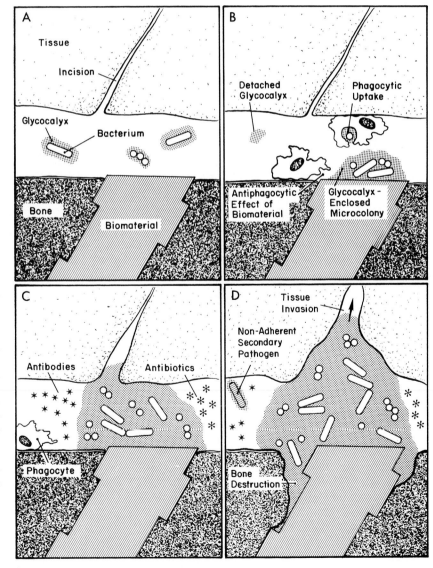

Figure 8–27. Diagrammatic evolution of a cryptic infection associated with a prosthetic biomaterial. Initially, bacteria are introduced into the wound *(A)*, and they express their natural tendency to adhere *(B)* to an inert surface, on which they are protected by the antiphagocytic effect of the biomaterial and on which they form as microcolonies within a biofilm that protects them from phagocytic uptake and from nonimmune antibacterial serum factors. When the bacterial microcolony has burgeoned to a greater size *(C)*, the ion-exchange function of its glycocalyx affords a measure of protection from antibiotics and appears to protect the bacteria from both bactericidal and opsonizing antibodies. In the later stages of this infection *(D)*, the pathogens may cause destruction of bone and other tissue changes, and the colonies may shed secondary pathogens that, being for some reason less adherent, are not necessarily representative in numbers or types or pathogenicity of the adherent colonies and may therefore confuse the diagnostic picture by dominating aspirates and other routine microbiologic samples. (From Gristina AG, Costerton JW: Bacterial adherence and the glycocalyx and their role in musculoskeletal infection. Orthop Clin North Am 15(3):528, 1984.)

Avascular Necrosis

Certain specific fractures are classically associated with this complication. Necrosis of the femoral head following femoral neck fracture, necrosis of the dome of the talus following fracture of the neck, and necrosis of the proximal pole of the scaphoid following fracture of the waist are all well recognized. The common thread seen in these injuries is the unique blood flow to the necrotic segment. Each of the fragments that becomes necrotic is supplied in a retrograde fashion, i.e., from distal to proximal. At the time of fracture, these segments are isolated from their normal circulation with the tragic consequence of a collapsing fragment of necrotic bone.

Reflex Sympathetic Dystrophy

This is an active, progressive, sympathetic mediated pain syndrome. It is characterized by severe pain, edema, and autonomic dysfunction. Although described in the hip and about the knee, it most frequently is seen following trivial trauma to the hand or foot. Even though psychological factors are usually implicated, the physiologic manifestations are obvious.

The exact mechanism of the abnormal sympathetic response is unknown. Injury activates an abnormal oscillation between increased sympathetic outflow, alternating with decreased sympathetic tone. Waves of vasoconstriction frequently alternate with periods of vasodilation. Abnormal feedback mechanisms have been described, and an atypical sympathetic reflex results. It is not unusual to see decreased bone density on the x-ray of the involved part. This is referred to as Sudeck's atrophy. In addition to the exquisite pain, clinically one sees mottled discoloration, hyperhydrosis, edema, stiffness, thermal sensitivity, and autonomic dysfunction. The treatment of this bizarre syndrome is difficult at best. Early recognition is key. Pulsed steroids, nonsteroidal anti-inflammatory drugs, occupational and physical therapy, intermittent splinting, relaxation techniques, mood modifying drugs, alpha blockers, and sympathetic interruption have all been employed with varying success. Early psychological evaluation and referral to a pain clinic can frequently obviate an otherwise very protracted course. The prognosis for these patients is guarded at best. Success hinges on early recognition and very aggressive management.

SUMMARY

The management of fractures and dislocations is the cornerstone of orthopaedic surgery. Reduction and immobilization techniques were known in antiquity. Knowledge has expanded rapidly over the years, often fueled by the sad lessons learned during wartime. New fixation devices, new surgical approaches, new antibiotics, and a rapidly progressing knowledge of the way bones heal appear to make the future promising. However sophisticated our current approaches seem to be, we must remember that we are still learning. Most of our present miracles are doomed to antiquity.

Selected Readings

Rhinelander F: Tibial blood supply in relation to fracture healing. Clin Orthop 1974;105:34–81.
    The classic article defining blood supply in diaphyseal bone. The injection studies have formed the basis for subsequent work, examining the changes that occur in cortical bone after fracture.
Salter R: Injuries involving the epiphyseal plate. J Bone Joint Surg 1963;45A:587–622.
    This article is the classic original description of a classification that has endured for almost 40 years. In addition, it provides information regarding the prognosis of these physeal injuries. A "must" read for orthopaedic residents.
Gazdag A: Alternatives to autogenous bone graft: Efficiency and indications. J Am Acad Ortho Surg 1995;3:1–8.
    Excellent review of the subject. This field is changing rapidly and current concepts reviews such as this assist in updating knowledge.
Frymoyer J: Multiple trauma: Pathophysiology and management. In Orthopaedic Knowledge Update, 4th ed. American Academy of Orthopaedic Surgery, 1993.
    Good review of the general principles of managing the polytrauma patient. Additional information regarding the underlying physiologic basis of trauma is provided.
Gustilo R: Problems in the management of type III open fractures. J Trauma 1984;24:742–746.
    Provides review of open fracture classification with emphasis on the severe injury.
Hansen S: Overview of the severely traumatized lower limb. Clin Orthop 1989;243:17–19.
    Addresses the issue of salvage versus amputation.
Charnley J: The Closed Treatment of Common Fractures. Edinburgh, Livingstone, Ltd., 1961.
    For those fortunate enough to have a copy of this classic text, extensive information is provided in the execution of this lost art.
Müller M: Manual of Internal Fixation. Berlin, Springer-Verlag, 1991.
    This is the classic technique manual of the AO group. In addition, information is provided regarding classification and indications for fracture management.

Chapter 9

Musculoskeletal Infections

Paul S. Cooper, M.D.
John N. Delahay, M.D.

Musculoskeletal infections include septic arthrosis and chronic osteomyelitis. Treatment of infected feet, spines, and total joints are covered in their respective chapters. Treatment of infections in adults requires a multidisciplinary approach involving the orthopedist, plastic surgeon, infectious disease specialist, and musculoskeletal radiologist. Successful management and eradication of the infectious process in the long bones and major joints require a thorough knowledge of the cause, the specific organisms involved, pathophysiology, diagnostic methods, and surgical management. An understanding of the virulence of the bacteria and of the growing resistance to antibiotics of certain organisms is essential to effective and timely eradication of the infection.

ADULT MUSCULOSKELETAL INFECTIONS

Adult Osteomyelitis

Treatment of chronic osteomyelitis presents a challenge to the orthopedic surgeon because of the difficulty of obtaining complete eradication of the infection. Management of osteomyelitis includes aggressive debridement of infected dead and ischemic tissue, use of culture-directed antibiotics, obliteration of dead space, and soft tissue coverage with well-vascularized tissue. The mainstays of successful management are the use of proper surgical techniques when resecting the osteomyelitic and surrounding infected soft tissues, sophisticated wound-coverage techniques using both local and free flaps, and aggressive, early bone grafting.

The diagnosis of osteomyelitis is based on clinical assessment combined with laboratory analysis, radiographic imaging studies, and tissue biopsy. A history of an open fracture, open reduction and internal fixation of an open or closed fracture, or hematogenous osteomyelitis that occurred decades earlier is relevant to diagnosis. Additionally, a patient may have a history of a previous purulent drainage that was treated with antibiotics or a chronic intermittent draining sinus. Recurrent redness, edema, and spontaneous drainage that "resolved" with a course of antibiotic therapy are commonly elicited. Pain-related symptoms are variable and may or may not be simultaneous with the activity of the osteomyelitis. Studies should include plain radiographs, nuclear medicine studies, sonograms, and computed tomography (CT). Plain radiographs of the extremity may confirm osteomyelitis by demonstrating periosteal elevation, se-

questrum formation, lysis, or a bony defect. A concurrent sonogram often shows the extension of the sinus tract and the extent of the infection. The technetium Tc 99m phosphate study relates to osteoblastic activity. This study is composed of an initial flow phase at the time of injection that creates a radionuclide angiogram demonstrating increased blood flow in the presence of musculoskeletal infection. The second, or intermediate, phase occurs approximately 15 minutes after injection and correlates with the distribution of the tracer in the extracellular space. Uptake in this phase that was not visualized in the delayed phase is usually consistent with a superficial cellulitic process. The third, or delayed, phase indicates osteoblastic uptake and is obtained 2 to 4 hours after injection. Indium 111–labeled leukocyte studies are more accurate than plain technetium Tc 99m or sequential technetium-gallium imaging in cases of suspected low-grade infections of long bone. White blood cells from the patient's blood are isolated, labeled with In 111, and reinfused. Studies are considered positive when local uptake exceeds normal adjacent bone activity. They are useful in the diagnosis of chronic low-grade osteomyelitis, especially that which is associated with prosthetic implants; the accuracy rate is 70 to 94%. Recently, In 111–labeled polyclonal antibodies prepared from pooled human serum gamma globulin have been found to be as effective as white blood cells, with a 92% sensitivity rate and a 95% specificity rate based on the minimal uptake by normal bone and normal marrow.

Magnetic resonance imaging (MRI) is considered superior to In 111–labeled leukocyte scans to define the extent of infection. MRI findings consistent with active osteomyelitis include an area of abnormal marrow with a low signal on T1-weighted sequences and a corresponding increased signal intensity on T2-weighted images. Unlike nuclear medicine scans, MRI scans are useful in determining the intramedullary extent of the osteomyelitis. Cellulitis may be differentiated on an MRI study as a diffuse area of intermediate signal in the soft tissues on T1-weighted images, with similar soft tissue areas displaying an increased signal on T2-weighted images. It should be noted, however, that MRI cannot differentiate between edema and bacteria-induced cellulitis. Similarly, MRI is unable to define the presence of a cortical osteomyelitis unless evidence of cortical disruption or medullary involvement is present.

Although no standardized classification and clinical staging system exist to describe chronic osteomyelitis, the most popular classification is a modification of the Cierny and Mater classification, which is based on the following parameters: the bone involved; the duration of infection (acute versus chronic); the mechanism (hematogenous versus exogenous); the site of involvement (periarticular, subchondral, metaphyseal, or diaphyseal); the extent of involvement (medullary versus superficial, localized versus diffuse); and host characteristics, which may range from normal to local or systemic compromise.

The initial surgical treatment of osteomyelitis is the excision of all necrotic, infected tissue. Follow-up management requires the treatment of the cavity, or dead space, with antibiotic-impregnated methacrylate beads, local or vascularized soft tissue flaps, autogenous bone grafts, vascularized bone grafts, or distraction osteogenesis. With aggressive debridement, appropriate antibiotics, and adequate management of dead space, chronic osteomyelitis can be eradicated in the majority of patients.

Crucial to successful outcome is the appropriate staging of the management. Initial management requires radical excision of the sinus tract, avascular scarring, and affected soft tissues to the level of active bleeding margins around the osteomyelitic region. Concern about the ability to perform a direct primary closure should not preclude adequate resection of necrotic margins. All necrotic bone and sequestrum must be resected even if instability or loss of bone continuity is created. This may be addressed adequately by using a bridging external fixator as a staged procedure for bony stabilization. All dead bone should be resected using sharp rongeurs or osteotomes and without excessive use of saws or burrs because of the risk of thermal necrosis. The intramedullary canal should be curetted to remove any associated necrotic debris, and the wound should undergo copious pulsed lavage with a mixture of antibiotics and normal saline. In cases of chronic diaphyseal osteomyelitis with marked sclerosis, recommendations have been made for intermedullary reaming, which is believed to diminish intraosseus pressure and assist in the revascularization of bone by improving the endosteal circulation (Fig. 9–1).

The use of local antibiotic beads created with a mixture of aminoglycoside and polymethyl methacrylate allows for the elution of high concentrations into the surrounding tissues, including bone. The use of high-dose local antibiotic beads avoids the possible toxicity associated with long-term intravenous aminoglycoside therapy. The antibiotic beads are placed in the dead space and left for approximately 4 to 6 weeks, with removal occurring during the staged grafting procedure. Wounds are typically packed, and wound closure is delayed to allow for further debridements every 24 to 48 hours to resect necrotic tissue and bone. Wounds are closed in a single layer without tension or require the use of either local rotation muscle flaps or free muscle flap transfers with split-thickness skin grafting.

Antibiotic therapy is based on cultures obtained intraoperatively from the deep zone of osteomyelitis, not from the superficial sinus tract. Prior to receiving the results of culture, a cephalosporin may be used postoperatively, as these antibiotics are generally effective against gram-positive and a number of gram-negative bacteria, excluding *Pseudomonas* species. When the organism is sensitive to penicillin, that is the treatment of choice, with 10 to 12 (million) units given per day. It should be noted, however, that in up to 70% of cases of infection by coagulase-

positive *Staphylococcus* species, the most common organism seen in chronic osteomyelitis, the bacteria are resistant to penicillin. Synthetic penicillins, such as oxacillin and methicillin, therefore, are the drugs of choice; in methicillin-resistant *Staphylococcus aureus*, the use of 1 g of vancomycin every 12 hours is effective. Long-standing open wounds and chronically draining sinuses often develop gram-negative rod infections or mixed infections of both gram-negative and coagulase-positive *Staphylococcus* species. The most common causal organisms noted in one study of cases in which chronic osteomyelitis had existed for a minimum of 2 years were species of *Pseudomonas*. Treatment involves the use of intravenous aminoglycosides or fluoroquinolone antibiotics such as ciprofloxacin, either intravenously or orally.

Hyperbaric oxygen (HBO) has been advocated as adjunctive therapy for the advanced stages of chronic diffuse osteomyelitis, especially in patients with local or systemic factors that compromise wound healing. HBO serves as a suppressive treatment of osteomyelitis in patients who are not candidates for surgical treatment, in those who refuse surgical intervention, and in those who have experienced suboptimal surgical outcomes. Additionally, HBO may be helpful in preventing the failure of difficult limb reconstructions that involve fasciocutaneous flaps, muscle flaps, or extensive bone grafts greater than 2 cm that may be compromised. Normal oxygen tension in healthy bone is 45 mmHg. However, in the typical osteomyelitic bone, the oxygen tension is noted to be 23 mmHg or less. HBO increases the oxygen tension in healthy, uninvolved bone to 322 mmHg and the tension in osteomyelitic bone to an average of 104 mmHg.

Increased oxygen tension has a direct lethal effect on strictly anaerobic organisms and on some microaerophilic aerobes but not on pure aerobes. During HBO therapy, an increase in oxygen tension leads to increased concentration of superoxides, including hydrogen peroxide, in the oxygen radicals produced, and anaerobic organisms are extremely sensitive to superoxides. HBO has a direct bacteriostatic or bactericidal effect on most *Clostridium* species, and it inhibits the production of clostridia alpha toxin. Although it does not demonstrate a direct lethal effect on aerobes, HBO improves the oxygen tension, so the environment is conducive to phagocytic function, thus killing many of the aerobic organisms; this function is normally diminished under the hypoxic conditions of infection. The least amount of phagocytic killing occurred at 23 mmHg (a tension found typically in osteomyelitic bone), whereas phagocytic ability increased with oxygen tensions that were raised to 45 mmHg or higher.

Adjunctive HBO has also been shown to enhance the effectiveness of vancomycin and tobramycin, which function poorly in the presence of low oxygen tension. Finally, the higher oxygen tension allows for better wound healing by improving the environment for fibroblastic proliferation, which has been shown not to synthesize collagen or to migrate in the presence of an oxygen tension less than 10 mmHg. Therefore, indirectly, HBO promotes collagen production, angiogenesis, and, ultimately, wound healing in ischemic and infected wounds.

Several options are available for addressing, as a staged procedure, the large defects left after debridement of major

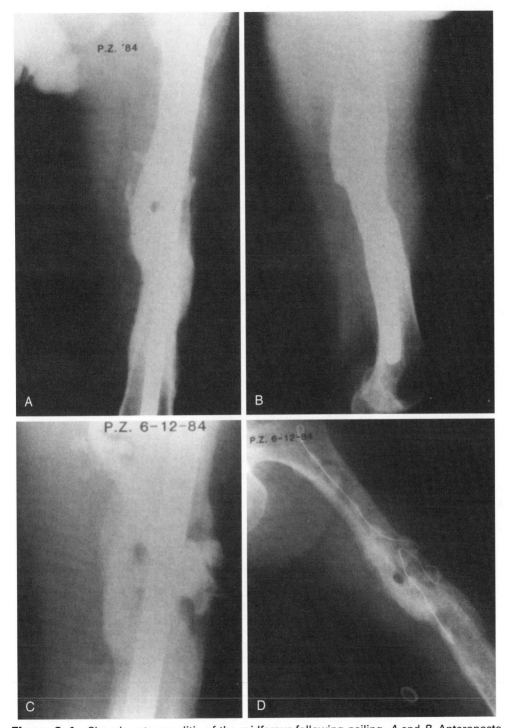

Figure 9–1. Chronic osteomyelitis of the midfemur following nailing. *A* and *B,* Anteroposterior (AP) and lateral radiographs show healed fracture with intramedullary nail. *C,* Sinogram shows extension of infection inside canal. *D,* The intramedullary nail was removed, and the entire medullary canal was reamed to bleeding bone. Tobramycin beads were inserted inside the intramedullary canal. The fracture healed.

Illustration continued on following page

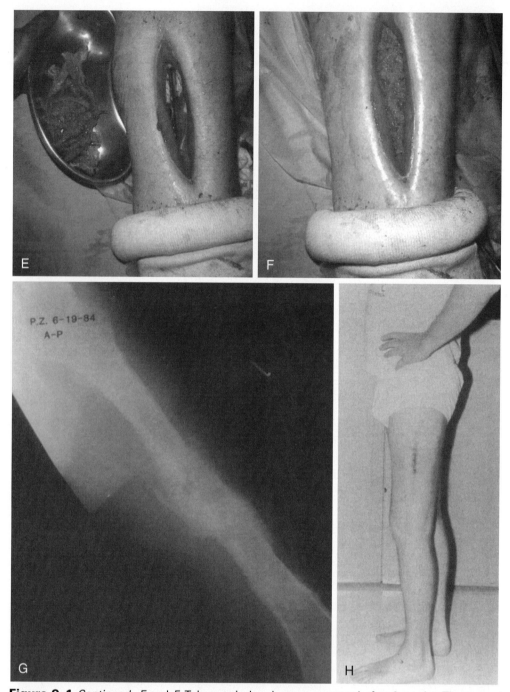

Figure 9–1 *Continued. E* and *F,* Tobramycin beads were removed after 2 weeks. The wound appeared clean and granulating. The cavity was filled with autogenous cancellous bone. *G* and *H,* Follow-up radiographs at 2 years show no evidence of recurrent sepsis. The fracture has healed. The patient is ambulating without support. (From Gustilo R, Gruninger RP, Tsukayama DT: Orthopaedic Infection: Diagnosis and Treatment. Philadelphia, WB Saunders, 1989, pp 158–159.)

long bones in which osteomyelitis is present. Early cancellous bone grafting is recommended when there is no evidence of purulent drainage and early and good granulation tissue has been produced. It may be performed as early as 5 to 10 days after initial debridement but often is staged at approximately 4 to 6 weeks following initial eradication of the osteomyelitis. In chronic osteomyelitis when there is inadequate soft tissue coverage and it is not possible to

close the skin directly, an alternative method of treatment advocated by Papineau and colleagues involves open excision and radical saucerization followed by cancellous bone grafting on granulation tissue. They achieved a 93% rate of good to excellent results in 39 cases of chronic osteomyelitis. Cancellous bone grafting is generally recommended as an adjunct to the treatment of osteomyelitis to (1) fill in the osteomyelitic cavity, (2) substitute for resected nonviable bone, and (3) promote union of a motion-associated septic nonunion. An alternative to autografted cancellous bone graft is the use of microvascular free tissue transfers. This procedure uses cortical struts from either the fibula or the iliac crest. It provides a vascularized graft, but these free transfers may take years to mature and thicken, which means a greater risk of refracture (Fig. 9–2).

The methods outlined by Ilizarov, which employ fine

wire fixator frames and bone transport, allow for greater and more radical resection and debridement of infected bones than do conventional techniques. His methods involve bilevel distraction-compression osteosynthesis utilizing a corticotomy through proximal healthy bone and soft tissues at a distance from the defect (Fig. 9–3). An intermediary fragment is thus created between the corticotomy and the defect. The fragment is gradually transported through

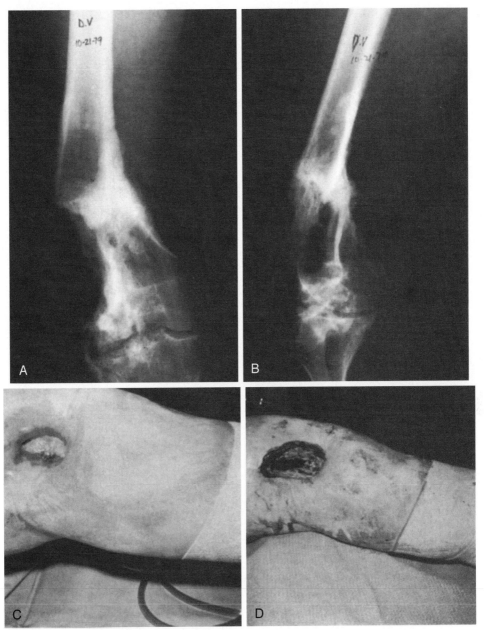

Figure 9–2. Chronic osteomyelitis of 10 years' duration after treatment of a type III open supracondylar fracture with vascular injury in a 31-year-old man. The fracture has healed but there is a chronic draining sinus and inadequate soft tissue coverage. A culture revealed *Pseudomonas aeruginosa*. *A* and *B,* Anteroposterior and lateral radiographs show complete healing of the fracture. However, there is a large area of lucency, with a sequestrum at the supracondylar area. Note the large concavity defect. *C,* Large, open, draining cavity with sinus tract formation. A culture revealed *P. aeruginosa*, which is sensitive to aminoglycoside antibiotics. *D,* Radical debridement of scarred tissue and dead bone, sequestrectomy, and copious irrigation were performed. The patient was given gentamicin intravenously for 10 days.
Illustration continued on following page

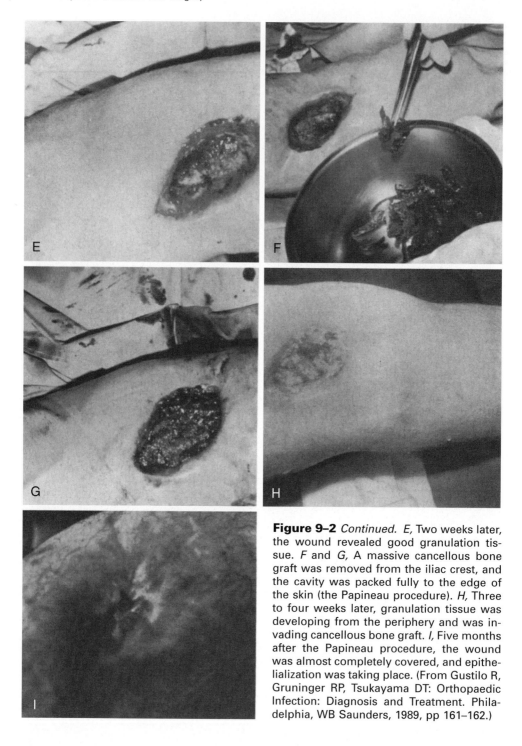

Figure 9–2 *Continued. E,* Two weeks later, the wound revealed good granulation tissue. *F* and *G,* A massive cancellous bone graft was removed from the iliac crest, and the cavity was packed fully to the edge of the skin (the Papineau procedure). *H,* Three to four weeks later, granulation tissue was developing from the periphery and was invading cancellous bone graft. *I,* Five months after the Papineau procedure, the wound was almost completely covered, and epithelialization was taking place. (From Gustilo R, Gruninger RP, Tsukayama DT: Orthopaedic Infection: Diagnosis and Treatment. Philadelphia, WB Saunders, 1989, pp 161–162.)

the limb with wires, which lengthens the corticotomy gap with cholestasis while simultaneously closing the segmental defect.

Early amputation is a viable option in specific cases of chronic osteomyelitis, including chronic, draining osteomyelitis of the tibia and an insensate foot. A below-knee amputation can be performed as salvage in a case involving massive bone exposure, a stiffened foot, or non-reconstructible soft tissue coverage with free flap due to significant arterial compromise.

In summary, the keys to managing chronic osteomyelitis include radical aggressive surgery with the use of appropriate intravenous and local antibiotics. Delayed and appropriate wound closure involving either primary closure or the use of local or free flaps to achieve soft tissue coverage is imperative. Optimal management requires a multidisciplinary team approach.

Adult Septic Arthritis

Septic arthritis in the adult continues to be a major health problem, especially in large medical centers, with the incidence figures ranging from .034 to .13% for nongonococcal cases. The rise in the incidence is related to the increasing

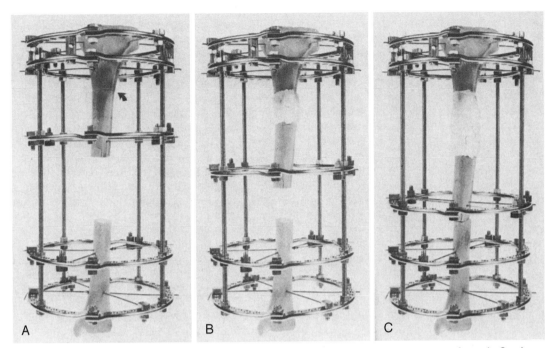

Figure 9–3. Bilocal distraction-compression osteosynthesis with a transport ring. *A,* Corticotomy through healthy tissues *(small arrow). B,* During transport, regenerate new bone forms at the corticotomy site while the defect closes. *C,* At the completion of the procedure, the docking of the moving fragment with the target fragment is seen. (From Esterhai J [ed]: Orthop Clin North Am 1991;22:517.)

age of the population associated with higher risk for developing diabetes, chronic illness, and other immunocompromised conditions.

Septic arthritis may be caused by hematogenous seeding secondary to bacteremia resulting from distant infection, by intravenous drug use, or by direct inoculation secondary to penetrating trauma or joint aspiration. Other routes include direct spread into the joint capsule from contiguous soft tissue infection, such as cellulitis or septic bursitis and joint contamination by periarticular osteomyelitis. Major predisposing factors include pre-existing joint disease, especially rheumatoid arthritis, closed trauma, direct penetration of the joint, intravenous drug use, and conditions that impair host defense mechanisms, including malignancy, steroid and cytotoxic drug use, diabetes, extreme age, and other chronic debilitating diseases.

There is an unusually high predisposition to adult joint sepsis in individuals with underlying rheumatologic conditions. In particular, patients with rheumatoid arthritis have the highest rate of septic arthritis, with a range of .3 to 3% of all patients. The majority of adult septic arthritis is monoarticular, but polyarticular septic arthritis may occur in approximately one fourth of cases. In polyarticular septic arthritis, typically three to four joints are involved, and 40% manifest extra-articular septic foci, including pulmonary infections, endocarditis, and subcutaneous abscesses. The greatest risk factor is the presence of a concurrent rheumatologic condition; this is the case in more than 50% of patients with polyarticular septic arthritis. The poor prognosis relates to the difficulty in distinguishing a rheumatoid flare from an acute infection, which results in delay in diagnosis. Overall fatality rates in polyarticular joint involvement range from 32 to 42%.

Another important risk factor for the development of infection is the presence of a joint prosthesis; approximately 1 to 2% of all hip and knee arthroplasties are complicated by infection. Patients with systemic lupus erythematosus constitute another subgroup at high risk for developing infections, including septic arthritis. Because of the depression of cell- and antibody-mediated immune responses resulting from the use of immunosuppressive therapy, patients with lupus have a high rate of chronic *Salmonella* carriage as well as infection. Similarly, patients with sickle cell anemia experience a higher than normal rate of infection, with salmonella making up more than 50% of all infections. Other individuals who are at increased risk for infection include those with the human immunodeficiency virus (HIV), those with diabetes mellitus, and intravenous drug users. Drug users are at special risk for gram-negative joint infection, with involvement uniquely of the sternoclavicular, sacroiliac, and manubriosternal joints as well as the symphysis pubis.

The knee is by far the most common joint involved; involvement occurs in 40 to 50% of all cases. Second in frequency of involvement is the hip joint at 20 to 25%, followed by the shoulder at 10 to 15%, the ankle at 10 to 15%, the elbow at 10 to 15%, and the hand at 5%.

Unique to adult septic arthritis is the potential for the coexistence of acute bouts of crystal-induced arthritis. The decreased pH level associated with infection in the joint decreases the solubility of urate or pyrophosphate crystals. Therefore, all patients with acute arthritis should be screened for both infectious and crystal-induced causes, and the presence of crystals does not rule out bacterial arthritis. There have been isolated reports of associated fungal and bacterial septic arthroses coexisting in individuals with HIV and frank AIDS. Additionally, septic arthritis may become a complicated picture in HIV-infected hemophiliacs. Any patient who develops fever and pain unresponsive to factor replacement should be assumed to have a septic joint and to require diagnostic arthrocentesis.

Diagnostic evaluation includes a history and physical examination and aspiration of joint fluid. Typical clinical features include fever, chills, arthralgia, malaise, anorexia, and local findings of joint pain, tenderness, swelling, erythema, and limited range of motion, especially with flexion. In immunocompromised patients, including the elderly, symptoms may be atypically mild. Decreased active and passive range of motion is one of the most consistent signs and is important in distinguishing septic arthritis from bursitis or cellulitis.

Diagnosis of septic arthritis must be ruled out with diagnostic aspiration of the joint fluid. Utilizing an aseptic technique, aspiration should be performed in an area free of infected skin or soft tissue. A large-bore needle, 18 gauge or larger, should be used to allow aspiration of the exudate. Fluid should be sent for a cell count differential, microscopic evaluation, glucose determination, and crystalline analysis. Suspect cultures should be sent for fungal and microbacterial analysis in addition to anaerobic and aerobic analysis. If aspiration of the joint is unsuccessful, non-bacteriostatic saline can be injected and aspirated for Gram stain and culture analysis. In joints that are difficult to reach, fluoroscope-, ultrasound-, or CT-guided aspiration may be performed. The use of a contrast medium can confirm joint entry. Further blood workup includes cultures, culturing at other sites, and a peripheral white cell count with a differential erythrocyte sedimentation rate. In general, a white blood cell count higher than 100,000 cells per mL in synovial fluid suggests the presence of infection. Overall, Gram stains of joint fluid are positive in 50 to 75% of patients with nongonococcal septic arthritis, yielding cultures that are positive in more than 85% of cases. Blood cultures are typically positive in approximately 50% of patients, in comparison with only 10% of patients with gonococcal infections. Other potential sources of infection, including skin lesions and urinary tract infections, should be cultured too.

Radiographic studies should include plain radiographs of the joint, which may reveal nonspecific joint effusion or joint space widening. Additionally, periarticular soft tissue swelling with displacement of the capsular fat pads may be seen. Subchondral bone erosions, periarticular osteopenia secondary to hyperemia or disuse, and joint space narrowing are typically seen in advanced stages, and cartilage destruction and joint subluxation indicating severe joint destruction are seen as late manifestations. Rarely, intra-articular gas resulting from previous aspiration may be identified. Ancillary radiographic studies may include radionuclide studies, MRI, and CT scanning. Radionuclide studies are not specific for infection, but they are sensitive and can rule out infection in a joint when results are negative. When a bone scan is positive, an In 111–labeled white blood cell scan, which is more specific for infection, may be indicated. MRI and CT are useful in the diagnosis and determination of the extent of infection. CT may show joint changes earlier than plain films reveal them, and it can indicate joint effusions within days of their onset. In cases of later-stage infections, CT may demonstrate bone destruction and abscess formation with high sensitivity. MRI is sensitive for the delineation of joint fluid, cartilage damage, and medullary bone destruction and shows high resolution of soft tissues. It is quite useful in delineating intramedullary osteomyelitis, which may occur concurrently. The hallmarks of treatment of adult septic arthritis include the use of parenteral antibiotics in conjunction with the drainage, decompression, and cleaning of the involved joint. The goals of treatment include sterilization of the joint; decompression; removal of all inflamed cells, enzymes, and debris; elimination of any destructive pannus; and return to full function. Methods of achieving the goals include antibiotic therapy, needle aspiration, open surgery, and arthroscopic drainage and lavage. The level of treatment is determined by the underlying medical conditions and the specific organism involved. In general, aggressive infections caused by *S. aureus* or gram-negative organisms require surgical drainage and lavage of the joint. Surgical drainage is also indicated for all joints that do not respond to antibiotic therapy, based on aspiration within 72 hours, and for joints in which the synovial fluid appears to be loculated and the major joints of the upper and lower extremities are involved.

Controversy exists about the use of oral versus intravenous antibiotics. Oral antibiotics have several advantages, including cost, convenience, comfort, and decreased length of hospitalization. The main issue is not the site of administration but adequate and consistent serum levels. A bactericidal lever that maintains titers of at least 1:8 may be achieved with either oral or intravenous therapy. It is generally recommended that antibiotic therapy continue for 2 weeks in cases of gonococcal arthritis and for 4 to 6 weeks in cases of nongonococcal infections. Adjunctive drainage and lavage, which aid in the elimination of bacteria, may serve to generate a sterilized environment sooner after treatment.

Methods of drainage and decompression are debated. The advantages of open drainage include the ability to fully debride the infected synovial tissue. The advantages of repeated arthrocentesis include shorter hospitalization, minimal wound-management problems, and decreased requirements for anesthesia. Proponents of open drainage procedures cite the inability of arthrocentesis to decompress purulent loculations and adhesions, the pain of repeated arthrocentesis, and the possible iatrogenic inoculation of bone with the arthrocentesis needle, in addition to the difficulty of aspirating certain joints, including the shoulder, wrist, and hip. Arthroscopy is a viable alternative in the decompression and lavage of the knee in particular. Arthroscopy allows visualization of all compartments of the knee and therefore facilitates more comprehensive decompression, cleaning, and debridement than does open arthrotomy. A lower rate of morbidity, which allows for a dramatically reduced hospital stay, is also cited as an advantage. Several authors have suggested that all elderly patients with septic arthritis undergo surgical decompression, either open or arthroscopic. The postoperative course involves the use of splinting during the acute phase of bacterial infection for initial relief, followed by early motion of diseased joints to prevent disuse osteoporosis, muscle atrophy, pain, and stiffness. Motion is especially essential in joints that have pre-existing arthrosis. The best management involves continual passive motion, which prevents adhesions and pannus formation and improves cartilage nutrition through increased effusion of synovial fluid.

Foot Infections in Diabetic Patients

Foot infections are a significant problem for individuals who have diabetes; at least one quarter of the admissions of diabetic patients to the hospital are because of foot infections, and they account for more than $300 million in direct hospital costs. The average hospital stay is longer than 1 month for 89% of patients and more than 3 months for 44% of patients. Infections may be more common among diabetics and once established, they are more severe and harder to treat. Approximately 5% of diabetic patients ultimately require amputation; these amputations make up more than half of all amputations performed in the United States each year. The typical diabetic patient is more than 135% above ideal body weight and has had diabetes for an average of 18 years; 71% have type I diabetes, 80% have neuropathy, 78% have nephropathy, and 67% have retinopathy.

Most foot infections in diabetic patients originate with breakdown of the plantar soft tissue by mechanical forces, which occurs because of the loss of normal protective sensation secondary to diabetic neuropathy. The autonomic component of the neuropathy causes dry, hyperkeratotic skin that develops fissures and ulcers and, in combination with the loss of protective sensation and altered immune mechanisms, creates a portal for infection.

Unlike painless plantar ulcerations secondary to mechanical breakdown, ischemic ulcers due to vascular insufficiency create pain and tissue gangrene. Atherosclerosis occurs more commonly in the diabetic, in whom marginal circulation is unable to meet the oxygen demands of infection, which increase fourfold. In addition, dorsal ulcerations on the sides of the foot are secondary to constant pressure from shoe wear rather than to the intermittent pressure of standing or walking. A complete medical history and physical examination are necessary. Evidence of redness, streaking, pain, fullness, or fluctuance should be determined. Ulcer calluses should be unroofed to define the margins and extent of the ulcer. The ability to proceed with a blunt probe down to the bone is indicative of osteomyelitis in more than 80% of cases. Vascular examination may be deceptive because bounding ankle pulses do not necessarily equate with healthy microcirculation. Ancillary Doppler and transcutaneous oxygen (TcO$_2$) studies can provide a more accurate picture of a wound's healing potential. Fever and leukocytosis may be deceptively normal, even in full sepsis, because of an immunocompromised state. Glucose level stability is a more sensitive finding for systemic involvement. Wagner's classification is a widely accepted system for grading diabetic ulcers. Grade 0 ulcers have intact skin; grade 1 ulcers extend down to subcutaneous tissue; grade 2 ulcers present with exposed tendons and deep structures; grade 3 is reserved for ulcers involving bone (osteomyelitis); grades 4 and 5 refer to ulcers that have variable degrees of gangrene. Outcome is related to the anatomic location of the ulcer: forefoot lesions result in higher limb salvage rates than do mid- and hindfoot lesions.

Unlike that found in other musculoskeletal infections, the microbiology in an infection in the foot of a diabetic patient is often polymicrobial. Both aerobic and anaerobic organisms should be cultured and often a typical combination includes gram-positive cocci, gram-negative enteric rods (coliforms), and anaerobes. Special culture and transport media designed for anaerobic organisms must be kept in the examination room in order to obtain cultures adequately. Often the organisms in a deep wound are not identical to those cultured from superficial swabs or draining sinuses. It is, therefore, essential to obtain deep-wound cultures or trocar biopsies intra-operatively through an incision other than the ulceration. Many patients have been partially treated with antibiotics, which clouds the picture. It is recommended that antibiotics be withdrawn 48 hours before the culture is taken so as to improve accuracy. The gas formation typically seen in the soft tissues of foot infections in diabetics is not associated with true gangrene gas caused by *Clostridium perfringens*. In a diabetic patient, certain aerobic organisms are gas producers within the soft tissues, including gram-positive cocci (i.e., *Streptococcus* species and enterococci) and mixed enteric gram-negative rods. It is important to obtain a stat Gram stain when gas is noted in the soft tissue spaces, however, because gas is also associated with necrotizing fasciitis as demonstrated by gram-positive rods within the tissues.

Diabetic patients with foot infections may present with few symptoms, which leads to a delay in treatment. Often, a fever or an increased insulin requirement may be all that is noted. Generally, the greater the size and depth of the ulcer, the greater the chance of underlying deep infection leading to osteomyelitis. A foul smell suggests the presence of anaerobes. Similarly, gangrene suggests a mixed infection. Difficulty in diagnosis exists when a patient has active, ongoing Charcot's arthropathy in addition to a plantar ulceration. It may be secondary to a superficial ulcer with concurrent Charcot's arthropathy or may involve extensive osteomyelitis of the involved joints.

Ancillary diagnostic studies include arterial Doppler ultrasound, blood work, and radiographic studies. Evaluation of the vascular status of the leg is essential; it is related to healing capacity and therefore to outcome. Generally, favorable prognostic indicators include biphasic and triphasic waveforms of the arteries, an ankle-to-brachial index greater than .45, toe pressures of 40 mmHg or higher, and TcO$_2$ levels over 40. Additional diagnostic studies include a white blood cell count and erythrocyte sedimentation rate. Radiographs typically show periosteal reaction, cortical erosions, or lytic lesions. Technetium Tc 99m bone scans are sensitive, but they are not specific for the detection of bony involvement. The addition of an In 111 leukocyte scan (Fig. 9–4) may increase specificity but can yield a false-negative result in the presence of prior antibiotic treatment or local soft tissue inflammation. MRI has greater sensitivity and specificity—80%—and accuracy is improved by using contrast enhancement. MRI is helpful in evaluating infections resulting from diabetes because of its superior ability to demonstrate marrow edema and soft tissue abscesses and its ability to detect the intramedullary extent of osteomyelitis.

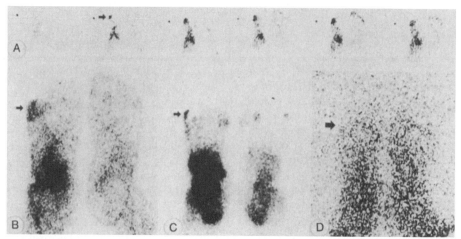

Figure 9–4. Combined three-phase bone scintigraphy (TPBS) and indium In 111–labeled white blood cell scintigraphy (WBCS) in the plantar projection (toes pointing to top) in a patient under evaluation for possible osteomyelitis of the right fifth toe *(arrows)*. *A,* This TPBS image shows increased blood flow. *B,* This image shows increased blood pool activity. *C,* This image shows increased bone tracer uptake in the right fifth toe and in the right tarsometatarsal (TMT) region. *D,* The WBCS image shows a physiologic pattern of radioactivity. This patient had both neuropathic joint disease of the right TMT region and degenerative changes affecting the toes. Pathologic examination of the right fifth toe after amputation did not show infection. (From Keenan AM, Tindel TL, Alavi A: Diagnosis of pedal osteomyelitis in diabetic patients using current scintigraphic techniques. Arch Intern Med 1989;149:2262–2266.)

Treatment principles include the initiation of culture-specific, high-level antibiotic coverage. Higher levels are required because of poor perfusion and impaired leukocyte function. For infections that do not threaten limbs, parenteral regimens include clindamycin, ampicillin, and trovafloxacin. Limb-threatening infections are managed by administering ticarcillin with clavulanate, cefoxitin, or cefotetan as well as piperacillin and fluoroquinolones. Debridement and drainage remain key in addressing diabetes-related foot infections. Plantar ulcers in general require aggressive debridement in the presence of infection and exposure of deep structures. Indications for surgical debridement include a draining sinus resulting from infected nongranulating ulcers, abscess, osteomyelitis, necrotic abscess formation, exposed nonviable tissue, and exposed nongranulated cartilage and bone surface. Basic principles include full debridement of all necrotic tissue back to bleeding margins. Skeletal shortening may be necessary for proper tension-free wound closure. In the central metatarsals, condylectomy, osteotomy, or resection arthroplasty of the metatarsal heads is performed. In plantar heel ulcers with osteomyelitis, a partial calcanectomy allows for tensionless wound closure (Fig. 9–5). Wounds are dressed twice a day initially, first with normal saline wet-to-dry dressings and then with wound gels. Sutures should remain in place for a minimum of 3 weeks.

PEDIATRIC MUSCULOSKELETAL INFECTIONS

In this section we discuss primary acute hematogenous osteomyelitis (AHO) and septic arthritis in children. These diseases are prevalent in the United States today and, unfortunately, cause significant disability in the pediatric

population when the diagnosis is delayed or the treatment is inadequate.

Acute Hematogenous Osteomyelitis

AHO is an inflammation of bone caused by bacteria, which typically reach the bone via the hematogenous route. In children this disease has a predilection for those in the first decade of life. Unlike adults, who usually have osteomyelitis in conjunction with other diseases, children typically manifest this condition as a primary disease. Characteristically, it affects the rapidly growing end of a long bone in the metaphyseal region and almost inexplicably has a greater predilection for the lower extremities of males. The fact that males are more commonly involved than females

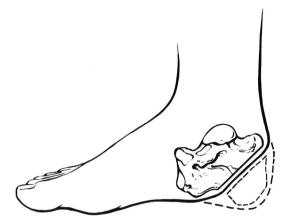

Figure 9–5. Partial calcanectomy. (From Gould J [ed]: Operative Foot Surgery. Philadelphia, WB Saunders, 1994, p 215.)

tends to indicate that trauma may play a provocative role. It has also been recognized that the incidence of AHO is slightly higher in climates in which high humidities are noted. This suggests that increased skin transport may play a role in the pathogenesis of this disease.

DEMOGRAPHIC DATA

Interestingly, as can be seen by reviewing the literature, there has been relatively no significant change in the number of cases per year over the past 15 years. Shortly after the introduction of penicillin, a decrease in the incidence of AHO was noted; however, numbers have rebounded to those of the pre-antibiotic era. This speaks to the emergence of resistant organisms in the causation of this disease. There has been a change in the presentation of the disease. The classic full-blown, fulminant infection is less commonly diagnosed. Currently, more subacute and atypical forms are seen. This has been attributed to the increased utilization of antibiotics for a wide range of pediatric illnesses.

In general, most cases of AHO are monostotic and involve a lower extremity. Typically, the disease affects the metaphysis of a long bone, especially the end with the greatest growth potential. Therefore, about 70% of cases affect the distal femur, proximal tibia, and proximal humerus.

BACTERIOLOGY

Over the years there has been relatively little change in which organisms cause this disease (Table 9–1). *Staphylococcus aureus* remains the primary offender; it is isolated in 70 to 90% of cases. If one were to look only at children 1 year of age and older, it would be seen that *S. aureus* causes 90% of cases. Beta hemolytic streptococcus accounts for 20 to 40% of cases, especially in infants under 1 year of age. It is now reported to be the most common cause of neonatal sepsis. The remaining cases typically are gram-negative in origin. At the present time, because of the eradication of *Haemophilus influenzae* by the vaccine, *Escherichia coli* is the most common gram-negative organism retrieved.

PATHOGENESIS

As mentioned earlier, a number of series implicate trauma as a predisposing factor in the etiology of AHO. Morrissy,

in his studies with the rabbit model, demonstrated the increased incidence of bacteremias after a traumatic event. This bacteremia may well serve as the herald of the development of AHO. Probably the single most important factor in the predisposition of children to this hematogenous disease is the unique anatomy of the circulatory system in the metaphysis. The arterioles in the metaphysis are configured in "hairpin loops," so by their very nature, they predispose the metaphysis to sluggish blood flow. In addition, the absolute physical boundary created by the physis creates fertile ground for bacterial engagement. The presence of these end-loop arterioles and the paucity of collaterals mean that the environment of the metaphysis is conducive to bacterial growth. Several studies have hinted at deficiencies in resistance of local tissue in the metaphysis such as the absence of normal macrophages in the tissue. If this is true, it is yet another factor that favors bacterial growth.

Once the focus of infection is established, the migration of white cells and the release of vasoactive substances, such as interleukins and prostaglandins, are seen. The effect is to increase osteoclastic activity, which results in the release of bone-damaging enzymes. Resorption of bone is the obvious net result. The earliest stages of infection have been compared to cellulitis of the bone with no evidence of pus accumulation. However, it is only a short time before pus drains through the Volkmann canals to the subperiosteal space, thereby elevating the periosteum and producing a subperiosteal abscess.

DIAGNOSIS

The diagnosis of AHO remains difficult despite current technology and, unfortunately, is frequently delayed. It goes without saying that the clinical picture is the most important factor in diagnosis. It is axiomatic that unexplained bone pain or pseudoparalysis plus fever should be considered diagnostic of osteomyelitis until proven otherwise. Failure to make this connection can be deleterious. In general, a child usually presents with a febrile illness of 1 to 2 days' duration. Typically, the child complains of pain in an extremity. Pseudoparalysis is common in a child younger than 1 year; a child older than 1 year limps or refuses to walk. The adjacent joint may appear swollen and may have an effusion. Occasionally, a child may also have an infection of the skin, ear, or throat.

In neonates and infants, the clinical picture can be confusing; physical findings are few and the presentation is more subtle. It is not uncommon to be presented with an infant who appears listless or restless, does not feed well, and has pseudoparalysis of a limb. It is important to avoid being misled by the absence of fever in this age group.

The laboratory evaluation of such children should include a complete blood count with differential, determination of the erythrocyte sedimentation rate, a C-reactive protein study, and blood cultures. Routine radiographs and aspiration of the bone are also necessary. The role of aspiration cannot be overemphasized. If osteomyelitis is a possibility in the differential diagnosis, aspiration of the area of maximal tenderness, using a large-bore needle, is an absolute must. This technique makes it possible to determine the presence of pus under pressure. Not only should the subperiosteal space be aspirated but also the

Table 9–1. Etiology of osteomyelitis by age group

Age Group	Causative Organism		
	Common	*Uncommon*	*Rare*
Neonates	S. aureus Group B streptococcus Enteric bacilli	H. influenzae	Candida
1 mo.–3 yr.	S. aureus streptococci	H. influenzae Pseudomonas species	Candida M. tuberculosis
>3 yr.	S. aureus streptococci	Pseudomonas species	M. tuberculosis Candida

From Tachdjian MO (ed): Pediatric Orthopaedics, 2nd ed. Philadelphia, WB Saunders, 1990, p 1094.

medullary canal should be entered to search for loculated pus. The retrieval rate of bone aspiration is reported to be as high as 80%; the rate of retrieval of organisms from blood cultures is approximately 50%. It has been reported by Canale and others that bone aspiration does not alter the results of a bone scan for a period of at least 72 hours.

Radiographic changes are often not helpful during the first 7 to 10 days. Other than deep soft tissue swelling, which is usually visible adjacent to the metaphysis in the first 72 hours, bone changes are commonly delayed (Fig. 9–6). Edema in muscle and obliteration of soft tissue planes may be seen 3 to 7 days after infection. Pus under the periosteum may also be apparent at this time. However, bone resorption and remodeling and the development of dead bone (sequestra) are commonly delayed until 10 to 14 days after metaphyseal seeding. The formation of new bone under the periosteum (involucrum) is not usually visible until 14 to 17 days.

Delay in diagnosis is not uncommon. It is often the result of the normal appearance of radiographs taken during the first several days; the normal erythrocyte sedimentation rate, which is seen in 25% of these children; the absence of fever (in a child younger than 1 year); the failure to attempt a bone aspiration; and the failure to retrieve organisms, which is not unusual today, considering the pervasive administration of antibiotics whenever a child appears to be ill.

SPECIAL STUDIES

Technetium Tc 99m bone scans are helpful in the evaluation of children with AHO (Fig. 9–7). Unfortunately, such studies are not always reliable and can often be equivocal. The reported sensitivity of a three-phase bone scan is 0.90 and the reported specificity is 0.80. The accuracy of bone scanning can be improved by repeating the study 72 hours later. White blood cell scans using indium In 111 labeling, although very helpful in evaluating an adult with chronic osteomyelitis, currently have relatively little, if any, application in the pediatric age group.

MRI scans are being used more commonly in the diagnosis of AHO (Fig. 9–8). They are currently reported to be 0.97 sensitive and 0.92 specific. It is usually a bright signal intensity on the T2-weighted image that is the indicator. This study is probably appropriate for atypical cases, such as those in the spine and the pelvis. However, they are rarely necessary for the more typical presentation in long bones.

Ultrasound is popular, but its use is controversial. It is said to be able to evaluate 2 to 3 mm of periosteum. This may be useful in localizing a needle for aspiration. There is current agreement that ultrasound is able to detect changes sooner than conventional radiographs can. In addition, the study is capable of localizing a subperiosteal abscess. Ultrasound is gaining popularity for evaluating and planning surgery for children with osteomyelitis.

TREATMENT

Overall, there has been a general change in philosophy concerning the management of children with osteomyelitis. There seem to be fewer indications for surgery because diagnosis, although delayed in some cases, is for the most part being made earlier. With early diagnosis, an excellent response to medical management can be anticipated as long as it is begun in the first 72 hours. Less than 10% of children require surgical treatment if diagnosis is made early.

Aggressive antibiotic management is the keystone of treatment. The antibiotic should be continued until the temperature is down and the clinical signs are consistent with subsidence and resolution. The choice of antibiotic in the absence of determination of the organism is based on an assumption concerning the most likely pathogen (Table

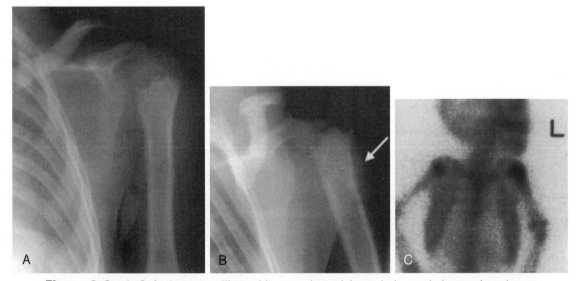

Figure 9–6. *A,* Soft tissue swelling with metaphyseal irregularity and destruction due to acute osteomyelitis of the left humerus in a 3-year-old boy. *B,* Two weeks later (without treatment) there is now further bony destruction and periosteal reaction *(arrow)* extending down the shaft of the humerus. *C,* Technetium Tc 99m bone scan shows increased uptake in the left humeral metaphysis and proximal shaft, which is consistent with osteomyelitis. (From Broughton NS: A Textbook of Paediatric Orthopaedics. London, WB Saunders, 1997, p 151.)

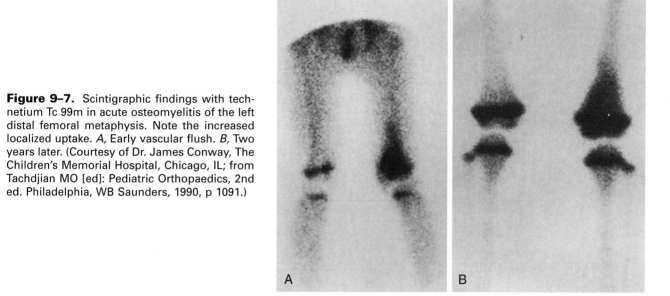

Figure 9–7. Scintigraphic findings with technetium Tc 99m in acute osteomyelitis of the left distal femoral metaphysis. Note the increased localized uptake. *A,* Early vascular flush. *B,* Two years later. (Courtesy of Dr. James Conway, The Children's Memorial Hospital, Chicago, IL; from Tachdjian MO [ed]: Pediatric Orthopaedics, 2nd ed. Philadelphia, WB Saunders, 1990, p 1091.)

9–2). Therefore, in children older than 1 year, nafcillin or a first-generation cephalosporin is the agent of choice. In the neonate, the common presence of Gram-negative organisms means that nafcillin plus gentamicin is an appropriate combination. Once the organism has been identified, antibiotic management should be tailored to the specific organism.

The route of delivery has been one of the most contentious issues for many years. All current authors agree that the initial management of a child should involve intravenous administration of the antibiotic. When to switch from intravenous to oral administration is the puzzle faced by most authors. The most commonly listed criteria for change of route include adequate response to intravenous treatment, ability to swallow medication, a compliant home environment, an established etiologic agent, and laboratory tests, which demonstrate bactericidal titers. The clinical problem relates to the evaluation of response.

Monitoring clinical response usually revolves around the defervescence of clinical findings; the normalization of the white blood cell count, erythrocyte sedimentation rate, and C-reactive protein level; and the absence of persistent tenderness in the area of the infection. Obviously, older children who have required surgical drainage may need a longer period of intravenous treatment.

The surgical treatment of osteomyelitis is primarily abscess drainage. The identification of loculated pus is accomplished by incising the periosteum and drilling a small hole into the metaphysis. These techniques have become standard practice. Aggressive stripping of the periosteum beyond the limits required for abscess drainage should be avoided.

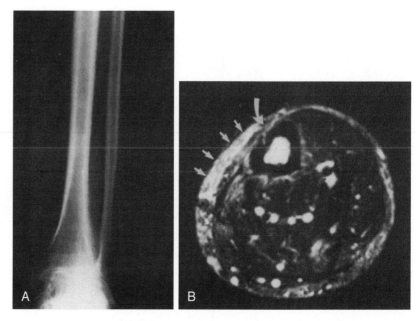

Figure 9–8. Diagnosis of osteomyelitis based on MRI in the setting of negative radiographs. *A,* Frontal view of the tibia and fibula is negative for osteomyelitis. *B,* Axial STIR MRI reveals high signal intensity (fluid) in the bone marrow of the tibia, in the cloaca penetrating the cortex *(curved arrow),* and in the subcutaneous fat *(arrows).* (From Boutin RD, Sartoris DJ [eds]: Musculoskeletal Imaging Update, Part II. Orthop Clin North Am 1998;29:52.)

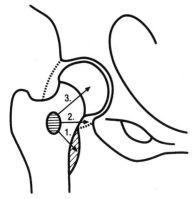

Figure 9–9. The spread of acute osteomyelitis. *1,* Formation of a subperiosteal abscess. *2,* Acute septic arthritis may develop if the metaphysis is intra-articular (e.g., hip and shoulder). *3,* In infants, infection may spread to the physis and epiphysis. (From Broughton NS: A Textbook of Paediatric Orthopaedics. London, WB Saunders, 1997, p 150.)

COMPLICATIONS

Despite early diagnosis and adequate treatment, some children do develop complications. Associated septic arthritis can occur in joints in which the metaphysis is intra-articular (Fig. 9–9), including the hip, the shoulder, the elbow (proximal radial metaphysis is intra-articular), and the ankle (a small portion of the distal tibia is intra-articular).

Metastatic seeding by the organism can occur. This complication, although rare, can result in pneumonia, pericarditis, and multifocal disease.

Pathologic fracture is perhaps the greatest risk (Fig. 9–10). Bony resorption and the replacement of dead and dying bone with involucrum, which is mechanically weak, predispose the infected bone to fracture. It is far easier to prevent these complications from occurring than to treat them once they have occurred. To this end, immobilization of the extremity during treatment is an integral part of the management of AHO. The development of chronic

Table 9–2. Initial antibiotic therapy for osteomyelitis in infants and children

Neonates	Probable Organism	Antibiotic
Neonates <2 months	Group B streptococcus, *S. aureus,* or gram-negative rods *H. influenzae*	Nafcillin + aminoglycoside Cefadyl + aminoglycoside Ceftriaxone or Cefotaxime Cefuroxime
Infants >2 months <3 years	*S. aureus* (90% of cases)	Cefuroxime
Children	*S. aureus* (90% of cases)	Nafcillin

From Tachdjian MO: Clinical Pediatric Orthopaedics: The Art of Diagnosis and Principles of Management. Stamford, CT, Appleton & Lange, 1997, p 205.

osteomyelitis (Fig. 9–11), although uncommon, does occur and is discussed in the subsequent section.

SUMMARY

The principles of managing osteomyelitis in children are simple and straightforward:

1. Early diagnosis of the disease
2. Identification of the organism
3. Selection of the appropriate organism-specific antibiotic
4. Choice of the appropriate route of antibiotic delivery to achieve necessary bactericidal levels in bone
5. Appropriate duration of antibiotic delivery
6. Drainage of sequestered pus
7. Avoidance of complications—specifically, pathologic fracture—by immobilizing the extremity.

By employing these simple principles, excellent results can be achieved when managing AHO. The current mortality rate in patients with this disease is less than 1%. Prior

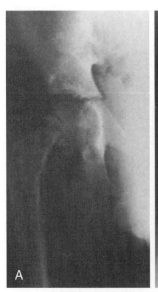
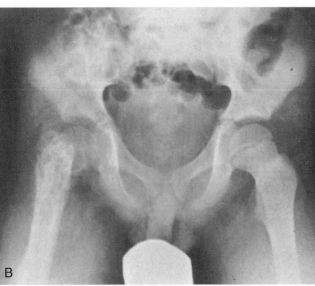

Figure 9–10. *A,* Radiogram of proximal femur showing extension of osteomyelitis to the femoral neck. *B,* Following minor trauma, the patient sustained a pathologic fracture to the neck of the femur. (From Tachdjian MO [ed]: Pediatric Orthopaedics, 2nd ed. Philadelphia, WB Saunders, 1990, p 1087.)

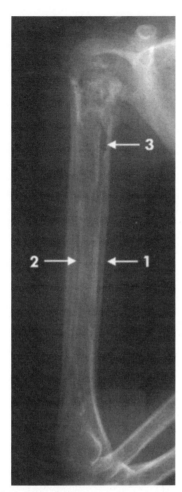

Figure 9–11. Chronic osteomyelitis in a 4-year-old girl. These images show classic appearances of chronic osteomyelitis. *1,* There is an envelope of new periosteal bone (involucrum) (1) involving most of the humerus. *2,* An extensive sequestrum has formed throughout the length of the shaft. *3,* There is a cloaca proximally and medially that discharged into the soft tissues and eventually out through a sinus. (From Broughton NS: A Textbook of Paediatric Orthopaedics. London, WB Saunders, p 157.)

to the use of penicillin, it approached 30%. Currently, the goal of management is not, as it once was, simply to save the child's life but to salvage a normally functioning extremity.

Variants of Acute Hematogenous Osteomyelitis

SUBACUTE OSTEOMYELITIS

With the use of antibiotics to treat a multiplicity of pediatric infections, a number of children have developed atypical and subacute osteomyelitis (Fig. 9–12). The child presents with an insidious onset of symptoms, few if any systemic signs, and perhaps the radiographic finding of a bone lesion. This bone lesion can be in either the epiphysis or the diaphysis of the long bone. In addition, the child may present with a limp and local tenderness at a specific point in the extremity.

The most important step in treatment is to establish the

diagnosis. The differential diagnosis of this condition is rather broad, so time is required to work it out. Once the diagnosis has been made, the management is relatively straightforward: antibiotics and occasional drainage procedures.

The term *Brodie's abscess* is still used to describe some types of subacute osteomyelitis. It is a localized metaphyseal lesion that is unassociated with systemic symptoms. These metaphyseal lesions are, in fact, the most common type of subacute osteomyelitis in children. Treatment is similar to that of any other subacute osteomyelitis.

EPIPHYSEAL OSTEOMYELITIS

Epiphyseal osteomyelitis (Fig. 9–13) may be acute or subacute. Most reported cases have been of the subacute variety. Both forms behave clinically much like their metaphyseal equivalents. It has been postulated that the lower incidence of epiphyseal disease may result from the presence of reticuloendothelial (RE) cells in the epiphysis. Biopsy is usually required for diagnosis. At the time of biopsy, debridement can be completed. Administration of antibiotics is similarly important in the management of this condition.

NEONATAL OSTEOMYELITIS

As previously mentioned, osteomyelitis in a neonate is a distinctly different disease from AHO in a child because of the involvement of different bacterial agents, the presence of transepiphyseal vessels, and the common occurrence of multifocal involvement. As mentioned before, group B streptococcal pathogens are the most common isolates, followed by *S. aureus* and gram-negative bacilli. Infection can follow invasive procedures, such as heel sticks, scalp monitors, and umbilical catheters. In the last case, *S. aureus* tends to be the predominant organism.

Transepiphyseal vessels (Fig. 9–14) are present before the secondary ossification centers appear. They are metaphyseal vessels that penetrate the chondroepiphysis directly. Therefore, a metaphyseal infection can spread directly through the epiphysis and subsequently break into the joint. The epiphysis is destroyed in the process. These vessels persist until a chid is 12 to 18 months of age. The long bones of the lower extremity are commonly affected. Also, there seems to be an unusual predilection for the facial bones. Of the long bones, the proximal femur is the most commonly involved. Infection here can cause destruction of the femoral head and resultant arrest of growth. Approximately 40% of affected neonates have infection at multiple sites.

Because of their immature immune systems, the response mounted by neotates is frequently weak, which results in rapid spread of the infection, with fewer clinical and laboratory findings. Aspiration of all suspicious sites is encouraged. A bone scan is the radiographic procedure of choice because it is able to image the whole body. Treatment principles are the same as those discussed for AHO. Sequestration and chronicity are rare; however, chondroepiphyseal destruction and growth problems are not.

Septic Arthritis

One of the most disastrous and dangerous musculoskeletal infections of childhood is septic arthritis of the hip (Fig.

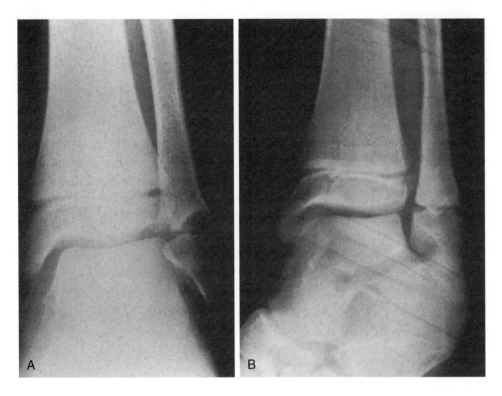

Figure 9–12. *A*, Pre-operative radiogram showing the area of metaphyseal radiolucency. There is no surrounding reactive bone. *B*, Postoperative radiogram following curettage and antibiotic therapy showing complete healing. (From Tachdjian MO [ed]: Pediatric Orthopaedics, 2nd ed. Philadelphia, WB Saunders, 1990, p 1101.)

9–15). It was recognized in 1874 by Thomas Smith, who reported on 21 infants, all of whom died or were severely disabled. Subsequent to this report, the disease was referred to as *Tom Smith's arthritis.* Septic arthritis in children has been reported to occur secondary to infection elsewhere. Meningitis, chicken pox, tonsillitis, and otitis have been mentioned as precursors to septic arthritis. In general, most discussions of septic arthritis exclude tuberculosis, even though that organism can certainly cause septic arthritis in children. The introduction of antibiotics has dramatically altered the prognosis and the mortality rate of the disease.

Emphasis is now placed on limb salvage and the minimization of complications resulting from the disease.

INCIDENCE DATA

Septic arthritis is an uncommon condition in children. In an active pediatric service, two to four cases per year can be expected. Approximately one third of these children will be younger than 2 years of age, and approximately half will be younger than 3 years of age. The joint most likely to be involved is the hip in infants and the knee in children. Approximately 10% of cases are polyarticular.

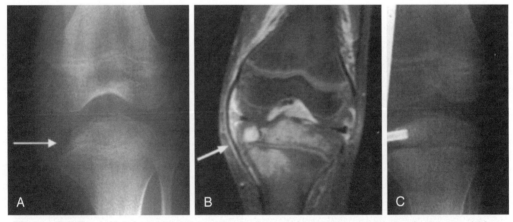

Figure 9–13. *A*, Epiphyseal osteomyelitis in the proximal tibial epiphysis of a 7-year-old boy. There is soft tissue swelling medially around the joint and cortical destruction of the medial aspect of the tibial epiphysis *(arrow)*. *B*, A T1-weighted MRI scan using fat suppression and the contrast agent gadolinium shows intense enhancement of the focal area of osteomyelitis *(arrow)* in the medial epiphysis. *C*, The patient failed to settle after 12 weeks of antibiotic treatment; therefore, biopsy and curettage of the lesion were performed. Appropriate antibiotics were then continued. (From Broughton NS: A Textbook of Paediatric Orthopaedics. London, WB Saunders, p 153.)

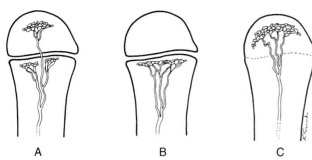

Figure 9–14. Normal vascular patterns of tubular bone in the infant, the child, and the adult. *A*, In the infant, some metaphyseal vessels may penetrate or extend around the open growth plate, ramifying in the epiphysis. *B*, In the child, the capillaries of the metaphysis turn sharply, without violating the open growth plate. *C*, In the adult, with closure of the growth plate, the vascular connection between the metaphysis and epiphysis is restored. (Adapted from Resnick D: Diagnosis of Bone and Joint Disorders, 3rd ed. Philadelphia, WB Saunders, 1995, p 2330.)

BACTERIOLOGY

As is the case with AHO, it is usually a consistent group of organisms that cause septic arthritis in children. When a child is younger than 1 year of age, *S. aureus*, group B streptococcal pathogens, and gram-negative bacilli can be expected to be present. When a child is older than 1 year of age, the organisms of concern are *S. aureus*, group B streptococcal pathogens, and a new isolate referred to as *Kingella kingae*. The last is a fastidious, hemolytic, gram-negative bacillus once considered to be an exceptional cause of the disease. However, it has emerged as an important pathogen in children. Because it is part of the commensal flora of the oropharynx, it is believed to gain access to the circulatory system during the course of an upper respiratory infection. In pre-adolescents and teenage children, *S. aureus* is by far the most likely isolate. In neonates, it is always important to consider *Candida* species as a possible cause of septic arthritis. This is particularly true in premature infants, who are kept in neonatal intensive care units for protracted periods and who have multiple indwelling lines.

A word about *Haemophilus influenzae* is appropriate. Prior to the development of the vaccine against it in the early 1990s, this organism was the most common isolate in children between 6 months and 4 years of age. Frequently, these cases were a complication of meningitis caused by *H. influenzae*, which was a particularly prevalent form of the disease. Since the immunization campaign, infections by *H. influenzae* have been virtually eradicated. Except in the occasional case of an unvaccinated child, it is unlikely that *H. influenzae* need be considered a significant cause of septic arthritis.

PATHOLOGY

The organism may enter the joint by three possible routes: hematogenously, from a distant site; contiguously, as a result of the spread of an adjacent metaphyseal osteomyelitis; and by means of direct inoculation. As noted earlier, septic arthritis following metaphyseal osteomyelitis is typically seen in the hip and the shoulder. In addition, in neonates, transepiphyseal vessels can take the organisms from the metaphysis through the chondroepiphysis and into the joint. The widespread use of femoral venipuncture accounts for the majority of cases of septic arthritis resulting from direct inoculation.

Once the organisms are present in the joint, the inflammatory process begins in the synovium, with massive vascular engorgement of the membrane and the accumulation of cellular-rich fluid. The articular cartilage and bone are damaged by a two-pronged attack. First, the mere increase of synovium and fluid within the joint distends the capsule to the extent that the small blood vessels, specifically those to the femoral head, can be collapsed, thereby causing ischemic necrosis of the head of the femur. The second prong of the attack results from a surge of enzyme-rich, bacteria-laden exudate in the joint. The enzymes produced by the white cells are chondrolytic in nature and, as such, can cause direct chondrolysis. It is important to remember that the presence of bacteria is not required for the process of chondrolysis to occur. Merely the presence of the white cells and their enzymes is enough to damage and destroy the articular cartilage. Destruction of cartilaginous ground substance is usually apparent within 5 days of infection.

CLINICAL CHARACTERISTICS

As with osteomyelitis, it is important to keep in mind that neonates present with symptoms different from those found in older children. The overall presentation in neonates is less fulminant; many times, only fever and pseudoparalysis are present, which may make it difficult to discover which joint is involved. Children, on the other hand, tend to be extremely sick. This is an acute illness that presents with fever, tachycardia, and pain in the joint. Indeed, exquisite pain is elicited with any attempt to move the joint passively. Muscle spasms and severe restriction of motion can be identified. Unlike those with osteomyelitis, these children show extensive systemic involvement.

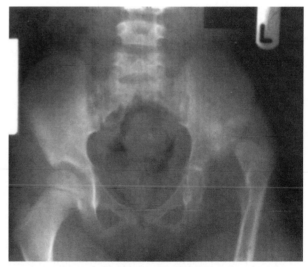

Figure 9–15. Dislocation of the left hip secondary to septic arthritis. There has been destruction on both sides of the joint resulting in a shallow acetabulum, almost complete destruction of the epiphysis, and subsequent dislocation. (From Broughton NS: A Textbook of Paediatric Orthopaedics. London, WB Saunders, p 155.)

DIAGNOSIS

The principles of diagnosis of septic arthritis are essentially the same as those enumerated for osteomyelitis. Appropriate laboratory studies and x-rays are mandatory. In addition, joint aspiration is the sine qua non of diagnosis. If septic arthritis is to be included in the differential diagnosis, it is imperative that the joint be aspirated. Unfortunately, aspiration of the joint in these small children is frequently difficult. Many physicians use a general anesthetic and perform it in the operating room. If the aspiration is positive, immediate arthrotomy is performed. Others prefer to use sedation and fluoroscopic control in a radiologic suite. Either way, it is important to confirm that the needle has entered the joint. Usually, a small amount of dilute contrast material is adequate for this purpose. Once placement of the needle has been confirmed and aspiration completed, microbiologic cultures and Gram stains can be performed. Making a count of the white blood cells in the fluid is important. A count above 100,000 should be considered diagnostic of septic arthritis; a count between 50,000 and 100,000, especially if it consists primarily of polymorphonuclear leukocytes (PMNs), should also be considered diagnostic of sepsis.

Standard radiography commonly shows joint distention and changes in soft tissue planes. In neonates, it is possible to see erosive changes in cases in which diagnosis has been delayed. It is important that a child be positioned symmetrically during radiography so that subtle changes such as alterations in soft tissue planes will be revealed. Bone scans may be helpful in answering the question "Where?" in cases of multiple site involvement. However, they are usually not helpful in the primary diagnosis when a solitary joint is affected. The use of ultrasound has become more popular in the initial evaluation of these children. The finding of fluid in a joint does not necessarily mean that it is pus; it may be nothing more than a sympathetic effusion adjacent to a metaphyseal osteomyelitis. None of these studies negates the need to perform a carefully planned joint aspiration.

A differential diagnosis includes such disorders as juvenile rheumatoid arthritis, Lyme arthritis, and, of course, toxic synovitis. It is important to keep in mind that toxic or transient synovitis does not occur in children prior to walking age. It is similarly critical to remember that toxic synovitis does not cause a child to be systemically ill.

TREATMENT

The treatment principles have been put forward by Patterson and others and can be summarized as follows:

1. Early diagnosis
2. Organism identification
3. Antibiotic delivery
4. Immediate arthrotomy
5. Immobilization of the joint.

Achieving the primary goal—saving the joint—requires aggressive treatment. It is extremely important to sterilize the joint and to evacuate all bacterial end products and debris. Otherwise, chondrolysis can occur, even in a sterile joint.

Surgical Drainage. Over the years, there has been a great deal of controversy among pediatricians, rheumatologists, and orthopaedic surgeons regarding the relative efficacy of joint aspiration, arthroscopy, and arthrotomy. Many articles have been put forward to support individual views. There is little doubt among authors, however, that the presence of pus within a joint for a period of 5 days or more can cause irreversible damage. By that time, the cartilage has been irrevocably affected, if not totally eradicated. All authors reach the same conclusion: pus must be removed from the joint as quickly and completely as possible. The controversy concerns the most efficient way of accomplishing this goal. In the minds of many surgeons, repeated joint aspiration in children is a criminal offense. The procedure is painful, it often must be performed on a daily basis, and the results of repeated aspiration in children are, for the most part, uncertain. Often, the pus is too thick to be adequately aspirated through the needle chosen and, to quote John Lloyd Roberts, "The misguided conservatism of the needle should yield to the conservatism of the knife."

The choice between arthroscopy and arthrotomy is made on the basis of the joint in question and the age of the child. Whereas arthroscopy may be appropriate for an older child with an involved knee, there is little question that the hip can be adequately drained only through an arthrotomy incision.

Surgical drainage is believed to be the treatment of choice for children with septic hips. In the past, the posterior approach was favored; however, reports of postoperative dislocation have led most authors to recommend the anterior approach. In addition, the anterior approach allows the surgeon to avoid the retinacular vessels. The scar is more cosmetically pleasing, as it follows the bikini line, and the risk of dislocation is significantly lower. Controversy also exists as to the use of a drain postoperatively. Patterson and others prefer no drain, whereas some choose to use a small Penrose drain for 48 hours. There is general agreement that postoperative immobilization in a Pavlik harness or a spica cast is reasonable.

Antibiotic Management. The use and delivery of antibiotics are similar to those discussed for AHO. In general, the duration of intravenous administration is somewhat shorter than that in AHO, assuming appropriate monitoring. The C-reactive protein level has become a popular method of following children with septic arthritis. This substance is an acute-phase protein and a specific marker for acute inflammation. Typically, it shows elevations within 6 hours of an inflammatory event and, similarly, defervesces over a much shorter period of time than does the erythrocyte sedimentation rate. When available, it is felt by most authors to be far more reliable in the monitoring of these children than is the sedimentation rate.

PROGNOSIS

Sir Dennis Patterson stated, "Every hour that an acute supurative process continues in a joint is of urgent significance to prognosis." This was an attempt to emphasize the need for aggressive and early arthrotomy when treating septic arthritis. Unfortunately, old traditions are slow to disappear. Despite the delay in diagnosis it causes, many still choose to treat this condition with antibiotics and repeated needle aspiration; only after cartilage has been destroyed are they willing to allow an arthrotomy. Unfortunately, arthrotomy cannot repair damage that has already been done. If the principles established by Patterson and others are observed—early diagnosis, immediate arthrotomy, immobilization, and administration of antibiotics—satisfactory results can be ensured in 90% of cases. Unfortunately, 50% of children who are not treated in this fashion are likely to experience poor results.

The sequelae of septic arthritis are disastrous for these children; long-term disability is common. The list of potential complications is long and includes the following:

1. Premature closure of the triradiate cartilage.
2. Acetabular dysplasia.
3. Leg-length discrepancy.
4. Premature or asymmetrical growth plate closure.
5. Pathologic dislocation of joints.
6. Necrosis of cartilage.
7. Necrosis of bone.
8. Pseudarthrosis of the femoral head and neck.
9. Complete dissolution of bony ends.

This list indicates the urgent need to manage these children aggressively and in a timely way. In addition, it also provides solace for the orthopaedic surgeon who occasionally opens a noninfected joint. As Dr. Gillespie stated, "There should be no remorse if, from time to time, we explore a hip needlessly."

Recommended Reading

Calhoun JH, Henry SL, Anger DM, et al: The treatment of infected nonunions with gentamicin-polymethacrylate antibiotic beads. Clin Orthop 1993;295:23–27.

Esterhai J: Orthopedic infection. Orthop Clin North Am 1991;22:3.
Evans RP, Nelson CL, Harrison BH: The effect of wound environment on the incidence of acute osteomyelitis. Clin Orthop 1993;286:289–297.
Gustilo R, Gruninger RP, Tsukayama DT: Orthopaedic Infection: Diagnosis and Treatment. Philadelphia, WB Saunders, 1989.
Lerner RK, Esterhai JL Jr, Polomano RC, et al: Quality-of-life assessment of patients with post-traumatic fracture nonunion, chronic refractory osteomyelitis, and lower extremity amputation. Clin Orthop 1993;295:28–36.

References

Canale ST, Harkness RM, Thomas PA, Massic JD: Does aspiration of bones and joints affect results of later bone scanning? J Pediatr Orthop 1985;5:23–26.
Choi I: Sequelae and reconstruction after septic arthritis of the hip in infants. J Bone Joint Surg 1990;72A:1150–1165.
  One of the few articles on the subject of long-term follow-up after hip sepsis. This is likely to be considered a classic.
Gillespie WJ: Musculoskeletal Infections. Melbourne, Blackwell Scientific Publications, 1987, p 35.
Green N: Bone and joint infections in children. Orthop Clin North Am 1987;18:555–576.
  Excellent summary of the spectrum of pediatric musculoskeletal sepsis. Complete bibliography.
Morrissy R: Acute hematogenous osteomyelitis. J Pediatr Orthop 1989;9:447–456.
  Classic article discussing the relationship of trauma and bacteremia. Good overview of the subject of etiology.
Patterson DC: Acute suppurative arthritis in infancy and childhood. J Bone Joint Surg 1970;52(B):474.
Shaw B, Kasser JR: Acute septic arthritis in infancy and childhood. Clin Orthop 1990;257:212–225.
  Review of all aspects of septic arthritis. Special emphasis is placed on treatment recommendations.
Watts H: Tuberculosis of bone and joint. J Bone Joint Surg 1996;78A:288–298.
  Excellent current summary of this timeless disease and its impact on the musculoskeletal system.

Chapter 10

Tumors of the Musculoskeletal System

George P. Bogumill, Ph.D., M.D.

Tumors of the musculoskeletal system are uncommon in comparison with tumors of the breast, uterus, lung, or skin. It is estimated that soft tissue sarcomas account for about 0.8 to 1.0% of all malignancies, and that 5000 to 5500 new cases are diagnosed per year. Osteosarcoma, although the most common primary malignant bone sarcoma, is even less common, with only 900 newly diagnosed cases being reported annually. This number is low in comparison with the 93,000 cases of lung carcinoma and 88,000 cases of breast cancer that are newly diagnosed each year. It has been calculated that primary malignant lesions of the skeleton will be seen by a primary care practitioner only two or three times in a lifetime of practice.

Primary tumors of bone and soft tissue are uncommon in the daily routines of even the busiest of orthopaedic surgeons. The majority of destructive skeletal lesions are metastatic carcinomas, and most of the soft tissue lesions are lipomas or a result of some inflammatory process. Because of this relatively infrequent occurrence of such malignancies, bone and soft tissue malignancies are often underdiagnosed and neglected by patient and physician. If a physician accepts the premise that any mass is abnormal and significant, early efforts can be made to ascertain the proper diagnosis. On occasion the workup will be more than is necessary for an innocent lesion, but a more serious lesion will not be neglected until too late for optimal treatment. Lesions regarded as potentially malignant should be referred to an oncology specialist for workup and treatment. The most important aspect of the initial evaluation of a patient with a musculoskeletal tumor is the recognition of its presence and potential. Musculoskeletal tumors should always be considered in the differential diagnosis of a patient with musculoskeletal symptoms or signs.

Orthopaedists and other scientists are fascinated by tumors of bone and soft tissue out of proportion to their incidence. Neoplasms frequently present a dramatic clinical picture, often in young people. The rapid onset and progression can cause extraordinarily devastating effects in the lives of the patients and their families. A major reason for the current intense interest of orthopaedists is the fact that over the past few decades remarkable strides have been made in the management of patients with such tumors. The ability to save lives and to leave patients with a useful extremity has been greatly enhanced. More is constantly being identified about the behavior of specific tumors, and new diagnoses with their specific behavior patterns are

continually being separated from the general mass of malignancies affecting the musculoskeletal system.

In the early 1960s, it was generally accepted knowledge that even with radical surgery, less than 20% of patients with osteosarcoma survived as long as 5 years. Ewing's sarcoma was so rapidly and uniformly fatal that surgery (amputation) was felt to be unnecessarily mutilating, and most patients were treated with radiation alone. In the late 1960s and early 1970s tumor centers were seeing some success with use of chemotherapeutic agents in treating the local lesion in these high-grade sarcomas, but more important, they were able to destroy the micrometastases invisible to standard imaging techniques and could thus markedly decrease the mortality rate. Use of multidrug protocols have enhanced the safety and efficacy of these agents bringing the 5-year survival rates of both osteosarcoma and Ewing's sarcoma to greater than 60%. Such therapies have provided surgeons greater latitude to perform limb-sparing surgery rather than amputations.

Use of radiotherapy in conjunction with surgery for local control of the primary sarcoma of bone or soft tissue, when coupled with appropriate chemotherapy for micrometastases, has enhanced the survival rates for patients with such tumors as lymphoma, myeloma, and Ewing's sarcoma. Radiotherapy to the local area given pre-, intra-, or postoperatively can reduce the incidence of local recurrence of soft tissue sarcomas to less than 5% after marginal or wide resection. Remarkable success has also been achieved in rendering patients with pulmonary metastases disease free by wedge resections of solitary or even multiple nodules, if not too numerous. For osteosarcoma and other high-grade malignancies, such pulmonary nodule resections may produce long-term survival without relapse in as many as 30% of patients.

A team composed of the surgeon, diagnostic radiologist, and a pathologist with a special interest and experience in the spectrum of tumors of the extremities is needed for proper diagnosis of such lesions. If any of the triumvirate is missing or inexperienced, misdiagnosis is common. Medical oncologists and radiotherapists are often necessary to provide the appropriate adjunctive treatment of tumors involving the extremities and spine.

DIAGNOSTIC EVALUATION

The diagnostic workup for the evaluation of musculoskeletal tumors is summarized in Figure 10–1. Every patient

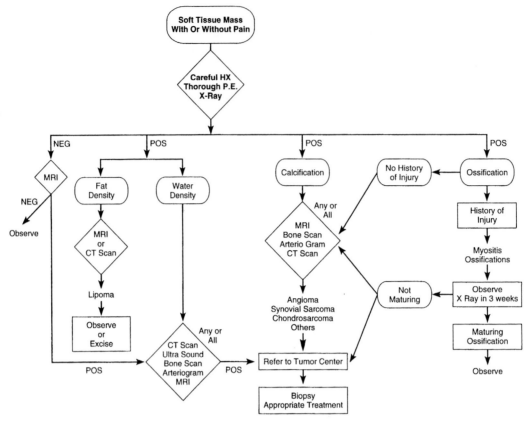

Figure 10–1. Algorithms for management of soft tissue tumors. (From Wiesel SW: Essentials of Orthopaedic Surgery, 2nd ed. Philadelphia, W.B. Saunders, 1997, p 119.)

with a soft tissue mass, with or without associated symptoms, or with radiographic evidence of a bone lesion, deserves thorough and careful evaluation. A good history must be the first step. The usual questions about when and how the mass was discovered, any change in size (either increase or decrease), a history of prior injury to the involved area, and a history of cancer should always be asked. A patient with a bone tumor often complains initially of pain or functional impairment of a part, whether or not there is a palpable mass. A history of a dull ache, not relieved by rest and present at night, is worrisome. On occasion, the incidental discovery of a radiographic abnormality may bring the patient to seek medical treatment. Occasional symptoms of anorexia, weight loss, or fever may be present. Age and sex may be helpful in narrowing the field of diagnostic possibilities. A pathologic fracture may be the first sign of a problem, and a history of pain prior to the fracture should raise suspicion that the lesion is malignant, either primary or secondary. A conventional radiograph of the region in question, when combined with the limited history and clinical findings, may suggest a differential diagnosis that is often quite accurate in the case of bone lesions, less so with soft tissue tumors.

Physical examination should include a general evaluation of the patient in addition to a careful examination of the part in question. Consideration should be given to the possibility of a metastatic lesion, especially in an older patient, because metastases are the most common malignant tumors in bone. A mass should be measured, and its location, shape, consistency, mobility in relation to adjacent tissues, tenderness and local temperature, atrophy of adjacent musculature, effusion of nearby joints with restricted motion, and skin changes such as telangiectasia all should be evaluated and recorded. Neurologic examination as well as evaluation of arterial and venous changes should be made. Although most primary musculoskeletal malignancies spread to the lung, some metastasize to regional or distant lymph nodes, which should be checked as part of the overall physical examination.

Routine laboratory studies include complete blood cell count, urinalysis, erythrocyte sedimentation rate and serum calcium, phosphorus, and alkaline and acid phosphatase; serum and urine electrophoresis may also be indicated. The studies generally have limited value in diagnosing or staging bone or soft tissue sarcomas. White blood cell count and erythrocyte sedimentation rate may be elevated in bone infections as well as Ewing's sarcoma, lymphoma, or bone metastases. They are nonspecific tests, as are most of the other routine blood or urine tests. Alkaline phosphatase may be elevated in osteosarcoma or giant cell tumor, and occasionally with bone metastases from carcinomas or soft tissue tumors.

The conventional radiograph is the key diagnostic imaging tool, giving information about the intraosseous location and extent of the tumor and position of the internal margins, the pattern of cortical destruction, and the periosteal response. Periosteal new bone formation may indicate the extent of intraosseous tumor (Fig. 10–2), as well as aiding in determination of whether the activity is episodic, allowing for some new bone formation in layers, showing the "onion skin pattern." Good quality radiographs in at least two planes at 90 degrees to each other often will provide most of the information necessary for an accurate diagnosis of a bone lesion. Although less helpful than in bone lesions, such films should also be done for patients with a soft tissue mass. Radiographs are noninvasive and economical, provide a gross anatomic image of a bone tumor, and often are diagnostic. The study should include the entire bone in question, as well as other sites from which symptoms may be referred (such as hip films for patients with knee pain). On reviewing the radiographs, the clinician should ask four questions:

1. *Where is the lesion?* This question refers to the anatomic location. L.C. Johnson and associates at the Armed Forces Institute of Pathology have long promoted the philosophy that both benign and malignant bone lesions occur in areas influenced by normal bone activity in that location (Fig. 10–3).

2. *What is the lesion doing to the bone?* Is the lesion causing resorption of bone, and if so, by what pattern? if the zone of transition is wide or has a permeative appearance, then the lesion is aggressive in its behavior, even though it may be a benign lesion, meaning that it will not metastasize. If the zone of transition is narrow (geographic, clear cut), the lesion is usually slow growing and more likely to be benign (Fig. 10–4).

3. *What is the bone doing to the lesion?* In slow-growing benign lesions, marginal ossification of the internal border of the lesion indicates there has been time to locally contain the lesion, and this feature is more suggestive of a benign lesion. Periosteal reactions can be quite varied, and like the internal margins, can suggest the aggressiveness of the lesion inside or on the surface of the bone (Fig. 10–5). The junction of the edge of the periosteal reaction with the bone (Codman triangle) is often productive of normal reactive bone and is not part of the tumor that has broken out of the bone and is therefore not a good site for biopsy.

4. *Are there any characteristics of the matrix that will suggest a diagnosis?* Internal characteristics of the matrix such as calcification, ossification, or pure osteolysis can be very helpful in pointing toward the correct tissue diagnosis (Fig. 10–6). Questions should always be asked about prior radiographs, because if they are available, they will give a history of the lesion over time. The surgeon should be knowledgeable about bone lesions and should continuously consider non-neoplastic entities when evaluating bone lesions to avoid excessive or inappropriate treatment. Tumors of the bone should be placed in one of three major groupings (benign primary, malignant primary, malignant metastatic).

Isotope scanning is a sensitive, readily available, efficient, cost-effective, nonspecific tool for diagnosis and staging of bone tumors. It helps determine the activity of a primary lesion, as well as exposing occult metastases, but is not specific for tumor type. Technetium-99m methylene diphosphonate is the most sensitive, cost-effective test for detection of bone metastases from carcinoma. It is an

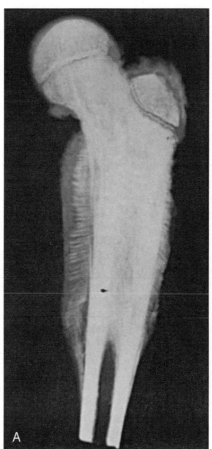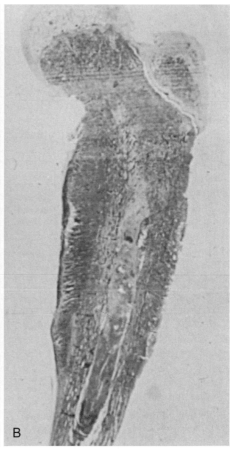

Figure 10–2. Ewing's sarcoma. *A*, Specimen radiograph of proximal femur with "hair-on-end" periosteal response, Codman's triangle, and intramedullary tumor filling canal. *B*, Macrosection of specimen indicating intramedullary extent of tumor matching extent of periosteal response. (From Madewell JE, Ragsdale BD, Sweet DE: Radiologic and pathologic analysis of solitary bone lesions: Part I. Internal margins. Radiol Clin North Am 19[1]:749–783, 1981.)

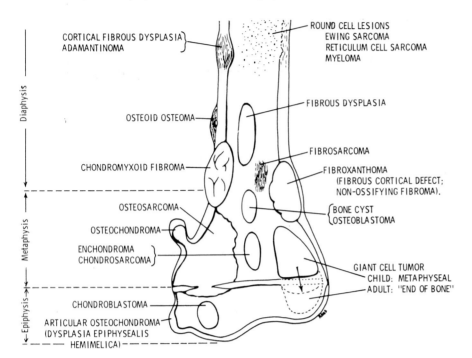

Figure 10–3. Diagram of typical locations of osseous lesions in long bones. (From Madewell JE, Ragsdale BD, Sweet DE: Radiology and pathological analysis of solitary bone lesions. Part I. Internal margins. Radiol Clin North Am 1981; 19[4]:715.)

avid bone-seeking isotope, with uptake in areas of bone formation and increased blood flow around the reactive margin of benign and malignant tumors. Lack of uptake indicates a benign process except in cases of multiple myelomas and histiocytosis X, which elicit less bone response. Gallium-67 scans may be useful, but take longer to accomplish than technetium-99m, and are more indicative of inflammation than tumor because the isotope is taken up by inflammatory cells. Isotope scans cannot distinguish between benign and malignant primary bone tumors. They have limited diagnostic or staging value in soft tissue tumors except those with bone metastases.

Conventional tomography has been very useful for obtaining further information about the bone alterations induced by the tumor. In most radiology departments, however, tomography has been replaced by computed tomography (CT scan), which can provide three-dimensional images with newer techniques. It is a superb tool to assess the extent and composition of an abnormal focus, particularly in bone, but also in soft tissue. CT scans provide better resolution of osseous structures than does magnetic resonance imaging (MRI), because calcification and ossification are seen better with the CT scan. However, MRI is equal or superior to CT in many cases, especially in evaluating soft tissue tumors where it outlines in several planes not only the lesion itself, but also normal structures such as joints, ligaments, nerves, and vessels showing both their location and their relation to the tumor. MRI can distinguish between tissues of different histologic types with similar radiographic densities. Intravenous gadolinium can help distinguish between tumor margins and edematous normal tissue, thus enabling better planning for surgical procedures. Disadvantages of MRI are the high cost, long examination times, and poor tolerance by claustrophobic patients, although open MRI machines have helped greatly in this regard. Small coils are also available and very

helpful in evaluating lesions of the peripheral parts of limbs, such as the hands and feet.

A chest radiograph is indicated in the evaluation of a patient with suspected malignancy. Routine CT scans of the lung provide more information, particularly for small metastatic foci in the lungs, but can be deferred until after biopsy of the primary site has proved the malignant nature of the lesion. CT scans, ultrasonography, MRI (with or without gadolinium), and radioisotope scans are often helpful in determining the extent of the tumor and help detect occult bone metastases or extent of bone involvement in the case of soft tissue tumors. The imaging is clearly helpful to the surgeon in developing a three-dimensional plot of the anatomic location prior to treatment. They can provide a sensitive method for determining the presence of pulmonary or osseous metastases either prior to treating the primary tumor or during the follow-up period.

Enneking and others have demonstrated convincingly the desirability of staging malignant musculoskeletal lesions for planning treatment methods and evaluating results. Staging also suggests the type of surgical procedure needed for local control of the tumor. Such staging should be done before any surgical procedure, including biopsy.

Unlike bone lesions, the clinical and radiographic evaluation of a soft tissue mass can be quite inaccurate. Soft tissue sarcomas are often painless, slow-growing and may persist for long periods. The routine radiographs of soft tissue tumors usually do not provide much diagnostic information, although they may occasionally have the radiodensity of fat, or contain calcifications to suggest cartilaginous or vascular tumors. Most soft tissue tumors have muscle or water density on routine radiographs, and thus may not visualize well. The clinical evaluation of soft tissue tumors is unreliable; they are often biopsied by a clinician who is not ultimately responsible for management of the patient. It is extremely important to be aware that improper or

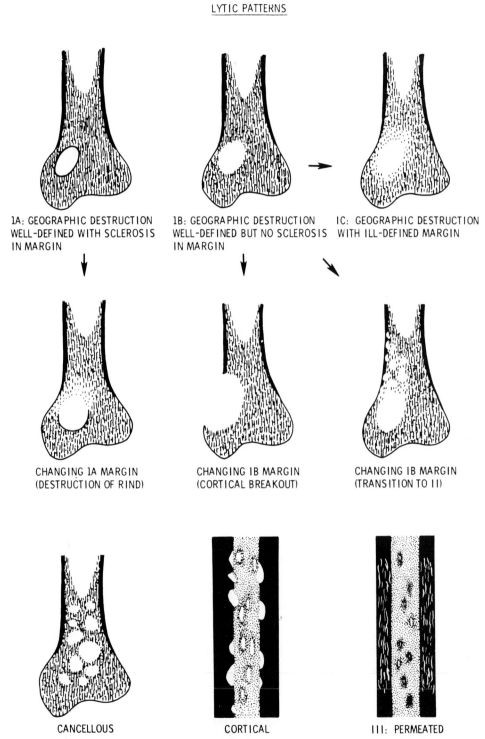

Figure 10–4. Diagram of tumor margin types. (From Madewell JE, Ragsdale BD, Sweet DE: Radiology and pathological analysis of solitary bone lesions. Part I. Internal margins. Radiol Clin North Am 1981; 19[4]:715.)

PERIOSTEAL REACTIONS

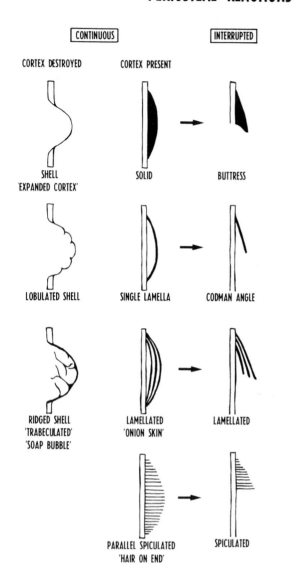
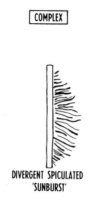
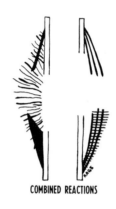

Figure 10–5. Diagram of periosteal reaction types. (From Ragsdale BD, Madewell JE, Sweet DE: Radiology and pathological analysis of solitary bone lesions. Part II. Periosteal reactions. Radiol Clin North Am 1981; 19[4]:749.)

careless biopsy technique may severely compromise subsequent surgical treatment and even patient survival.

Biopsy

The biopsy is exceeded in importance only by the definitive surgery itself. Most orthopaedic oncologists prefer a diagnostic approach that involves staging of the lesion before biopsy is done; thus, biopsy should follow all indicated imaging studies. Proper planning is imperative to prevent complications, which could lead to unnecessary amputation or death. The number and type of tests in a given case depend on the consideration by an experienced clinician of the diagnostic possibilities the patient presents and should be done in a cost-effective manner. Obtaining diagnostic tests before biopsy is much more informative in regard to anatomic locus than getting such tests after the lesion has been altered by a biopsy, however well planned. If such preoperative planning is utilized, definitive surgery often can be carried out under the same anesthetic if frozen

section of a biopsy specimen provides a clear diagnosis that confirms the prebiopsy suspicion.

Biopsy is the ultimate diagnostic study for evaluation of neoplasms. Needle aspiration is more useful in evaluating soft tissue than bone lesions but in any case requires experienced personnel using image intensifier to localize the placement of the needle, and capable histologists or cytologists to interpret the material obtained. Preparations for open biopsy, whether incisional or excisional, should be as deliberate and detailed as preparations for a major surgical procedure. Biopsy should be planned with consideration of the possible next surgical procedures and treatments. Biopsy of a suspected malignancy should be done in such a manner that a minimum of normal tissue is contaminated by tumor spill or hematoma, preferably staying in one compartment, avoiding neurovascular planes, and obtaining meticulous hemostasis. Avoid undermining the skin, and place drains, if deemed necessary, through the wound and not through a separate incision.

A tourniquet, if used, should be released prior to closure

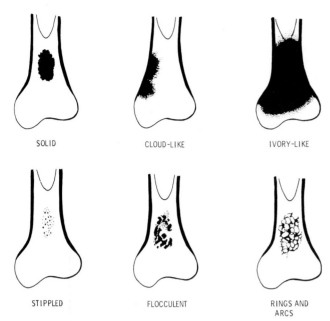

SOLID CLOUD-LIKE IVORY-LIKE

STIPPLED FLOCCULENT RINGS AND ARCS

Figure 10–6. Diagram of matrix patterns of osseous lesions. (From Sweet DE, Madewell JE, Ragsdale BD: Radiology and pathological analysis of solitary bone lesions. Part III. Matrix patterns. Radiol Clin North Am 1981;19[4]:785.)

of the biopsy incision to minimize hematoma formation. Also if a tourniquet is used, the limb should not be exsanguinated by wrapping prior to inflation to avoid pushing tumor cells into the vascular system of the tumor where they can be washed out into the general circulation upon release of the tourniquet.

Placement of the incision for biopsy should be planned carefully, and should almost always be longitudinally oriented so that the biopsy tract can be removed completely during subsequent surgical treatment of the tumor. Frozen section evaluation and interpretation should always be done on the biopsied tissue to be certain that the tissue obtained is viable, representative of the tumor, and adequate in volume. Bacteriologic culture should be obtained of any lesion that has open biopsy (also any infection operatively treated should have a biopsy of the tissue obtained).

Ideally, the biopsy and definitive procedure should be done in the same institution by a surgeon experienced in the care of such tumors. Mankin and associates have shown that inappropriate biopsy is a major problem for the patient and the subsequent treating surgeon. If specific lesions are not treatable at a given institution, the biopsy should be deferred and the patient should be referred to a facility where definitive management can be done. Excisional biopsy generally should be reserved for small benign lesions. Bone marrow aspiration may be helpful in diagnosis of round cell lesions (myeloma, Ewing's sarcoma, lymphoma, leukemia).

Staging of Sarcomas

A number of staging methods have been developed over the years. The one proposed by Enneking and coworkers for both bone and soft tissue sarcomas has gained wide acceptance among orthopaedic oncologists and the Muscu-

loskeletal Tumor Society. Staging a tumor requires incorporation of three elements, surgical grade (G), surgical site (T), and presence or absence of detectable metastases (M). The surgical grade is based on evaluation of tissue from the lesion by the orthopaedic surgeon and pathologist, combined with knowledge of the preoperative clinical and radiographic evaluation. Grade is considered either low (G1, less than 25% likelihood of metastases) or high (G2, more than 25% chance of spread). The surgical site is determined by preoperative studies and confirmed by operative studies as being intracompartmental (A) or extracompartmental (B). Thus, a tumor can be stage I or II, depending on grade, and A or B, depending on site. Any metastases will place the tumor in stage III (Table 10–1).

Surgical Techniques—Bone

In the surgical removal of bone tumors, one must consider the margins achieved by the various methods. Enneking and coworkers have provided a useful guide to planning surgical treatment by discussing the tumor margins through which the excision occurs and their effect on the outcome.

Intralesional margins are those in which the dissection passes through tumor tissue, as occurs in curettage of bone lesions. Debulking is another term for treatment of lesions with this type of margin. Curettage is considered an intralesional excision without margins, and thus is reserved for benign lesions of bone. The lesions are approached through a cortical window, which should be longer and wider than the lesion whenever possible so that the entire extent of the lesion can be visualized directly and lesional tissue will not be hidden by overhanging edges of bone. When thorough curettage has been accomplished, the walls of the cavity may be further treated by a high speed burr, or thermal cautery with liquid nitrogen or methyl methacrylate; the use of concentrated phenol (89% or a 50% suspension), followed by absolute alcohol, is the preferred technique of the author to kill cells hidden in the interstices of the internal tumor margin.

Many benign bone tumors can be treated successfully by curettage with or without bone grafting, depending on site or size of the lesion. Lesions in the upper limb, particularly the hand, usually can be treated without bone grafting unless such grafting is needed to provide support to the subchondral plate of a major bone. Filling an excavated cavity is more important in the lower limb because of the necessity for weight bearing. Various materials to fill such cavities are autograft or allograft bone, methyl methacrylate, or calcified materials such as prepared coral. Bone morphogenic proteins are being used in conjunction with various grafted materials.

Table 10–1. Staging of tumors by grade, site, and metastases

Stage	Grade	Site	Metastases	
IA	G1	T1	M0	Low grade, intracompartmental
IB	G1	T2	M0	Low grade, extracompartmental
IIA	G2	T1	M0	High grade, intracompartmental
IIB	G2	T2	M0	High grade, extracompartmental
III	Any	Any	M1	With metastases

Marginal margins result when soft tissue tumor is "shelled out" through the pseudocapsule forming the periphery of the specimen. Both intralesional and marginal resections invariably leave behind microscopic remnants of the tumor.

Wide margins are achieved when the entire dissection is carried out entirely through normal tissue outside the reactive capsule, although "skip metastases" may be left by this method.

Radical margins are achieved when all the tissues of one or more compartments are removed from origin to insertion. Wide local resections are used more often than radical resections at present because protocols involving chemotherapy and radiation therapy are proving to be effective in aiding limb preservation and improved function.

Tumor-removing procedures not involving amputation are termed limb-sparing or local resections. Margins similar to those achieved by local resections may occur with amputations, with much the same potential for leaving tumor remnants behind, depending on the relation of amputation level to the tumor. Enneking and coworkers have pointed out that amputation does not necessarily achieve radical margins, and in fact may be debulking, marginal, wide, or radical, depending on the level of the amputation in relation to the lesion.

A combination of treatment modalities is commonly used in the treatment of malignant musculoskeletal lesions. The most predictable local control is achieved by appropriate surgery, with adjuvant therapies used to gain systemic control. It has become common to use chemotherapy or local radiotherapy after biopsy and before definitive surgery to help shrink the tumor and diminish the active margins of the tumor so that residual tumor is less likely to be left behind during definitive surgery for tumor removal.

BENIGN TUMORS OF BONE

Benign Bone-Forming Tumors

Bone and soft tissue tumors vary widely in type. The simplest approach is to categorize them on the basis of tissue type or common attributes and then distinguish between benign and malignant entities.

Osteoid Osteoma. Osteoid osteoma is a benign growth of uncertain etiology, seen most often in young males. It can affect any bone in intramedullary, intracortical, or subperiosteal location. Malignant change has not been reported. The clinical picture is so characteristic that the diagnosis is rarely missed. Typically the patient has severe, poorly localized, aching pain, which is worse at night and relieved dramatically by aspirin but less well by NSAIDs. It is often said that osteoid osteoma should be suspected in a child with a painful scoliosis, because idiopathic scoliosis is painless. The sclerosis induced by the small nidus is often extensive enough to hide the nidus on plain radiographs, although computed or plain tomography will often clearly identify it. MRI and angiography are not as useful. Because the lesions are usually less than 1.0 cm in diameter, the cuts of the tomograms must be thin to avoid missing the nidus. Technetium-99m bone scans are useful in localizing the site of the lesion because the active osteoid formation shows an affinity for the isotope. The lesions usually show little or no growth in size over long periods. Grossly, the nidus is reddish brown, reflecting its vascularity. Microscopic examination of the lesional tissue shows osteoid formation by nonmalignant cells in a highly vascular, loosely arranged fibrous tissue. They are well supplied by nerves. Block excision is the usual recommended treatment, although it does pose the risk of subsequent fracture.

Osteoblastoma. Osteoblastoma is a rare, benign, bone-forming tumor that has histologic resemblance to osteoid osteoma but is usually larger and progressive. From 80 to 90% of patients are younger than 30 years of age; males predominate 2:1 over females (Fig. 10–7). The posterior elements of the spine, as well as the pelvis, femur, tibia, and mandible, account for 75% of lesions. The lesions are painful but lack the characteristic night pain and often the dramatic response to salicylates seen in osteoid osteoma. Radiographic appearance is quite variable. In long bones they are usually diaphyseal or metaphyseal, often eccentrically placed and at times subperiosteal. Size ranges from 2 to 10 cm, and they are variably mineralized and often almost purely osteolytic on radiographs. Grossly, the tissue is reddish purple, reflecting its vascularity, and feel gritty on palpation or when cutting with scalpel. Histologically, the lesions are similar to osteoid osteoma with abundant osteoblasts producing irregular spicules of osteoid and bone in a highly vascularized, loosely arranged fibrous tissue. Neoplastic cartilage is not found in osteoblastoma or osteoid osteoma. At times it can be difficult to distinguish from low-grade osteosarcoma. Behavior is erratic and unpredictable. Most pursue a benign course, and some even resolve after incomplete removal. Others recur after what is considered thorough resection or curettage, and still others appear to undergo malignant change. Radiation therapy should not be used unless absolutely necessary to control or eradicate the tumor because of the risk of postirradiation sarcoma.

Benign Tumors of Cartilage

Benign cartilage tumors of bone can create a major problem in diagnosis and management. They may arise from within the bone or on the surface. Management of a patient

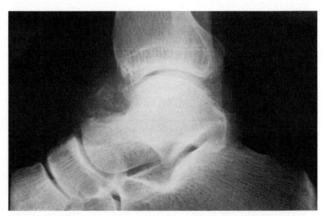

Figure 10–7. Osteoblastoma of talus. This 28-year-old man has had this tender, enlarging mass anterior to ankle joint for months.

with a benign cartilage lesion can be treacherous. Malignant potential must always be considered and demands accurate diagnosis and evaluation by the oncology team of surgeon, pathologist, and radiologist. Even with experience, differentiation of benign from malignant cartilage is difficult because both may exist in the same lesion, if large, and location of the biopsy is critical. Discussion with a diagnostic radiologist prior to the biopsy may lead the surgeon to sample the appropriate areas of the tumor and avoid misdiagnosis. Principal among the methods of diagnosing the lesions are good radiographic studies in multiple planes. CT enables identification of the reactive margination of benign enchondromas and chondroblastomas as well as demonstrating cortical breakthrough. MRI is superior in defining the intramedullary extent of the lesions. Bone scans are helpful in diagnosis. Benign lesions show significant variability in active isotope uptake. Malignant cartilage tumors, in addition to often being painful, show significant uptake of the isotope on bone scans. Thus, a hot scan does not differentiate between benign or malignant, but a "cold" scan is strong evidence of a benign lesion. No laboratory tests are specific for cartilage tumors.

Solitary Osteochondroma. Solitary osteochondroma, a cartilage-capped protuberance growing outward from the surface of a normal bone, is the most common benign tumor of bone. Regarded as developmental anomalies rather than true tumors, they originate in the metaphysis and grow most rapidly during growth spurts. After puberty they mature with gradual ossification of the cartilage cap. Continued growth beyond puberty is highly suggestive of malignant change. They generally are discovered during such growth spurts and then stop growing when skeletal maturity is reached. Discovery is incidental; they usually cause no symptoms other than the presence of a firm immobile mass. Radiographically they present as either stalked lesions or broad-based (sessile) bone masses. Of considerable diagnostic importance is the absence of subjacent cortex at the attachment site of the exostoses. Typically the cortex and medullary cavity of the parent bone are continuous with those of the osteochondroma. The lesion is capped by cartilage which is usually only a few millimeters thick, irregular, and radiolucent unless there are calcifications within it. A bursa frequently overlies the tumor. A rare form of osteocartilaginous exostosis is dysplasia epiphysealis hemimelica, in which an osteochondroma-like lesion arises from an epiphysis, usually protruding into the knee or ankle joint.

Treatment of osteochondroma is indicated when the lesion is unsightly or causes symptoms from pressure on adjacent structures, or when there is rapid growth after skeletal maturity. Surgical treatment is excision of the entire lesion en bloc down to the level of the cortex of the host bone, taking a rim of normal bone around the base of the stalk. Recurrences are uncommon, and are probably due to incomplete excision of the entire cartilage cap. Malignant transformation of solitary osteochondromas is uncommon, probably less than 1%. When it does occur it usually presents as chondrosarcoma.

Multiple Osteochondromas. Multiple osteochondromatosis appears to be an anomaly of skeletal development rather than an accumulation of neoplasms. The most striking feature is the presence of many exostoses along with disturbances of growth such as abnormal tubulation of bones, broad and blunt metaphyses, and curvatures of long bones. There is a familial tendency in about half the offspring of an involved parent (autosomal dominant). Exostoses may be numerous or relatively few, they are most conspicuous about the knees, ankles, and wrists. The physical and radiographic appearances of multiple lesions are similar to the solitary ones. Because "cure" cannot be obtained, surgical treatment is not routinely indicated, but may be required to remove painful or rapidly growing lesions, particularly if possible malignant change is suggested by the continued growth occurring after cessation of overall growth of the patient (Fig. 10–8). Pressure on adjacent structures, such as nerves or vessels, or blockage of joint motion are surgical indications in either solitary or multiple osteochondromas. Surgical correction of deformities may also be indicated.

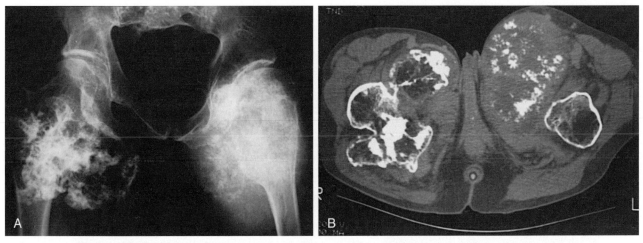

Figure 10–8. Malignant degeneration in 58-year-old man with long-standing osteochondromatosis. *A*, Bilateral large cartilaginous mass arising from both proximal femurs. Left mass has shown fairly rapid enlargement with pain during past 6 months. *B*, CT scan of proximal femurs showing large soft tissue component on left.

Propensity of malignant change is significantly higher in multiple than in solitary lesions; thus, these patients should be watched throughout life, and they should be warned to promptly report to a physician if any lesion appears to be growing.

Enchondromas. Enchondromas probably represent genetic errors with retention of embryonic cartilage anlage rather than true benign tumors of mature hyaline cartilage. Central location in the diaphysis or metaphysis is more common than an eccentric position (Fig. 10–9). They appear to grow during the period of growth in skeletal length, and exhibit little or no growth after skeletal maturity. Less common than osteochondromas, they are usually discovered during the patient's second, third, or fourth decades, often as an incidental finding on radiographs taken for trauma or pain.

Enchondroma is the most common tumor of the small tubular bones of the hands and feet. Solitary enchondromas rarely exhibit aggressive behavior. In the absence of fracture, pain is an ominous presenting symptom, suggesting possible malignant transformation. The radiographic appearance depends on the location and amount of intralesional calcification. In small tubular bones the lesion is usually diaphyseal with thinned, expanded overlying cortex (Fig. 10–10). Small foci of flocculent calcification may be seen and help in radiographic diagnosis. Differentiation of benign and malignant cartilage tumors is difficult even for pathologists experienced in reviewing bone lesions.

Histologic examination shows formation of mature hyaline cartilage with cells of small and relatively uniform size. Aggressive appearing lesions with atypical cells may be found in the hands or feet and may behave in a benign

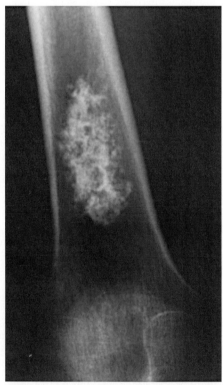

Figure 10–9. Typical benign calcifying enchondroma in distal femur.

fashion, whereas lesions in larger bones may have a more benign histologic appearance but act aggressively and recur after surgical excision. Indications for surgery are related to maintenance of skeletal integrity, correction of deformity, treatment of fractures, or concern regarding potential malignancy.

Thorough curettage with or without bone grafting is the usual treatment, although occasionally excision of lesions in bones that can be spared may be preferred. Most solitary enchondromas can be treated by an intralesional approach of curettage and treatment of the resulting cavity walls with concentrated phenol and absolute alcohol. Care must be taken to avoid spill of tumor cells into the soft tissues, where they can take up independent growth. Surgery for recurrences should include removal of the previous surgical tract. Recurrences commonly look more aggressive than the original tumor; whether this represents malignant transformation or underdiagnosis of the original lesion may be difficult to determine.

Multiple enchondromatosis (Ollier's disease) is an uncommon entity in which many cartilage lesions appear in both large and small tubular bones and in the flat bones. It is caused by failure of normal enchondral ossification. There is considerable variability in presentation; the lesions may be found in epiphyses and metaphyses of many or only a few bones, with more extensive involvement of one side of the body, although usually not to the total exclusion of the other side. Growth abnormalities are common with impairment of longitudinal growth and shortening, bowing of long bones, and broadening of metaphyses. Multiple lesions of the small bones of the hands may cause considerable deformity and disability (Fig. 10–11A and B).

The lesion tissue consists of masses of hyaline-like cartilage present within the medullary cavity. The masses may be confluent or separate, with varying amounts of calcification or enchondral ossification. Bones without prior cartilage model are seldom involved. The facial bones or base of the skull may be involved, with foraminal encroachment or distortion of facial appearance. When associated with venous hemangiomas of the overlying soft tissues, the name Maffucci is attached to the syndrome (see Fig. 10–11C). The individual lesions in Ollier's disease are quite similar to solitary enchondromas, but the cellularity is more bizarre and malignant transformation is more common. Surgical treatment is undertaken for the same reasons as in the solitary variety. Patients with the syndromes of multiple lesions should be watched carefully throughout their lifetime. Estimates of the frequency of malignant deterioration in this syndrome are as high as 50% but are more than likely in the 25 to 35% range.

Chondroblastoma. Chondroblastoma is uncommon, but 90% of patients are in the age range of 5 to 20 years; males predominate 3:2 over females. Knee, hip, and shoulder epiphyses, along with the tarsal bones, are most common sites, although apophyses are also involved on occasion (Fig. 10–12). Pain is the usual first symptom, and because these tumors occur near a joint, patients may present with limitation of movement. Radiographs are often quite characteristic, but biopsy is necessary to confirm the diagnosis.

The histologic picture consists of sheets of cells identified as chondroblasts; polygonal cells with clear, somewhat

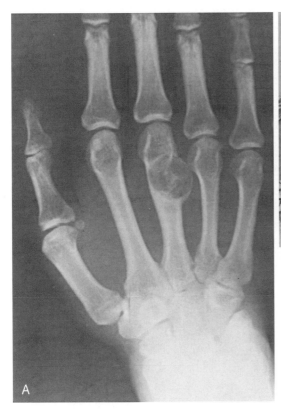

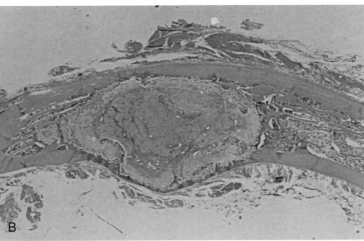

Figure 10–10. Enchondroma. *A,* Typical eccentric location in small tubular bone with expansion of the bone. *B,* Macrosection of benign enchondroma of a rib with expansion of the bone eccentrically but cortical bone present over the lesion.

bluish cytoplasm with a centrally placed, rounded nucleus; and a modest amount of matrix of atypical cartilage. Giant cells may be sparse, or may be found in large enough numbers to confuse the diagnosis with giant cell tumor. Calcification may present as small rounded foci or may surround the margins of each cell, producing the "chicken wire" pattern.

Thorough curettage followed by phenol and alcohol cautery of the cavity wall (unless there is significant danger of damage to the epiphyseal cartilage by the phenol) and packing of the cavity with autologous or allograft bone to support the articular surface is usually curative. Recurrences average about 15 to 20% and can be resected or curetted again. Occasional malignant or aggressive behavior of chondroblastomas have been reported, as have metastases, which may have benign histologic appearance. Radiation therapy should be reserved for the very few cases in which surgery is impossible.

Chondromyxoid Fibroma. Chondromyxoid fibroma is rare, usually found in second or third decades of life, although a wide age range is possible. Most are found in the metaphyses of long bones of the lower extremities. Usually the lesion presents as an eccentrically placed, oval or rounded radiolucency, sometimes with a thin cortical shell overlying it. Histologically the chondromyxoid fibroma shows an extraordinary merging of the three elements of the tumor in low-power field. A hyaline chondroid focus may blend into a myxoid area with a few stellate cells, or an adjacent focus of whorled fibrous tissue. All the elements are benign, although malignant forms have been described. Treatment is similar to that for chondroblastomas, consisting of

resection where feasible and curettage if resection would result in loss of too much function.

Juxtacortical Chondroma. Juxtacortical chondroma (parosteal chondroma, periosteal chondroma) is a very rare lesion of young adults or adolescents, seen most often in the proximal humerus. These tumors appear to have no relation to the physis; rather, they may be diaphyseal. They are extraosseous, although they may cause some erosion or scalloping of the underlying cortex with periosteal new bone around the site. There may be some calcification within the matrix of the lesion, as well as extension of the lesion into the soft tissues. Treatment consists of surgical excision with removal of the underlying cortex, the overlying soft tissues, and the reactive periosteal bone in the periphery.

Fibrous Lesions

Fibrous cortical defect and cortical desmoid are asymptomatic irregularities in the cortical surface. They usually present in the posteromedial aspect of the distal femoral metaphysis in boys 10 to 15 years of age. Oblique radiographs with the limb externally rotated 20 to 45 degrees present a typical picture. The lesions are benign and require no treatment, but often are not recognized as such by doctors not familiar with the entity and may be overtreated.

Nonossifying Fibromas. Nonossifying fibroma (fibroxanthoma), the most common benign bone tumor in children or adolescents, is larger than the cortical lesions, but the histologic appearance is similar, with xanthoma cells (his-

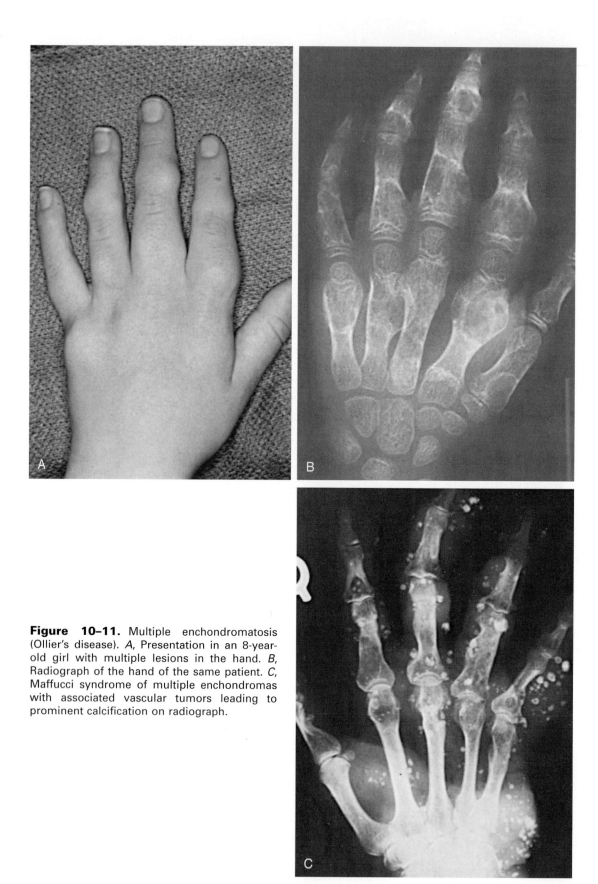

Figure 10–11. Multiple enchondromatosis (Ollier's disease). *A*, Presentation in an 8-year-old girl with multiple lesions in the hand. *B*, Radiograph of the hand of the same patient. *C*, Maffucci syndrome of multiple enchondromas with associated vascular tumors leading to prominent calcification on radiograph.

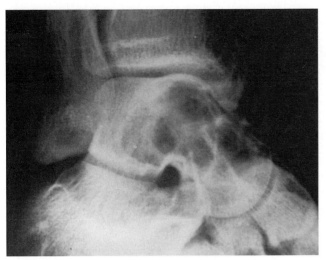

Figure 10–12. Chondroblastoma of the talus in 24-year-old female. Tarsal bones are a common location.

tiocytes) and giant cells intermingled with fibrous stroma. The radiographic appearance is quite characteristic with an eccentric location in long bones, sclerotic internal border, and "soap bubble" appearance; the lesions usually heal slowly without treatment by ossification progressing from the diaphyseal side toward the physis (Fig. 10–13). Surgery is indicated if there is doubt about the diagnosis, or if the lesion is so large that fracture is imminent or has occurred. Curettage, with or without bone grafting, is the preferred surgical treatment.

Fibrous Dysplasia. Fibrous dysplasia is considered to be a developmental anomaly rather than a neoplasm; it may exist in monostotic or polyostotic form. The microscopic pattern is characterized by benign fibrous stroma stippled with bony islands of metaplastic woven-type bone, in so-called "alphabet soup" or curlycue patterns. Associated endocrine abnormalities may be present, resulting in precocious sexual development, abnormal skin pigmentation, intramuscular myxoma (Fig. 10–14A), and thyroid disease. The radiographic appearance is usually characteristic, with well-defined radiolucency, or possibly a "ground-glass" appearance of the matrix, depending on the amount of calcification of the osteoid spicules contained in the fibrous stroma (Fig. 10–14B).

Surgery may be indicated in some cases for diagnosis or treatment of significant deformity, pathologic fracture, or pain. Pathologic fracture occurs in the majority of patients. The process tends to become inactive after puberty, but may become active again with pregnancy. Lesions are adequately treated by curettage, with or without bone grafting or internal fixation for skeletal support. Deformities and fractures are corrected by osteotomy, curettage of the abnormal tissue, and internal fixation. Extensive polyostotic disease may result in major deformities of the proximal femur (shepherd's crook deformity), skull, and facial bones, as well as any of the long bones. Recurrence is uncommon after adequate surgical treatment. Radiotherapy is contraindicated because of the risk of sarcomatous change.

Ossifying Fibroma. Ossifying fibroma (osteofibrous dysplasia) is a rare lesion, usually affecting the tibia. The initial appearance generally occurs in the first decade of life with enlargement and anterior bowing of the tibia. Radiographs show eccentric intracortical osteolysis with expansion of the cortex. Alteration of this lesion over time into adamantinoma has been suggested. The natural course of the lesion is unpredictable, and spontaneous regression has been reported; the lesion frequently recurs after curettage or subperiosteal resection. Campanacci and Laus recommend that surgical treatment be delayed until age 15 or later and that fractures be treated nonsurgically by cast immobilization.

Desmoplastic Fibromas. Desmoplastic fibroma is a rare, densely collagenized tumor of fibrous tissue histologically similar to soft tissue desmoid tumors. It can occur at any age, although it tends to affect adolescents or young adults, and has no sexual preference. Long tubular bones are most commonly involved. Radiographs show a well-defined lytic defect centrally located in the bone with minimal bone reaction to it. The primary form of treatment is surgical, and en bloc wide local excision is preferred. The tumor is benign, local recurrences are common, and metastases are highly unlikely.

Cystic Lesions

Unicameral bone cyst is probably not a true neoplasm, and its pathologic origin remains unknown, although malignant transformation arising in the cyst wall has been reported. Bone cysts usually occur in the first 2 decades of life, and males predominate 2:1 over females. In a large series, 53%

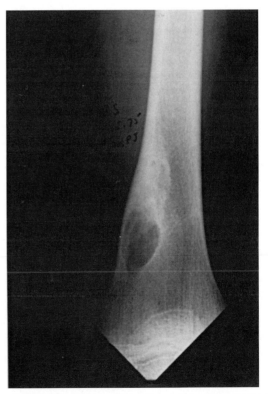

Figure 10–13. Nonossifying fibroma in 12-year-old boy. Lesions typically ossify from the diaphysis toward the physis and eventually disappear without treatment.

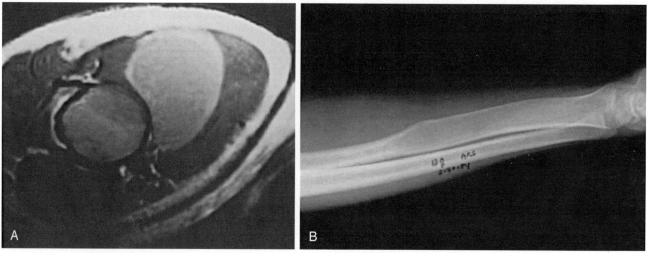

Figure 10–14. Fibrous dysplasia. *A*, Myxoma adjacent to proximal humerus in 33-year-old male was discovered on radiographs during workup for shoulder mass. Further workup revealed extensive involvement of multiple bones with fibrous dysplasia. *B*, Expanded bone with typical "ground-glass" appearance in 13-year-old girl.

occur in the proximal humerus and 19% in the proximal femoral metaphysis. They are usually called to attention by pathologic fracture, which has been reported in 82% of proximal humeral cysts. The commonly held belief that these cysts will heal spontaneously after fracture is often mistaken. Indications for surgery are thinning of cortical bone and the threat of repeated fractures.

Recurrence after treatment is more common in cysts, which are in contact with the growth plate, termed active cysts (Fig. 10–15*A*), than in those in which the physis has grown away from the cyst, leaving normal cancellous bone between the physis and cyst. Recurrence is also more common in children under 10. Curettage and bone grafting, with or without treatment of the cavity wall with phenol, has not reduced the recurrence rate of approximately 25%.

Scaglietti and coworkers and Capanna have reported good results in 80 to 90% of cases treated with injections of methylprednisolone into the cyst cavity at intervals of 2 months. Three fourths of patients require more than one injection. The lesion cavity is typically filled with xanthochromic fluid, and the lining contains numerous vascular channels, fibrous tissue, some giant cells, and foam (xanthoma) cells (see Fig. 10–15*B* and *C*).

Aneurysmal bone cyst is probably a non-neoplastic, vasocystic lesion engrafted on either previously normal bone or a pre-existing lesion (Fig. 10–16). It may occur in any bone; vertebral involvement is not uncommon. Curettage is followed by recurrence in about 25% of cases. Radiation therapy is rarely indicated because of the danger of malignant transformation.

Ganglion cysts of bone occur typically in subchondral regions of long bones in middle-aged men. The author regards these as degenerative cysts because they have the gross and histologic appearance of resorption cavities seen in proximity to osteoarthritic joints. If treatment is indicated, it consists of curettage and resection of adjacent soft tissues.

Epidermoid cysts are filled with keratinaceous material and lined with flattened squamous epithelium. They are found most commonly in the skull or in the phalanges of the fingers. They usually appear to be encroaching on the bone from outside and are seen as osteolytic defects surrounded with sclerotic bone.

Tumors of Peripheral Nerve Tissue

Neural tumors of bone are quite rare. On radiographs neurilemmomas appear as discrete osteolytic lesions. The microscopic appearance mimics similar lesions of soft tissue. Neurofibromas also appear in bone, especially in von Recklinghausen's disease. In this condition, multiple lesions are present, and problems such as gigantism, kyphoscoliosis, congenital bowing, and pseudoarthroses of long bones occur.

Tumors of Blood Vessels

Unlike neural tumors, vascular tumors are common in bone. Hemangiomas are seen most frequently in the vertebrae (Fig. 10–17). Surgical treatment is occasionally needed if compromise of spinal cord or nerve roots is present or threatened. Massive osteolysis (disappearing bone disease) is fortunately very rare. It usually affects children with involvement of one or more adjacent bones; progression is unpredictable, and some cases are self-limited, but deaths have been reported from respiratory compromise when the shoulder girdle and chest wall have been involved.

Tumors of Fat

Fatty marrow seldom produces intraosseous lipoma. They are usually discovered incidentally on radiographs taken for other reasons. Cure is obtained by curettage with or without bone grafting.

Giant Cell Tumor of Bone

Giant cell tumor of bone is a relatively uncommon (approximately 5% of bone lesions), most often benign, though

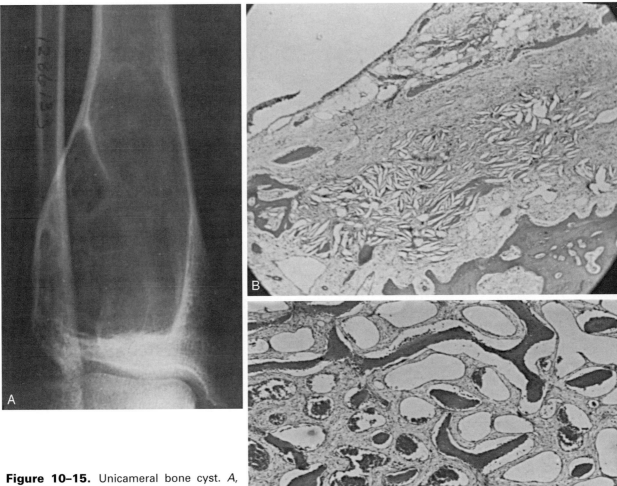

Figure 10–15. Unicameral bone cyst. *A,* Expanded bone with lucent area in metaphysis of distal tibia. Note abutment to growth plate. *B,* Cyst wall with thin epithelium, fat cells, fibrous dysplastic type bone, and numerous cholesterol clefts. *C,* Portion of cyst wall with angiomatoid presentation.

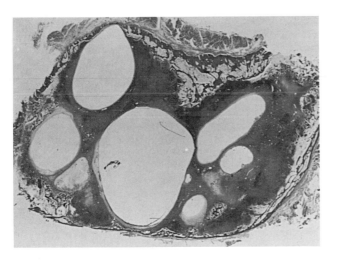

Figure 10–16. Extensive cystic change in an osteoblastoma of a rib. Such changes are often diagnosed as aneurysmal bone cyst if emphasis is placed on the cavities and not on the tissue composing the basis of the lesion.

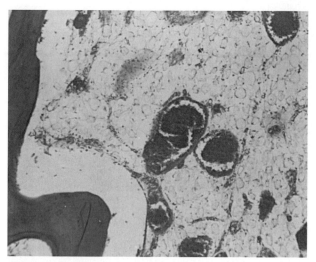

Figure 10–17. Hemangioma of bone. Such lesions are commonly found in the vertebrae but may occur in any bone, including the skull.

locally aggressive tumor of young adults and has a slight female predominance. About 50% occur around the knee, others are seen in the distal radius or proximal humerus, but any bone can be involved. Most patients present with pain or disability or both. The radiograph is usually so characteristic that the diagnosis may be made on the plain films (Fig. 10–18). The lesion begins eccentrically located in the end of long bones. Prior to growth plate closure the geographic center is in the metaphysis (see Fig. 10–18*B* and *C*), although it will expand to underlie the subchondral bone after closure of the physis.

On plain radiographs the lesion is radiolucent without matrix densities. It has a narrow transitional zone, producing a geographic border without a rim of reactive endosteal bone. Perforation of the cortex occurs in 25%, although penetration of the periosteum or subchondral bone with extrusion into the soft tissues or joint is uncommon. Reactive periosteal new bone formation, though very active, is unable to keep up with the osteolysis produced by the tumor. Increased uptake on technetium bone scan is the rule, with "hot" periphery and "cool" center. CT scanning has replaced plain tomography and angiography in evaluating most bone tumors, especially this one. It is the best method of assessing the intraosseous extent of the tumor, the relation to the subchondral bone, the degree of cortical erosion and expansion, and the presence of soft tissue extension.

Biopsy is necessary to establish the diagnosis, but the high level of suspicion provided by the radiograph usually allows definitive treatment at the time of biopsy if frozen section is confirmatory. Grossly the lesion confirms the radiographic picture as regards extent in the bone and relation to the subchondral plate. The tumor is friable and vascular, variable in color from white to brown, reddish brown, or yellow. There are often blood-filled cavities within the tumor which can lead to a misdiagnosis of aneurysmal bone cyst (see Fig. 10–18*D*). Microscopically the tissue is filled with two cell populations (see Fig. 10–18*E*). The giant cells are thought by many to be osteoclasts, justifying the British name of osteoclastoma, and

consistent with the osteolysis, which is the major response to the tumor. The stromal cell is a round to oval cell with easily seen nucleus but ill-defined cytoplasm and no discernible intracellular substance. Normal mitotic figures are common in nearly every lesion. The nuclei of the giant cells are indistinguishable from those of the stromal cells. Pulmonary metastases occur in approximately 10%; histologic grading of either the primary or secondary deposits has little proven value in predicting outcome. Pulmonary deposits have been seen to stabilize after adequate treatment of the primary.

Treatment remains controversial, although most authors agree that they are best treated surgically. Curettage must be aggressive; with or without bone grafting in early lesions, curettage is followed by recurrence within 18 to 24 months in an unacceptably high percentage up to 65%. With delay in treatment leading to more extensive involvement by the tumor, or following recurrence, resection is the preferred treatment. Liquid nitrogen cryosurgery has reduced the recurrence rate, as has high-speed burring of cavity margins, or phenol and alcohol treatment of the cavity. Some authors report that filling the cavity with polymethyl methacrylate after thorough curettage has resulted in lower recurrence rate and satisfactory joint function in many cases. Marginal or wide resection replaced with massive allografts for arthrodesis or retention of some joint function is being used by some surgeons as primary treatment. Use of the proximal fibula after resection has been used with good success for distal radius or proximal humerus. Primary amputation should seldom be necessary except in cases of extreme neglect leading to massive soft tissue extension. Radiation therapy should rarely, if ever, be used except in inaccessible lesions such as the sacrum where resection may cause significant functional loss.

Histiocytosis X

Histiocytosis X is a complex of syndromes whose clinical and radiographic appearance depends on the age of the patient at presentation. The basic disease process appears to be accumulations of non-neoplastic histiocytes with varying proportions of eosinophils and other chronic inflammatory cells. This has led some experts to conclude that this is some form of infection rather than neoplasm. Eosinophilic granuloma presents with pain or a mass occurring in the patient's second decade. Multiple eosinophilic granulomas, Hand-Schüller-Christian disease, and Letterer-Siwe syndrome occur at progressively younger ages and with increasing risk to life. Eosinophilic granulomas can occur in any bone; skull, spine, rib cage, pelvis, and proximal portions of the limbs are sites most commonly reported. The lesion is often diaphyseal. Biopsy is necessary to establish the diagnosis. Curettage with or without bone grafting, low-dose radiotherapy, and corticosteroid injections all have been used successfully. Solitary lesions have a benign course, but occasionally alteration to the disseminated form has occurred, usually within 1 year after treatment of the primary.

MALIGNANT TUMORS OF BONE

Chordoma

Chordoma is a rare and unusual tumor that may occur anywhere along the spinal axis from the base of the skull

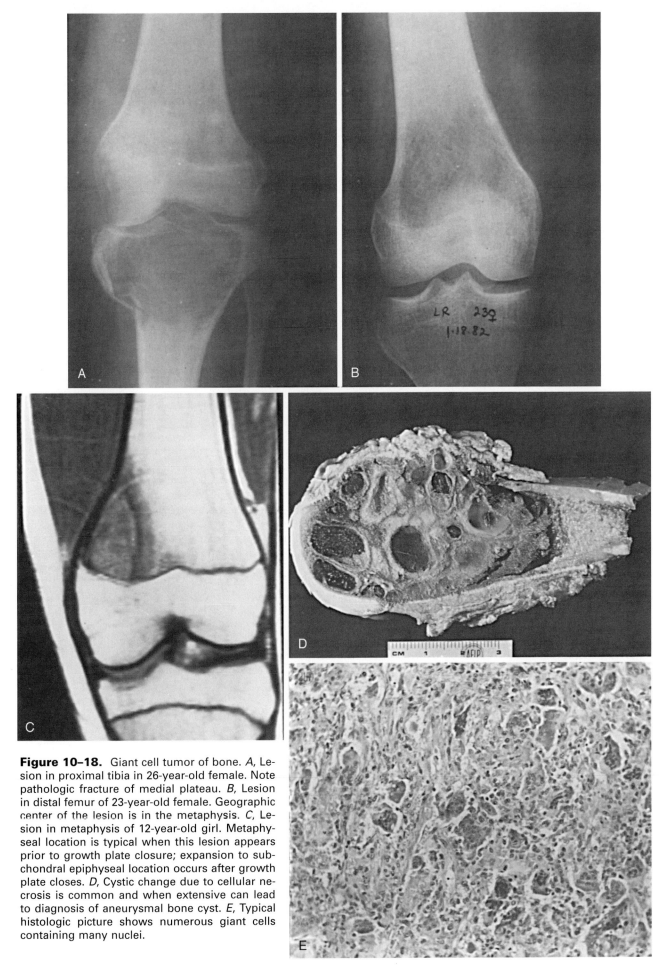

Figure 10–18. Giant cell tumor of bone. *A*, Lesion in proximal tibia in 26-year-old female. Note pathologic fracture of medial plateau. *B*, Lesion in distal femur of 23-year-old female. Geographic center of the lesion is in the metaphysis. *C*, Lesion in metaphysis of 12-year-old girl. Metaphyseal location is typical when this lesion appears prior to growth plate closure; expansion to subchondral epiphyseal location occurs after growth plate closes. *D*, Cystic change due to cellular necrosis is common and when extensive can lead to diagnosis of aneurysmal bone cyst. *E*, Typical histologic picture shows numerous giant cells containing many nuclei.

to the coccyx. It is believed to arise from notochordal remnants; thus, it is usually centrally located in vertebral bodies or sacrum, unlike giant cell tumor, which is more eccentrically placed, or like osteoblastoma, which favors the posterior elements of the vertebra. The tumor grows slowly, infiltrates widely in the bone and surrounding tissues, and metastasizes late if at all. Symptoms are pain, sciatica or other neurologic symptoms, often bowel and bladder disturbances. A presacral mass may be felt on rectal examination, and radiographs show local destruction of the bone. CT is helpful in localization and planning surgery. If cure is to be obtained, wide resection with surrounding normal tissue margin is necessary, even if neurologic deficit will result. Radiation therapy offers significant palliation in unresectable or recurrent lesions. Grossly, the tumor appears lobulated, soft, grayish, and semitransparent. The histologic hallmark is the physaliphorous cell, a large cell containing numerous vacuoles filled with mucus droplets. Mucus is often extruded from the vacuoles into the extracellular spaces. Anterior and posterior approaches may be necessary, utilizing a team approach for sacral lesions. Death usually results from local invasion rather than metastases.

Osteosarcoma

Osteosarcoma is a highly aggressive, rapidly growing malignant tumor of bone, which has often spread beyond its site of origin before it is diagnosed, decreasing the possibility of cure. Estimated tumor doubling time is 34 days. The basic tenet is production of osteoid or bone by pleomorphic malignant cells. Calcification of the osteoid is usually prominent and seen as sclerosis on radiographs. Classical osteosarcoma is slightly more common in males than females, and accounts for approximately 20% of all primary malignant bone tumors. The peak incidence is late teens and early 20s; a second peak may occur in later life, usually associated with Paget's disease of bone.

The tumor is usually found in the metaphyses of the most rapidly growing long bones (Fig. 10–19) and thus is most common (approximately 50%) about the knee. Steadily progressive low-grade pain existing over a period of months along with a palpable mass are the usual presentation. More than 95% have violated the cortex by the time of diagnosis (stage IIB). Up to 20% may have evidence of metastatic disease, usually to the lung, when first diagnosed (stage III). Radiographs typically show a metaphyseal lesion with intermingled areas of bone destruction and production. The aggressive behavior of the tumor is evident by the moth-eaten or permeative pattern of cortical destruction, by growth of the tumor into the soft tissues with characteristic ossification, and with a periosteal reaction often in a "sunburst" pattern. Codman's triangle of normal reactive bone appears at the ends of the periosteal reaction.

Treatment is controversial. Prior to the advent of adjuvant chemotherapy in the 1970s the primary treatment was amputation, with a 5-year survival rate of about 20%. Even now, aggressive surgery for local control is usually recommended, consisting of either wide or radical excision of the primary site with allograft or prosthetic replacement, or transmedullary amputation (wide margin) or disarticulation through the joint above (radical margin). Resection of

pulmonary metastases unless too numerous is also recommended. Sequential thoracotomies may be needed. Adjuvant radiotherapy or chemotherapy combined with surgery has brought the 5-year cure rate from 10 to 15% with radical surgery alone up to 50 to 80% in some series. It is common now for chemotherapy to be administered for two to three courses prior to definitive surgery in an attempt to "stun" the primary tumor or kill micrometastases before they have had a chance to take root at a distance from the primary site. In any event, osteosarcoma from biopsy onward should be treated in centers where large numbers of malignancies are managed and where experience in various forms of surgical treatment can ensure expert care by experienced medical, surgical, and radiotherapy oncologists whose combined talents and experience are available to optimize the care of the individual patient. Death usually occurs by pulmonary metastases, often within 6 months of relapse.

Parosteal Sarcoma

Parosteal sarcoma has a wide age range and is more common in females. The distal femur is the site for many of these tumors, though the humerus, tibia, and fibula are also common sites (Fig. 10–20A and B). It is frequently underdiagnosed on biopsy by pathologists who seldom see bone tumors. The usual course is one of slow growth of a hard, painless mass that may interfere, by its bulk, with the adjacent joint. If inadequately excised, they invariably recur, and given time, they will invade the medullary cavity of the metaphysis and then begin to behave more like the classic intramedullary osteosarcomas (see Fig. 10–20C). Plain radiographs often are diagnostic, and CT scans usually confirm that, unlike classic osteosarcoma or osteochondroma, the lesion is originating from altered cortical bone without change of the medullary contents (see Fig. 10–20B).

Resection through the apparent cleavage plane seen on routine films leads to recurrence in almost all cases. Recurrences are often more aggressive than the original tumor, and often are found to have grown inward into the medullary canal, necessitating more drastic surgery (see Fig. 10–20C). Wide resection with a margin of normal soft tissue overlying the tumor and the cortical and medullary bone surrounding the tumor are necessary for surgical cure. The basic tissue may be predominately bone-forming, although others may be made up of malignant cartilage or fibrous tissue (see Fig. 10–20D).

Chondrosarcoma

Chondrosarcoma is about half as common as osteosarcoma. Diagnosis is difficult to establish but hinges on (1) tissue that resembles hyaline or other types of cartilage, (2) malignant cells that appear to be producing the cartilage matrix, and (3) a matrix having histologic and biochemical characteristics of the normal cartilage tissues of body. By definition it is composed of chondroid produced by malignant cartilage cells. Although enchondral ossification may occur, osteoid or bone arising from malignant cells makes up only a small portion of these often large tumors. Typical chondrosarcomas may be central (intramedullary) or pe-

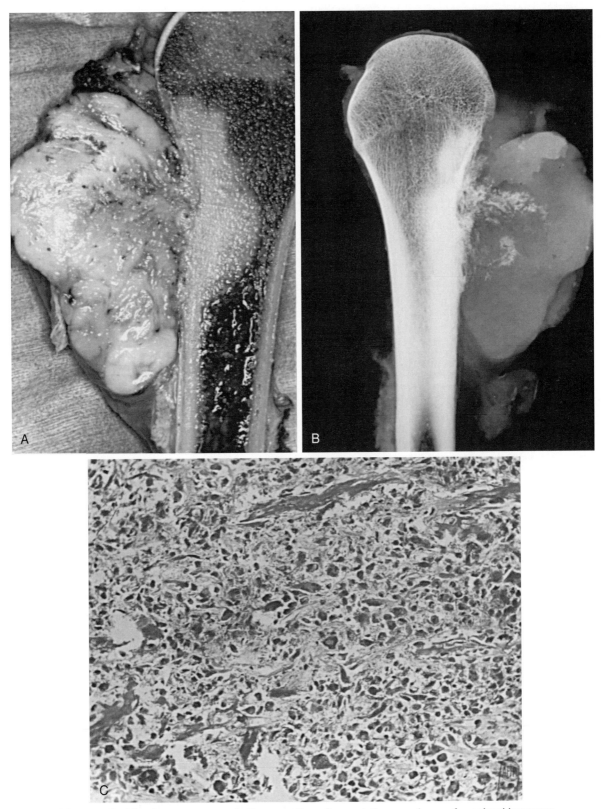

Figure 10–19. Osteosarcoma. *A,* Gross section of amputation specimen of proximal humerus from 22-year-old man. Extraosseous extent of tumor raised a question of possible parosteal sarcoma with backgrowth. *B,* Specimen radiograph of lesion, intraosseous portion heavily ossified, periphery of soft tissue mass growing so fast that ossification is minimal. *C,* Histologic examination of the lesion reveals its pleomorphic nature with minimal osteoid production. Patient died within 6 months.

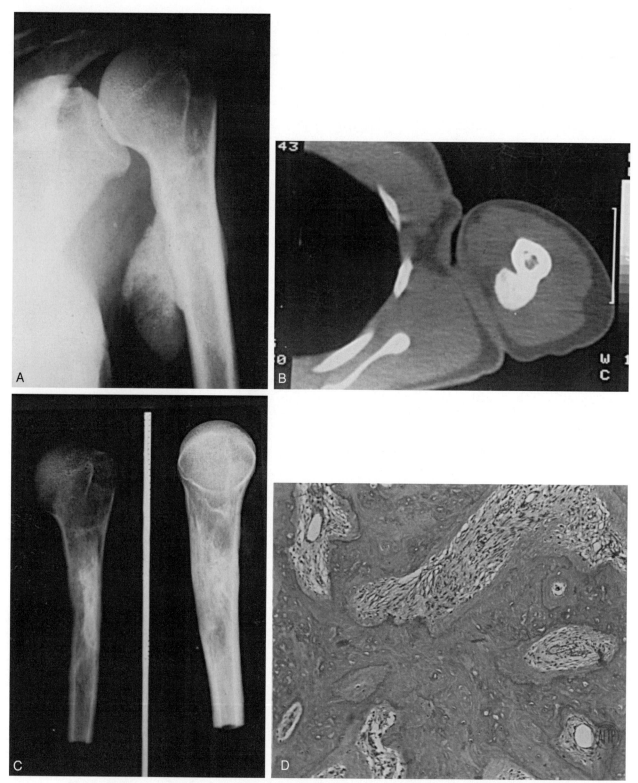

Figure 10–20. Parosteal osteosarcoma. *A*, Radiograph of shoulder of 22-year-old female who presented with a hard painless mass in axilla. Note apparent cleavage plane between the mass and altered underlying cortex. *B*, CT demonstrates that mass is originating from the cortex without medullary involvement. *C*, Lesion had been resected through the apparent cleavage plane (and thus through the tumor). When this is done, the recurrence rate is 100%. Backgrowth into medullary cavity is evident on the specimen radiographs. *D*, Typical histologic picture demonstrates relatively benign appearing, but abnormal, bone and medullary contents. Such deceptive benign appearance leads to frequent underdiagnosis unless the pathologist and surgeon are familiar with the entity.

ripheral, and may be primary or secondary to a pre-existing benign lesion, such as enchondroma or osteochondroma. Chondrosarcomas usually occur in adults aged 30 to 60 years, although they can occur in childhood, usually secondary to multiple osteochondromatosis or Ollier's disease. Patients with multiple benign cartilage lesions run a relatively high risk of eventually developing malignant change, especially when involving bones near the central axis of the body. The femur, pelvis, humerus, scapula, and ribs (bones near the axial skeleton or limb girdles) are most common sites. Primary chondrosarcomas often grow very large before the patient presents for treatment (see Fig. 10–8); this makes surgical extirpation extremely difficult. A wide spectrum of behavior is exhibited and can be predicted to some extent by the histologic picture.

Even for pathologists with great experience in bone tumors, histologic diagnosis may be difficult, and grading may be even more so. This problem has led to a simplified approach to grading into benign, low-grade, and high-grade lesions. Because the tissue in large lesions is not uniform, a generous incisional biopsy with sampling of a number of areas of the tumor may be necessary. Preoperative guidance by an experienced diagnostic radiologist may be very helpful in locating appropriate tissue. The diagnosis is based on the most differentiated portion; the prognosis is determined by the least differentiated area, and the relative amounts of each. Proper staging requires adequate study preoperatively with plain radiographs, CT and bone scans, and MRI and vascular studies to determine the anatomic setting and extent of the tumor to assist in planning appropriate surgery (Fig. 10–21B). Low- and intermediate-grade lesions require wide margins; high-grade lesions should have radical margins, often requiring radical amputation (see Fig. 10–21C and D). Wide excision of any soft tissue mass should include the surgical tract of any previous biopsy or attempted resection. High-grade lesions should also be treated with systemic chemotherapy.

There are several variants of chondrosarcoma. *Clear cell chondrosarcoma* is a low-grade lesion usually located in the ends of long bones of young adults, often epiphyseal in location. The tumors are composed of sheets of plump chondrocytes with distinct cell borders, which has led in past to diagnosis of "atypical chondroblastoma." They are slow-growing, low-grade lesions that can be treated by en bloc resection rather than more radical surgery. *Periosteal chondrosarcoma* is a low-grade lesion of young males, most commonly seen in the distal femur. *Mesenchymal chondrosarcoma* is a high-grade, lethal lesion with biphasic histologic appearance; sheets of small round or oval cells resembling Ewing's sarcoma are mingled with lobules of cartilage appearing benign and well differentiated. *Dedifferentiated chondrosarcoma* is a high-grade transition of a low-grade chondrosarcoma into a lethal lesion of different histologic type such as fibrosarcoma, malignant fibrous histiocytoma, or osteosarcoma (see Fig. 10–21F). Such dedifferentiation has been found to occur in approximately 10% of chondrosarcomas. Prognosis has been uniformly poor.

Chondrosarcoma in general is not very responsive to adjuvant radiotherapy or chemotherapy, so the primary treatment remains surgical extirpation by whatever means necessary. The surgeon must be aware that chondrosarcoma can infiltrate between normal trabeculae and can destroy these structures. The tumor replaces the normal marrow but not the bone (see Fig. 10–21E), making the margins deceptive on radiograph. The extent of the tumor is more evident on MRI, which should be done routinely to help in planning the operation. Survival of the patient is directly related to the extent of the surgical procedure. Death occurs by local invasion of vital structures or by pulmonary metastases.

Fibrosarcomas

Fibrosarcoma of bone is diagnosed less often at the present time; most such tumors are included in the category of malignant fibrous histiocytoma. Fibrosarcomas arise from spindle cells, which produce collagen but no osteoid. Microscopically, one sees interwoven bundles of spindle cells with narrow tapering nuclei and ill-defined cytoplasmic borders, often in a "herring-bone" pattern. It is a tumor of adults involving the femur, tibia, and humerus most commonly. The biologic behavior can be predicted by the histologic grade. Patients present with pain or mass or both. Radiographs show a bone lesion that is primarily osteolytic. Biopsy is necessary for diagnosis. Wide resection may be adequate for low-grade lesions, radical surgery is necessary for high-grade lesions. Radiotherapy may be helpful for palliation.

Malignant Fibrous Histiocytoma

Malignant fibrous histiocytoma is a relatively rare, malignant tumor of bone. These tumors are believed to arise from histiocytes, and they can occur at any age, but are seen most often in older adult males, with the femur, tibia, and humerus being the most frequent sites. They are seldom found in the axial skeleton. Patients complain of a mass and pain; occasionally they have a pathologic fracture. Radiographs show areas of osteolysis in a motheaten pattern. The lesion must be biopsied for diagnosis. Histologic grade predicts biologic behavior. The tumor is often associated with a pre-existing lesion, such as bone infarct or Paget's disease. Surgical treatment is determined by staging, but almost all are stage IIB and require resection with radical margins. High-grade lesions probably should be treated by systemic chemotherapy as well as surgery. It differs on histologic appearance from fibrosarcoma in that its cells show striking nuclear pleomorphism and abundant cytoplasm. The mononuclear cells are fibroblastic and show a cartwheel or storiform growth pattern. Tumor necrosis and mitoses are variable, sometimes extensive. Radiotherapy and chemotherapy have not shown clear-cut benefit.

Adamantinoma

Adamantinoma is a rare, slowly growing, primary malignant bone tumor, usually of the tibia. Age range is wide, and sex predominance is absent. Patients may present with mild pain or a mass or both, present for prolonged period before diagnosis. Radiographs show an irregular lytic lesion with multiple, sharply outlined defects of different sizes involving primarily the cortical bone for varying lengths. Radiographic appearance has been confused with fibrous dysplasia or ossifying fibroma. Histologic examination shows a biphasic pattern with islands of neoplastic cells in columnar or palisading, almost alveolar, pattern, encased in a fibrous stroma. Progression is indolent, but recurrences are common if surgery does not provide wide margins. Local recurrence after wide resection should be treated promptly with amputation. Metastases eventually occur in inadequately treated tumors. Adjunctive therapy has not been shown to have any value.

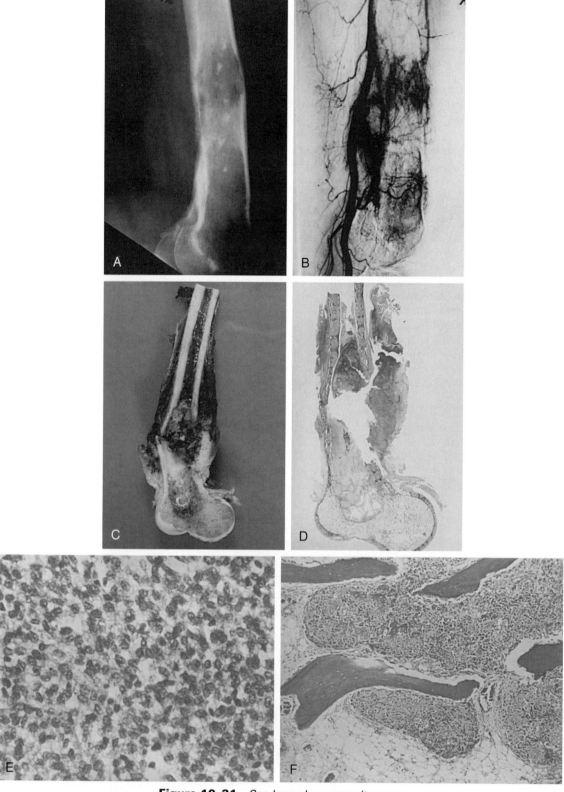

Figure 10–21. *See legend on opposite page*

Liposarcoma

Liposarcoma is relatively common as a soft tissue tumor but is quite rare as a bone tumor. Radical resection or amputation is advised. Most have acted in a highly malignant fashion.

Hemangioendothelioma

Hemangioendothelioma is a rare malignant tumor originating from endothelial cells. Lesions can occur in any bone with quite variable course and wide age range. Pain is the usual symptom, and occasionally swelling is seen in superficial locations. Radiographs show purely osteolytic, often multifocal lesions that are not distinctive, although calcifications may indicate their vascular nature. Periosteal reaction is rarely observed. Biopsy is required for diagnosis. Grossly, the lesions are soft and velvety in texture and bleed readily, often dramatically. Grading varies from grade I (borderline), which may be hard to distinguish from rapidly growing capillary hemangiomas, to grade II (low-grade), grade III, or grade IV (high-grade varieties appropriately called angiosarcomas). Local resection for grades I and II lesions is appropriate, with radical resection or amputation advised for grade III or IV. Radiotherapy is helpful when less than appropriate margins are obtained. Grades I and II have an indolent course with occasional metastases from grade II. Grades III and IV tend to have a very aggressive and rapid course with early metastases to lungs, amputation stump, viscera, and skeleton. Aggressive multimodal systemic chemotherapy probably should be used and is often given preoperatively, followed by wide or radical surgery. These tumors are moderately radiosensitive.

Lymphoma

Lymphoma and leukemia may produce bone changes because the bone marrow is an organ for production of blood elements. Lymphomas may involve bone either primarily (approximately 40%) or as a manifestation of disseminated disease. Primary lymphomas occur in middle-aged or elderly adults, but rarely in children. Primary lymphomas (formerly termed reticulum cell sarcoma) of bone are potentially curable. Secondary lymphomas are usually fatal and interest orthopedists mainly when treatment for pathologic fractures becomes necessary. The pelvis and diaphyses of long bones are the chief sites of involvement.

Pain, swelling, or pathologic fractures may be the pre-senting features; involvement of the spine may cause neurologic symptoms. Finding enlarged regional lymph nodes suggests disseminated disease. Lesions in the bone are often fairly large, involving most of the diaphysis. They are irregularly osteolytic, producing a mottled appearance with indistinct margins on radiographs. Periosteal new bone formation may not be as exuberant as in Ewing's sarcoma. Extension of the lesion into the soft tissues is not unusual, and may be associated with pathologic fracture. Grossly, the tissue is soft and grayish white, and on microscopic examination the large reticulum cells have vesicular, ovoid, or folded nuclei. The cytoplasm is irregular, and nucleoli may be prominent. Reed-Sternberg cells may be present, as may a reticulin network around the cells. Reticulin stains may be helpful in demonstrating this.

Treatment of the bone lesion is almost always radiotherapy unless surgery is needed for pathologic fractures. Systemic chemotherapy is also useful in disseminated disease. Sometimes a leukemic picture may develop in fatal cases.

Multiple Myelomas

Multiple myeloma (plasmacytoma) is a malignant neoplasm derived from plasma cells, and is usually associated with abnormalities of protein synthesis. It is the most common primary malignancy of bone. It arises in the diaphysis of long bones or in other bones with red marrow. The disease is rarely found before the fifth decade, and men are affected more than women. Usually the bone marrow of much or all of the skeleton is involved, making bone marrow biopsy or aspiration diagnostic.

The radiographic picture may be quite suggestive, with punched-out osteolytic lesions that have not stimulated significant reactive bone production (Fig. 10–22A). This lack may be the explanation for the absence of positive bone scans, as well as the difficulty in getting pathologic fractures through myeloma deposits to heal. Diffuse osteoporosis without localized destruction is sometimes seen. Ribs, vertebrae, pelvis, and skull are most often involved because they are the locations of red marrow in the adult (see Fig. 10–22B).

Myeloma may be diagnosed with accuracy by laboratory tests. Serum and urine protein electrophoresis may be diagnostic, showing a sharp peak in the electrophoretic pattern suggesting monoclonal gammopathy. Grossly, the tumors are soft, cellular, gray, and friable. Masses of amyloid may be seen, occasionally in extraosseous locations. Microscopically, the tumor consists of sheets of closely packed cells with little stromal material (see Fig. 10–22C). Typically, the

Figure 10–21. Chondrosarcoma of distal femur in 60-year-old female. Patient had been unaware of lesion until several months prior to evaluation when she developed aching pain in thigh. *A,* Lateral radiograph of distal femur demonstrates aggressive appearance of lesion proximally and distally, with central location which looks less so. *B,* Arteriogram show several areas of differing activity. Note posterior displacement of popliteal artery by soft tissue mass. *C,* Longitudinal section of amputation specimen. Three distinct areas are noted in the bone, which had sustained pathologic fracture. *D,* Macrosection of distal femur. Distal tumor was well-differentiated chondrosarcoma in conjunction with enchondroma. Proximal portion of tumor is most aggressive, dedifferentiated tumor. *E,* Histologic specimen of tissue from dedifferentiated portion of tumor. *F,* Histologic specimen from another case illustrating invasion and replacement of normal fatty marrow without much change in trabeculae, making it difficult to determine extent of tumor on plain radiographs.

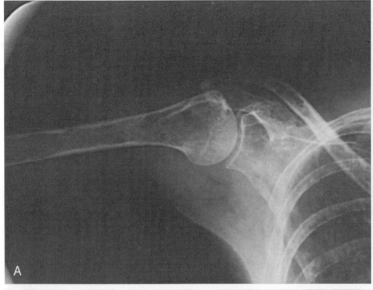

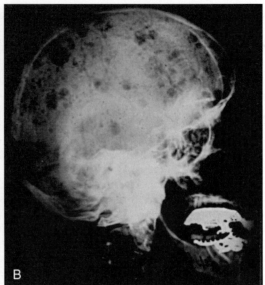

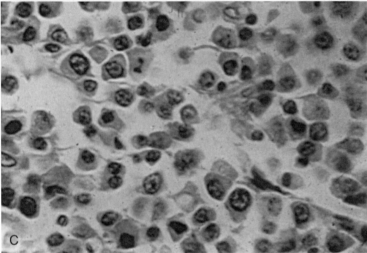

Figure 10–22. Multiple myeloma. *A*, Humerus demonstrating multiple osteolytic lesions with no periosteal reaction. *B*, Multiple "punched-out" lesions in the skull, a fairly typical location. *C*, Histologic appearance of focus of multiple myeloma with varied presentation of plasma cells with eccentrically located nuclei within the cells, some with "clock face" appearance, prominent cytoplasm, and mitotic figures.

cells have an eccentric nucleus with clumped chromatin, abundant basophilic cytoplasm due to a high content of ribosomes producing protein, and a clear area near the nucleus, which is the Golgi apparatus. The so-called clock face nucleus is uncommon.

Overall treatment is similar to that of metastatic carcinomas, consisting of treatment of anemia, hypercalcemia, impaired renal function, increased susceptibility to infections, amyloidosis, and coagulation defects. Physical therapy, judicious bracing, and other measures to keep the patients ambulatory and functional are important modalities of care. Solitary myelomas may be a precursor of widespread disease. Early aggressive treatment with radiotherapy and chemotherapy constitute the treatment of choice for solitary lesions, although dissemination and fatality is a frequent sequel. Radiation therapy to painful lesions in the bones is effective in relieving pain.

Ewing's Sarcoma

Ewing's sarcoma is a primary malignant tumor of bone of uncertain histogenesis. This tumor occurs most commonly in males in their second decade of life, grows rapidly, and

spreads to the lungs early in its course. Any bone, including the spine, may be affected; diaphyses of the long bones of the lower limb and pelvis are most frequent sites. Patients usually have progressively worsening pain followed by the appearance of a mass. Systemic symptoms of low-grade, intermittent fever, malaise, elevated white blood cell count, and erythrocyte sedimentation rate may mimic infection. Duration of symptoms before diagnosis is relatively short, often less than 2 months.

Radiographs usually show irregular, diffuse bone destruction and production in a mottled, moth-eaten pattern, often involving large areas of the bone (Fig. 10–23*A*, *B*, and *C*). Reactive subperiosteal new bone formation in "onion-skin" or "hair-on-end" patterns indicates the extent of the lesion in the bone and intermittency in growth pattern, not unlike osteomyelitis (see Fig. 10–2). Biopsy is necessary to establish a diagnosis. The gross appearance may at times be semiliquid and simulate pus. Histologic examination shows small round cells with limited cytoplasm and very little stromal tissue; areas of necrosis are common (see Fig. 10–23*D* and *E*).

Recommended treatment consists of radiation and chemotherapy. Heavily radiated limbs in children are some-

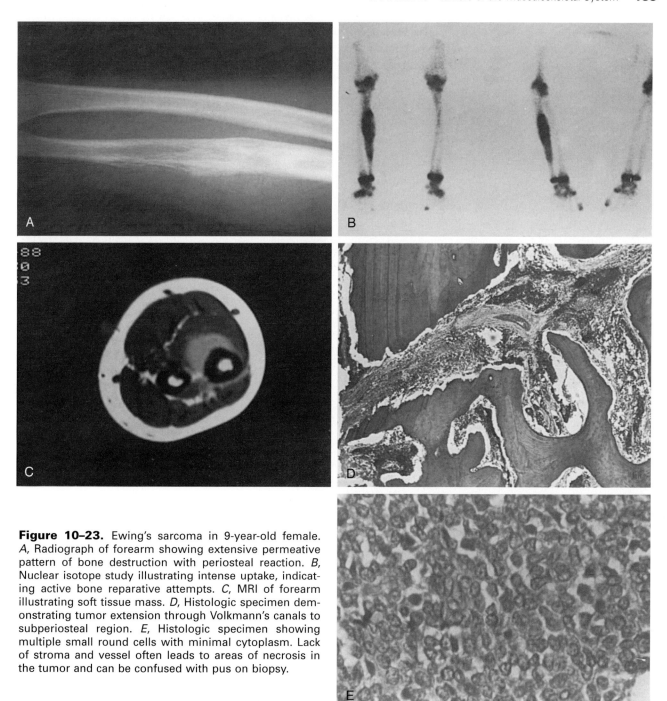

Figure 10–23. Ewing's sarcoma in 9-year-old female. *A,* Radiograph of forearm showing extensive permeative pattern of bone destruction with periosteal reaction. *B,* Nuclear isotope study illustrating intense uptake, indicating active bone reparative attempts. *C,* MRI of forearm illustrating soft tissue mass. *D,* Histologic specimen demonstrating tumor extension through Volkmann's canals to subperiosteal region. *E,* Histologic specimen showing multiple small round cells with minimal cytoplasm. Lack of stroma and vessel often leads to areas of necrosis in the tumor and can be confused with pus on biopsy.

times less functional than prostheses, and thus, amputation in younger children with growth plate alterations may be desirable. Amputation is also advisable when the lesion is large or there is a pathologic fracture. Most series are reporting 50 to 60% survival rates with current treatment methods. Ewing's sarcoma tends to metastasize to the lungs and to other bones; the majority of patients with Ewing's sarcoma die of metastatic disease.

Metastatic Tumors

Metastatic tumors are by far the most common malignant tumors of bone. They usually present in one of three ways:

(1) a patient has spine or extremity pain as the initial manifestation of the disease process; (2) a patient appears with a pathologic fracture; (3) a patient with pain in the spine or an extremity has a known primary malignancy. The patient is usually in middle or late life when presenting with metastases to bone. The bone scan is the most sensitive method of detection; radiographs alone probably miss 20 to 25% of metastatic deposits. Needle biopsy in experienced hands results in 80 to 90% positive results. Often the primary site can be inferred from the biopsy of an osseous lesion. In 22% of cases a biopsy of a bone lesion is the first indication that the patient has a primary carcinoma. For this reason, early biopsy during the workup may

be helpful in locating the primary tumor. The most common primary sites are breast, prostate, kidney, thyroid, and lung.

Treatment is often a two-pronged process: medical and surgical. General systemic support with pain medications, physical therapy, assistive devices for ambulation, and nutritional support is helpful. The principal treatment for osseous metastases is radiotherapy, which relieves pain, stops progression of bone destruction, and helps avoid pathologic fracture. Surgical treatment by prophylactic nailing of long bones containing metastases to prevent pathologic fracture is controversial. When metastatic deposit causes significant pain, especially after radiotherapy, or if 50% or more of the cortex is destroyed, or if a femoral lesion is larger than 2.5 to 3.0 cm in diameter, prophylactic nailing and postoperative radiotherapy are indicated. Treatment is directed toward providing support of the skeleton, usually by internal fixation or prosthetic replacement. Operative methods of internal fixation using methyl methacrylate provide the patient with pain relief, allows many to avoid prolonged bed rest, and does not interfere with radiotherapy of the area because there is no secondary ionization of the bone cement. The radiation does not cause changes in the mechanical properties of the methacrylate.

An algorithm for the evaluation of bone lesions is shown in Figure 10–24.

BENIGN TUMORS OF THE SOFT TISSUES

Masses in the musculoskeletal soft tissues are seen more frequently than lesions in the skeleton. They can originate in any mesenchymal tissue; thus, we can see lesions of fat, fibrous tissue, blood vessels, synovium, and occasionally muscles. Peripheral nerves can also be the source of benign and malignant soft tissue tumors. The masses are often discovered incidentally during a shower or when the patient looks in the mirror and notes an asymmetry. Pain is seldom present to a major degree. Thus, the tumor may become quite large before the patient seeks attention (Fig. 10–25).

Plain radiographs are not very helpful when the lesion does not involve calcified tissue because radiographically many of the lesions are isodense with muscle. Exceptions are tissues with a high fat content, or those vascular lesions containing calcification. CT scans can assist in delineation of these lesions, but MRI has been the most helpful diagnostic tool in evaluation of soft tissue tumors.

Anatomic localization of any soft tissue tumor, benign

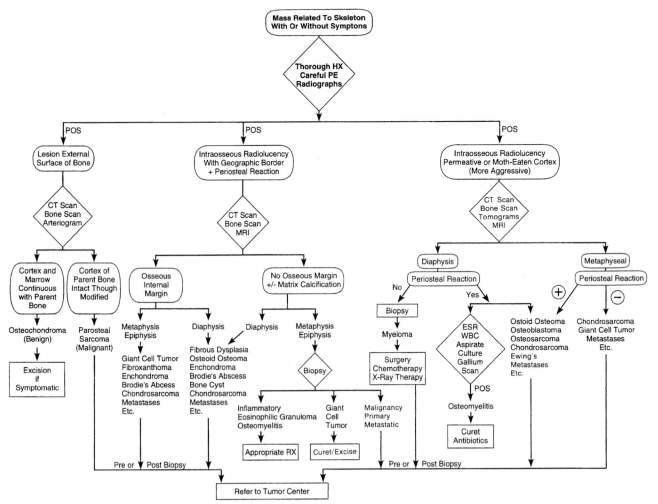

Figure 10–24. Algorithm for management of skeletal tumors. (From Wiesel SW: Essentials of Orthopaedic Surgery, 2nd ed. Philadelphia, W.B. Saunders, 1997, p 115.)

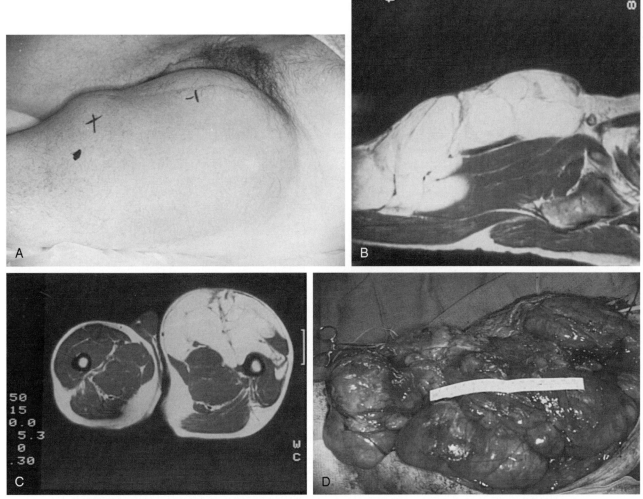

Figure 10–25. Lipoma in thigh of 67-year-old man. He had been aware of, but had neglected to treat, a slowly enlarging, painless mass in the thigh for years. *A*, Photograph of left thigh. *B*, MRI of thigh demonstrates lobular nature of large mass with clear definition from muscle. *C*, Axial MRI of mass. *D*, Photograph of excised tumor. Ruler is 15 cm in length.

or malignant, is the most important factor to consider in surgical management. One must know the precise anatomic extent of tissue change in order to plan surgical removal through normal tissue. The appearance of encapsulation is deceptive because clusters of tumor cells have pseudopod-like extensions beyond the apparent pseudocapsule and can be left behind if the lesion is simply "shelled out" by marginal excision.

Tumors of Fibrous Tissue

Fibroma is a rare, nonmetastasizing, self-limiting neoplastic lesion that some authors regard as a reactive process rather than a tumor. Fibromas can appear at any age, usually are found in the subcutaneous tissues, are slow-growing and painless. They appear to be well encapsulated, and their consistency varies from firm and gritty when cutting to soft or even semisolid. Grossly, they are glistening white to gray on cut section, glistening to myxoid in appearance. Composition varies from dense fascicles of acellular hyalinized collagen to loosely arranged myxoid matrix with few to moderate numbers of cells. Marginal resection usually is curative.

Pseudosarcomatous reactions consist of cellular tissue, often with bizarre cells and numerous mitotic figures, that clinically have not behaved in a malignant fashion. Nodular fasciitis (pseudosarcomatous fasciitis) consists of proliferating fibroblasts, often in a myxoid matrix with prominent vascular pattern. Typically, a young adult patient becomes aware of a painful mass in the forearm or leg which rapidly increases in size over a few weeks. This lesion can appear at any age and in either sex. The deep fascia is often involved, with the lesion protruding into the subcutaneous tissue or occasionally into the muscle. At its periphery the lesion contains many capillaries and inflammatory cells and resembles granulation tissue. Numerous mitotic figures are present but are not atypical, as would be seen in a malignancy. Simple excision seems to suffice for this benign, self-limited lesion.

Fibromatoses are a disparate group of nonmalignant fibrous lesions that frequently recur after removal but do not metastasize. A keloid is a benign tumor of the skin in which the process of repair after injury fails to cease spontaneously. It may be unsightly, become quite large, and tend to recur after excision.

Palmar and plantar fibromatoses are common. They are usually seen in adults, in men more often than women, and in caucasians more than African Americans, Native Americans, or Asians. There is often a positive family history, and a higher incidence in epileptics, diabetics, and alcoholics. The lesions start as painless subcutaneous nodules in the palm or sole; contractures in the hand develop later with the appearance of more nodules and bands (Dupuytren's contracture). Contractures are uncommon in the feet. Grossly, the lesions blend with the fibrous and fatty tissues of the hands and feet, are grayish white, and gritty when cut and may adhere into the deeper layers of the skin. Microscopically, early in the course the nodules are quite cellular, filled with proliferating, immature, spindle-shaped fibroblasts with scanty collagen. The margins of the nodules are indistinct, blending with the surrounding fibrous tissue. Mitoses are not a big component. With maturation of the lesion, increased amounts of dense collagen appear, and the cellularity is considerably less.

Desmoid tumors are relatively common, benign, locally aggressive, fibroblastic lesions that develop in mesenchymal tissues, particularly muscle. They frequently recur locally, even after wide excision, although they do not metastasize. They were initially described in the abdominal muscles of women who have borne children; those occurring in other regions (termed extra-abdominal desmoids) actually are more common and may occur in any mesenchymal tissue. Nearly all patients are young adult males who present with a deep-seated, firm, poorly circumscribed mass; approximately one third of patients also have pain. Delay of a year or more before presentation to a physician is not unusual. These tumors may occur at any age from infancy to senility. The regions about the shoulder or pelvic girdles may contain many of these lesions. Plain radiographs are not helpful, nor are many CT evaluations; MRI is extremely useful in defining the precise location and extent of the lesion and its relationship to surrounding structures. It is the examination of choice for evaluating these lesions. Grossly, these tumors have the look and feel of scar tissue; they are dense, hard, rubbery, and grayish white and are relatively avascular. The margins of the tumor are quite indistinct, blending imperceptibly into the surrounding muscle or fibrous tissues. Histologically, they are highly collagenized, sparsely cellular, infiltrating the muscle in which they develop. Mitotic figures are infrequent. In spite of their benign histologic appearance, they tend to aggressively recur after excision and may infiltrate any of the surroundings tissues widely, but they do not metastasize.

Treatment requires wide local excision. Intralesional or marginal excisions have a high rate of recurrence, 90% at the Mayo Clinic. Even with wide local excision their recurrence rate was 50%. Approximately two thirds of patients undergoing a local excision have a recurrence within 2 years. The role of radiation therapy in treating this lesion is still to be determined.

Fibromatosis colli (congenital torticollis) occurs in the sternocleidomastoid muscle of infants. They usually develop during the first or second week of life as a hard, white, fibrous mass located within the lower third of the muscle, producing shortening, causing the wry neck. Microscopically, the lesion is characterized by proliferating fibroblastic tissue infiltrating the muscle bundles. It varies from poorly cellular, resembling the desmoid, to quite cellular, resembling other fibromatoses.

Juvenile aponeurotic fibroma is a rare, distinctive lesion found in young children, usually in the hand or foot. Microscopically, the fibrous mass consists of plump fibroblasts, less elongated or spindled than in other fibrous tumors. Lesions may have foci of calcification or ossification, or may have a peculiar palisade pattern with occasional areas of chondroid material. Treatment is marginal resection, repeated if necessary. There is a definitive tendency to recur after excision.

Tumors of Fatty Tissue

Lipoma is probably the most common benign tumor of soft tissue. It occurs at any age, in either sex, but is more common in women in the middle decades of life. They usually present subcutaneously but may involve deeper structures. Clinically they are soft, movable, circumscribed masses that grow slowly and are painless, so they are often neglected by the patient until they are quite large (see Fig. 10–25A, B, and C). On radiographs the larger ones have a discrete radiolucent presentation. Grossly, they present as a lobulated, well-circumscribed, yellow mass of normal-appearing fat tissue (see Fig. 10–25D). Larger lipomas may undergo calcification or even metaplastic ossification (Fig. 10–26). Lipomas may be intermuscular or intramuscular and cause pain by expansion; nerve compression syndromes can occur, particularly in the anterior forearm, around the elbow or at the wrist. Microscopically they are composed of mature fat cells. Some lipomas have a prominent vascular component, and are called angiolipomas. Focal areas with finely vacuolated cells of brown fat may be found, particularly around the shoulder girdle or supraclavicular region or in the groin (the so-called hibernoma). They are thought to originate from fetal fat remnants or lipoblasts. Some lipomas infiltrate between muscle bundles and may suggest malignancy, but the tumor is usually readily controlled. Lipomas are treated by marginal resection.

Tumors of Muscle

Leiomyoma is a benign tumor of smooth muscle most often found in the uterus and GI tract. Occasionally they are found in the skin and subcutaneous tissue; in these cases they are thought to arise from blood vessels or arrectores pilorum. They are composed of interlacing bundles of smooth muscle intermingled with varying amounts of fibrous tissue. Simple excision is the treatment of choice.

Tumors of Blood Vessels

Hemangiomas and other vascular malformations are common; some types are present at birth. The type composed of closely packed endothelial cells with many mitotic figures is often called strawberry hemangioma or benign hemangioendothelioma. It is found at birth, is deep red, grows

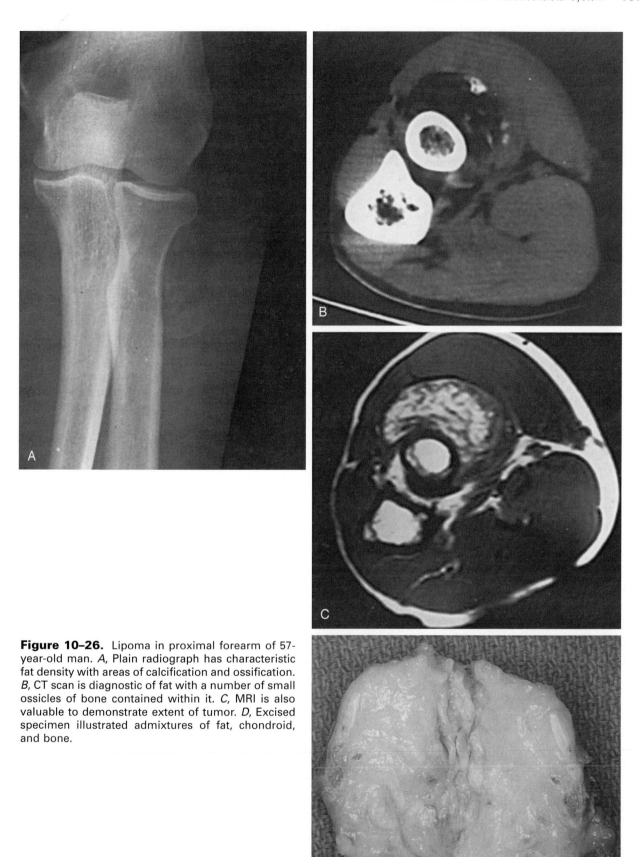

Figure 10–26. Lipoma in proximal forearm of 57-year-old man. *A*, Plain radiograph has characteristic fat density with areas of calcification and ossification. *B*, CT scan is diagnostic of fat with a number of small ossicles of bone contained within it. *C*, MRI is also valuable to demonstrate extent of tumor. *D*, Excised specimen illustrated admixtures of fat, chondroid, and bone.

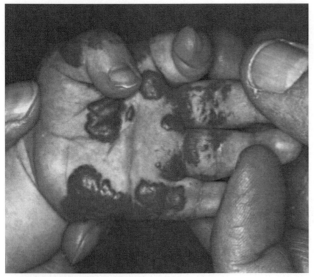

Figure 10–27. Hemangiomas in 3-month-old female. Such lesions often shrink and disappear over time and do not usually require treatment.

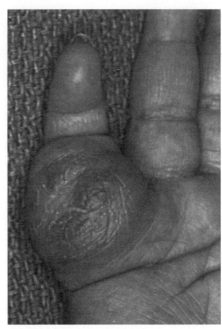

Figure 10–28. Cavernous hemangioma in finger of 10-month-old male. Mass regrew rapidly after previous excision. Such lesions can involve adjacent soft tissues and bone, making total extirpation difficult without significant functional impairment.

rapidly during first few months of life, and then stops growing spontaneously (Fig. 10–27); in most cases, it eventually disappears. It seldom requires surgery. The port wine stain often occurs on the face, neck, or upper trunk and is also present at birth. It grows at about the same rate as the patient and may become quite large and unsightly. It usually persists, and removal is quite difficult.

Classification of hemangiomas is difficult and unsatisfactory at present. It is customary to distinguish capillary and cavernous types. Capillary hemangiomas are the most common and are composed of a network of newly formed capillaries. The cavernous variety are composed of widely dilated blood vessels and spaces lined by thin walls (Fig. 10–28). Hemangiomas may occur deep in skeletal muscle and other soft tissue of extremities and trunk. The patients complain of an ache in the muscle, aggravated by exercise. There is not usually a discrete mass, which makes excision difficult. Recurrence is usual unless completely removed, which involves removal of the muscle in which they occur.

Cavernous hemangiomas may occur in joints, particularly the knee. Part or all of the synovial membrane and surrounding soft tissues may be involved. Children and young adults are most often affected. Patients may have intermittent hemarthroses. Angiography and arthrography may aid in diagnosis. Osteolytic lesions in the bones on both sides of the joint may be evident.

Glomus tumors are uncommon but painful lesions. The skin and subcutaneous tissue of the hands and feet are the usual locus, but a tumor may develop in any location in which a glomus body is found. Exquisite, sharply localized point tenderness is invariably present. Many appear beneath the nail. Diagnosis is often delayed because the lesions are tiny, and the entity is not considered in the differential diagnosis. Microscopically, the lesion consists of sheets of uniform cells that appear somewhat epithelial in nature and lie along the course of abundant vessels. Nonmyelinated nerve fibers are plentiful and can be demonstrated by special stains. The tumors are cured by excision.

Hemangiopericytoma is said to arise from the pericytes of Zimmerman. Biologic behavior is quite variable from benign to aggressively malignant (Fig. 10–29). It may occur at any age but is seen most often during fourth or fifth decades. Histologic grading can help with predicting future behavior. Borderline and malignant forms are best treated with wide resection or wide amputation and systemic chemotherapy.

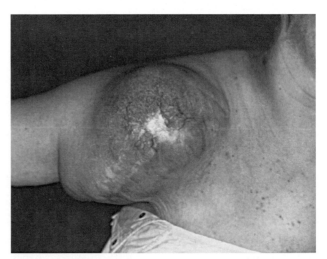

Figure 10–29. Angiosarcoma in axilla of 24-year-old female. Biopsy of a golf ball–sized mass was done during the second month of pregnancy, but the patient refused further surgery at the time, fearing it would affect the pregnancy. This photograph was taken shortly after delivery of a full-term infant. The patient died within 6 weeks.

Tumors of Synovial Tissue

A ganglion is a thin-walled cystic lesion arising from a joint capsule or tendon sheath. It has a predilection for wrists, fingers, and feet. It may be the result of myxoid degeneration of the fibrous tissue of the joint capsule or tendon sheath. It is usually a globular mass with smaller adjacent "daughter" cysts. The lumen is filled with colorless viscous fluid that apparently comes from the joint via an intermittent one-way valve effect. This may be the reason that the mass fluctuates in size. Pain may precede the appearance of the cystic mass. Transillumination of larger cysts or aspiration of the viscous, almost gelatinous fluid content with collapse of the cyst is diagnostic. Surgical treatment is seldom necessary, but if undertaken can be a marginal excision with a rim of normal capsule or tendon sheath at the base to include any small marginal cysts.

Synovial chondromatosis is an uncommon process of cartilaginous or osteocartilaginous metaplasia within the synovial membrane of joints, tendon sheaths, or bursae. Patients typically have a long history of pain, swelling and limited joint motion. There may be episodes of locking or buckling of the joint because of loose bodies getting caught between the joint surfaces. This metaplastic change is most common at the knee; less commonly, the shoulder, elbow, or wrist may be involved. Radiographs characteristically show multiple calcified and ossified bodies in the joints or bursae, irregularly sized and shaped, particularly in the recesses. Microscopically, small nests of hyaline cartilage are found in the synovial lining of the joint. Enchondral ossification may be seen if an adequate blood supply to the nodule is available. Loose bodies in the joint can continue to grow, being nourished by synovial fluid. Surgical treatment is total synovectomy and removal of all loose bodies, but this can seldom be accomplished. Although recurrence is not uncommon, the clinical course can be one of prolonged symptom-free function.

Pigmented villonodular synovitis (PVNS) is an uncommon joint malady of the synovium of joints, particularly the larger joints. Similar histiocytic lesions arising from the small joints or tendon sheaths of the digits have been given the inclusive term giant cell tumor of tendon sheath (GCTTS). PVNS expresses itself as a slowly progressive, monarticular arthritis, particularly about a large joint such as the knee, hip, shoulder, ankle, or elbow. Periodic serosanguinous effusions, pain, and limited function that worsens over several years are common.

The lesions grow slowly and are often relatively painless until late in the course. Grossly, the mass is shaggy, reddish brown, villous, and nodular, invading surrounding soft tissues and adjacent bone. Radiographs may show such erosions of the bone from without, which develop as a result of local destruction of bone from the basic hyperemia of the lesion. Delay in diagnosis is common, particularly for large lesions in the hip, and their size can make complete excision difficult. Treatment is "total" synovectomy; however, total excision is rarely accomplished, and the recurrence rate approaches 50%. Radiotherapy may be justified if surgery fails to control the process. If significant bone erosion has occurred (hip or shoulder), joint reconstruction may be necessary.

GCTTS is a relatively common benign tumor, usually involving the tendon sheaths of the fingers in adults. These tumors initially appear as painless, slowly enlarging masses. Occasionally radiographs show bony erosion from without. Histologic examination shows characteristic foam cells, which are thought to be histiocytes and are called xanthoma cells. Fibrous stroma, giant cells, and hemosiderin deposits are usually present in varying proportions. Vascularity may be a prominent feature, and may be responsible for the bone erosion that is occasionally seen. Treatment is marginal excision, which may be difficult to obtain completely in larger lesions, or those with poor encapsulation; in such cases, recurrence is possible.

Tumors of Peripheral Nerves

Neurilemoma (schwannoma) is a solitary, benign, encapsulated tumor of Schwann cell origin that may undergo cystic change when it is as large as 3 to 4 cm in diameter. It usually involves one of the larger peripheral nerves and is well encapsulated, causing splaying of the nerve fibers. Even when the tumor is large there is usually little or no neurologic deficit. The presence of a mass may be the initial complaint (Fig. 10–30A). Percussion of the mass often elicits a positive Tinel's sign. Microscopically, the tumor is biphasic with Antoni A tissue showing spindle cells, some of which show marked palisading. Antoni B tissue is myxomatous and often contains cystic spaces and thick-walled blood vessels (see Fig. 10–30B). The tumor usually separates the nerve fibers and can be dissected carefully out of the nerve after incision of the epineurium with minimal neurologic disturbance or section of any axons (see Fig. 10–30C). Often, cystic degeneration in the center of the tumor may be extensive enough to hide the true nature of the lesion.

Neurofibroma is characterized by a greater production of collagen than the neurilemoma, although both are Schwann cell tumors. It may occur as a solitary lesion, but more often it is part of a more generalized process. It can arise from within a larger nerve, or from a nerve branch too small to be identified. Neurofibromas can become malignant, and usually should be excised unless they are so numerous as to make excision impractical. Generalized neurofibromatosis (von Recklinghausen's disease) presents with many such tumors, and they may be accompanied by skin changes (café-au-lait spots) and various other lesions. Spinal lesions on the nerve roots can be seen with vertebral changes and scoliosis. Localized gigantism may also accompany the generalized form.

Amputation neuroma and Morton's neuroma are non-neoplastic tumor masses of nerves. Traumatic (amputation) neuroma occurs after nerve section, and is due to proliferation of Schwann cells and axons from the cut end of the nerve to form a mass mixed with fibrous tissue scarring. Some are quite painful and bothersome to the patient and need to be excised. Morton's interdigital neuroma results from perineural fibrosis with secondary degeneration of a nerve.

Tumors of Uncertain Origin

Myxoma of soft tissue is seen in the thigh muscles of women and rarely attains much size. It is a soft, mucoid

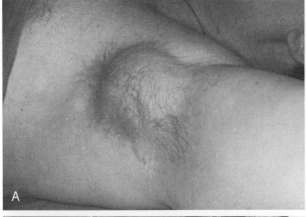

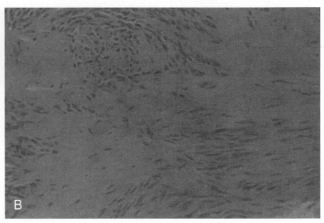

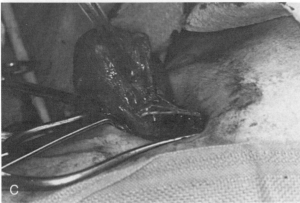

Figure 10–30. Neurilemoma in axilla of 37-year-old male. *A,* Mass was most prominent with arm abducted. The patient experienced no pain, and the mass was not tender. *B,* Typical histologic appearance with cellular Antoni A areas and less cellular areas of myxomatous appearing tissue, which may undergo cystic degeneration. *C,* Appearance at excision of the mass from the musculocutaneous nerve. Paralysis of the biceps and brachialis with anesthesia of radial aspect of forearm to wrist was present postoperatively but recovered within 6 months.

growth containing a few loosely arranged stellate cells in a matrix of gelatinous material of acid mucopolysaccharides, presumably secreted by the stellate cells. Blood vessels are few, and there are minimal connective tissue fibers. Wide or marginal excision is appropriate treatment; recurrences are uncommon. An unusual correlation of myxoma with fibrous dysplasia has been reported.

MALIGNANT TUMORS OF SOFT TISSUES

Malignant tumors of the soft tissues are three to four times more common than malignancies of bone. Careful physical examination of the tumor, the involved part, and regional lymph nodes is necessary. Plain radiographs usually are not helpful but may demonstrate the characteristic radiolucency of lipomas, or abnormal calcification as seen in synovial sarcomas or vascular lesions (Fig. 10–31A and B). CT, ultrasonography, and arteriography are all useful, but MRI has proved to be the most helpful diagnostic tool in documenting tumor size and the relationship to contiguous structures. Isotope scans often are useful to rule out involvement of nearby bone. When malignancy is suspected, CT scan of the lungs is indicated.

Biopsy of a suspected malignancy can be done by needle or by open incision and must be planned in such a manner that the biopsy tract can be removed widely at any subsequent definitive surgery. If the tumor is benign, the proper biopsy technique may be excisional, which often constitutes definitive treatment as well. After biopsy and before definitive treatment, malignant tumors must be staged; Enneking's staging system is useful. Definitive surgical procedures are classified by the margins they achieve (intralesional, marginal, wide, radical). Amputations are also classified by the margin achieved.

Staging does not involve naming the tumor or detecting the presumed cell of origin, but rather is based upon the aggressiveness of the individual tumor, both on radiographic and histologic studies. A small lesion in the thigh can be resected with minimal loss of function. The same-sized lesion in the foot often requires amputation to get adequate margins. A number of recent protocols utilize neoadjuvant (preoperative) radiotherapy to shrink the tumor, especially at the active margins, to allow for less extensive resection of normal tissue. High-grade lesions should receive adjuvant chemotherapy or radiotherapy, often given after biopsy but before surgical resection. This may permit marginal resections followed by further radiotherapy for the tumor bed and chemotherapy for any apparent or potential micrometastases. Thoracotomy for pulmonary metastases has increased the cure rate unless the metastases are too numerous to allow resection without compromising pulmonary function excessively.

Malignant Fibrous Lesions

Dermatofibrosarcoma protuberans is a rare neoplasm that arises just beneath the epidermis as one or several nodules, which may grow slowly into sizable masses that demonstrate infiltrative growth. The overlying skin may become atrophic and easily injured. It occurs more often on the trunk than on the extremities, usually in later life. Microscopically, the tissue is well differentiated but cellular; the

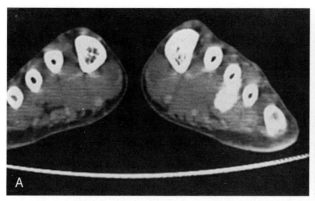 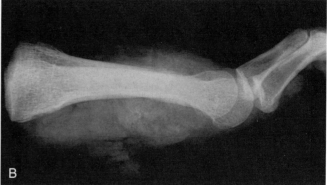

Figure 10–31. Synovial sarcoma in 19-year-old male. *A,* Lesion presenting into sole of foot is heavily calcified. *B,* Specimen of resected third and fourth metatarsals with tumor shows calcification throughout the soft tissue tumor.

cells resemble fibroblasts. Treatment of choice is wide resection. Local recurrence is common, but metastases are rare.

Fibrosarcoma is used as a diagnostic label at present; most cases currently are categorized as malignant fibrous histiocytoma. Fibrosarcoma is generally a disease of older age groups, most common in adults 30 to 50 years of age, with equal sex distribution. Most patients present with a mass, occasionally with low-grade, persistent pain. Congenital fibrosarcoma is a variant which may occur in infants or very young children in the distal parts of the extremities and present very difficult problems in diagnosis and treatment (Fig. 10–32). Fibrosarcoma may occur anywhere in the body where fibrous tissue is found. Grossly, the tumor appears as a solitary mass of soft to firm consistency, white to gray. Smaller ones appear well circumscribed and even encapsulated. Larger ones often are poorly defined with microscopic extensions into the surrounding tissues, which makes resection difficult. The microscopic appearance is one of rather uniform spindle-shaped cells that are separated by bundles of collagen in a herring-bone pattern. Mitotic activity varies, but the biologic behavior, and thus treatment, depends on the histologic grade of tissue obtained on incisional biopsy. Low-grade lesions require wide margins, and high-grade lesions require radical margins. Combined modalities may be used with less extensive surgery. Systemic chemotherapy is probably indicated for high-grade lesions. Death occurs within 5 years in two thirds of patients with high-grade lesions.

Malignant fibrous histiocytoma is currently the most frequently diagnosed soft tissue malignancy of late adult life. Most occur in men 50 to 70 years of age, but there is a wide age range. Less aggressive forms have been seen in children. Clinically, the lesions of the extremities present as a painless, enlarging mass of a few months duration. Grossly, the lesions are lobulated, solitary, fleshy masses, grayish white on cut section (Fig. 10–33*A*). Hemorrhage and necrosis are common features of this tumor, probably related to the varied vascularity (see Fig. 10–33*B*). The characteristic histologic picture shows plump, pleomorphic, spindle cells arranged in short fascicles in a whorled (storiform, cartwheel) pattern with large and bizarre multinucleated giant cells scattered in the fields (see Fig. 10–33*C*). Bizarre mitotic figures may be scattered throughout the

tumor. The biologic behavior is predicted by histologic grade rather than by variants such as fibrous, giant cell, myxoid, angiomatoid, or inflammatory. Tumors located deep in the soft tissues have a poorer prognosis than more superficial tumor that are unlikely to metastasize. Surgical treatment should follow Enneking's principles, with wide margins for low-grade lesions and more radical resections or amputations for high-grade lesions. Combined treatment with radiotherapy or systemic chemotherapy may allow less aggressive surgery. Death is most often due to pulmonary metastases.

Alveolar soft tissue sarcoma is a rare malignant tumor arising in the muscles of the extremities. It occurs in adolescents or young adults, usually in the lower limb, particularly the anterior thigh. When it occurs in children, it is more commonly found in the head and neck. It usually presents as a slow-growing mass without associated functional impairment and the diagnosis may therefore be delayed. They are highly vascular, and massive bleeding during surgical removal is not uncommon. Grossly, they tend to be poorly circumscribed, often with large areas of necrosis or hemorrhage. Metastasis usually occurs early in the course of the disease. The mortality rate with standard surgical resection has been high and recommended treatment at this time is radical resection with adjuvant chemotherapy.

Epithelioid sarcoma is an unusual, slow-growing, malignant, soft tissue tumor usually occurring in young adults. Males predominate. Most tumors are in the extremities, with the upper extremity having the highest incidence. The tumor occurs in the subcutaneous or deeper tissues as a firm, painless nodule. Those in the skin frequently ulcerate and fail to heal, even with aggressive treatment of presumed infectious process (Fig. 10–34*A* and *B*). Deeper lesions tend to be larger, less well defined, and firmly fixed to tendons or fascial structures. The tumor has varied histologic characteristics, which lead to frequent misdiagnosis as a chronic inflammatory process, necrotizing granuloma, or benign or other malignant tumors. Microscopic features are the presence of malignant cells with epithelioid or spindled appearance, often in a nodular pattern. A distinct biphasic appearance is lacking. Inflammatory cells and necrosis are common features. Because of the frequent long intervals, often years, between the appearance of the

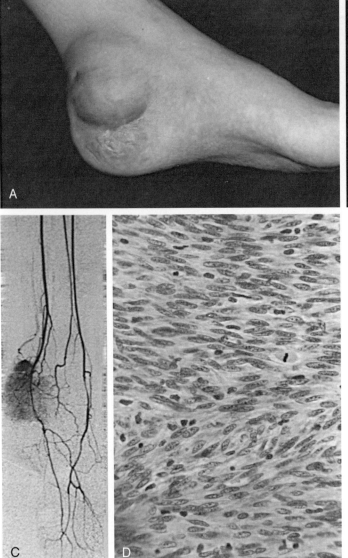

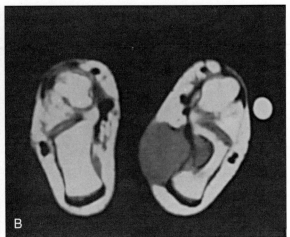

Figure 10–32. Congenital fibrosarcoma in foot of 12-year-old boy. *A*, Photograph of medial aspect of foot showing recurrent mass in region of scar of previous resection done prior to age 2. A probable diagnosis of fibrosarcoma as made at that time, but no further investigation was done. *B*, MRI of foot illustrating soft tissue mass and intraosseous invasion. *C*, Arteriogram shows typical tumor blush of malignancy. *D*, Histologic specimen of the lesion with spindle-shaped nuclei with minimal stroma and a number of mitotic figures. Pulmonary metastases were found at the time of this evaluation, so no amputation was done.

lesion and its proper diagnosis, the aggressive nature of the tumor is often minimized, but is evidenced by a recurrence rate up to 85% and a 30% metastasis rate. Spread of the disease is by contiguous surface or invasive growth, vascular emboli to lungs, or regional lymph nodes. The interval between diagnosis and death may be a matter of a few months. Recommended treatment is radical resection or amputation, followed by radiotherapy in various permutations and multidrug chemotherapy.

Liposarcoma is the second most common malignant tumor of mesodermal soft tissue, constituting 15 to 20% of all soft tissue sarcomas, exceeded in incidence only by malignant fibrous histiocytoma. It occurs in both sexes equally, usually after age 50, and is rare in children or persons under 20. The tumor is found most often in the retroperitoneum or lower extremities. Symptoms are related to the mass, and pain comes later. Although an occasional anaplastic tumor may grow rapidly, most grow slowly, and are often quite large before the patient presents for diagno-

sis and treatment. Physical examination reveals a mass that may be well defined or have indistinct boundaries. Radiographs may show a lucency in the soft tissues if the tumor is well differentiated; otherwise, water or muscle density is more common. MRI is the study of choice for defining the anatomic extent of the lesions, its relations to surrounding structures, and its degree of homogeneity. Grossly the tumors appear encapsulated, large, and lobulated. The apparent encapsulation is deceptive, however, with permeation of pseudopod-like extensions of neoplastic cells beyond the thin, often discontinuous pseudocapsule into the surrounding tissues or fascial spaces. Grossly, the tumor can be soft and gelatinous, greasy or fatty, firm and fibrous. Areas of different colors are due to necrosis, fibrous septa, and hemorrhage (Fig. 10–35).

Microscopically liposarcomas vary greatly. Most common are the low-grade, well-differentiated (30% of cases), or myxoid (30 to 40%) types resembling embryonal fat. These tumors contain prominent sinusoidal capillaries and

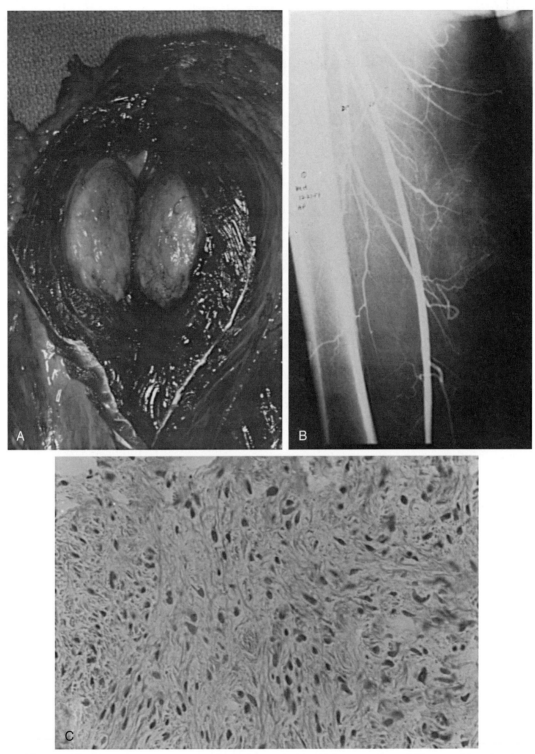

Figure 10–33. Malignant fibrous histiocytoma in hamstring muscles of 39-year-old male. *A,* Section through lesion illustrates apparent encapsulation without invasion of surrounding muscle. *B,* Arteriogram shows tumor blush of well-defined lesion. *C,* Histologic examination shows pleomorphic cellular pattern with moderate amount of stroma.

large quantities of acid mucopolysaccharides in "puddles." Mitotic figures are absent. They grow slowly and recur locally, metastasizing late, if at all.

The *round cell type* (10%) is highly cellular with an excessive proliferation of uniform round cells with foamy cytoplasm and atypical but not highly bizarre nuclei. These tumors are always high grade and often metastasize.

Pleomorphic liposarcomas (20%) are characterized by a very disorderly growth pattern, extreme degrees of cellular pleomorphism, and highly bizarre giant cells. This variant

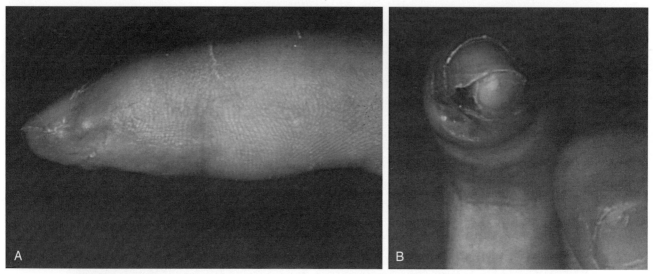

Figure 10–34. Epithelioid sarcoma in finger pulp of 21-year-old male. Lesion had been present for 2 years and had been incised twice for presumed pulp space infection. No pus was obtained, and no biopsy of the tissue was done. *A,* Deformity of end of finger with tumor replacing most of pulp tissue. *B,* End-on view of finger.

is very malignant and tends to metastasize early. Many liposarcomas are mixed and have areas of transitions to any or all of the patterns just described. The behavior depends not only on the different cell patterns but also on their proportions in any given tumor.

The well-differentiated *lipoma-like liposarcomas* resemble a lipoma and are often misdiagnosed until they have recurred several times. Aggressiveness of treatment of liposarcoma depends on grading; one may need to sample several areas of large tumors to get a true picture for staging. High-grade lesions require the more aggressive

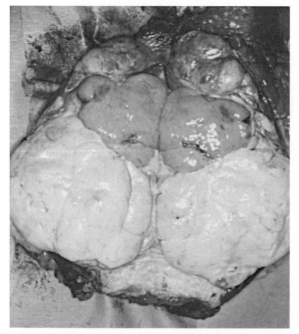

Figure 10–35. Liposarcoma from 43-year-old male illustrating the varied nature of portions of the tumor.

surgery, and should be followed with systemic chemotherapy or radiotherapy or both. Metastases to lungs or liver are common but rarely extend to lymph nodes. Five-year survival rate varies from 18 to 85%, depending on histologic type of tumor and completeness of surgical excision.

Leiomyosarcoma arises occasionally in the skin, but more often in deeper soft tissues. Grossly, these tumors appear encapsulated but the temptation to enucleate them must be avoided. The tumor cells have elongated nuclei with blunt ends, and occasional myofibrils may be seen. Only presence of significant mitotic activity distinguishes the malignant variant from benign leiomyoma. They are locally aggressive and metastasize early; treatment is based on histologic grade and anatomic setting. Those in subcutaneous or cutaneous locations have a much more favorable prognosis than the more common and frequently larger tumors in the retroperitoneum.

Rhabdomyosarcoma is the malignant tumor of striated muscle whose cells show characteristic cross striations on microscopy. There are three microscopic types—embryonal, alveolar, and pleomorphic; some are mixed. Embryonal and alveolar forms are found in children and adolescents and are among the more common malignant tumors of these age groups. The *embryonal type* is soft and gelatinous with long spindle cells containing hyperchromatic nuclei and abundant cytoplasm. Myxoid areas may be prominent. *Alveolar rhabdomyosarcomas* usually occur in the head, neck, or extremities, and are typically firmer and less myxoid than the embryonal type. They have often spread with regional and distant disease present before the patient appears before the physician. Regional lymph node involvement is present in approximately 20% and must be searched for during the staging process. Microscopically the predominant cell is round with scanty eosinophilic cytoplasm. Occasionally, giant cells are present.

The morphologic characteristics of the *pleomorphic type* has led in the past several decades to their redesignation as malignant fibrous histiocytoma, leaving most rhabdomyosarcomas as a childhood entity. Microscopically, the pleomorphic type is composed of spindle-shaped cells in parallel and interlacing bundles. They are the most malignant of the soft tissue sarcomas in children. Treatment is wide resection when possible, but marginal and even intralesional resections may be acceptable when combined with adjuvant radiotherapy and prolonged systemic polychemotherapy. Patient survival and cure rates have markedly improved with the multidisciplinary approach now in use for childhood rhabdomyosarcomas. With favorable staging of the tumor, adequate local tumor resection, and no evidence of regional lymph node involvement, over 80% survive for a long time.

Synovial sarcoma is a malignant soft tissue tumor arising near, but not usually in, a joint. The typical patient is a young adult who presents with a mass, or pain, or both. It is not unusual for a patient to have known of a mass for years without significant change, and then experience a sudden increase in growth over a few months (Fig. 10–36A, B, and C). Radiographs may show soft tissue calcification. The microscopic appearance usually is biphasic with pseudoglandular (epithelial) areas interspersed with spindle cell elements. Slit-like spaces suggest formation of primitive joints or bursae (see Fig. 10–36D). Some tumors may have

the spindle-cell element making up the major part of the tumor, others have predominant areas of undifferentiated round cells. The most common pathway of spread is via blood vessels to the lungs, but lymph node metastases are seen with this tumor more than with most soft tissue sarcomas. Reports indicate no improved survival rate with lymph node dissection. Radical resection or amputation has provided 5-year survival rates of 35 to 50%. Wide resection is followed by radiotherapy to achieve local control of the tumor, and multidrug adjuvant chemotherapy provides systemic control. Even with more aggressive surgical and adjuvant therapy, the overall prognosis is poor. Local recurrences or metastases have been reported to occur after long periods (months to years) of apparent disease-free intervals.

Malignant schwannoma is the malignant counterpart of neurofibroma (Fig. 10–37). Approximately 25% of patients with this tumor have neurofibromatosis and appear to have a worse prognosis than patients with isolated malignant schwannoma. Microscopic diagnosis of malignant change in a neurofibroma may be difficult. Wide surgical margins should be obtained, and frozen sections of the margins are advisable because the tumor does not have clear-cut encapsulation. Combined modalities of treatment are indicated (wide resection plus radiotherapy and chemotherapy).

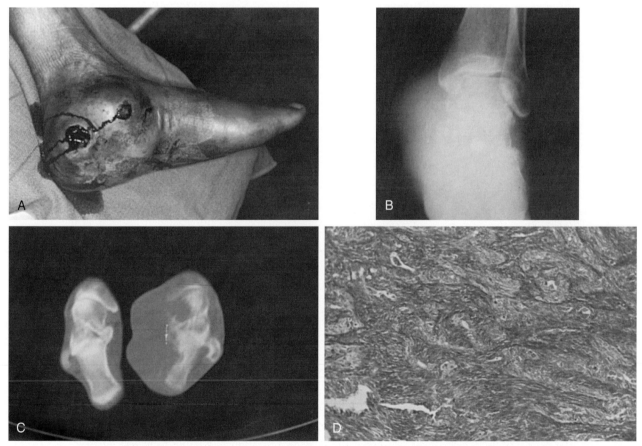

Figure 10–36. Synovial sarcoma in foot of 41-year-old male. Incision and drainage were done on two occasions without improvement or diagnosis. *A,* Incision sites failed to heal, and biopsy was done of tumor extruding through the openings in the skin. *B,* Radiograph demonstrated large soft tissue mass without calcification. *C,* CT shows soft tissue mass with extensive destruction of the underlying bone. *D,* Histologic examination shows the biphasic nature of the tumor with pseudoglandular areas, some with slitlike spaces, interspersed with spindle elements. Either component can predominate.

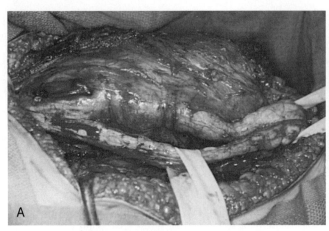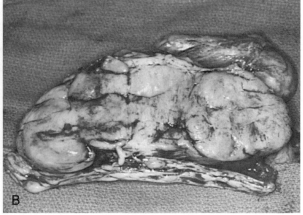

Figure 10–37. Malignant schwannoma (neurosarcoma) arising in peroneal portion of sciatic nerve of 21-year-old female. *A,* Marginal resection was done to preserve function in the tibial portion of the nerve. *B,* Resected specimen showing lobular nature of the tumor.

Unclassified Sarcoma

Occasionally a tumor may be so undifferentiated that the pathologist cannot place it in any recognized category. These tumors are invariably highly malignant with a poor prognosis. Treatment should be radical resection or amputation with adjuvant therapy consisting of limb perfusion, radiotherapy, and systemic chemotherapy.

Non-Neoplastic Conditions Simulating Bone Tumors

Paget's disease is an entity of unknown cause characterized by osteoclastic resorption of bone. Attempts at simultaneous aggressive osteoblastic repair result in poor quality, woven bone. The process may result in (1) a radiographic appearance simulating malignant tumor of bone, (2) deformity, or (3) pathologic fracture. Biopsy may be needed to establish the diagnosis. Histologicaly, numerous osteoclasts in Howship's lacunae, osteoblasts lined up on remaining or newly formed trabeculae, and a vascular fibrous stroma result in numerous reversal lines and a mosaic appearance to the bone. Intraosseous arteriovenous shunts may develop and lead to impressive bleeding during operative procedures on involved bone. Deformity may make fracture fixation difficult. Sarcomatous change in pagetoid bone is not uncommon; such tumors are usually high grade and involve the pelvis, femur, and humerus. The tumor types are as expected from the cell types seen in the bone; thus, giant cell tumors, osteosarcomas, less commonly chondrosarcomas, or malignant fibrous histiocytomas occur. The prognosis of these sarcomas arising in Paget's disease is uniformly poor.

Myositis ossificans is a generic term for a class of lesions characterized by extraskeletal metaplasic ossification in muscle or other mesenchymal soft tissues, usually following trauma. The process can be divided into three stages. The first stage, lasting 4 to 6 weeks, is known as the "pseudosarcomatous stage" because of the massive tissue necrosis with a response of extremely cellular proliferation of tissue with numerous mitotic figures suggesting sarcoma. A second stage is a period of differentiation, followed by a third stage of maturation. The clinical history is essential, but is often misleading because the patient cannot recall any injury, or may not want to relate the circumstances surrounding an injury. Radiographic and clinical features in the initial stage are primarily a tender soft tissue mass that later shows bone production at the periphery of the lesion during the second stage. Localized forms must be distinguished from osteosarcoma. Myositis ossificans is usually situated outside the diaphysis of long bones, while osteosarcoma is intraosseous, usually in the metaphysis. In myositis ossificans the pain and mass decrease with time, whereas the opposite is true with osteosarcoma. In myositis ossificans radiographs demonstrate intact underlying cortex, whereas the cortex is usually violated in osteosarcoma. If at least 10 days are permitted to elapse after onset of symptoms, biopsy of the mass in myositis ossificans can often demonstrate a definite zonal pattern. The least differentiated portion of the lesion is the center, where the muscle damage is the greatest, and the most differentiated portion of the lesion with the most recognizable and mature ossified tissue is at the periphery. This is usually the opposite of the pattern in a malignancy in which the least differentiated tissue is at the periphery. Finding such zones on microscopy confirms the diagnosis, and watchful waiting until radiographic follow-up shows maturation of the periphery of the lesion would be proper treatment. With a good history and clinical examination, the lesion can be watched for a period of up to 3 weeks to see if radiographic examination will demonstrate ossification at the periphery of the mass, indicating its benign nature. Progressive myositis ossificans is a rare genetic entity, usually does not follow trauma, and is readily diagnosed.

Patients with Gaucher's disease usually present to the orthopedist with avascular necrosis of the femoral head and a painful hip, or with pathologic fracture of proximal femur. The surgeon should be aware that these patients are prone to postoperative infections.

Bone infarcts occur in caisson workers or divers, in patients with sickle cell anemia, or in patients on steroids for variable, usually lengthy, periods. The diagnosis is usually not difficult, but occasionally lesions are noted in the metaphyseal region of long bones that resemble cartilage tumors on radiographs. Such lesions do not show increased uptake on technetium bone scan. Biopsy shows mineralization of necrotic marrow elements. No treatment is required. Malignant fibrous histiocytomas arising from old bone infarcts have been recorded.

"Brown tumors" of hyperparathyroidism result from increased circulating parathyroid hormone produced by parathyroid glands that are overactive from tumor or hyperplasia. Symptoms may be chiefly renal, psychiatric, or skeletal. The initial symptom may be peptic ulcer. When the disease is discovered early, diffuse demineralization is the first skeletal finding. Only rarely does the process become focal and produce a "brown tumor" that resembles a giant cell tumor of bone. The diagnosis of hyperparathyroidism is readily established by determinations of serum calcium, phosphorus, and alkaline phosphatase. Biopsy of the tumor shows smaller giant cells occurring in a somewhat nodular arrangement and stromal cells, which are more spindle-shaped and delicate than in the classic giant cell tumor of bone. Evidence of osseous metaplasia within the stroma is prominent. The bone surrounding the lesion may show intense osteoclastic and osteoblastic activity associated with intratrabecular fibrosis ("dissecting osteitis").

Osteomyelitis can at times simulate tumors with osteoblastic and osteolytic changes. Occasionally Ewing's sarcoma can mimic infection with increased erythrocyte sedimentation rate and elevated white blood cell count. Such an abundance of plasma cells may occur in infection, and multiple myeloma must be considered. Malignant change can occur in chronically draining sinuses of long duration; both squamous cell carcinoma and fibrosarcoma have been reported.

Fracture callus or stress reactions producing periosteal new bone, with or without actual fracture, may simulate osteosarcoma. When biopsy is done the microscopic picture may be difficult for the inexperienced pathologist to distinguish from sarcoma. The florid callus seen in osteogenesis imperfecta may also simulate osteosarcoma radiographically.

Bibliography

Aaron AD, Bogumill GP: Tumors of the musculoskeletal system. *In* Wiesel SW, Delahay JN (eds): Essentials of Orthopaedic Surgery, 2nd ed. Philadelphia, W.B. Saunders, 1997, Chapter 5.

Bogumill GP, Schwamm HA: Orthopaedic Pathology: A Synopsis with Clinical and Radiographic Correlation. Philadelphia, W.B. Saunders, 1984.

Bogumill GP, Fleegler EJ (eds): Tumors of the Hand and Upper Limb. Edinburgh, Churchill Livingstone, 1993.

Campanacci M, Laus M: Osteofibrous dysplasia of the tibia and fibula. J Bone Joint Surg 1981; 63A:367.

Capanna R, Dal Monte A, Gitelis S, Campanacci M: The natural history of unicameral bone cyst after steroid injection. Clin Orthop 1982; 166:204.

Crenshaw AE (ed): Campbell's Operative Orthopaedics, 7th ed. St. Louis, C.V. Mosby, 1987, Chapters 30–34.

Enneking WF, Spanier SS, Goodman MA: Current concepts review: The surgical staging of musculoskeletal sarcoma. J Bone Joint Surg 1980; 62A:1027.

Enneking WF: Staging Musculoskeletal Tumors. *In* Enneking WF (ed): Musculoskeletal Tumor Surgery. New York, Churchill Livingstone, 1983, p 87.

Johnson LC, Vetter H, Putschar WG: Sarcoma arising in bone cysts. Virchows Arch 1962; (A) 335:428.

Madewell JE, Ragsdale BD, Sweet DE: Radiology and pathological analysis of solitary bone lesions. Part I: Internal margins. Radiol Clin North Am 1981; 19(4):715–748.

Mankin HJ: Section 11: Bone and soft tissue tumors. *In* Evarts C McC: Surgery of the Musculoskeletal System, 2nd ed. New York, Churchill Livingstone, 1990.

Mankin HJ, Lange TA, Spanier SS: The hazards of the biopsy in patients with malignant primary bone and soft tissue tumors. J Bone Joint Surg 1982; 64A:1121.

Ragsdale BD, Madewell JE, Sweet DE: Radiology and pathological analysis of solitary bone lesions. Part II: Periosteal reactions. Radiol Clin North Am 1981; 19(4): 749–783.

Scaglietti O, Marchetti PG, Bartolozzi P: Final results obtained in the treatment of bone cysts with methylprednisolone acetate (Depo Medrol) and a discussion of results achieved in other bone lesions. Clin Orthop 1982; 165:33.

Sweet DE, Madewell JE, Ragsdale BD: Radiology and pathological analysis of solitary bone lesions. Part III: Matrix patterns. Radiol Clin North Am 1981; 19(4):785–814.

Chapter 11

Metabolic Bone Disease

John N. Delahay, M.D.
Brian G. Evans, M.D.

GENERAL CONCEPTS

The disease states considered within the category of metabolic bone disease are varied and their pathogenesis is complex. More often than not, the skeleton is merely a mirror reflecting abnormalities in hormonal balance. An understanding of the principles of skeletal homeostasis is necessary to order these diverse disease states. There is a constant turnover of bone in the skeleton. As bone is removed by the osteoclasts, it is replaced by the osteoblasts in an ongoing cycle of bone remodeling.

First and perhaps most important to appreciate is the *relationship between bone formation and bone resorption* (Fig. 11–1). As discussed elsewhere in this text, bone formation and bone resorption are normal processes in the skeleton. On a day-to-day basis, portions of bone are removed by normal osteoclastic activity and replaced by normal osteoblastic activity. This flux is necessary for skeletal rejuvenation and homeostasis. As a result of metabolic aberrations, there is frequently either an increase in bone resorption or an increase in bone formation, or both. It is critical to recognize that it is the *net effect* of these changes that is important. For example, in hyperparathyroid states, bone resorption dramatically increases. There is also a compensatory rise in bone formation; however, this rise is minimal relative to the amount of bone resorption that is occurring. Therefore, the net effect is bone loss. Further, the relationship between bone formation and bone resorption is frequently said to be *coupled*; that is, if one goes up the other will also go up and, conversely, if one is depressed, so is the other. Obviously, they change in varying degrees in relation to each other. There are relatively few disease states in which one sees an *uncoupling* of this bone remodeling mechanism. Perhaps most notable is the effect that glucocorticoids have on skeletal remodeling. Typically, they dramatically increase bone resorption and at the same time suppress bone formation. Hence, the overall net effect is severe bone loss.

A second important concept is the *relationship between mineral and matrix* (Fig. 11–2). As noted earlier, there is a fixed ratio of bone mineral to bone matrix. This is determined by the steric influences of the collagen quarter-stagger arrangement. Hence, only a specific amount of mineral may be deposited into a given amount of matrix. Various disease states can alter the ratio of mineral to matrix. Osteoporosis is a decrease in bone mass. However, despite a substantial decrease in bone volume, the ratio of mineral to matrix is maintained at normal levels. Conversely, in osteomalacic states, in which there is an inadequate amount of mineral available to deposit into the matrix, the ratio of mineral to matrix is significantly altered. Because of a marked increase in the amount of unmineralized matrix, the ratio is much less than normal. Thus, one must be cognizant of this relationship when evaluating the effect of vitamins, hormones, and other extrinsic factors on skeletal mass.

Third, it is imperative to recognize the *significance of serum calcium levels*. Many feel that the major role of the skeleton is to act as a reservoir for elemental calcium and to release this stored calcium when it is needed to meet normal homeostatic demands. Calcium is absorbed from the intestine. Subsequently, it is incorporated into the skeleton as apatite or is excreted at the renal level. There is a continuous ongoing exchange of calcium in and out of the skeleton throughout life. Needless to say, ionic calcium is required for normal cellular functioning at multiple levels. To meet these metabolic demands, there is minute-to-minute exchange between the calcium held in the skeleton and the ionic calcium in the blood. The serum calcium level however, is rarely representative of skeletal activity. Considering that more than 95% of the body's calcium is stored in bone apatite, it is understandable that the 180 mg of ionized calcium represents literally the "tip of the iceberg." Peripheral sampling of the serum calcium provides only a remote clue to the true content of skeletal apatite. It does, however, provide a convenient means of classifying metabolic bone diseases. Using serum calcium levels, one classification scheme is as follows:

- *Eucalcemic states*, for example, osteoporosis
- *Hypercalcemic states*, for example, parathyroid bone disease
- *Hypocalcemic states*, for example, rickets and osteomalacia

One other suggested grouping for metabolic bone diseases is simply to classify them based on an identifiable cause. For example, *primary metabolic bone diseases* have no apparent or identifiable cause. One such example that is frequently mentioned is Paget's disease of bone. Conversely *secondary metabolic diseases* usually result from a demonstrated abnormality extrinsic to bone, such as deficiencies of hormones and vitamins.

This chapter reviews the important metabolic bone diseases and discusses the way in which they affect skeletal

Four Mechanisms of Bone Mass Regulation

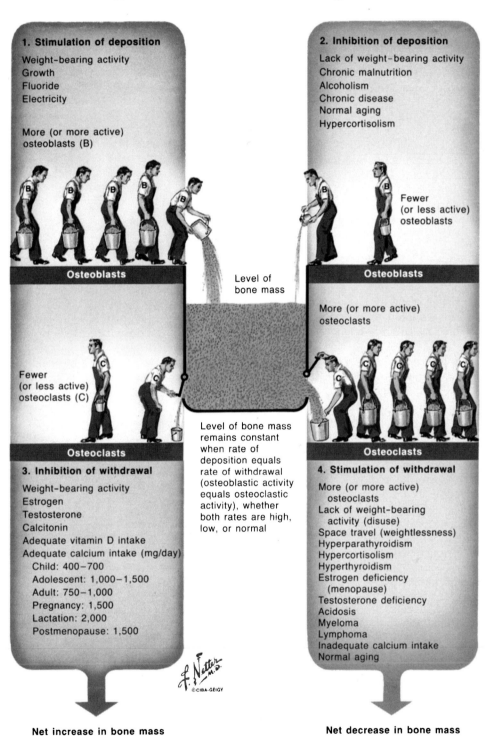

Figure 11–1. Four mechanisms of bone mass regulation. (From Netter FH: The Ciba Collections of Medical Illustrations. Volume 8: Musculoskeletal System. Part 1: Anatomy, Physiology, and Metabolic Bone Disease. Summit NJ: Ciba Geigy Publications, 1987, p 181.)

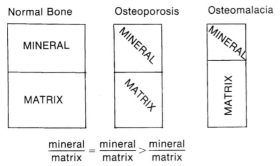

$$\frac{\text{mineral}}{\text{matrix}} = \frac{\text{mineral}}{\text{matrix}} > \frac{\text{mineral}}{\text{matrix}}$$

Figure 11–2. Ratio of mineral to matrix in normal and abnormal metabolic states: normal = osteoporosis > osteomalacia.

homeostasis. For ease of discussion, they are grouped using the former classification rather than the latter. A section is included at the end of the chapter on the endocrine effects on bone, specifically those that are responsible for some of the secondary metabolic bone diseases.

EVALUATION OF THE PATIENT WITH METABOLIC BONE DISEASE

Evaluation of the patient with metabolic bone disease involves a combination of laboratory, radiographic, and pathologic analyses. Serum calcium and bone metabolism are rigidly controlled by several hormones and are influenced by a wide variety of factors. The use of appropriate laboratory studies can greatly assist in the analysis of the patient with altered bone metabolism.

Calcium

The majority of the body's calcium, 99%, is stored within bone tissue. However, the 1% in solution within the serum and tissues is meticulously controlled. There is a complex hormonal feedback system to control the serum calcium level between 8.8 and 10.4 mg/dL. Calcium in solution is essential for many metabolic activities in cells. If the calcium level is significantly altered, it can lead to significant changes in muscle function, alter cellular energy production and metabolism, and alter neural impulse transmission and coagulation.

Approximately 50% of the serum calcium is in a free ionic form. The remainder is bound to plasma proteins, mainly albumin. The amount of calcium in free ionic form can be estimated by subtracting 1 mg/dL for every 1 g/dL serum albumin less than 4 g/dL of serum albumin. Alteration in the serum calcium has profound physiologic effects. Low serum calcium results in perioral paresthesias, muscle irritability, bronchospasm, and a prolonged Q-T interval on electrocardiography. Increased serum levels of calcium result in decreased appetite, nausea, vomiting, constipation, and subsequent lethargy and coma.

The average intake of calcium is 600 to 1000 mg/day. The USRDA for adults is 1200 mg/day for adolescents and young adults and 800 mg/day for adults. In postmenopausal women, however, the suggested dietary intake is 1200 to 1500 mg/day. Vitamin D and its metabolites are required

for the absorption of calcium from the gut. The majority of calcium is absorbed in the proximal small intestine. Therefore, processes that result in impaired small bowel function, or small bowel resection, can create a calcium-deficient state.

Both the bowel and the kidney excrete calcium. The calcium excreted by the bowel (approximately 60 to 120 mg/day) is poorly regulated. The majority of calcium excretion is performed by the kidney, which is limited in its ability to control the calcium level. Normal calcium excretion for adults with an average calcium intake is between 100 and 400 mg/day. In calcium-deficient states, the rate of renal excretion can be as low as 200 mg/day. In normal individuals, variation in calcium intake has little effect on the rate of calcium excretion. A negative or positive calcium balance with bone maintains the serum calcium level. In patients with chronically reduced calcium intake, the serum calcium level is maintained by a negative calcium balance and mobilization of calcium from bone.

Phosphorus

Phosphorus is another major component of bone. The level of phosphorus is not as meticulously controlled as that of calcium. The normal serum level is 2.8 to 4 mg/dL. The majority of serum phosphorus is in the ionic form. Less than 15% of serum phosphorus is protein bound. Serum phosphorus is in several ionic forms in solution. The relative amount of each form is controlled by the serum pH. The level of phosphorus can be decreased significantly after eating and should therefore be measured in the fasting state. Ingestion of non-absorbable antacids also reduces the serum phosphorus level. Few symptoms are noted with hyperphosphatemia. However, if the level remains high for a long time, ectopic calcifications may be noted. Hypophosphatemia, however, can lead to anorexia, dizziness, and muscle weakness. In severe hypophosphatemia, elevated creatine phosphokinase (CPK) levels may be elevated, indicating rhabdomyolysis. In chronic hypophosphatemia, osteomalacia results.

Phosphorus is efficiently absorbed from the gut. If the intake of phosphorus is reduced, the small intestine can absorb approximately 80 to 90% of the available phosphorus. In a normal state, approximately 70% of the phosphorus is absorbed. The kidney is responsible for maintaining the serum phosphorus level. The majority of the phosphorus is filtered at the renal glomerulus and is then reabsorbed in the proximal and distal renal tubule. In the normal circumstance, only 10 to 15% of the filtered phosphorus is excreted. The amount of excreted phosphorus is directly related to the amount filtered to allow control of the serum phosphorus level. Thus, the amount of excreted phosphorus is related to the amount ingested.

Vitamin D and its Metabolites

Vitamin D is actually a group of fat-soluble sterol vitamins including ergocalciferol and cholecalciferol. They are either ingested via vitamin D–fortified products such as milk or are formed as the result of a reaction to ultraviolet sunlight on exposed skin. The USRDA for vitamin D is 400 to 800 IU. Vitamin D undergoes hydroxylation in the liver to form

25-hydroxyvitamin D. This is a pro-vitamin form that is weakly active physiologically and is a storage form of vitamin D. The serum level of 25-hydroxyvitamin D is an excellent indicator of the body's vitamin D reserves.

The next step in the activation of vitamin D occurs in the kidney. Here the 25-hydroxyvitamin D again undergoes hydroxylation to form 1,25-dihydroxyvitamin D. This is the active form of vitamin D. The enzyme controlling the hydroxylation, 25-hydroxyvitamin D-1α-hydroxylase is stimulated by parathyroid hormone (PTH). 1,25-dihydroxyvitamin D affects the intestinal absorption of calcium and phosphate. In addition 1,25-dihydroxyvitamin D activates bone resorption by aiding in the recruitment of pre-osteoclasts.

Parathyroid Hormone

PTH is a peptide hormone formed by the parathyroid glands on the posterior surface of the thyroid gland. The hormone is released in response to a reduction in the serum calcium level. It affects several organ systems to increase the serum calcium level. PTH directly stimulates the resorption of bone by increasing the osteoclast activity and directly and indirectly recruiting pre-osteoclasts. As already mentioned, PTH activates the hydroxylation of 25-hydroxyvitamin D to 1,25-dihydroxyvitamin D in the kidney. In addition, PTH stimulates the reabsorption of filtered calcium in the renal tubule in the kidney and reduces the reabsorption of phosphate. Although PTH has no direct effect in the gut, by stimulating the production of 1,25-dihydroxyvitamin D, it assists in stimulating intestinal absorption of calcium. In the end, the effects result in an increase in the serum calcium level and a decrease in the serum phosphate level. The amount of PTH produced is strongly affected by the serum calcium level, and the primary source of calcium is from bone, leading to a negative bone balance with more calcium being removed than is deposited.

PTH has a short serum half-life. The intact peptides are cleaved and the inactive fragments have a longer half-life in the serum. The half-life can be further extended in patients with renal insufficiency. Measurement of PTH is performed by radioimmunoassay, usually for the C terminus. This results in sampling both the active and the more prevalent inactive cleaved form. Thus, the results need to be interpreted in conjunction with the serum calcium level.

Calcitonin

Calcitonin is also a peptide hormone. The parafollicular cells in the thyroid gland produce calcitonin. The release of this hormone is mediated by an increase in the serum calcium level. The hormone has an effect on osteoclastic activity. It inhibits bone resorption and can lead to a reduction in the serum calcium level. Calcitonin does not appear to have an effect on either the kidney or the gut. However, calcitonin is not essential for control of the serum calcium level or the maintenance of bone metabolism. Patients who undergo thyroidectomy for malignancy do not manifest any aberration in bone metabolism when replacement therapy with thyroxine only is provided.

Each of the preceding factors can be involved in both the normal physiology of bone and a pathologic process. In normal bone metabolism, the rate of bone formation is linked to bone resorption. In young adults and children, more bone is deposited than is taken away. In older patients, generally more bone is removed than is laid down. This results in an increase in bone mass for children and young adults and, as patients age, a gradual reduction in bone mass. The peak bone mass is determined by the patient's dietary status, genetic predisposition, certain disease states, and activity level (see Fig. 11–1).

Radiographic Assessment of the Patient with Metabolic Bone Disease

ROUTINE RADIOGRAPHY

Routine radiography is helpful in the assessment of patients with metabolic bone disease because there are patterns within the bone that can be associated with various types of metabolic bone disease. The routine radiographs should be assessed to determine the location of the bone loss, that is, focal, regional, or generalized. Patients with focal bone loss may have a localized tumor that is either benign or malignant. Malignant lesions can be primary, originating within the bone, or can metastasize to bone. The majority of tumors that produce bone metastases are lung, thyroid, renal cell, prostate, and breast. Primary malignancies are less common that metastatic disease. Malignancies of the hematopoietic system can also lead to bone lesions and focal radiographic lesions.

Regional bone lesions can result from processes involving an entire extremity, such as bone loss associated with immobilization. This can occur in patients who are placed in a plaster cast for the treatment of a fracture for a prolonged period with restriction of weight bearing. The lack of the weight-bearing stimulus to bone results in the bone becoming diffusely osteopenic. This bone loss can be restored with return to weight bearing. Regional bone loss can also result from processes such as Paget's disease of bone, transient osteoporosis of the hip or reflex sympathetic dystrophy.

Generalized bone loss results from a generalized metabolic process such as osteoporosis or osteomalacia. The assessment of bone loss or bone quality by plain radiography is at best difficult.

The qualitative assessment of bone density with plain radiographs can be obtained by several techniques. In general, osseous structures with a plain radiographic appearance of significantly reduced bone density are referred to as osteopenic. The general impression of reduced bone mass on plain radiography can lead to misleading interpretation. The assessment of cortical thickness and cortical or trabecular bone density is highly subjective and sensitive to changes in radiographic technique. To produce a visible reduction in bone density by plain radiograph, the bone density must be reduced by approximately 50%. However, a fair qualitative assessment can be made in patients who have advanced changes with pronounced cortical thinning, loss of density in the trabecular bone, and loss of the normal endosteal architecture.

The traditional method of qualitatively assessing bone density on plain radiographs was described by Singh (Fig.

11–3). He described an index based on the visualization of the tension and compression trabeculae within the proximal femur and femoral neck. The index went from I to VI, with I having the lowest density and VI demonstrating all the trabeculae normally found within the proximal femur. This index has been found difficult to use because of large interobserver variability. Also, the technique suffers greatly with variation in the technique used to expose the radiographic film.

A second method used to assess bone density is to place aluminum step blocks on the radiographic film next to the osseous structures (Fig. 11–4). The relative bone density can then be compared with the density of the various layers of the aluminum step wedge. This can assist in comparing the technique and relative bone density of two radiographs taken at two different times with the same step wedge. The precision of this technique can be improved by using a quantitative measurement of the "gray scale" brightness of the osseous structure in question. This measurement can then be normalized with the use of the aluminum step wedge. This normalized assessment of the "gray scale" can then be compared with similar measurements from other radiographs taken using the same aluminum step wedges. However, even with the use of uniform wedges,

the assessment of bone density with plain radiographs is essentially a qualitative ranking.

Other techniques are available to obtain a more quantitative assessment of bone density in a non-invasive fashion. Quantitative computed tomography (CT) scans of the lumbar spine were used for a short period. This is similar to the approach with plain radiographs using phantoms of known radiographic density in the same image as the spine (Fig. 11–5). The density of the lumbar vertebral body could then be calculated based on the relative gray scale radiographic density of the phantoms relative to that of the bone. This technique involved significant radiation exposure and expense.

Currently, the most common technique for the assessment of bone density is the dual energy x-ray absorptiometry (DEXA) scan (Fig. 11–6). This technique allows the accurate measurement of the real density of bone in the axial skeletal. Commonly, measurements are made in the lumbar spine and in the intertrochanteric region of the hip. These measurements are then compared with a normal curve with two standard deviations of density indicated (Fig. 11–7). If the patient's bone density is less than two standard deviations from the normal bone density for an age- and sex-matched group, they are considered signifi-

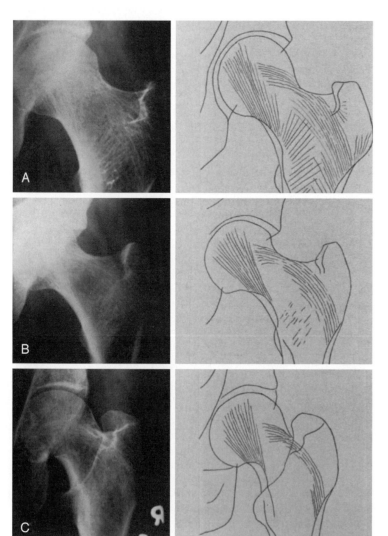

Figure 11–3. Singh's index of osteoporosis. *A*, Grade VI: All the normal trabecular groups are visible and the upper end of the femur seems to be completely occupied by cancellous bone. *B*, Grade V: The structure of principal tensile and principal compressive trabeculae is accentuated. Ward's triangle appears prominent. *C*, Grade VI: Principal tensile trabeculae are markedly reduced but can still be traced from the lateral cortex to the upper part of the femoral neck.

cantly osteopenic and at risk for fracture. These patients should be evaluated for the cause of the osteopenia and treatment instituted to maintain and attempt to increase bone density.

Error in the measurement of bone density with DEXA can occur in patients with extensive calcification in the overlying blood vessels or in patients with significant lumbar degenerative disease or those who have had prior surgery in either the lumbar spine or hip.

BONE HISTOMORPHOMETRY

Bone histomorphometry is a quantitative technique used to analyze undecalcified bone tissue obtained by bone biopsy. This is a powerful tool that can provide a definitive analysis and differentiation between osteoporosis and osteomalacia as the cause of decreased bone density and osteopenia (Fig. 11–8). To maximize the information gained about the bone physiology, the bone needs to be labeled at two time points. This is commonly done with the tetracycline antibiotics, which have two significant advantages. First, they become incorporated into any exposed immature bone. Second, they fluoresce when exposed to ultraviolet light. The label-

ing protocols are usually performed over a 4-week period. The antibiotics are administered for 3 days followed by a 2-week interval after which a second tetracycline antibiotic is administered for 3 days followed by a second 2-week interval after which the biopsy is performed. The biopsy must be done in a specific fashion to allow for the quantification of the bone mass. The iliac wing is sampled in an area that has not been violated by previous surgery or trauma. The specimen is taken approximately 3 to 4 cm posterior to the anterior-superior iliac spine and 3 to 4 cm below the level of the iliac crest. A 7 to 9-mm trephine is used to obtain a solid core of bone. It is essential to obtain both the inner and outer cortices of the iliac wing to allow for the quantification of the bone mass. The specimen should also be transported in 70 to 100% alcohol (not formalin) to maintain the tetracycline staining. The specimen must be labeled with the specific dates the tetracycline antibiotics were administered and the date of the biopsy to allow accurate assessment of the rate of bone metabolism. The specimen is then imbedded in polymethylmethacrylate plastic to allow processing and cutting of the undecalcified tissue. This imbedding process takes approximately 1

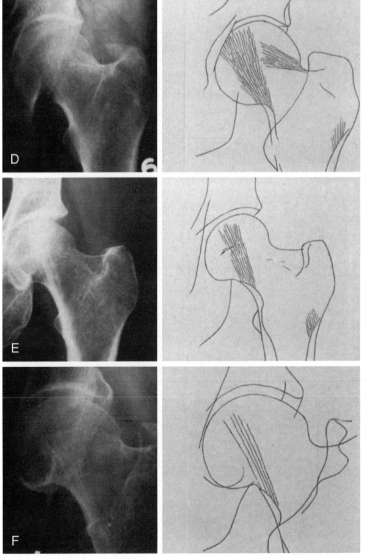

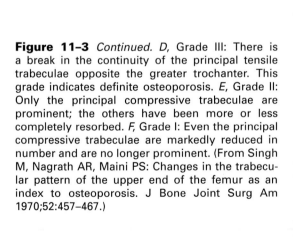

Figure 11–3 *Continued. D,* Grade III: There is a break in the continuity of the principal tensile trabeculae opposite the greater trochanter. This grade indicates definite osteoporosis. *E,* Grade II: Only the principal compressive trabeculae are prominent; the others have been more or less completely resorbed. *F,* Grade I: Even the principal compressive trabeculae are markedly reduced in number and are no longer prominent. (From Singh M, Nagrath AR, Maini PS: Changes in the trabecular pattern of the upper end of the femur as an index to osteoporosis. J Bone Joint Surg Am 1970;52:457–467.)

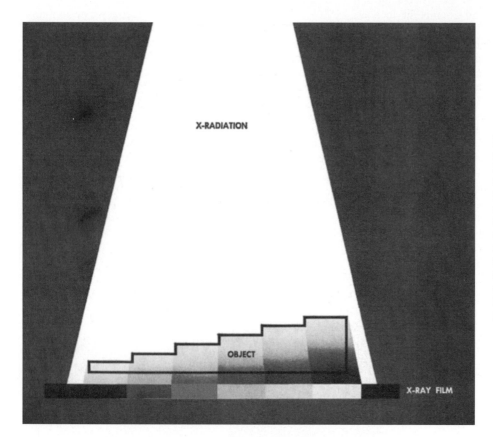

Figure 11–4. If the object is an aluminum step wedge, the thicker the wedge, the greater the absorption of the x-rays and the less exposure of the radiographic film. If the same wedge is used on each film, the radiodensity of the wedge can be used to compare different films taken on different days. (From Squire LF: Fundamentals of Radiology, 3rd ed. Washington, DC: Howard University Press, 1982, p 7.)

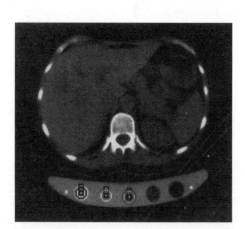 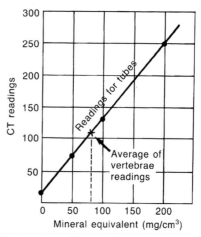

Figure 11–5. Transverse CT scans made through T12, L1, L2, L3, and L4 with phantom included. Computer gives readings for specific areas of each vertebral body and phantom tubes. Readings are averaged CT readings for known mineral values of tubes. Average of readings for vertebrae gives vertebral mineral content in milligrams per centimeter cubed. (From Netter FH: The Ciba Collections of Medical Illustrations. Volume 8: Musculoskeletal System. Part 1: Anatomy, Physiology, and Metabolic Bone Disease. Summit NJ: Ciba Geigy Publications, 1987, p 224.)

k = 1.240 d0 = 121.5(1.000H) 6.213

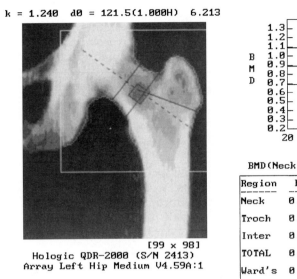

[99 × 98]
Hologic QDR-2000 (S/N 2413)
Array Left Hip Medium V4.59A:1

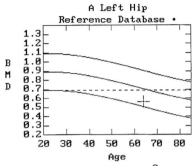

A Left Hip
Reference Database ◆

BMD(Neck[L]) = 0.553 g/cm²

Region	BMD	T		Z	
Neck	0.553	−3.41	62%	−1.52	78%
		(22.0)			
Troch	0.540	−2.02	75%	−0.76	89%
		(30.0)			
Inter	0.820	−2.34	71%	−1.10	84%
		(29.0)			
TOTAL	0.696	−2.32	71%	−1.02	85%
		(28.0)			
Ward's	0.329	−4.25	41%	−1.54	66%
		(20.0)			

◆ Age and sex matched
T = peak bone mass
Z = age matched

Figure 11–6. Dual x-ray absorptiometry (DEXA) bone mineral density measurement in the proximal femur of a postmenopausal woman. The patient's bone density is compared with both the mean young normal bone density and age-matched and gender-matched controls. The T-score and Z-score represent the number of standard deviations below young normal and age-matched controls, respectively. Because the bone density provides a gradient of risk of fracture, therapies may be instituted to prevent the development of osteoporosis or to treat patients at increased risk for a fracture. (Modified from LeBoff MS, El-Hajj Fuleihan G, Brown EM: Osteoporosis and Paget's disease in bone. *In* Branch WT [ed]: Office Practice of Medicine, 3rd ed. Philadelphia: WB Saunders, 1994, pp 700–714. Reprinted from Kelley WN, Harris ED Jr, Ruddy S, Sledge CB: Textbook of Rheumatology, 5th ed, Vol 2. Philadelphia: WB Saunders, 1997, p 1566.)

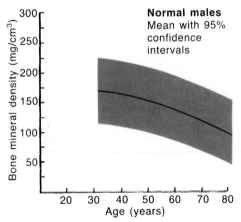

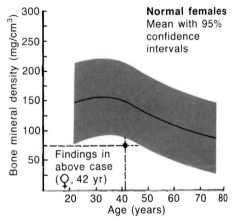

Figure 11–7. Results compared with normal values by age and sex. (From Netter FH: The Ciba Collections of Medical Illustrations. Volume 8: Musculoskeletal System. Part 1: Anatomy, Physiology, and Metabolic Bone Disease. Summit NJ: Ciba Geigy Publications, 1987, p 224.)

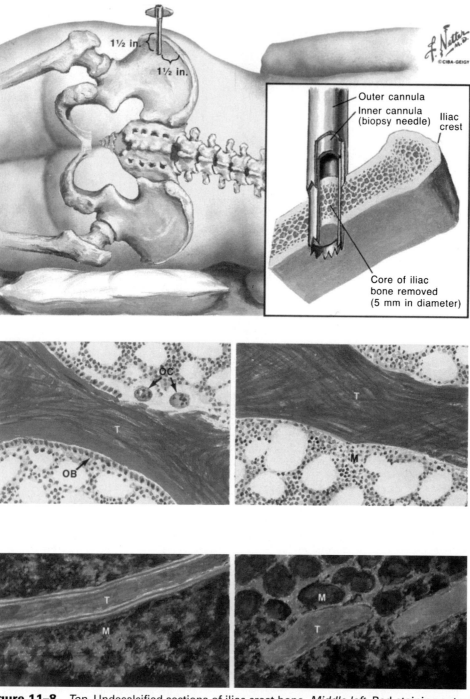

Figure 11–8. *Top*, Undecalcified sections of iliac crest bone. *Middle left*, Red-staining osteoid seams (hypomineralized matrix) lined with osteoblasts (OB). Osteoclasts (OC) in resorption bays (Masson's trichrome). *Middle right*, Section shows few osteoid seams, osteoblasts, or osteoclasts, indicating little bone formation or resorption. *Bottom left*, Yellow lines (tetracycline deposition at mineralization front), seen on fluorescent microscopy after two courses of tetracycline, indicate normal mineralization. *Bottom right*, Absence of tetracycline-labeled lines indicates lack of bone formation. T, trabecular bone; M, marrow. (From Netter FH: The Ciba Collections of Medical Illustrations. Volume 8: Musculoskeletal System. Part 1: Anatomy, Physiology, and Metabolic Bone Disease. Summit NJ: Ciba Geigy Publications, 1987, p 225.)

month and cannot be rushed. In most laboratories, the total time from the specimen's arrival until the result is available is approximately 6 weeks. Bone histomorphometry measures the metabolic activity of the bone sampled in a quantitative fashion. The area of bone resorption (osteoclastic activity) and bone formation (osteoblastic activity) can be measured. The distance between the two lines of the tetracycline labeling can determine the rate of bone formation. Also, the pattern of the label line can be helpful. In normal bone formation, the lines of labeling should be narrow and well defined. In some forms of osteomalacia, the label lines are broad and less distinct, indicating a defect in normal bone formation.

The volume of bone within the specimen expressed relative to the total volume of the specimen can be used as an indicator of osteopenia. In patients with osteoporosis, there is a normal appearance of bone but a reduced volume of bone within the specimen. In patients with osteomalacia, there may be a normal amount of bone or a decrease or, in some circumstances, an increase in the volume of bone. However, the metabolic activity and the patterns of bone formation and resorption will not be normal. Thus, bone histomorphometry can give a great deal of detailed information about the metabolic activity and pattern of bone formation and resorption. However, the underlying disease process involving the bone can frequently be diagnosed by the history, physical examination, and laboratory studies.

HYPERCALCEMIC STATES

Parathyroid bone disease is the prototype condition within the group of hypercalcemic states; it results when there is an elevated level of circulating PTH. Typically, hyperparathyroidism can be either primary or secondary.

Primary Hyperparathyroidism

Primary hyperparathyroidism was originally described by Fuller Albright as "the disease that results from more parathormone being secreted than is necessary for maintenance of normal serum calcium." Primary hyperparathyroidism is a relatively common cause of hypercalcemia, with the incidence suggested to be as high as 1 in 700. It ranks third to diabetes and hyperthyroidism in the listing of endocrine disease. It is caused by a benign solitary *adenoma* in approximately 80% of cases. The adenoma is made up of *chief cells* surrounded by a rim of normal tissue. *Hyperplasia* of the four parathyroid glands accounts for approximately 15 to 20% of primary hyperparathyroidism cases, with *carcinomas* accounting for less than 1%. The pathophysiology of the disease is based on the insensitivity of the parathyroid gland to the extracellular calcium level. Normally, the glands respond to subtle fluctuations in serum calcium. In primary disease, however, the normal feedback loop controlling the secretion of PTH is lost. Hence, PTH continues to be secreted even in the face of hypercalcemia.

Early, the *clinical manifestations* can be somewhat protean. The disease is usually discovered after the finding of asymptomatic hypercalcemia. The patients however, present with severe bone pain or pathologic fractures, that

have occurred through pre-existent brown tumors (described further on). In addition, patients often complain of loss of appetite, nausea, vomiting, and malaise. Ultimately, these patients suffer from renal lithiasis, peptic ulcer disease, and pancreatitis. Hence, many remember this disease using the old cliche, "stones, bones, stomach groans, and psychic moans."

Laboratory studies classically show a fasting hypercalcemia with a compensatory hypophosphatemia. Completing the picture, one finds elevated urine calcium and urine phosphate levels. The alkaline phosphatase level is frequently increased. The measurement of PTH is the most specific way of making this diagnosis. Elevated levels of PTH in the presence of hypercalcemia virtually establishes the diagnosis.

The *radiographic features* of the disease are typical. Unfortunately, they tend to occur late in the course and are florid in only 30 to 40% of patients. Subperiosteal resorption, especially on the radial side of the middle phalanx, and simultaneous resorption of the distal tuft in the hand are typical findings (Fig. 11–9). In addition, one may also see dystrophic calcification of the small vessels in the hand. Resorption of the distal clavicle has been said by many to

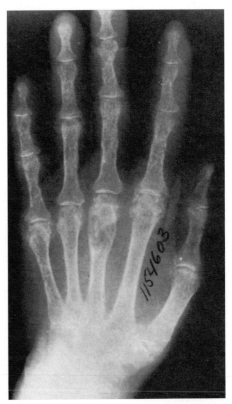

Figure 11–9. Hyperparathyroidism. Radiograph of the hand with extensive subperiosteal resorption of numerous phalanges. Note the fuzzy margin, which reflects subperiosteal bone formation and removal. The cyst-like expansion in the third metacarpal is a brown tumor. Subperiosteal resorption of the phalanges is a classic, easily demonstrable bony manifestation of parathyroid disease. (From Metabolic diseases of bone. *In* Bogumill GP, Schwamm HA [eds]: Orthopaedic Pathology: A Synopsis with Clinical Radiographic Correlation. Philadelphia: WB Saunders, 1984, p 255.)

be pathognomonic of the disease. The trabecular resorption seen within the medullary bone of the skull is referred to as the "salt and pepper skull" (Fig. 11–10).

In the long bones, small resorption cavities that result from the activity of osteoclasts slowly coalesce into larger cystic lesions; these are referred to as *brown tumors*. Within these lesions one can identify accumulations of fibrous tissue and giant cells in addition to the hemosiderin pigment, which stains the tissue brown. These cystic lesions are usually quite apparent on radiographs and may be complicated by a pathologic fracture. In addition, the osteoclasts will dissect within the cortex of a long bone. Pathologically, this is referred to as *dissecting osteitis*. Radiographically, this can be seen as tunneling within the cortex of a long bone (Fig. 11–11).

Histologically, the parathyroid effect is usually obvious. There is evidence of marked bone resorption with an increase in the number of osteoclasts. The osteoclasts are located on many bony trabeculae, either actively resorbing those trabeculae or leaving their footprint (Howship's lacuna) behind as a mark or their activity as they disengage from the trabeculum. The presence of osteoclasts and osteoblasts on the same trabeculum of bone is said to be a histologic hallmark of hyperparathyroidism. It is seen in only two other disease states: hyperthyroidism and Paget's disease. The *dissecting osteitis* (Fig. 11–12) and coalescing osteoclastomas or brown tumors are also apparent histologically. Spindle cells and giant cells are present within these brown tumors.

Obviously, the *management* of primary hyperparathyroidism is surgical. If the cause is an adenoma, excision is appropriate. Typically for hyperplasia, 3½ of the glands are resected. It is important to remember that post-operatively a "hungry bone" syndrome can result in a significant hypocalcemia. As one would expect, there is an intense

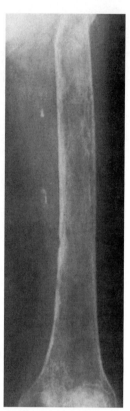

Figure 11–11. Radiograph of femur in patient with severe hyperparathyroidism. Note osteoporosis and cancellization of cortex. The soft tissue calcification is due to arteriosclerotic vasculature; the patient does not have renal disease. (From Metabolic diseases of bone. *In* Bogumill GP, Schwamm HA [eds]: Orthopaedic Pathology: A Synopsis with Clinical Radiographic Correlation. Philadelphia: WB Saunders, 1984, p 255.)

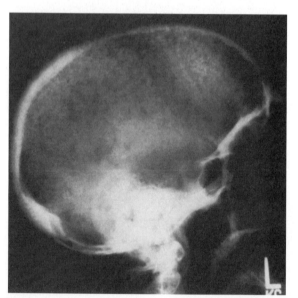

Figure 11–10. Lateral radiograph of "salt and pepper" in the skull of a patient with hyperparathyroidism. (From Metabolic diseases of bone. *In* Bogumill GP, Schwamm HA [eds]: Orthopaedic Pathology: A Synopsis with Clinical Radiographic Correlation. Philadelphia: WB Saunders, 1984, p 256.)

need for calcium and phosphorus by the skeleton; hence, rapid skeletal uptake of these ions can deplete their circulating numbers in the short term.

Secondary Hyperparathyroidism

Although there are multiple causes of secondary hyperparathyroidism, the common denominator is a tendency toward hypocalcemia. In the United States today, the most common cause of secondary hyperparathyroidism is chronic renal failure. Uremia produces hypocalcemia via two mechanisms (Fig. 11–13):

1. Phosphate retention occurring at the renal level results in hyperphosphatemia and hypocalcemia results to maintain the solubility product.
2. The necrosis of the renal parenchyma significantly impairs the activation of vitamin D. The net result is a decrease in calcium absorption at the intestinal level and a resulting hypocalcemia.

This two-pronged hypocalcemic drive dramatically stimulates the parathyroid glands, forcing them to secrete large quantities of PTH. The skeletal effects are essentially the same as those seen in the primary form of the disease. The radiographic effects, however, suggest a more extreme

Figure 11–12. Histologic section of more extensive dissecting osteitis in trabecular bone. Note the adjacent normal marrow, separated from the fibrovascular tissue. (From Metabolic diseases of bone. *In* Bogumill GP, Schwamm HA [eds]: Orthopaedic Pathology: A Synopsis with Clinical Radiographic Correlation. Philadelphia: WB Saunders, 1984, p 249.)

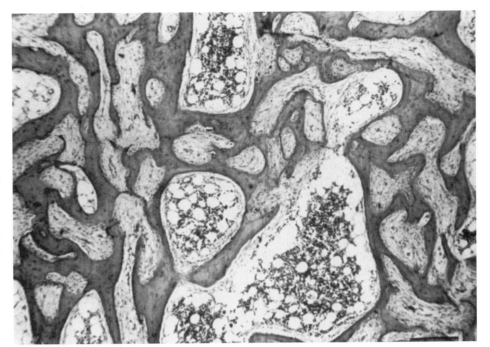

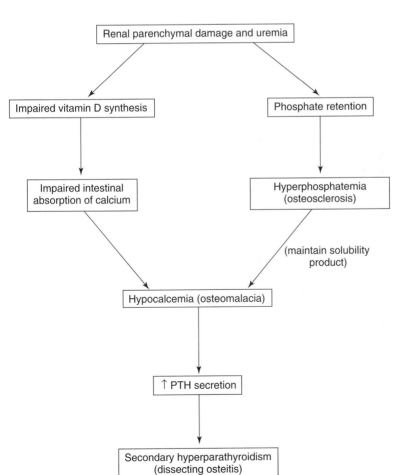

Renal parenchymal damage and uremia

Impaired vitamin D synthesis → Impaired intestinal absorption of calcium

Phosphate retention → Hyperphosphatemia (osteosclerosis)

(maintain solubility product)

Hypocalcemia (osteomalacia)

↑ PTH secretion

Secondary hyperparathyroidism (dissecting osteitis)

Figure 11–13. Progression from renal parenchymal damage and uremia to secondary hyperparathyroidism (dissecting osteitis).

bone resorptive process: larger cystic cavities and more erosive changes are typical in secondary hyperparathyroidism. Histologically, bone resorption is a striking feature. Intense cellular activity and fibrous replacement of the marrow is more pronounced than in primary hyperparathyroidism. In addition to these parathyroid effects, the relative paucity of vitamin D results in a superimposed osteomalacic state.

The bone disease resulting from chronic renal failure is frequently referred to as *renal osteodystrophy*. Since there are multiple metabolic aberrations, the histologic changes seen in the bone are a collage of hyperparathyroidism, osteomalacia, and osteosclerosis.

The cause of the hyperparathyroid changes has already been discussed. The osteomalacic changes result from the low levels of active vitamin D. The subsequent mineralization defect is manifested histologically by the finding of large areas of unmineralized matrix on the trabeculae (osteoid seams). The osteosclerosis is usually attributed to the hyperphosphatemia that results from renal retention of phosphate.

Other conditions that have been reported to cause a hyperparathyroid state include sarcoidosis, multiple endocrine neoplasia, and the hypercalcemia of malignancy.

Tertiary Hyperparathyroidism

Tertiary hyperparathyroidism follows the correction of a renal defect (i.e., transplantation). Patients may manifest so-called pseudoadenomatous functioning of the parathyroid glands. It is thought that the chronic stimulation of the parathyroids, in the absence of renal function, results in an altered setting of the "calcistat." Hence, the glands are more sensitive to minimal changes in serum calcium levels. In these patients, correction of the renal abnormality is not adequate to reset this mechanism. Thus, the parathyroids continue to secrete high levels of PTH even in the face of relative normocalcemia. This, in turn, causes ongoing skeletal disruption.

Hypoparathyroidism

Hypoparathyroidism is primarily iatrogenic. It has been estimated that hypoparathyroidism can complicate as many as 50% of thyroidectomies. Biochemically, these patients are mildly hypocalcemic and hyperphosphatemic. The latter results from the lack of a PTH effect on the kidney; calcium is lost and phosphate is retained. Despite these chemical abnormalities, most patients are asymptomatic. Diagnosis depends on identifying the excessive response to an exogenous dose of PTH. This typically results in a dramatic increase in urinary phosphate excretion and urinary cyclic adenosine monophosphate (cAMP) excretion. Histologically, it is noted that bone resorption decreases as expected in the face of less PTH; it is matched by a decrease in bone formation. The resulting net effect is a minimal change in bone mass.

Pseudohypoparathyroidism

Pseudohypoparathyroidism is a congenital condition or *resistance syndrome*, as it has often been called. It is charac-

terized by hypocalcemia and hyperphosphatemia. In addition, elevated levels of PTH can be measured, and anatomically the parathyroid glands are enlarged. All of this is caused by a peripheral nonresponsiveness to the biologic effects of PTH. Hence, the excessive PTH excretion and hyperplasia of the parathyroid glands, which characterize hypoparathyroidism, result from an effort to effect a peripheral response by gland overactivity. Fuller Albright actually demonstrated this lack of response to an administered dose of parathyroid extract. He suggested that this was not a deficiency of PTH but rather a resistance of the target organs, specifically bone and kidney, to the effects of the hormone.

It is well known that PTH activates its target cells (kidney and bone) by increasing cellular levels of cAMP. The latter is often referred to as the *second messenger*. This second messenger, in turn, activates a protein cascade, bringing about a physiologic effect. In this syndrome, there is a defect in the enzyme complex that synthesizes cAMP. Although PTH binds to the cell, it fails to produce the anticipated effect because of the lack of a second messenger.

Affected patients classically have a short stature and often are characterized by shortened metacarpals and metatarsals (commonly the fourth). Mental retardation is present but mild.

The term *pseudo pseudo-hypoparathyroidism* is rarely used any more but refers to the patient who has a PTH resistance syndrome without abnormal biochemistry. Hence, the phenotypic appearance is the same in the face of normal calcium and phosphorus levels.

EUCALCEMIC STATES

Osteoporosis

Osteoporosis is a clinical condition that results from a reduction in bone density with normal histological appearance. This is the most common form of bone disease in the elderly. Osteoporosis is diagnosed in patients with a reduction of bone mass below two standard deviations of the mean bone mass of a normal age- and sex-matched control group. The bone physiology is normal on bone histomorphometry. There is simply less volume of bone present. The reduction in the volume of bone tissue also leads to structural weakness and an increased risk of fracture. As the weight-bearing long bones age, the form of the bone changes. The cortex becomes thinner and the outside diameter of the bone increases. In addition, the cortical bone that is present is more porous than that in the young adult.

In the normal coupled physiology of bone formation and resorption, there is a constant remodeling of bone. In normal children and young adults, the amount of bone deposited exceeds the amount of bone reabsorbed. This pattern continues until approximately the age of 35 years. At that point, most patients have achieved their peak bone mass. For a short period the rate of deposition equals the rate of resorption. After the age of 40 years in most patients, the rate of bone resorption exceeds the rate of bone formation. This results in a gradual reduction in the bone mass. This reduction in bone formation results in type II or age-related osteoporosis.

A person's peak bone mass is determined by several factors. Significant osteoporosis is more commonly noted in people of northern European descent compared with those of African descent. Also, if there is a strong family history of osteoporosis, the patient is at risk for significant bone loss. Genetic disorders such as osteogenesis imperfecta and homocystinuria also result in osteoporosis.

Diet and activity also play a significant role in the determination of a patient's peak bone mass. Patients with a diet that is deficient in calcium, protein, and vitamin C will not optimize their peak bone mass and are at risk for the development of osteoporosis. Chronic alcoholism results in reduced intestinal absorption of calcium and these patients also usually have a poor diet. Young adults (more commonly women) may suffer from anorexia nervosa and bulimia, which may prevent them from obtaining adequate dietary intake of nutrients for bone formation, resulting in a reduction in bone mass.

Certain medications will also affect the bone mass and bone formation. Generally, medications that affect bone mass are taken for years, resulting in a cumulative effect on bone. Methotrexate, a folic acid inhibitor, is given to patients with rheumatoid arthritis as a disease-modifying agent. This medication can inhibit calcium absorption in the bowel by causing atrophy of the intestinal mucosa. Glucocorticoids result in a significant reduction in bone mass if used chronically. These medications affect bone in several ways. They cause the intestinal mucosa to atrophy.

This, in turn, impairs the ability of the gut to absorb calcium. In addition, there is a direct negative effect on the bone, impairing bone formation. The combination of these two factors leads to a reduction in bone mass.

Activity level also has a role to play in increasing the bone mass. Bone mass responds to weight-bearing forces. Patients put to bedrest commonly lose bone mass and demonstrate an increased rate of calcium excretion. Patients who have significant metabolic disease or musculoskeletal disease that significantly impairs mobility lose bone mass. Patients with rheumatoid arthritis, for example, undergo an extensive assault on their bone mass. The arthritis limits their activity and they are commonly treated with glucocorticoids and methotrexate, both of which can cause a reduction in bone mass.

Conversely, patients who increase their activity demonstrate bone remodeling and an increase in bone mass. An example of this would be the metatarsal stress fracture in a new military recruit. These patients experience a dramatic increase in activity. The bone responds to this activity. To increase the bone mass, the bone undergoes remodeling. First, bone is removed and then new stronger bone is deposited. The bones therefore go through a period of weakening prior to growing stronger. It is in the weakened state that the bone fails and a stress fracture occurs. However, for the majority of bones that do not fracture, the bone becomes stronger and increases in mass.

The most common form of osteoporosis is involutional (Table 11–1), type I, postmenopausal osteoporosis. The latter is related to a significant reduction in the level of

Table 11–1. Involutional Osteoporosis

	Postmenopausal (Type I)	Age-Related (Type II)
Epidemiologic Factors		
Age	55 to 75	>70 (F); > 80 (M)
Sex ratio (F/M)	6:1	2:1
Bone Physiology or Metabolism		
Pathogenesis of uncoupling	Increased osteoclast activity ↑ resorption	Decreased osteoblast activity ↓ formation
Net bone loss	Mainly trabecular	Cortical and trabecular
Rate of bone loss	Rapid/short duration	Slow/long duration
Bone density	>2 standard deviations below normal	Low normal (adjusted for age and sex)
Clinical Signs		
Fracture sites	Vertebrae (crush), distal forearm, hip (intracapsular)	Vertebrae (multiple wedge), proximal humerus and tibia, hip (extracapsular)
Other signs	Tooth loss	Dorsal kyphosis
Laboratory Values		
Serum Ca^{2+}	Normal	Normal
Serum P_i	Normal	Normal
Alkaline phosphatase	Normal (↑ with fracture)	Normal (↑ with fracture)
Urine Ca^{2+}	Increased	Normal
PTH function	Decreased	Increased
Renal conversion of 25(OH)D to 1,25(OH)$_2$D	Secondary decrease due to ↓ PTH	Primary decrease due to decreased responsiveness of 1-α-OH$_{ase}$
Gastrointestinal calcium absorption	Decreased	Decreased
Prevention		
High-risk patients	Estrogen or calcitonin supplementation Calcium supplementation Adequate vitamin D Adequate weight-bearing activity Minimization of associated risk factors	Calcium supplementation Adequate vitamin D Adequate weight-bearing activity Minimization of associated risk factors

circulating gonadal hormones. It is noted in patients between the ages of 55 and 75 years. The reduction can occur as a result of age-related changes in the production of these hormones or surgical removal of the ovaries. This removes the negative effect of estrogen on osteoclasts and there is rapid bone resorption in the perimenopausal period. This continues for approximately 5 to 10 years. The rate of bone loss then slows and approximates the rate of age-related bone loss. However, because of the accelerated bone loss in the early perimenopausal period, patients have a significantly reduced bone mass compared with those who do not have this accelerated bone loss. Type I osteoporosis is far more common in females than in males (6:1, F:M). This can be reduced by the use of hormone supplementation in the perimenopausal period. However, if the hormone supplementation is discontinued in the future, the rapid bone loss will occur at that time.

Type II osteoporosis is age-related osteoporosis. It reflects the age-related decrease in osteoblast activity and is found in patients older than 70 years. This results in a gradual bone loss over years. It is also more common in females than in males (2:1, F:M). This results in a decrease in bone mass. At a bone mass of two standard deviations below normal, the patient is considered to have osteoporosis. However, treatment to prevent osteoporosis or minimize bone loss should be instituted prior to that point if the condition is identified.

In both type I and type II osteoporosis the calcium, phosphate, and alkaline phosphatase levels are normal. The serum PTH level may be slightly increased in type I and slightly decreased in type II osteoporosis. In type I osteoporosis, there can be an increase in the urinary excretion of calcium during the period of rapid bone loss.

These patients are usually diagnosed with normal laboratory test results, as noted previously, and a decrease in bone mass noted on a DEXA scan. However, in some cases, the laboratory test results may be slightly abnormal or the level of bone loss may be severe. In these cases, bone histomorphometry may be helpful. In type I and type II osteoporosis, the bone histomorphometry is essentially normal except for a decrease in the volume of bone present within the specimen.

Osteoporosis and the resulting decrease in bone density are also affected by a variety of endocrine conditions. The most common endocrine abnormality is hypogonadism, which results in type II osteoporosis. Other endocrine abnormalities can also result in a reduction in bone mass. Hyperthyroidism can result in an increased rate of bone turnover, with resorption exceeding formation. Over time, this results in a net decrease in bone mass. This can also result from excessive replacement therapy for patients with hypothyroidism or after thyroidectomy. Hyperadrenalism or Cushing's disease results in a chronic excess of glucocorticoids, leading to decreased calcium absorption from the gut, which causes an increase in the serum PTH to maintain the serum calcium levels. The released PTH restores the calcium level by quickly mobilizing calcium from bone. Over time, this results in a significant loss of bone.

Osteoporosis can be detected by screening medical evaluation and with the use of a bone density evaluation. However, the most common clinical presentation of osteoporosis is a fracture. The most common areas for fracture are the proximal femur, distal radius, proximal humerus, and the lumbar or thoracic vertebral bodies. These fractures usually occur as a result of low-energy trauma. The plain radiographs can show a variable degree of comminution, but the bone density is usually noted to be significantly decreased. Fractures through osteoporotic bone heal in about the same length of time as do fractures in patients without osteoporosis. However, a patient with one fracture due to osteoporosis is at risk to develop other fractures. Therefore, attempts should be made to treat these patients and to attempt to reduce their risk for falls and fractures in the future.

The most common mechanism for fracture in the osteoporotic population is a simple fall. The risk for falls is increased in the elderly because of their slow reaction times, reduced visual acuity, weakness due to reduced activity level, and possible motor or sensory neurologic deficits due to medical problems such as diabetes or cerebrovascular accident. Altering the patient's environment can minimize falls. Removal of area rugs and cluttered furniture can remove sources of tripping. Patients can maintain balance and optimize muscle reaction time with a regular low-impact exercise program.

TREATMENT OF OSTEOPOROSIS

The treatment of osteoporosis involves a combination of supplements, prescription medications, and changes in activity level and lifestyle. The most important first steps in the treatment and prevention of osteoporosis is to increase or maintain an exercise program with weight-bearing exercise, such as walking, racquet sports, golf (without a cart), or walking on a treadmill. These activities expose the osseous structures of the spine and lower extremities to the stress of resisting gravity, and the bones are stimulated to maintain and possibly increase the bone mass. Patients who are sedentary either because of medical conditions or by choice are at a significantly increased risk for the development or exacerbation of osteoporosis.

In addition to changes in activity, there are changes to the diet and dietary supplements that can be helpful in maintaining bone mass. A daily intake of 1000 to 1500 mg of elemental calcium per day should be consumed. This can be accomplished with approximately five to six glasses of milk per day or with use of over-the-counter calcium supplements. Calcium should also be taken with vitamin D, particularly for patients who cannot tolerate dairy products or who are not exposed to sunlight. The recommended dose is not to exceed 800 IU of vitamin D per day. It is important to remember that the active form of vitamin D is 1,25, dihydroxyvitamin D, which is formed by controlled enzymatic reactions in the liver and kidney. Patients with impairment in vitamin D metabolism may require treatment with parenterally administered 1,25-dihydroxyvitamin D. Excessive vitamin D intake can result in hypercalcemia and hypercalciuria and a reduction in bone mass.

Estrogen and Hormone Replacement Therapy: Hormone supplementation has many effects for the postmenopausal woman, not the least of which are the effects on bone. The reduction in estrogen that occurs in the perimenopausal period results in a release of the inhibition in osteoclast function. This release results in a period of rapid bone loss, which continues for 5 to 10 years after menopause. Supplementation with estrogen in the early menopausal period can preserve bone mass. However, this supplementation needs to continue long term for the beneficial effects on the bone to be preserved. If the hormone replacement therapy is discontinued, the period of rapid bone loss will begin at the time the replacement therapy is discontinued. Hormone replacement should include both estrogen and progesterone for patients who have not had a hysterectomy. Estrogen can be used alone for patients who have had a hysterectomy.

The use of estrogen has been shown to maintain bone mass and reduce the rate of both vertebral and hip fractures. In addition to the bone effects, estrogen has been shown to reduce the incidence of coronary artery disease and relieve some of the symptoms of menopause such as hot flashes and genitourinary tract atrophy. However, estrogen use has also been associated with an increased risk of endometrial cancer and breast cancer. In fact, the use of estrogen replacement therapy increases the risk of breast cancer by as much as 30%. This factor has led many women away from hormone replacement therapy in the postmenopausal period.

Tamoxifen and several of the other antiestrogenic agents have been found to be effective at maintaining bone mass and do not appear to increase the rate of breast cancer. Tamoxifen, in fact, has been used in the treatment of patients with breast cancer. Recent studies have demonstrated that this medication will also have a beneficial effect in maintaining skeletal mass. Tamoxifen appears to be 70% as effective as estrogen. However, tamoxifen also increases the risk of uterine cancer and therefore continues to have limitations in its usefulness. Several new selective estrogen-receptor agents are in clinical trials and may have a role to play in maintaining bone mass—hopefully without an increased risk of endometrial, uterine, or breast carcinoma.

Calcitonin: Calcitonin is a peptide hormone that acts on osteoclasts. The hormone provides an inhibitory effect, reducing the number and activity of osteoclasts. Calcitonin has been isolated from several species. However, salmon calcitonin is the most commonly used. Calcitonin can be administered subcutaneously, rectally, or via nasal spray. Calcitonin inhibits osteoclast activity, which should result in stabilized bone mass. It has been shown to be effective at reducing the rate of vertebral fractures. However, it does not appear to have any benefit for reducing hip fractures. The long-term use of the medication has not been well studied. Salmon calcitonin can become antigenic, with up to 22% of patients developing resistance to the medication over time. It has been shown to have an analgesic effect, which can be beneficial in the early period after a vertebral fracture. Few data exist to demonstrate any beneficial effect for the reduction in hip fractures.

Bisphosphonates: Bisphosphonates are analogs of pyrophosphate and are effective through their ability to bind to the surface of hydroxyapatite crystals. This binding inhibits bone resorption and bone formation. Etidronate, an early bisphosphonate, had a significant effect on the inhibition of both formation and resorption of bone. New bisphosphonates have separated the inhibition of bone formation and resorption so that the effect on bone resorption is 1000 times as effective as the inhibition of bone formation at normal therapeutic doses. These new agents appear to have a significant beneficial effect on bone mass. An additional concern with these medications is their effect on fracture healing. The process of fracture healing and the maturation of bone callus involves both bone formation and bone resorption. A similar process is bone ingrowth into a porous surface to obtain fixation of a joint replacement implant. The effect on human fracture healing or bone ingrowth has not yet been delineated. Without data, it should be recommended that the therapy be discontinued during the period of fracture healing or in the early period after the use of a porous ingrowth joint replacement implant. Alendronate, a new form of a bisphosphonate, has been shown to reproducibly maintain, and in some cases increase, the bone mass of osteoporotic patients. The recommended dose is 10 mg per day. However, a dose of 5 mg per day has been found to have 85% of the efficacy of the full dose. Therefore, for patients with a greater than two standard deviations from normal decrease in bone mass, a dose of 10 mg per day is recommended. For patients who have a risk for osteoporosis between one and two standard deviations of normal, a dose of 5 mg per day is appropriate. Alendronate has been found to have a beneficial effect at reducing the rate of fractures and stabilizing the bone mass.

The common side effects with the medication are gastrointestinal: dyspepsia, nausea, and diarrhea. Patients also report bone pain with therapy. This effect can be minimized with the administration of calcium. However, the calcium and alendronate should be given at different times because the calcium inhibits the absorption of the alendronate if administered simultaneously.

The drug has a long (10-year) half-life in bone. Therefore, it is not recommended for use in children or women of childbearing age. An additional effect of the long skeletal half-life is that there have been some regimens of 10 mg every other day that appear to be at least as effective as 5 mg daily. Also, the period of rapid bone loss is not noted after cessation of alendronate, as is seen with estrogen. However, the long-term effects of this medication are not known as yet.

The current treatment alternatives center on the use of calcium, vitamin D, and weight-bearing exercise for the prevention and treatment of osteoporosis. In addition, there may be a role for the use of a new-generation bisphosphonate such as alendronate. For patients with a painful thoracic or lumbar compression fracture, there is a role for calcitonin, both for its effects on bone mass and as an analgesic.

HYPOCALCEMIC STATES

The history of rickets and osteomalacia dates back to the 1600s, when Whistler was credited with one of the initial descriptions of this disorder. Subsequently in the late eighteenth century, it was recognized that a substance, cod liver oil, could prevent many of the symptoms of rickets. In the early twentieth century, Schmorl and others recognized a relationship between rickets and sunlight. It was in 1924 that McCollum and his associates were able to identify vitamin D as the protective factor against rickets and osteomalacia. Further studies by Albright in the 1930s described additional forms of vitamin D deficiency, specifically the so-called resistant forms.

Rickets

The *pathogenesis* of rickets and osteomalacia is based on a paucity of calcium. Normal levels of calcium and phosphate are required for normal mineralization of the skeleton. Hence, any pathologic state that results in hypocalcemia or hypophosphatemia will significantly disrupt these normal mineralization pathways. Adequate levels of activated vitamin D are required to maintain normal calcium homeostasis. In vitamin D deficiency syndromes there is inadequate calcium available for normal skeletal mineralization. Hence, rachitic syndromes can result from virtually any cause of vitamin D deficiency.

The classic cause of rickets is, of course, dietary vitamin D deficiency. In the United States today it is extremely rare to see children with rickets from dietary deficiency. The fortification of milk with vitamin D has all but eradicated deficiency rickets in the United States. Unfortunately, in developing countries or in cultures whose traditions do not permit sunlight to activate vitamin D in the skin, deficiency syndromes are more commonly seen.

Other causes of vitamin D deficiency include malabsorption states, renal tubular and renal glomerular disease, chronic hepatic disease, as well as a number of rare inborn errors of metabolism.

The *clinical manifestations* of rickets vary with the age of the individual at onset as well as the severity of the vitamin D deficiency. The clinical features, however, are generally considered to be stereotypic and therefore do not allow one to differentiate one form of rachitic syndrome from another. Deficiency rickets, malabsorptive rickets, and renal rickets can all look the same. Children with these conditions generally are apathetic and irritable. They show a certain degree of muscular weakness and ligamentous laxity. They typically are found to be in the first or second percentile in height and the twentieth to thirtieth percentile in weight. The skull in these children is said to be characteristic, demonstrating the manifestation of *craniotabes*. This phenomenon is due to a certain degree of calvarial softening and frontal bossing. As one might expect, dental defects occur because adequate levels of calcium and vitamin D are essential for normal dentinogenesis.

The thorax tends to be somewhat constricted in these children, and there are bulbous enlargements at the costochondral junctions anteriorly, giving the child the classic *rachitic rosary*. As a consequence of the thoracic constriction and the pectus carinatum, there is usually a prominent abdomen (rachitic potbelly) noted. The appendicular skeleton is characterized by enlarged joints, frequently associated with bowing of the extremity. The incidence of pathologic fractures is said to be increased.

Histologically, rickets manifests most characteristically in the physis. In fact physeal changes are said to be pathognomonic. Calcium is typically incorporated at the level of the zone of provisional calcification. Because of the lack of calcium, the zone of provisional calcification is all but absent, causing significant distortion of the zone of hypertrophy above it (Fig. 11–14). Within the zone of hypertrophy, the cells become enormous, and their normal regular arrangement becomes grossly distorted. As one might expect, this distortion can also alter the architecture within the other zones of the plate. Below the zone of provisional calcification, where orderly primary spongiosa bone is typically seen, similar disorganization results. The bony trabeculae, which are laid down on the cartilage bars in the zone of primary spongiosa, are rudimentary at best in rickets (Fig. 11–15).

The long bones are osteopenic with prominent cortical thinning, and a marked decrease in the amount of medullary trabecular bone is seen. Perhaps the classic histologic finding is the presence of *unmineralized osteoid* on the trabeculae of bone. The paucity of calcium makes normal mineralization of the matrix impossible; hence, the unmineralized matrix or osteoid will be obvious in areas where bone is to be made. Normally the *osteoid seam* (Fig. 11–16) adjacent to a trabeculum is less than 15 μm. In rachitic syndromes, the width can be doubled or tripled.

The *radiographic manifestations* simply mirror these histologic changes (Fig. 11–17). The cortices of the long bones are thin and the trabeculae are indistinct. Osteopenia is the hallmark of rickets in the child. Since there is no zone of provisional calcification with the resultant "pile-up" of hypertrophic zone cells, the axial height of the

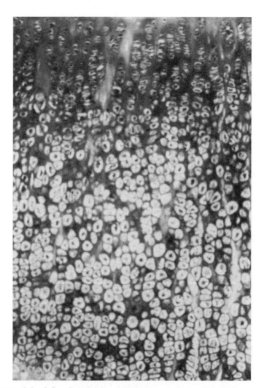

Figure 11–14. Rachitic epiphyseal plate. Resting and proliferative zones are normal. There is widening of the hypertrophic zone with loss of normal columnar arrangement of chondrocytes. The zone of provisional calcification is inadequately calcified, and vascular invasion is irregular. The zone of primary spongiosa is not shown. (From Doppelt SH: Vitamin D, rickets, and osteomalacia. Orthop Clin North Am 1984, 15:678.)

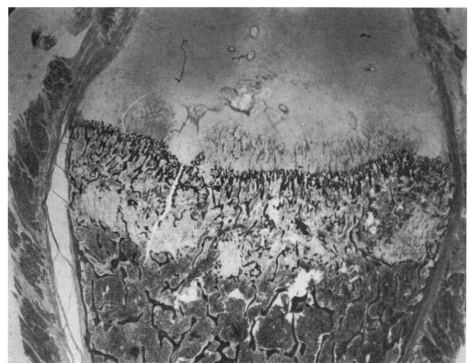

Figure 11–15. Macrosection of rachitic rib responding to therapy. The line of cartilage bars in the zone of provisional calcification exhibits extensive calcification. Note the large masses of cartilage that were formed earlier. They have not matured and persist between the growth plate and bone formed before the onset of rickets. (From Metabolic diseases of bone. *In* Bogumill GP, Schwamm HA [eds]: Orthopaedic Pathology: A Synopsis with Clinical Radiographic Correlation. Philadelphia: WB Saunders, 1984, p 259.)

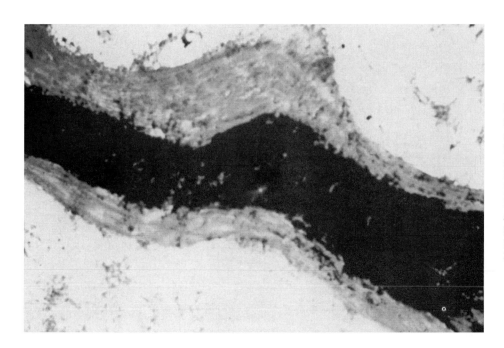

Figure 11–16. Osteomalacia. Section of undecalcified trabecula exhibiting a central mineralized portion and a large unmineralized osteoid seam. (From Metabolic diseases of bone. *In* Bogumill GP, Schwamm HA [eds]: Orthopaedic Pathology: A Synopsis with Clinical Radiographic Correlation. Philadelphia: WB Saunders, 1984, p 263.)

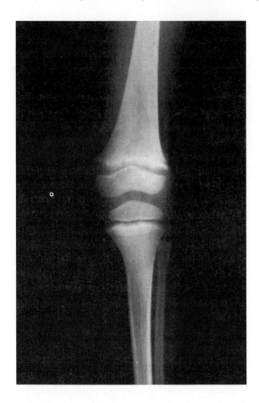

Figure 11–17. Anteroposterior radiograph of the knee of a child with rickets. There is generalized osteopenia. The epiphyseal plates are increased in height. There is increased metaphyseal flaring of the distal femur and proximal tibia. There is also some cupping of the metaphysis, seen best here at the distal femur. (From Doppelt SH: Vitamin D, rickets, and osteomalacia. Orthop Clin North Am 1984, 15:679.)

physis is increased. Similarly, the classic *cupping* or *trumpeting* of the metaphysis is noted to occur from the stunting of the plate growth centrally while normal peripheral appositional growth of the perichondral ring continues. It should be remembered that, above all, rickets is a disease of growth. If, for whatever reason, growth slows down or stops, the radiographic changes will "appear" to improve. This phenomenon has been referred to as the "paradox of rickets." Deformities in the extremities result from soften-

ing of the bones, alterations in long bone growth, and the application of eccentric load. Genu varum in the lower extremities is perhaps the most typical of the angular deformities associated with rickets.

The *biochemical changes* (Table 11–2) typical of deficiency rickets include low or low-normal calcium levels as well as hypophosphatemia and elevated levels of alkaline phosphatase. The urine calcium level is similarly decreased.

Table 11–2. Chemical Abnormalities in Metabolic Bone Disease

	Ca	P	Alk P	iPTH	25(OH)D	1,25(OH)$_2$D	UCa	T$_m$P/GFR	U Hpro
Osteoporosis									
Postmenopausal	nl	nl	nl	nl	nl	nl	nl	nl	nl
Hyperthyroidism	nl, ↑	nl	nl, ↑	nl, ↓	nl	nl, ↓	nl, ↑	nl, ↑	nl, ↑
Hypercortisolism	nl	nl	nl	nl, ↑	nl	nl, ↑	nl, ↑	nl, ↓	nl
Malignancy									
Bone metastases, MM	nl, ↑	nl	nl, ↑	nl, ↓	nl	nl, ↓	↑	nl, ↑	nl
Humoral syndrome	↑	nl, ↓	nl	nl, ↓	nl	nl, ↓	↑	↓	nl
Immobilization	nl, ↑	nl	nl	nl, ↓	nl	nl, ↓	nl, ↑	nl, ↑	nl
Osteomalacia									
Vitamin D deficiency	nl, ↓	↓	↑	↑	↓	nl, ↑, ↓	↓	↓	nl
VDDR, type I	nl, ↓	↓	↑	nl, ↑	nl	↓	nl, ↓	nl, ↓	nl
VDDR, type II	nl, ↓	↓	↑	nl, ↑	nl	nl, ↑	nl, ↓	nl, ↓	nl
VDRR	nl	↓	↑	nl	nl	nl, ↓	nl	↓	nl
Oncogenic	nl	↓	↑	nl	nl	nl, ↓	nl	↓	nl
Osteitis Fibrosa Cystica									
Primary hyperparathyroidism	↑	↓	nl, ↑	↑	nl	nl, ↑	nl, ↑	↓	nl, ↑
Renal insufficiency	nl, ↓	↑	nl, ↑	↑	nl	↓	nl	↓	nl
Paget's Disease	nl	nl	↑	nl	nl	nl	nl, ↑	nl	↑

Ca = serum calcium; P = fasting serum phosphorus; Alk P = serum alkaline phosphatase; iPTH = serum immunoreactive parathormone level; 25(OH)D = serum 25-hydroxyvitamin D level; 1,25(OH)$_2$D = serum 1,25-dihydroxyvitamin D level; UCa = 24-hour urine calcium; T$_m$P/GFR = renal phosphate threshold; U Hpro = 24-hour urine hydroxyproline; MM = multiple myeloma; VDDR = vitamin D-dependent rickets; VDRR = vitamin D–resistant rickets; nl = within normal limits.
From Burtis W, Lang R: Chemical abnormalities. Orthop Clin North Am 1984, 15(4):653.

Again, it should be kept in mind that the specific cause of the histologic and radiographic findings is often not readily apparent. These manifestations reflect the hypocalcemic state and are not indicative of a specific cause.

Osteomalacia

Essentially, osteomalacia is the rachitic syndrome of adults. The growth plates being closed preclude changes within those structures. However, vitamin D deficiency in the adult certainly produces a mineralization defect. This defect in the adult is characterized by the finding of multiple fractures, spinal kyphosis, generalized osteopenia, generalized bone pain, and the unique finding of *pseudofractures* (Looser's zones). These painless pseudofractures represent areas of unmineralized osteoid that have accumulated in several unique locations within the skeleton. They are pathognomonic of the disease. Always symmetrical, they are located on the concave side of long bones, the axillary border of the scapula, the inferior pubic ramus, the ribs, the femoral neck, and occasionally in the subtrochanteric region (Fig. 11–18). These pseudofractures have the potential to become real fractures with the application of persistent load. As one would expect, the bones that are especially at risk are the femoral neck and subtrochanteric region of the proximal femur.

In the United States, dietary causes of osteomalacia are certainly more prevalent than they are for rickets. Elderly women who place themselves on restricted diets frequently can convert a pre-existent osteoporosis into a florid osteomalacia by depriving themselves of adequate calcium intake. It is generally believed that the vast majority of osteomalacic syndromes are in fact superimposed on pre-existing osteoporosis. Most patients with osteomalacia manifest hypocalcemia and hypophosphatemia. In addition, there is usually an elevated alkaline phosphatase level. Although the clinical manifestations tend to be subtle, careful evaluation of the osteoporotic patient will frequently uncover an unexpected osteomalacia. Iliac crest biopsy will confirm the diagnosis of osteomalacia in the vast majority of these patients. As with rickets, the finding of *widened osteoid seams* is the diagnostic histologic appearance.

Renal Disease

ACQUIRED RENAL GLOMERULAR DISEASE (HYPERPHOSPHATEMIC RICKETS)

A number of acquired diseases damage the renal parenchyma and glomerulus. As a result, there is an inability to filter phosphate, and the patient becomes *hyperphosphatemic*. In addition, the damage to the renal parenchyma dramatically alters the patient's ability to synthesize vitamin D. The net effect of this renal parenchymal damage is a severe depression in serum calcium levels. As discussed previously in the section on hypercalcemic states, this will result in a secondary hyperparathyroidism, with all of its associated effects (see Fig. 11–7). In addition, the depression of vitamin D synthesis produces a mineralization defect and a secondary osteomalacic state. The third unique finding in *renal osteodystrophy* is the hyperphosphatemia that somewhat idiosyncratically causes metastatic calcification in numerous tissues. In the skeleton, osteosclerosis results from the hyperphosphatemia. In summary, renal glomerular disease results in the syndrome referred to as renal osteodystrophy. The bone changes mirror the multiple metabolic abnormalities (Fig. 11–19):

1. *Decreased vitamin D* produces an osteomalacic state with widened osteoid seams.
2. *Hyperphosphatemia* causes hypocalcemia and osteosclerosis.
3. *Hypocalcemia* causes a secondary hyperparathyroidism with dissecting osteitis and bone resorption (Fig. 11–20).

RENAL TUBULAR DISEASE (HYPOPHOSPHATEMIC RICKETS)

Abnormalities at the renal tubular level are generally the result of inborn errors of vitamin D metabolism. These hereditary defects result in a rachitic syndrome. Although a number of defects have been identified, only a few are reviewed here.

Hypophosphatemic Vitamin D–Resistant Rickets (VDRR): This syndrome was first described by Fuller Albright. At that time, it was recognized as an inborn error of vitamin D metabolism associated with an X-linked dominant trait. Advances in molecular biology have localized the mutant

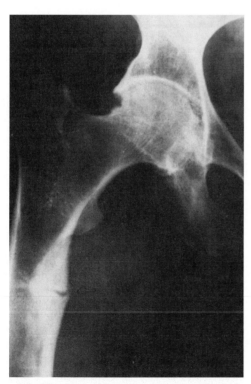

Figure 11–18. Pseudofracture of subtrochanteric region of the femur *(arrow)*. It appears as a ribbon-like radiolucency on the concave side of the femur, extending through one cortex and part of the medullary canal. There is some adjacent sclerosis but no periosteal new bone formation. (From Doppelt SH: Vitamin D, rickets, and osteomalacia. Orthop Clin North Am 1984, 15[4]:681.)

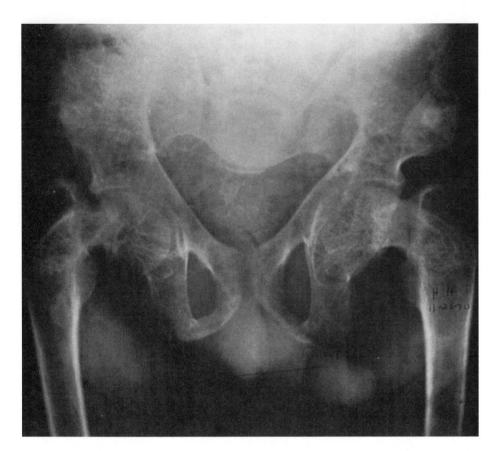

Figure 11–19. Radiograph of patient with long-standing renal osteodystrophy. Marked osteoporosis due to secondary hyperparathyroidism is evident. There is bowing of the proximal femurs, marked lordosis, and pelvic tilt. The deformity of the pelvis is commonly seen in osteomalacia, but it does not usually occur in primary hyperparathyroidism. (From Metabolic diseases of bone. *In* Bogumill GP, Schwamm HA [eds]: Orthopaedic Pathology: A Synopsis with Clinical Radiographic Correlation. Philadelphia: WB Saunders, 1984, p 270.)

Figure 11–20. Renal osteodystrophy. Histologic section of bone exhibiting wide osteoid seams. These are seen in patients with primary renal disease, but they are not present in patients with primary hyperparathyroidism because the osteoid produced in primary hyperparathyroidism is normal. (From Metabolic diseases of bone. *In* Bogumill GP, Schwamm HA [eds]: Orthopaedic Pathology: A Synopsis with Clinical Radiographic Correlation. Philadelphia: WB Saunders, 1984, p 269.)

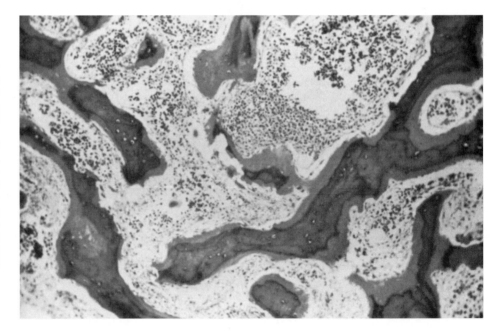

gene to the distal end of the short arm of the X chromosome. This has led to the current nomenclature of X-linked hypophosphatemia (XLH). It is now recognized that this is a primary inborn error of phosphate transport at the level of the proximal tubule in the nephron. As a result of this defect, there is a renal phosphate leak; hence, the resulting hypophosphatemia and hyperphosphaturia. In patients with chronic hypophosphatemia, the physeal changes are similar to those seen in the rickets of vitamin D deficiency. The accumulation of unmineralized osteoid, typical of a mineralization defect, is usually apparent. However, since these patients are usually normocalcemic, there is no secondary hyperparathyroidism. Since no significant osteoclastic resorption occurs, bone mass is generally unchanged. Phenotypically, these patients manifest stunting of growth, deformities in the lower extremities, and hypophosphatemia.

Vitamin D–Dependent Rickets (VDDR): This syndrome should not to be confused with resistant rickets. The dependent form is a rare inborn error of metabolism, which at present is classified into type I and type II forms. The term *pseudodeficiency rickets* was used in the past for this syndrome. Both types demonstrate the typical clinical and radiographic manifestations of deficiency rickets, despite a normal intake of vitamin D. Classically, however, these patients respond to only extremely high doses of exogenous vitamin D. These findings suggest a relative end-organ insensitivity to the patient's own vitamin D. This insensitivity has been said to affect both gut and kidney.

Type I VDDR is inherited as an autosomal recessive trait; the presumed defect is a deficiency in 25-hydroxyvitamin D_1-hydroxylase. This enzyme is important at the renal level to complete the second hydroxylation step in the activation of vitamin D. Hence, its deficiency results in a decrease in circulating levels of active vitamin D.

Type II VDDR is actually the result of an intracellular receptor defect. The receptor is felt to be important for active vitamin D binding, but beyond that its exact mechanism remains to be elucidated.

The clinical manifestations seen in these patients are essentially identical to those of rickets and osteomalacia. A feature that is peculiar to these syndromes is alopecia. As one might expect, a history of parental consanguinity and intermarriage is frequently obtained from these patients.

Fanconi's Syndrome: Renal Fanconi's syndrome is typified by a generalized defect in the renal proximal tubule. This defect is more global than that seen in VDDR, in that there is impaired reabsorption of glucose, amino acids, uric acid, bicarbonate, and phosphate. In addition, the resorption of low molecular weight proteins is also affected. These defects result in hypocalcemia and the anticipated bony changes.

Renal Tubular Acidosis (RTA): This syndrome is felt to be inherited as an autosomal dominant trait. In the classic form of the disease, there is a wasting of bicarbonate at the tubular level. As a result of this failure to acidify the urine, there is a resultant hyperchloremic metabolic acidosis.

At present, the classification of RTA still includes four types, even though type III RTA is no longer believed to exist. Currently, most feel it is a hybrid of types I and II. The extent of bicarbonate wasting varies among the legitimate remaining three. When all is said and done, renal tubular acidosis results in metabolic changes that produce a rachitic syndrome.

ENDOCRINE EFFECTS ON BONE AND SECONDARY METABOLIC BONE DISEASE

As seen in the preceding sections, bone is a metabolically active tissue. It responds to many hormonal factors. Growth hormone, also known as somatotropin, can be either over- or underproduced. The anterior pituitary, under control of the hypothalamus, produces growth hormone. This hormone affects a wide variety of visceral and connective tissue and provides a positive stimulus for protein and nucleic acid synthesis. Growth hormone increases bone mass by supporting net bone production. Growth hormone in skeletally immature persons also has effects on the growth plate and the stimulation of growth in the skeleton. In skeletally mature persons, insufficiency in the secretion of growth hormone alone has little effect. However, it is more common to have an insufficiency in all the hormones secreted by the anterior pituitary. This leads to a spectrum of symptoms such as amenorrhea (or testicular atrophy), hypoglycemia, and hypotension. If, however, there is an excess of growth hormone (known as *acromegaly*) there will be continued growth in bone diameter as well as cortical thickening and an increase in bone mass. Patients will note this by an increase in shoe, glove, and hat size. The facial features will slowly become more prominent. Erosion of the articular surfaces can occur, and osteoarthritis is common. The diagnosis can be made by an elevation in the circulating growth hormone levels. Treatment is directed at eliminating the source of the elevated growth hormone. Most commonly, this involves a pituitary adenoma that is treated with either surgery or irradiation.

Thyroid hormone has a stimulatory effect on many metabolic processes. It results in increased protein synthesis and increased oxygen consumption in almost every organ system. Clinically, the patient notes agitation, tachycardia and palpitations, tremors, and insomnia. In bone it exerts a stimulatory effect on bone turnover. In hypothyroidism, there is a decreased rate of bone turnover. This tends to stabilize bone mass and has little effect on the structure of the skeleton. In hyperthyroidism, the rate of bone turnover is accelerated. However, the rate of bone resorption exceeds the acceleration of bone formation. Over time, this leads to a net loss of bone mass. Hyperthyroidism can also occur in excessive supplementation with Synthroid. This may lead to an increase in serum calcium levels; however, the increased rate of bone turnover can be documented by an increase in hydroxyproline levels in the urine. If treated by chemical or surgical thyroidectomy, the bone effects can reverse. Glucocorticoids can exert a significant effect on the skeleton. Reduced glucocorticoid levels can cause hypoglycemia, hypotension, fatigue and weakness, and cold intolerance. There can be chronic skin changes. However, there is little effect on the skeleton from a chronic reduction in cortisol. Increased secretion of glucocorticoids can have a significant impact on the skeleton. The effects on the body and skeleton are similar for both endogenous overproduction, such as in Cushing's disease, and from externally administered glucocorticoids, such as prednisone used for inflammatory conditions. Increased levels have profound effects. Patients develop moon facies, truncal obesity, muscle wasting and weakness, thin atrophic skin that bruises easily, and difficulty in wound healing. The skeletal effect is osteoporosis. The density and total mass of bone is reduced. On histologic analysis, the bone appears normal; however, there is less bone present. The rate of bone turnover is also reduced; however, the resorption exceeds formation, leading to decreased bone mass. In addition, the lining of the gut is atrophied, and the absorption of calcium from the gut is impaired. This leads to an increase in PTH and bone resorption to maintain the serum calcium level. The increased production of PTH leads to an increased excretion of phosphate and subsequently to the formation of renal calculi. The first step in treatment is to determine the source of the increased glucocorticoid levels. The elevation can be caused by a primary tumor in the adrenal cortex or by overstimulation of the adrenal cortex by corticotropin from the pituitary. Once the source is identified, appropriate treatment can be instituted. If the source of glucocorticoid is from exogenously administered hormone, the patient's need for the medication needs to be weighed against its systemic effects. The dosage should be minimized as much as possible to reduce the systemic effects. Hypogonadism, which occurs in women after menopause and in both men and women as they age, can have a significant impact on the skeleton and bone mass. Follicle stimulating hormone (FSH) and luteinizing hormone (LH) are found both in males and females and have a role in supporting the normal growth, development, and function of the testes and ovaries. The anterior pituitary also secretes these hormones, and their release is governed by the release of gonadotropin-releasing hormone from the hypothalamus. As a patient ages, the levels of these hormones decrease and the end organs atrophy to some extent. In women, this occurs over a relatively short period at menopause. This results in a sudden lack of estrogen. In men, the process occurs much more slowly. There is a decrease in testosterone despite an increase in LH.

The end result of the decrease in these hormones on the skeletal system differs for males and females. In women, estrogen exerts an inhibition of osteoclasts. This tends to promote bone formation over resorption. However, with the rapid decline in estrogen in menopause, there is a release in this inhibition. This results in a period of rapid bone loss over 5 to 10 years following menopause. After the period of rapid bone loss, there is continuous bone loss due to age-related or involutional osteoporosis. In males, the gradual decrease in testosterone results in a gradual loss of bone. In both sexes, if the mean bone mass falls below two standard deviations from normal, the patient has osteoporosis and should be treated. Significant reductions in bone mass, regardless of the cause, increase the risk for fracture.

The effects of a reduction in gonadal hormones can be reversed to some degree with supplementation. However, hormone supplementation can increase the risks for thromboembolic phenomenon and can promote some forms of cancer. Therefore, hormone supplementation should be undertaken carefully under the guidance of a physician. In addition, many elderly patients at risk for osteoporosis have a diet insufficient in calcium and vitamin D. Therefore, the first step is prevention by advising patients as young adults to maintain a balanced diet with calcium supplementation and weight-bearing activity. As patients age, physicians should encourage them to maintain both the diet and exercise to minimize the risk of osteoporosis. If osteoporosis does develop, patients may benefit from treatment with bisphosphonates in addition to calcium and vitamin D.

MISCELLANEOUS METABOLIC BONE DISEASES

Paget's Disease

Osteopetrosis, osteogenesis imperfecta, and osteoporosis have been discussed elsewhere in the text. That leaves Paget's disease as the remaining primary metabolic bone disease yet to be reviewed. In fact, many authors believe that Paget's disease would best be grouped with infectious diseases of the skeleton. However, on a historical basis, Paget's disease is usually considered as a primary metabolic bone abnormality and a disease of bone turnover. Described in 1876 by Sir James Paget, this condition was originally referred to as *osteitis deformans*. At present, Paget's disease has an incidence of about 3 to 4% in the middle age group and about 15% in the elderly. There are racial and geographic variations in the incidence of the disease. It is common in the United Kingdom, in the United States, and in Western Europe; it is rare in Japan, China, the Middle East, and Africa. In addition, significant familial clustering of the disease is often reported.

It is the clustering geographically and familially that has led many to suspect that a slow virus is the causative factor. Further, the finding of intranuclear inclusions in the osteoclasts has led many researchers to conclude that indeed a viral cause should be suspected (Fig. 11–21). These inclusions are said to resemble the nucleocapsids of the paramyxoviruses. To date, no viral particles have been isolated from the bone of these patients.

Essentially, Paget's disease is a focal disorder of bone turnover. The initial event is increased osteoclastic activity resulting in increased bone resorption. This is typically followed by an osteoblastic phase, which is considered compensatory. The histologic and radiographic changes mirror these remodeling effects.

The *histologic pattern* of the bone reflects the repetitive waves of bone resorption and bone formation. *Mosaic bone* (Fig. 11–22) is the result of osteoclastic bone removal followed by cyclic osteoblastic activity. This bone, although dense, is mechanically weak because of the presence of multiple and irregular cement lines. In addition to the finding of mosaic bone, individual trabeculae of bone can be found with both osteoblastic and osteoclastic cell lines on the same trabeculum (Fig. 11–23). As noted elsewhere, this finding is seen only in Paget's disease, hyperparathyroidism, and hyperthyroidism.

Radiographically one of the earliest findings is a "flame sign" or "a blade of grass sign" (Fig. 11–24). This finding

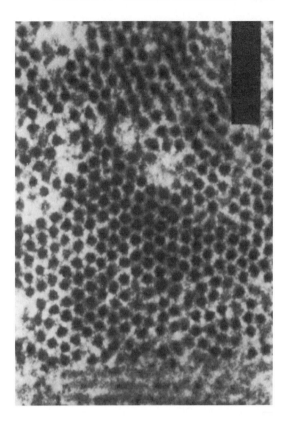

Figure 11–21. Viral particles located in osteoclasts within pagetoid bone have been implicated as a causal factor. (From Merkow RL, Lane JM: Paget's disease of bone. Orthop Clin North Am 1990, 21[1]:172.)

is seen uniquely in the long bones, especially the tibia. This sign reflects a wave of osteolysis moving down the long bone. As the process evolves over time, there is an overall enlargement in individual bone size and mass, as well as a prominent coarsening of the trabecular pattern. Many have used the term *caricature* of normal to describe the trabeculae of the involved bones (Fig. 11–25).

Clinically, the sites of involvement most commonly include the spine and sacrum followed by the femur, skull, sternum, pelvis, and bones of the foot. Monostotic and polyostotic involvement can be seen. When the skull is involved, an unusual pattern of patchy areas of sclerosis mixed with lucent regions produces the classic osteoporosis circumscripta cranii (Fig. 11–26).

Bone pain is the most prominent symptom suffered by these patients. It is deep and aching in quality and tends to be worse with weightbearing. It is frequently associated with pagetoid arthritis of the hips and knees. Vascular shunting through these active remodeling bones is often mentioned; this phenomenon can on occasion lead to high-output cardiac failure. Most series report this in fewer than 20% of patients.

Skeletal deformity results from the alteration in skeletal mechanics. The increased size and shape of the affected

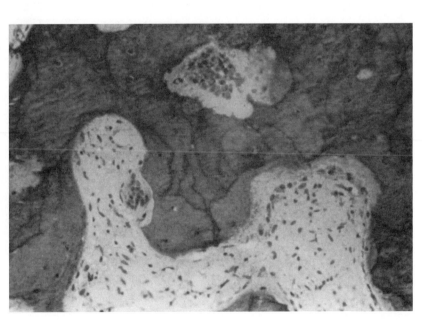

Figure 11–22. Photomicrograph of a pagetic bone affected by long-standing disease. There is increased cellular activity and a prominent "mosaic pattern" of irregularly arranged cement lines. (Courtesy of P. Bullough. From Merkow RL, Lane JM: Current concepts of Paget's disease of bone. Orthop Clin North Am 1984, 15:752.)

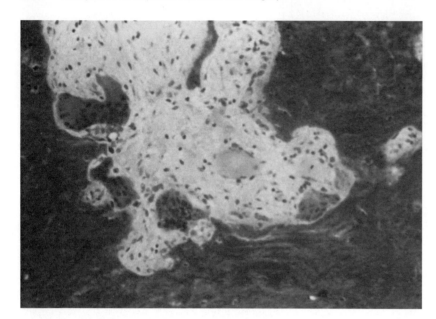

Figure 11–23. Photomicrograph of a bone affected by active Paget's disease. There is increased cellularity, numerous osteoblasts, and multinucleated osteoclastic giant cells. (Courtesy of P. Bullough. From Merkow RL, Lane JM: Current concepts of Paget's disease of bone. Orthop Clin North Am 1984, 15:751.)

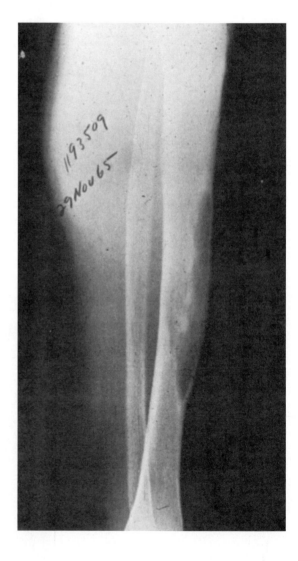

Figure 11–24. Clinical radiograph of a patient with Paget's disease exhibiting "blade of grass," a sharply circumscribed process usually limited to the cortex. This is often the first manifestation of Paget's disease. There is localized expansion of bone diameter in the involved area. (From Circulatory disturbances. *In* Bogumill GP, Schwamm HA [eds]: Orthopaedic Pathology: A Synopsis with Clinical Radiographic Correlation. Philadelphia: WB Saunders, 1984, p 180.)

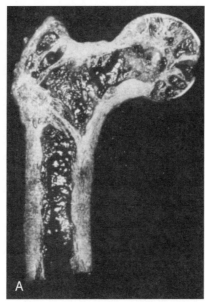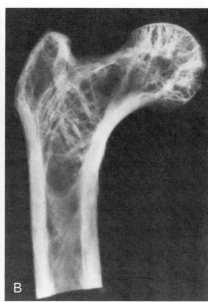

Figure 11–25. *A*, A coronal section of a gross specimen from the proximal femur. Note the varus deformity, thickened cortices, and coarse, scant trabeculae. *B*, Radiograph of the same specimen demonstrating thickening of cortical bone and a distorted architectural pattern. (Courtesy of P. Bullough. From Merkow RL, Lane JM: Current concepts of Paget's disease of bone. Orthop Clin North Am 1984, 15:750.)

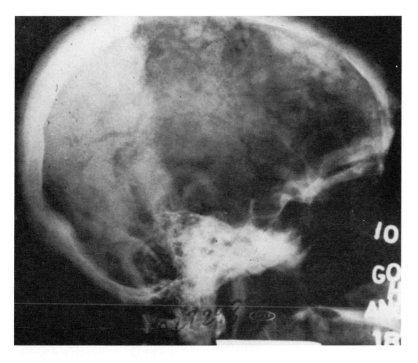

Figure 11–26. Lateral skull radiograph of patient with Paget's disease exhibiting marked osteolytic destruction of skull with patchy refill. Such removal of large areas of skull is termed *osteoporosis circumscripta*. (From Circulatory disturbances. *In* Bogumill GP, Schwamm HA [eds]: Orthopaedic Pathology: A Synopsis with Clinical Radiographic Correlation. Philadelphia: WB Saunders, 1984, p 184.)

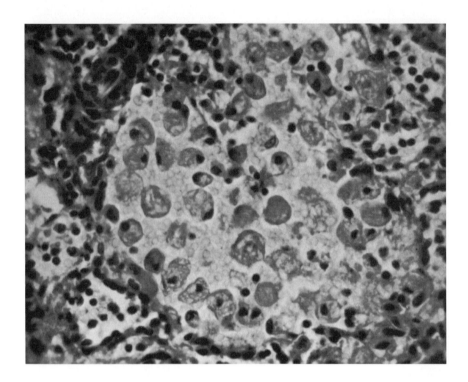

Figure 11–27. Gaucher's cells, characteristic of Gaucher's disease. Hematoxylin and eosin, ×400. (From Bone. *In* Tachdjian MO: Pediatric Orthopedics, 3rd ed. Philadelphia: WB Saunders, 1990, p 883.)

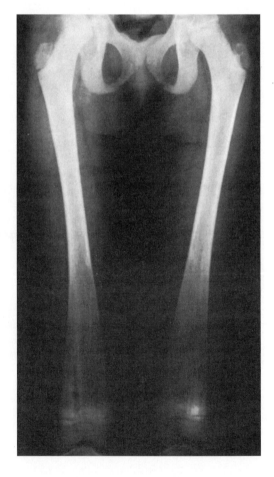

Figure 11–28. Bilateral "Erlenmeyer flask" deformity of the femora in Gaucher's disease. (From Bone. *In* Tachdjian MO: Pediatric Orthopedics, 3rd ed. Philadelphia: WB Saunders, 1990, p 884.)

bones, the enlargement of the skull, and the bowing of the femurs and other long bones are typical in the pagetoid patient. *Pathologic fracture* is seen in approximately 30% of patients and typically involves the subtrochanteric region of the femur, the femoral neck, and the tibia.

Spinal involvement and secondary neurologic complications are also fairly common. Encroachment on the neural elements resulting from a *spinal stenotic syndrome* has been reported. In addition, *foraminal encroachment* at the base of the skull frequently results in eighth nerve palsy and neurosensory deafness. *Hypercalcemia* and hypercalciuria are often reported and, as one would expect, these conditions result in renal stones as well as the other complications of hypercalcemia.

Lastly, *malignant transformation* in Paget's disease has been reported to occur in fewer than 1% of pagetoid patients. These pagetoid sarcomas account for 25% of bone sarcomas in the elderly. Although frequently described as a type of osteogenic sarcoma, these sarcomas are better referred to as pagetoid sarcomas because of their unique histologic appearance and biologic behavior.

Laboratory findings (see Table 11–2) include an elevation in the alkaline phosphatase level and an elevation in urinary hydroxyproline levels. In addition, hypercalcemia is especially common in pagetoid patients who are placed at bedrest for a variety of reasons, but especially for fracture care.

Treatment includes both medical management of the disease and surgical management of its complications. Various agents have been used in an effort to decrease the bone pain, slow the progress of deformity, and manage neurologic compromise. *Calcitonin* can be shown to inhibit osteoclastic bone resorption. However, the problem of "osteoclastic escape" after a time has been similarly reported. *Diphosphonates*, such as etidronate (Didronel) and alendronate (Fosamax), have also been used in Paget's disease in an effort to "freeze" the skeleton and halt bone turnover. Most protocols recommend monitoring alkaline phosphatase levels with the initiation of drug therapy. Once the alkaline phosphatase level returns to normal, the medications can be withdrawn and restarted as the alkaline phosphatase level begins to climb. The severity of the bone pain tends to parallel the alkaline phosphatase levels. It is also important to remember to discontinue any pharmacologic agent that retards bone formation when the patient is being treated for a fracture or has had an osteotomy to correct deformity. Obviously, bone healing will be adversely affected in these circumstances if these drugs are continued.

Surgical options are available for the management of arthritis, fracture, deformity, and malignant transformation. Suffice it to say that corrective osteotomies can be used to correct long bone deformity. Arthroplasty can be used to correct pagetoid arthritis of major weight-bearing joints, and fracture fixation devices are frequently used to deal with this complication.

Storage Diseases

Another heterogeneous group of syndromes that is often considered with the metabolic bone diseases are the storage diseases. Loosely defined, these entities result from the deposition of a metabolic end product into bone cells and other tissues. Two major subsets of storage diseases are described here: reticuloendothelial (RE) storage diseases and the mucopolysaccharidoses (MPS).

RETICULOENDOTHELIAL STORAGE DISEASES

The RE storage diseases can be further subdivided based on the product stored. The RE system has cells in multiple organs; therefore, storage of the metabolite occurs not only in bone but also in liver, spleen, lung, and skin.

The *secondary forms* of RE storage diseases are often referred to as the sphingolipidoses. These conditions result from a defect in lipid metabolism, usually a deficiency in a specific lysosomal enzyme. The result is a block in a metabolic pathway and the resulting storage of the blocked metabolite. Examples are listed, along with the stored metabolite:

Tay-Sachs disease (gangliosides)
Niemann-Pick disease (sphingomyelin)
Metachromatic leukodystrophy (cerebroside)
Fabry's disease (cerebroside)
Gaucher's disease (glucocerebroside)

Primary forms of RE storage diseases are often called *lipid histiocytoses*. These are primary idiopathic inflammatory lesions of bone and other tissues, demonstrating cholesterol stored in the histiocytic cytoplasm. They include:

Letterer-Siwe disease (acute form)
Hand-Schüller-Christian disease (subacute form)
Eosinophilic granuloma (chronic form)

Gaucher's Disease

Gaucher's disease is the storage disease with the most typical bony involvement and therefore is a good representative of the group. It is a common familial condition characterized by an abnormal accumulation of glucocerebroside in the RE cells. There is a lysosomal enzyme defect, as is the case in most of these syndromes. The glucocerebroside arises from the breakdown of complex sphingoglycolipids (usually from white blood cells and red blood cells). Glucocerebroside is insoluble; if not degraded further, it will accumulate in tissues. The RE cells, once they engulf this metabolite, are transformed into an extremely large cell with wrinkled cytoplasm containing fibrillar material and an eccentric nucleus called a *Gaucher cell* (Fig. 11–27). The finding of these cells in a bone marrow aspirate permits easy diagnosis.

Although several clinical forms of the disease occur, it is the adult form that is most typical. It occurs in any age group and in both sexes; 75% of patients demonstrate radiographic changes, especially in the femur, pelvis, and spine. The femur, which is the most common bone affected, has an "Erlenmeyer flask" configuration at the distal end (Fig. 11–28). The bulk of stored material in the region blocks normal "cut-back" by the osteoclasts. Proximally, the stored material tamponades the small vessels of the intraosseous arterial system to the femoral head, causing

Table 11–3. Differential Diagnosis of Mucopolysaccharidosis

Type	Enzyme Defect	Increased Urinary Excretion of Acid Mucopolysaccharide	Inheritance	Age at Which Features Present	Facies	Corneal Clouding
Hurler syndrome MPS I	Deficient α-L-iduronidase	Dermatan sulfate ++ Heparan sulfate +	Autosomal recessive	First few months May appear normal at birth	Grotesque Gargoyle	Present
Hunter syndrome MPS II	Low sulfoiduronate sulfatase	Heparan sulfate ++ Dermatan sulfate +	Sex-linked recessive All patients male	6–12 months	Similar to Hurler; less severe	Absent
San Filippo syndrome MPS III	Low N-heparan sulfatase or α-acetyl-glucosaminidase	Heparan sulfate ++	Autosomal recessive	Early childhood	Not coarse	Absent
Morquio syndrome MPS IV	N-Ac-Gal-6 sulfate sulfatase	Keratin sulfate ++ (diminishes with age)	Autosomal recessive	2–4 years	Not coarse Wide mouth Prominent maxilla	Present, slowly progressive
Scheie syndrome MPS I-S	α-L-Iduronidase	Heparan sulfate + Dermatan sulfate ++	Autosomal recessive	Late childhood	Somewhat coarse	Present
Maroteaux-Lamy syndrome MPS VI	N-Ac-Gal-4-sulfatase	Dermatan sulfate ++	Autosomal recessive	Early to late childhood	Coarse	Present, poor vision

From Bone. *In* Tachdjian M (ed): Pediatric Orthopaedics, 3rd ed. Philadelphia: WB Saunders, 1990, p 875.

Table 11–3. *Continued*

Deafness	Hepato-splenomegaly	Cardiovascular Abnormality	Stature	Skeletal Changes	Mental Retardation	Prognosis
Present	Present	Present	Normal at birth, later may be moderately short	Moderate dorsolumbar kyphosis Anterior-inferior beaking of body of L2 or L1	Severe	Progressive disease; usually death by 10 years of age due to heart disease or respiratory infection
Frequent	Present	Present Pulmonary hypertension	Normal at birth; later may be moderately short	Moderate, absence of lumbar kyphosis	Late in onset, less severe than in Hurler	Survival usually into the third decade of life Eventual death from cardiopulmonary disease
Present	Minimal or moderate	Absent	Normal	Minimal widening of clavicles at medial ends, no kyphosis	Severe	Survival to third or fourth decade
Present	Usually absent	Minimal, if present, aortic regurgitation	Markedly short (< 4 ft.)	Severe and diffuse platyspondyly with central tongue Capital femoral epiphyses irregular, eventually disappear	Absent	Normal longevity Respiratory failure due to rib cage rigidity
Present	Absent	Present; aortic valve disease	Normal	Small epiphysis on hands	Absent	Normal longevity
Present	Hepatomegaly rather than splenomegaly	Absent	Normal at birth, later markedly short	Severe (same as Hurler)	Absent	Guarded, death from cardiovascular complications

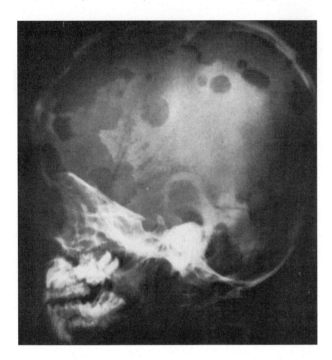

Figure 11–29. Hand-Schüller-Christian disease. Radiograph of skull. Note multiple sharply defined radiolucent holes. (From Bone. *In* Tachdjian MO: Pediatric Orthopedics, 3rd ed. Philadelphia: WB Saunders, 1990, p 1280.)

avascular necrosis (AVN). The AVN is usually bilateral and typically results in whole head involvement. Weakening of the dead bone in the region of the neck can lead to pathologic fracture; if this complication occurs, it is best managed with arthroplasty rather than open reduction with internal fixation.

Extraosseous involvement occurs in the form of hepatosplenomegaly, intra-abdominal and intrathoracic adenopathy, and hematologic manifestations. The latter result primarily from marrow displacement, although a hemolytic anemia has been reported.

Lipid Histiocytoses

The acute form of the disease, *Letterer-Siwe disease*, affects children younger than 2 years of age. Males are more commonly affected than females. Despite profound involvement of the vascular system (petechiae, purpura, and anemia), bony lesions are rare. Unfortunately, this is because these children do not live long enough to develop osseous involvement. If present, aggressive histiocytes can be observed in the lesions of long bones and skull.

Hand-Schüller-Christian disease, the subacute form, was placed in this grouping in 1935. Before that time, it was thought to be a type of Gaucher's disease. The classic triad that defines the disease is diabetes insipidus, exophthalmos, and bony lesions. Usually, only 10% of affected individuals demonstrate the triad. The bony lesions can be seen in the long bones and the skull. When affected, the skull demonstrates a "map-like" or "geographic" appearance because of multiple, round, punched-out holes that are coalescing (Fig. 11–29). The lesions contain masses of histiocytic "foam" cells containing cholesterol. When these cells degenerate, they leave behind cholesterol clefts.

Eosinophilic granuloma (the chronic form) was described in 1940 by Jaffe and Lichtenstein. As with the other forms of lipid histiocytoses, the common denominator is the histiocyte. The more material that is stored in a given cell, the more foamy the cytoplasm will appear. This lesion is monostotic and associated with pain. In the child it appears highly aggressive, causing it to be confused with infection or Ewing's sarcoma. This is especially true if it is located in the supra-acetabular region of the pelvis. In the adult, the lesion has a benign appearance, which is often described as a solitary, round, punched-out lesion with a sclerotic margin especially in the skull. When located in a vertebral body, the typical pattern is *vertebra plana*. Histologically, the lesion contains monotonous sheets of benign eosinophils. Since this lesion is rare after 20 years of age, one must consider lymphoma if a similar lesion, containing histiocytes, is seen in an older patient.

MUCOPOLYSACCHARIDOSES

The mucopolysaccharidoses are a group of inherited lysosomal storage diseases characterized by the accumulation of mucopolysaccharides or, as they are currently referred to, glycosaminoglycans (GAGs). In 1910, Hunter and Hurler reported on the syndromes in this group, which bear their names. It was not until the 1960s that the concept of a lysosomal storage disease evolved. All are inherited as autosomal dominant traits with the exception of Hunter's syndrome (mucopolysaccharidosis [MPS] II), which is X-linked recessive.

GAGs are large polymers of repeating disaccharide units. These substances are degraded sequentially by removing sugar and sulfate groups. Thus, a deficiency in any one of the glycosidases or sulfatases results in the accumulation of undegraded GAGs.

Although the severity and location of the lesions vary with the specific enzyme defect, certain features are common to most of these syndromes (Table 11–3). The GAGs accumulate in connective tissue cells, mononuclear phagocytes, endothelial cells, neurons, and hepatocytes. Hence, the important lesions in these syndromes can be anticipated. Central nervous system involvement results in extensive loss of neurons, gliosis, and cortical atrophy. GAGs accumulate in the chondrocytes and disrupt normal enchondral ossification. Cardiac lesions are often severe and include distorted heart valves and endocardial hypertrophy. Hepatosplenomegaly is common, as is corneal clouding.

The classification of these syndromes is a work in progress as the techniques of molecular biology are applied to the identification of the gene defects. The syndromes of orthopedic significance follow (list includes enzyme defect and stored material):

MPS I Hurler's syndrome (iduronidase deficiency) dermatan sulfate and heparan sulfate stored

MPS II Hunter's syndrome (iduronate sulfatase deficiency) dermatan sulfate and heparan sulfate stored

MPS IV Morquio's disease (galactosamine-6-sulfatase deficiency) keratan sulfate stored

SUMMARY

Metabolic bone diseases are a varied and complex group of entities. This chapter has used the simple classification of metabolic bone disease based on serum calcium levels. The *hypercalcemic states*, which primarily result from excess levels of PTH, result in a generalized skeletal dissection due to the overactivity of osteoclasts. The *hypocalcemic syndromes* are typified by rickets and osteomalacia and the histologic finding of unmineralized osteoid. Certainly, osteoporosis is the most important *eucalcemic disease*. This classic metabolic disease results in an overall decrease in skeletal mass, without altering the ratio of mineral to matrix. It is one of the most common diseases in the United States today. A working familiarity with these diseases can assist the physician not only in diagnosis but also in an approach to management. Often, unique solutions are required to deal with the fractures and deformities seen in these patients with dynamic, rapidly changing skeletal systems.

C h a p t e r 12
Rheumatic Disorders

Daniel J. Clauw, M.D.
Frank Petzke, M.D.

THE IMMUNE SYSTEM

The immune system serves many vital functions, including defense against foreign organisms and surveillance against tumors. But function, or dysfunction, of the immune system also plays a significant role in many rheumatic diseases. In some cases, the damage caused by the immune system is an inevitable consequence of killing invading microorganisms (e.g., polymorphonuclear cells attacking bacteria in a septic joint). In other instances, hyperactivity of the immune system is the primary problem, as occurs in autoimmune disorders in which self-antigens are recognized as foreign, such as rheumatoid arthritis (RA) or systemic lupus erythematosus (SLE). And in yet other settings, an initial injury can be followed by an inflammatory response that is responsible for continued symptoms (e.g., tendinitis or bursitis).

Thus, to understand the diagnosis and management of rheumatic disorders, it is crucial to understand the basic organization of the immune system. The focus of this review is to introduce the basic concepts of immunology and immunopathology as they relate to rheumatic disorders. As with any attempt to make an extremely complex system simple, important details are necessarily omitted, and for this information the reader is encouraged to consult more detailed reviews of these subjects.

The immune response can be divided into two broad categories: specific and nonspecific. The nonspecific immune response includes mucosal barriers of defense, some types of immune cells, and the alternative pathway of complement activation. The specific immune response involves a sophisticated afferent system to recognize self from nonself.[1, 2] After the immune system has distinguished self from nonself, there are a set of specific effector agents that act to target and destroy external agents, hopefully with the least damage possible to host tissues. Defects in the function of this system lead to most of the classic autoimmune disorders.

Components of the Immune System

General Concepts. During fetal development, hematopoietic cells move from the yolk sac to the bone marrow and other tissues to begin differentiating into lymphoid and myeloid cell lines. Myeloid cells are widely distributed in many tissues, whereas lymphoid cell lines concentrate in hematopoietic organs such as the thymus, spleen, lymph nodes, and bone marrow. The development of lymphoid cells is particularly complex. Although all lymphoid cells are produced in the bone marrow, one type of cell line migrates to the thymus (the T cell) for further development. The thymus plays a crucial role, being particularly important for the development of the ability to recognize self from nonself (tolerance) by these cell lines. Mature T lymphocytes then direct the immune role of self-recognition and regulate both cell- and antibody-mediated (humoral) immunity.[3] In early development cells that will eventually become B cells (so named because of the involvement of a bursa in this process in birds) mature independently of the thymus. These cells develop cell surface markers such as surface immunoglobulins, and their major function is to produce antibodies.

An important concept for understanding the function of both T and B cells is the process of clonal expansion. In early development, the immune system has cells that could theoretically respond to virtually any possible antigen. The subsequent interaction of that person with the environment will largely determine which of these cell lines are stimulated to expand and replicate (i.e., clonal expansion) and which are deleted (because they react with self-antigens). This latter concept that describes the loss of reactivity to self-antigens is termed *immune tolerance*.

Antigen-Presenting Cells. The first step in the specific immune response is the interaction between antigen and antigen-presenting cells (APCs) (Fig. 12–1).[4] There are a number of cell types that are capable of acting as APCs, including B cells, tissue macrophages, and site-specific cells such as dendritic cells in the skin or Kupffer cells in the liver. In general, these cells first process antigen by internalizing protein and digesting this into peptides and then present these peptides on the cell surface for recognition by other types of cells.

T Cells. T cells (particularly the CD4+ subset of T cells, also called T helper cells) are responsible for the recognition of antigens on APCs in a T cell–dependent antibody response. When the immune system is functioning properly, T cells will respond to foreign antigens but not to self-antigens. This process occurs primarily in the thymus and involves the positive selection of clones of cells that respond to foreign antigens, as well as the elimination of clones that respond to self-antigens.

When a CD4+ T cell binds to an antigen on an APC,

Processed antigen is presented to T cells in association with class II molecules

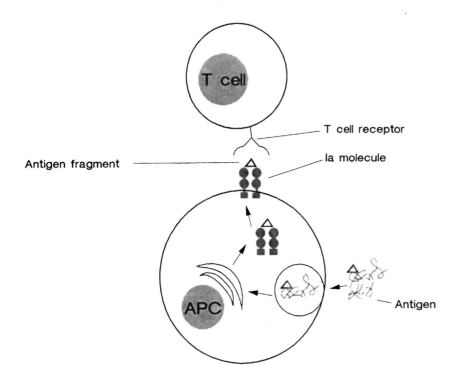

Figure 12–1. Schematic representation of the processing and presentation of an antigen molecule. The particular antigenic determinant of interest is represented as Δ and is situated on the antigen molecule, shown as composed of several polypeptide chains. A fragment of the antigen molecule containing this determinant is produced by processing and is expressed on the cell surface in association with a major histocompatibility complex molecule. In this case a class II molecule was used to illustrate presentation, but similar events occur with class I molecules. APC, antigen-presenting cell. (From Kelley WN, Harris ED Jr, Ruddy S, Sledge CB: Textbook of Rheumatology, 3rd ed. Philadelphia, WB Saunders, 1989, p 104.)

several processes occur. The T cell becomes activated and expresses a different set of cell surface receptors, and the T cell also produces a number of soluble molecules (cytokines) that can cause both local and distant effects on immune and nonimmune functions. A prominent function of these cytokines is to attract the new macrophages to the tissue. These new macrophages that were not involved in the initial antigen presentation are more effective at phagocytosis and killing microorganisms.

The other major class of T cells is the CD8+ (T suppressor) cell (Table 12–1).[5] These cells have quite different functions than their CD4+ counterparts, having no role in the humoral antibody process but instead being responsible for T cell killing. This mechanism of direct cell killing is particularly important in defense against viruses and intracellular organisms. These cells have speci-

ficity for antigens associated with the major histocompatibility complex (MHC) class I products, the HLA-A, HLA-B, and HLA-C antigens, in contrast to the class II product specificity of CD4+ cells.

In addition, the CD4+ and CD8+ cells play an essential role in regulating the overall function of the immune system. Immunoregulatory cytokines include interleukins 2, 4, 5, 7, 9, 10, and 11 and interferon gamma, are released by T lymphocyte subsets, and exert both positive and negative effects on the overall activity of the inflammatory response.

Within the classic autoimmune disorders, some are characterized by a relative excess of activity of CD4+ cells (e.g., SLE, RA) whereas others (e.g., ankylosing spondylitis, reactive arthritis) are characterized by a relative CD8+ excess. This runs in parallel to our understanding of the immunogenetic risk factors for these types of disorders (Tables 12–2 and 12–3). For example, the seronegative spondyloarthropathies (e.g., ankylosing spondylitis) are strongly associated with the presence of the HLA-B27 (or related, e.g., B7, Bw22, B42) haplotypes, and CD8+ cells have specificity for these MHC class I products. In contrast, the immunogenetic risk for developing disorders such as SLE or RA is conferred by certain MHC class II haplotypes (e.g., HLA-DR4), again in parallel with the more prominent role of CD4+ cells in the pathogenesis of these disorders. This phenomenon of reciprocal roles of CD4+ and CD8+ cells also appears to be evident when persons with autoimmune disorders become infected with the human immunodeficiency virus (HIV). The lowering of the CD4+ count associated with infection with this virus frequently leads to an improvement in CD4+-dependent disorders such as

Table 12–1. Major peripheral T cell subsets

Phenotype	CD4+/CD8−	CD4−/CD8+	CD4−/CD8−
Proportion	60%	35%	5%
Antigen receptor	α/β	α/β	γ/δ
MHC restriction	Class II	Class I	?
Function	Predominantly helper/inducer	Predominantly cytolytic/suppressor	?
mAb defining heterogeneity	Anti-CD11	9.3	

From Kelley WN, Harris ED Jr, Ruddy S, Sledge CB: Textbook of Rheumatology, 3rd ed. Philadelphia, WB Saunders, 1989, p 155.

Table 12–2. Summary of common associations of MHC alleles with rheumatic diseases: class I alleles

Disease	HLA Allele	Relative Risk	Patients (% Positive)	Controls (% Positive)
Seronegative spondyloarthropathy				
Ankylosing spondylitis	B27	69.1	89	9
Pauciarticular peripheral arthritis	B27	15.6	69	9
Isolated sacroiliitis	B27	20.4	62	9
Reactive arthritis				
Salmonella species	B27	35.5	85	10
Shigella flexneri	B27	28.7	85	14
Campylobacter jejuni	B27	13.8	71	14
Yersinia species	B27	21.4	77	11
Inflammatory bowel disease (ankylosing spondylitis)	B27	10.2	52	10
Psoriatic arthritis				
Axial arthropathy	B13	3.9	16	5
Axial arthropathy	Bw16	7.8	26	5
Axial arthropathy	B17	2.2	13	7
Axial arthropathy	B27	10.8	47	8
Axial arthropathy	B38	10.3	23	3
Peripheral arthropathy	B13	2.4	12	7
Peripheral arthropathy	Bw16	2.1	10	7
Peripheral arthropathy	B17	3.1	25	7
Peripheral arthropathy	B27	2.0	14	10
Peripheral arthropathy	B38	3.5	15	3
Behçet's syndrome: "East"	B5(w51)	7.2	69	23
"West"	B5(w51)	3.8	31	12
Whipple's disease	B27	4.6	30	8

Adapted with modifications from Tiwari JL, Terasaki PL: HLA and Disease Associations. New York, Springer Verlag, 1985.

Table 12–3. Class II alleles (DR haplotypes)

Disease	HLA Allele	Relative Risk	Patients (% Positive)	Controls (% Positive)
Rheumatoid arthritis	DR1	1.4	20	17
	DR2	−2.2	13	25
	DR3	−1.4	16	21
	DR4	2.7	47	25
	DR5	−3.1	7	19
	DRw6	−3.1	2	6
	DR7	−1.7	14	22
After recalculation for DR4 increase	DR1	1.7	20	13
Systemic lupus erythematosus	DR2	2.3	44	25
	DR3	2.5	40	21
Sjögren's syndrome	DR2	5.2	73	33
	DR3	3.6	56	26
Takayasu's arteritis	B5	3.3	63	36
	DRw52	5.0	45	14
	DR2	2.4	60	36
Lyme arthritis, chronic	DR4	4.1		
After recalculation for DR4 increase	DR3			

Adapted in part and with modifications from Tiwari JL, Terasaki PL: HLA and Disease Associations. New York, Springer Verlag, 1985, and from data provided by A. G. Steere.

Table 12–4. Human immunoglobulin classes

	IgG	IgM	IgA	IgE	IgD
Molecular weight (kD)	150	950	160 or polymer	180	160
Sedimentation constant	6.6S	19S	7S, 9S, 11S, 14S	8S	7S
Carbohydrate (%)	3	10	8	13	9
Serum concentration (mg/mL)	10–15	0.5–1.25	0.5–2.1	0.000015–0.002	0.003–0.3
Half-life (days)	23	5	6	2.5	3
Valence	2	5 or 10	2 (monomer)	2	2
Molecular formula	γ_2,L_2	$(\mu_2,L_2)_5$	$(\alpha_2,L_2)_n$	ϵ_2,L_2	δ_2,L_2

From Kelley WN, Harris ED Jr, Ruddy S, Sledge CB: Textbook of Rheumatology, 3rd ed. Philadelphia, WB Saunders, 1989, p 170.

SLE or RA but a marked worsening of CD8 + -dependent disorders such as the seronegative spondyloarthropathies. Different types of antigens also elicit different types of immunologic responses. For example, some antigens, such as *Mycobacterium* and fungi, elicit exclusively a cell-mediated response, whereas most pathogens elicit a mixed response.

B Cells. Once activated, the major function of the B cell is to produce antibodies. This activation can occur by means of T cell–dependent or T cell–independent mechanisms.[6] In the T cell–dependent system, the CD4 + cell is activated through an interaction with a specific APC. Some antigens are capable of directly interacting with B cells, independent of T cells, and lead to a less specific immunoglobulin response.

Immunoglobulins. Immunoglobulins are the product of activated, mature B cells. There are nine classes of immunoglobulins, each of which consists of two heavy chains and two light chains (Table 12–4 and Fig. 12–2). For each type of immunoglobulin, there is a constant region that is largely responsible for the physiologic functions of the immunoglobulin molecule (e.g., complement activation) and a variable domain that is largely responsible for the antigen specificity of that particular immunoglobulin. Each of the subclasses of immunoglobulins serves different functions (Table 12–5).

Autoantibodies are immunoglobulins directed against self-antigens.[7] The two most commonly considered autoantibodies are antinuclear antibodies (ANAs) and rheumatoid factor. ANAs are antibodies directed against various components of the cell nucleus. Several factors need to be considered before ordering this test. First, a substantial percentage of the general population (as high as 30%) will have a positive result for this assay using newer, more sensitive techniques.[3] Because of the low specificity of this test, it should be ordered only when there is a high pretest probability that the person has a disease characterized by a positive ANA test (Table 12–6). If this test is found to be positive, then further testing for extractable nuclear antigens can be considered (e.g., anti-Ro [SSA], anti-La [SSB], anti-Sm, anti-RNP, anti-dsDNA), because these are much less commonly present as false-positive tests in normal individuals.[8]

Rheumatoid factors (RFs) represent a heterogeneous group of antibodies directed against the Fc portion of IgG. As with the ANA test, an RF test should only be ordered in persons with a high pretest probability of RA, because approximately 80% of persons with RA will have a positive value. Although the rate of false-positive RF is lower than for ANA, ordering this test in persons without evidence of synovitis or elevated inflammatory indices will lead to far more false-positive results than true-positive results (Table 12–7). It is important to recognize that the serum levels of RF and ANA do not correlate with the level of disease activity, so that once these tests are ordered and known to be positive, there is little value to following these values longitudinally in an individual.

Neutrophils. The cell most active in the initial stages of an inflammatory response is the neutrophil. Neutrophils may

Table 12–5. Some biologic properties of human immunoglobulin isotypes

	IgG1	IgG2	IgG3	IgG4	IgA1	IgA2	IgM	IgD	IgE
Complement fixation									
Alternative pathway					+	+		±	±
Classical pathway	+ +	+	+ +	−	−	−	+ +	−	−
Placental transport	+	+	+	+	−	−	−	−	−
Binds to									
Mast cells or basophils	−	−	−	−	−	−	−	−	+
Macrophages	+	±	+	±	−	−	−	−	−
Lymphocytes	+	+	+	+	−	−	+	−	±
Platelets	+	+	+	+	−	−	−	−	−
Polymorphonuclear leukocytes	+	+	+	+	+	+	−	−	−
Staphylococcal protein A	+	+	−	+	−	−	−	−	−

From Kelley WN, Harris ED Jr, Ruddy S, Sledge CB: Textbook of Rheumatology, 3rd ed. Philadelphia, WB Saunders, 1989, p 172.

Table 12–6. Fluorescent antinuclear antibody in various conditions

	SLE (662)*	RA (201)	Scleroderma (91)	MCTD (57)	Myositis (30)	Arteritis (79)
Positive tests (%)	95	52	55	95	40	33
Titer of test Mean	298	142	338	508	173	50
Percentage with						
Titer ≥ 1:40	34	72	46	7	50	90
Titer = 1:80	17	8	9	5	10	10
Titer = 1:160	19	10	18	14	10	0
Titer = 1:320	20	6	13	48	17	0
Titer ≥ 1:640	10	4	14	26	13	0
Pattern of fluorescence						
Diffuse (%)	64	73	29	10	27	51
Speckled (%)	30	22	58	86	17	33
Nucleolar (%)	3	5	13	4	56	16
Peripheral (%)	3	0	0	0	0	0

*Number of observations in parentheses.
From Fries JF: Systemic Lupus Erythematosus: A Clinical Analysis. Philadelphia, WB Saunders, 1975.

be attracted to the site of inflammation by many factors, including proinflammatory cytokines (e.g., tumor necrosis factor-α, interleukins 1, 6, and 8) released by mononuclear immune cells, immune complexes, and components of the complement cascade. Once present, a neutrophil will attempt to phagocytose individual particles or microorganisms by internalizing and then digesting the foreign material. Alternatively, in some settings the neutrophils degranulate and release the contents of their lysosomal enzymes into the tissue environment, and this process can be responsible for extensive tissue damage. A related toxic effect of neutrophils, both to microorganisms as well as tissues involved in inflammation, is the release of oxygen free radicals.

Monocytes/Macrophages. Monocytes are circulating unstimulated macrophages. In addition to the previously described role of these cells as APCs, macrophages also play a vital role in control of the inflammatory response. It has been estimated that there are more than 100 products produced and released by macrophages, including cyto-

kines, complement components, coagulation factors, and bioactive lipids such as cyclooxygenase and lipooxygenase products.[9]

Complement. The complement system consists of a series of proteins that are involved in mediating a variety of inflammatory effects.[10] As with other components of the immune system, this system is vital in protecting the organisms against infection (particularly bacterial pathogens) but can be responsible for tissue damage in rheumatic disorders.

Two separate pathways of complement activation have been identified: the classical pathway and the alternative pathway (Figs. 12–3 and 12–4). Although these pathways are activated in different manners, the terminal event in both sequences is the cleavage of C3 to C3a and C3b. There are a number of components of the complement cascade that are responsible for the biologic consequences of complement activation (Table 12–8). C3a as well as

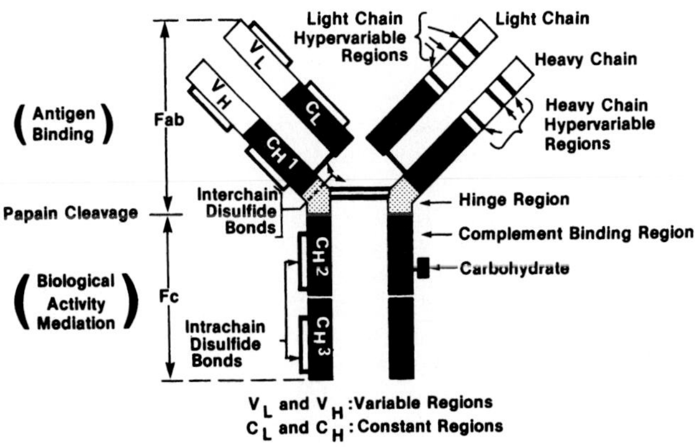

Figure 12-2. A prototype IgG monomer. (Modified from Wasserman RL, Capra JD: Immunoglobulins. *In* Horowitz MI, Pigman W [eds]: The Glycoconjugates. New York, Academic Press, 1977, p 323.)

Table 12–7. Diseases commonly associated with rheumatoid factor

Rheumatic diseases: rheumatoid arthritis, systemic lupus erythematosus, scleroderma, mixed connective tissue disease, Sjögren's syndrome
Acute viral infections: mononucleosis, hepatitis, influenza, and many others, after vaccination (may yield falsely elevated titers of antiviral antibodies)
Parasitic infections: trypanosomiasis, kala-azar, malaria, schistosomiasis, filariasis, etc.
Chronic inflammatory diseases: tuberculosis, leprosy, yaws, syphilis, brucellosis, subacute bacterial endocarditis, salmonellosis
Neoplasms: after irradiation or chemotherapy
Other hyperglobulinemic states: hypergammaglobulinemic purpura, cryoglobulinemia, chronic liver disease, sarcoid, other chronic pulmonary diseases

From Kelley WN, Harris ED Jr, Ruddy S, Sledge CB: Textbook of Rheumatology, 3rd ed. Philadelphia, WB Saunders, 1989, p 22.

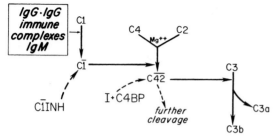

Figure 12–3. The classical pathway for complement activation. (From Kelley WN, Harris ED Jr, Ruddy S, Sledge CB: Textbook of Rheumatology, 5th ed. Philadelphia, WB Saunders, 1997, p 234.)

several other products of the classical complement cascade act as anaphylatoxins. These substances lead to the degranulation of mast cells and basophils, releasing a variety of mediators that are responsible for smooth muscle contraction, local edema, and increased vascular permeability. C3b begins a series of steps leading to the formation of membrane attack complex (MAC), which is capable of leading to damage or death of a number of different types of cells by insertion into the cell membrane.

Homozygous deficiencies of complement may lead either to an increased incidence of infection (especially of organisms such as *Neisseria* that are killed by MAC) or to autoimmune disorders.[11] The paradoxic development of autoimmune disorders in individuals with hereditary complement deficiencies has been perplexing because many autoimmune diseases are characterized by complement consumption.[12] The best supported theory for this phenomenon is that complement is vital for the normal clearance of immune complexes in the circulation and that these deficiency states are characterized by ineffective immune complex clearance and subsequent complement activation.

Complement measurements can sometimes be useful in assessing an individual for the presence of, or activity of, an autoimmune disorder.[13] The CH50 is an assay of the total hemolytic complement activity and is a useful screening test if a homozygous complement deficiency is suspected. Assays for individual complement levels (C3 and C4 are the most available commercially) can sometimes be helpful to assess for activity of autoimmune disorders characterized by complement consumption (e.g., immune

complex–mediated disorders such as SLE, RA, cryoglobulinemia). However, in many instances these values are difficult to interpret, because complement is produced in increased quantities by the liver as an acute phase reactant. Thus, in many autoimmune disorders characterized by complement consumption, a normal plasma value can still occur because of increased liver synthesis.

Immunoregulation and Immunopathology

Immunoregulation involves a tenuous balance of reacting to pathogens without harming the host. There are several levels of immunoregulation, beginning in early development with establishing tolerance. Once the organism can appropriately identify nonself antigens, the response to these challenges must be appropriate to potential danger of the challenge. An inflammatory response that is not localized to the area of infection, or that persists after the infection has been cleared, will cause undue damage to the organism.

Classically, four types of specific immunopathologic mechanisms have been identified:

Type I. *IgE mediated.* The combination of an IgE antibody binding to the Fc receptor of a basophil or mast cell, and an antigen binding to that antibody, leads to stimulation of these cells. Products contained in basophilic granules include histamine, serotonin, bradykinins, and other substances. This type of reaction is most prominent in allergic diseases.

Type II. *Direct antibody-mediated effects on cells.*

Table 12–8. Biologic activities of the products of complement activation

Product	Activity
C4, C2 kinin	Increase in vascular permeability; putative mediator of edema in hereditary angioedema
C3bBb	Chemotaxis of polymorphonuclear leukocytes
Bb	Spreading of monocytes
C3a	Anaphylatoxin; releases histamine from basophils and mast cells, serotonin from platelets, contracts smooth muscle, suppresses B lymphocyte responses
C5a	Anaphylatoxin; same activities as C3a on mast cells, marked chemotactic effect for monocytes and polymorphonuclear leukocytes
C3b	Multiple effects, depending on cell bearing receptor: phagocytosis enhancement, triggers cycling of alternative pathway amplification loop (see Fig. 12–4)
iC3b	Binding to glomerular, monocyte complement receptors
C3dg	Binding to lymphocyte complement receptors, inducing activation
C567	Active complex capable of binding to "innocent bystander" cell membranes and initiating formation of C5b–C9
C5b-C9	Membrane attack complex: forms transmembrane channels leading to cytolysis

From Kelley WN, Harris ED Jr, Ruddy S, Sledge CB: Textbook of Rheumatology, 3rd ed. Philadelphia, WB Saunders, 1989, p 246.

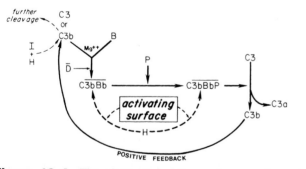

Figure 12–4. The alternative pathway for complement activation. (From Kelley WN, Harris ED Jr, Ruddy S, Sledge CB: Textbook of Rheumatology, 5th ed. Philadelphia, WB Saunders, 1997, p 234.)

Autoantibodies binding to self-antigens on a cell or tissue can cause complement fixation and/or direct cytotoxic killing of that particular cell. An example occurs in some types of hemolytic anemia, when red blood cells are destroyed when autoantibodies bind to cell surface antigens. This type of reaction is relatively uncommon.

Type III. *Immune complex formation.* In contrast to type II reactions, in which antibody binds to antigens on a cell or tissue surfaces, in this instance soluble antigens bind to antibodies in the circulation. These immune complexes may bind to cell surface receptors or activate complement and cause an inflammatory process in the tissue(s) where they are deposited. Many classic systemic autoimmune disorders, such as SLE, are characterized by the presence of circulating and tissue immune complexes. However, it remains unclear how much of the disease process is actually caused by these immune complexes.

Type IV. *Direct cell injury.* Several types of immune cells, including both T cells and CD8+ cells, can cause direct cell injury, whereas other types of cells such as CD4+ cells can effect cell injury by attracting other types of cells. This mechanism is probably operative in a number of autoimmune and other rheumatic disorders.

EVALUATION OF THE PATIENT WITH ARTHRITIS

History

The important elements of the history in the patient with suspected arthritis are the same as for other orthopaedic problems, although here there is more of an emphasis on certain features. These include elucidating the pattern and timing of joint involvement, differentiating inflammatory from noninflammatory processes, and determining whether extra-articular symptoms are present or absent.

The pattern of involvement can be particularly helpful when evaluating the patient with arthritis. Examples of such patterns are whether the arthritis is monoarticular or polyarticular (Table 12–9). Although this distinction is rarely absolute, as with any clinical pearl this can be helpful.

Another critical point in the evaluation of the patient with joint pain is how the symptoms began. Extremely rapid onset of symptoms (e.g., over seconds), especially if accompanied by trauma, suggests a mechanical process (e.g., fracture, loose body). Acute onset of symptoms over hours or days may occur in a number of types of arthritis and is especially common in inflammatory arthropathies (e.g., infectious, crystal-induced). The onset of symptoms is less helpful if the process is chronic or evolves over days to weeks, because this can occur with many different forms of arthritis.

Both the history and physical examination are helpful in differentiating whether the patient is suffering from an inflammatory or noninflammatory arthritis. Elements of the history that suggest an inflammatory process include prominent morning stiffness, improvement with exercise or activity (or worsening by prolonged immobility), or a his-

Table 12–9. Differential diagnosis of monoarticular arthritis

Usually Monoarticular	Often Polyarticular
Common	
Septic arthritis	Rheumatoid arthritis
Bacterial	Osteoarthritis
Tuberculous	Psoriatic arthritis
Fungal	Reactive arthritis
Lyme disease	Calcium pyrophosphate
Gout	deposition disease
Internal derangement	Chronic articular hemorrhage
Ischemic necrosis	Most JRA and juvenile
Hemarthrosis	spondylitis
Coagulopathy	Erytherma nodosum/sarcoid
Warfarin (Coumadin)	Serum sickness
Trauma/overuse	Acute hepatitis B
Pauciarticular JRA	Rubella
Neuropathic	Henoch-Schönlein purpura
Congenital hip dysplasia	Systemic lupus erythematosus
Osteochondritis dissecans	Lyme disease
Reflex sympathetic dystrophy	Parvovirus
Hydroxyapatite deposition	Dialysis arthropathy
Hemoglobinopathies	
Loose body	
"Pallindromic rheumatism"	
Paget's disease involving	
joint	
Stress fracture	
Osteomyelitis	
Osteogenic sarcoma	
Metastatic tumor	
Synovial osteochondromatosis	
Rare	
Pigmented villonodular	Undifferentiated connective
synovitis	tissue disease
Plant thorn synovitis	Relapsing polychondritis
Familial Mediterranean fever	Enteropathic disease
Synovioma	Ulcerative colitis
Synovial metastasis	Regional enteritis
Intermittent hydrarthrosis	Bypass arthritis
Pancreatic fat necrosis	Whipple's disease
Gaucher's disease	Chronic sarcoidosis
Behçet's disease	Hyperlipidemias types II and IV
Regional migratory	Still's disease
osteoporosis	Pyoderma gangrenosum
Giant cell arteritis/	Pulmonary hypertrophic
polymyalgia rheumatica	osteoarthropathy
Sea urchin spine	Chondrocalcinosis-like
Amyloidosis (myeloma)	syndromes due to ochronosis,
	hemochromatosis, Wilson's
	disease
	Rheumatic fever
	Paraneoplastic syndromes

From Kelley WN, Harris ED Jr, Ruddy S, Sledge CB: Textbook of Rheumatology, 3rd ed. Philadelphia, WB Saunders, 1989, p 443.

tory of warmth, redness, or swelling of the affected region(s). Pain that is worse after exercise or activity, on the other hand, is suggestive of a noninflammatory arthritis.

The presence or absence of nonarticular features can also be helpful in diagnosing the person presenting with arthritis. Nonarticular features are common in a number of conditions, especially systemic autoimmune disorders, where the joint is but one tissue that is being targeted by the inflammatory process (Table 12–10).

And, although the person who presents with the complaint of joint pain may indeed have a process localized to the joint, it is equally important to recognize the plethora of periarticular or nonarticular syndromes that frequently may present in this manner (Table 12–11).

Physical Examination

Both a general physical examination and a musculoskeletal examination are important in the person who presents with arthritis. As noted earlier, there are a number of nonarticular features that can accompany arthritis.

In the musculoskeletal examination of the person with joint pain, the goal of the evaluation is to (1) determine the extent of involvement, (2) localize the anatomic structure(s) involved, and (3) determine whether the process is inflammatory or noninflammatory. To determine the extent of involvement, it is important to perform a generalized examination of the joints and soft tissues, even if the person presents with a localized complaint. The patient with a systemic inflammatory process will very frequently present with the complaint of pain in a single joint. Limiting the focus to that joint will lead to an improper diagnosis and ineffective treatment.

The best manner to localize the anatomic structure(s) involved is to perform the musculoskeletal examination by palpating with firm pressure (enough to blanch the examiner's fingernail) over both joints and soft tissues, first in regions of the body where the person is not complaining of pain and finally in the affected region. This type of examination accomplishes several objectives. One is to obtain an assessment of the patient's overall pain threshold. If an individual has tenderness over bones and soft tissues in a number of regions in the body, he or she may suffer from a generalized disturbance in pain processing (e.g., fibromyalgia) rather than a process localized to a specific region. This type of examination also will detect whether periarticular structures (e.g., at tendon insertions, bursae) are involved. Finally, this procedure will identify the individual who may have more than one process that is co-expressed and responsible for symptoms (e.g., the patient with osteoarthritis of the hip or knee and concurrent trochanteric or anserine bursitis involving those same regions, respectively).

By the use of this technique, special attention is paid to the joints, and in particular examining the joint for evidence of synovitis. To the unskilled examiner, an enlarged joint represents arthritis. But with experience, palpation of enlarged joints can differentiate the firm and less painful bony proliferation secondary to osteophytes (as occurs with Heberden's and Bouchard's nodes in the distal and proximal interphalangeal joints of the hands in osteoarthritis) from the tender, boggy swelling seen in chronic inflammatory arthritis due to synovial proliferation and/or joint effusions.

Diagnostic Testing

Again, the evaluation of the patient with arthritis parallels that of the patient with other orthopaedic problems, although certain points bear emphasis.

Table 12–10. Systemic features of monoarticular arthritis

System	Diagnosis
Skin	Febrile-onset juvenile chronic arthritis
	Psoriatic arthritis
	Reactive arthritis
	Enteropathic arthritis
	Sarcoid arthritis
	Familial Mediterranean fever
	Septic arthritis (esp. *Neisseria gonorrhoeae* and *N. meningitidis*)
	Hyperlipoproteinemia
	Hemochromatosis
	Fat necrosis due to pancreatic disease
	Amyloidosis
	Lyme arthritis
	Systemic lupus erythematosus
	Serum sickness
	Sporotrichosis
Nasopharynx and ear	Reactive arthritis
	Gout
	Relapsing polychondritis
Eye	Juvenile rheumatoid arthritis
	Reactive arthritis
	Relapsing polychondritis
	Sarcoidosis
Gastrointestinal tract	Crohn's disease
	Whipple's disease
	Hemochromatosis
	Fat necrosis due to pancreatic disease
	Ulcerative colitis
	Bypass arthritis
	Ulcerative colitis
Heart and circulation	Amyloidosis
	Reactive arthritis
	Relapsing polychondritis
	Endocarditis
	Lyme arthritis
	Ankylosing spondylitis
	Systemic lupus erythematosus
Respiratory tract	Sarcoidosis
	Relapsing polychondritis
	Whipple's disease
	Tuberculosis
Nervous system	Meningococcal arthritis
	Neuropathic arthropathy
	Lyme arthritis
	Systemic lupus erythematosus
Genitourinary system	Systemic lupus erythematosus
	Amyloidosis
	Gout
Hematologic	Coagulopathies
	Gaucher's disease
	Hemochromatosis
	Myeloma/amyloid
	Leukemia

From Kelley WN, Harris ED Jr, Ruddy S, Sledge CB: Textbook of Rheumatology, 3rd ed. Philadelphia, WB Saunders, 1989, p 947.

Perhaps the most important point to emphasize is that the history and physical examination typically yield far more useful information for evaluating the person with joint pain than laboratory studies. This can be stated in two different ways: (1) if you don't have a good idea of the

Table 12–11. Regional periarticular syndromes

Region	Periarticular Syndrome	Nonarticular Syndrome
Jaw	Temporomandibular joint dysfunction	Temporal arteritis Molar dental problems Parotid swelling Preauricular lymphadenitis
Shoulder	Subacromial bursitis Long head bicipital tendinitis Rotator cuff tear	Pancoast's tumor Brachial plexopathy Cervical nerve root injury
Elbow	Olecranon bursitis Epicondylitis	Ulnar nerve entrapment
Wrist	Extensor tendinitis (including de Quervain's tenosynovitis) Gonococcal tenosynovitis	Carpal tunnel syndrome
Hand	Palmar fasciitis (Dupuytren's contracture) Ligamentous/capsular injury	
Hip	Greater trochanteric bursitis Adductor syndrome Ischial bursitis Fascia lata syndrome	Meralgia paresthetica Deep infection Paget's disease Neoplasm
Knee	Anserine bursitis Prepatellar bursitis Meniscal injury Ligamentous tear—laxity Baker's cyst	Neoplasm Osteomyelitis
Ankle	Peroneal tendinitis Subachilles bursitis Calcaneal fasciitis Sprain Erythema nodosum	Tarsal tunnel syndrome
Foot	Plantar fasciitis	Morton's neuroma Vascular insufficiency Cellulitis

From Kelley WN, Harris ED Jr, Ruddy S, Sledge CB: Textbook of Rheumatology, 3rd ed. Philadelphia, WB Saunders, 1989, p 444.

correct diagnosis before ordering the laboratory tests, it is unlikely that such testing will be helpful, and (2) it is rarely appropriate to perform an extensive laboratory evaluation when a person initially presents with joint pain.

There are several reasons for the strong note of caution regarding diagnostic testing in patients who present with joint pain. Unfortunately, there are virtually no diagnostic tests that can be ordered in this setting that function well as screening tests; most of the laboratory studies done in the evaluation of a person with joint pain have a relatively low positive or negative predictive value unless they are ordered in the appropriate setting. Luckily, however, in most rheumatic disorders it is not necessary to make a definitive diagnosis before initiating treatment. This combination of poor diagnostic utility of frequently ordered tests, and the fact that treatments can be initiated before diagnoses are established, is somewhat unusual in other fields of medicine.

A suggested diagnostic approach to the patient with joint pain is to first consider whether the patient may have an infection or malignancy causing the symptoms. It is important to recognize that it is unusual for persons who are not immune compromised (e.g., HIV infection, malignancy) or without some recent surgical event or trauma to a joint to develop septic arthritis. The exceptions to this are disseminated gonococcal infection, Lyme disease, and tuberculous arthritis, which can occur in persons with intact immune systems and no other risk factors. If a septic joint is suspected, then the study of choice is to perform an arthrocentesis and synovial fluid analysis. And, if a malignancy is suggested—for example, because of weight loss or other systemic symptoms—then imaging studies of that region should be performed immediately, followed by a biopsy in most settings.

Once those individuals with infection and malignancy have been identified, the next consideration is whether the person may have a life-threatening (or organ-threatening) autoimmune disorder. These individuals rarely present with nonspecific symptoms and mild impairment but instead will appear and feel very ill. In this setting, the workup should be guided by the presenting symptoms, with particular attention to detecting organ involvement (e.g., cardiopulmonary, central nervous system, renal) that may require specific and aggressive intervention. This is also the setting in which extensive diagnostic testing for the presence of autoantibodies, complement, and other studies (e.g., antineutrophil cytoplasmic antibodies for systemic vasculitides) is likely to be helpful in rapidly establishing a diagnosis and initiating aggressive treatment.

If the history and physical examination suggest that a person may suffer from a systemic autoimmune disorder, then a general set of screening laboratory studies can be

Table 12–12. Synovial fluid and associated laboratory findings in monoarticular arthritis

Synovial Fluid White Blood Cell Count	Predominant Cells	Appearance	Viscosity	Micro-organisms	Crystals	RBC	Glucose	Protein	Complement	Cartilage Debris	Other
0–200											
Normal	M	Clear	↑	–	–	–	90%	1.5–2.0	–	–	Small amounts not demonstrable on physical examination
0–2000											
Osteoarthritis	M	Clear	↑	–	+/– occ. occ. CPPD	–	–	–/↑	–	+	Radiographs positive in advanced disease; synovial fluid findings variable
Structural	M	Clear	↑	–	–	+/–	–	–/↑	–	+	MRI, arthrogram (knee) arthroscopy
Internal derangement						+/–					
Neuropathic						+ + +/–					Marked x-ray changes MRI, CT scan
Osteochondritis dissecans						–					
Ischemic necrosis						–					MRI, bone scan, x-ray in advanced cases
Traumatic	RBC	Cloudy bloody	↑	–	–	+ + +	–	↑/↑ ↑ ↑			X-ray
2000–10,000											
Pigmented villonodular synovitis	RBC	Brown bloody	↓	–	–	+ +	→	↑ ↑ ↑		–	Synovial biopsy
Amyloid	M	Sl turbid		–	–						Congo red: synovial fluid Monoclonal gammopathy

Disease	M/P	Appearance								Diagnostic findings
Enteropathic arthritis	M/P	Sl turbid	—	—	—	—	—		—	+ stool occult blood; Lee cells
Systemic lupus erythematosus	M	Sl turbid	↑	—	—	—	—		—	Serum autoantibodies
6000–50,000										
Juvenile rheumatoid arthritis	P	Sl turbid	→	—	—	↑/↑ ↑	—	—/↓	—	Synovial fluid leukocytes may be ≥ 100,000; Serum: + ANA (50%) + rheumatoid factor (<20%)
Sarcoidosis		Sl turbid	→	—	—	—	—		—	Chest radiographs, slit lamp examination
Reactive arthritis	P	Sl turbid	→	—	—	↑/↑ ↑	—	↑	—	Negative rheumatoid factor, ANA
Psoriatic arthritis	P	Sl turbid	→	—	—	—	—		—	
Rheumatoid arthritis	P	Turbid	→	—	—	↑/↑ ↑ ↑	—	→	—	Serum: (+) rheumatoid factor (50–80%) + ANA
Tuberculous arthritis	M	Turbid	→ →	+/−	—	↑ ↑/ ↑ ↑	—	→	—	PPD usually positive unless anergic; Synovial biopsy essential

ANA, antinuclear antibodies; CT, computed tomography; MRI, magnetic resonance imaging; PPD, purified protein derivative.

helpful. A reasonable choice would include a complete blood cell count, renal and hepatic studies, urinalysis, and screen for acute phase reactants. The most commonly ordered tests that assess acute phase reactants are the erythrocyte sedimentation rate (ESR), and the C-reactive protein (CRP) (see later).[14] As noted previously, tests for ANA and RF, and for other autoantibodies, should generally be reserved for persons with objective features suggesting autoimmune disorders, or in whom this initial screening indicates abnormalities.

The ESR is a nonspecific measure of inflammation that is inexpensive and easy to measure, but the results of this test must be interpreted with caution. The rate at which red blood cells settle in anticoagulated blood depends on many factors, but in most settings this is closely related to the plasma concentration of acute phase proteins, with fibrinogen being the most important. Although a Westergren sedimentation rate of greater than 20 mm/hour is generally considered to be abnormal, there are many factors, such as normal aging, that may cause mild elevations in this value. Other noninflammatory factors that can influence the ESR include anemia (increase), pregnancy (increase), drugs (heparin and valproic acid increase), or changes in shape of red blood cells (decrease). Very high levels of the ESR (e.g., more than 100 mm/hour) are typically only seen in inflammatory disorders, infection, and malignancy.

The CRP is a plasma protein that is produced in the liver in response to various types of tissue injury.[15] The advantage of measuring this protein instead of the ESR is that there are fewer noninflammatory stimuli that cause an elevation of the CRP, and this value will rise and fall more rapidly in response to inflammatory stimuli. The normal CRP value is less than 1 mg/dL. Values between 1 and 10 mg/dL are seen in a variety of inflammatory states, whereas values above 10 mg/dL are usually (but not always) indicative of infection.

Synovial Fluid Analysis

The aspiration of an involved joint and analysis of extracted synovial fluid can be particularly helpful in assessing the person with arthritis. In addition to a cell count and differential, the appearance and viscosity of the fluid should be assessed and the protein and glucose concentrations in the fluid should be determined. Table 12–12 indicates how this information can be used, together with the history, physical examination, and other diagnostic tests, in assessing the patient with arthritis.

RHEUMATOLOGIC DISORDERS

A brief overview of a number of rheumatic disorders that may present as orthopaedic problems is given in the following section. Space constraints severely limit both the breadth and depth of this section, and the reader is referred to several excellent rheumatology textbooks for a more extensive overview of these and other rheumatologic disorders.

Rheumatoid Arthritis (RA)

RA is the most common form of chronic, systemic inflammatory arthritis. It is estimated than 1 to 2% of the population worldwide suffers from this disorder. Population-based studies may overestimate the prevalence of true RA, because many people identified in such studies may have self-limited forms of inflammatory arthritis (e.g., postviral arthritis) or may not have inflammatory arthritis at all. Nonetheless, this is likely the most common autoimmune rheumatic disease. As with most autoimmune disorders, females are affected more commonly than males, with a ratio of approximately 2.5:1. RA can strike at any age from youth to the elderly.

As with most autoimmune disorders, the cause of RA is unknown. Genetic risk factors play some role, in that monozygotic twins show an 11-fold risk over dizygotic twins, and the majority of individuals who develop this disorder have either the HLA-DR4 and/or HLA-DR1 epitope. But genetic factors play a relatively small overall role, because even individuals with a positive family history of RA and one of the putative HLA epitopes have a low *absolute* risk of developing this disorder. It has long been suspected that both the combination of these genetic immune risk factors and the subsequent exposure to infectious agents lead to the development of disease. But there are no infectious agents that have been clearly identified as being causative in RA.

The hallmark of RA is the presence of a chronic polyarticular, inflammatory arthritis (Table 12–13).[16] This can begin either abruptly, or more indolently, and can begin in small or large joints. The presence of inflammatory arthritis can be documented by the finding of synovitis on examination, the finding of inflammatory (white blood cell count > 2000 cells/mm³) synovial fluid, or the radiographic appearance of characteristic erosions (not present until later in the course of the illness). If the diagnosis of RA is made primarily on the basis of the physical examination, then it must be clear that there is synovial proliferation present, not just tenderness over the joint.

The 1988 revised American Rheumatological Association (ARA) criteria for the classification of RA include some of the most important clinical features of this disorder (Table 12–14). Although prolonged morning stiffness occurs in nearly all cases of RA, this is seen in a number of other inflammatory and noninflammatory disorders and is not specific for this diagnosis. Three of the criteria are related to the fact that RA usually involves the small joints of the hand and typically is relatively equally distributed on both sides of the body (i.e., symmetrical). The joints initially and ultimately involved in RA are listed in Table 12–15.

In the person with polyarticular inflammatory arthritis, laboratory and radiographic testing can be helpful to make a specific diagnosis. RF is found in approximately 80% of persons with RA. The presence of RF is helpful because it makes it much more likely that RA is the most likely diagnosis, and RA patients who are RF positive are more likely to have severe disease, as well as extra-articular features such as rheumatoid nodules, interstitial lung disease, and Felty's syndrome. But once an RF is found to be positive, there is no reason to order the test sequentially, because the titer does not correlate with disease activity. Another test that is helpful in this setting is testing for the IgM titer for parvovirus infection (especially if the person has been exposed to ill children), because an acute parvovi-

Table 12–13. Onset of rheumatoid arthritis in 300 patients with definite or classic disease

Characteristic		Percentage
1. Mode of onset	Rapid* (days or weeks)	46
	Insidious	54
2. Site of onset	Small joints	32
	Medium-sized joints	16
	Large joints	29
	Combined	26
3. Pattern of onset	Monoarticular	21
	Oligoarticular	44
	Polyarticular	35

*This time frame includes patients described in other studies as having "intermediate" onset.
From Fallahi S, Halla JT, Hardin JG: Clin Res 31:650A, 1983.

rus infection in adults can cause an inflammatory arthritis that resembles RA but remits in several months. In areas that are endemic for Lyme disease, this may be a helpful test, especially in those with a history of a tick bite or rash, or in persons with monoarticular or oligoarticular large joint involvement.

Early in RA, radiographs are not likely to show the characteristic erosions seen late in the disease. The most common radiographic finding in early RA is a normal film, with soft tissue swelling, and then periarticular osteopenia, being the next most common findings.

The involvement of certain joints by RA bears special mention. Cervical spine involvement is relatively common and the source of significant morbidity and mortality.[17] The most serious involvement involves C1 (particularly the transverse ligament) and C2 (especially the odontoid process), leading to C1–C2 instability. This should be considered in any patient with established RA who presents with neck pain and/or myelopathic symptoms or findings. Patients with long-standing RA who are undergoing surgery that would involve intubation should probably also be screened for this complication. These persons should have flexion-extension radiographs of the cervical spine and those with a preodontoid space of greater than 5 mm, an inadequate space available for the cord, or instability should be considered for surgical intervention.

Hand involvement is very common in RA. Although the distal interphalangeal joints are rarely involved in this disorder, nearly all other hand joints are commonly involved. The characteristic deformities seen in the digits (e.g., swan-neck deformity [Fig. 12–5], boutonnière deformity [Fig. 12–6], and ulnar deviation at the metacarpophalangeal joints [Fig. 12–7]) are due to a combination of joint destruction and ligament and tendon laxity. Tenosynovitis commonly can lead to clinical symptoms in RA, especially as trigger fingers when the flexor tendons of the digits are involved.

Extra-articular manifestations of RA are common, especially in persons with a positive serum RF. These nodules most commonly occur on the extensor surfaces of the arm in the olecranon region, but they can occur nearly anywhere in the body, particularly on other extensor surfaces (Fig. 12–8). The formation of nodules can become accelerated

Table 12–14. 1988 Revised American Rheumatological Association criteria for classification of rheumatoid arthritis

Criteria	Definition
1. Morning stiffness	Morning stiffness in and around the joints lasting at least 1 hour before maximal improvement
2. Arthritis of three or more joint areas	At least three joint areas have simultaneously had soft tissue swelling or fluid (not bony overgrowth alone) observed by a physician. The 14 possible joint areas are (right or left): proximal interphalangeal, metacarpophalangeal, wrist, elbow, knee, ankle, and metatarsophalangeal joints
3. Arthritis of hand joints	At least one joint area swollen as above in wrist, metacarpophalangeal, or proximal interphalangeal joint
4. Symmetrical arthritis	Simultaneous involvement of the same joint areas (as in 2) on both sides of the body (bilateral involvement of proximal interphalangeal, metacarpophalangeal, or metatarsophalangeal joints is acceptable without absolute symmetry)
5. Rheumatoid nodules	Subcutaneous nodules, over bony prominences, or extensor surfaces, or in juxta-articular regions, observed by a physician
6. Serum rheumatoid factor	Demonstration of abnormal amounts of serum "rheumatoid factor" by any method that has been positive in less than 5% of normal control subjects
7. Radiographic changes	Radiographic changes typical of rheumatoid arthritis on posteroanterior hand and wrist x-rays, which must include erosions or unequivocal bony decalcification localized to or most marked adjacent to the involved joints (osteoarthritis changes alone do not qualify)

For classification purposes, a patient is said to have rheumatoid arthritis if he or she has satisfied at least four of the above seven criteria. Criteria 1 through 4 must be present for at least 6 weeks. Patients with two clinical diagnoses are not excluded. Designation as classic, definite, or probable rheumatoid arthritis is *not* to be made.

in persons with RA given methotrexate, although the reason for this is not clear.

There are a variety of forms of pulmonary disease in RA. As with many cardiopulmonary manifestations in persons with autoimmune disorders, this occurs in nearly all RA patients in autopsy series but is less commonly clinically apparent. Interstitial fibrosis preferentially involving the basilar regions is most commonly seen. Pleural involvement, nodules in the lung (especially fulminant in coal

Table 12–15. Joints involved in rheumatoid arthritis*

	Percentage Initially Involved[55]			Percentage Ultimately Involved[50]
	Right	Left	Bilateral	
Metacarpophalangeal	65	58	52	87
Wrist	60	57	48	82
Proximal interphalangeal	63	53	45	63
Metatarsophalangeal	48	47	43	48
Shoulder	37	42	30	47
Knee	35	30	24	56
Ankle	25	23	18	53
Elbow	20	15	14	21

*Other joints (e.g., distal interphalangeal joints) are not tabulated here.
From Kelley WN, Harris ED Jr, Ruddy S, Sledge CB: Textbook of Rheumatology, 3rd ed. Philadelphia, WB Saunders, 1989, p 947.

miners and termed *Caplan's syndrome*), and bronchiolitis obliterans are also seen.

Cardiac involvement may include pericarditis, myocarditis, and cardiac conduction defects (perhaps due to rheumatoid nodules involving the conduction system) can be seen rarely in RA. Vasculitis may also occur in persons with RA, and in this setting is termed *rheumatoid vasculitis*. This can involve both small and medium-sized vessels of the skin, peripheral nerves, and visceral organs. Felty's syndrome is the combination of RA, splenomegaly, ischemic leg ulcers, and neutropenia. These persons also commonly exhibit lymphadenopathy and thrombocytopenia, and sometimes splenomegaly is necessary for effective treatment.

The natural history of RA has become better understood recently and has led to consideration of different treatment paradigms.[18] It has become increasingly clear that much of the joint damage in RA occurs in the first several years of the illness. Thus, old pyramid treatment strategies that slowly added one drug at a time have been replaced by more aggressive paradigms. Also, until approximately 10

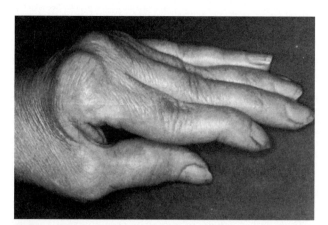

Figure 12–5. Early swan-neck deformity in rheumatoid arthritis. Synovial proliferation and early subluxation of the metacarpophalangeal joints are present as well. (Courtesy of G. Uribarri and the Ministerio de Sanidad y Consuma, Madrid, Spain. From Kelley WN, Harris ED Jr, Ruddy S, Sledge CB: Textbook of Rheumatology, 3rd ed. Philadelphia, WB Saunders, 1989, p 961.)

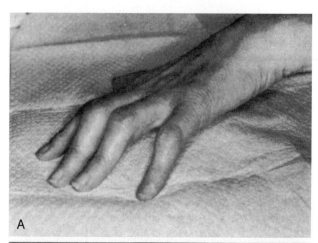

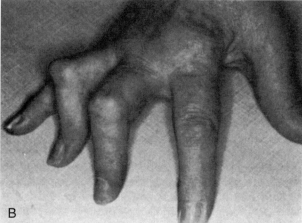

Figure 12–6. Early (A) and late (B) "boutonnière" deformity of the phalanges in rheumatoid arthritis. In B, moderate soft tissue swellings at the second and third metacarpophalangeal joints are visible. (From Kelley WN, Harris ED Jr, Ruddy S, Sledge CB: Textbook of Rheumatology, 3rd ed. Philadelphia, WB Saunders, 1989, p 962.)

years ago, RA had been considered an indolent, debilitating disorder characterized by the slow progressive course and eventual remission in some. It is now clear that patients with RA have significantly increased mortality and die 10 to 15 years earlier than expected.[19] This excess mortality appears to be multifactorial, including an increased risk of infections, cardiovascular disease, and pulmonary and gastrointestinal complications.

There is no unanimity on how exactly to treat RA, but nearly all persons without a contraindication to taking a nonsteroidal anti-inflammatory drug (NSAID) will benefit from taking this class of medication. It is unusual for RA to be controlled with this agent alone, and in milder disease a logical step is then to add hydroxychloroquine (200 mg twice daily).[20] The principal concern with this agent is retinal toxicity. Because of this, twice-yearly ophthalmologic examinations are typically recommended. For patients with more aggressive disease, or who fail hydroxychloroquine, weekly methotrexate is a logical next choice. This medication is typically given orally once weekly, beginning at 7.5 mg per week and escalating as high as 20 mg or more per week. Folic acid is typically coadministered at 1 mg/day to help avoid gastrointestinal toxicity. Short-term

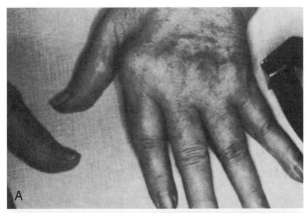

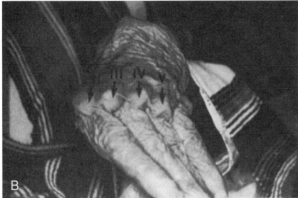

Figure 12–7. *A,* Early ulnar deviation of the metacarpophalangeal joints without subluxation. Extensor tendons have slipped to the ulnar side. The fifth finger, in particular, is compromised with weak flexion, causing loss of power grip. *B,* Complete subluxation with marked ulnar deviation at the metacarpophalangeal joints of a 90-year-old woman with rheumatoid arthritis. *Arrows* mark the heads of the metacarpals, now in direct contact with the joint capsule instead of the proximal phalanges. (Courtesy of James L. McGuire, M.D.)

side effects of this medication include diarrhea, nausea, fatigue, and stomatitis, whereas the more serious toxicities are liver disease and hypersensitivity pneumonitis. For patients who fail methotrexate, new agents such as leflunomide and anti–tumor necrosis factor agents are extremely effective. When and where to use corticosteroids in the chronic treatment of RA remains controversial, with some data suggesting that long-term, low-dose (e.g., <10 mg/day) prednisone is both helpful and relatively free of side effects.

Osteoarthritis

Osteoarthritis (OA) likely represents a number of different pathologic processes all characterized by progressive loss of articular cartilage and by new bone formation in the subchondral region (sclerosis) and the joint margins (osteophytes). OA is the most common joint disease, affecting the majority of people older than age 65 and nearly all people older than age 80.[21, 22] Although increasing age is the single largest risk factor for OA, other genetic and environmental factors play a role, especially for certain joints. For example, genetics plays a significant role in OA

of the hands, especially in women. In the knee, genetic factors play a minor role. For this joint, obesity, decreased muscle strength in the quadriceps, and a history of major trauma to this joint are the most consistently identified risk factors for OA. Although major trauma to any joint can lead to OA, and certain occupations have an increased incidence of OA, in general, use, and even mild overuse, is not a risk factor for OA. Finally, some joints rarely develop OA, such as the elbow, wrist, and shoulder.

The precise pathologic mechanisms leading to osteoarthritis are unclear. Most believe that this disease process is a result of an interaction between abnormal biology of cartilage and bone and/or abnormal forces being applied to the joints. With respect to biology, one of the earliest changes seen in OA is *increased* cartilage thickness. This early increase in thickness is likely due to increased water content of the cartilage due to disruption of the collagen network. Chondrocytes respond to this process by increasing proteoglycan synthesis. This early phase of hypertrophy of cartilage is followed by loss of cartilage and a decrease in proteoglycan synthesis. Figure 12–9 demonstrates the progressive nature of the process from this point forward. In the early stages of cartilage loss there is the development of small crevices or clefts in the cartilage and, with contin-

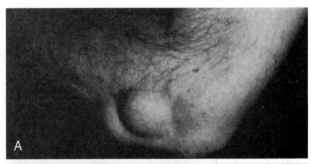

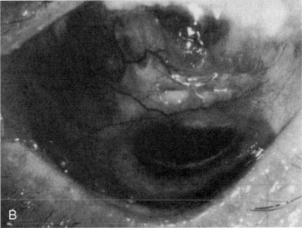

Figure 12–8. Manifestations of increased reactivity of mesenchymal tissue in rheumatoid arthritis appearing *(A)* as nodules on the elbow and *(B)* within the sclera of the eye. The eye lesion represents scleral perforation associated with a granulomatous scleral reaction. Treatment was placement of a scleral patch graft. Note the great increase in the vascularity of the sclera. The dark areas represent scleral thinning with exposure of the uveal pigment. (Patient of Drs. S. Arthur Bourchoff and G. N. Fouhls. Photograph courtesy of Marty Schener.)

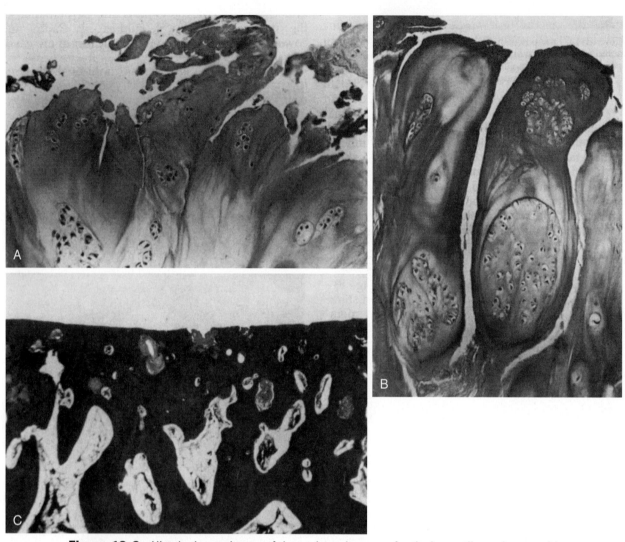

Figure 12–9. Histologic specimens of the various degrees of articular cartilage change with advancing degrees of osteoarthritis. *A,* The surface from a site on the femoral head with osteoarthritis, demonstrating surface irregularities, early cloning of the cells, and altered matrix staining (H & E, ×200). *B,* The changes of more advanced disease, demonstrating the deepening of the clefts to the radial zone, altered matrix staining, and large clones of cells (H & E, ×200). *C,* The appearance of end-stage disease with complete denudation of the surface and eburnation and sclerotization of the underlying bone (H & E, ×95). (From Kelley WN, Harris ED Jr, Ruddy S, Sledge CB: Textbook of Rheumatology, 3rd ed. Philadelphia, WB Saunders, 1989, p 1486.)

ued time and use, these clefts deepen and widen and the chondrocytes cluster, forming clones of cells. Finally, there is complete loss of cartilage and denudation of the bone. Bone responds in a number of ways to the cartilaginous changes that occur in OA. Appositional bone growth occurs in the exposed subchondral regions, leading to sclerosis. At the joint margins, bone and cartilage grow and lead to the formation of osteophytes (Fig. 12–10).

Abnormal forces can lead to the development of OA, even if biology is not abnormal. The examples of OA caused by trauma or repetitive activities are evidence of this phenomenon. Once OA has begun, whether the initial problem is biologic or mechanical, abnormal forces usually play a role. This is particularly true in weight-bearing joints.

The diagnosis of OA is based on appropriate symptoms and radiographic findings. The most common symptom of OA is pain. The pain is frequently deep, aching, and poorly localized. Early in the course of the illness the pain will typically be primarily with use of the affected joint, whereas later in the disease the pain may occur even at rest. Because OA is not an inflammatory condition, there is minimal (i.e., less than 30 minutes) morning stiffness. Other symptoms may include crepitus, limitation of motion, and giving way of joints.

Plain radiographs remain the gold standard for diagnosing OA, although there are several caveats necessary to interpret this information correctly. The classic findings in OA are joint space narrowing (in many cases asymmetrical), sclerosis of subchondral bone, and the formation of marginal osteophytes and cysts. Studies that have compared the results of radiographs with the findings on arthroscopy

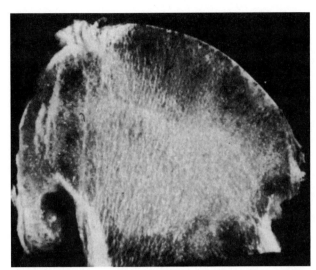

Figure 12–10. Cut section of an osteoarthritic femoral head showing the large osteophyte arising from the lateral aspect of the cartilaginous surface. (From Kelley WN, Harris ED Jr, Ruddy S, Sledge CB: Textbook of Rheumatology, 3rd ed. Philadelphia, WB Saunders, 1989, p 1482.)

have demonstrated that mild changes of OA may be visualized by arthroscopy before any radiographic abnormalities are present. This is not of substantial clinical consequence because most of these persons are asymptomatic. A larger problem with interpreting radiographs is that a minority of people with radiographic evidence of OA will be symptomatic. The reason for this disparity between radiographic changes and the presence of pain and disability is not clear, and this discrepancy is not only seen in OA but in nearly any chronic pain condition.[23] Nonetheless, this points out that nonmechanical mechanisms may be operative in many persons who present with pain and are found to have osteoarthritis. In individual patients, in whom there is a poor relationship between symptoms and pathology, treatments such as those described for nonanatomic pain syndromes such as fibromyalgia should be considered.

The management of osteoarthritis is primarily nonsurgical, until very late in the disease. Several nonpharmacologic therapies have been shown to be effective in randomized controlled trials, including patient education, weight loss (in persons who are obese, particularly for the knee), strengthening exercises (again, especially for the knee), and aerobic exercise.[24] The Arthritis Foundation has established many of these programs and is a valuable resource for this type of patient information.

In persons who do not respond to nonpharmacologic therapy, acetaminophen is the drug of choice.[25] In patients who fail acetaminophen alone, topical capsaicin cream or intra-articular corticosteroids can be considered, especially for the knee joint. If these treatments are ineffective, then low doses of NSAIDs, followed by high doses of NSAIDs, are a reasonable option (see Pharmacologic Therapy). Several new therapies for OA of the knee have recently emerged, but their place in the treatment algorithm remains unclear. Some small randomized controlled trials studies have suggested that glucosamine and chondroitin sulfate may be effective in relieving pain in OA of the knee.

Large-scale studies are now being conducted to confirm these findings. Also, the U.S. Food and Drug Administration has approved two intra-articular hyaluronic acid preparations for use in knee OA. Both of these products must be given with a series of injections and were shown to be more effective than sham injection and the use of acetaminophen. This treatment modality may be most effective in those who have a contraindication to using an NSAID or who have failed a trial of several NSAIDs.

Fibromyalgia and Regional Soft Tissue Rheumatism

Fibromyalgia is the second most common rheumatic condition in the United States after osteoarthritis. It affects approximately 2% of the population, women much more than men. In the classic form, this condition is characterized by widespread musculoskeletal pain and diffuse soft tissue tenderness. The American College of Rheumatology criteria for this illness require that a person have pain throughout the entire body, as well as in 11 of 18 tender points, but many persons with the clinical diagnosis of fibromyalgia will only exhibit pain in a few regions of their body or have fewer than 11 tender points.[26]

This diagnosis should be suspected when a person presents with multifocal pain and there is no evidence of inflammation or damage to peripheral structures on physical examination and/or further diagnostic workup. Other clinical features that occur commonly in the setting of fibromyalgia are fatigue, insomnia, memory or concentration difficulties, headaches, and irritable bowel symptoms. It is also common to find a lifetime history of chronic pain in other regions of the body, such as the neck, back, or temporomandibular joint. Routine laboratory testing will be normal in this condition, and imaging studies will either be normal or detect abnormalities of uncertain clinical significance (e.g., mild degenerative changes, bulging disks).

There is considerable evidence that the pain in fibromyalgia occurs because of a disorder in the central nervous system processing of sensory stimuli, and thus this condition typically does not respond to analgesics that act primarily in the periphery such as acetaminophen and NSAIDs. Low doses of tricyclic drugs such as cyclobenzaprine (Flexeril) and amitriptyline (Elavil) given at bedtime can be effective analgesics in this setting. These drugs should be initiated at very low doses (e.g., 10 mg), given several hours before bedtime, and escalated slowly (e.g., 10 mg every 1 to 2 weeks). The maximum dose is 40 mg of cyclobenzaprine, or approximately 70 mg of amitriptyline, but side effects of dry eyes and mouth, morning sedation, constipation, and weight gain sometimes prevent dose escalation. Other drugs such as tramadol (Ultram) and venlafaxine (Effexor, using the extended-release form once in the morning) can also be beneficial. In addition to pharmacologic therapy, other treatment modalities may be helpful. Low-impact aerobic exercise can be particularly useful, but as with the tricyclic drugs this should be started very slowly and increased very gradually. Cognitive behavioral therapy or other structured pain management programs are also very beneficial.

Table 12–16. Contrasting clinical features between rheumatoid arthritis and ankylosing spondylitis

Feature	Rheumatoid Arthritis	Ankylosing Spondylitis
Joint distribution	Polyarthropathy Symmetrical Small and large Upper > lower limb	Oligoarthropathy Asymmetrical Large > small Lower > upper limb
Sacroiliac	−	+
Spine involvement	Cervical	Total: ascending
Nodules	+	−
Eyes	Sicca syndrome Scleritis Scleromalacia perforans	Uveitis
Aortic regurgitation	−	+
Lungs	Caplan's syndrome Effusions	Upper lobe pulmonary fibrosis

Seronegative Spondyloarthropathies

The four classic seronegative spondyloarthropathies are ankylosing spondylitis, reactive arthritis, inflammatory bowel disease–associated arthropathy, and psoriatic arthritis. These disorders are considered together because they share an immunologic predisposition (HLA-B27) that leads to (1) similar articular features (an inflammatory arthritis involving the axial skeleton) and (2) common extra-articular features (e.g., inflammatory eye disease, cardiac conduction defects, aortic valve disease).[27–29] Even the approximately 80% of individuals who are HLA-B27 positive but do not develop a seronegative spondyloarthropathy have an independent risk of developing the classic extra-articular features seen in this spectrum of illness.

ANKYLOSING SPONDYLITIS

Ankylosing spondylitis is the prototypical disease in this category. The characteristic features of this illness are contrasted to RA in Table 12–16. The earliest joint involved in most persons with this disorder is the sacroiliac joint. Clinically, these individuals will complain of indolent onset of morning stiffness and pain involving the low back that typically improves with exercise. Other characteristic features of the pain seen in ankylosing spondyltitis, as well as the symptoms that help differentiate mechanical back disease from inflammatory back disease, are shown in Tables 12–17 and 12–18. On physical examination, individuals with sacroiliac involvement will usually demonstrate limited motion in this area of the body. The most commonly performed test to demonstrate this is the modified Shober test.[30] In this test, a mark is made on the skin overlying the spine where an imaginary line would connect the left and right posterior iliac spines. Another dot is placed 10 cm higher, and the patient is asked to maximally flex forward. The distance in normal individuals should increase to at least 15 cm, and if it does not, it suggests that there is some limitation of motion in this region.

The classic radiographic findings of ankylosing spondylitis include sacroiliitis, enthesopathy (periostitis at tendon and ligament insertions), and ankylosis (fusion) (Figs. 12–11 and 12–12).[31] In the spine, the initial change seen is a loss of concavity of vertebral bodies due to enthesopathic disease, eventually followed by fusion, leading to the classic bamboo spine (Figs. 12–13 through 12–15). It is important to differentiate this finding from that of diffuse idiopathic skeletal hyperostosis, in which the hyperostoses are thicker and typically only involve the right side of the

Table 12–17. Characteristic features of back pain (or discomfort) in ankylosing spondylitis

1. Age at onset younger than 40 years
2. Insidious onset
3. Duration greater than 3 months
4. Association with morning stiffness
5. Improvement with exercise

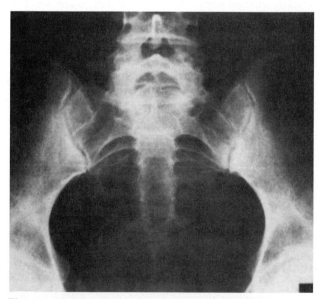

Figure 12–11. Minimal sacroiliitis (grade II). Note juxta-articular sclerosis, blurring of joint margin, minimal erosions, and some joint space narrowing in this 35-year-old woman. (From Kelley WN, Harris ED Jr, Ruddy S, Sledge CB: Textbook of Rheumatology, 3rd ed. Philadelphia, WB Saunders, 1989, p 1029.)

Table 12–18. Differential history in back symptoms of mechanical and inflammatory type

	Mechanical	Inflammatory
Past history	±	+ +
Family history	−	+
Onset	Acute	Insidious
Age (years)	15–90	<40
Sleep disturbance	±	+ +
Morning stiffness	+	+ + +
Involvement of other systems	−	+
Effect of exercise	Worse	Better
Effect of rest	Better	Worse
Radiation of pain	Anatomic (S1, L5)	Diffuse (thoracic, buttock)
Sensory symptoms	+	−
Motor symptoms	+	−

thoracic spine. In addition to an inflammatory arthritis involving the axial skeleton, patients with ankylosing spondylitis may also develop peripheral joint involvement. Women may be more likely than men to have primarily peripheral joint involvement, as well as isolated cervical involvement.[32]

The extra-articular manifestations of ankylosing spondylitis are similar to those that can occur in the other seroneg-

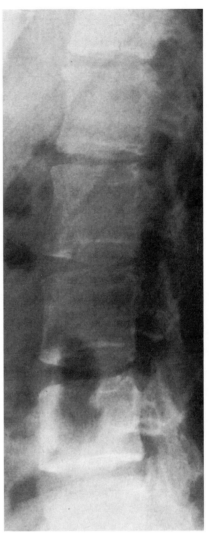

Figure 12–13. Ankylosing spondylitis. Note loss of concavity of lumbar vertebra due to enthesopathic disease. (From Kelley WN, Harris ED Jr, Ruddy S, Sledge CB: Textbook of Rheumatology, 3rd ed. Philadelphia, WB Saunders, 1989, p 1031.)

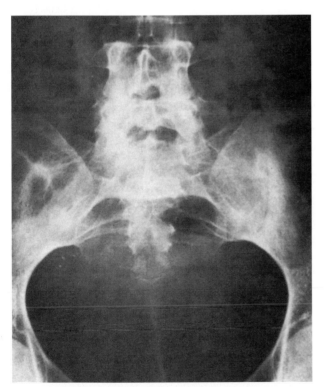

Figure 12–12. Moderate sacroiliitis (grade III) on the left side; note juxta-articular sclerosis and further loss of joint space. Right side shows total ankylosis (grade IV) in this 40-year-old woman. (From Kelley WN, Harris ED Jr, Ruddy S, Sledge CB: Textbook of Rheumatology, 3rd ed. Philadelphia, WB Saunders, 1989, p 1029.)

ative arthropathies. Inflammatory anterior eye disease (uveitis or iritis) typically presents as unilateral eye pain, photophobia, and blurred vision. Cardiac conduction defects may occur in up to 7% of patients with long-standing disease, and aortic insufficiency may occur in 10% of patients with chronic disease. Interstitial lung disease in this illness has an unusual predilection for the upper lobes. Neurologic involvement is rare but can be catastrophic, usually when a patient with a fused spine is involved in trauma, and may present as paresis.

Laboratory testing is generally unhelpful, except in some cases to rule out other disorders. Inflammatory indices such as the ESR and CRP may be elevated. In persons with inflammatory peripheral arthritis, an RF (which will be negative, thus the term *seronegative spondyloarthropathy*) is useful. Testing for HLA-B27 is rarely indicated, because this haplotype is seen in about 6% of whites (lesser percentages of Asians and blacks) and only about 20% of those who are positive will develop this disorder.

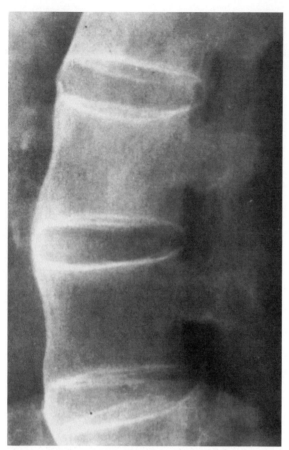

Figure 12–14. Ankylosing spondylitis. Note syndesmophyte formation (ossification in anterior fibers of annulus fibrosus). (From Kelley WN, Harris ED Jr, Ruddy S, Sledge CB: Textbook of Rheumatology, 3rd ed. Philadelphia, WB Saunders, 1989, p 1031.)

The first-line treatment of the seronegative spondyloarthropathies is with the NSAIDs. There is some evidence, primarily anecdotal, that indomethacin is the most effective of the commonly used NSAIDs, especially when given at 150 mg/day. Patients should be encouraged to remain active and to routinely do stretching exercises to maintain chest expansion, cervical extension, and lumbar flexion. Sulfasalazine is typically the slow-acting antirheumatic drug chosen to control symptoms of this illness unresponsive to NSAIDs. This drug is typically begun at 1000 mg twice daily, with the maximum dose being a total of 4 g per day.

REACTIVE ARTHRITIS

Reactive arthritis is classically described by the clinical triad of arthritis, urethritis, and conjunctivitis. Since the initial description, it has become clear that there are several variations on this theme, with some individuals having only two of three manifestations (i.e., incomplete reactive arthritis) and others having colitis instead of urethritis. This syndrome typically develops in a genetically susceptible host after the infection of the genitourinary or gastrointestinal tract with organisms such as *Chlamydia, Salmonella, Shigella, Yersinia,* or *Campylobacter.* The term *reactive arthritis* is used to refer to this phenomenon.

The arthritis that occurs in reactive arthritides is typically an asymmetrical, oligoarticular, inflammatory arthritis that has a predilection for the large joints of the lower extremities. Occasionally, the synovial fluid cell counts in this disorder can be very high, in the range normally only seen in septic arthritis. In addition to the joint involvement, inflammation of tendinous insertion into bone is common, such as the Achilles tendon or plantar fascia. Another characteristic finding related to the presence of an enthesopathy is the finding of a sausage digit, a diffusely swollen toe or finger due to the presence of both synovitis and enthesopathy (Fig. 12–16). In addition to the peripheral arthritis that accompanies the acute illness, some persons with reactive arthritis will develop a spondyloarthropathy similar to ankylosing spondylitis. This process is typically less symmetrical than ankylosing spondylitis, and the syndesmophytes are usually larger.

Other clinical features may commonly be seen on initial presentation (Table 12–19). Urethritis is more likely to be symptomatic in males than in females, and involvement of other portions of the urogenital tract (e.g., cystitis, prostatitis) may also occur. Eye disease is most commonly conjunctivitis, but uveitis and iritis may also be seen. There

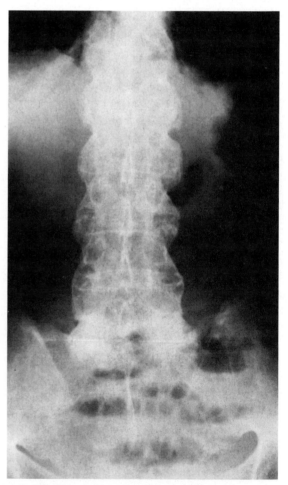

Figure 12–15. Ankylosing spondylitis. Late stage. Note paraspinal ossification and fused sacroiliac joint. (From Kelley WN, Harris ED Jr, Ruddy S, Sledge CB: Textbook of Rheumatology, 3rd ed. Philadelphia, WB Saunders, 1989, p 1032.)

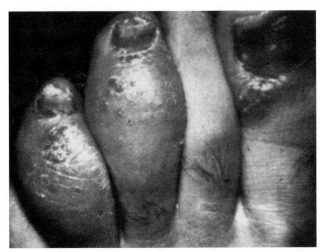

Figure 12–16. Reactive arthritis. Note two "sausage" digits (dactylitis) and typical nail changes. (From Kelley WN, Harris ED Jr, Ruddy S, Sledge CB: Textbook of Rheumatology, 3rd ed. Philadelphia, WB Saunders, 1989, p 1043.)

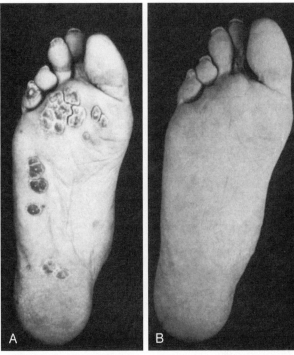

Figure 12–17. Reactive arthritis. *A*, Keratoderma blennorrhagicum on sole of foot. Note hyperkeratotic lesions. *B*, Same foot as shown in *A*, 6 weeks later. Note total healing of lesions. (From Kelley WN, Harris ED Jr, Ruddy S, Sledge CB: Textbook of Rheumatology, 3rd ed. Philadelphia, WB Saunders, 1989, p 1043.)

are a variety of distinctive mucocutaneous features that can be seen, including stomatitis, keratoderma blennorrhagicum (Figs. 12–17 and 12–18), circinate balanitis (Fig. 12–19), and nail changes (Fig. 12–20).

In the patient who presents with the classic triad of findings, the diagnosis of reactive arthritis is straightforward. With atypical presentations, other diagnoses must be considered, including gonococcal arthritis, Lyme disease, rheumatic fever, and crystal-induced arthropathies. The similarities and differences between reactive arthritis and gonococcal arthritis are particularly important and are listed in Tables 12–20 and 12–21.

Just as with the other seronegative spondyloarthropathies, NSAIDs are the treatment of choice, and indomethacin is the drug most frequently used. In cases of acute reactive arthritis unresponsive to indomethacin, phenylbutazone may be helpful. Anecdotal evidence suggests that

Table 12–19. Characteristics of 131 consecutive patients with reactive arthritis, at initial visit

Total (n = 131)	%
Arthritis	100
Monoarthritis	4
Polyarthritis	96
Urethritis/cervicitis	90
Diarrhea	18
Eye disease	63
Back pain	72
Heel pain	56
Tendinitis	52
Balanitis	46
Stomatitis	27
Keratoderma	22
Nail lesions	6

From Kelley WN, Harris ED Jr, Ruddy S, Sledge CB: Textbook of Rheumatology, 3rd. ed. Philadelphia, WB Saunders, 1989, p 1042.

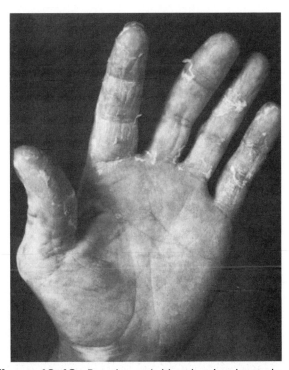

Figure 12–18. Reactive arthritis, showing keratoderma blennorrhagicum. Note scaling lesions on palms. (From Kelley WN, Harris ED Jr, Ruddy S, Sledge CB: Textbook of Rheumatology, 3rd ed. Philadelphia, WB Saunders, 1989, p 1044.)

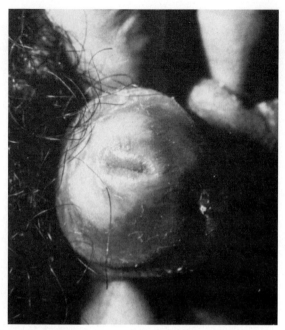

Figure 12–19. Reactive arthritis, showing circinate balanitis. Note superficial ulceration. (From Kelley WN, Harris ED Jr, Ruddy S, Sledge CB: Textbook of Rheumatology, 3rd ed. Philadelphia, WB Saunders, 1989, p 1045.)

Table 12–20. Similarities between reactive arthritis and gonococcal arthropathy

Feature	Reactive Arthritis	Gonococcal Arthropathy
Oligoarthritis	+	+
Tenosynovitis	+	+
Conjunctivitis	+	+
Urethritis	+	+
Skin lesions	+	+
Fever	+	+
Urethral cultures for gonococcus	? +	? +
Sexual activity	+	+
Synovial fluid	Variable	Variable

From Kelley WN, Harris ED Jr, Ruddy S, Sledge CB: Textbook of Rheumatology, 3rd. ed. Philadelphia, WB Saunders, 1989, p 1048.

like antibiotics have improved the course of this illness, a prolonged course of antibiotics may be considered in the acute phase.[33] Some patients with reactive arthritis will have an acute self-limited course, but most will develop chronic symptoms. These patients with chronic disease may benefit from the addition of drugs such as sulfasalazine or methotrexate.

PSORIATIC ARTHRITIS

Psoriatic arthritis shares many features with reactive arthritis, and in some instances these two conditions are indistinguishable. The presence of psoriasis is necessary for the diagnosis of psoriatic arthritis (although in some

the acute phase of this illness is less responsive to systemic corticosteroids than other types of inflammatory arthritis, but topical corticosteroids may be helpful for extra-articular features. Because of the infectious triggers of this illness, and because some trials have suggested that tetracycline-

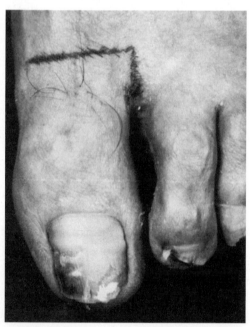

Figure 12–20. Reactive arthritis, showing nail lesions. Note typical destructive nature of changes with subungual hyperkeratotic accumulation of material. (From Kelley WN, Harris ED Jr, Ruddy S, Sledge CB: Textbook of Rheumatology, 3rd ed. Philadelphia, WB Saunders, 1989, p 1045.)

Table 12–21. Differences between reactive arthritis and gonococcal arthritis

Feature	Reactive Arthritis	Gonococcal Arthritis
Sex distribution	Males > females	Males < females
Personal or family history of arthritis	+	−
Uveitis	+	−
Gonococcus culture		
Joint	−	? +
Skin	−	? +
Pharynx	−	? +
Rectum	−	? +
Back pain	+	−
Migratory arthralgias	−	+
Joint distribution	Lower > upper	Lower < upper
Achilles tendinitis	+	−
Plantar fasciitis	+	−
Massive recurrent knee effusion	+	−
Stomatitis	+	−
Balanitis	+	−
Keratoderma blenorrhagicum	+	−
Response to penicillin	−	+
HLA-B27 (%)	80	5
Course	Recurrent/chronic	Acute

From Kelley WN, Harris ED Jr, Ruddy S, Sledge CB: Textbook of Rheumatology, 3rd. ed. Philadelphia, WB Saunders, 1989, p 1048.

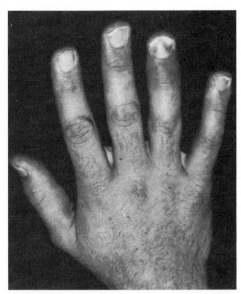

Figure 12–21. Hand showing prominent psoriatic nail involvement of fourth finger and swelling of the fourth distal interphalangeal joint. (From Kelley WN, Harris ED Jr, Ruddy S, Sledge CB: Textbook of Rheumatology, 3rd ed. Philadelphia, WB Saunders, 1989, p 1055.)

instances the arthritis antedates the rash). However, only about 5% of individuals with psoriasis develop psoriatic arthritis. The axial skeleton involvement, and extra-articular features, are similar in psoriatic arthritis and reactive arthritis. One distinctive feature of psoriatic arthritis is more extensive involvement of the distal interphalangeal joints and the relationship between this feature and nail pitting (Fig. 12–21). Only about 20% of persons with psoriasis have nail pitting, but 80% of persons with psoriatic arthritis have nail pitting. Other unusual articular features seen in some patients with psoriatic arthritis are resorption of the tufts of the distal phalanges, peripheral joint ankylosis, and characteristic pencil-in-cup deformities (Fig. 12–22).

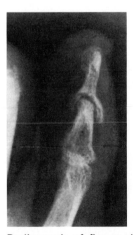

Figure 12–22. Radiograph of finger showing pencil-in-cup deformity. (From Kelley WN, Harris ED Jr, Ruddy S, Sledge CB: Textbook of Rheumatology, 3rd ed. Philadelphia, WB Saunders, 1989, p 1059.)

ARTHROPATHY ASSOCIATED WITH INFLAMMATORY BOWEL DISEASE

Enteropathic arthritis is the term commonly used to describe the arthritides associated with inflammatory bowel disease. The two main forms of enteropathic arthritis are (1) acute episodes of peripheral oligoarticular arthritis that resemble reactive arthritis and are typically associated with flares of the colitis, and (2) an axial spondyloarthropathy that is closely related to HLA-B27 positivity and follows a slow, indolent course that is largely independent of the bowel disease.

Crystal-Induced Arthropathies

There are three types of crystal-induced arthropathies that will be discussed: (1) gout, (2) calcium pyrophosphate deposition disease (CPPD), and (3) hydroxyapatite deposition disease (HADD). Nearly any crystalline or particular substance that can somehow be introduced into the joint or soft tissues (e.g., injected corticosteroid, fragments from prostheses, plant thorns) can lead to a localized inflammatory response.[34]

GOUT

Although gout refers to the disease process that occurs when monosodium urate crystals deposit in various tissues in the body, only the articular manifestations will be emphasized. The serum uric acid concentration largely determines whether monosodium urate crystals will deposit in tissues. Purine metabolism is largely genetically determined, but male gender, increased age, increased body weight, high purine diet, diabetes, hypertension, and alcohol and other drugs (e.g., diuretics, cyclosporine) will raise the serum concentration of uric acid.[35] The higher the serum uric acid concentration, the more likely an individual will develop gout. It is important to recognize, however, that only a small percentage of hyperuricemic individuals ever develop gout.

Rheumatic features of gout include some combination of acute attacks of monoarticular or polyarticular arthritis and more indolent changes caused by accumulation of uric acid crystals (tophi). The first metatarsophalangeal joint of the foot is the most commonly involved joint during the first gout attack.[36] Other peripheral joints in the lower extremity (e.g., other metatarsophalangeal joints, midfoot, ankle, knee) are next most commonly involved, followed by peripheral joints in the hand (e.g., distal or proximal interphalangeal, metacarpaphalangeal, wrist). The predilection for peripheral joints farthest from the core of the body is likely due to temperature. Uric acid solubility decreases considerably as temperature decreases; thus, in the setting of a high serum (and thus tissue) uric acid value, crystal formation and deposition occur in these cooler areas of the body. For this same reason, acute gout is rarely seen in the axial skeleton. This temperature-related decrease in solubility may also explain why acute attacks of gout frequently occur at 2 or 3 o'clock in the morning, abruptly awakening an individual from sleep. During this time period, a person's core body temperature falls slightly due to diurnal changes and the inactivity of the extremity also contributes to decreased blood flow and cooler peripheral temperatures.

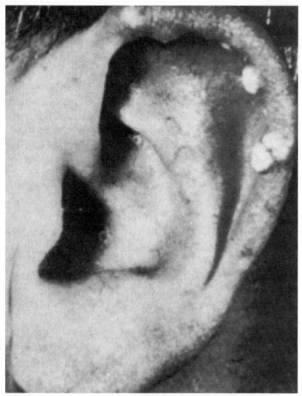

Figure 12–23. Multiple tophi of the helix of the ear. (From Kelley WN, Harris ED Jr, Ruddy S, Sledge CB: Textbook of Rheumatology, 3rd ed. Philadelphia, WB Saunders, 1989, p 1399.)

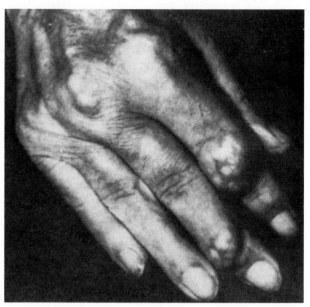

Figure 12–24. Tophi of dorsal aspects of index and second fingers, over distal interphalangeal joints. Subcutaneous urate deposits are easily visible. (From Kelley WN, Harris ED Jr, Ruddy S, Sledge CB: Textbook of Rheumatology, 3rd ed. Philadelphia, WB Saunders, 1989.)

An acute gout attack will usually begin as a monoarticular process, and with chronicity it may become polyarticular. Men are much more likely to be affected than women, largely because at any given age men have higher serum uric acid levels. Postmenopausal females may develop gout, but even then this usually occurs because of other risk factors (e.g., alcohol or medication use). During an acute attack, a person may be febrile, and there is typically an acute inflammatory response evident over the involved region. This inflammatory response is so pronounced that it is common for the skin overlying an attack to desquamate after the attack has subsided. This acute inflammatory response can also resemble cellulitis, especially when it occurs in the mid- or hindfoot or dorsum of the wrist. In addition to articular involvement and soft tissue inflammation, an acute bursitis can sometimes occur, especially in the olecranon region.

When a 50-year-old man presents with acute onset of metatarsophalangeal joint arthritis, the diagnosis of gout is straightforward. In many settings, other clinical information is necessary to establish the diagnosis. The presence of tophi is helpful. Tophi may occur in various locations in the body, including the helix of the ear (Fig. 12–23), fingers (Fig. 12–24), or olecranon region (Fig. 12–25). Laboratory testing is not typically useful. Most people with gout will

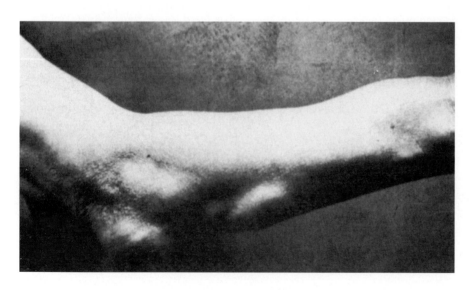

Figure 12–25. Lumpy tophi of olecranon bursa, ulnar surface, and wrist. (From Kelley WN, Harris ED Jr, Ruddy S, Sledge CB: Textbook of Rheumatology, 3rd ed. Philadelphia, WB Saunders, 1989, p 1401.)

have an elevated uric acid level during an acute attack, but some will not. Many persons will exhibit a leukocytosis, or elevations in inflammatory indices, but these will not help differentiate the patient with gout from those with other types of inflammatory arthritis. Radiographs during an acute attack will typically be normal or just reveal soft tissue swelling; in chronic tophaceous disease, radiographs will show evidence of sclerotic marginal erosions, typically with preservation of the joint space until late in the disease.

The detection of monosodium urate crystals in the joint fluid is the most definitive way to establish the diagnosis of gout. Uric acid crystals are thin, needle-shaped crystals that are approximately the same length as a leukocyte, and in fact they may be seen inside leukocytes. Under a polarizing microscope, the crystals will appear bright yellow and blue, depending on the axis of polarization. This is in contrast to calcium pyrophosphate crystals, which are pleomorphic in both size and shape, are less intensely birefringent, and thus appear pale yellow and blue.

The management of gout can be divided into treatment of the acute attack and prophylaxis against future attacks. The goal in treating the acute attack is to inhibit the ability of white blood cells to phagocytize the crystals. The most effective drugs in this setting are the NSAIDs, and indomethacin is a preferred agent because of the rapid onset of action and potent anti-inflammatory properties. Any other NSAID can also be used, but those with a rapid onset of action are preferred. Colchicine can also be helpful during an acute attack of gout, although the gastrointestinal intolerance of this medication frequently limits the effectiveness. Typically, the patient is instructed to take 0.6-mg tablets once hourly until the attack subsides, until side effects occur, or until a total of 10 tablets is taken. Colchicine, and to a lesser extent NSAIDs, is much more effective when treatment is begun rapidly. The likely reason for this is that these anti-inflammatory regimens (especially colchicine) act in part by inhibiting chemotaxis of leukocytes to the joint; once this has occurred, these agents are much less effective. In persons with contraindications to colchicine (renal or hepatic impairment) or NSAIDs, corticosteroids can be effectively used to treat acute gout attacks. These can be administered intra-articularly (if there is monoarticular involvement) or systemically. When these are given systemically, the person typically needs to receive treatment for several days to avoid a rebound effect (alternatively, a single intramuscular dose of a depot form of corticosteroids can be given).

When persons have frequent attacks of gout, or when there is evidence of tophaceous (or extra-articular) disease, therapy directed toward lowering the serum uric acid level should be considered. A low purine diet, or avoiding alcohol use, is sometimes all that is necessary to lower serum uric acids. If behavioral modifications are ineffective, then either uricosuric drugs or allopurinol can be used. These drugs should not be used in the setting of an acute attack, because this can paradoxically precipitate a worsening of the attack. Probenecid is the most commonly used uricosuric drug; it can be started at 500 mg/day and increased to 2 g/day and is given in divided doses. This drug is effective only in persons with relatively normal renal function and should not be used in those with a history of nephrolithiasis, and patients must be counseled to maintain a high fluid intake. Alternatively, allopurinol can be given beginning at doses ranging from 100 mg (in the elderly or those with impaired renal function) to 300 mg once daily. The principal concern with this drug is hypersensitivity reaction, so patients must be warned to stop this medication immediately if they develop a rash or pruritus. About 5% of individuals taking allopurinol will develop a pruritic maculopapular rash that resolves when the medication is stopped. However, a small percentage of these patients will go on to develop a serious and sometimes fatal hypersensitivity reaction reminiscent of a Stevens-Johnson reaction. An alternative approach to prophylaxis against gout attacks is to use a low dose of colchicine (e.g., 0.6 mg twice daily in persons with normal renal and hepatic function) or an NSAID chronically.

CALCIUM PYROPHOSPHATE DEPOSITION DISEASE

CPPD crystals can be deposited in a number of articular structures, including cartilage, synovium, tendons, and ligaments. In most cases there is no clear reason why a person has CPPD deposition (i.e., idiopathic), whereas in other instances this occurs as a hereditary disorder or secondary to another disease process (Table 12–22).[37] Having CPPD is not necessarily associated with any disease, because a significant percentage of persons with this finding will be asymptomatic. For instance, it is estimated that nearly 50% of individuals have CPPD of the knees by the time they reach age 80. In other instances, CPPD deposition is associated with disease. The disease processes commonly seen in association with CPPD include episodes of acute or chronic inflammatory arthritis (pseudogout), as well as an accelerated chronic degenerative arthritis (pseudo-osteoarthritis).

CPPD is diagnosed with a combination of appropriate clinical findings, radiographs, and synovial fluid analysis.

Table 12–22. Classification and possible disease associations of CPPD

Sporadic (idiopathic)
Hereditary
Secondary
Association strong
　Hyperparathyroidism
　Hemochromatosis
　Hypomagnesemia
　Aging
Association likely
　Osteoarthritis
　Amyloid disease
　Barter's syndrome
　Hypermobility syndrome
　Hypocalciuric hypercalcemia
　Hypothyroidism
Association weak
　Ochronosis
　Paget's disease
　Wilson's disease
　Acromegaly
　Diabetes mellitus
　Gout

From Kelley WN, Harris ED Jr, Ruddy S, Sledge CB: Textbook of Rheumatology, 3rd ed. Philadelphia, WB Saunders, 1989, p 1450.

The joint distribution of CPPD overlaps somewhat with similar disorders (e.g., gout, osteoarthritis), but the overall pattern of involvement can be helpful in differentiating these disorders. The knees, hips, symphysis pubis, and wrist are all common locations for CPPD deposition, and radiographs of these regions will commonly show the typical chondrocalcinosis (i.e., calcification of cartilage) (Figs. 12–26 and 12–27). In the knee, chondrocalcinosis may be seen in either the tibiofemoral joint or the patellofemoral joint, with the latter sometimes being preferentially involved. Another clinical clue to the presence of CPPD is more aggressive destruction of the joint than would otherwise be expected in osteoarthritis. Synovial fluid analysis identifying the characteristic rod-shaped (and pleomorphic) crystals of CPPD is helpful.

The treatment of CPPD depends somewhat on the mode of presentation. If CPPD is secondary to a metabolic disorder, then this obviously should be addressed. If CPPD presents as pseudogout, the treatment is very similar to that of gout noted earlier. Both NSAIDs and corticosteroids can be used to manage acute attacks, and colchicine is even somewhat efficacious, although less so than for gout. Both NSAIDs and colchicine can be used prophylactically against the acute attacks of pseudogout, as well as for the pseudo-osteoarthritis presentation.

HYDROXYAPATITE DEPOSITION DISEASE

Hydroxyapatite may be deposited in soft tissues, periarticular structures, or joints. As with other crystal deposition syndromes, hydroxyapatite deposition may either occur as an asymptomatic finding or be associated with disease. Soft tissue calcification usually occurs as a result of illnesses such as scleroderma, dermatomyositis, and chronic renal insufficiency. In some instances where the calcification is extensive and causes troublesome symptoms, surgical intervention is necessary. Much more com-

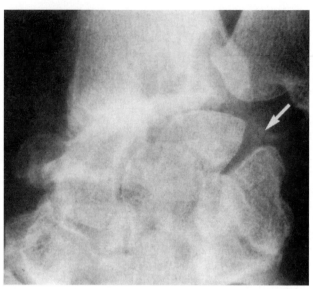

Figure 12–27. Wrist in calcium pyrophosphate deposition disease. Calcification of the triangular fibrocartilage is noted *(arrow)*. In addition, pyrophosphate arthropathy characterized by narrowing of the radionavicular joint, subchondral sclerosis, and cysts in the distal radius and carpal bones are readily seen. (From Kelley WN, Harris ED Jr, Ruddy S, Sledge CB: Textbook of Rheumatology, 3rd ed. Philadelphia, WB Saunders, 1989, p 1456.)

monly, hydroxyapatite may be deposited in the periarticular tissues. This usually occurs at tendon insertions, especially in the shoulder, hands, hip, and knee (Fig. 12–28). When symptomatic this can be treated with NSAIDs or corticosteroid injections, although the use of crystalline corticosteroid preparations may in some instances exacerbate the problem. HADD involving the joints is uncommon. McCarty and colleagues coined the term *Milwaukee shoulder* to describe an aggressive degenerative process of the entire shoulder region primarily affecting older women (Fig. 12–29).[38] A similar process may uncommonly affect other joints.

Systemic Lupus Erythematosus

SLE is the prototypical systemic autoimmune disorder. A systemic response by the body against various self-antigens leads to inflammation, immune complex deposition, and damage to blood vessels throughout the body. Women are affected approximately five times more commonly than men, and the peak incidence is in the third and fourth decades of life.

SLE can affect nearly any organ or tissue in the body. The frequency of clinical symptoms in this disorder is listed in Table 12–23. The musculoskeletal features bear special emphasis, because these are the manifestations that may bring the patient to an orthopaedist. Nearly all patients with this illness eventually have either arthralgias or arthritis. The distinguishing characteristics of these symptoms in patients with SLE are listed in Table 12–24 and this illness is contrasted to RA. The main difference from RA or other types of inflammatory arthritis is that there is little synovitis or joint destruction seen in SLE, although the joints may

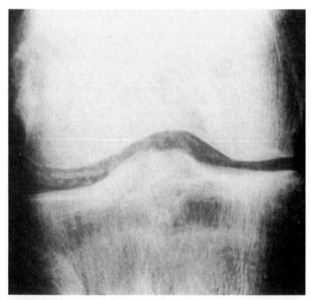

Figure 12–26. Punctate calcification of fibrocartilage in knee meniscus of patient with CPDD. (From Kelley WN, Harris ED Jr, Ruddy S, Sledge CB: Textbook of Rheumatology, 3rd ed. Philadelphia, WB Saunders, 1989, p 1456.)

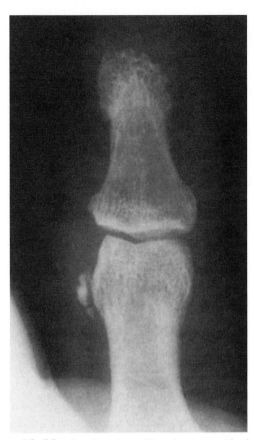

Figure 12–28. Apatite deposition in para-articular soft tissue of the finger in this patient led to an acute inflammatory reaction suggesting septic arthritis. (From Kelley WN, Harris ED Jr, Ruddy S, Sledge CB: Textbook of Rheumatology, 3rd ed. Philadelphia, WB Saunders, 1989, p 1462.)

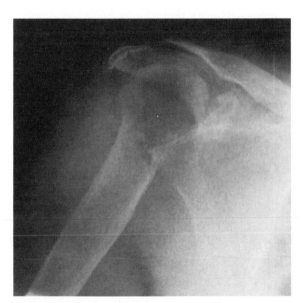

Figure 12–29. Classic roentgenographic appearance of shoulder in patient with "Milwaukee shoulder" syndrome. Destructive arthritis is characterized by bony erosions, cyst formation, and loss of joint space, noted particularly at the inferior aspect of the joint. (From Kelley WN, Harris ED Jr, Ruddy S, Sledge CB: Textbook of Rheumatology, 3rd ed. Philadelphia, WB Saunders, 1989, p 1462.)

be very painful. Also, some patients with SLE develop ulnar deviation of the fingers, swan-neck deformities, and other changes that appear very similar to those seen in RA. On examination, however, these deformities are all reducible, and this entity has been termed *Jacoud's arthropathy*. This seems to occur because of tendon laxity rather than destruction of joints, and radiographs will reveal normal joints. Another orthopaedic problem encountered relatively frequently in SLE is avascular necrosis (AVN). Corticosteroid therapy is probably the biggest reason for this complication, although AVN has been noted in patients with SLE who were not treated with corticosteroids (especially those with a positive anticardiolipin antibody).

The diagnosis of SLE is based on a combination of clinical and laboratory features. The ARA diagnostic criteria for SLE are helpful in this setting (Table 12–25). Persons who have four or more of these features are likely to have SLE. The ANA element of the criteria is particularly important, because nearly all patients with SLE will have a positive result of an ANA test.

The treatment of SLE is based on the symptoms and site of involvement.[39] Generally, skin and musculoskeletal involvement is treated nonaggressively with NSAIDs, topical corticosteroids, and/or hydroxychloroquine. Hematologic involvement, serositis, and severe constitutional

Table 12–23. Frequency of clinical symptoms in systemic lupus erythematosus

Symptoms	Percentage
Fatigue	80–100
Fever	>80
Weight loss	>60
Arthritis, arthralgia	~95
Skin	>80
Butterfly rash	>50
Photosensitivity	>55
Mucous membrane lesion	27–41
Alopecia	~70
Raynaud's phenomenon	17–30
Purpura	15
Urticaria	8
Renal	~50
Nephrosis	18
Gastrointestinal	38
Pulmonary	0.9–98
Pleurisy	45
Effusion	24
Pneumonia	29
Cardiac	46
Pericarditis	8–48
Murmurs	23
ECG changes	34–70
Lymphadenopathy	~50
Splenomegaly	10–20
Hepatomegaly	25
Central nervous system	25–75
Functional	Most
Psychosis	5–52
Convulsions	52–20

ECG, electrocardiographic.
From Kelley WN, Harris ED Jr, Ruddy S, Sledge CB: Textbook of Rheumatology, 3rd ed. Philadelphia, WB Saunders, 1989, p 1102.

Table 12–24. Musculoskeletal manifestations in systemic lupus erythematosus (SLE) and rheumatoid arthritis (RA)

	SLE	RA
Arthralgia	Common	Common
Arthritis	Common	Deforming
Symmetry	Yes	Yes
Joints involved	PIP > MCP > wrist > knee	MICP > wrist > knee
Synovial hypertrophy	Rare	Common
Synovial membrane abnormality	Minimal	Proliferative
Synovial fluid	Transudate	Exudate
Subcutaneous nodules	Rare	35%
Erosions	Very rare	Common
Morning stiffness	Minutes	Hours
Ulnar deviation	Rare	Common
Myalgia	Common	Common
Myositis	Rare	Uncommon
Osteoporosis	Variable	Common
Avascular necrosis	5–50%	Uncommon
Deforming arthritis	Uncommon	Common
Swan-neck	10%	Common
Ulnar deviation	5%	Common

MCP, metacarpophalangeal; PIP, proximal interphalangeal.
From Kelley WN, Harris ED Jr, Ruddy S, Sledge CB: Textbook of Rheumatology, 3rd ed. Philadelphia, WB Saunders, 1989, p 1103.

symptoms are usually managed with corticosteroids, typically with corticosteroid-sparing drugs given concurrently (e.g., azathioprine, methotrexate, hydroxychloroquine) employed to minimize the long-term complications of these drugs. Renal and central nervous system involvement is treated very aggressively, in many instances with both corticosteroids and cytotoxic drugs such as cyclophosphamide.

Infectious Arthritis

BACTERIAL AGENTS

Septic arthritis from common pathogens is covered in other sections of this book. Such processes usually occur in an immunocompromised host, or as the result of bacteremia or direct bacterial inoculation of a joint. However, there are a few types of infectious (or postinfectious) arthritis that can occur without such risk factors. Rheumatic fever and gonococcal infections are specific examples.

The arthritis associated with rheumatic fever does not occur because the joint is infected with the causative organism but rather because of an immunologic reaction to the group A *Streptococcus*.[40] For reasons that are unclear, only pharyngeal infections with this organism are associated with rheumatic fever. The classic manifestations of rheumatic fever are described by the Jones criteria and may follow the pharyngitis by several days to weeks. The major clinical findings include polyarthritis, carditis, chorea, erythema marginatum, and subcutaneous nodules; minor findings include fever, arthralgia, and previous rheumatic fever. The arthritis associated with rheumatic fever is unique in that this is one of the few arthritides that are truly migratory; that is, the arthritis moves from one joint to the next. The most commonly involved joints are the large peripheral joints. The onset is typically abrupt and severe, and myal-

gias and fever commonly coexist. Although this disorder is uncommon in adults, in adults the articular features may predominate the clinical picture, with an absence of extra-articular features. Also, in adults the arthritis may be more additive than migratory and be less responsive to salicylates or NSAIDs than it is in children.

Gonococcal arthritis can follow a gonococcal infection involving the urethra, cervix, pharynx, or rectum.[41] Typically, an individual will initially experience several days of fevers, chills, multiple skin lesions, and polyarthralgias or tenosynovitis. If untreated in this stage, it will typically progress to involve just a few joints or tendons. Individuals with such a clinical picture should be started immediately on an antibiotic such as ceftriaxone and should have cultures taken of all orifices, any affected synovium, and any skin lesions. These cultures should be plated at the bedside on Thayer-Martin medium or chocolate agar. The persons in the early phase are most likely to have positive blood cultures, whereas those in the later phase are more likely to have positive synovial or skin lesion cultures.

NONBACTERIAL AGENTS

Less commonly, joints (or soft tissue structures) can become infected with nonbacterial agents such as tuberculosis or fungi. With the exception of tuberculosis, which can cause a septic arthritis in persons with normal immune function, most persons who have joint infections with these types of organisms have an underlying defect in immune function.

VIRAL AGENTS

Nearly all viral agents can lead to the development of a postviral arthritis in a small percentage of affected individuals. It appears as though the most common cause of postinfectious arthritis in persons who seek medical attention is that associated with parvovirus B19 infections. This

Table 12–25. Revised criteria for classification of systemic lupus erythematosus

Criterion	Definition
Malar rash	Fixed erythema, flat or raised, over the malar eminences, tending to spare the nasolabial folds.
Discoid rash	Erythematous raised patches with adherent keratotic scaling and follicular plugging; atrophic scarring may occur in older lesions.
Photosensitivity	Rash as a result of unusual reaction to sunlight, by patient history or physician observation.
Oral ulcers	Oral or nasopharyngeal ulceration, usually painless, observed by a physician.
Arthritis	Nonerosive arthritis involving two or more peripheral joints, characterized by tenderness, swelling, or effusion.
Serositis	Pleuritis—convincing history of pleuritic pain or rub heard by a physician or evidence of pleural effusion *or* Pericarditis—documented by electrocardiogram or rub or evidence of pericardial effusion.
Renal disorder	Persistent proteinuria > 0.5 g/day or greater than 3+ if quantitation not performed *or* Cellular casts—may be red cell, hemoglobin, granular, tubular, or mixed.
Neurologic disorder	Seizures—in the absence of offending drugs or known metabolic derangements; e.g., uremia, ketoacidosis, or electrolyte imbalance *or* Psychosis—in the absence of offending drugs or known metabolic derangements, e.g., uremia, ketoacidosis, or electrolyte imbalance.
Hematologic disorder	Hemolytic anemia—with reticulocytosis *or* Leukopenia < 4000/mm total on two or more occasions *or* Lymphopenia < 1500/mm on two or more occasions *or* Thrombocytopenia < 100,000/mm in the absence of offending drugs.
Immunologic disorder	Positive lupus erythematosus cell preparation *or* Anti-DNA: antibody to native DNA in abnormal titer *or* Anti-Sm: presence of antibody to Sm nuclear antigen *or* False-positive serologic test for syphilis known to be positive for at least 6 months and confirmed by *Treponema pallidum* immobilization or fluorescent treponemal antibody absorption test.
Antinuclear antibody	An abnormal titer of antinuclear antibody by immunofluorescence or an equivalent assay at any point in time and in the absence of drugs known to be associated with "drug-induced lupus" syndrome.

From Kelley WN, Harris ED Jr, Ruddy S, Sledge CB: Textbook of Rheumatology, 3rd ed. Philadelphia, WB Saunders, 1989, p 1123.

virus is common in children, leading to fifth disease (erythema infectiosum).[42] In affected children, cutaneous manifestations predominate, with the characteristic "slapped cheeks" appearance, as well as a serpiginous rash affecting the torso or extremities. Adults who develop this infection have less prominent cutaneous features and more prominent articular features. The articular features closely resemble those of RA, so closely in fact that up to 50% of these persons will meet criteria for the diagnosis of RA. The diagnostic test of choice is an IgM titer for parvovirus B19, which will be positive at the time joint symptoms begin and last approximately 2 months. Although this illness typically has a self-limited course and is not associated with joint damage, these patients are quite uncomfortable and debilitated and may need treatment with NSAIDs or even low doses of corticosteroids for several months.

LYME DISEASE

Lyme disease is a multisystem illness caused by the tick-borne spirochete *Borrelia burgdorferi*. Within days to weeks of a bite by an infected tick, there is typically the development of a characteristic lesion. This lesion is termed *erythema chronicum migrans* and evolves into an annular lesion with a central clearing. Once the organism becomes hematogenously spread, a variety of manifestations can occur, including similar annular lesions in other regions of the body, fever, lymphadenopathy, myalgias, arthralgias, and fatigue. This early phase, even if untreated, typically evolves into an intermediate phase, characterized by arthritis, cardiac, and/or neurologic involvement. The true arthritis of Lyme disease (in contrast to the arthralgia and myalgias that occur early) develops months after the exposure. This will usually begin as intermittent episodes of inflammatory arthritis involving the large joints and, over years, will progress to become a constant monoarticular or oligoarticular arthritis involving large joints. The knees are frequently involved, and in severe cases joint erosions and damage may occur.

Polymyalgia Rheumatica

Polymyalgia rheumatica (PMR) is a common syndrome occurring almost exclusively in persons older than age 50 and is characterized by stiffness and pain in the proximal muscles.[43] The onset may be abrupt or indolent. Patients will have prominent "gelling" whenever they are inactive for prolonged periods. In some persons there is swelling and/or synovitis of the hands associated with this condition. In a subset of individuals PMR coexists with temporal arteritis, which can be associated with visual symptoms, headaches, jaw claudication, and alopecia. Patients with these symptoms or with temporal artery tenderness on palpation should have one or more temporal artery biopsies to determine if this may be present because more aggressive treatment regimens are used for this subset of patients.

In the appropriate clinical setting, the diagnosis of PMR is confirmed by finding a markedly elevated ESR. Other diagnoses that should be considered are fibromyalgia and hypothyroidism. Another diagnostic test is treatment with intermediate doses of corticosteroids, usually 20 mg of prednisone per day for several weeks with a rapid taper to 5 to 10 mg per day. In patients who do not respond rapidly and completely to corticosteroids the diagnosis should be questioned. Typically, patients will need to stay on corticosteroids at least 1 to 2 years, and sometimes much longer.

PHARMACOLOGIC THERAPY

The basic principle of pharmacologic therapy for any disorder is to use the least toxic and least expensive medication for the illness being treated. This is particularly true for the rheumatic diseases, in which there are several relatively nontoxic and inexpensive drugs (e.g., acetaminophen, over-the-counter NSAIDs) available that are effective for many conditions.

There are two important factors that need to be considered when choosing the most appropriate pharmacologic therapy for a patient with a rheumatic problem. The first is whether the problem is local or systemic, and the second is whether the process is inflammatory or noninflammatory. For local problems, topical analgesics or injections may be considered instead of systemic therapy. And for noninflammatory conditions, analgesics such as acetaminophen can be considered instead of NSAIDs or other potentially more toxic regimens.

Analgesics

Acetaminophen is an effective and safe analgesic for many noninflammatory rheumatic conditions. For example, in osteoarthritis, several randomized controlled trials have suggested that this compound is as effective as either the over-the-counter or prescription-strength NSAIDs.[44] The principal toxicity of acetaminophen is hepatic, although this typically occurs in persons either consuming concurrent hepatotoxins (especially alcohol) or exceeding the recommended dose. Tramadol is a relatively new non-narcotic analgesic that can be considered in persons who require an analgesic but do not respond to acetaminophen. Finally, narcotics can be effective in both the short- and long-term management of pain, although both tolerance and addiction are potential problems.

NSAIDs

The NSAIDs represent one of the most commonly prescribed classes of drugs. Aspirin is the original and prototypical NSAID. These drugs all act largely by inhibiting cyclooxygenase, the enzyme that transforms arachidonic acid into prostaglandins, prostacyclin, and thromboxane (Fig. 12–30); the clinical relevance of the effects of NSAIDs on lipid metabolism, granulocyte migration, and bradykinin synthesis is less well understood.[45] Although there are now dozens of NSAIDs available, newer drugs in this class are not necessarily more effective than aspirin but are generally better tolerated. The main differences between NSAIDs are (1) half-life, (2) relative potency at the prescribed dose, (3) tolerability, and (4) cost.

When considering the appropriate NSAID, several factors should be considered in regard to half-life. If a drug is to be used to treat an acute inflammatory conditions (e.g., an attack of gout), a drug with a short half-life and rapid onset of action, such as indomethacin, should be considered. On the other hand, when prescribing NSAIDs for elderly patients, who comprise the subset of NSAID users who experience nearly all of the major gastrointestinal hemorrhages and death from this class of drugs, compounds with long half-lives should generally be avoided.

With respect to potency, there again are several factors to consider. The first is that for most NSAIDs the recommended prescription dose has an anti-inflammatory effect, and one half to one third of that dose (the dose that is typically available over the counter) has an analgesic effect. One of the most important principles in prescribing this class of drugs is to use the lowest dose possible, because the gastric and renal side effects of these compounds are directly related to the ability of these compounds to block cyclooxygenase. Thus, if one chooses to treat a noninflammatory condition such as osteoarthritis with this class of drugs, a dose lower than the typical prescription dose usually will be just as efficacious and safer. It is difficult to directly compare the relative potency of one NSAID with another, because there are no established in vitro assays that predict the relative potency of this class of compounds. Generally, however, NSAIDs that have been marketed more recently are tested and released at relatively less potent doses than older compounds. The reason for this is that the manufacturers of more recently released compounds generally were attempting to demonstrate a safety advantage over the older NSAIDs. There is general agreement that the most potent NSAID in routine clinical practice in the United States is indomethacin (phenyl-

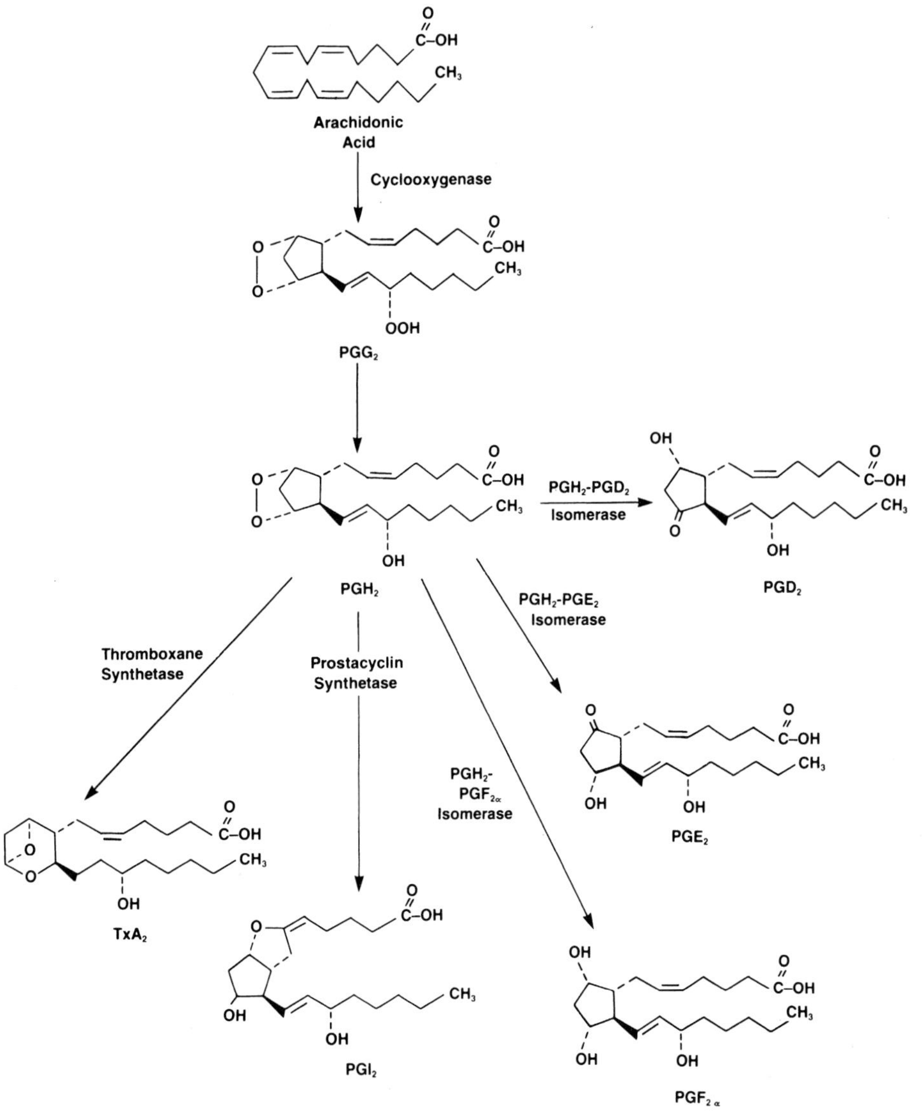

Figure 12–30. The cyclooxygenase pathway. (From Kelley WN, Harris ED Jr, Ruddy S, Sledge CB: Textbook of Rheumatology, 3rd ed. Philadelphia, WB Saunders, 1989, p 255.)

butazone is probably even more potent but is rarely used because of the [albeit low] risk of aplastic anemia), whereas the nonacetylated salicylates such as magnesium choline salicylate and salsalate are the least potent (and thus useful alternatives for persons with relative contraindications to other NSAIDs).

Tolerability is an important issue with respect to NSAIDs and should not be confused with toxicity. There is a general misconception than when a person takes an NSAID and develops dyspepsia, heartburn, or other gastrointestinal side effects that this person may be developing peptic ulcer disease. Innumerable studies have demonstrated that there is a poor relationship between the *symptoms* (i.e., tolerability) that a person develops when they consume an NSAID and the development of peptic ulcer disease. Most persons who develop a major gastrointestinal hemorrhage from NSAIDs have no symptoms that antedate the hemorrhage, and, in fact, *symptomatic* persons taking NSAIDs are actually *less likely to have a peptic ulcer* than asymptomatic persons. The reason for this appears to be that the tolerability of an NSAID may be influenced by local factors such as acidity in the gastrointestinal tract

(and thus is improved by taking antacids or histamine-2 blockers, or by enteric coating of tablets), whereas the development of peptic ulcer disease is due to a systemic effect of the NSAID on the production of prostaglandins in the stomach. For this reason, NSAIDs that are administered parenterally (e.g., ketorolac) are just as likely to cause peptic ulcer disease as orally administered compounds. The only drug currently approved to be used prophylactically against NSAID-induced gastropathy is misoprostol, a prostaglandin analog (although recent studies suggest that very high doses of histamine-2 blockers, or proton pump inhibitors, may be as effective).

The primary toxicities of the NSAIDs are gastrointestinal, coagulation, and renal. The gastrointestinal side effects were reviewed earlier. A difficult issue in clinical practice is to decide which patients who are prescribed NSAIDs should also receive prophylaxis against peptic ulcer disease. It is first important to understand who is at increased risk of developing this complication. The factors that place a person at higher risk of developing a gastrointestinal hemorrhage include a prior history of peptic ulcer disease, chronic use of antacids or histamine-2 blockers, cigarette smoking, alcohol use, anticoagulant use, concomitant corticosteroid therapy, and being older than age 65. The more of these risk factors a person has, the more likely they are to develop a major gastrointestinal hemorrhage. Arguably, however, the most important risk factor is being elderly. Although elderly persons taking NSAIDs are only approximately one and one-half times as likely to develop a gastrointestinal hemorrhage than a younger person, nearly all of the mortality from NSAID-associated gastrointestinal hemorrhages occurs in persons older than age 65. The reason for this appears to be that younger persons tolerate gastrointestinal hemorrhages better than the elderly, who commonly will develop a myocardial infarction, cerebrovascular accident, or some other major event in association with a gastrointestinal hemorrhage.

The coagulation effects of NSAIDs are also widely misunderstood in clinical practice. Aspirin *irreversibly* binds to cyclooxygenase, so that the inhibition of platelet function that occurs after consuming aspirin lasts until all of the platelets that were exposed to the drug die (approximately 2 weeks). However, all other NSAIDs *reversibly* bind to cyclooxygenase, so the antiplatelet effects of these drugs only last while they are in the circulation (i.e., several half-lives). There is no need to stop nonaspirin NSAIDs more than a few days before a surgical procedure to avoid the antiplatelet effects of these drugs.

By far the most common renal side effect of the NSAIDs is a reversible decline in renal function. This almost always occurs in persons who have diminished baseline renal blood flow (e.g., in patients with low cardiac output states, renal artery stenosis, or pre-existing renal disease). The reason for the selective occurrence of this side effect in these persons is probably that vasodilatory prostaglandins are only produced by the kidney as a compensation for low renal blood flow. Administering these medications in this setting will decrease local prostaglandin synthesis in the kidney, decrease renal blood flow, and worsen renal function. In some instances this decline in renal function can be permanent, so NSAIDs should be prescribed with caution in this setting.

A new class of drugs that selectively inhibit the type two isoform of cyclooxygenase has been developed and is available in the United States. Because these drugs have substantially less inhibitory activity on the type 1 isoform of cyclooxygenase that is present in the gastrointestinal tract, these new compounds have less toxicity than the older NSAIDs.[46] Because of this, these new compounds may have the greatest utility in persons who need to take an NSAID but are at risk of gastrointestinal or bleeding complications from the current compounds.

Corticosteroids

Because of the potent anti-inflammatory effects of corticosteroids, these drugs are useful for the treatment of a number of local and systemic inflammatory conditions.[47] A thorough review of the mechanism(s) of actions of these drugs is not possible, but these drugs likely act by a variety of mechanisms, including interference with cell adhesion and migration into inflammatory sites, interruption of cell-cell communication, impairment of prostaglandin, leukotriene, and neutrophil superoxide production, and impairment of antigen opsonization and immune complex clearance.

The short-term use of systemic corticosteroids is relatively well tolerated, even at higher doses. Uncommon but serious side effects in this setting may include avascular necrosis, psychosis or less serious mood disturbance, hyperglycemia, hypertension, and electrolyte disturbances. In contrast, the long-term use of corticosteroids, even at low doses, is associated with a plethora of side effects, including osteoporosis, accelerated atherosclerosis, infections, cataracts, skin changes, and so on. Because of this, and because of the fact that corticosteroids represent by far the most effective medications to bring inflammatory processes under rapid control, most clinicians attempt to use high doses initially for short periods of time, followed by as rapid a taper as possible, either with complete discontinuation or to chronic regimens (e.g., less than 7.5 mg of prednisone per day, or alternate-day dosing) that minimize toxicity.

Another significant problem with chronic corticosteroid usage is suppression of the hypothalamic-pituitary-adrenal axis. This can occur with as little as 1 week of high-dose corticosteroid treatment and occurs in nearly all individuals who receive daily corticosteroid treatment. This is important because persons with a suppressed hypothalamic-pituitary-adrenal axis need to receive exogenous corticosteroids when exposed to stressors, such as undergoing a major surgical procedure. There is no "correct" regimen in this setting, but administering 100 mg of hydrocortisone parenterally on call to the operating room and 50 mg every 6 hours for 24 hours, then 25 mg every 6 hours for another 24 hours, is more than sufficient (less aggressive regimens may also be used).

Slow-Acting Antirheumatic and Cytotoxic Drugs

A number of slow-acting antirheumatic and cytotoxic drugs are used in the management of patients with autoimmune disorders. These medications are commonly used in a variety of settings, sometimes as single agents in less aggressive disease (e.g., hydroxychloroquine in mild RA, sulfasalazine in reactive arthritis) or as corticosteroid-sparing drugs (to minimize the usage of long-term corticosteroids) in illnesses such as SLE and vasculitis.

The main reason that the practicing orthopaedist needs to be aware of these medications is because of their effects on wound healing and infections (especially perioperative). Although it is commonly believed that many of these drugs (e.g., high-dose corticosteroids, methotrexate) may increase the rate of perioperative infections, the data to support this are largely anecdotal. Nonetheless, most clinicians will attempt to stop methotrexate for 1 week before, and 2 weeks after, major surgical procedures. With respect to corticosteroids, there is typically an attempt to get the patient to the lowest dose possible before surgery.

References

1. Sprent J: Immunological memory. Curr Opin Immunol 1997;9:371–379.
2. Zinkernagel RM, Bachmann MF, Kundig TM, et al: On immunological memory. Annu Rev Immunol 1996;14:333–367.

3. Croft M: Activation of naive, memory and effector T cells. Curr Opin Immunol 1994;6:431–437.

4. Blum JS, Ma C, Kovats S: Antigen-presenting cells and the selection of immunodominant epitopes. Crit Rev Immunol 1997;17:411–417.

5. Carter LL, Zhang X, Dubey C, et al: Regulation of T cell subsets from naive to memory. J Immunother 1998;21:181–187.

6. Klinman NR: The cellular origins of memory B cells. Semin Immunol 1997;9:241–247.

7. Fritzler MJ: Autoantibodies: Diagnostic fingerprints and etiologic perplexities. Clin Invest Med 1997;20:50–66.

8. Cabral AR, Alarçon-Segovia D: Autoantibodies in systemic lupus erythematosus. Curr Opin Rheumatol 1997;9:387–392.

9. Vilcek J: Forty years of interferons, forty years of cytokines. Cytokine Growth Factor Rev 1997;8:239–249.

10. Sheerin NS, Sacks SH: Complement and complement inhibitors: Their role in autoimmune and inflammatory diseases. Curr Opin Nephrol Hypertens 1998;7:305–310.

11. Walport MJ, Davies KA, Morley BJ, Botto M: Complement deficiency and autoimmunity. Ann NY Acad Sci 1997;815:267–281.

12. Liszewski MK, Farries TC, Lublin DM, et al: Control of the complement system. Adv Immunol 1996;61:201–283.

13. Ahmed AE, Peter JB: Clinical utility of complement assessment. Clin Diagn Lab Immunol 1995;2:509–517.

14. Kushner I, Rzewnicki DL: The acute phase response: General aspects. Baillieres Clin Rheumatol 1994;8:513–530.

15. Trautwein C, Boker K, Manns MP: Hepatocyte and immune system: Acute phase reaction as a contribution to early defence mechanisms. Gut 1994;35:1163–1166.

16. Grassi W, De Angelis R, Lamanna G, Cervini C: The clinical features of rheumatoid arthritis. Eur J Radiol 1998;27(Suppl 1):S18–S24.

17. Rawlins BA, Girardi FP, Boachie-Adjei O: Rheumatoid arthritis of the cervical spine. Rheum Dis Clin North Am 1998;24:55–65.

18. Harris ED: Rheumatoid arthritis: Pathophysiology and implications for therapy. N Engl J Med 1990;322:1277–1289.

19. Pincus TA, Callahan LF: Early mortality in RA predicted by poor clinical status. Bull Rheum Dis 1992;41:4.

20. Machold KP, Eberl G, Leeb BF, et al: Early arthritis therapy: Rationale and current approach. J Rheumatol Suppl 1998;53:13–19.

21. Felson DT, Zhang Y: An update on the epidemiology of knee and hip osteoarthritis with a view to prevention. Arthritis Rheum 1998;41:1343–1355.

22. Ettinger WHJ: Physical activity, arthritis, and disability in older people. Clin Geriatr Med 1998;14:633–640.

23. Felson DT, Naimark A, Anderson J, et al: The prevalence of knee osteoarthritis in the elderly: The Framingham osteoarthritis study. Arthritis Rheum 1987;30:914–918.

24. Brandt KD: The importance of nonpharmacologic approaches in management of osteoarthritis. Am J Med 1998;105:39S–44S.

25. Lane NE, Thompson JM: Management of osteoarthritis in the primary-care setting: An evidence-based approach to treatment. Am J Med 1997;103:25S–30S.

26. Claw DJ: Fibromyalgia: More than just a musculoskeletal disease. Am Fam Phys 1995;52:843–851.

27. Olivieri I, Barozzi L, Padula A, et al: Clinical manifestations of seronegative spondylarthropathies. Eur J Radiol 1998;27(Suppl 1):S3–S6.

28. Nuki G: Ankylosing spondylitis, HLA B27, and beyond. Lancet 1998;351:767–769.

29. Arnett FC, Chakraborty R: Ankylosing spondylitis: The dissection of a complex genetic disease [editorial; comment]. Arthritis Rheum 1997;40:1746–1748.

30. Moll JMH, Wright V: Normal range of spine mobility: An objective clinical study. Ann Rheum Dis 1971;30:281.

31. Helliwell PS, Hickling P, Wright V: Do the radiological changes of classic ankylosing spondylitis differ from the changes found in the spondylitis associated with inflammatory bowel disease, psoriasis, and reactive arthritis? Ann Rheum Dis 1998;57:135–140.

32. Ostensen M, Ostensen H: Ankylosing spondylitis—The female aspect. J Rheumatol 1998;25:120–124.

33. Sieper J, Braun J: Treatment of reactive arthritis with antibiotics [editorial]. Br J Rheumatol 1998;37:717–720.

34. Schumacher HR: Crystal-induced arthritis: An overview. Am J Med 1996;100:46S–52S.

35. Wise CM, Agudelo CA: Gouty arthritis and uric acid metabolism [see comments]. Curr Opin Rheumatol 1996;8:248–254.

36. McGill NW: Gout and other crystal arthropathies. Med J Aust 1997;166:33–38.

37. Pritzker KP: Calcium pyrophosphate dihydrate crystal deposition and other crystal deposition diseases. Curr Opin Rheumatol 1994;6:442–447.

38. McCarty DJ, Halverson PB, Carrera GF, et al: "Milwaukee shoulder": Association of microspheroids containing hydroxyapatite crystals, active collegenase and neutral protease with rotator cuff defects. Arthritis Rheum 1981;24:464–473.

39. Strand V: Approaches to the management of systemic lupus erythematosus. Curr Opin Rheumatol 1997;9:410–420.

40. Hutchison SJ: Acute rheumatic fever. J Infect 1998;36:249–253.

41. Cohen M: Gonococcal arthritis. Bull Rheum Dis 1998;47:4–6.

42. Naides SJ: Rheumatic manifestations of parvovirus B19 infection. Rheum Dis Clin North Am 1998;24:375–401.

43. Swannell AJ: Polymyalgia rheumatica and temporal arteritis: Diagnosis and management. BMJ 1997;314:1329–1332.

44. Bradley JD, Brandt K, Katz BP, et al: Comparison of an anti-inflammatory dose of ibuprofen, an analgesic dose of ibuprofen, and acetaminophen in the treatment of patients with osteoarthritis of the knee. N Engl J Med 1991;325:87–91.

45. Simon LS: Biology and toxic effects of nonsteroidal anti-inflammatory drugs. Curr Opin Rheumatol 1998;10:153–158.

46. Bolten WW: Scientific rationale for specific inhibition of COX-2. J Rheumatol Suppl 1998;51:2–7.

47. van Vollenhoven RF: Corticosteroids in rheumatic disease: Understanding their effects is key to their use. Postgrad Med 1998;103:137–142.

Chapter 13

Principles of Sports Medicine

Benjamin Shaffer, M.D.

Few areas of orthopaedic subspecialization can claim both the historic tradition and the contemporary interest experienced in the field of sports medicine. As long ago as 2500 BC, the Smith papyrus, humankind's oldest written document, chronicled shoulder instability. Hippocrates himself wrote extensively about the treatment of many injuries seen and treated during athletic endeavors. And Galen, the true forefather of sports medicine and perhaps the first recognized "team physician," cared for the warrior gladiators of ancient Rome.

Yet sports medicine today is no longer defined by its storied ancestry. Scientific advances and social changes have led to a revolution that would render the field unrecognizable to earlier physicians. Technologic development in imaging such as magnetic resonance imaging (MRI) and arthroscopy have led the way. Just in the past decade, MRI has permitted better understanding of joint structure and function and has rendered noninvasive diagnostic imaging possible. Arthroscopy has changed the way we see and understand joint structure and made minimally invasive complex reconstructive procedures possible.

Parallel changes in the social arena have also contributed to the explosive interest in sports from a medical perspective. First, interest and participation in fitness have led to an exponential increase in the number of individuals engaged in athletic activities, ranging from the occasional recreational enthusiast, to the weekend warrior, to the elite competitive athlete. And these "athletes" participate at all ages, beginning when they are very young (Tiger Woods first swung a club when he was 3 years old!) and continuing until they are very old (marathons routinely have several octogenarians). The second social factor has been our society's unprecedented (and increasing) financial compensation of elite and professional athletes. As society's value on these athletes' accomplishments has increased, so too have the stakes for rendering swift and precise diagnosis, treatment, and prompt return to activity. The financial and career risks associated with injury leave little room for diagnostic uncertainty or therapeutic imprecision. This emphasis on minimizing "down time" has spurred the development of sophisticated diagnostic and therapeutic techniques used today.

And society's thirst for detailed information regarding the diagnosis, treatment, and outcome of athlete's injuries at times seems unquenchable. The daily sports section is replete with injury reports, speculations on dates for return to play, and in-depth articles on the reconstructive procedure(s) that have allowed the player to return. Medicine's ability to return athletes to their preinjury level of activity has become a mainstream concept. Not surprisingly, less elite athletes have come to expect the same level of attention, care, and outcome in treating their own orthopaedic problems.

Since its early inception in Greco-Roman times, sports medicine seems to have come a long way. But the principles are in fact the same as those practiced by Galen, and include the prevention, diagnosis, and treatment of athletic injury, emphasizing return to the athletes to their preinjury level of activity with little or no risk. Although the majority of injuries are musculoskeletal, this field is by no means the isolated purview of the orthopaedist, but is shared by many other skilled and trained professionals. Examples of some of the other sports medicine health care providers whose unique expertise qualifies their contribution include coaches, fitness trainers, motivational speakers, psychologists, exercise physiologists, certified athletic trainers, nutritionists, physical and occupational therapists, and nonorthopaedic physicians. Although each of the aforementioned areas of expertise affects care of the athlete, the most common injuries involve the musculoskeletal system. This chapter will therefore emphasize evaluation and management of orthopaedic problems seen in sports medicine.

EVALUATION OF COMMON SPORTS INJURIES

The principles of evaluation include a thorough history and physical examination, supplemented by appropriate radiographic evaluation and other testing as necessary. One consideration that is somewhat unique to sports injuries is the frequent presence of others in attendance at the time of the injury, including coaches, parents, other players, or the team trainer or physician. This opportunity often lends considerable insight into the mechanism and severity of injury. Evaluation *at the time of injury* not only enhances diagnostic accuracy but allows assessment prior to the onset of soft tissue swelling, joint stiffness, muscle spasm, and reflex guarding. On-the-field or sideline evaluation is part of the reason for game and event coverage by athletic trainers and team physicians. Delaying the evaluation by even a few hours may preclude early diagnosis, which in turn may obligate more sophisticated (and more expensive) diagnostic tests or inadvertently delay definitive treatment while awaiting resolution of pain and swelling. Competitive athletes, who cannot afford a lengthy and unpredictable recovery, poorly tolerate a "wait and see" approach.

History

In acute injuries, the history is usually pretty straightforward. The patient may have twisted an ankle when coming down from a rebound, felt the shoulder "go out" when colliding with another player, or felt a "pop" in the knee after planting and cutting cross-field to evade a tackler. Although the injury may seem obvious, ask about symptoms at the time of injury. For example, the patient may admit to transient numbness or tingling of the arm following an anterior shoulder dislocation (suggesting possible axillary nerve injury). Inquire about pain, the sense of "instability," and mechanical catching or clicking or the presence of radiating pain or numbness. The patient may indicate that the knee was at a "funny angle" and required manipulation at the sideline. Such a history indicates the possibility of an actual knee dislocation.

Ask about associated symptoms. There may be burning sensations, such as "stingers," in which traction injury to the brachial plexus may lead to radicular pain. Stingers are common among contact sport athletes such as football and lacrosse players. Anterior shoulder subluxation (partial dislocation of the glenohumeral joint) may present with the "dead arm syndrome" experienced when the arm is in the cocking position of throwing.

Determine if the problem ever occurred before, and if so, how did it occur, what type of treatment was rendered, and what was the outcome. Previous problems may offer an alert to the need for a different treatment approach (i.e., treatment of a first-time dislocation differs from treatment of recurrent shoulder instability).

Some sports medicine problems are not related to a specific event. The patient may report a gradual onset of pain, stiffness, weakness, giving way, or instability. Problems related to so-called microtrauma or overuse injuries are common, particularly in the unconditioned athlete (the weekend warrior) in whom demands outstrip their supply.

For example, shin splints, which is common among runners, are usually insidious in onset. Symptoms are usually due to training errors. Ask about changes in mileage or intensity, shoe wear, or training circumstances (track to road, flat surface to uneven terrain). The same principle of trying to determine what may contribute to injury in running applies to other repetitive activities in other sports (baseball, softball, volleyball, tennis, and swimming). Determining when during the course of a throw or swim stroke an athlete experiences symptoms may help the examiner identify the cause of symptoms.

Typically, overuse injuries are symptomatic with activity and improve with rest. When symptoms persist at rest or lead to nocturnal awakening, underlying structural injury or systemic disorder should be considered. The most common overuse injury of that type is a stress fracture.

Find out if there are specific activities that cause symptoms. In the athlete with intermittent knee symptoms, pain in the front of the knee with stair-climbing and prolonged sitting suggests problems of the patellofemoral joint. Symptoms that occur predictably only with pivoting and cutting activities, accompanied by swelling and giving way, suggest an internal derangement such as a torn meniscus or ligament (usually the anterior cruciate ligament).

Determine if the condition has been previously treated, and if so, how. Has the athlete taken any medication or modified the level or type of activity? How did the symptoms respond? In the athlete whose symptoms persist or have recurred despite "adequate" treatment, the specific details of previous treatment are important to elicit. Many athletes will insist they have already tried rest or some type of rehabilitation. But further inquiry is warranted to ensure both the patients' compliance and the adequacy of previous treatment. Did they truly rest? How did they modify their activities during this time? What specific exercises did they do and how frequently? Have they been on an anti-inflammatory medication, and if so, was it effective? Did they receive any corticosteroid injections and if so, what was the result? Nothing should be taken for granted in any patient. This is especially true when considering possible surgical intervention for the athlete in whom previous treatment has been seemingly ineffective.

Physical Examination

The standard musculoskeletal physical examination involves inspection, palpation, and assessment of range of motion, strength, ligament stability, and neurovascular status of the affected area. In addition, each anatomic region and some orthopaedic conditions have pertinent "special" tests. As a general principle, take advantage of the body's symmetry. When inspecting, palpating, assessing range of motion, strength and stability, use the opposite limb for comparison.

Inspection should be performed under both static and dynamic conditions. During static inspection, examine for skin changes such as ecchymoses (bruising), abrasions, lacerations, and swelling. Look for evidence of asymmetry or atrophy with respect to the opposite extremity. In the patient with an acute AC (acromioclavicular) separation, for example, inspection usually reveals a visibly prominent distal clavicle and drooped shoulder girdle (Fig. 13–1). After palpation of the soft and skeletal tissues for tenderness, palpate for tissue integrity, looking for evidence of any defects in underlying fascia, muscle tendon, or bone. For example, examination of the distal calf following an achilles rupture will yield a palpable defect at the site of the tear.

Static inspection, however, is insufficient for evaluating many conditions. Dynamic evaluation may be necessary to appreciate abnormal motion or alignment. For example, the runner with shin splints may appear normal when seated, but upon walking may demonstrate a tendency to pronate (become exaggeratedly flatfooted). In the athlete with shoulder pain or dysfunction, failure to inspect the shoulder during normal elevation (raising of the arm) may preclude identification of scapular winging due to weakness of the serratus anterior (Fig. 13–2).

Examine the affected joint for active (performed by the patient) and passive (measured by the examiner) range of

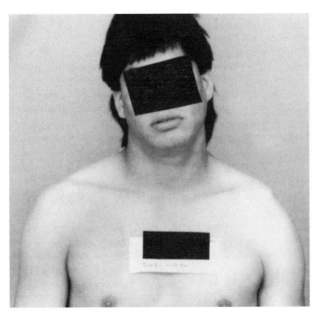

Figure 13–1. Note the asymmetry of the left shoulder, with prominence of the acromioclavicular (AC) joint due to a complete (grade III) AC separation. (From DeLee JC, Drez D: Orthopaedic Sports Medicine. Philadelphia, WB Saunders, 1994, p 487.)

motion. Remember to compare motion to the opposite side. Active motion may be decreased for a number of nonspecific reasons, including pain, swelling, injury to the muscle-tendon unit, mechanical block due to interposed tissue, or nerve injury. Passive motion restriction, however, is less common, and is more likely due to actual mechanical interference with normal joint kinematics. One common example of passively restricted joint motion is the adolescent or young adult athlete with a "locked knee" due to an interposed "bucket-handle" meniscus tear (Fig. 13–3). Another example of passive restricted motion can be seen in the adolescent with foot and ankle pain and a rigid hindfoot, known as tarsal coalition, in which persistent fusion between the bones of the hindfoot restricts motion and causes pain with activity.

Ligament assessment is probably the most difficult part of the examination. Although some ligaments can be assessed by palpation for tenderness and integrity, all require the application of a specific force across the joint to determine ligament injury. Evaluations differ for each ligament. Variability in individual joint laxity (some people are "loose" jointed, others are "tight"), mandates comparison to the opposite normal side. Distinguishing normal from pathologic laxity can be challenging and improves with experience.

Ligaments that are subcutaneous and can be palpated for tenderness include the ligaments of the AC joint, medial collateral ligament of the knee and elbow, lateral collateral ligament of the knee, and the anterior talofibular ligament of the ankle. Examination in almost all cases is limited to eliciting tenderness rather than integrity. Only the lateral collateral ligament of the knee can be palpated for integrity. When placed in the "figure of four" position, the lateral collateral ligament of the knee stands out in taut relief between the lateral epicondyle and the fibular head (Fig. 13–4).

Ligament integrity usually depends upon joint motion

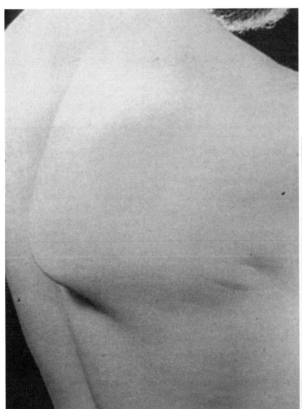

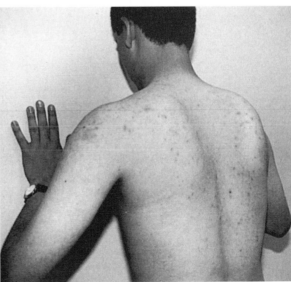

Figure 13–2. Scapula winging is demonstrated in this patient, who has weakness of the serratus anterior. Note the prominent scapulae, exacerbated on performing a wall push-up. (From Richwood CA Jr, et al: The Shoulder. 2nd ed. Philadelphia, WB Saunders, 1998, p 172.)

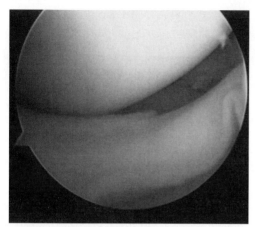

Figure 13–3. In this arthroscopic photo, the torn medial meniscus has become interposed between the joint surfaces and prevents normal knee extension. Its configuration is referred to as a "bucket handle" tear pattern.

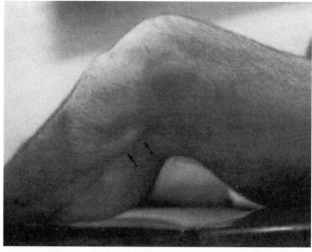

Figure 13–4. The lateral collateral ligament (LCL) can be easily felt and seen as a distinct taut band on the lateral aspect of the knee *(arrows),* when placed in the "figure of four" position. (From Reider B: Sports Medicine: The School-Age Athlete. Philadelphia, WB Saunders, 1996, p 325.)

or translation that reproduces the patients' symptoms or is greater than the opposite side. Common examples of abnormal laxity include the Lachman test, named for the Temple University professor who described abnormal anterior tibial translation relative to the femur in patients with anterior cruciate ligament (ACL) insufficiency (Fig. 13–5). Another example is the "opening up" of the medial aspect of the elbow when applying a valgus stress to the slightly flexed elbow in the athlete with medial collateral ligament (MCL) insufficiency. Testing for a complete tear of the anterior talofibular ligament (ATFL) is performed using the anterior drawer test, performed by grasping the heel and anteriorly translating it in relation to the tibia (Fig. 13–6).

Some instability patterns are not detected by applying stresses. For example, recurrent anterior shoulder instability may be best detected by provocatively placing the shoulder in the "throwing" position. This throwing position, in which the shoulder is placed in abduction and external rotation, is the position in which the shoulder is most vulnerable to anterior instability. When so positioned, the

athlete may observe that the shoulder feels like it is "going to come out of place," and this manipulation is known as the apprehension test.

During strength assessment, weakness may be due to pain, guarding, or muscle-tendon or nerve injury. The opposite side must be examined for comparison. Nerve injury is not uncommon, and requires familiarity with motor, sensory, and reflex testing. Although uncommon, vascular injury should always be considered during assessment, with attention to capillary refill and pulses. However, it must be kept in mind that the presence of a seemingly normal pulse does not preclude vascular injury! This is especially true in managing a patient with a knee dislocation, in which the incidence of vascular injury approaches 20% in some series.

The physical examination is completed with special examination techniques specific to the region examined

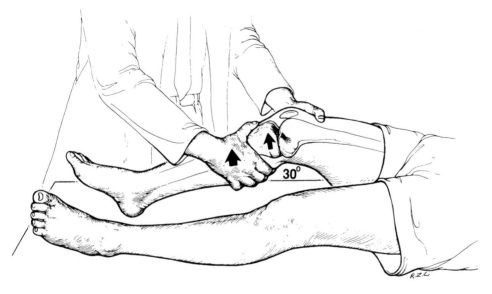

Figure 13–5. The Lachman test is performed by attempting to anteriorly translate the tibia in relation to the fixed femur. Increased translation, combined with a poor quality "end point," suggests anterior cruciate ligament (ACL) injury. (From Fu FH, et al: Knee Surgery, Vol 1. Baltimore, Williams & Wilkins, 1994, p 261.)

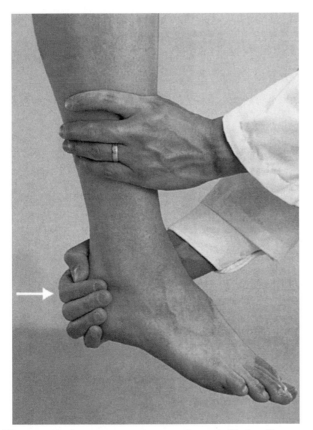

Figure 13–6. Injury to the anterior talofibular ligament (ATFL), the most commonly sprained ankle ligament, is assessed by attempting to anteriorly translate the talus. The calcaneus is grasped and translated anteriorly in relation to the fixed tibia, determining both the amount of motion and the quality of the "end point," compared to the opposite side. (From Reider B: The Orthopaedic Physical Examination. Philadelphia, WB Saunders 1999, p 294.)

and the suspected diagnosis. Examples of such special tests include the impingement signs in patients with shoulder pain, apprehension tests for patients with glenohumeral or patellar instability, and Tinel's sign in the evaluation of entrapment neuropathies.

Radiographic Evaluation

Radiographs should always be obtained in evaluating any athlete or patient with a history of trauma. Problems that are insidious in onset or that have been present for sometime, such as lateral epicondylitis (tennis elbow) or iliotibial band friction syndrome (runner's or cyclist's knee), rarely have positive x-ray findings, so radiographs usually are not necessary, at least at the time of the first evaluation.

Plain films must include two views perpendicular to the joint or bone of interest. When obtaining views of long bones, the joint above and below should be imaged so that pathology is not missed. The exact films ordered depend upon the suspected diagnosis, physical findings, and the specific anatomic area.

STRESS VIEWS

Stress x-rays are occasionally useful in assessing ligament integrity. The most common examples are for evaluation

of the acromioclavicular (AC) joint, the medial collateral ligament of the elbow, and the anterior talofibular ligament of the ankle. In testing for the severity of AC joint injury, weight is secured to the patient's wrist and comparison views are obtained. The weights must be secured rather than held by the patient, because holding the weights can bypass the AC joint and fail to show true joint separation (Fig. 13–7).

BONE SCAN

X-rays are very effective screening tools and are particularly helpful in identifying fractures or dislocations from traumatic injury. However, many sports injuries are due to overuse and do not involve a discrete traumatic event. Tests to detect pathology not visible on x-ray include the use of technetium bone scan in which radioisotope-labeled dye (technetium pyrophosphate) enhances the detection of soft tissue and bone injury. This test reflects physiology rather than static bone anatomy. Dye is injected intravenously, and the area of interest is then scanned for distribution of the dye. Increased tracer uptake may indicate the presence of a stress reaction or fracture. It is important to recognize that the results of the bone scan test are nonspecific; any condition that leads to increased blood flow to the bone or joint can cause a bone scan to be positive. For example,

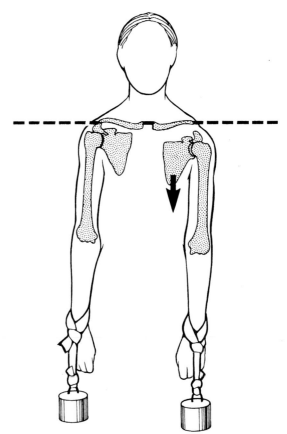

Figure 13–7. Stress views of the acromioclavicular (AC) joint demonstrate increased distance between the clavicle and acromion as well as an increased space between the coracoid and clavicle. These findings confirm a complete (type III) AC separation. (From Richwood CA Jr, et al: The Shoulder, 2nd ed. Philadelphia, WB Saunders, 1998, p 216.)

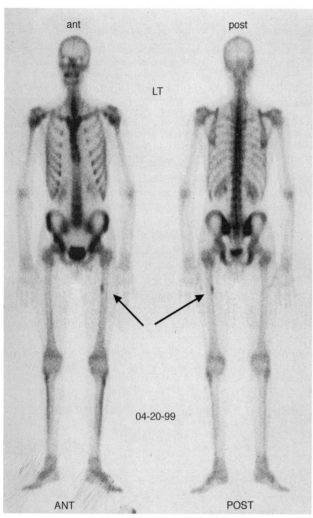

Figure 13–8. In this college runner, persistent groin and thigh discomfort, pain even at rest, and inability to walk without a limp led to a bone scan, which confirmed a proximal femur facture. Plain radiographs were negative.

increased uptake can be due to fracture, infection, inflammation, or tumor. Because of the nonspecificity of this test, results must be interpreted in the context of the patient's presentation and examination findings. One of the most common indications for use of a bone scan is in the runner with persistent leg pain, with suspected "shin splints" that has not yielded to treatment. Increased focal uptake on the bone scan confirms the suspected "stress fracture" common in this athletic population (Fig. 13–8).

Magnetic Resonance Imaging

Revolutionizing our ability to noninvasively visualize soft tissue, cartilage, and bone, magnetic resonance imaging (MRI) is a remarkable diagnostic tool. MRI demonstrates precise anatomic detail and provides a physiologic window with which to identify various pathologic conditions. Software manipulation allows the radiologist and clinician to distinguish scar from normal soft tissue, identify effusions (fluid in joints), and assess ligament and muscle tendon integrity (Fig. 13–9). Newer techniques even permit assess-

ment of articular cartilage. MRI, however, is expensive, and must be used judiciously in today's climate of cost effectiveness in health care.

Electrodiagnostic Tests

Electrodiagnostic testing is helpful in the evaluation of nerve function. Electromyography (EMG) involves the insertion of electrodes within specific muscles and recording the electrical signal generated at rest and with activity. Abnormal patterns of activity can reflect various pathologic states, such as denervation (loss of normal nerve input, such as may occur when a nerve is injured), or disease (neuropathy such as may occur with diabetes or neurologic disorder). Another test performed during electrodiagnostic testing is for nerve conduction velocity (NCV). This test involves recording the speed of conduction of nerve impulses along a specific nerve pathway, comparing it to the opposite (presumably normal) side or normal control values. A common example of nerve conduction velocity testing involves assessment of the ulnar nerve in patients with suspected entrapment behind the medial epicondyle of the elbow (cubital tunnel syndrome). Through analysis of the exact pattern of electrical activity and nerve speed, inference regarding etiology and site of nerve involvement is possible.

Arthroscopy

Arthroscopy, derived from the words *oscopy* (visualization) and *arthros* (joints), refers to the technique of imaging a joint's interior. Most commonly applied to the knee, shoulder, ankle, and elbow, arthroscopy is the gold-standard diagnostic tool for evaluation of joint problems and injuries. In addition to decreasing the need for of open joint surgery (complications like pain, stiffness, infection, nerve injury), arthroscopy provides visualization that is actually superior to conventional open techniques (Fig. 13–10) because of the precision and magnification afforded by the optics. In situ evaluation permits direct visualization of the normal anatomic relationships not otherwise appreciated during with more conventional open procedures (arthrotomy). Despite these benefits, however, diagnostic arthroscopy is an invasive technique and is an expensive surgical resource. It should be considered only when other evaluative methods have not successfully afforded the diagnosis.

PATTERNS OF SPORTS INJURIES

Sports medicine problems can be thought of as due to macrotrauma or microtrauma. Macrotrauma, injury due to a specific traumatic event, accounts for injuries during contact and collision sports, such as football, rugby, lacrosse, hockey, and downhill skiing. Microtrauma occurs as a consequence of repetitive stresses that lead to structural breakdown, most commonly seen during noncontact, endurance sports such as running, cycling, swimming, and throwing. These overuse injuries can occur whenever imposed demands exceed structural integrity.

Macrotrauma

Discrete macrotraumatic events may result from collision, contact, or sudden and abrupt deceleration. When applied

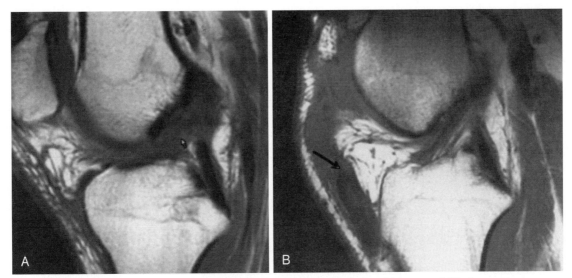

Figure 13–9. This 19-year-old suffered an acute knee injury, which upon MRI demonstrates a complete tear and absence of the normally present anterior cruciate ligament (ACL) *(A)*. Note in comparison *(B)* the normal striated discrete fibers seen in a normal patient's MRI. (From Miller MD, et al: MRI—Correlative Atlas. Philadelphia, WB Saunders, 1997, p 39.)

to bone, trauma can cause a contusion or fracture. When applied to soft tissue, the specific injury depends upon the structure involved and the degree of stress.

Ligaments

Acute trauma to ligaments can cause *sprains*. A sprain refers to a tear of the organized discrete fibrous structures that connect one bone to another. The severity of the sprain is determined by the degree of injury, and is generally graded from I to III (Fig. 13–11). In a grade I (mild) sprain, only a few ligament fibers are torn. The injury is accompanied by a small amount of hemorrhage and edema, with overall ligament integrity intact. The most common example is a mild ankle sprain, in which the anterior talofibular ligament (ATFL) is partially torn.

In a grade II (moderate) sprain, some of the fibers are macroscopically disrupted, with interstitial stretching of

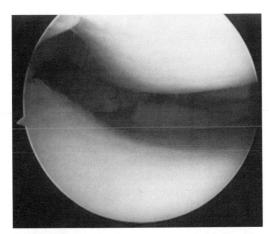

Figure 13–10. In this arthroscopic close-up view, note the anatomic detail of the articular surface and the meniscus, which in this patient was torn and required partial excision (meniscectomy).

some of the remaining ligament. The amount of pain, swelling, ecchymoses, and disability is greater than with a grade I sprain. Overall, however, some fibers remain intact. A common moderate sprain involves the knee's medial collateral ligament (MCL), strained during an acute valgus stress (directed toward the body's midline) to the knee. Testing the integrity of the ligament by applying a valgus stress to the slightly flexed knee allows assessment of the degree of injury, and in a grade II sprain, the knee will "open up" in comparison with the opposite side. However, the ligament will have an "end point," and overall remains intact (Fig. 13–12).

A grade III (severe) sprain implies a complete tear of the ligament. The amount of force at the time of injury is often considerable, leading to a greater degree of pain, ecchymoses, swelling, stiffness, and disability. Physical examination of the injured joint usually reveals compromise of the normal ligaments' integrity. Grade III sprains are relatively common, and are seen in the shoulder (tear of the anterior inferior glenohumeral ligament complex), the knee (anterior cruciate ligament tear), elbow (medial or ulnar collateral ligament tear), and ankle (anterior talofibular ligament tear). Complete ligament tears render these joint potentially unstable. Despite this vulnerability, some complete ligament (grade III) tears demonstrate excellent healing potential. Such is the case routinely following injuries to the knee MCL and the ankle ATFL.

PATHOPHYSIOLOGY OF LIGAMENT HEALING

The pathophysiology of ligament healing has been well studied. Early following injury, a fibrin clot forms and within 2 to 3 days leukocytes, platelets, macrophages, and chemotactic factors infiltrate the region. Early angiogenesis brings in further growth factors and fibroblasts deposit collagen into the tear site. The first several weeks are notable for the angiogenesis, synthesis of collagen (primarily type I), and extracellular matrix. Cellular proliferation and metabolic activity continue for the first 6 weeks, pro-

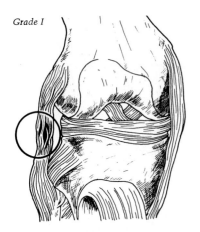
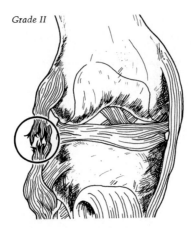
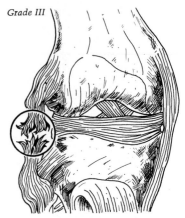

Grade I *Grade II* *Grade III*

Figure 13–11. In these illustrations, grade I sprain of the lateral collateral ligament shows microscopic tearing. In grade II, LCL sprain reveals a more significant tear, but the ligament remains in continuity. In grade III, sprain shows complete ligament disruption. (From Southmayd W, Hoffman M: Sports Health: The Complete Book of Athletic Injuries. New York, Perigree Books, Putman Publishing Group, 1981, p 84.)

ducing a somewhat disorganized cellular scar. Initially inadequate in structural properties, this scar progressively remodels over time with macrophage and fibroblast activity into a more organized parallel-oriented collagen structure. Such maturation may take up to 1 year following injury.

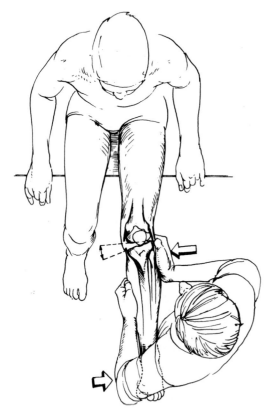

Figure 13–12. Medial collateral ligament integrity is assessed by the application of valgus stress and determination of the degree and quality of the opening. (From Hoppenfeld S: Physical examination of the knee. *In* Physical Examination of the Spine and Extremities. Appleton-Century-Crofts, 1976, p 185.)

Despite this well chronicled sequence of healing, some ligaments have poor healing potential, which may then predispose to joint instability. Common examples of poor healing potential and likely recurrent instability include injury to the anterior inferior glenohumeral ligament of the shoulder (recurrent anterior shoulder instability) and the anterior cruciate ligament (ACL) of the knee (recurrent anterolateral knee instability). The reasons for failure of these ligaments to heal may be related to their intra-articular environment, which precludes formation of a stable fibrin clot.

Because ligaments contribute substantially to joint stability, injury to these structures accounts for joint instability patterns. Instability is classified as either subluxation or dislocation. In a dislocation, there is complete separation of the joints' articular surfaces. Reduction of the joint is often necessary. The most common dislocation involves the glenohumeral joint of the shoulder. Subluxation is a "partial" dislocation, with incomplete separation of the joint surfaces. Subluxation involves transient separation of the joint surfaces followed by spontaneous reduction, and more commonly occurs in the patellofemoral joint.

MUSCLES AND TENDONS

Muscles and their tendon insertions can be injured by either direct (blunt or sharp force) or indirect (tension or torsional load) trauma. Direct injury results in a bruise, contusion, or laceration of the muscle, whereas indirect injury usually leads to a tear of the muscle, muscle-tendon junction, tendon, or site of the tendon's bony attachment.

Direct injury to a muscle results in a contusion. Quadriceps contusions are particularly common. The location of the quadriceps muscles directly anterior in an unprotected position places them at considerable risk during contact sport activities, particularly football, rugby, and lacrosse. Damage to the muscle usually occurs in the region directly anterior to the femur, with muscle fiber disruption, hemorrhage, and edema formation.

Treatment involves RICE (rest, ice, compression, elevation), with the application of ice and a compressive wrap immediately following the injury. Immobilization for a short period of time has been shown to be effective in decreasing the duration of symptoms, with use of a knee immobilizer or brace and crutches for the first few days. Cold whirlpool baths are effective at decreasing the swelling and pain, and helping achieve motion. When the patient is able to bend the knee 90 degrees and has reasonable quadriceps control, he or she is allowed off crutches and encouraged to begin normal ambulation. Return to activity is variable, depending on the severity of the initial injury and response to treatment. In a severe quadriceps contusion, the athlete may be out 3 weeks or more.

The most significant complication of muscle contusion is *myositis ossificans*. A blow to the muscle (usually the quadriceps) stimulates differentiation of normally reparative mesenchymal cells into osteoblasts, which generate bone (Fig. 13–13). Bone formation in an abnormal soft tissue location results, and leads to a disquieting hard lump in otherwise normal muscle. Occasionally this same phenomenon can occur in the anterior soft tissues (brachialis) of the elbow following trauma. Usually this condition is treated nonoperatively, with expectant management as outlined for muscle contusions. The formation of heterotopic bone may be followed with serial x-rays and often takes 6 months to a year to mature. Other than protective padding there is no indication to remove the mass unless motion is restricted or the mass is unusually prominent and uncomfortable. In such circumstances it may be excised, but only after confirming its maturity. Most commonly this is carried out by performing a bone scan to assess activity. The best treatment for myositis is preventive. Indomethacin has been shown effective in prophylaxis against heterotopic

bone formation and is recommended following significant muscle contusion.

Tear of a muscle is known as a muscle strain, and is the most common type of muscle injury. A strain usually results from a strong eccentric contraction that exceeds the intrinsic strength of the muscle itself, most commonly occurring at the musculotendinous junction. Strains are most common in muscles that cross two joints, such as the hamstring, rectus femoris, adductor longus, and gastrocnemius. As the muscle is working to accelerate one joint, for example, the hamstrings contracting to move the hip, the distal (knee) joint is relatively fixed. Not surprisingly, rapid knee extension, such as experienced during sprinting, may lead to hamstring failure due to its relative inflexibility.

Patients will note the acute onset of pain or may feel something "pull" at the time of activity. They may note a popping sensation at the time. Running thereafter (in the case of a hamstring strain) is painful, and even walking may be uncomfortable. There is often tenderness on palpation over the injured area, accompanied by swelling and not infrequently ecchymoses. Pain on range of motion, both active and passive, may be present. Strains are classifiable into three grades based on severity. Grade I describes a mild strain, in which there may be pain and local tenderness but no actual palpable defect in the muscle belly and little in the way of weakness. A grade II (moderate) strain is more severe, with compromise of some fibers, but overall continuity remains intact. In a grade III strain, there is complete disruption of the muscle, which usually occurs at the muscle-tendon junction (rather than within the muscle belly or at the tendon attachment to bone). In a grade III injury, the athlete may not be able to actively move the joint normally powered by the affected muscle. Complete tears of the gastrocnemius-Achilles complex, the pectoralis major muscle, and the quadriceps muscle are common examples seen clinically.

Diagnosis and classification of strains are fairly straightforward. However, differentiation of complete muscle-tendon tears versus tendon detachments may be clinically difficult and require further diagnostic evaluation. For example, in cases of seemingly complete pectoralis major ruptures, MRI has been found useful in distinguishing a complete tear at the muscle-tendon junction versus a tear of the tendon (usually from the bone attachment). This distinction has clinical implications because muscle-tendon tears are usually treatable nonoperatively, whereas tendon detachment usually mandates surgical repair.

In general, the treatment of muscle-tendon strains is frustrating in that they are slow to heal. Healing of muscle tendons relies on the same principles outlined above for ligament sprains, involving ingress of blood and plasma, formation of hematoma, deposition of cellular elements with formation of extracellular matrix, and eventual reorganization along the lines of stress.

Tears within the substance of the muscle, or at the muscle tendon junction are usually treated nonoperatively. Common examples include strains of the hamstring and gastrocnemius. The key to treatment is prevention through effective warm-up and flexibility exercises. However, once a strain has occurred, treatment involves RICE (consisting of rest, a comfortable compressive wrap, ice, and elevation). As symptoms subside, return to normal activity (such

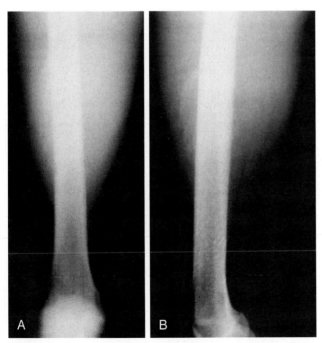

Figure 13–13. AP *(A)* and lateral *(B)* radiographs of the femur show ossification within the quadriceps mechanism following injury to the front of the thigh. (From Slanitski CL, et al: Pediatric and Adolescent Sports Medicine. Philadelphia, WB Saunders, 1994, p 139.)

as walking) and stretching in the pain-free range are allowed. Activities are advanced as the motion improves and pain decreases.

Disruptions of tendon from at or near its bony attachment, on the other hand, are usually (but not always) treated surgically. Such examples include rupture of the pectoralis major tendon (from the insertion along the proximal humerus), the distal biceps tendon (from the radial tuberosity of the elbow), the distal quadriceps tendon (from the superior patella), and the Achilles tendon (from the distal insertion on the calcaneus).

PERIARTICULAR STRUCTURES

Trauma can affect any of the periarticular structures. Structures common to all synovial joints include the articular cartilage, synovial lining, and the surrounding neurovascular structures. Some structures are unique to their particular joint, including the fibrocartilage medial and lateral menisci of the knee, the circumferential fibrous labrum of the shoulder, and the fibrocartilage disk of the AC joint.

CARTILAGE

Chondral (cartilage) and osteochondral injuries can occur in any joint, but are most common in the lower extremities, where compressive and shear stresses from weight bearing are high. The most common locations are the femoral condyles of the knee following a twisting injury and the patella following patella dislocation.

Chondral damage is reflected in the form of softening, fibrillation, cracks and fissures, or actual detachment of fragments, with or without the underlying bone. Cartilage lesions may lead to swelling following activity, or occasionally mechanical catching or "locking" episodes. If the damage is purely chondral, x-rays will be negative. Although MRI is usually able to detect full-thickness cartilage lesions, or those that have become detached, it is less sensitive in reliably demonstrating partial thickness cartilage lesions.

Cartilage lesions have been classified based on their appearance. The most common classification scheme is that described by Outerbridge, based on size and thickness of chondral injury (Fig. 13–14). In grade I chondral damage, there is softening of the normally firm and smooth articular surface. Grade II lesions demonstrate some surface roughening, with fibrillation and shaggy texture. Grade III changes are deeper and often involve areas of cracks or fissures, but are only partial in thickness. In grade IV injury, there is full-thickness articular cartilage loss down to exposed subchondral bone. Other more useful classification schemes have been introduced, and they describe the location of the lesions in addition to the chondral appearance.

Sometimes the chondral injury will include trauma to the underlying subchondral bone. This type is known as an *osteochondral* injury, and is most common in the knee, but can occur in any synovial joint. These lesions are more commonly recognized than purely chondral lesions because they can be seen on x-ray (Fig. 13–15). The lesion (chondral or osteochondral) may be part of the overall presentation following joint trauma (pain, swelling, joint stiffness). Osteochondral injuries have been classified by Berndt and Hardy based on the fragment's relationship to the bone from which it arises (Fig. 13–16). Grade I lesions are incomplete, without actual complete fracture from the underlying subchondral bed into the joint. In grade II, a fracture line extends from the subchondral bone to the joint, but the fragment remains within the bed. In grade III lesions the fragment is loose within its bed. In grade IV injury the fragment has become detached and is free within the joint.

Treatment of these injuries varies according the patients' symptoms, classification, and findings. Most joint injuries do not demonstrate evidence of chondral injury by x-ray. Even MRI fails to reveal many articular cartilage lesions. Most patients with joint injuries are therefore treated on the basis of their associated injuries and are not routinely treated differently because they have a suspected articular cartilage lesion. If the lesion is detected, then treatment is

Grade I	Softening and swelling of the cartilage, "closed chondromalacia," note pitting edema of articular cartilage in foreground
Grade II	Fissuring and fragmentation, 1.2 cm diameter or less.
Grade III	Fissuring and fragmentation, greater than 1.2 cm diameter.
Grade IV	Erosion to bone, eburnated bone.

A

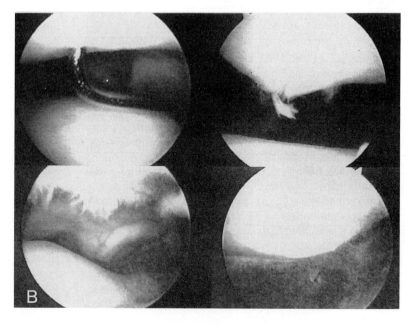

Figure 13–14. The most common classification scheme of cartilage injury is the Outerbridge classification *(A)*, graded based on lesion size and depth *(B)*. (From Fu FH, et al: Knee Surgery, Vol 1. Baltimore, Williams & Wilkins, 1994, p 1003.)

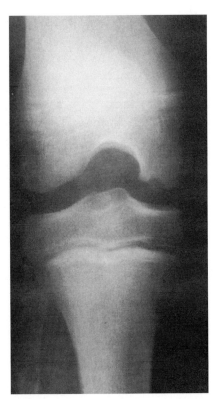

Figure 13–15. Osteochondritis dissecans is seen on this AP radiograph of the medial femoral condyle. (From Fu FH, et al: Knee Surgery, Vol 1. Baltimore, Williams & Wilkins, 1994.)

based on its severity, location, and degree of displacement. Incomplete lesions (grades I and II) will often respond to activity modification. Conversely, complete osteochondral injuries (grades III and IV) usually require operative intervention. Grade III lesions may be treated by in situ fixation. Grade IV lesions are usually removed, although rarely, they may be reimplanted into the bed where they originated.

SYNOVIUM

The highly innervated synovial lining may be pinched or torn due to trauma. The pain, swelling, and disability may be difficult to distinguish from that seen in a capsular or ligament sprain. Synovial injuries heal and do not require operative treatment. However, occasionally a synovial band may become thickened following a traumatic injury. This problem is most commonly found in the knee, where an otherwise normal synovial band may then become symptomatic and cause snapping or clicking, occasionally associated with pain. Known as plicae, these bands are normal vestigial remnants of development, but when prominent they can become interposed between joint surfaces and cause irritation, leading to symptoms. Usually this problem will resolve with nonoperative means, but occasionally arthroscopic evaluation and resection of the prominent pathologic plica is necessary (Fig. 13–17).

MENISCUS

Although the knee is the most common site of meniscal injury, menisci are located in several other areas of the body, including the temporomandibular joint (TMJ), the acromioclavicular (AC) joint, and the sternoclavicular (SC) joint. Each of these menisci serve the same protective function to their respective joints, and are made of fibrocartilage attached to the joint's periphery. There are medial and lateral crescent-shaped rings of fibrocartilage in each knee. These menisci play important roles in normal knee mechanics, with their most significant contribution in distributing normal load across the joint surfaces. Other less important functions include increased stability through enhanced joint congruency, "shock absorption" during loading, and enhancement of articular cartilage nutrition.

Meniscus tears can result from a specific traumatic event, such as a twist, squat, or an awkward landing. With age, the meniscus fibrocartilage becomes less flexible, and tears may occur with seemingly innocuous injuries, such as stepping down from a curb, or squatting down. Tears are usually accompanied by pain in the area of the tear (most commonly over the medial meniscus) and admitted difficulty with twisting or turning activities or squatting. The pain is usually related to activity, and there are few symptoms at rest. Sometimes the athlete will feel a clicking or catching sensation in the vicinity of the discomfort, a consequence of a torn fragment that is intermittently interposed in the joint.

A somewhat less common but distinct presentation of a meniscus tear is that of a "locked" knee due to a "bucket handle" configuration meniscus tear (see Fig. 13–3). The athlete will note inability to straighten the knee following a specific traumatic event. Most commonly the patient will have been playing a sport involving twisting or pivoting, felt something happen, and was then unable to straighten the knee. Walking with a bent-knee gait, motion is restricted both actively and passively, with inability to extend the knee comparable to the opposite (normal) knee. Tenderness is present directly over the joint line.

The diagnosis of meniscus tears is pretty straightforward, and depends upon a careful history and physical examination. Although further diagnostic imaging is not usually necessary, MRIs are extremely reliable when indicated. The accuracy rate varies according to location, with medial meniscal tears more accurately detected (95%) than those of the lateral meniscus of the knee (90%). Treatment of meniscus tears depends upon the athletes' symptoms, activity level, and type and location of the tear. Because most meniscus tears do not have inherent healing potential, they will usually remain symptomatic or become recurrently symptomatic with activity. Although the pain may improve with a period of rest, return to sports often reactivates the injury and causes recurrent pain. For this reason, most meniscus tears are treated operatively. With the arthroscope, the tear is identified, and the torn portion is resected (Fig. 13–18). The historical treatment of meniscus tears was removal of the entire meniscus. However, increasing appreciation of the meniscus' contribution to normal function, combined with the development of the arthroscope (ushered into clinical use in the 1970s) has led to attempts to remove only the smallest amount of meniscus necessary for elimination of pain and return to function. This trend toward meniscal preservation has been further advanced in the 1980s and 1990s with efforts to repair the meniscus using sutures or other fixation devices. Despite the appeal of repair, however, most meniscus tears are not

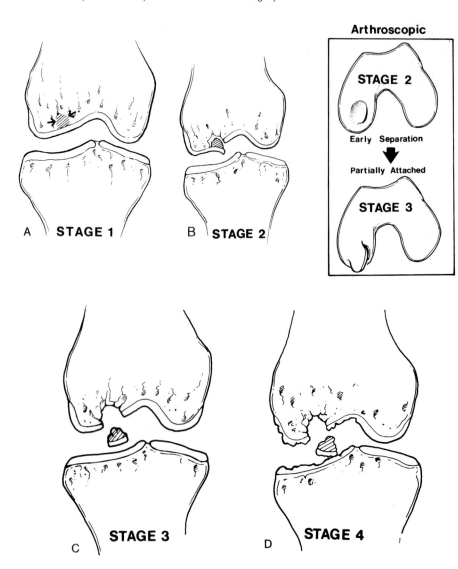

Figure 13–16. The Berndt and Hardy classification of osteochondritis dissecans begins with grade (here called *stage*) I, in which there is a stable articular surface, and extends to grade IV, with complete fragment separation. (From Scott WN: Arthroscopy of the Knee: Diagnosis and Treatment. Philadelphia, WB Saunders, 1990, p 180.)

reparable. Injuries that are best candidates for repair are longitudinal in orientation (rather than radial, oblique, or horizontal) and located near the periphery of the meniscus (only the peripheral or outer third is well vascularized and therefore predictably capable of allowing a healing response). Emphasis on the meniscus' importance has contributed to current efforts at replacement using synthetic and biologic scaffold substitutes.

LABRUM

The labrum is a distinct structure that enhances joint stability by increasing the depth of the "socket." Found in the shoulder and the hip, both ball-and-socket joints, the labrum is a strong fibrous thickening, which parallels the glenoid rim and the acetabular rim, respectively. In the shoulder, the presence of the labrum increases the "depth" of the glenoid process by a substantial 50%! Injury to the labrum can lead to joint complaints, including pain, swelling, and mechanical catching or clicking.

Labral injuries are decidedly less common than those to the menisci, but when they occur they are more difficult to diagnose. Symptoms are somewhat vague and nonspecific, and there are few reliable physical findings that implicate the labrum specifically. In the shoulder, labral tears usually present with a history of specific trauma, such as landing on the outstretched hand or feeling a distinct pain or pop during a particular throw. In the hip, labral tears are even more uncommon, and are almost always related to a specific injury. Symptoms in both joints are brought on by activity and relieved by rest.

Unlike meniscal injuries of the knee, imaging tests are rarely helpful in diagnosing labral injury. Labral tears are not well seen even on MRI, and definitive diagnosis is made by arthroscopic examinations. Treatment involves arthroscopic débridement (removal of the unstable torn fragment) or repair (most common in the shoulder).

Injury Due to Microtrauma (Overuse)

The second type of injury seen in athletes involves microtrauma. Rather than a specific event sufficient to damage normal structures, microtrauma involves repetitive stresses that are individually insufficient to harm tissue, but cumulatively can lead to injury. Overuse injuries can affect all tissues but most commonly affect muscles, tendons, and bones.

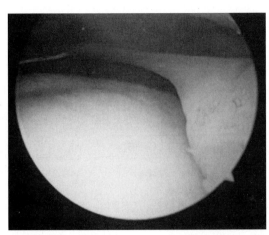

Figure 13–17. Note the medial synovial plica, a normal variant in most knees, which on occasion can become symptomatic.

Responsible for perhaps the majority of sports-related injuries, overuse occurs whenever the degree of stress generated by the activity exceeds the body's ability to tolerate the stress. Overuse can occur in both the highly trained athlete and the poorly conditioned "weekend warrior" nonathlete. It most commonly occurs in the poorly conditioned recreational athlete who neglects warm up, stretching, and then proceeds to do in 1 hour what he or she has not done for months. Repetitive stresses subject various structures to cyclic loading and eventually fatigue failure.

STRESS FRACTURES

In bone, repetitive stresses can result in structural failure of the bone. An example is that of a stress fracture seen commonly in runners. Most commonly, stress fractures occur in the proximal tibia or the metatarsals, but they have been described in many areas, including the femur, fibula, foot (navicular and sesamoid), spine (pars interarticularis), ribs, and even the humerus. Typically, the athlete presents with pain that does not go away after activity and persists at rest, and sometimes at night. The pain is worsened by activity, and thus interferes with the ability to continue to participate in sports. A careful history usually points to a change in recent activity level. For example, patients training for a marathon may often indicate a rather dramatic jump in their weekly mileage. Or there may be a change in the terrain, from soft track to hard pavement. Sometimes a change in the frequency of the activity can be sufficient to cause an overuse injury, even if the distance itself has not substantially increased. A change in equipment can also lead to increased stress, such as new shoes in a runner. The history should be thorough, investigating anything that is "different."

Physical examination reflects findings expected of a fractured bone. This may include tenderness to palpation in bones that are subcutaneous (tibia/fibula/metatarsals, navicular) or pain with passive joint motion for bones that are not easily palpable (back extension with pars defect, pain with internal or external range of motion of the hip for femora neck stress fractures). X-rays are usually initially negative, but with time may show indirect evidence of

fracture, such as callus formation (Fig. 13–19). Definitive diagnosis is made by either bone scan or MRI. A positive bone scan shows increased focal uptake of the dye correlating to the area of suspected injury. The more diffuse uptake of dye without specific focal uptake suggests the more benign condition of "stress reaction," which is considered a precursor of stress fracture.

Fortunately, treatment for suspected and even proven stress fractures requires little more than activity modification. Most stress injuries will eventually resolve, allowing return to previous activity. How long this takes varies with the patient, the fracture site, and the duration and severity of symptoms. In general, stress fractures will usually heal within the approximate 6-week time frame noted for other fractures. However, this does not mean the athlete will be able to return at that time to the previous level of activity. Often the athlete needs to return gradually and build up conditioning. The athlete should be reassured that nearly all stress fractures will heal if just given the opportunity to do so. Getting the athlete to "buy into" this diagnosis and understand how it happened in the first place will increase the probability of compliance with the activity modification program and the likelihood of successful asymptomatic return to full activity.

TENDON INJURIES

Repetitive tensile stresses in tendon can also lead to a similar breakdown of tissue, known generally as tendonitis.

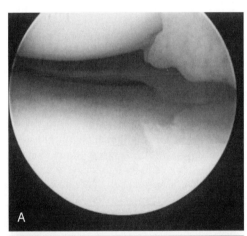
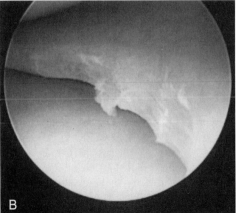

Figure 13–18. The tear shown in this arthroscopic photograph *(A)* was resected to a smooth stable base *(B)*, relieving the patient's symptoms and permitting return to activity.

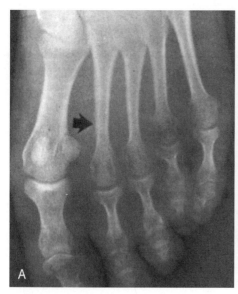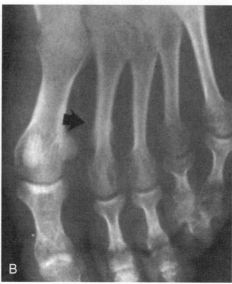

Figure 13–19. Callus is seen in the vicinity of the second metatarsal in this runner, whose symptoms and focal tenderness suggested a stress fracture, but whose x-rays demonstrated only the healing callus, confirming the suspected stress fracture when repeated 4 weeks *(B)* after the first negative films were obtained *(A)*. (From Perrin DH: The Injured Athlete. Philadelphia, Lippincott-Raven, 1999, p 422.)

Although specific inflammatory reaction is not usually found with these entities, the term "tendonitis" has gained widespread use and general acceptance. Some have tried to encourage use of the term "tendinopathy" or "tendinosis" instead. Regardless of the specific nomenclature used, tendon overuse injuries manifest themselves in ways that are similar to those of stress injuries to bone. The common presentation is pain related to activity. Often there is a history of overuse, such as playing three sets of tennis in one day after not having played for months beforehand. At other times, there doesn't appear to be any relationship between symptom onset and activity. The most common conditions involving tendons are those afflicting the elbow (medial and lateral epicondylitis, or tennis elbow), hip (trochanteric bursitis), knee (patellar tendonitis), ankle (Achilles tendonitis), and foot (plantar fasciitis).

Physical examination findings include the presence of tenderness to palpation directly over the tendon insertion. In tennis elbow, for example, the athlete will complain of pain over the lateral aspect of the elbow. Examination reveals localized tenderness over the lateral epicondyle, at the site of origin of the extensor-supinator muscle group. Pain is reproduced with wrist extension or forearm supination against resistance. X-rays are negative in most patients, with about 25% showing ossification or calcification at the site of tendon origin.

Treatment of overuse tendinopathies includes activity modification and a short course of a nonsteroidal anti-inflammatory drug (NSAID) (assuming no GI intolerance, reaction or allergy, history of peptic ulcer disease, pregnancy, or concomitant medication with which it cannot be taken). Activity modification refers to avoiding the abusive activities that provoke the symptoms. In the tennis player with lateral epicondylitis, this means avoidance of tennis. In the non–tennis player, it may mean stopping the other offending activities of daily living such as shaking hands, carrying briefcases, opening and closing doors (turning door knobs), and lifting things. The use of a brace or orthotic can often be very helpful. In the patient with patellar tendonitis for example, use of a special Chopat strap can decrease the irritation in the tendon itself. Simi-

larly, a counterforce brace (tennis elbow brace) seems to help patients with tennis elbow purportedly by decreasing the strain in the muscle-tendon's origin. A small heel lift and heel cup are helpful for patients with Achilles tendonitis and plantar fasciitis, respectively. Persistent symptoms usually require formal intervention in the form of physical therapy, incorporating stretching, strengthening, and other modalities. Occasionally, use of cortisone proves a helpful adjunct in treating overuse injuries.

Corticosteroids are thought to work by suppressing the inflammatory response early in the inflammatory cascade, and are known to reduce the chemotactic factors influencing the infiltration of leukocytes. Cortisone can be applied in two ways, via topical application or via injection. In physical therapy, cortisone is topically applied and penetrated into the affected tissue via ultrasound (phonophoresis) or via electricity (iontophoresis). Direct injection of corticosteroid is a safe and effective alternative, as long as it is not injected into the tendon itself. Perhaps the most common injection site is the elbow, where corticosteroid is infiltrated into the vicinity of the lateral epicondyle's extensor supinator origin in the treatment of tennis elbow (lateral epicondylitis). Although a single injection may be sufficient to cure the symptoms, repeated injections may be necessary. As a general rule, no more than three injections over a 6-month period are administered. Beyond this use, alternative treatments are probably preferable to avoid the risk of tissue damage or infection. Because cortisone has been shown to temporarily weaken collagen tissue, athletic activities must be temporarily modified. Because of risk of tendon rupture, cortisone injections are infrequently indicated in the treatment of patellar tendon or Achilles tendon disorders. When refractory to treatment, tendinopathies may require surgical treatment with excision of the pathologic tissue.

TREATMENT OF SPORTS INJURIES

Whether the injury is macrotraumatic or microtraumatic, the goals of treatment are to reduce pain, inflammation, and swelling; prevent atrophy and stiffness; and return the athlete to normal function and activity. Treatment can be divided into three distinct but overlapping phases: immediate, early, and definitive.

Traumatic Injuries

IMMEDIATE

Immediate treatment begins at the time of injury and involves RICE (rest, ice, compression, and elevation). Rest means the cessation of activity that causes or exacerbates the symptoms, and protects the extremity or joint from further injury. After an acute twisting injury to the knee, for example, the person may be unable to bear weight and may require crutches. Ice should be used immediately, applying it directly to the affected area. Because of the possibility of local frostbite, ice should be applied intermittently, for example, a half-hour on and a half-hour off. Ice is particularly effective during the first 24 hours when bleeding and swelling occur. Compression and elevation further decrease local tissue edema, swelling, and pain.

EARLY

Early treatment involves minimizing the complications of trauma (joint stiffness and muscle atrophy) and establishing a working diagnosis. Muscular atrophy occurs rapidly in the absence of normal physiologic stress and should be avoided by instituting weight bearing and exercise as soon as possible. Instituting early gentle active motion, sometimes assisted by a trainer or physical therapist, is often helpful in preventing progressive joint stiffness. The key in the early stage of treatment is to decrease swelling, atrophy and restore motion.

DEFINITIVE TREATMENT

Definitive treatment of most traumatic sports injuries is nonoperative and includes rest, NSAIDs, and some rehabilitation to restore normal motion and strength. Physical therapy in which local treatments (modalities) and exercises are instructed is an integral part of most athletes' recovery. Specific indications for operative management vary with the injury, its natural history, patient goals, activity level, and response to nonoperative treatment. Surgery may involve traditional open or newer arthroscopic techniques.

Microtraumatic (Overuse) Injuries

IMMEDIATE TREATMENT

When treating overuse injury, rest is the key. But rest does not necessarily mean use of a sling or crutches. It means temporary modification of the activity responsible for the symptoms. This means no running for the track athlete with unrelenting shin splints and no tennis for the player with recurrent tennis elbow (lateral epicondylitis). The tissues must be allowed to recover and heal, and this is only achievable through a temporary interruption of the repetitive stress pattern. However, it does not mean the end of all activity. For example, even with stress fractures,

athletes are able to cross-train, with swimming and cycling, for example. A water vest allows runners to run in the deep end of the pool, thereby maintaining fitness, while avoiding stress on the vulnerable areas.

EARLY TREATMENT

During the period of activity modification a number of techniques can be helpful to further relieve pain and inflammation and to restore function. This can begin immediately with the use of NSAIDs. Various modalities (local agents such as ice, heat, electrical stimulation, and massage) are often useful in decreasing pain, inflammation, and swelling.

DEFINITIVE TREATMENT

Although rest in and of itself is sometimes the mainstay of treatment, symptoms frequently recur on resumption of activity. Definitive treatment usually involves a rehabilitation program. The goal of rehabilitation is to restore normal function, including flexibility, motion, strength, conditioning, and endurance. Supervised by a physical therapist or a trainer, specific phases of treatment include local modalities to the affected area, followed by passive (by the therapist/trainer) and active (by the patient) stretching and strengthening techniques. As symptoms resolve, surrounding muscles are strengthened and the mechanics of the sport are examined. Alignment problems are often identified in this phase and corrections can be made. For example, the fabrication of a shoe lift orthotic may correct a previously unrecognized leg-length discrepancy, or a medial arch support may correct pronation during gait. Sometimes videotape analysis of the activity or technique is helpful to identify, correct, and change poor mechanics.

Occasionally, despite rest, modalities, NSAIDs, and rehabilitation, symptoms persist. In these instances, injection of a corticosteroid preparation may be effective. Again, care is taken to avoid intratendinous injection because of potential weakening of the collagen and subsequent rupture. For this reason, cortisone is rarely, if ever, injected near the Achilles or patellar tendons.

Occasionally, overuse injuries do not respond to nonoperative measures, and surgical intervention may be necessary. Some conditions seem to be more refractory to rehabilitation than others. Conditions that will occasionally lead to operative treatment include lateral epicondylitis (tennis elbow) and rotator cuff impingement (shoulder tendonitis). Rarely, stress fractures will fail to heal with rest or immobilization, and require fixation surgically.

SUMMARY

As the number of active individuals continue to grow, so too does the demand for knowledgeable and skilled care of the recreational and elite level athlete. Sports medicine emphasizes injury prevention, comprehensive care of the athlete, and prompt treatment and return to activity without risk of reinjury. The two most common mechanisms of injury involve acute trauma and overuse. In acute injury, treatment strategies include RICE, early exercises to avoid atrophy and stiffness, and definitive treatment through rehabilitation; occasionally, surgery is necessary. Overuse injuries occur from repetitive stresses, which outstrip the body's structural integrity and are usually successfully treated with activity modification, identification and treatment of underlying malalignment or mechanics, and return to activity.

Bibliography

DeLee J, Drez D Jr: Orthopaedic Sports Medicine: Principles and Practice, Vols. 1–3. Philadelphia, W.B. Saunders, 1994.

Kibler WB: ACSM's Handbook for the Team Physician. Baltimore, Williams & Wilkins, 1996.

McGinty JB: Operative Arthroscopy, 2nd ed. Philadelphia, Lippincott-Raven, 1996.

Reider B: Sports Medicine: The School-Age Athlete. Philadelphia, W.B. Saunders, 1991.

C h a p t e r   14

Wound Management in the Orthopaedic Patient

Christopher E. Attinger, M.D.

Wound healing progresses in an orderly fashion that involves hemostasis, chemotaxis, phagocytosis, mitogenesis, angiogenesis, collagen synthesis, and neoepithelialization (Fig. 14–1). Understanding the process and the factors that aid or disrupt it is essential for the successful treatment of open wounds. More complete knowledge over the last 20 years has spurred new treatment modalities including topical growth factors, hyperbaric oxygen, a wide array of dressing regimens, and soft tissue coverage techniques. These modalities have made it possible to treat chronic wounds far more successfully than in the past. Finally, applying current wound healing principles before, during, and after surgery is critical to ensure successful healing more effectively and with fewer complications.

THE WOUND HEALING MODULE

Coagulation Phase

Wound healing[1] occurs in an orderly fashion after an injury to the tissue has occurred (Fig. 14–2). The injury begins when the microcirculation is damaged by a surgical incision, blunt or sharp trauma, burn, radiation, cold injury, ischemia, infection, antigen-antibody reaction, etc. Blood extravasates into the surrounding tissue and is exposed to the underlying collagen matrix. This triggers the coagulation phase: blood vessels go into vasospasm, the coagulation cascade is activated, platelets aggregate, and a number of chemotactants are activated. The end product of the coagulation cascade, fibrinogen, is converted into fibrin to form a lattice-like framework at the wound site, entrapping platelets, proteins, and cells. The vasoconstrictive phase lasts 10 to 15 minutes after the initial wound. That phase is followed by vasodilation due to platelet and endothelial release of histamines, complement, kinins, and prostaglandins. The combination of decreased blood flow (secondary to clotting) and increased diffusion distance between tissue and open blood vessels (secondary to edema) causes a sharp drop in both the pH at the wound edge (from 7.4 to 7.25 to 7.35) and in the local Po_2 (60 mm Hg to 20 mm Hg).

Inflammatory Phase

The inflammatory phase, which follows the coagulation phase, encompasses the wound's defense against infection (early phase) and initiation of cell growth for repair (late phase). Platelets aggregate on the fibrin matrix and release a number of chemotactants, vasoactive amines, and growth factors to initiate this phase. The alpha granules[2] of the platelets release platelet-derived growth factor (PDGF), transforming growth factor-β (TGF-β), and platelet factor 4. These products serve as chemotactants for granulocytes, fibroblasts, and macrophages and activate macrophages, endothelial cells, and fibroblasts. In addition, complement C5a from the coagulation cascade and formyl methionyl peptide products from bacteria attract granulocytes (polymorphonuclear neutrophils, or PMN). The granulocytes adhere to the cell wall, in a process called margination, and migrate through the vessel wall toward the wound site in a process called diapedesis. The granulocytes infiltrate the wound within 24 to 48 hours and are there principally to destroy bacteria and remove foreign debris. In the process they consume local oxygen and produce lactate and CO_2, all of which contribute to the local hypoxia and acidity.

The late phase of the inflammatory phase is marked by the migration of blood monocytes and tissue macrophages to the wound site. They become the predominant cells in the area within 48 to 72 hours and replace granulocytes as the main scavenger. Their principal function, however, is to produce the necessary growth factors needed to direct the repair of the wound. Macrophages are activated by endothelial integrins, fibrin, lactate, hypoxia, foreign bodies, and some growth factors. They produce insulin-like growth factor (IGF-I), leukocyte growth factor, interleukins (IL-1 and IL-2), transforming growth factor (TGF), and vascular endothelial growth factor. The growth factors stimulate the fibroblasts to synthesize and deposit the extracellular matrix, the endothelial cells to create new vessels, the smooth muscle cells to proliferate, and the epithelial cells to differentiate and form new epithelium.

Angiogenesis

Angiogenesis[3] is growth and movement of endothelial cells to create new vascular channels. Angiogenesis is promoted in three successive stages. Platelets are the first to secrete angiogenic factor when they release PDGF, TGF, IGF-I, etc. The second stage occurs when fibroblast growth factor (FGF) is released from normal binding sites in the connec-

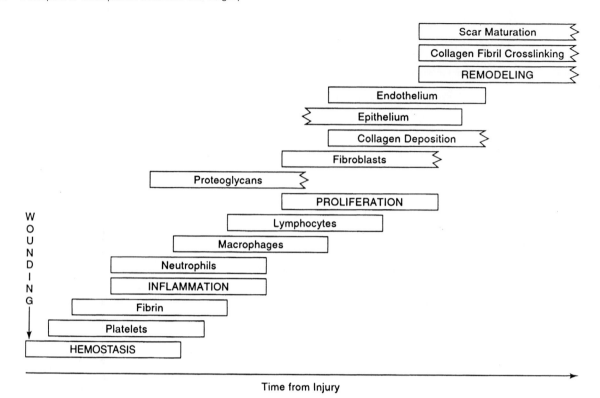

Figure 14–1. The temporal relationship of the sequential phases of wound healing is shown. Note the specific time frame at which the important cells and their by-products become a factor in the wound-healing response. (From Mast BA: The skin. *In* Cohen IK, Diegelman RF, Lindblad WJ [eds]: Wound Healing: Biochemical and Clinical Aspects. Philadelphia, W.B. Saunders, 1992, p 347, Fig. 22–2.)

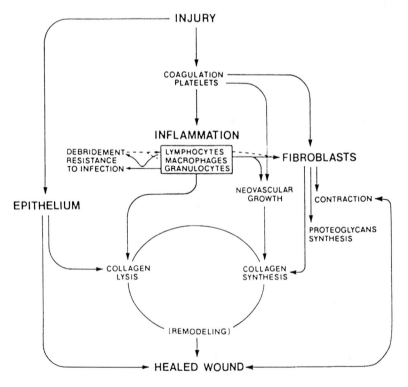

Figure 14–2. This wound-healing module outlines the principal phases of and cellular interactions in wound healing. (From Barbul A: Immune aspects of wound repair. Clin Plast Surg 1990;17:434.)

tive tissue. The third stage occurs with the release of vascular endothelial growth factor (VEGF) from the macrophage as well as the stimulus of hypoxia and high lactate concentrations. However, there has to be sufficient oxygen at the potential site of new vessel formation to allow angiogenesis to occur. The exact process in which hypoxia, high lactate, and growth factors interact to stimulate angiogenesis is not yet well understood.

Fibroplasia

Fibroplasia is the growth, replication, and migration of fibroblasts to the wound site for the production of collagen and proteoglycans at the wound site. The stimulus for fibroblast differentiation is oxygen tension, chemoattractants, and a variety of growth factors. They become the predominant cells at the wound site by day 7, although they start producing collagen and proteoglycans by day 5. This increases linearly for the next 2 to 3 weeks. The stimulus for collagen synthesis is growth factors and lactate concentration. Lactate concentrations and growth factors regulate the synthesis of collagen mRNA, whereas Po_2 controls the posttranslational modifications of collagen.

Fibronectins are the first matrix proteins secreted in the extracellular space by the fibroblasts, epithelial cells, and macrophages and provide the necessary scaffolding for the laying down of collagen. Their role is to aid in cell-to-cell interactions and cell matrix interactions. Fibroblasts also secrete core protein and four types of polysaccharides called glycosaminoglycans. The first glycosaminoglycan produced is nonsulfated hyaluronic acid, and the three others (chondroitin sulfate, heparan sulfate, keratan sulfate) are sulfated. The glycosaminoglycans (GAGs) are covalently linked to the core protein and form proteoglycans to create a charged and hydrated environment that facilitates cell mobility.

The synthesis of collagen begins with the translation of two procollagen α_1-chains (chromosome 17) and one procollagen α_2-chain (chromosome 7). The α-chains bind to one another through the hydroxylation of proline and lysine and form a triple helix (tropocollagen). The cofactors that are necessary for the hydroxylation of the α-chains are oxygen, ferrous oxide (Fe^{2+}), α-ketoglutarate, and ascorbic acid (Fig. 14–3). The tripeptide tropocollagen molecule has registration peptides attached to both the carboxy terminal and the amino terminal of the molecule. Before the tropocollagen molecules can aggregate to form collagen fibrils, the carboxy and amino terminal peptides have to be cleaved by procollagen peptidases. This is done as the tropocollagen molecule is exported out of the cell via secretory vesicles.

The loss of the terminal peptides makes tropocollagen insoluble so that it begins to spontaneously precipitate outside the cell wall. The aggregating cleaved tropocollagen molecules are further linked to one another via a hydroxylysine to hydroxylysine covalent cross-link (keto-imine) or via a hydroxylysine to lysine cross-link (Schiff base). Copper (Cu^{2+}) is a necessary cofactor in the deamination of the hydroxylysine or lysine molecule so that the covalent cross-links can form. The tropocollagen molecules (15 Å in diameter and 3000 Å in length) are linked to one another in staggered fashion so that each adjacent row is displaced by approximately one quarter of the length of the basic unit (Fig. 14–4). The tropocollagen molecules thus combine in staggered fashion to form filaments with a diameter of 200 Å. These filaments then form fibrils that are 2000 Å in diameter, and they then coalesce to form primitive fibers with a diameter of 20,000 Å. The primitive fibers then form the final thick fiber that is 100,000 Å in diameter.

As mentioned earlier, the laying down of collagen is the dominant activity in a wound from days 7 to 42. Type III collagen is the initial collagen formed. Because of the matrix proteinases, collagen is being simultaneously degraded. Equilibrium between synthesis and degradation is reached by the twenty-first day and continues for the life of the patient. During that process, type III collagen is gradually replaced by type I collagen. The healed remodeled wound, however, will reach only to a maximum 80% of the prewound skin strength (Fig. 14–5).

Epithelialization

The epithelial basal cell layer begins to mobilize at the wound's edge and, if still present, along deeper dermal structures (at the base of hair follicles). The basal epithelial cells enlarge, flatten, and begin to migrate over the wound. The leading edge of the epithelial cells dissolves the base of any clot or scab by secreting proteolytic enzymes. As the cells migrate to the center, the cells further back begin to undergo mitosis, and those that were at the initial wound's edge start migrating upward.

If the epithelial cells migrate over a sutured wound, the epithelial cells begin to migrate over the defect before there is an underlying wound matrix. They bridge the gap within 48 hours and then start mitosis and vertical migration. The epithelial cells also start to migrate down the suture tracts. When the epithelium begins to keratinize along a suture tract and remains exposed to connective tissue, it often invokes a violent inflammatory reaction. Although often labeled as a stitch "abscess," cultures are negative.

When epithelial cells migrate over an open wound, they need a base over which to migrate. Granulation tissue formed by new connective tissue and new vessels provides the base for the epithelial migration. The true rete pegs of normal skin never re-form so that the number of cells in the basal cell layer is far reduced. The attachment of this new skin is therefore never as thick or as strong as that of normal skin.

Factors that speed up epithelialization are wounds that do not require debridement, wounds in which the basal layer is intact, and wounds that are well oxygenated and moist.

GROWTH FACTORS

Growth factors modulate the inflammatory response at every step. They are proteins secreted by cells and directly affect the secreting cell, the neighboring cell, or those of a given type. Their exact role and importance within the complicated wound-healing cascade is still being defined. However, their identification and current clinical application signify that major strides in understanding wound healing have occurred in the last 10 years.

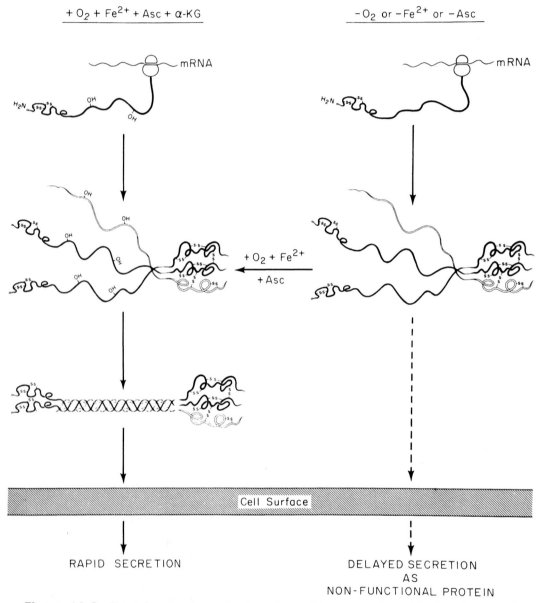

Figure 14–3. The left side of the drawing shows the posttransitional hydroxylation and helical confirmation of procollagen in the presence of adequate oxygen (O_2), ferrous ions (Fe^{2+}), ascorbic acid (Asc), and α-ketoglutarate (α-KG). Note that without oxygen, ferrous oxide, and ascorbic acid, the hydroxylation and helical confirmation cannot occur. Secretion is delayed and the product is a nonfunctional protein. This sequence is shown on the right side of the figure. (From Peacock EE: Wound Repair, 3rd ed. Philadelphia, W.B. Saunders, 1984, p 68, Fig. 4–13.)

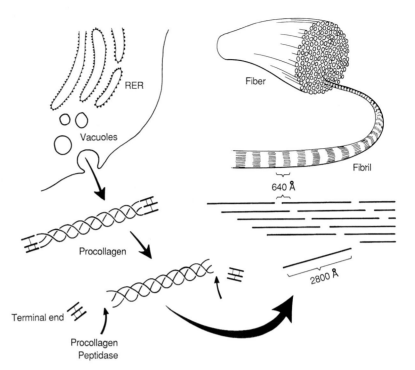

Figure 14–4. This diagram shows the secretion of procollagen and its assembly into collagen fibers in the extracellular matrix. Note that the procollagen carboxy and amino terminal peptides are cleaved so that the molecules can be linked to one another in a staggered fashion. The filaments then assemble to form fibrils, which in turn form primitive fibers, and then mature fibers. (From Peacock EE, Cohen IK: Wound healing. *In* McCarthy JG [ed]: Plastic Surgery. Philadelphia, W.B. Saunders, 1990, p 170, Fig. 5–6.)

PDGF attracts and activates neutrophils and macrophages. PDGF also serves to attract fibroblasts and stimulates their proliferation and their collagen production. PDGF also stimulates angiogenesis. When platelets degranulate, epithelial growth factor (EGF) is released, and it attracts and stimulates epithelial cells, endothelial cells, and fibroblasts. EGF also stimulates angiogenesis and collagenase activity. Platelets also secrete TGF-β, which stimulates monocytes to secrete other growth factors and attracts macrophages and fibroblasts. TGF-β also stimulates

fibroblast proliferation and production of collagen and proteoglycans.

A multitude of growth factors is produced by other cells, including the macrophages, lymphocytes, endothelial cells, fibroblasts, and smooth muscle cells. For example, IL-1 is chemotactic for epithelial cells, monocytes, and lymphocytes. It stimulates fibroblast proliferation, collagen synthesis, and collagenase activity. Transforming growth factor-α (TGF-α) stimulates mesenchymal, endothelial, and epithelial cells and is a cofactor for TGF-β to stimulate fibroblast proliferation. Tumor necrosis factor-α (TNF-α) is produced by macrophages and stimulates fibroblasts, collagen synthesis, and collagenase activity.

HYPERBARIC OXYGEN

The role of oxygen is crucial throughout the wound-healing process. The oxygen gradient between the center of the wound and its edge initiates wound healing. Oxygen is necessary for the neutrophil-mediated killing of bacteria (Fig. 14–6), as well as being in and of itself bactericidal for anaerobic bacteria (e.g., *Clostridium perfringens*). Oxygen is also one of the essential components in collagen synthesis and in angiogenesis. Hyperbaric oxygen therapy[4] is used to stimulate wound healing by increasing the tissue oxygen level. A patient within an oxygen chamber breathes oxygen at 2 atm of pressure. The resulting tissue oxygen tension rises to 400 to 500 mm Hg. This elevation of transcutaneous oxygen pressure (TcPo$_2$) at the periphery of the wound accentuates the oxygen gradient between periphery and the center of the wound. The sharpness of this gradient determines the wound-healing response. This gradient becomes especially important in wounds with low TcPo$_2$ at the wound periphery (below 40 mm Hg).

Hyperbaric oxygen is effective as long as arterial inflow to the area is adequate. If the local TcPo$_2$ fails to rise after

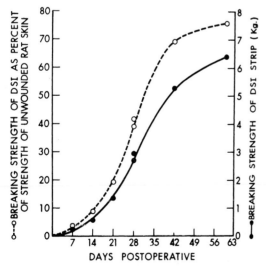

Figure 14–5. The breaking strength of a healing wound will achieve only 80% of the strength of normal skin. The dotted line represents the breaking strength as the percentage of the strength of unwounded rat skin, and the solid line represents the breaking strength of the healing wound. (From Peacock EE: Wound Repair, 3rd ed. Philadelphia, W.B. Saunders, 1984, p 108, Fig. 5–7.)

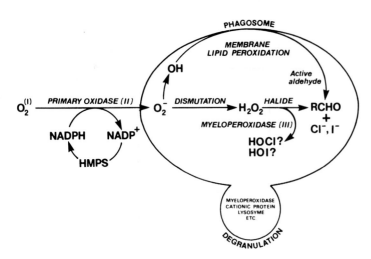

Figure 14–6. The reduction of dissolved molecular oxygen is the key to the oxidative bacterial killing mechanism. If the P_{O_2} falls below 30 mm Hg, the process of oxygen reduction is remarkably decreased so that oxidative bacterial killing becomes ineffective. (From Hunt TK, Hussain Z: Wound microenvironment. *In* Cohen IK, Diegelman RF, Lindblad WJ [eds]: Wound Healing: Biochemical and Clinical Aspects. Philadelphia, W.B. Saunders, 1992, p 280, Fig. 16–3.)

a trial with hyperbaric oxygen, then the inflow to the area is suspect, and hyperbaric oxygen will not help unless the arterial vascular supply is improved. Hyperbaric oxygen treatment is effective when factors other than poor inflow account for low TcPo$_2$ levels. Hyperbaric therapy is effective in radiation wounds, osteomyelitis, gas gangrene, ischemic flaps, ischemic wounds with good arterial supply (sickle cell), etc.

For example, the local blood flow in an irradiated wound is severely compromised because of the direct damage to the soft tissue and the resultant hypovascular scarring. TcPo$_2$ often falls below 20 mm Hg in such wounds. This problem can be addressed by removing all the scarred tissue until only normal tissue remains. Often the options of wide resection are limited because the scarred tissue involves too large an area to resect, a very difficult area to reconstruct (face), or vital structures (carotid artery or mediastinal structures). Hyperbaric oxygen then becomes a useful adjunct in the treatment of an irradiated wound by potentiating neutrophil-mediated bacterial killing and by stimulating local angiogenesis to increase the local TcPo$_2$. This then results in increasing collagen synthesis and neoepithelialization.

DEBRIDEMENT

The most important step in treating any wound is removing all nonviable or unhealthy tissue until only clean and healthy tissue remains (debridement). This establishes a healthy base for wound healing by (1) ensuring that the wound is free from gross infection and (2) ensuring that there is no dead or necrotic tissue left behind to inhibit healing. The debridement differs slightly in acute trauma and in acute or chronic infection.

Acute Trauma

The patient should receive a tetanus shot if his or her tetanus status is unknown or not up to date (within 5 years). The wound is stabilized and cleansed of contaminants and dead tissue as soon as possible. This procedure may have to be done in the emergency room if there may be any delay (more than 2 hours) in bringing the patient to the operating room. The emergency room debridement can be facilitated by using Xylocaine (lidocaine) without epinephrine for a peripheral nerve block. The actual cleaning of the wound is best done with pulsed lavage[5] of the wound using several liters of saline. Samples[6] of the actual debrided tissue and loose bone fragments should be cultured, as these have been shown to best correlate with future cultures of osteomyelitis if the latter were to develop. The wound is then dressed with a sterile, moist normal saline and cotton gauze dressing while the patient awaits surgery.

Once the cultures have been sent, the patient should be started on broad-spectrum antibiotics, which can reduce the rate of infection from 24% to 4.5%. In the case of gross contamination such as may occur with garbage truck or farm injuries, penicillin and an aminoglycoside or more potent combination should be added to better cover anaerobes and gram-negative infection. Antibiotics can then be adjusted for more specific coverage when the initial wound culture results are back.

In the operating room, initial debridement is best accomplished by removing all obviously dead muscle and skin and leaving questionable tissue behind to reevaluate in 24 hours. If the skin and subcutaneous tissue is avulsed, there is an overwhelming chance that most of it will die if is tacked back in place. One should trim the avulsed tissue until actual bleeding is seen. Cultures of the wound are again obtained. The anatomic damage should be fully evaluated, including avulsed nerves and or tendons. Cut nerves should be tagged with a fine monofilamentous suture so that they do not become lost in the subsequent soft tissue swelling. The wound should then be cleansed with pulse lavage to remove all foreign debris. Pulse lavage has a tendency to cause tissue swelling, and therefore, untagged nerves are easily lost. The wound should be dressed in a continuously moist, nonirritating bandage that keeps exposed tendons and bone moist.

Serial debridements every 24 to 48 hours are recommended until the wound is stable. By "stable" it is implied that the wound contains only viable tissue, is soft, is without erythema, and is minimally painful. It is important to get the wound ready for reconstruction within 7 days from the injury to minimize complications.[7] However, one can still obtain good results after that time provided that the wound is clean and fully debrided to normal tissue at the time of reconstruction.

The Acutely or Chronically Infected Wound

In the infected wound, it is important to know the source and extent of the infection. Obtaining an x-ray of the area underlying the wound is helpful in knowing if bone is involved and if gas exists in the soft tissue. If gas is seen on the x-ray, then one is usually dealing with gas gangrene, a surgical emergency. The gas is a by-product of anaerobic bacteria (usually *C. perfringens*), which travel along the fascial planes. The wound needs to be debrided very aggressively and immediately to prevent limb loss or death. Hyperbaric oxygen should be considered postoperatively to ensure that the anaerobic infection is controlled.

It is important to assess whether there is sufficient blood supply to eradicate the infection. Insufficient blood flow inhibits the body from delivering the necessary white blood cells and antibiotics to the wound site to fight the infection. Palpable pulses usually signify sufficient inflow. Otherwise noninvasive vascular studies should be performed. If the flow is deemed insufficient, the affected extremity should be revascularized. Unless there is gas gangrene or a rapidly ascending infection in an ischemic ulcer, debridement should be limited until the limb with the wound in question has been revascularized.

It is important to obtain a culture of the wound as soon as possible. One has to obtain a deep piece of tissue to send for aerobic and anaerobic culture because a swab or superficial tissue culture is contaminated with surface flora. Broad-spectrum antibiotics can be started after the deep tissue culture has been obtained. When surgically debriding the infected wound, ensure that all eschar, nonviable tissue, and debris are removed. Burr bone down to bleeding bone. Remove all stringy, soft, or limp tendon and leave healthy tendon behind. Remove all nonbleeding soft tissue. The presence of clotted veins suggests that the local capillary bed is no longer functional and the tissue containing the clotted vein should be debrided. It is important to explore the normal tracts along which an infection can spread to determine the extent of the infection. The infections usually spread along fascial planes (necrotizing fasciitis) or along tendon sheaths.

The edge of the erythema around the wound is then marked with an indelible ink marker and followed closely. If the redness subsequently extends beyond the drawn margins, either the broad-spectrum antibiotic is insufficient or the wound has not been adequately drained. The antibiotics are then changed and the wound is explored to ensure that it is completely drained. Hydrogen peroxide, 1% Dakin solution, povidone iodine, and chlorhexidine tend to harm normal tissue while sterilizing the wound and should therefore be used sparingly. Silver sulfadiazine is often used because it controls gram-negative and gram-positive bacteria while minimizing damage to normal tissue. It is gentle enough on the underlying tissue to stimulate epithelialization.

Once the wound is clean and noninfected, the wound care should focus on providing the optimal environment for wound healing. The guiding principle therefore should be "Do not place anything on the wound that cannot safely be placed on the eye." This ensures that the local environment is optimized so that the collagen deposition, angiogenesis, epithelialization, and wound contracture can rapidly ensue. For this to occur, the wound should remain hydrated, oxygenated, and at an adequate temperature. Wound dressing regimens that provide such an environment usually include a combination of occlusion and absorption. For heavily secreting wounds, one can also add a filler product (honey, gels, powders, beads, granules, or pastes) to the wound to help absorb the exudate while keeping the environment moist and clean. In addition, these dressings tend to decrease the pain for reasons that are poorly understood.

RECONSTRUCTION

Reconstruction is guided by the principle that coverage of a wound should be done as quickly and efficaciously as possible. Once the wound is clean, the reconstructive ladder encompasses the following reconstructive options: (1) allowing the soft tissue defect to heal by secondary intention, (2) closing the wound primarily, (3) applying a split-thickness (STSG) or full-thickness skin graft (FTSG), (4) rotating or advancing a local random flap, (5) transferring a pedicled flap, or (6) transplanting an autogenous microvascular free flap (Fig. 14–7). The solution is guided by the patient's health, the state of the wound, the location of the wound, and the surgeon's experience. For example, infected incisions in total knee replacements are best treated by pedicled gastrocnemius flaps with skin graft

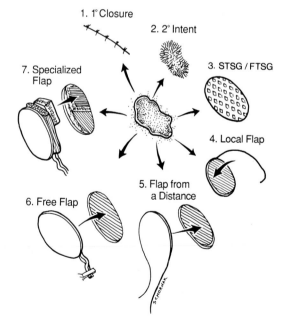

Figure 14–7. Seven different options exist when determining how to close a wound. Note that as one goes clockwise, the degree of complexity increases. However, the more complex procedure is often the less radical procedure because it may carry a higher chance of success. (From Daniel RK, Kerrigan CL: Principles and physiology of skin flap surgery. *In* McCarthy JG [ed]: Plastic Surgery. Philadelphia, W.B. Saunders, 1990, p 280, Fig. 9–4.)

because they have the highest chance of success, although simpler solutions are possible.

Healing by Secondary Intention

Healing by secondary intention (allowing the wound to heal by itself) is the way that most small wounds heal. It is also used for larger wounds when the patient is too sick to undergo another operation. It takes time and can be expensive because it may require months of visiting nursing care and dressing supplies. While the wound is open, there is always the risk that a new infection may develop, so close monitoring is required. Pain is also a frequent component of this type of healing because the raw wound surface remains exposed. This adds to the stress that the patient may feel. New dressing regimens, hyperbaric oxygen, and topical growth factors can speed this timetable by 25 to 30%.

The healed wound usually leaves the patient with a stiff noncompressible scar that is subject to future breakdown. After 10 to 20 years, the scar can develop a Marjolin's ulcer (an aggressive squamous cell cancer). If bone, joint, tendon, or the neurovascular bundle is left exposed during the long healing phase, function of the extremity may be subsequently permanently impaired. If the wound and the resulting scar lie over a joint or tendon, tethering of that joint can occur. Allowing larger wounds to heal by secondary intention are far from ideal but should strongly be considered as a viable option, especially in the very sick patient.

Delayed Primary Closure

Delayed primary closure (direct reapposition of the wound skin edge) should be attempted if it can be done without excessive skin tension. With low-velocity injuries, there is usually minimal swelling and little to no loss of the surrounding soft tissue so that primary closure is usually possible. Signs of excessive skin tension are pallor at the suture line that does not resolve by the time the wound is closed, loss of distal pulses by Doppler, and compartment pressures greater than 30 mm Hg. Wounds tend to swell postoperatively and add to the existent tension. Therefore, if any questions about the resultant skin tension exist, it is best to hold off closing the wound. Obviously, with high-velocity or crush injuries, there is usually so much soft tissue necrosis and swelling that primary closure is not advisable. To minimize the risk of infection when primary closure is done, it should be done with minimally reactive suture (monofilament polyglycolic acid, nylon or prolene) and with no buried sutures. Indeed, deep sutures should be used only to approximate structures (tendon, capsule, vessels, nerve, paratenon) and not to close dead space.

Skin Graft

Skin grafting consists of harvesting epidermis with varying thicknesses of accompanying dermis and placing it on a recipient base (Fig. 14–8). The anatomy of the skin is such that the epidermis represents 5% of the skin thickness and 95% of the dermis. A split-thickness skin graft (STSG) includes epidermis and a portion of dermis. As more dermis

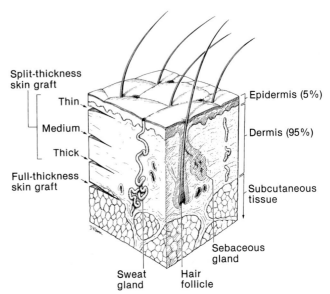

Figure 14–8. This diagram of a cross section of the skin shows the differences between the various thicknesses of split-thickness skin grafts and a full-thickness skin graft. The thinner the skin graft, the higher its percentage of take, the more the wound will contract, the less natural lubrication it will have, and the more it will hyperpigment. When the skin graft is thicker, more dermis is incorporated and the reverse will occur. (From Attinger CE: Soft tissue reconstruction for lower extremity trauma. Orthop Clin North Am 1995;26:300, Fig. 3.)

is included, the graft obviously becomes thicker. A full-thickness skin graft (FTSG) includes epidermis and all the dermis. Although the dermis contains sebaceous glands, nerve endings, and terminal capillaries, it is otherwise relatively acellular. It is made up principally of elastin, collagen, and collagen matrix. The subcutaneous tissue contains the sweat glands and hair follicles. The blood supply arises out of a vascular network that lies on top of fascia and sends vertical branches up through the subcutaneous tissue to the dermis. The vessels arborize along the way and terminate as capillary buds between dermal papillae.

The choice of whether to use a STSG or FTSG depends on the recipient bed and the desired quality of the healed graft. The thinner the harvested graft, the higher the chances of a successful take. This may in part be due to the higher number of transected blood vessels through which primary revascularization is established. The thinner the graft is, the more it will shrink as it heals because the decreased amount of dermis is less effective in inhibiting secondary contraction. In contrast, full-thickness dermis is believed to prevent contraction by inhibiting both myofibroblast proliferation and prolyl hydroxylase activity. The thinner the graft, the greater the chance for hyperpigmentation. Finally, the thinner the graft, the more susceptible it is to trauma because of the absence of anchoring rete pegs and the loss of lubricating sebaceous glands. Although the thickness of the harvested STSG can vary between 0.004 and 0.030 inch, it is usually harvested at 0.015 inch. The thickness of the FTSG depends on where it is harvested because the skin can vary in thickness from 0.015 inch (upper eyelid) to 0.150 inch (back).

PREPARATION OF RECIPIENT SITE

In order to have a successful graft, it is important that the recipient site be clean and well vascularized. If the wound is a fresh surgical wound, then one can graft directly onto dermis, fat, fascia, paratenon, or periosteum but not onto fresh cortical bone or tendon. If the area to be grafted is a chronic wound, then the bacterial count of the recipient bed should be less than 100,000 organisms per gram of tissue before successful grafting can be undertaken.[8] This can be accomplished by serial surgical debridement followed by topical Silvadene dressings. New granulation tissue should be allowed to appear before considering skin grafting because it demonstrates that adequate vascularity exists throughout the recipient site and that infection is under control. More expensive biologic dressings (pigskin or amniotic membrane) changed every 24 hours will achieve the same result.

The recipient bed can be judged ready to accept a skin graft if there is red granulation tissue, the pH is at 7.4, the $TcPo_2$ is above 40 mm Hg, and there is neoepithelialization at the wound edges. Because granulation tissue itself contains bacteria within its interstices, its superficial layer should be removed from the recipient bed before the skin graft is actually placed on it. One cannot generally graft on denuded cortical bone or tendon; intact periosteum and paratenon are required. However, if the exposed tendon or bone is less than 0.5 cm wide, then surrounding tissue will provide enough support to allow the skin graft over the denuded tissue to survive.

TECHNIQUE

Appropriate donor sites for split-thickness skin grafts include thighs, buttocks, and calves and for smaller grafts the dorsum of the foot or instep. If cosmetic considerations are important, care should be used to harvest the graft from a location where it can be concealed by a normal bathing suit.

Although older techniques exist to harvest skin, the Zimmer air-driven dermatome or the electrically driven Padgett dermatome are the easiest to operate and most reliable. One has to set the desired width of the graft by placing the correct width guard (2.5 cm, 5 cm, 7.5 cm, or 10 cm). The thickness between the blade and the guard is set (usually at 0.015 inch). The donor site, which was shaved preoperatively, is lubricated with mineral oil and then placed under tension using a tongue blade. The dermatome is set in motion and approaches the donor site much like a plane landing. Constant pressure is maintained as it harvests skin. When sufficient skin is harvested, the dermatome is lifted off the donor site. The skin graft is then stored in a saline soaked cotton gauze until it is ready to be used.

The donor site bleeding can be minimized by placing topical thrombin or a dilute concentration of epinephrine (1:200,000) on the donor site. The old-fashioned dressing of the donor site consists of placing Xeroform or scarlet red on the site. The site is then treated with repeated heat lamp treatments of 20 minutes each to dry out the site. One then trims the nonattached covering daily until re-epithelialization is complete. This dressing is labor intensive and painful. One can also use an occlusive dressing (Aquaphor gauze with Adaptic, Op-Site, or Tegaderm) or a semipermeable dressing such as Biobrane. These dressings minimize the donor site pain and speed up the re-epithelialization of the donor site. One, however, has to be careful that the fluid that collects under the dressing does not become infected because this will significantly delay the re-epithelialization of the donor site.

Improved adherence of the graft and control of the bleeding at the just prepared recipient site is achieved by spraying topical thrombin on the site prior to grafting. If the bleeding at the recipient site cannot be adequately controlled to prevent potential hematoma, skin grafting should be delayed. A sterile dressing is placed on the recipient site and the harvested skin graft is placed back on the donor site.

One then has to decide whether to mesh the harvested skin graft or not before placing it on the recipient site (Fig. 14–9). The advantage of meshing is that hematomas or seromas cannot build up underneath because the meshed graft interstices allow fluid to escape before a fluid collection can build up. Unless skin is in short supply, there is no advantage to meshing at a ratio greater than 1.5:1 or to stretching the mesh far apart. The only advantage to not meshing is that the resultant crisscross pattern is avoided when the graft heals.

Insetting the graft has to be done carefully. It is usually inset loosely and tacked into place by staples or a running 5-0 monofilament stitch along its periphery. The graft is then covered with a petroleum gauze, bacitracin, cotton roll, and Ace bandage. To prevent shearing of the graft off the recipient site, one can either wrap the extremity in an Unna boot or splint the extremity until the graft has taken (usually 2 weeks). In areas where it is difficult to ensure graft take, an additional bolster (Fig. 14–10) can be placed over the graft, which is held in place with strategically placed bolster sutures. The bolster is built by first placing Xeroform and then normal saline–soaked cotton. The water is forced out of the cotton as the bolster stitches are tied down. This allows the skin graft to conform exactly to the recipient site. The extremity is then placed in a splint to prevent motion and resultant shearing of the skin graft off its bed. A gentle ace wrap holds it all together. The dressing can be removed at 5 to 7 days, as will be detailed later.

PHYSIOLOGIC PHASES IN SKIN GRAFT SURVIVAL

The biologic step for graft survival begins with a plasmatic imbibition phase that lasts 48 hours. The graft is ischemic during this time, passively taking up fluid while the underlying bed proliferates. Although split-thickness skin grafts can tolerate this ischemia for up to 5 days, full-thickness skin grafts can do so for only 3 days. Therefore, a graft threatened by an underlying hematoma or seroma can be salvaged if the clot or fluid is removed before the graft's tolerance for ischemia is exceeded. Evacuation of the hematoma or seroma reestablishes contact of the graft with the underlying bed so that revascularization of the graft can proceed.

The inosculatory and capillary growth phase starts after 48 hours when capillary budding from the recipient bed makes contact with the graft vessels. Whether an anastomo-

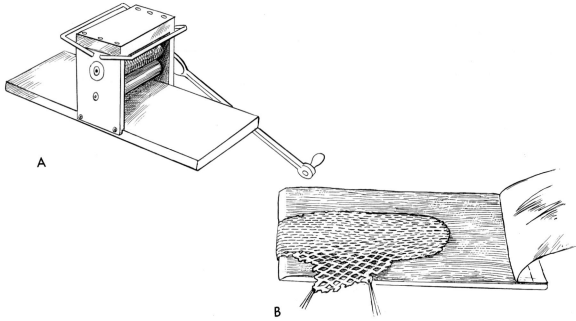

Figure 14–9. A skin graft is meshed by placing it on a scored plate and then running it through the meshing machine. This imprints a mesh pattern on the skin graft, which allows extra fluid and blood to escape through the graft interstices. This prevents fluid build-up underneath the graft that could inhibit its take. (From Rudolph R, Ballantyne DL: Skin grafts. *In* McCarthy JG [ed]: Plastic Surgery. Philadelphia, W.B. Saunders, 1990, p 238, Fig. 8–13.)

sis occurs between host and recipient vessels or whether the graft is revascularized via an ingrowth of recipient vessels is unclear. Circulation of the graft, however, begins between day 4 and 7. The flow initially consists only of inflow which leads to venous congestion and swelling. Venous outflow and lymphatic drainage is established by day 6 and the graft begins to lose the accumulated water by day 9.

A skin graft on an extremity should be kept elevated for at least 7 days until venous drainage is fully established and graft venous stasis can be avoided. The use of a compressive Unna boot over the graft allows for far earlier dependency. A meshed graft is usually first examined at 5 to 7 days, by which time it should have "taken." Obviously, it should be examined sooner if potential infection is likely. If the graft is unmeshed and unbolstered, it is important to examine it at 48 hours to ensure that there is no fluid collection between the graft and its bed that could inhibit its revascularization. As mentioned earlier, if the collection exists, it should be aspirated with a needle.

FULL-THICKNESS SKIN GRAFT

A full-thickness skin graft (FTSG) is a skin graft that includes the epidermis and all the underlying dermis. The donor site therefore has to be closed because it will not spontaneously re-epithelialize. The principal advantage of a FTSG is that there is no wound contracture (important over joints). In addition, the lubrication of the skin is normal (sebaceous glands are preserved) and there is no change in skin color or texture. The return of sensation that occurs reflects the innervation of the underlying bed and returns in the following order: pain, light touch, and temperature. Sensory recovery starts at 4 weeks and can take up to 1 to 2 years to complete.

The best donor sites for FTSG are flexor surfaces such as the groin, the antecubital fossa, and the popliteal fossa. These harvesting sites can easily be closed primarily and leave a thin scar. An accurate pattern of the recipient site is made and then encompassed within a lenticular pattern with a length-to-width ratio of at least 3:1 (this ratio ensures that no dog-ears are created when the wound is closed). That lenticular pattern is then drawn out with the long axis parallel to the flexor crease. The actual FTSG pattern is first cut out and the fat trimmed from its underside with a sharp scissors (Fig. 14–11). It will shrink up to 40% of its preharvest size because of the elastin within the dermis. It is then stored in a normal saline soaked sponge. The remaining lenticular pattern is then excised and the skin edges are undermined and closed with an interrupted deep dermal stitch and a running superficial dermal stitch.

The stored graft is then placed on the recipient site and sewn into place with a running 4-0 nylon. It stretches back out to its original size as it is sewn in place. It is important to place several small perforations in the FTSG to allow fluid to escape and thus avoid a seroma or hematoma. The 4-0 nylon stay sutures are strategically placed along the edges and then tied tightly over a Xeroform and soaked wet cotton bolster. This ensures excellent coaptation of the graft on the recipient site by helping prevent hematoma, seroma, or shearing.

It is more difficult to achieve 100% take with a FTSG because the revascularization is more tenuous. Primary revascularization can be interrupted if the initial contact between the graft and the underlying dermis is disturbed by hematoma, seroma, or shearing. That portion of the graft not revascularized by primary revascularization (day 4 to 7 after skin graft) must then receive its blood supply via a slower process involving neovascularization. This

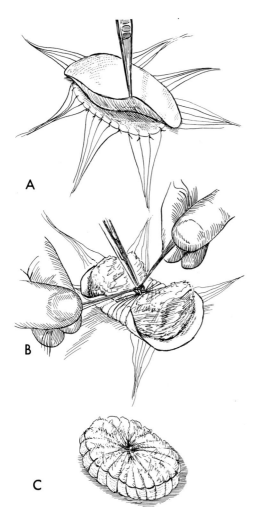

Figure 14–10. Bolster dressings are used to immobilize full-thickness and split-thickness skin grafts over the recipient site to prevent shearing. Bolster stitches are placed around the edges of the wound and serve to hold the graft in place as well *(A)*. The graft is then covered with petrolatum gauze. Wet un-wrung cotton is placed over the petrolatum gauze *(B)*. The bolster stitches are then tied over the dressing, applying direct pressure to the underlying graft *(C)*. (From Rudolph R, Ballantyne DL: Skin grafts. *In* McCarthy JG [ed]: Plastic Surgery. Philadelphia, W.B. Saunders, 1990, p 241, Fig 8–18.)

process is triggered by the anaerobic metabolism of the skin graft itself releasing vasoactive substances to stimulate capillary growth. The prolonged ischemia the skin graft faces causes an initial loss of the epidermis and capillary dermis, which then are replaced by a thin capillary dermis and attenuated epidermis. The resulting graft is smooth, fibrotic, tight skin with a silvery sheen.

COMPLICATIONS OF SKIN GRAFTING

Hematoma is the most common cause of graft failure. It prevents the capillary buds from the underlying bed from making contact with the skin graft. For this reason, it is suggested that if there is excessive bleeding, the placement of the graft should be delayed 24 to 48 hours. A useful adjunct is the use of topical thrombin, which not only helps stop the bleeding but also acts as glue to hold the graft in

place. Obviously meshing the skin graft will help in preventing a hematoma from forming between the skin graft and underlying bed. Pressure from an Unna boot dressing or bolster also is helpful.

Infection is the second most frequent cause of graft failure. The key to preventing infection is to skin graft *only* when the recipient bed has been debrided to normal tissue and is relatively sterile (less than 100,000 bacterial colonies per gram of tissue). The presence of bacteria (especially β-hemolytic streptococcus or *Pseudomonas*) can be lethal to the graft. They produce a high level of proteolytic enzymes and plasmin which together dissolve the fibrin holding the graft to the recipient bed.

Seroma also leads to graft failure and is more prominent in areas where a confluence of lymphatic channels meet: groin or axilla. Meshing the graft in those areas can be very helpful. Atraumatic tissue handling will likewise minimize the amount of necrotic tissue left behind. A bolster dressing is also helpful.

Shearing of the graft from the underlying bed occurs with movement of the underlying bed and leads to rupture of the tenuous attachments that lead to revascularization of the graft. It is therefore important to immobilize the graft on the bed and prevent movement of the underlying bed by splinting the leg extremity. Similarly, it is important to keep the extremity elevated so that the venous hydrostatic pressure does not inhibit outflow from the just revascularized graft.

Flaps

Flaps are blocks of tissue that are rotated into existing soft tissue defects. They can include any combination of skin, subcutaneous fat, fascia, muscle, and bone. The flap can be random (without identifiable blood supply), pedicled or axial (with a blood supply that extends from the flap's base to its tip), or free (detached with its blood supply interrupted and then moved to a distant site where blood flow is reestablished using microsurgical technique).

The random skin flap, whose design was based on a length-to-width ratio, is a viable but outmoded concept that has existed for millennia because of a lack of understanding

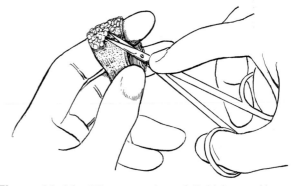

Figure 14–11. When preparing a full-thickness skin graft, it is critical to remove all subcutaneous tissue from the graft to ensure better take. This can be done by placing the full-thickness skin graft on the finger and defatting it with scissors. (From Rudolph R, Ballantyne DL: Skin grafts. *In* McCarthy JG [ed]: Plastic Surgery. Philadelphia, W.B. Saunders, 1990, p 239, Fig 8–16.)

of cutaneous blood flow. The accepted ratios of length to width to ensure flap viability were based on experience and were 3:1 on the face, 2:1 on the trunk, and 1:1 on the extremity. This principle guided flap design until 1970 when Milton wrote a landmark paper[9] proving that it was not the length-to-width ratio but rather the presence of an artery at the base of a flap that determined its success. The rediscovery and refinements by Ian Taylor[10] of Manchot's (1889) and Solomon's (1939) treatises on cutaneous blood flow now enable surgeons to design flaps based on vascular anatomic principles. That knowledge, combined with the expanded use of the delay principle, now enables surgeons to design complex flaps with the full confidence that they will survive.

ANATOMIC PRINCIPLES OF FLAPS

A specific area of skin can receive blood from one of three principal sources: directly from a cutaneous artery, from musculocutaneous perforating arteries, or from fasciocutaneous arteries. An angiosome defines the specific cutaneous territory and its underlying tissue supplied by a given source artery (Fig. 14–12). Angiosomes are connected to one another by choke vessels that open when blood flow to a single angiosome is compromised. The source artery of a given angiosome will thus be able to supply blood to a neighboring angiosome via choke vessels. However, it will not carry the angiosome beyond the neighboring one

unless a delay procedure is employed. Delaying a flap[11] is a surgical method to increase the blood flow to the distal end of the flap by interrupting its intermediate blood supply. This gives sufficient time for two sets of choke vessels to open so that the distal angiosome can now survive (Fig. 14–13). The territory that is drained by a given set of named veins is called a venosome. Venosomes are linked to one another by valveless oscillating veins that allow redirection of flow when the normal drainage has been interrupted. The oscillating veins are located in the same area as the choke vessels and therefore angiosomes and venosomes overlap and indeed together comprise an angiotome.

Direct cutaneous arteries run in subcutaneous fat parallel to the skin. They are usually accompanied by two venae comitantes, and these veins drain the area supplied by the cutaneous artery. Flaps based on this direct blood supply have a far larger length-to-width ratio than traditional random flaps.[12] They are traditionally known as axial pattern flaps and can be used as a pedicled flap (the flap has its base dissected free of most of the tissue surrounding the artery and veins for added mobility), as an island flap (when the vascular pedicle is dissected completely free for a certain length and the flap is then transferred to a local site separate from the donor site while the pedicle is buried under the intervening tissue), or as a free flap (in which the pedicle is totally detached and then reconnected to

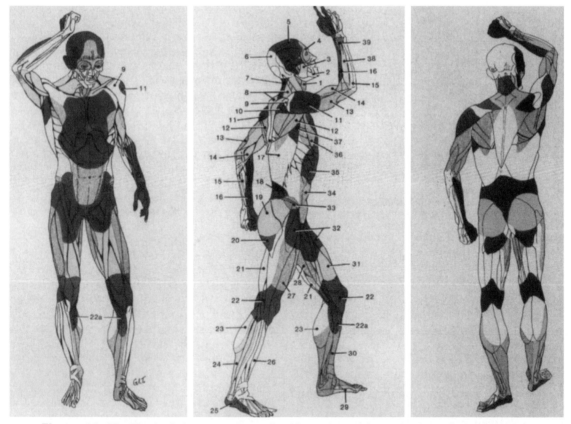

Figure 14–12. The body is compartmentalized into 40 vascular territories called angiosomes as delineated by Ian Taylor in his classic study. Each angiosome is a three-dimensional block of tissue fed by a source artery. (From Taylor I, et al: The vascular territories of the body (angiosomes) and their clinical application. *In* McCarthy JG [ed]: Plastic Surgery. Philadelphia, W.B. Saunders, 1990, p 343, Fig. 10–10.)

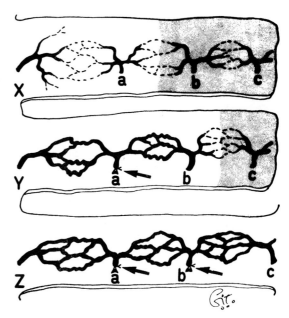

Figure 14–13. These three diagrams illustrate how flap delay works using the principles of vascular territories. *Top,* Source artery X feeds its own territory as well as the adjacent territory a via the choke vessels between them. Therefore, if vessels a, b, and c were to be ligated at the same time, the line of necrosis would be along the choke vessels between territories a and b. *Middle,* With source artery Y, vessel a has been previously tied off to allow the choke vessels between a and b to open. Thus, vessel Y can now carry three angiosomes: its own and those formerly fed by arteries a and b. *Bottom,* Vessels a and b have been sequentially tied off, allowing source artery Z to carry the angiosomes previously fed by a, b, and c. (From Attinger CE: Soft tissue reconstruction for lower extremity trauma. Orthop Clin North Am 1995;26:308, Fig. 10.)

recipient vessels anywhere on the body utilizing microsurgical technique).

Musculocutaneous flaps consist of muscle, fascia, subcutaneous fat, and skin.[13] The muscle receives its blood supply according to one of the five patterns (Fig. 14–14). They include type I (one vascular pedicle, e.g., tensor fascia lata muscle), type II (one dominant vascular pedicle entering at or near the origin with minor pedicles entering the muscle belly more distally, e.g., gracilis muscle), type III (two major vascular pedicles from separate regional arteries, e.g., gluteus maximus muscle), type IV (segmental minor vascular pedicles along the entire length of the muscle, e.g., sartorius muscle), type V (one dominant vascular pedicle at the origin with several smaller secondary segmental pedicles at the insertion, e.g., latissimus dorsi muscle). The skin is more likely to receive blood from

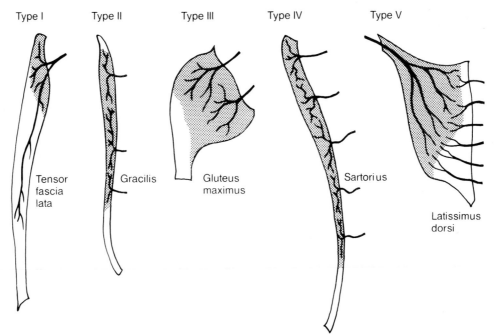

Figure 14–14. The predominant patterns of the vascular anatomy of the muscles of the body are shown here. Type I has a single vascular pedicle. Type II has one dominant pedicle and several minor pedicles. Type III has two dominant pedicles. Type IV has segmental minor pedicles. Type V has one dominant pedicle and secondary segmental pedicles. A muscle with a dominant pedicle (I, II, III, V) can be utilized as a pedicled flap. Because type IV muscles have only minor pedicles, they are difficult to use as pedicled flaps. (From Mathes SJ, Eshima I: The principles of muscles and musculocutaneous flaps. *In* McCarthy JG [ed]: Plastic Surgery. Philadelphia, W.B. Saunders, 1990, p 381, Fig. 11–2.)

musculocutaneous perforators if the muscle is broad rather than thin. The skin paddle obviously must overlie the muscle and, without utilizing delay procedures, can only extend beyond the edge of the muscle.

The fasciocutaneous system is the third source of blood supply to the skin. It is fed by a major regional artery via perforators that pass along the fascia between muscle bellies and then fan out at the level of the deep fascia. There these perforators form a plexus of vessels that ascend through the subcutaneous tissue to the overlying dermis. Classical examples include the fasciocutaneous systems that arise along the long axis of the three arteries of the leg: anterior tibial artery, posterior tibial artery, and peroneal artery. The medial and lateral plantar arteries supply the sole of the foot in much the same way.

It is important to ensure that blood supply to the flap is not compromised by extensive tension, kinking of the pedicle, external pressure, hematoma, infection, or decreased systemic flow due to vasospasm or decreased cardiac output. Tension can best be detected when pallor develops anywhere along the flap as it is inset. Kinking of the pedicle usually affects venous return first and occurs when the flap or its pedicle is sharply angulated. External pressure can develop from tight external bandages or poor positioning. Hematoma causes damage not only by a volume effect but also by the free radicals that it releases. Infection likewise can be disastrous because the inflammatory response causes edema that leads to compromised venous blood flow and tissue destruction.

It is therefore important to preplan the flap exactly. Knowing the vascular anatomy of the area in question helps ensure the safe design of flaps based on anatomic principles. The term random flap with its obligate 1:1 length-to-width ratio in the extremity is a flap based on unknown vascular anatomy and therefore has limited utility. An axial pattern flap has identifiable blood flow at its base and has a viable area that depends on the angiotome that the artery serves. This flap must be preplanned using Doppler technique, and its area can be extended beyond its defined angiotome using delay principles.

LOCAL FLAPS

Local flaps are adjacent to the defect and are either rotated on a pivot point or advanced forward from their base to cover the defect. They include at a minimum the epidermis, dermis, and subcutaneous tissue. They can include the underlying fascia or muscle. The donor site is either closed primarily or skin is grafted. It is important to carefully preplan the flap by determining the size of the defect after debridement and then using a slightly larger pattern to ensure adequate fit. When moving the pattern from its base to cover the defect, it is important that the flap move without tension.

Local flaps can be either random or pedicled (axial). If it is a random flap, then the length-to-width ratio in the extremity should be no more than 1:1 to ensure flap viability. If those dimensions are exceeded, then a Doppler has to be used to make sure that sufficient blood supply exists at the base of the flap. Atraumatic technique[14] is a necessary prerequisite when dissecting the flap (bipolar cautery, sharp dissection rather than cautery dissection, grasping flap with skin hooks rather than pickups, etc.) and when

insetting the flap (half buried horizontal mattress or simple vertical stitch with nonreactive suture).

Flaps That Rotate Around a Pivot Point. These random flaps rotate around a single pivot point and therefore need to be planned carefully to avoid excessive tension along the radius of the arc of rotation.

The rotation flap is designed when a pie-shaped triangle defect is created to remove a lesion or pre-existent defect (Fig. 14–15). The base of the triangle lies along the circumference of a semicircular flap that is drawn so that it can be rotated into the defect. The outline of the flap is then cut and includes skin and subcutaneous tissue. If vascular anatomic considerations dictate, it can include fascia and/or muscle.

Transposition flaps are rectangular with rounded edges and can be rotated up to 90 degrees (Fig. 14–16). The end of the flap has to be longer than the distance between the pivot point and edge of the defect so that when the flap is rotated it can fit in without tension. Preplanning with gauze is key to avoid excessive tension. It is wise to ensure that perforators exist at the base of the flap, especially if the length-to-width ratio is to exceed 1:1. The donor site can usually be closed primarily. Otherwise, it may require skin grafting.

Z-plasty is a type of rotation flap that is extensively used to both lengthen existing scars and to reorient them along lines of minimal tension (Fig. 14–17). The key is to have loose skin around the existing scar. The Z-plasty consists of three limbs of equal length in the shape of a Z. The angle between the limbs can vary from 30 to 90 degrees, and the wider the angle, the more the theoretical gain in length. Clinically the 60-degree angle has been

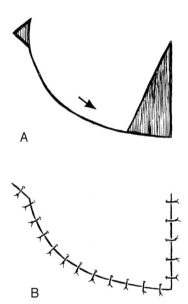

Figure 14–15. A standard rotation flap is designed so that it can cover a triangular defect. Note that, at the distal end of the flap, a Burrow's triangle has been cut out *(A)*. This avoids the normal dog ear that occurs when the flap is rotated into position *(B)*. (From Daniel RK, Kerrigan CL: Principles and physiology of skin flap surgery. *In* McCarthy JG [ed]: Plastic Surgery. Philadelphia, W.B. Saunders, 1990, p 290, Fig. 9–19.)

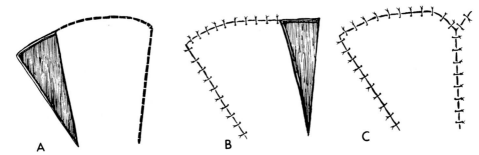

Figure 14–16. A transposition flap shows a rectangular flap being swung into a triangular type defect *(A)*. Either the resultant donor deficit can be closed primarily or it can be skin grafted *(B)*. In this case, it has been closed using a V-Y advancement principle *(C)*. (From Daniel RK, Kerrigan CL: Principles and physiology of skin flap surgery. *In* McCarthy JG [ed]: Plastic Surgery. Philadelphia, W.B. Saunders, 1990, p 290, Fig. 9–17.)

found to be most useful and yields a theoretical 75% gain in length. The actual gain is anywhere from 28 to 45% less than calculated. The length of the center limb also determines the amount of length gained, and the longer the center limb, the larger the gain in length. The theoretical gain in length is the difference between the long and short diagonal and the combination of wider angle and longer limb yields the greatest gain in length.

The center limb changes its orientation 90 degrees after the flaps are rotated. It is important that the new central limb be oriented along the lines of minimal tension so that as it heals there will be minimal tension on it and hence less propensity for hypertrophic scarring and contracture. The lines of minimal tension always lie perpendicular to the line of pull of underlying muscle or tendons and are parallel to naturally occurring wrinkles. Therefore, the incisions over joints should always be parallel to the joint line to preserve full range of motion and avoid tethering. Although the resulting Z-plasty scar is now three times the

length of the original scar, the central limb, now reoriented along the lines of minimal tension, serves to release the original tethering scar.

Advancement Flaps. Advancement flaps are moved directly forward to fill a defect without rotation or lateral movement (Fig. 14–18). A rectangle of skin is dissected out and should include, at a minimum, skin and subcutaneous tissue. The flap is advanced into the defect. This may create folding of the tissue (dog ears) at both ends of its base, which can be removed (Burrow's triangles) so that the skin can be sutured together without causing any irregularities in the contour. It is also important that the tension on the flap is adjusted so that there is no blanched area when it is in its new position.

A V-Y flap is a V-shaped flap that, when advanced, forms a Y (Fig. 14–19). The V-Y flap depends on direct underlying perforators to stay alive. For that reason, no undermining whatsoever can be done when dissecting out

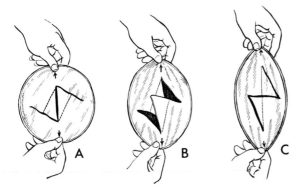

Figure 14–17. A Z-plasty is a method of elongating a given area. In the first drawing, the central limb is the scar that needs to be lengthened. Therefore, side limbs of equal length are drawn at opposite ends at approximately 60 degrees off the central limb *(A)*. The flaps are cut out and transposed *(B)* and are then sewn in place. The resultant transposition has lengthened the central scar area *(C)*. Note that the circle is now elliptical and that the central limb is longer than it was prior to the transposition. (From McCarthy JG: Introduction to plastic surgery. *In* McCarthy JG [ed]: Plastic Surgery. Philadelphia, W.B. Saunders, 1990, p 56, Fig. 1–59.)

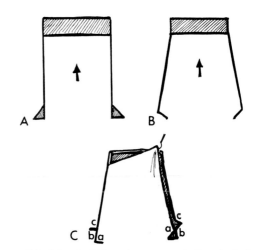

Figure 14–18. *A*, This advancement flap is being designed to fill an existing rectangular defect. Note that Burrow's triangles have been cut out at the base of the flap so that dog ears *(B)* can be avoided when the flap is advanced. *C*, A Z-plasty can also be used to avoid dog ears. (From Daniel RK, Kerrigan CL: Principles and physiology of skin flap surgery. *In* McCarthy JG [ed]: Plastic Surgery. Philadelphia, W.B. Saunders, 1990, p 288, Fig. 9–15.)

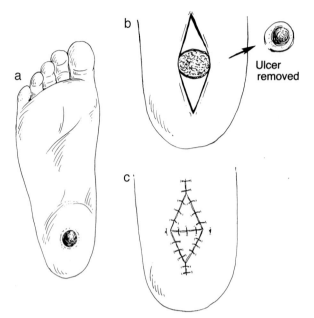

Figure 14–19. A double V-Y advancement flap will be used to fill a 3-cm diameter defect *(A)*. Two flaps were used in this instance because a single V-Y flap on the sole of the foot can only be advanced 1.5 cm *(B)*. It is very important when dissecting these flaps to avoid any undermining as the flap is being mobilized *(C)*. (From Attinger CE: Soft tissue reconstruction for lower extremity trauma. Orthop Clin North Am 1995;26:327, Fig. 26.)

this flap. It is important to realize that the maximum advancement is limited to 1 to 2 cm. Therefore, if the defect is larger, double opposing V-Y flaps can be used to close defects of up to 3 to 4 cm wide. The flap is especially useful for small defects on the sole of the foot.

INTERPOLATION AND ISLAND FLAP

An interpolation flap has a soft tissue pedicle with a distal skin island that is rotated into a defect that is close to but not adjacent to the donor site (Fig. 14–20). If the pedicle is to be buried underneath the skin between the donor and recipient site, a tunnel is created and the bridge is de-epithelialized. If the bridge is to lie over the skin, it should

be tubed so that the pedicle undersurface is protected from infection or desiccation. At 10 to 14 days, the pedicle is separated from the flap and can be returned to the donor site. Indeed from 1916 to the late 1970s this was the principal way in which flaps were transferred from one part of the body to another.

An island flap is a specialized interpolation flap in which the only link between the cutaneous flap and its bed is the neurovascular bundle (Fig. 14–21). Littler first used this flap in 1955 to give sensation to an insensate thumb by taking an island flap from the fourth digit and transferring it to the thumb. This type of flap can be very useful in the hand or foot because one can create a sensory island flap based on the digital vessels. An island flap is clearly a very elegant way to transfer a flap because the result is aesthetic and sensate and can be very functional. The donor site can be closed primarily or with a skin graft.

LOCAL MUSCLE AND MUSCULOCUTANEOUS FLAPS

A simple muscle or muscle with overlying soft tissue can be transferred to cover a soft tissue defect. It is obviously critical to know both the anatomic blood supply to the muscle as well as that of the overlying skin. It is also important to assess whether atherosclerotic disease has altered the normal pattern of blood flow and to adjust the plan accordingly. One then has to be able to judge whether the planned arc of rotation will allow the flap to adequately fill the defect (Fig. 14–22). The distal end of the rotated muscle can be small and narrow, and flap planning should consider this. If the blood supply to the skin overlying the planned muscle flap is not dependable, then it is preferable to transfer the muscle without skin and then skin graft the muscle. This allows one to close the donor defect without skin grafting.

Muscle flaps are very useful when dealing with osteomyelitis. The blood flow is three to five times that of a fasciocutaneous flap. It delivers the white blood cells and antibiotics necessary to cure osteomyelitis (assuming the infected bone has been previously removed). Muscle is also very useful to fill deep defects because it conforms well to an irregular outline.

Useful muscles in the upper extremity are limited because patients tolerate sacrifice of function poorly. For the upper arm, the pectoralis muscle or latissimus muscles are

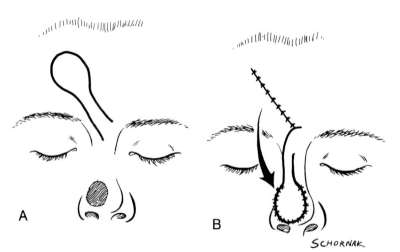

A   B

SCHORNAK

Figure 14–20. Interpolation flap requires two stages. The first stage is elevation of the flap *(A)* and rotating it into the defect. Note that the vascular pedicle stays above normal skin *(B)*. The second stage involves the division and removal of the flap pedicle. This can safely be done 10 to 15 days later when the flap circulation has connected itself to the peripheral circulation. (From Daniel RK, Kerrigan CL: Principles and physiology of skin flap surgery. *In* McCarthy JG [ed]: Plastic Surgery. Philadelphia, W.B. Saunders, 1990, p 291, Fig. 9–21.)

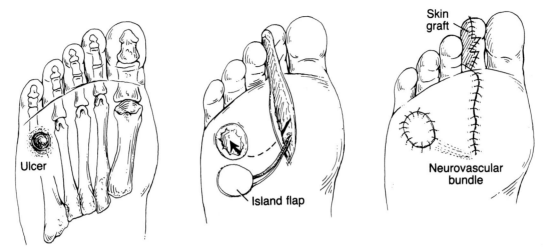

Figure 14–21. In an island flap, the skin and subcutaneous tissue as well as the neurovascular bundle are dissected out. The island flap is then placed in its new location while the neurovascular pedicle is buried underneath. The donor site is then skin grafted. (From Attinger CE: Soft tissue reconstruction for lower extremity trauma. Orthop Clin North Am 1995;26:312, Fig. 13.)

useful. For the lower arm or hand, microsurgical free flaps or fasciocutaneous pedicled flaps are more useful because function is not sacrificed.

Useful muscles in the thigh include the sartorius muscle for infected femoral distal bypasses, the tensor fascia lata, rectus femoris, or vastus lateralis muscle for groin, trochanteric, or acetabular defects. The gastrocnemius muscle is useful for knee or top third tibial defects. The soleus

muscle is useful for middle third defects. The distal third of the leg has few options because the lower leg muscles are all type 4 muscles with segmental blood supply and do not lend themselves well to transposition. Therefore, muscles from other parts of the body usually have to be harvested and transferred as free flaps to the lower third of the leg to obtain adequate coverage. For small ankle defects, the extensor digitorum brevis muscle, abductor digiti

Figure 14–22. The arc of rotation of a muscle determines its usefulness to fill distal defects. Shown here are the possible arcs of rotation when a latissimus dorsi muscle is elevated on its dominant pedicle. (From Mathes SJ, Eshima I: The principles of muscle and musculocutaneous flaps. *In* McCarthy JG [ed]: Plastic Surgery. Philadelphia, W.B. Saunders, 1990, p 382, Fig. 11–3.)

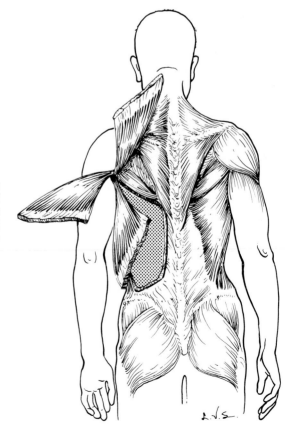

minimi, or abductor hallucis muscle can be used. For heel defects, the flexor digiti minimi, abductor digiti minimi, or abductor hallucis muscles are useful.

SKIN AND FASCIOCUTANEOUS FLAPS

Skin flaps receive a direct blood supply, whereas the fasciocutaneous flaps receive their blood supply either directly or via perforators that rise to the surface along fascial septa that separate muscle compartments or between muscle bellies. The advantage of these flaps is that they are thin, pliable, and reliable. They can be used to cover exposed bone or tendon but usually not to fill a large dead space. In addition, the use of these flaps means that function is not sacrificed and that the aesthetic result is superior to that of muscle flaps with skin grafts. The donor site either can be closed primarily or may require a skin graft.

Around the elbow, a reverse flow lateral arm flap or antegrade radial forearm flap works well. For defects around the wrist or hand, the reverse radial or ulnar flap is very useful. Island flaps are ideal for finger pulp defects.

Along the upper thigh the anterolateral thigh flap is very functional. Around the knee the sural artery flap, the antegrade peroneal flap, or the Ponten flap can be used. Around the ankle, the retrograde peroneal flap, the lateral malleolar flap, the medial plantar flap, the supramalleolar flap, or the dorsalis pedis flap works well. The heel and midfoot is best covered with a medial plantar flap. For the forefoot, the reverse dorsalis pedis flap can be used.

MICROSURGERY

The advent of microsurgery and free flaps has revolutionized our ability to cover soft tissue defects. Free flaps can include fasciocutaneous, musculocutaneous, muscle, osteocutaneous, and osteomusculocutaneous flaps. In experienced microsurgical centers they can be performed with a 96% success rate. Because of the numerous options, the donor site morbidity can be minimal. However, the free flap requires adequate arterial inflow. If the artery is not palpable, an angiogram should be obtained to make sure there is adequate inflow. Venous drainage should also be assessed by using Doppler visualization of the deep and superficial veins in question.

The free flap arterial anastomosis, whenever possible, should always be done end to side so that the distal blood flow is not compromised. The end-to-side patency rate is superior to the end-to-end patency rate. The vein grafts should be end to end, and two veins should be used whenever possible. It is best to ensure that the free flap pedicle is of adequate length so that no intervening vein graft is needed. The patency rate drops precipitously if an interposition vein graft is required. Perioperative anticoagulation was initially thought to be essential in the past, but it has been established that good technique is all that is necessary to ensure patency. Heparin can be used postoperatively if the surgeon is at all concerned about the quality of the vessels or anastomoses. For a more thorough discussion of microsurgical technique, the reader is referred to four recent excellent texts on the subject.[15–18]

We now have the ability to specifically tailor each free flap to the particular defect so that the rebuilt defect ends up with a normal soft tissue envelope. The microsurgeon should have a repertoire of very reliable flaps that can be used with confidence as well as a thorough understanding of possible recipient vessels. The flaps that are most often used are the following: muscle flaps with or without overlying skin include the latissimus muscle, the serratus muscle, the rectus abdominis muscle, the rectus femoris muscle, the vastus lateralis muscle, and the gracilis muscle. The skin and fasciocutaneous flaps that are frequently used include the lateral arm flap, the radial forearm flap, and the anterolateral flap.

Should osteocutaneous flaps be required, the flap of choice is the fibular flap. Should the vascular supply of the donor leg be inadequate, other choices include the radial forearm osteocutaneous free flap, the iliac crest graft, or the parascapular osteocutaneous free flap. The advantage of using vascularized bone is that the risk of infection is diminished and the bony union is more rapid and reliable.

SUMMARY

Soft tissue reconstruction in orthopaedic soft tissue defects can be successfully performed with superior functional and aesthetic results if the following precepts are followed: (1) the conditions are optimized to allow for adequate wound healing, (2) excellent surgical technique is used to minimize tissue damage, (3) vigorous debridement is performed until only healthy tissue remains, (4) the surgeon possesses a thorough knowledge of anatomy to ensure successful harvest of a given flap, and (5) the surgeon uses a thoughtful approach in choosing the mode of reconstruction so that the optimal functional result occurs.

Bibliography

1. Hunt TK, Hopf HW: Wound healing and wound infection. Surg Clin North Am 1977;77:587–606.
   One of the foremost researchers in wound healing, T.K. Hunt defined the wound-healing module and delineated the importance of oxygen in the process. This article summarizes these findings.
2. Glat PM, Longaker MT: Wound healing. In Grabb and Smith's Plastic Surgery, 5th ed. Philadelphia, Lippincott-Raven, 1998, pp 3–12.
   This chapter nicely delineates the role of growth factors in wound healing by M.T. Longaker, a foremost expert in the field.
3. Knighton DR, Silver IA, Hunt TK: Regulation of wound healing angiogenesis—Effect of oxygen gradients and inspired oxygen gradients. Surgery 1981;90:262–270.
   This paper explains the importance of oxygen in wound healing
4. Tibbles PM, Edelsberg JS: Hyperbaric oxygen therapy. N Engl J Med 1996;334:1642.
   This excellent review article details the usefulness of hyperbaric medicine in wound healing, carbon monoxide poisoning, bends, and similar situations.
5. Rodeheaver GT, Pettry D, Thacker JG, et al: Wound cleansing by high pressure irrigation. Surg Gynecol Obstet 1975;141:357–362.
   This critical paper delineates the importance of pulsed lavage in the treatment of wounds to reduce the rate of infection.
6. Gustilo RB, Anderson JT: Prevention of infection in the treatment of 1025 open fractures of long bones. J Bone Joint Surg 1976;58A:453–458.
   This landmark paper discusses the prevention of infection in orthopaedic trauma.
7. Byrd HS, Spicer TE, Cierny G III: Management of open tibial fractures. Plast Reconstr Surg 1985;76:719.
   The argument for early closure of an orthopaedic trauma is elegantly made in this article by three of the leaders in the field.
8. Krizek TJ, Robson MC: The evolution of quantitative bacteriology in wound management. Am J Surg 1975;130:579.
   This key paper shows that the number of bacteria per gram of tissue

predicts with relative accuracy the chances of successful skin graft take. The same criteria can be used for other types of closure. Unfortunately, few hospitals actually run this test, so its predictive usefulness has not been realized.

9. Milton SH: The fallacy of the length to width ratio. Br J Surg 1970;57:502.

   This critical paper in the evolution of our understanding of flap viability established that it was the direct blood flow to the flap rather than an arbitrary length-to-width ratio that determined flap survival.

10. Taylor GI, Palmer JH: The vascular territories (angiosomes) of the body: Experimental studies and clinical applications. Br J Plast Surg 1990;43:1.

    Taylor summarizes and reorganizes all the previous century's work on our understanding of how blood supplies bone and soft tissue. To do so, he develops the key concept of angiosomes (blocks of tissue fed by named arteries).

11. Callegari PR, Taylor GI, Caddy CM, et al: An anatomic review of the delay phenomenon: I. Experimental studies. Plast Reconstr Surg 1992;89:397.

    In this paper Taylor uses the angiosome concept to give the first intelligible explanation of the delay phenomenon.

12. Cormack GC, Lamberty BGH: The Arterial Anatomy of Skin Flaps, 2nd ed. London, Churchill Livingstone, 1994.

    This superb volume delineates the vascular anatomy of the skin as well as all the possible skin flaps that can be dissected out.

13. Mathes SJ, Nahai F: Classification of the vascular anatomy of muscles: Experimental and clinical correlation. Plast Reconstr Surg 1981;67[2]:177.

    This classic paper delineates the vascular supply of muscles. The authors have since published the second edition.

14. Edgerton MT: The Art of Surgical Technique. Baltimore, Williams & Wilkins, 1988.

    This is the classic text on developing superb atraumatic surgical technique. This book is a must for any surgeon!

15. Serafin D: Atlas of Microsurgical Composite Tissue Transplantation. Philadelphia, W.B. Saunders, 1998.

    Excellent text on microsurgery.

16. Strauch B, Yu HL, Chen ZW: Atlas of Microvascular Surgery: Anatomy and Operative Approaches. New York, Thieme Medical Publishing, 1993.

    Another excellent text of microsurgery.

17. O'Brien BMcC, Morrison WA: Reconstructive Microsurgery. New York, Churchill Livingstone, 1987.

    Another excellent text on microsurgery.

18. Mathes SJ, Nahai F: Reconstructive Surgery: Principles, Anatomy, and Technique, 2nd ed. New York, Churchill Livingstone, 1999.

    Another excellent text on microsurgery.

GWENT HEALTHCARE NHS TRUST
LIBRARY
ROYAL GWENT HOSPITAL
NEWPORT

Section IV
Pediatric
Orthopaedics

Chapter 15

General and Regional Problems in Children

John N. Delahay, M.D.

Children are very different from adults. This concept is obvious but is sometimes overlooked. Yet, it is critically important to recognize this central fact in order to successfully diagnose and treat orthopaedic problems in this age group. Within this rather broad range of ages, there are dramatic differences among the specific subsets of neonate, child, and adolescent.

These differences are not only biologic but also physiologic, social, and emotional, and it is inappropriate to focus only on one aspect of these differences when treating children. For example, it would be unwise to ignore a young child's activity level when treating a fracture—inadequate immobilization or premature cast removal will have disastrous results. The treatment of this special age group actually gave orthopaedics its name. The word "orthopaedics" means literally "straight child" in Latin, and alludes to the interest and time spent correcting deformities in children. These deformities can result not only from injury but also from systemic and local disease states, both congenital and acquired. As a result of the continued growth of the child, these diseases produce anatomic and physiologic effects not expected in the adult. Thus, before discussing specific entities, it would be appropriate to review some of the biologic differences of the child's musculoskeletal system, including influences that can act on the immature skeleton.

PHYSIOLOGIC DIFFERENCES IN CHILDREN

Biologic Differences

GROWTH

The fact that the child's skeleton is actively growing, both longitudinally and latitudinally, positions it uniquely for damage due to the adverse effects of trauma and disease. The extent of this damage is a reflection of the rate of growth and the immaturity of the skeleton. Hence, a given insult will have a greater impact, if applied at a time of more rapid growth (a growth spurt) or when the skeleton is very immature (the neonatal period).

REMODELING

The immature skeleton can remodel to a much greater degree than that of the adult. Because of the presence and activity of multiple cell populations, damage to the skeleton can be repaired more extensively than one should anticipate in the adult. The challenge for the physician is to be able to recognize the limitations of this remodeling process and to work within the boundaries of this potential.

VARIATIONS IN ANATOMIC STRUCTURE

The bone of a child is histologically similar to adult bone. There is a lamellar pattern throughout much of the skeleton, even though some areas of immature bone can be seen. However, from a mechanical standpoint, the bone of a child is far more "biologically plastic." This allows the bone to bend without breaking. In point of fact, it is responsible for some of the unique fracture patterns that are seen in the pediatric age group, such as torus and greenstick fractures. In addition, the mechanical properties of a child's bone vary from those of the adult. The differences in such characteristics as modulus of elasticity, ultimate tensile strength, and yield point all reflect the elasticity and plasticity unique to this age group. However, the overall strength tends to be less than that of the adult in certain modes of loading, such as tension and shear.

Ligament is one of the most age-resistant tissues in the human body. The tensile strength of ligament in children and adults is very similar. Although the strength of bone, cartilage, and muscle tends to change, the ligaments show relatively consistent mechanical behavior throughout life. Hence, any given injury pattern will likely be reflected differently in different age groups depending on which tissue—bone, physeal cartilage, or ligament—is weakest.

PERIOSTEUM

The outer covering of bone is a dense fibrous membrane. The periosteum of a child is actually composed of two layers: an inner cambial (osteogenic) layer and an outer fibrous layer. Unlike the mature periosteum of the adult, the child's periosteum confers both mechanical strength as well as biologic activity. The effect of this biologic difference is far reaching when treating fractures in children. Because of the thickened periosteum, pediatric fractures do not tend to displace to the degree seen in adults. The intact periosteum can be used as an aid in fracture reduction and maintenance. In addition, pediatric fractures heal significantly faster than similar injuries in the adult because all the cellular precursors are already present. The osteogenic layer supplies active osteoblasts ready to make bone for the fracture callus. The generation of these precursor elements in adults takes a longer period of time; thus, fracture healing is prolonged.

CARTILAGE

Large portions of the skeleton develop embryologically within a cartilage model. Hence, at birth, large portions of any given bone remain largely cartilaginous. Unfortunately, cartilage is not seen on standard x-rays. The cartilage anlages are very labile and dramatically affected by external influences, such as mechanical loading. It is important to realize, when examining a child's x-ray, that what is not seen (cartilage) is more important than what is. Otherwise, one can be falsely reassured that all is normal. Aberrant cartilaginous growth will drastically affect the ultimate shape of bones and, more important, joints. The best example is the proximal femur; most of the upper end is cartilaginous for a rather lengthy period of postnatal life. Adverse influences due to eccentric loading, such as seen in developmental dysplasia of the hip, can have far-reaching effects when applied to the immature cartilage of the neonatal hip.

THE PHYSIS

Perhaps no biologic structure better defines the pediatric age group than the presence of a growth plate. The histology and physiology of this structure have been discussed in the chapter on growth and development. Its importance in the growth of the skeleton is axiomatic. Unfortunately, its presence creates a mechanical flaw in the long bone. The physeal cartilage is extremely vulnerable to shear load. Certainly other modes of loading such as compression and tension are also capable of causing significant damage to the plate. Perhaps the greatest challenges in pediatric orthopaedics are (1) to be aware of the effect of injury and disease on the physis, (2) to anticipate these potential complications, and (3) to plan management strategies to appropriately deal with them.

FACTORS AFFECTING SKELETAL GROWTH

Numerous intrinsic and extrinsic factors affect the way in which the skeleton develops.

Genetic Impact

Inborn errors of metabolism, such as renal rickets, as well as chromosomal alterations, such as Down's syndrome, can cause phenotypic variations in the development of the skeleton. Abnormal histology, aberrant growth, and variational development all will affect the unique shape and behavior of the skeleton.

Nutrition

Vitamins, minerals, and proteins are required for normal skeletal development, and without appropriate intake, abnormalities will occur. Rickets, for example, will alter the shape of the metaphysis of a long bone in addition to disrupting normal physeal development.

Endocrine Effects

Hormonal influences play a significant trophic (permissive) role in the development of the skeleton. Deficiencies or excesses, therefore, will disrupt the way in which the skeleton matures. Thyroid hormone is a typical example. Absent or low levels of this critical hormone cause disruption of normal epiphyseal development and result in aberrant growth of the epiphysis.

Environmental Factors

Mechanical effects as well as environmental toxins and drugs can adversely affect the way in which the skeleton develops. Fetal alcohol syndrome and the use of illicit narcotics by the mother are just two examples of how externally applied toxins can cause skeletal aberrations.

Coexistent Disease

The neuromuscular diseases, which will be discussed shortly, such as cerebral palsy, poliomyelitis, and muscular dystrophy, provide excellent examples of the secondary effects seen in the skeleton due to extrinsic disease. In these examples the final common pathway in the pathophysiology of the deformities is muscle imbalance. Hence, eccentric and aberrant mechanical loading of the immature skeleton produce changes such as joint dislocations and deformity.

GENERAL AFFLICTIONS OF THE SKELETON

Normal Variations and "Nondisease"

If one is to appreciate abnormalities in skeletal growth, then knowledge of normal growth and development is required. Before one can diagnose and effectively treat diseases of the pediatric musculoskeletal system, one needs to be comfortable in the evaluation and management of nondisease. The term *nondisease* was coined by Dr. Mercer Rang, an eminent Canadian orthopaedist, to emphasize the fact that frequently children present to an orthopaedist for evaluation of phenomena that are essentially normal variational patterns. Torsional and angular changes in the lower extremity are among the most common reasons for referral of a child. The complaint of toeing-in or toeing-out as well as knock-knees and bowlegs are a major preoccupation of parents and grandparents alike. The simple fact is that the vast majority of these children, well over 90%, are normal children who are simply reflecting modest variational changes in growth and development. It is incumbent upon the orthopaedist to be comfortable in the recognition of these physiologic variations and in the treatment of nondisease. Clearly, as Dr. Rang points out, there is a difference between doing nothing and nontreatment for nondisease. The physician evaluating the child must be able to reassure the family that these are indeed normal variations. Education of the family both verbally and with the use of appropriate handouts, careful physical examination, and the offer of regular follow-up visits will frequently be appropriate nontreatment for these children.

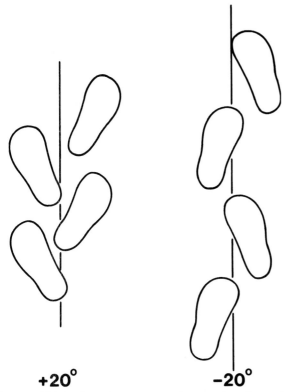

Figure 15–1. The foot-progression angle. A positive value denotes out-toeing *(left)* and a negative value denotes in-toeing *(right)*. (From Benson MKD, Fixsen JA, MacNicol MF: Children's Orthopaedics and Fractures. Edinburgh, Churchill Livingstone, 1994.)

The physical examination of these children focuses primarily on the so-called *torsional profile*. One needs to determine the foot-progression angle (Fig. 15–1) when observing the child walk. Normally, the foot should be slightly externally rotated from the line of progression by approximately 10 to 25 degrees. Evaluation of the foot for any abnormalities such as metatarsus adductus and a prehensile hallux are important to note. Examining the child prone with the hip extended and the knee flexed allows the examiner to use the leg itself as a goniometer in measuring internal and external rotation of the hip (Fig. 15–2). Frequently, as is the case in children with femoral anteversion, excessive internal rotation can be observed. Examining the child in the seated position and placing the patella in a neutral direction allows one to carefully evaluate the alignment of the transmalleolar axis (Fig. 15–3). Normally, the transmalleolar axis will lie approximately 15 to 30 degrees external to the coronal plane of the leg.

Once a torsional profile has been developed, one can consider the diagnoses appropriate for the condition. For example, the differential diagnosis of toeing-in is primarily metatarsus adductus, internal tibial torsion, or femoral anteversion. The out-toed gait is likely to be caused by calcaneovalgus feet, external tibial torsion, or physiologic external rotational contractures of the hip.

The specific age at the time of presentation can often give a clue as to the specific cause of the in-toeing. For example, when presented with a child under 18 months of age, the frequent cause of in-toeing will be internal tibial torsion. A child over age 2 years will frequently have metatarsus adductus or a prehensile toe with overpull of

TORSIONAL VARIATIONS OF THE LIMB

Torsional deformity generally refers to variations in axial rotation along the long axis of the limb. The child is frequently brought in for evaluation of either an in-toed or out-toed gait. More often than not, variations in axial rotational alignment are due to mechanical forces applied in utero. Large babies frequently will have rotational changes in the lower extremity. Similarly, sleeping positions postnatally can affect the overall alignment of the limb.

Remodeling of torsional variations can be anticipated over time. A number of factors will determine the rate of normalization. Mechanical factors such as positioning, gravity, and body weight clearly play a role. In addition, ethnic and racial factors have also been demonstrated to be influential. The timing of correction varies rather widely, but for the most part, ranges have been determined from the analysis of many normal children.

When presented with a child with a torsional deformity, it is first appropriate to take a history, seeking information regarding the birth, including weight, mode of delivery, and the presence or absence of complications such as oligohydramnios. If the child is walking, it is important to know the age at which independent walking began. It is also helpful to ask about similar variations in siblings or parents. The old adage that the "acorn does not fall far from the tree" is clearly a factor when one considers the likelihood of spontaneous correction of these deformities.

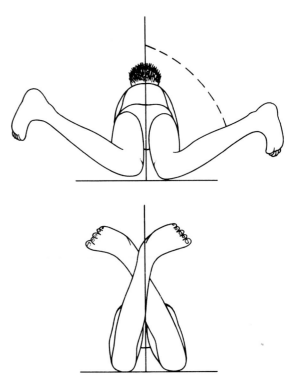

Figure 15–2. Hip rotation measured prone. *Top,* Internal rotation. *Bottom,* external rotation. (From Benson MKD, Fixsen JA, MacNicol MF: Children's Orthopaedics and Fractures. Edinburgh, Churchill Livingstone, 1994.)

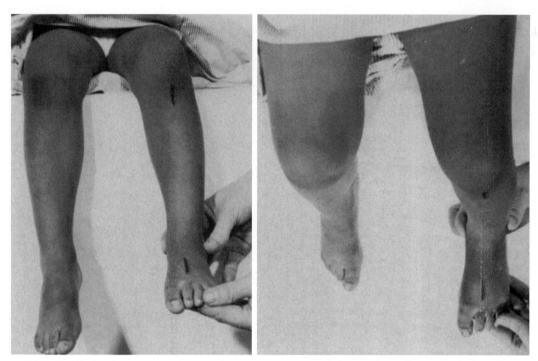

Figure 15–3. Practical clinical method of measuring tibial torsion. (From Tachdjian MO: Pediatric Orthopedics, 2nd ed. Philadelphia, WB Saunders, 1990.)

the abductor hallucis. Typically, when evaluating a pigeon-toed child over the age of 3, one should consider femoral anteversion as the most likely cause. Because torsional variations are so common, and in the vast majority of cases are categorized as nondisease, one must be very cognizant to exclude pathologic conditions. For example, the child with femoral anteversion may actually have a dysplastic hip. External tibial torsion can occasionally be confused with Blount's disease, and it is always critical to be aware of the child with asymmetric torsion. Frequently, spasticity as seen in the child with cerebral palsy will cause in-toeing on one side and not on the other.

TIBIAL TORSION

Axial rotation of the tibia is extremely common. Many children are born with a modest degree of internal tibial torsion. Clinical evaluation of the transmalleolar axis is notoriously unreliable. However, the use of sophisticated studies such as the CT scan is gross overkill in the evaluation of variational patterns. The simple use of the prone thigh-foot axis allows for the most efficient measurement of tibial torsion. Typically, internal torsion is more common than external and the vast majority of abnormal torsion will correct by age 3 years. Obviously, the appearance of the child with internal tibial torsion is only made worse if the child has coexistent femoral anteversion or genu valgum. Internal tibial torsion is of no functional significance; therefore, treatment should be minimized. Parent reassurance and education are usually all that is necessary. The occasional use of night splints for the child with skeptical parents is not unreasonable. However, it is important to be sure that the rotation is tibial in origin prior to the application of the splint. If it is primarily femoral, the use of a night splint will only accentuate the abnormal torsional

pattern. External tibial torsion is far less common and also less likely to resolve spontaneously. Similarly, it tends to produce more of a functional deficit for the child. Frequently, it is associated with planovalgus feet; the combination of the two often makes the child clumsy. Therefore, the use of splints and, in rare situations, tibial osteotomy have been suggested by some for extreme degrees of torsion with functional deficits.

FEMORAL TORSION

Typically, the lower limb rotates medially during the eighth week of fetal life. This rotation brings the great toe to the midline. Normally, at birth, the plane of the femoral neck is externally rotated, in relation to the coronal plane of the distal femur, by approximately 30 to 40 degrees. This external rotation of the plane of the neck is referred to as femoral anteversion. With growth and development the normal anteversion gradually decreases to an adult angle of about 10 to 15 degrees. The remodeling rate is approximately 2 to 3 degrees per year. Numerous x-ray techniques have been described to accurately measure femoral anteversion. Most, however, recommend simple use of physical examination as mentioned previously. It is important in examining these children to ask the simple question, "Where is the patella?" With excessive anteversion it is not uncommon to see external tibial torsion. The combination of internal femoral torsion (femoral anteversion) and external tibial torsion has been referred to a "skew leg." In this complex deformity the patella frequently tracks far laterally; patellar subluxation can then be anticipated. The vast majority of children with femoral anteversion correct spontaneously by age 8 years. Those who are delayed in this spontaneous correction should be evaluated carefully for ligamentous laxity. In addition, persistent sitting in the

FEMORAL TORSION

The cause of femoral torsion is unknown. Femoral torsion is usually most severe when the child is about 5 or 6 years old. Most children outgrow this condition

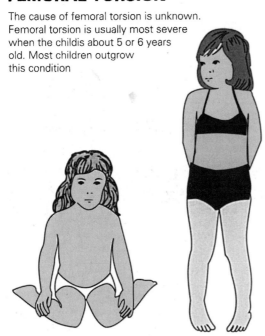

Shoe modifications and braces do not work for femoral torsion. They can make the child uncomfortable, self-conscious and hamper play.

Figure 15–4. Femoral torsion. (From Staheli LT: Fundamentals of Pediatric Orthopaedics. New York, Raven Press, 1992.)

so-called "TV" or "W" position will delay spontaneous correction. There is no indication for the use of night splints in the management of femoral anteversion (Fig. 15–4). The rare child who does not spontaneously correct usually has a familial predisposition to this configuration.

It is important to reassure the family that femoral anteversion is not a functional deformity but a cosmetic one. There has been no evidence to suggest an increase in osteoarthritis in these hips and no evidence to suggest any alteration in agility. The use of femoral osteotomy to correct benign excessive version of the femur is frowned upon. The old adage, "Think osteotomy—think twice," should be respected. The complications of femoral osteotomy are well recognized and, should they occur, defeat the entire purpose of a purely cosmetic procedure.

FEMORAL RETROVERSION

External femoral torsion is far less common. It is generally not viewed as a bony deformity but rather an external rotational contracture of the hip joint itself. When seen in a child under 1 year, spontaneous correction is the norm. Persistent external femoral torsion is frequently associated with external tibial torsion. The child with both of these torsional variations will very frequently be clumsy. As is the case with most of these patterns, spontaneous correction remains the norm. Unfortunately, one may need to wait 5 to 7 years before complete correction is achieved.

ANGULAR MALALIGNMENT

Frontal plane deformities such as knock-knees and bowlegs are other common causes for orthopaedic referral. As is the case with torsional variations, angular variations are most frequently benign. There are, however, some pathologic states to be considered. The Salenius diagram (Fig. 15–5) has been very helpful in evaluating angular deformity. In general, the neonate will demonstrate a modest amount of genu varum at birth. The varus pattern persists through the first year of life with spontaneous correction anticipated by 18 months of age. Beginning about age 2, valgus alignment is expected. Maximum knock-knee is usually present in the 5- to 6-year-old age group, with rapid spontaneous correction thereafter. Therefore, knowledge of the normal variation in development assists one in determining the etiology of the deformity in a given child.

A history of familial deformity is obviously important. In addition, because rickets can cause genu varum, a nutritional history of the child is likewise noteworthy. The finding of ligamentous laxity and screening by comparison against routine growth charts should be reported.

As is the case in torsional deformity, angular deformities are for the most part physiologic and resolve spontaneously. Bowlegs are usually normal; however, one should consider Blount's disease (infantile tibia vara), rachitic states (vitamin D deficiency), and the chondrodystrophies. Conversely, the differential diagnosis of genu valgum includes multiple epiphyseal dysplasia, pseudoachondroplasia, some rachitic states (renal rickets), and of course, the "idiopathic" variant. When evaluating a child with unilateral varus or valgus, the possibility of posttraumatic deformity must be considered. The classic proximal metaphyseal fracture of the tibia has been well known to result in late valgus deformity.

Finally, it is important to recall that occasionally the valgus is more apparent than real. Diagnosis of obese children with fat thighs, children with excessive joint laxity, muscle hypotonia, and excessive femoral anteversion can all be confused with true valgus deformity at the knees. An efficient and usually reproducible way of monitoring resolution of deformity is fingerbreadth measurements between the adductor tubercles for varus and the medial malleoli for valgus.

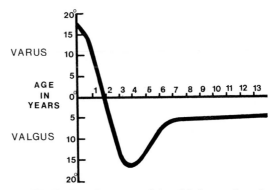

Figure 15–5. Development of the tibiofemoral angle during growth. (From Tachdjian MO: Pediatric Orthopedics, 2nd ed. Philadelphia, WB Saunders, 1990.)

TOE-WALKING

More often than not the complaint of toe walking in a child qualifies as nondisease. This is a common variation in normal children. Unfortunately, some children who are seen for toe-walking may have a neurologic cause. Therefore, it is incumbent upon the physician to exclude pathologic states prior to resolving the diagnosis as *habitual toe-walking*. Careful physical examination including muscle testing, reflex evaluation, and strength testing are important to exclude neurologic causes. Such problems as cerebral palsy, muscular dystrophy, tethered cord syndrome, and autism have all been associated and, indeed, diagnosed in the child who initially presents with toe-walking.

The habitual toe-walker (physiologic toe-walker) typically will show spontaneous improvement at about age 5 years. Examination of these children fails to show a fixed contracture of their gastrocnemius-soleus complex. Unfortunately, the etiology and natural history have remained clouded; therefore, various treatment recommendations have been put forward. Serial casts, ankle-foot orthoses, and physical therapy modalities are frequently employed in the management of these children. Rarely, but occasionally, surgical lengthening of the heel cord is indicated for the unresponsive child.

ARTHRITIS

Juvenile Rheumatoid Disease

In 1897 George Still, an English pediatrician, identified this disease in the pediatric age group. It is currently estimated that there are 350,000 children afflicted with this disease in the United States. Approximately three new cases per year are diagnosed per 100,000 children under the age of 13. Typically, two incidence peaks have been described: one group under 6 years of age and the other between 10 and 15 years of age.

Juvenile rheumatoid arthritis (JRA) can actually present in one of three onset modes: systemic disease, polyarticular disease, or monarticular (pauciarticular) disease. The *systemic form* of juvenile rheumatoid disease is an acute febrile illness representing approximately 20% of the total patients involved. These children consistently manifest a fever with an intermittent pattern and a rash, which are seen in virtually all these children. This rash is nonpruritic and evanescent; 85% will demonstrate hepatosplenomegaly. The differential diagnosis includes systemic lupus erythematosus, leukemia, and rheumatic fever, among others.

Polyarticular disease is seen in approximately 50% of the involved children (Fig. 15–6). Although chronically ill in appearance and stunted in their growth, these children do not manifest the generalized systemic symptoms seen in the previous group. Characteristically, multiple large joints (classically the knees) are involved. Flaring of four joints in under 6 months is usually considered diagnostic. Rheumatic fever must be considered in the differential diagnosis.

The *monarticular form* (pauciarticular) of the disease is seen in approximately 30% of the affected children. This is by far and away the most benign of the three forms. Typically, the onset is insidious and occurs in an otherwise healthy child. Effusion most commonly occurs in the knee,

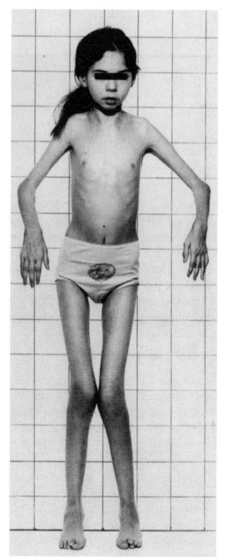

Figure 15–6. This 12-year-old patient developed seronegative polyarthritis at 2 years of age. She has had multiple joints affected, some of which are still swollen (such as the fingers), while others have developed contractures. Note the underdeveloped jaw, rigid cervical spine, contractures, and deformities of the arm joints. There are adduction and flexion contractures of the hips associated with femoral neck anteversion. The patellae are squinting and there is a secondary lumbar lordosis. Genu valgum has developed together with secondary external tibial torsion. The feet are rigid and in varus. (From Benson MKD, Fixsen JA, MacNicol MF: Children's Orthopaedics and Fractures. Edinburgh, Churchill Livingstone, 1994.)

followed in frequency by the elbow and ankle. The small joints are universally spared. Usually joint aspiration and synovial analysis are required, if for no other reason than to rule out sepsis. The monarticular involvement of JRA can be identical to that seen in tuberculosis in the child.

PATHOGENESIS

The exact etiology of the disease is unknown. Occasional references have been made to an association with an initiating traumatic event. Despite the underlying etiology, the immunologic response in the synovium is the common thread that relates this entity to the adult form of rheumatoid disease. Synovial proliferation and the release of lysosomal enzymes cause the characteristic progressive joint destruction. In addition, the thickened pannus and the resultant effusion cause ligamentous stretching and mechanical damage to the joint. Unlike in the adult, the hypervascular granulation tissue causes secondary effects on the physis. Stimulation of the growth plate frequently causes overgrowth of epiphyseal nuclei. This overgrowth clearly can alter joint mechanics.

DIAGNOSIS

The diagnosis of juvenile rheumatoid arthritis is frequently problematic, because of the lack of specific diagnostic tests. The radiographic changes are similar to those seen in an adult. Early soft tissue swelling is not unusual; later, the findings of osteoporosis, decrease in the joint space, articular erosions, and local periostitis are common. The laboratory studies may demonstrate a low-grade anemia and a mildly elevated erythrocyte sedimentation rate. Leukocytosis is frequently seen in the systemic form of the disease. However, the rheumatoid factor is elevated in only 10 to 15% of patients. A constellation of physical findings, radiographic changes, and abnormal laboratory values is usually required for diagnosis.

CLINICAL FEATURES

Iridocyclitis is the most common cause of disability in these children. The smoldering eye changes impair vision as a result of adhesions (synechiae) and band keratopathy. Frequently, the ocular changes may occur before joint involvement or coincident with it. Because iridocyclitis is seen in 20% of children with monarticular disease, routine slit lamp examination at 6-month intervals is critical.

Hepatosplenomegaly and lymphadenopathy may be mild to severe. As mentioned earlier, these changes are seen in the acute form of the disease. Associated with this, alterations in liver function tests are typical. Occasional lymphadenopathy can be seen both centrally and subcutaneously, but rarely to the point of symptom production.

Joint involvement can be generalized. In the systemic and polyarticular forms of the disease, essentially no joint is immune from the rheumatoid process. However, certain joints are more typical of the disease. The temporomandibular joint will be involved in one third of patients. These children frequently complain of earache. In addition, because of alteration in mandibular growth, these children have a micrognathic appearance and orthodontic problems.

The cervical spine is involved in 50% of the children and classically C1–C2 subluxation is seen. The stretching of the transverse ligament of C1 results from chronic synovial proliferation in the small bursa between the posterior aspect of the dens and the anterior surface of the transverse ligament. A flexion lateral view of the cervical spine is usually adequate to diagnose C1–C2 instability. The finding of an ADI (atlantodens interval) greater than 4 mm is frequently used as a diagnostic test for JRA. The management of C1–C2 instability in the asymptomatic child frequently presents a treatment dilemma.

Involvement of the joints of the upper extremity occurs less frequently than those of the lower. The shoulder is one of the few joints usually spared in the juvenile rheumatoid process. Elbow changes, on the other hand are extremely common, and the clinical and radiographic picture is reminiscent of hemophilia. Overgrowth of the radial head and other growth changes about the elbow are frequently seen. Bony resorption and cystic changes are seen in the juxta-articular region. Changes in the hand begin with early fusiform swelling of the interphalangeal (IP) joints followed by late subchondral erosions, joint subluxation, flexion contractures, and degenerative changes. Typically, radial deviation of the carpometacarpal (CMC) joint and ulnar drift of the fingers are characteristic.

In the lower extremity, although the knee is more commonly involved, disease in the hip joint is the major cause of severe disability. Loss of joint motion with coincident collapse of the joint space and progression to subluxation are not uncommon. Protrusio acetabuli is believed by many to be a pathognomonic finding of the disease (Fig. 15–7). The knee is the most commonly involved joint in JRA. Flexion contractures, chronic synovial thickening, joint swelling, and condylar enlargement are characteristic. Alterations of growth with angular deformities and leg length inequality have also been reported.

The foot and ankle complex is also commonly involved in this disease process. In fact, the subtalar joint is a unique target of JRA. It is not uncommon to make the diagnosis in a child who presents initially with pain and stiffness vaguely described about the hindfoot. Frequently, the child complains of fatigue and discomfort during sports. Confusion with tarsal coalition and the resultant peroneal spastic flatfoot are not uncommon. Careful physical evaluation of the foot can frequently trigger the diagnostic workup for JRA.

TREATMENT

Nonsurgical treatment for children with JRA includes rest, therapeutic exercise, splinting, corrective casting, bracing, and pharmaceutical agents. Aspirin remains the mainstay in management. The use of corticosteroids remains controversial; clearly, they can be used to decrease the acute inflammatory reaction but unfortunately have the dual effect of causing iatrogenic damage. The immunosuppressive agents frequently used in adults are rarely indicated in children.

Surgical treatment such as synovectomy and soft tissue releases have their place in the treatment armamentarium for these children. Occasional corrective osteotomies for late angular deformities will restore the alignment in an extremity. Similarly, the judicious use of arthrodesis for the child with a severely involved subtalar joint can produce significant symptomatic improvement. In general, total joint arthroplasty is reserved for the adolescent or adult with severe recalcitrant joint involvement.

PROGNOSIS

It is important to recognize that one third of affected children have pauciarticular disease. This population will have minimal, if any, long-term disability. In point of fact, in many children with polyarticular JRA the disease will burn out with relatively little joint involvement. Therefore, in most collected series, 50% of children with JRA have minimal residual disease, if any, and no disability. Another

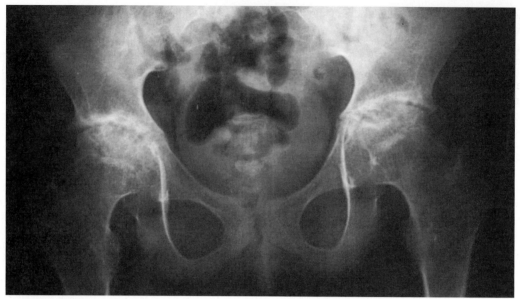

Figure 15–7. This 13-year-old developed polyarthritic onset arthritis at the age of 3 years. X-rays show erosive changes and narrowing of the joint space. (From Benson MKD, Fixsen JA, MacNicol MF: Children's Orthopaedics and Fractures. Edinburgh, Churchill Livingstone, 1994.)

25% have slight disability, which does not affect their ability to walk and run or perform the vast majority of activities of daily living. Another 20% will go on to severe crippling and possible blindness. Fewer than 5% die prematurely; death is usually due to persistent hepatosplenomegaly, proteinuria, or amyloid renal disease.

As is so often the case, early diagnosis and appropriate nonsurgical and surgical management can frequently obviate some of the residual problems that these children experience.

Lyme Arthritis

Lyme disease is a tick-borne inflammatory disorder caused by a spirochete, *Borrelia burgdorferi*. It is vectored by the deer tick, *Ixodes dammini*. The disease got its name from the town in Connecticut where one of the initial outbreaks occurred. "Lyme arthritis" was a term used to denote an unusual clustering of children with inflammatory arthropathy reported in 1975 in the vicinity of Lyme, Connecticut. It was this increased incidence of childhood arthritis, and the suspicion of an infectious etiology, that led to the actual discovery of the spirochete responsible for Lyme disease. The disease is endemic to the northern Atlantic coastal region. On the Pacific coast another endemic area is seen; however, the vector is *Ixodes pacificus*. The upper Midwest, the third endemic region, shares the same vector as that seen in the northern Atlantic region, *Ixodes dammini*. As one would expect, the highest rates of the disease occur in the summer and the fall and coincide with high deer activity and high outdoor activity by humans.

Typically, the disease presents in three stages. The *first stage* lasts days to weeks and is typified by systemic symptoms and the classic erythema chronicum migrans (ECM). This is an expanding, macular erythematous rash with a central clearing area. It is often seen on the thigh, groin, or axilla. Occasional migratory musculoskeletal symptoms can be seen during this stage. The *second stage*, which lasts weeks to months, is typified by cardiac and neurologic involvement. The cardiac sequelae include varying degrees of heart block and myocarditis, and the neurologic findings include meningitis, encephalitis, chorea, and Bell's palsy. The *third (chronic) stage*, which can persist from months to years, is characterized by frank arthritis. Intermittent attacks of asymmetrical joint swelling and pain, primarily in the large joints (especially in the knee), are typical. These joints are hot, swollen, and very painful. When aspirated, the fluid will typically show elevated white blood cell (WBC) counts in the range of 25,000 to 50,000 cells/ml. Attempts at culture, when positive, are clearly diagnostic of the disease, but retrieval of organisms is very low. An indirect immunofluorescent assay is available; however, the ELISA (enzyme-linked immunosorbent assay) test demonstrates better specificity. The radiographic changes about the joint are similar to those seen in rheumatoid disease: soft tissue swelling, juxta-articular osteopenia, and occasional peripheral calcification. Late changes are similar to those seen in any osteoarthritic joint.

Lyme disease in children typically follows a course somewhat different from that in the adult. ECM is seen in less than 50% of cases. Children also are more susceptible to the acute symptoms of Lyme disease, but usually are spared the chronic joint changes. In children, the differential diagnosis includes juvenile rheumatoid disease, septic arthritis, and toxic synovitis.

Antibiotic treatment for Lyme disease is largely determined by the stage. Early Lyme disease is usually treated effectively using doxycycline for the adult and amoxicillin for the child. Once neurologic or cardiac manifestations are seen, additional protocols are used in an effort to control the disease. As of this writing, vaccines have been developed that, optimistically, will markedly decrease the incidence, if not eradicate, this disease in the future.

SHORT STATURE AND SKELETAL DYSPLASIAS

Not infrequently, children are referred to an orthopaedic surgeon for evaluation of short stature. It is initially important to determine whether the short stature is pathologic or physiologic. The conditions causing short stature are a very heterogeneous group. In this section, the evaluation of these individuals will be explored. In addition, a working classification of skeletal dysplasias will be provided, and several of the more common skeletal dysplasias and skeletal dystrophies will be discussed. Once it has been determined that the short stature is pathologic, the correct diagnosis must be established when possible in order to provide appropriate medical care for these patients, to provide genetic counseling to the patient and family, and to provide information regarding prognosis.

Short stature is a relative phenomenon, and individual heights vary widely, making it all the more difficult to differentiate between pathologic and physiologic stature. Growth curves and growth tables do provide some normative information that allows the examiner to compare a given individual to his or her peers. The normal child grows very rapidly while in utero. Upon delivery there is a rapid deceleration in growth, followed by a relatively constant linear growth period during childhood. With the onset of puberty, there is almost an exponential rise in linear growth, which ceases at the time of physeal closure. At each stage there are variations in the distribution of size and shape. For example, at birth the head is relatively large, achieving about 70% of its mature circumference at the time of delivery. During infancy, the growth of the trunk predominates. During childhood, the rapid growth of the lower limbs dominates the growth pattern.

Linear growth velocity is a reliable indicator of the basic health of the child. Serial measurements and the comparison to standard tables give the examiner a rapid assessment of any aberrant growth. In general, growth is considered aberrant when it falls below two standard deviations (± 2 SD) for age. This would place a given child in the third percentile. Arguably, normal individuals can fall within this range. However, it should stimulate the examiner to more carefully and assiduously pursue a diagnosis before assuming the child to be "physiologically short."

EVALUATION OF THE PATIENT

Family history is perhaps the most essential piece to be retrieved during the history taking. Many skeletal dysplasias have a genetic basis, and frequently similar aberrations can be discovered in the pedigree. Additionally, one should inquire about any history of stillbirths in the immediate or extended family. Certain severe dwarfing syndromes, such as achondrogenesis, frequently cause the fetus to be stillborn. A history of mental retardation tends to move the diagnostic emphasis toward endocrine or chromosomal defects rather than true skeletal dysplasias. Dysplasias rarely are complicated by mental retardation.

The *physical examination* can yield a great deal of information that is helpful in the evaluation of short stature. Body proportions are key in the diagnosis and differentiation of short stature. The use of the *upper body/lower body segment ratio* is most helpful in determining proportionality. The upper body segment is defined as the total height of the individual minus the distance measured from the symphysis to the floor. The lower body segment is obviously the remaining measurement—that is, the symphysis pubis to the floor. The ratio of the upper body segment to the lower body segment can be compared against standard tables. White infants typically have a ratio of 1.7, which decreases to 1.0 by age 8 to 10 years. After puberty it falls below 1. By adulthood, the average white has an upper/lower segment ratio of 0.92 and the average black has a ratio of 0.82. The finding of a disproportion between limb segments and trunk segment leads one to the diagnosis of disproportionate short stature. Virtually all the skeletal dysplasias result in disproportionate dwarfism. Should it be determined that the short individual is proportionate, then the diagnostic focus is on endocrine, metabolic, nutritional, or other nonskeletal causes.

Another rough index of limb versus trunk length is based on the *arm span measurement*. The measurement from the tip of the long finger from one arm to the other with the arms fully abducted usually falls within a few centimeters of the total height. At this point, one should be able to determine the proportionality of the short stature syndrome. Proportionate short individuals have a normal ratio and their arm span equals height. Disproportionate syndromes demonstrate an abnormal ratio and an altered arm span relationship to height. Moreover, these measurements allow the grouping of short-statured, disproportionate individuals into two groups: (1) *short-limbed dwarfs*, who have an abnormally high upper body segment/lower body segment ratio and an arm span less than their height, and (2) *short-trunked dwarfs*, who have an abnormally low upper body segment/lower body segment ratio and an arm span greater than their height. Short-limbed dwarfs account for 30% of the total, while the remaining 70% are short-trunked dwarfs. One other easy screening method is to look at the *fingertip to thigh ratio*. In normal individuals, the fingertip of the long finger will reach roughly to the midthigh region. In individuals who are short-limbed disproportionate dwarfs, the fingertips will rarely reach below the level of the greater trochanter. Conversely, in individuals who are short-trunked dwarfs, the fingertip will reach to the knee.

Among short-limbed dwarfs are three subsets. The first group consists of those who have shortening primarily in the proximal segment of the limb. They are called *rhizomelic* short-limbed dwarfs, and an example is achondroplasia. When the middle segment of the limb (forearm and leg) is short, the categorization is that of *mesomelic* shortening. If the distal segments (hands and feet) demonstrate the shortening, this is referred to as *acromelic* shortening.

Once a careful history and physical examination have been completed, appropriate radiographs are extremely helpful. Several specific x-rays are most valuable when evaluating a child with a skeletal dysplasia. A specific survey in these children should include a lateral view of the skull, anteroposterior (AP) and lateral views of the spine, an AP view of the pelvis, and AP views of the hands and feet. These specific six x-rays will provide the information most often required to assist in making an accurate diagnosis. The skeletal structures projected in these films provide insight into the type of enchondral and intramembranous bone formation, which are frequently affected adversely in these dysplastic syndromes. In addition, specific epiphyseal nuclei and adjacent physeal regions are visible to allow classification for diagnostic purposes as well.

HISTOLOGIC EXAMINATION

Histologic analysis is becoming an increasingly helpful tool in the differentiation of various dysplastic states. In recent years, a number of articles have been published specifically outlining the physeal and epiphyseal changes in a given dysplastic condition, making the value of biopsy increasingly important. In addition, newer glycol methacrylate embedding techniques with the application of special stains are rapidly improving the ability to better define cellular detail.

NOMENCLATURE AND CLASSIFICATION

For many years, skeletal dysplasias were named for the individual who initially described the syndrome. Unfortunately, many eponyms still persist in the lexicon of short-statured states. It was not until Phillip Rubin published his classic work in 1964 entitled "The Dynamic Classification of Bone Dysplasias" that any semblance of order was forced upon the widespread and varied descriptions of

seemingly unrelated syndromes that had previously been published. Rubin's work was a milestone in the classification of skeletal dysplasias. He grouped these disease states into categories based on the segment of the skeleton that appeared to be most affected by the syndrome. For example, he described epiphyseal dysplasias, physeal dysplasias, metaphyseal dysplasias, and diaphyseal dysplasias (Fig. 15–8). Further, within each group he described hyperplastic syndromes and hypoplastic syndromes (Fig. 15–9). Most current authors are uncomfortable with Rubin's rigid classifications, and many reject it completely. However, it does provide a framework and a basis upon which to sensibly order and characterize a huge group of seemingly unrelated diseases. For that reason many still prefer to loosely group the dysplastic syndromes within these broad categories: epiphyseal, physeal, metaphyseal, and diaphyseal.

In the late 1970s, following an international symposium in France, a consensus was reached by many groups to rearrange the dysplastic syndromes; thus, the Paris Nomenclature was developed. Suffice it to say, at the present time there is still a significant amount of confusion regarding the classification of this multitude of syndromes. For the most part, many of the eponyms previously used have been dropped. The techniques of molecular biology and molecular genetics have now provided new information that allows the classification of these diseases based on more scientific principles related to their genetic defects.

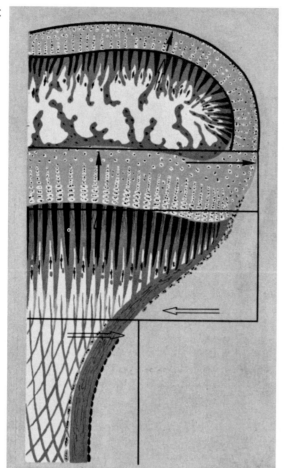

PHYSIOLOGIC ANATOMIC

Hemispherization — Epiphysis

Growth — Physis

Funnelization — Metaphysis

Cylindrization — Diaphysis

Figure 15–8. Proposed terminology for normal bone modeling (anatomic-physiologic correlation). (Adapted from Rubin P: Dynamic Classification of Bone Dysplasias. Chicago, Year Book Medical Publishers, 1964.)

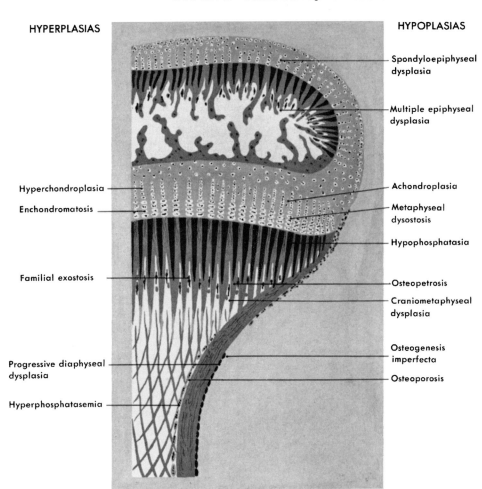

HYPERPLASIAS   HYPOPLASIAS

Spondyloepiphyseal dysplasia

Multiple epiphyseal dysplasia

Hyperchondroplasia ———   ——— Achondroplasia

Enchondromatosis ———   ——— Metaphyseal dysostosis

——— Hypophosphatasia

Familial exostosis ———   ——— Osteopetrosis

——— Craniometaphyseal dysplasia

——— Osteogenesis imperfecta

Progressive diaphyseal dysplasia ———   ——— Osteoporosis

Hyperphosphatasemia ———

Figure 15–9. Dynamic classification of bone dysplasias. (Adapted from Rubin P: Dynamic Classification of Bone Dysplasias. Chicago, Year Book Medical Publishers, 1964.)

CLINICAL PROBLEMS IN SHORT STATURE

Before looking at several specific and important skeletal dysplasias, it is appropriate to mention some of the clinical manifestations that are seen in these children in general.

During the *neonatal period*, intra-abdominal herniations have frequently been identified as life-threatening abnormalities. Esophageal atresia and tracheoesophageal fistulas frequently have mandated prompt surgical repair. Omphaloceles, perforations of the stomach, and intestinal obstruction due to duodenal atresia and malrotation similarly have been reported.

During *infancy*, some nonorthopaedic problems that require immediate care are cleft palate, inguinal hernias, dextrocardia, and coarctation of the aorta with transposition of the great vessels. The orthopaedic problems frequently observed are clubfeet, joint deformity, contractures, and spinal abnormalities. Both sagittal and coronal plane deformities can be seen and frequently present significant challenges in treatment. The clubfeet are typically rigid and require early surgical treatment.

During *childhood*, the nonorthopaedic problems mandating care include hearing loss, chronic middle ear infections, ear deformities, aberrations of the nasal bridge, and occasionally chronic cardiac abnormalities. The orthopaedic problems, however, become the most important in this age group. Odontoid hypoplasia and C1–C2 subluxation must be considered in any child undergoing surgery. In fact, most of the neuromuscular disturbances in these children,

all well described in the older literature, were actually due to failure to recognize C1–C2 subluxation, which is a classic problem in the dwarfing syndromes. The abnormalities of the occiput and C1–C2 complex are critical to evaluate early, lest severe damage be done when these children are anesthetized for various surgical procedures. In addition to odontoid hypoplasia, significant ligamentous laxity can compound the problem of C1–C2 subluxation. The management of this problem is similar to that in children with Down syndrome and juvenile rheumatoid arthritis who share this unfortunate abnormality. Depending on the degree of subluxation, the management may be nonsurgical, such as activity restriction; should the subluxation be severe, surgical fusion is almost always the recommended course of action. Because of abnormalities in the ring of C1, the fusion usually is extended to the occiput.

Hip dysplasia in this age group is well known. It is critical to recognize that the standard treatment protocols used for the child with developmental dysplasia of the hip are not applicable to these children. In fact, many dwarfs can function well with dislocated hips; therefore, it is frequently best to leave the hips subluxed or dislocated. Reconstructive procedures can cause severe stiffness and increased disability.

Dysplastic changes about the knee such as genu varum and genu valgum, flexion contractures, recurvatum deformity, and frank dislocations have all been seen. It is absolutely critical when evaluating angular deformity of the knee in dwarfing syndromes to carefully differentiate between ligamentous laxity and true bony deformity. In point of fact, most of these angular changes are the result of severe ligamentous laxity. That being the case, osteotomy of the femur or tibia will not correct the deformity. Rather, it would be better to manage the problem with orthotics. Unfortunately, even in the presence of skeletal deformity, corrective osteotomies are frequently complicated by recurrence of the deformity. The *adolescent* with short stature is most frequently compromised by the problem of obesity. Not only does the obesity dramatically and profoundly increase the psychosocial problems of these patients, but it can dramatically accentuate problems such as scoliosis and hip dysplasia. Currently, there is increased interest in leg lengthening procedures to increase the height of these short patients. However, because significant complications can be encountered with this type of leg-lengthening surgery, these procedures and techniques are controversial at best.

By the time most of the children reach *adulthood*, they have compensated for most of their physical impairments. Orthopaedic procedures in the adult dwarf are rarely required. Current interest centers on the management of their joint deformities and late osteoarthritis. Newer developments in prosthetic design have sparked some enthusiasm for the use of total joint arthroplasty in this unique population. Long-term results are unavailable at this time.

DEFINITIONS

A *skeletal dysplasia* is a disease in which the predominant error is in bone modeling; therefore, the error is intrinsic to the skeletal system. As such, it affects all bones, and the distribution is generalized. Depending on the degree of growth inhibition, the words aplasia, hypoplasia, and hyperplasia are frequently used.

A *bone dystrophy*, on the other hand, is a disease that arises from faulty metabolism or a nutritional defect. Therefore, the error is extrinsic to bone. Hyperthyroidism and rickets are two extrinsic bone dystrophies. The changes in the skeleton simply mirror the underlying endocrine or nutritional defect.

A *skeletal dysostosis* is a bit more difficult to define. In the broadest sense, these disorders represent a disturbance of ossification or malformation of individual bones, singly or in combination. Their distribution is largely unpredictable, because they follow a defect in ectodermal or mesodermal tissues. These entities are frequently isolated or unilateral conditions.

SPECIFIC MODELING ERRORS OF BONE

Epiphyseal Modeling Errors

At the onset, it should be recognized that the epiphysis is a *secondary ossification center*. The physiologic role of the epiphysis is the process of "hemispherization" (see Fig. 15–8). Essentially, this means that it is responsible for shaping the normal end of a long bone. Conversely, if the dysplastic condition adversely affects the epiphysis, one can anticipate a misshapen epiphyseal end of the bone. Several specific entities reflect such modeling errors. The two most important in this group are multiple epiphyseal dysplasia and spondyloepiphyseal dysplasia.

MULTIPLE EPIPHYSEAL DYSPLASIA

These children are short-limbed dwarfs with spinal sparing and are usually not diagnosed until late childhood. They usually achieve the adult height of between 54 and 60 inches. The more benign (tarda) form has frequently been referred to as Fairbank's disease. As mentioned, these children are symptom-free for most of their childhood years.

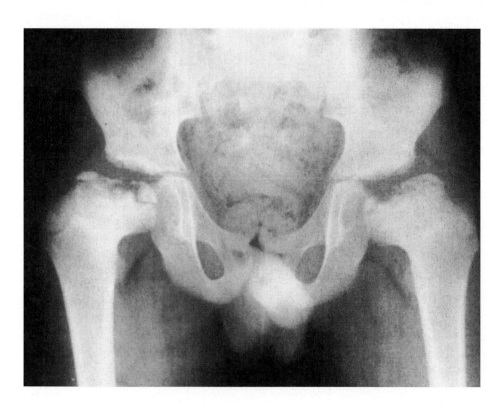

Figure 15–10. Multiple epiphyseal dysplasia. Radiograph of pelvis at 6 years of age showing abnormal ossification of femoral heads and short, broad femoral necks. This patient developed incongruous hips with premature osteoarthritis. (From Benson MKD, Fixsen JA, MacNicol MF: Children's Orthopaedics and Fractures. Edinburgh, Churchill Livingstone, 1994.)

They have normal IQs and normal muscle tone. The key feature is the aberration in growth of the epiphyseal nuclei. As a result, the misshapen, "cobblestoned" condylar ends of long bones lead to the characteristic precocious osteoarthritis.

The children have a normal head and neck. Their vertebral bodies are virtually normal with the exception of some arterior rounding at the corners. Their extremities manifest the brunt of the disease. The hips are usually the most severely involved joints, with coxa magna and coxa breva being present early, followed by the development of osteoarthritis in the young adult (Fig. 15–10). In the child, the radiographic changes in the hips may suggest the diagnosis of bilateral Perthes' disease. In the knees, one can notice a sloping of the tibial condyles, which is said to be very characteristic. Similarly, the most diagnostic feature in the ankle is a sloping of the mortise into a valgus position. This feature is seen in about 50% of these children. Common findings in the upper extremity include dislocation of the radial head with compensatory capitellar enlargement and deformities of the fingers.

SPONDYLOEPIPHYSEAL DYSPLASIA

As the name implies, these children not only have dysplastic epiphyses, but they also manifest changes in the spine. Recall that the ring apophyses of the vertebrae are, in point of fact, secondary ossification centers. This condition not only affects the appendicular skeleton but also the axial skeleton. This syndrome is frequently evident at birth, because these children are short-trunked dwarfs. Exaggerated kyphosis in the thoracic spine and lumbar lordosis are frequently seen (Fig. 15–11). Because of the hip changes, a waddling gait is prominent. Several different inheritance patterns have been identified, some sex-linked and others autosomal.

The clinical features are more profound than in multiple epiphyseal dysplasia. Ocular changes, such as myopia and retinal detachment, are seen in 50% of the affected children. In addition, C1–C2 instability is a hallmark of this disease. It is due to a combination of odontoid hypoplasia and ligamentous laxity. The trunk is characterized by a pectus carinatum and the prominent abdomen reflects the constricted chest wall. The rib cage tends to be horizontal due to the classic changes seen in the spine. The syndrome is characterized by the marked platyspondylisis ("canoe paddle vertebra") seen throughout the spine. Disk height is frequently increased, even in the face of severe truncal shortening. It is very important to note that the interpedicular distance is normal, which is not the case in achondroplasia.

The appendicular changes in the skeleton are very similar to those seen in multiple epiphyseal dysplasia. The joints clinically appear "knobby," due to aberrant epiphyseal ossification. Articular surfaces tend to be irregular, resulting in precocious osteoarthritis. Generalized ligamentous laxity only compounds the breakdown of the diarthrodial joints.

The syndrome described as Morquio's disease is similar to spondyloepiphyseal dysplasia, with the exception that these children have an identifiable mucopolysaccharidosis. One is able to measure abnormal levels of keratosulfate in

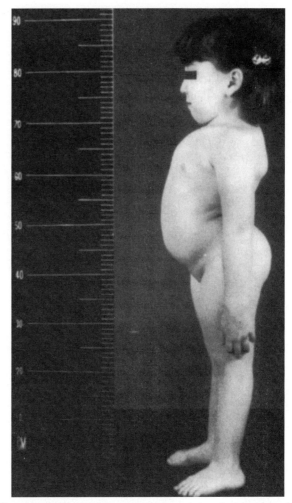

Figure 15–11. Spondyloepiphyseal dysplasia congenita. Clinical appearance at 3 years of age showing short stature, short trunk, and relatively long limbs. This patient has excessive lumbar lordosis and prominence of the sternum. (From Benson MKD, Fixsen JA, MacNicol MF: Children's Orthopaedics and Fractures. Edinburgh, Churchill Livingstone, 1994.)

the urine. Otherwise, many of the phenotypic patterns look very similar to those seen in spondyloepiphyseal dysplasia.

CRETINISM

This bone dystrophy adversely affects the epiphyseal growth. Deprivation of thyroid hormone at birth causes these changes. These children demonstrate a generalized delay in ossification, which radiographically appears as if the epiphyseal nucleus is ossifying from multiple centers. The exact role of thyroid hormone in the production of these changes has yet to be defined. A number of suggestions point at a basic abnormality in mucopolysaccharide metabolism. A failure to degrade one of the normal glycosaminoglycans has been suggested. The resulting accumulation of this material appears to inhibit chondroblast activity.

DIASTROPHIC DWARFISM

This syndrome is a dysostosis, primarily affecting the epiphyseal center (Fig. 15–12). This is a complex chondrodys-

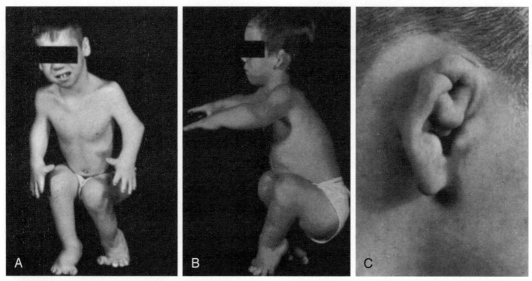

Figure 15–12. Diastrophic dysplasia. *A and B*, Clinical appearance of a patient with the typical deformities. Note the severe flexion contractures of the hips and knees and the equinovarus deformities of the feet. "Hitchhiker's thumb" is a principal feature. *C*, The deformed ears have thickened lobes, are furrowed, and have a narrow external auditory canal. (From Tachdjian MO: Pediatric Orthopedics, 2nd ed. Philadelphia, WB Saunders, 1990.)

trophy characterized by short limbs, progressive scoliosis, hand anomalies, severe rigid clubfeet, hip dysplasia, joint contractures, and malformation of the external ear. The overall pattern, although variable, is primarily that of a rhizomelic short-limbed dwarf. The inheritance pattern is primarily autosomal recessive; however, significant variability has been reported.

The clinical features, which typify the diastrophic dwarf, are the finding of a "cauliflower" ear and cleft palate. The severe resistant clubfeet are certainly one of the most challenging of the orthopaedic problems. The "hitchhiker thumb," due to hypoplasia of the first metacarpal (triangular metacarpal), is probably the most pathognomonic finding in diastrophic dwarfism.

Physeal Modeling Errors

The role of the physis is singular: linear bone growth. With that in mind, physeal defects can be expected to produce the most severe shortening. The epiphyseal nucleus and resultant condylar modeling are normal in this group. Some secondary changes in the metaphysis, such as flaring or "cupping," can be seen radiographically. However, the most dramatic impact of these syndromes is on physeal growth.

ACHONDROPLASIA

Achondroplasia is the most common skeletal dysplasia. It is inherited in an autosomal dominant fashion; however, 75% of children with this disorder have a negative family history. Thus, achondroplasia most commonly results from spontaneous mutations. The only associated finding is increased paternal age. This syndrome essentially defines rhizomelic short-limbed dwarfism. It is a defect in normal enchondral bone growth, primarily affecting and altering the proliferating zone of the growth plate. It is important

to remember that intramembranous bone growth is *not* affected.

The clinical manifestations of the disease reflect the aberrations in bone growth. Recalling that the calvarial portions of the skull grow intramembranously, whereas the basilar portions of the skull grow enchondrally, one can then realize why the head and neck have such a typical appearance (Fig. 15–13). The facial retrusion and saddle-nose deformity are simply the result of an underdeveloped basilar skull. The calvarium is of normal size, thereby causing the skull to appear disproportionate. Prognathism and frontal bossing complete the picture. Essentially, every long bone in the body is short. This includes the ribs, causing the chest wall to be small and somewhat constricted, which results in a protuberant abdomen. The spine typically is hyperlordotic in the lumbar region with a concurrent increase in thoracic kyphosis. Most important in the achondroplastic spine is the decrease in interpedicular distance. This decrease is most obvious in the lumbar region. This change is in contrast to the normal interpedicular distance seen in spondyloepiphyseal dysplasia. As a result, a spinal stenotic syndrome can result, with cord compression likely. Scoliosis is also seen in approximately one third of these children; however, the curvature is usually mild.

The radiographic appearance of the pelvis is classic in achondroplasia (Fig. 15–14). Remember that the height of the pelvis is a function of the enchondral bone growth from the triradiate cartilage. In achondroplasia, one sees a flattened pelvis with a "champagne glass" outlet. (The normal pelvic outlet is frequently described as being "wine glass" in configuration.) These changes are merely a reflection of overall decrease in pelvic height. Unlike the epiphyseal dysplasias, in which precocious arthritis is the hallmark, in achondroplasia, joint contractures and angular deformity tend to be more prominent. In fact, arthritic

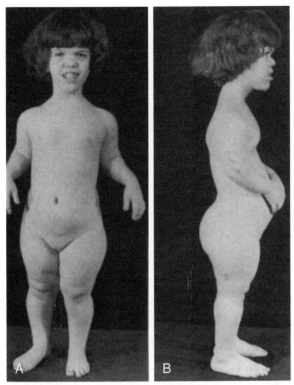

Figure 15–13. Achondroplasia in an 8-year-old girl. *A and B*, Clinical appearance of a patient with typical deformities. (From Tachdjian MO: Pediatric Orthopedics, 2nd ed. Philadelphia, WB Saunders, 1990.)

joints are rarely seen. Flexion contracture of the elbow, the hip, and the knee are frequently present. Genu varum, which is considered the major orthopaedic problem in the paediatric age group, appears to be primarily due to fibular overgrowth in relation to that of tibia. Management of this

problem by fusion of the proximal fibular growth plate reportedly has been successful. As is so often the case, the changes in the hand frequently become pathognomonic for the syndrome. In achondroplasia, the "trident hand" (Fig. 15–15) is a classic finding, frequently permitting early diagnosis.

As these children age, obesity becomes a major problem. It will aggravate their back problems, as well as the angular deformities of their knees. In addition, these patients complain of multiple myofascial and bursal syndromes. Similarly, cord compression in the adult needs to be recognized, especially in any patient complaining of easy fatigability, gait disturbances, or impotence in the males.

MUCOPOLYSACCHARIDOSES

These syndromes are frequently cited as bone dystrophies, involving the physeal portion of the long bone. The accumulation of end products, such as chondroitin sulfate and keratin sulfate, frequently accumulate in and around the growth plate. In doing so, normal physeal growth is disrupted, and histologic changes in the proliferating and hypertrophic zones are seen. Children with mucopolysaccharidoses have foreshortened extremities among the other classic findings, which are listed in Table 15–1.

ELLIS–VAN CREVALD SYNDROME

Chondroectodermal dysplasia, as this syndrome is also called, is identified as a dysostosis, primarily affecting the physeal portion of the bone. The classic *triad* of acromelic limb shortening, manual polydactyly, and ectodermal dysplasia is typical in these children. Approximately half of the patients have a congenital heart defect, such as a single atria with or without a cleft mitral valve. This syndrome is reportedly autosomal recessive. Clinical features include

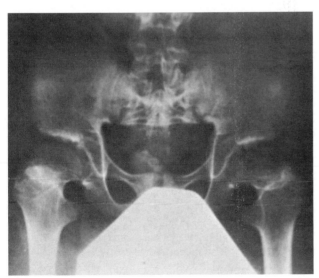

Figure 15–14. Achondroplasia in a 10-year-old boy. Anteroposterior radiograph of the pelvis. Note the typical appearance of the inner pelvic contour and the squaring off of the iliac wings. (From Tachdjian MO: Pediatric Orthopedics, 2nd ed. Philadelphia, WB Saunders, 1990.)

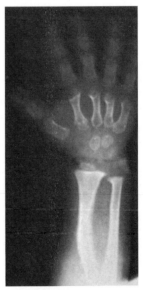

Figure 15–15. Achondroplasia in a 10-year-old boy. Anteroposterior radiograph of the hand. Note the short thick metacarpals and phalanges. The long and ring fingers are spread apart, forming a V-shaped space ("main en trident"). (From Tachdjian MO: Pediatric Orthopedics, 2nd ed. Philadelphia, WB Saunders, 1990.)

Table 15–1. Main features of the mucopolysaccharidoses (MPS)

Classification	Enzyme Deficiency	Excreted Glycosaminoglycan	Main Organs Affected	Appearance	Mental State
IH Hurler	α-L-Iduronidase	Dermatan sulfate Heparan sulfate	CNS, skeleton, viscera	Hurler ("gargoylism")	Rapid deterioration
IS Scheie	α-L-Iduronidase	Dermatan sulfate Heparan sulfate	Skeleton, viscera	Coarse features	Normal
IH/S Hurler/Scheie	α-L-Iduronidase	Dermatan sulfate Heparan sulfate	Intermediate phenotype	Coarse features	Variable
II Hunter	Iduronate sulfate sulfatase	Dermatan sulfate Heparan sulfate	CNS, skeleton, viscera	Like Hurler	Variable deterioration
III A Sanfilippo–III D	4 distinct biochemical types; identical phenotypes	Heparan sulfate	CNS	Not characteristic	Severe mental deterioration
IV Morquio	Galactosamine-6-sulfatase	Keratan sulfate	Skeleton, severe deformities, flat, beaked vertebrae, thoracolumbar gibbus, odontoid hypoplasia	Not diagnostic	Normal
VI Maroteaux–Lamy	N-acetylgalactos-amine-4-sulfatase	Dermatan sulfate	Skeleton	Like Hurler	Variable
VII	β-glucuronidase	Dermatan sulfate Heparan sulfate	CNS, skeleton Viscera	Like Hurler	Variable

Note that all these disorders are inherited as autosomal recessive disorders with the exception of MPS II (Hunter's syndrome), in which the enzyme deficiency is inherited as an X-linked recessive.

There are common skeletal abnormalities in this group of disorders (referred to as dysostosis multiplex); these are seen typically in Hurler's syndrome (MPS I). Specific features occur in MPS IV (Morquio's syndrome).

In MPS I, there is a large skull, with J (shoe)-shaped pituitary fossa; in the spine, persistence of infantile biconcave vertebrae gives way to a thoracolumbar kyphosis; in the thorax the ribs are paddle-shaped; in the hands the phalanges are pointed distally ("bullet-shaped"), and the metacarpals proximally.

In MPS IV, excessive joint mobility combines with typical skeletal deformity. The spine initially resembles MPS I. Later, platyspondyly with an anterior projecting central tongue is typical. The odontoid is small or absent. There is gross deformity of the chest, shortening of the spine, and genu valgum. The small bones of the hand are well modeled.

From Benson MKD, Fixsen JA, MacNicol MF: Children's Orthopaedics and Fractures. Edinburgh, Churchill Livingstone, 1994.

sparse, thin hair, hypertelorism, cleft palate, and hairlip with delayed dentition. Pectus carinatum and scoliosis are common, and as one would expect in most dysostotic states, there is an ectodermal component; frequently, deformed nails and extra digits occur.

Metaphyseal Modeling Errors

The physiologic role of the metaphysis is to cut back the widened end of a long bone into a more cylindrical diaphysis. Rubin has referred to this process as "funnelization." In order for this to occur, osteoblasts on the endosteal side of the metaphysis and osteoclasts on the periosteal side must be active. This pattern of cell distribution is exactly the opposite of that seen in the diaphyseal region. Subjacent to the growth plate, one typically sees primary spongiosa bone, which is primitive bony trabeculae adherent to cartilage bars. As development progresses, the cartilage bar is resorbed, leaving behind bony trabeculae. Once this occurs these bony bars, devoid of cartilage, are referred to as secondary spongiosa.

OSTEOPETROSIS (MARBLE BONE DISEASE)

In 1907, Albers-Schoenberg described this syndrome in the German literature. Obviously, at that time the basic defect had not been identified. Presently, osteopetrosis is believed to be one of the "sick cell syndromes." The *osteoclasts*

are normal in number but abnormal in function. As a result, they do not remove the primary spongiosa bone in the metaphysis; this failure to resorb these primary bony trabeculae leaves behind a dense pile of primitive trabeculae with cartilage cores in the metaphysis. This accumulation of material makes it impossible for the metaphysis to cut back, or funnelize, the end of the long bone. Hence, one will see a dilated metaphysis, typical in this group of modeling errors ("Erlenmeyer flask" femur) (Fig. 15–16).

The basilar portions of the skull are sclerotic. Inadequacy of cranial nerve foramen and the foramen magnum can cause cranial nerve palsy and hydrocephalus, respectively. In addition, the supraorbital ridge is dense and occasionally prominent.

The vertebrae frequently demonstrate a "bone within a bone" pattern (Fig. 15–17). Additionally, endplate sclerosis with normal density of the centrum leads to the radiographic pattern referred to as "sandwich vertebrae." In the appendicular skeleton, the metaphyses are abnormally widened. Frequently, translucent bands are seen subjacent to the growth plate and transverse fractures are due to the general mechanical weakness of osteopetrotic bone. Despite its density, the bone is very poorly integrated and, as a result, subject to mechanical failure. One should not confuse increased density with increased mechanical strength.

The management of fractures in these patients can be a

challenging problem. Often, only closed treatment is required; however, if open treatment is necessary, implant fixation is frequently difficult to achieve. Finally, the marked displacement of bone marrow by the retained abnormal bone causes a myelophthistic anemia, resulting in hepatosplenomegaly as extramedullary sites of hematopoiesis are stimulated.

SCURVY

This nutritional defect is a classic bone dystrophy that largely affects the metaphyseal region. The extrinsic defect is well known to be a deficiency in vitamin C. Vitamin C is a cofactor in the normal synthetic pathway of bone collagen synthesis. In its absence, the resulting collagen is poorly cross-linked and thus, mechanically deficient. As a result, the clinical state is a mirror of this deficient collagen. "Slipping" of the epiphyseal plates with minimal, if any, trauma is a hallmark of the disease. With physeal displacement, hemorrhage occurs under the periosteum. This results in stripping of the adjacent metaphyseal periosteum and subsequent subperiosteal bone formation. The petechial hemorrhages seen in these children are merely another reflection of deficient collagen. In this case, the basement membrane collagen is defective and allows these spontaneous hemorrhages to occur.

Diaphyseal Modeling Errors

The role of the diaphysis is to create a normal tube of bone. Rubin again has characterized this role using the word "cylinderization." It will be recalled that periosteal bone growth is essentially intramembranous in nature; therefore, diseases that impact on enchondral bone growth have no effect on the diaphysis of a long bone directly.

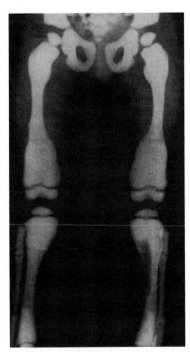

Figure 15–16. Osteopetrosis. Anteroposterior radiograph of both lower limbs. (From Tachdjian MO: Pediatric Orthopedics, 2nd ed. Philadelphia, WB Saunders, 1990.)

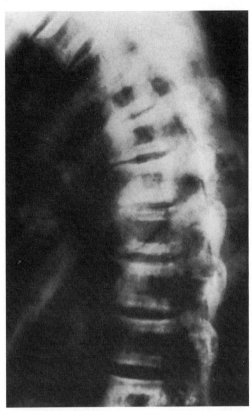

Figure 15–17. Vertebrae in osteopetrosis. (From Tachdjian MO: Pediatric Orthopedics, 2nd ed. Philadelphia, WB Saunders, 1990.)

Conversely, diseases that are primarily aberrations of intramembranous bone formation will have a severe impact on the development of a long bone.

OSTEOGENESIS IMPERFECTA

Osteogenesis imperfecta is the prototype dysplasia of this group. Described in 1849 by Rollick, this is clearly the epitome of aberrant intramembranous bone growth (Fig. 15–18). Most cases are transmitted in an autosomal dominant fashion, yet over one third arise as spontaneous mutations. This disease is also considered by some to be a "sick cell syndrome." In this case, *osteoblast* numbers are normal but their activity is aberrant. As a result, the "impotent osteoblasts" are unable to adequately form bone in an intramembranous fashion. Thus, the normal cylinderization of long bones does not occur, leaving behind thin stenotic diaphyses as the hallmark of this disease (Fig. 15–19).

Classically, the skull manifests wormian bones, which are said to be a radiographic hallmark of the disease. These bones are isolated lakes of bone typically found in and around the sutures. Changes in the basilar portions of the skull frequently result in otosclerosis; however, it is the calvarium that is most prominently affected. The discrepancy between the calvaria and basilar portions of the skull causes the child to have a triangular face. The teeth are small and fragile due to abnormal dentinogenesis. Perhaps the most classic finding in the head and neck region is the presence of blue sclera. Due to the collagen dysplasia, which causes the sclera to be very thin, one can see a reflection through this thin sclera of the retina behind. Typically, this gives the sclera its bluish tint.

The spine in these children is typically osteoporotic with the development of both coronal and sagittal plane deformity. The surgical management of the spinal deformities in these children is complicated by the soft bone, which makes implant fixation at best problematic. The extremities tend to be short, due not to an aberration in physeal growth but rather to the multiple fractures that characterize this syndrome. As mentioned earlier, the long bones are markedly thin and osteoporotic. The diaphyseal caliber is strikingly narrowed to such a degree that the medullary canal appears almost obliterated. Depending on the penetrance of the genetic material, the child with severe osteogenesis imperfecta will sustain multiple fractures throughout life. In point of fact, the most common cause of premature death in these children is skull fractures with resultant subdural or epidural hematomas.

Pathologic fracture in osteogenesis is the hallmark of the disease (Fig. 15–20). Frequently, these fractures can be treated closed, using simple splints or casts. Occasionally, they can be a "fortunate fracture," which occurs in an already deformed bone, thus allowing correction of the deformity. Interestingly enough, the healing time of fractures in these children is usually normal.

Severe deformities in the lower extremities are not infrequent. This often makes ambulation difficult, if not impossible, for these children, with or without braces. The presence of severe deformities in the long bones of the lower

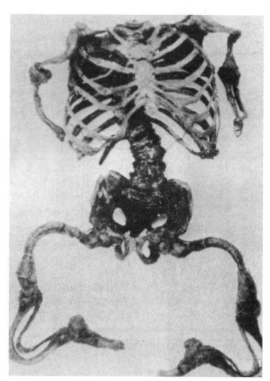

Figure 15–19. Skeleton in osteogenesis imperfecta. (From Bullough PG, Davidson DD, Lorenzo JC: The morbid anatomy of the skeleton in osteogenesis imperfecta. Clin Orthop 159:42, 1981. Reprinted by permission.)

extremity can frequently be treated with a Sofield fragmentation osteotomy. By achieving axial alignment of the limb, improved ambulatory ability can be anticipated. The Sillence classification of osteogenesis imperfecta is based on the various phenotypic patterns and is outlined in Table 15–2.

CLEIDOCRANIAL DYSOSTOSIS

Cleidocranial dysostosis is a unique condition, often grouped with the diaphyseal modeling errors. Considered as a germ plasm defect, this is an error in intramembranous bone formation. The syndrome is inherited primarily in an autosomal dominant fushion. The typical findings are a large brachycephalic skull with a small face, cleft palate, and delayed dentition. The wormian bones seen in the skull seem to validate this entity as a defect in intramembranous formation. Certainly, the hallmark of this syndrome is the aplastic or hypoplastic clavicles, which clinically result in dropped shoulders and winged scapulae. These children are frequently able to literally oppose their shoulders in front of them. There are frequently some ectodermal changes evidenced by nail changes in the hands and feet and hypoplastic distal phalanges.

Summary

Many dysplastic syndromes of the skeleton still largely defy classification. Despite attempts to organize these very disparate syndromes, there still remains a great deal of confusion and overlap in the literature. The technologic advances in molecular biology and genetics have in some ways only compounded the problem. Syndromes and dis-

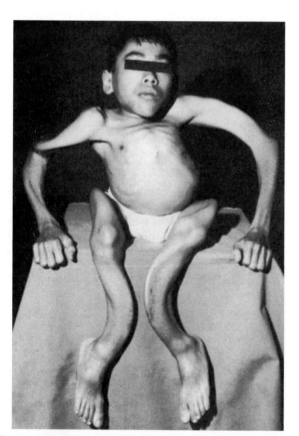

Figure 15–18. Osteogenesis imperfecta type III. This patient presented with multiple deformities and minimal previous treatment.

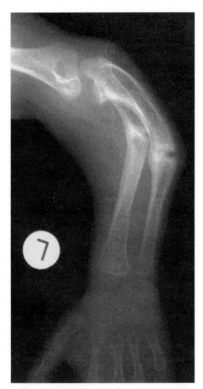

Figure 15–20. Upper limbs of a child with type IV osteogenesis imperfecta. Multiple fractures and increasing deformity are typical throughout growth. Both forearm bones have suffered recent fractures, and there is marked bowing of the forearm secondary to previous fractures. (From Broughton NS: A Textbook of Paediatric Orthopaedics. London, WB Saunders, 1997.)

eases once thought to be similar have been shown to be quite dissimilar by these techniques. Therefore, a great deal of work remains in the research arena before true characterizations can be completed. Until then, the diagnosis is primarily based on phenotypic appearance and radiographic changes. This is likely to remain the norm in the near future. Finally, it is important to recognize that approximately 60% of children referred for the evaluation of a dysmorphic syndrome defy classification at the completion of their workup.

NEUROMUSCULAR DISEASE

Children afflicted with neuromuscular diseases frequently manifest severe musculoskeletal abnormalities. Not only

do they suffer from the intrinsic effects of the neuropathic or myopathic abnormalities, but they are usually profoundly affected by the secondary bone and joint deformities that result from these diseases. In addition, the impact on bone growth with subsequent aberrant changes cannot be overestimated. For management to be effective, it is important that the physician recognize the basic differences between the various neuromuscular diseases. The differentiation between central neurologic disease and peripheral neurologic disease is critical to understanding the neuromuscular effects that are manifested. Moreover, certain, diseases affect only the motor component of the nerve, whereas others affect both the sensory and the motor components. Cerebral palsy, for example, is a central neurologic defect with resulting spasticity in the periphery. These children typically have reasonable sensation. In contrast, myelodysplasia affects the spinal cord and adjacent nerve roots, leaving the child flaccid in the extremities and insensate. The historically classic motor neuron disease, poliomyelitis, is different in that it affects the anterior horn cell neurons and results in motor paralysis but spares the dorsal root ganglion, preserving sensation. Similarly, spinal muscle atrophy is a degenerative condition of the anterior horn cells with significant secondary muscle denervation. Muscular dystrophies (Duchenne and others) affect the end organ, causing significant myopathic change. The nerves typically are unaffected. Arthrogryposis, a bizarre neuromuscular disease of unknown etiology, causes a typical syndrome complex. In fact, there is debate as to whether the arthrogrypotic syndromes are myopathic, neuropathic, or mixed. As can be seen, the variation in pathogenesis of neuromuscular disease is wide-ranging; nevertheless, the frequently encountered musculoskeletal abnormalities often show some similarities of involvement.

Cerebral Palsy

This syndrome is often referred to as Little's disease, following John Little's original description. Cerebral palsy is especially important because it is relatively common. Cerebral palsy is not one disease, but a syndrome of motor disorders resulting from insults to the immature brain. These insults may occur prenatally, postnatally, or at the time of delivery. The name, cerebral palsy, has been referred to by some as an "administrative convenience," because it allows the family access to government-provided services. Perhaps the two characteristics that best typify these syndromes are that (1) they result from an *injury to the immature brain* and (2) they are *static neuromuscular*

Table 15–2. Classification of osteogenesis imperfecta

Type	Features	Inheritance
I (dominant, blue sclerae)	IA: Bone fragility, blue sclerae and normal teeth IB: Same as IA but with dentinogenesis imperfecta	Autosomal dominant
II (lethal, perinatal)	Severe porosis with multiple fractures and malformed skeleton	Autosomal dominant
III (progressive, deforming)	Multiple fractures at birth with progressive deformities, normal sclerae, and dentinogenesis imperfecta	Autosomal recessive
IV (dominant, white sclerae)	IVA: Bone fragility, white sclerae, and normal teeth IVB: Similar to IVA but with dentinogenesis imperfecta	Autosomal dominant

From Benson MKD, Fixsen JA, MacNicol MF: Children's Orthopaedics and Fractures. Edinburgh, Churchill Livingstone, 1994.

deficits without progression. At the present time, the incidence of cerebral palsy is approximately 2 to 4 per 1000 live births. It is without a doubt the most common neuromuscular problem of childhood, and approximately 25,000 new cases are reported each year.

ETIOLOGY

Fifty percent of affected children have an identifiable cause. Prenatal causes such as the infections toxoplasmosis, rubella, cytomegalic inclusion virus, herpes, and syphilis have been reported. Maternal use of drugs and alcohol and congenital cerebral malformations have also been implicated. Perinatal causes such as birth trauma and anoxia are well known. In point of fact, the most common perinatal factor related to cerebral palsy is prematurity. Infants less than 1500 g have a 25 times greater risk of manifesting the syndrome. This latter group typically presents with spastic diplegia. On the other hand, children who suffer traumatic deliveries usually sustain global cerebral anoxia, which manifests as spastic quadriplegia. Postnatal causes such as head trauma, intraventricular hemorrhage, and meningitis also result in the syndrome.

CLASSIFICATION

In general, cerebral palsy (CP) can be classified in one of two ways. Physiologic grouping is based upon the movement disorder seen. The most common type is *pyramidal tract disease.* Typically these children are spastic with increased stretch reflexes, clonus, and muscle spasticity. This is the most common form and is typically associated with prematurity, anoxia, and prenatal sepsis. The other physiologic type is *extrapyramidal disease* (dyskinetic syndromes), which is characterized primarily by movement disorders such as athetosis, chorea, ballismus, and rigidity. Of these, the most common is athetosis, even though it is seen far less frequently than it was 40 years ago. At that time, Rh incompatibility and the resultant basal ganglia involvement was the most common cause of athetoid CP. Some mixed forms have been reported but are generally uncommon.

The other method used in classifying these children is by geographic grouping. The three most common types are hemiplegia, diplegia, and quadriplegia. The *hemiplegic* child (Fig. 15–21) is the most minimally involved and is frequently not diagnosed until after the age of walking. These children walk at the normal age. They may manifest a mild limp or asymmetric torsion in the lower extremities. Initial evaluation may suggest spasticity that is dominant on one side. Similarly, be alert to handedness manifested prior to 2 years of age. This may suggest involvement on the side of the nondominant hand. Frequently, there is some delay in speech and perceptional skills but these defects tend to be mild. Seizure disorders are well recognized in these children. Fortunately, the vast majority of these children will walk.

Diplegia (Fig. 15–22) is the most common form of cerebral palsy in the United States today. It is the type associated with prematurity. These children demonstrate delay of all milestones, but most will be able to walk by age 7. Many have normal intelligence, although some have low IQs. Typically, the pattern of involvement is such that

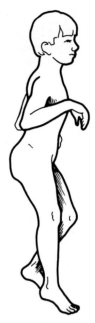

Figure 15–21. Hemiplegic posture: flexed elbow, wrist, and fingers; foot and ankle equinus position. (From Bleck EE: Orthopaedic Management of Cerebral Palsy, Vol 2. Philadelphia, WB Saunders, 1979.)

the lower extremities are more affected than the upper extremities.

Quadriplegia (the totally involved child) usually follows an episode of global anoxic damage (Fig. 15–23). Frequently, the infant is floppy and will not suck. All motor milestones are delayed, and all areas of brain function are affected. In the neonatal period, the major cause of death

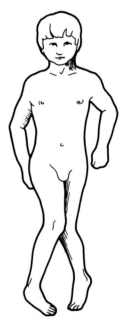

Figure 15–22. Diplegic posture: upper limbs grossly normal; flexed, internally rotated, and adducted hips. (From Bleck EE: Orthopaedic Management of Cerebral Palsy, Vol 2. Philadelphia, WB Saunders, 1979.)

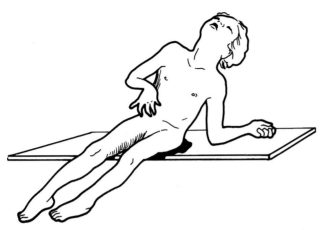

Figure 15–23. Total body involvement—spastic or athetoid or mixed quadriplegia—usually a predominant extensor postural pattern. (From Bleck EE: Orthopaedic Management of Cerebral Palsy, Vol 2. Philadelphia, WB Saunders, 1979.)

is aspiration, and the death rate is about 17 times normal. These children manifest a wide spectrum of involvement, and fewer than 30% achieve ambulation by age 7.

It is important to recognize that all extremities tend to show some involvement. The use of these descriptive terms is meant merely to identify the predominant pattern. For example, the term "diplegia" is used rather than paraplegia to emphasize the fact that the upper extremities are involved, but to a lesser degree than the lower.

PATHOPHYSIOLOGY

The impaired motor control manifested in these children results from damage to the central nervous system. As a result, the usual inhibitory role of the central nervous system is suppressed, thereby resulting in a heightened response to the stretch reflex. These abnormal stretch reflexes heighten muscle tone and result in decreased joint motion. Over time, the spasticity in the extremity results in contracture and joint deformities. Initially, the contractures may be dynamic, but over time they will become fixed.

It is important to remember that cerebral palsy is a fixed neurologic deficit. This implies that uninvolved areas will not subsequently become affected. With this in mind, one needs to beware of apparent neurologic progression. The child who is getting progressively worse should be carefully evaluated for other neurologic etiologies. Specifically, evidence of brain or spinal cord tumors, vascular anomalies, metabolic storage diseases, or syringomyelia should be carefully sought.

GENERAL FEATURES

These children have a number of characteristics in common despite variation in etiology and geographic type. They all manifest some deficits in development, learning, vision, perception, communication, and locomotion. Their ability to perform the activities of daily living (ADLs) is highly variable. It is also critical to remember that the child and young adult affected with these syndromes may have treatment goals different from those of the family or physi-

cian. When questioned about their needs, affected children list communication skills as their most important need. Their next need concerns normal sitting balance, followed by independence in ADLs. Only when these needs have been addressed do these children request assistance with improved ambulation. It is important for the physician not to lose sight of what is important to the child.

EVALUATION

Birth history and the development of motor milestones are important facts to elicit from the child's parents. Aberrations in gait and the use of the upper extremities may also be helpful in identifying etiology.

In the child under 1 year, careful evaluation of primitive reflexes (infantile autisms) can suggest a great deal of information related to prognosis. The five primitive reflexes, which should disappear in the normal child by 6 months to 1 year of age, are the Moro reflex (Fig. 15–24), the asymmetric tonic neck reflex (Fig. 15–25), the symmetric tonic neck reflex (Fig. 15–26), the extensor thrust (Fig. 15–27), and the neck righting response (Fig 15–28). In addition, two reflexes should appear by age 1 year: the parachute response (Fig. 15–29) and the foot placement response (Fig. 15–30). Eugene Bleck has developed a score to allow the examiner to determine the prognosis for walking. At 1 year of age, the child is examined for the presence or absence of these reflexes. One point is allowed for each persistent primitive reflex that should have disappeared and for the absence of each reflex that should be present. A

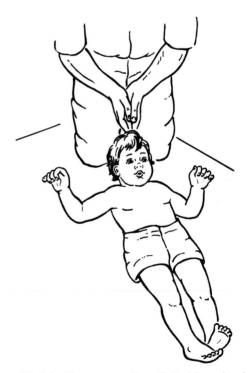

Figure 15–24. The Moro reflex elicited by a loud noise, by a jar of the examining table, by 20 to 30 degrees extension of the head, or sometimes by pinching the upper abdominal skin. The complete response is abduction of the upper limbs followed by the embrace. (From Bleck EE: Orthopaedic Management of Cerebral Palsy, Vol 2. Philadelphia, WB Saunders, 1979.)

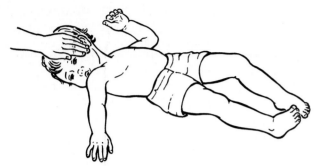

Figure 15–25. Asymmetrical tonic neck reflex. With head turning, the limbs on the skull (occipital) side flex and those on the face side extend. (From Bleck EE: Orthopaedic Management of Cerebral Palsy, Vol 2. Philadelphia, WB Saunders, 1979.)

score of 0 equates to certainty of ambulation. Two points essentially proves to the family that the child will not walk (within a 95% certainty). One point leaves the prognosis for walking in doubt.

Further physical features of importance are standing posture, which allows the examiner to note any spinal deformity; pelvic obliquity; and leg length inequality. Equilibrium reactions are significant in that they suggest the potential need for ambulatory assistive devices such as crutches or a walker. When observing the child sitting, the clinician should note whether or not the child requires the use of an upper extremity to maintain sitting balance. Finally, one of the most important findings is to observe

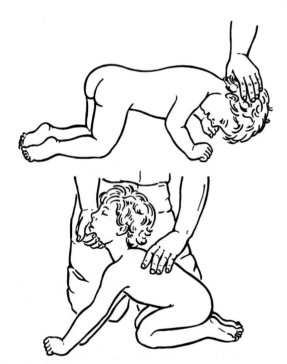

Figure 15–26. Symmetrical tonic neck reflex. With flexion of the head, the upper limbs flex and the lower limbs extend. With extension of the head, the upper limbs extend and the lower limbs flex. (From Bleck EE: Orthopaedic Management of Cerebral Palsy, Vol 2. Philadelphia, WB Saunders, 1979.)

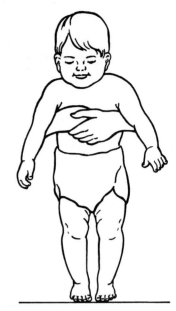

Figure 15–27. Extensor thrust. The child is held erect and the feet are lowered to the floor or table top. Progressive extension of the lower limbs upward toward the trunk is an abnormal response. (From Bleck EE: Orthopaedic Management of Cerebral Palsy, Vol 2. Philadelphia, WB Saunders, 1979.)

the child kneeling tall. Kneeling with the knees flexed 90 degrees and the hips extended eliminates the effect of a tight Achilles tendon, tight hamstrings, and to some degree tight hip flexors. If the child is unable to assume this position, the central balance is so poor that it is unlikely he or she will be able to walk. The recognition of short muscle groups around given joints will be discussed in the individual sections.

PRINCIPLES OF TREATMENT

In general, the goals of treating the CP spastic child are aimed at preventing deformity, correcting deformity, and

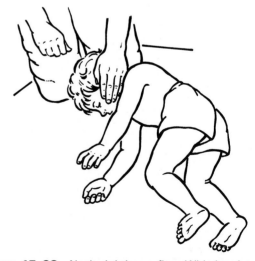

Figure 15–28. Neck righting reflex. With head turning, the entire trunk and all limbs turn to the same side. (From Bleck EE: Orthopaedic Management of Cerebral Palsy, Vol 2. Philadelphia, WB Saunders, 1979.)

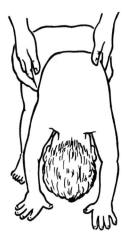

Figure 15–29. Parachute reaction. The prone child is lifted by the trunk and suddenly lowered or tipped to the tabletop. The normal response is automatic extension of the upper limbs and placement of the hands on the surface of the table. (From Bleck EE: Orthopaedic Management of Cerebral Palsy, Vol 2. Philadelphia, WB Saunders, 1979.)

improving function. It is important, when discussing plans with the parents, to help them realize that the goals are limited. Patients are improved by surgery, but they are not made normal. It is well recognized that spastics (as opposed to the extrapyramidal types) will benefit the most from

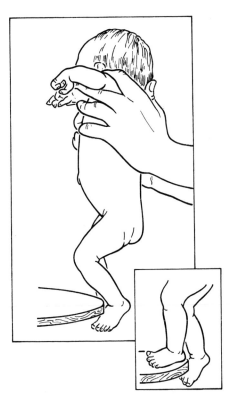

Figure 15–30. Foot placement reaction. The child is lifted by the axillae so that the dorsa of the feet come up against the underside of a tabletop or chair. Symmetric or asymmetric placement of the feet on the surface is the normal response. (From Bleck EE: Orthopaedic Management of Cerebral Palsy, Vol 2. Philadelphia, WB Saunders, 1979.)

surgical intervention. Appropriate exercise programs and night splinting are important modalities in preventing deformity early and in maintaining corrected position following surgical procedures. It is equally important that the surgical procedures be integrated into an ongoing program of exercise, education, and conservative treatment. To simply perform a procedure and inadequately follow the child will ensure failure.

It is similarly necessary to integrate the surgical procedures into the child's life experience. It is helpful to complete all procedures necessary prior to the age of 6 or 7, if possible. After that time, frequent hospitalizations and surgical procedures significantly affect the child's psychosocial development.

In general, the child should be old enough to cooperate with a postoperative regimen and should have adequate balance to ensure an upright posture. Obviously, it is helpful if the child's IQ is adequate to allow postoperative training. Certainly there are times when severely retarded children require surgical procedures for positioning and custodial care. As a general principle, fixed deformities respond best to surgical intervention. It is very difficult to anticipate the result of correcting dynamic deformities. As one can imagine, the result of surgery depends upon the patient selection and postoperative care.

THE HIP IN CEREBRAL PALSY

Despite what many may think, the "marquee" pediatric hip diseases (Perthes, slipped capital femoral epiphysis, and developmental dysplasia of the hip (DDH) do not approximate the incidence of cerebrospastic hip disease. In fact, surgery on the cerebrospastic hip accounts for the largest number of procedures performed on the pediatric hip. These children have significant hip disease initiated by muscle imbalance, the development of soft tissue contractures, subsequent bony deformity, and ultimately hip subluxation and dislocation. The contractures involve the hip flexors (psoas and rectus femoris) and the hip adductors. With progressive contracture, the axis of hip rotation is altered and secondary osseous changes develop. Femoral anteversion is present at birth, remains persistent in these children, and accentuates the rate at which hip subluxation and dislocation occur. Similarly, pelvic obliquity and fixed spinal deformity cause the femoral head on the high side of the obliquity to be uncovered, predisposing it to early subluxation (Fig. 15–31).

Adduction contracture is the most common deformity and is frequently associated with contracture of the flexors. The simplest screening test for tight adductors is to abduct the hips with the child supine and the hips extended. Normally, the composite angle of abduction should be 90 degrees, or 45 degrees for each hip. Rapid stretching (fast test) of the adductors will permit testing for dynamic contracture, whereas gentle stretching (slow test) of the muscles is more appropriate to evaluate fixed deformity.

Flexion contracture frequently coexists with that of adduction. The iliopsoas is most often affected. It typically externally rotates the proximal femur while the adductors internally rotate the shaft, thereby accentuating the femoral anteversion. The *Thomas test* (Fig. 15–32) is easily performed with the child supine. Flexing the opposite hip to lock the pelvis allows the examiner to measure a hip flexion contracture on the side to be tested. The rectus

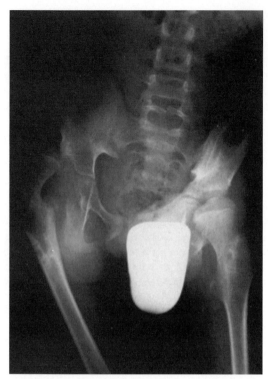

Figure 15–31. Paralytic dislocation of the left hip in severe spastic cerebral palsy is shown in this radiograph. (From Tachdjian MO: Pediatric Orthopedics, 2nd ed. Philadelphia, WB Saunders, 1990.)

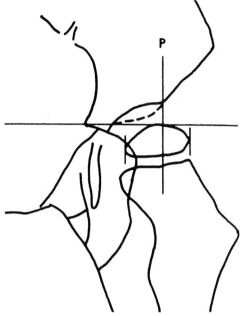

Figure 15–33. Reimer's migration index is the part of the femoral head extending beyond Perkins' line (P) expressed as a percentage of the entire width of the head measured in the horizontal plane. (From Benson MKD, Fixsen JA, MacNicol MF: Children's Orthopaedics and Fractures. Edinburgh, Churchill Livingstone, 1994.)

femoris also contributes to hip flexion contracture. It is best evaluated using the *prone rectus test* (Ely test). With the child positioned prone and the hip extended, the knee is flexed slowly and the effect of a tight rectus femoris is appreciated by observing a buttock rise.

Femoral anteversion is normally present in the neonate. Progressive correction is anticipated in the normal child. In cerebrospastic children, this normal correction does not occur. As a result, the rotational axis of the hip is altered. Radiographs of the cerebrospastic hip frequently are misinterpreted as demonstrating significant valgus, when in fact they are demonstrating anteversion. As the angle between the femoral neck and Hilgenreiner's line approaches 90 degrees, the hip becomes progressively more unstable. In general, the configuration and alignment of the child's hips

by age 4 can be assumed to be permanent. No correction is likely to occur following that age. In addition to causing hip instability, uncorrected anteversion tends to precipitate external tibial torsion.

Subluxation and dislocation of the hip is the ultimate result of fixed deformity. It is important to realize that these children are born with normal hips, and the subsequent changes are the result of neuromuscular imbalance. Therefore, the standard treatment modalities discussed for DDH are not applicable to the cerebrospastic hip. Over time, the hips become progressively more unstable with disruption of Shenton's line, loss of normal joint contours, increased acetabular index, and uncovering of the femoral head. This latter phenomenon frequently is measured using Reimer's migration index (Fig. 15–33). Dislocation of the hip has been reported in 50% of those with spastic quadriplegia and athetoid disease, and 30 to 40% of those with

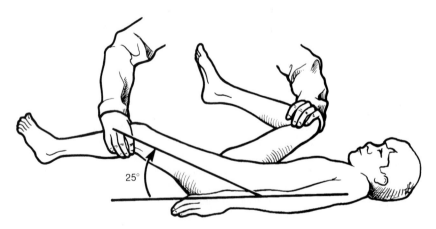

Figure 15–32. The Thomas test for hip flexion contracture. (From Bleck EE: Orthopaedic Management of Cerebral Palsy, Vol 2. Philadelphia, WB Saunders, 1979.)

spastic diplegia. It is rare for the hip to dislocate in the hemiplegic child.

A great deal of study has been directed toward the natural history of spastic hip dislocation. There seems to be general agreement that the dislocated hip has a 50% chance of becoming painful. It is this observation, and the benefits of improved peroneal care, improved gait, and improved seating position, that make the best argument for reduction of the subluxed or dislocated hip. Many authors make a strong case for keeping the femoral head in the acetabulum, regardless of the severity of cerebral palsy.

TREATMENT

Clearly, there is a role for physical therapy and prolonged splinting in an effort to minimize the rate of contracture development as well as the magnitude of the contracture. However, once it becomes apparent that the contractures are fixed and excessive, or if there is radiographic evidence of subluxation, surgical treatment is indicated. Adductor tenotomy or transfer, with or without anterior obturator neurectomy, is appropriate when the adduction deformity is excessive. Neurectomy is usually reserved for the non-ambulatory child. Similarly, release of hip flexion contractures, either intrapelvic or extrapelvic (for nonambulator), is required if the contracture exceeds 45 degrees. Once subluxation or dislocation has occurred, additional procedures may be required to relocate the femoral head and perhaps provide additional acetabular coverage. The use of varus derotation osteotomies of the hip, with or without acetabular procedures such as a Dega osteotomy, will relocate the femoral head and hopefully achieve a concentric reduction of the hip. It is important to remember that symmetric surgery is the norm rather than the exception; therefore, both hips should be surgically treated. The use of internal fixation devices when osteotomies are performed is mandatory in these spastic children. In addition, the postoperative application of a spica cast will usually be required to maintain position and also minimize postoperative pain.

The management of the older child or adult with a fixed spastic dislocation is problematic. Total hip replacement has been reportedly successful in very selected cases, but for the most part, arthroplasty is not considered appropriate. The use of resectional type arthroplasties, such as proximal femoral resection with soft tissue interposition, has reportedly been successful in some select series. It is important to remember that the hips should not be viewed as an isolated problem. Rather, surgical procedures on these hips need to be integrated into the management of knee and spine deformity. The so-called "evil triad" of hip dislocation, pelvic obliquity, and scoliosis still remains one of the unanswered problems in the management of cerebral palsy. The belief that the dislocated hip is the cause of the other two is entirely too simplistic.

DEFORMITY OF THE KNEE

Integrated care of knee deformity is critical, especially if surgery on the hip and foot and ankle is to be successful. Hamstring contracture and the subsequent development of *knee flexion deformity* are common problems in the spastic child. The contracture of the hamstrings cannot be underestimated when evaluating the child who stands and walks with a crouched gait. Hip flexion contracture, knee flexion deformity with tight hamstrings, and calcaneus deformity of the foot can operate singly or in combination to produce the crouched posture. Knee flexion deformity is the most common deformity seen about the knee. The evaluation of hamstring contracture is best done with the child supine and the hip flexed 90 degrees (Fig. 15–34). Placing the child's knee initially at 90 degrees, the examiner attempts to extend the knee against the flexed hip and the point at which the hamstrings block further extension is the measure of *popliteal angle*. Significant contracture of the hamstrings is best treated by hamstring tenotomy. Remember that a hamstring contracture is aggravated by a flexion deformity of the hip, again emphasizing the importance of not viewing joints in isolation.

Angular deformity of the knee is not terribly common in children with cerebral palsy; however, rotational deformity of the tibia is frequently seen. As is the case with femoral anteversion, internal tibial torsion tends to persist in these children. If unresolved by age 4, supramalleolar osteotomy of the tibia with coincident fibular osteotomy is an appropriate solution.

Patellofemoral pain syndrome is common in adolescents with cerebral palsy. Coexisting spasticity of the rectus femoris and hamstrings results in a stiff-legged gait, frequently with the knee flexed. These children are said to be in the jump or crouch position. If allowed to remain in this position for protracted periods, the patella will actually be high riding (patella alta). Patellofemoral pain syndrome is best managed by hamstring tenotomy to decrease the crouched posture of the child.

FOOT AND ANKLE DEFORMITIES

Foot and ankle deformities occur frequently in cerebral palsy. *Equinus deformity* of the ankle is probably the most

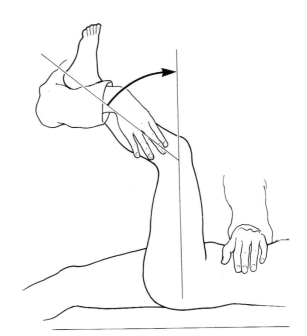

Figure 15–34. Popliteal angle. (From Benson MKD, Fixsen JA, MacNicol MF: Children's Orthopaedics and Fractures. Edinburgh, Churchill Livingstone, 1994.)

common deformity. Typically, its severity depends on the severity of the neurologic damage, the age of walking, and imbalance between the dorsiflexors and triceps surae (gastrocnemius, soleus, and plantaris) group. Most cerebrospastic children begin ambulation as toe-walkers. An ankle-foot orthosis (AFO) will generally not prevent the development of the deformity but may certainly alter its rate. In addition, the use of the AFO in the young child who is beginning to walk frequently improves the child's proprioceptive ability to achieve balance. The *Silverskiold test* (Fig. 15–35) is generally used to evaluate the degree of equinus deformity. First, the ankle is dorsiflexed with the knee flexed to negate the effect of the gastrocnemius muscle. Then the knee is extended, bringing the gastrocnemius into play, and the test is repeated. If there is a significant difference between ankle dorsiflexion in these two positions, the implication is that the contracture of the gastrocnemius is the primary offender. Should ankle dorsiflexion be essentially the same in both knee positions, the implication is that the gastrocnemius and soleus are contributing equally to the deformity.

Fixed contracture of the heel cord is best treated by lengthening of the triceps surae group. This can be accomplished either by formal heel cord lengthening or gastrocnemius recession, done in the midportion of the calf. Again,

it is important to coordinate heel cord lengthening with other procedures that may be required, such as hamstring lengthening and hip flexor releases. Postoperative bracing is essential in maintaining the corrected position achieved and in preventing recurrence of the deformity. The most important complication of heel cord lengthening procedures is overlengthening and a resultant *calcaneus deformity*. This deformity can have a severe impact on the child's ability to walk. Indeed, if the heel cords are lengthened in the face of an uncorrected hamstring contracture, the crouch position will be worsened.

Equinovarus is another typical deformity in the spastic foot. Characteristically, this is the foot position seen in hemiplegic children and is thought to be due to overactivity of the posterior tibialis muscle in the presence of weak peroneal muscles. Occasionally, however, the anterior tibialis is the offending agonist. Early equinovarus deformity is generally supple and can be managed conservatively with a brace or surgically with a transfer of the anterior tibial tendon or the posterior tibial tendon, depending on which is the major offender. Once the equinovarus deformity becomes fixed, bony procedures will be required for correction.

Planovalgus is the common foot deformity seen in diplegic and quadriplegic children. At first, there is liga-

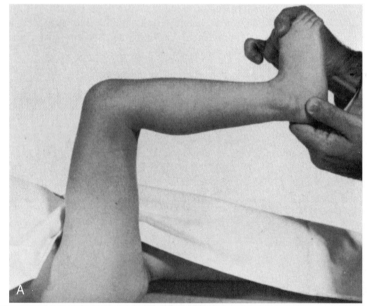
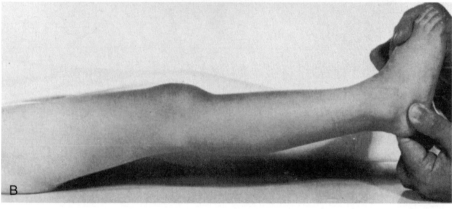

Figure 15–35. Testing spasticity and contracture of triceps surae muscle by passive dorsiflexion of the ankle. *A,* With the knee in flexion, the gastrocnemius muscle is relaxed and equinus deformity is caused by contracture of the soleus muscle. *B,* With the knee in extension, the parts played by both the gastrocnemius and soleus are tested. (From Tachdjian MO: Pediatric Orthopedics, 2nd ed. Philadelphia, WB Saunders, 1990.)

mentous laxity and a contracture of the heel cord. As the deformity progresses, the posterior tibialis stretches and becomes nonfunctional. These factors allow the foot to collapse through the arch. In long-standing deformity, a midfoot break can actually be seen. The treatment of the planovalgus foot depends on its severity. Frequently, in the young child, an Achilles tendon lengthening and subsequent AFO will suffice. The addition of a peroneus brevis lengthening may be helpful. However, most often these procedures are not adequate to stabilize the hindfoot. If that is the case, the young child is best managed by some type of subtalar stabilization procedure such as a subtalar stapling procedure or a formal subtalar arthrodesis. The once-popular Grice procedure (extra-articular fusion) is rarely used at the present time. Once the planovalgus foot has become rigid, triple arthrodesis may be the only alternative.

Spastic bunion deformity commonly complicates the planovalgus foot. It develops from two mechanisms: (1) the equinovalgus forcing the medial border of the foot against the floor and (2) the spasticity of the adductor hallucis muscle. Most authors feel that standard bunion procedures, whether they are soft tissue procedures done distally or metatarsal osteotomies, are ineffective to correct the spastic bunion. Most prefer arthrodesis of the first metatarsophalangeal (MTP) joint as a definitive procedure to correct this deformity.

DEFORMITIES OF THE UPPER LIMB

Frequently, the physician is asked to improve the child's hand function. However, treating deformities of the upper extremity is fraught with more frustration than managing the deformities of the lower. Selectivity becomes extremely important when the physician is contemplating surgical care in the upper limb. In general, surgical treatment should be confined to the hemiplegic group. All these children will walk and generally have reasonable hand function. When initially faced with requests to correct hand function, careful evaluation of the upper extremity and its functional abilities is critical prior to beginning surgical intervention. Perhaps no other deficit is more important to remember than the sensory privation, which precludes good functional results. Typically, protective sensation and touch remain, but more sophisticated stereognosis is lacking. Jacqueline Perry has reminded us that "the key to muscle action is sensory feedback." Lacking such feedback, a normal-functioning upper extremity is impossible to achieve.

Assessment of function is important prior to planning surgical intervention. Watching the child use the hand at play is an important clue to cognition. Observe the upper extremity for involuntary movements that will complicate any anticipated correction. Similarly, test the child's *control* by asking him or her to throw a ball or similar small object. Evaluation of *placement* can be accomplished by the simple test of asking the child to first touch the head and then touch the knee. He or she should be able to accomplish this task of hand to knee to head and back in under 10 seconds. If unable to so, the child's placement is so poor that any functional improvement is unlikely. Finally, evaluate the hand for *grasp and release*. Despite early reports, grasp is rarely the problem. The major motor problem of the hand is the inability to relax the flexors and

release objects once they are grasped. Sensation can be evaluated using two-point discrimination, object identification, graphesthesia testing, and texture appreciation.

The goals in treating the upper extremity are to improve its function as a helping hand, perhaps as an object stabilizer; to improve its gross function in grasping, pinching, and releasing; and to improve its appearance. Surgical approaches are available to correct the thumb-in-palm deformity, the instability of the first metacarpophalangeal joint, and the instability of the carpometacarpal joint of the thumb. Wrist flexion deformity has been managed by tendon transfers, tenodesis, and wrist fusion. Controversy exists as to the best approach to this problem. Deformities of the fingers are similarly treated either by contracture releases, tendon transfers, or joint stabilization procedures. Finally, in the severely involved patient, who is cognizant enough to be self-conscious about the appearance of his hand, appropriately selected tenotomies can improve its overall appearance. The physician must be very careful in the selection of patients for upper extremity surgery and warn parents and patients of the expected limited results. The use of molded splints is speculative at best. Children, left to their own devices, will rarely use them. This suggests that in the child's view they are not helpful. Some therapists believe they are important in delaying the onset of contracture; however, many see little benefit from their use.

Adjunctive techniques are available primarily for the management of spasticity. *Dorsal column rhizotomy* has been reported to produce mixed results. The principle of this neurosurgical procedure is to interrupt the reflex arcs by cutting the dorsal roots. By disrupting the reflex arc, there is a theoretic decrease in peripheral end-organ spasticity. With careful patient selection and careful neurosurgical technique, some of the results with this procedure have been impressive. In general, the optimal patient is a severely spastic, mentally high-functioning diplegic child who has excellent potential for ambulation.

The *oral muscle relaxants* such as dantrolene (Dantrium), diazepam (Valium), and baclofen have been used with varying results. At present, there is increasing enthusiasm for the use of the *baclofen pump*. This device is inserted into a pocket created in the anterior abdominal wall, much like that for a pacemaker. The reservoir is refilled regularly with the drug, which is, in turn, slowly released into the spinal canal. Initial results have been encouraging. Many children show a significant decrease in spasticity.

The use of *botulinum toxin* (Botox), phenol, or alcohol to block the motor end plate has enjoyed a somewhat checkered history. These substances have all been shown to produce a reversible neuromuscular blockade for a variable period of time. At present, there appears to be a role for Botox injections to decrease dynamic spasticity and contractures in isolated muscle groups. Once fixed contractures develop, one cannot expect improvement with the use of these injectable agents.

SUMMARY

The management of the cerebrospastic child is complex and is best accomplished as a team effort. The orthopaedic surgeon who operates in a vacuum is not serving the child's best interests. Developmental pediatricians, neurologists, physical therapists, and orthotists all must participate in the overall decision-making process. With time, patience, and appropriately planned operative procedures, these children can clearly be improved functionally.

Myelodysplasia (Spina Bifida)

Neural tube defects were recognized as early as the 1700s. However, their etiology still remains relatively obscure. Von Recklinghausen suggested that spina bifida resulted from a true failure of the neural tube to close. However, Morgagni in 1769 preferred the theory that the neural tube closed and then secondarily ruptured in utero. Certainly at the present time most authors favor the former theory of neural tube defects. Tragically, the neural tube failure occurs during the fourth week of fetal life. The mother is usually not even aware of her pregnancy at that time. Typically, myelodysplasia involves the lower portion of the spine. However, many cases are complicated by additional damage elsewhere in the neural axis. Such defects as hydrocephalus, hydromyelia, and Arnold-Chiari malformation are reported in these children. As indicated earlier, this neuromuscular disease is primarily an abnormality of the spinal cord, although different types of spina bifida are seen (Fig. 15–36). Although the lower extremity involvement is generally flaccid nature, it is not unusual for these children to develop some spasticity in the lower extremities later in life.

At the present time in the United States, it is estimated that the incidence of spina bifida is 1 per 1000 live births. In Britain and Ireland, the incidence is twice as great but is decreasing. Both genetic and environmental factors have been implicated in this syndrome. Most recently, the etio-

logic role of maternal folic acid deficiency has received a great deal of attention. The prenatal diagnosis of spina bifida is now relatively straightforward. The identification of alpha-fetoprotein in the maternal blood (sampled at 15 to 16 weeks) will frequently trigger an amniocentesis. This study is quite definitive for the diagnosis of open neural tube defects. Ultrasound has also been shown to be reasonably sensitive in the diagnosis of some open neural tube defects. The current widespread use of prenatal diagnostic studies and optional termination have made the previous discussion of selection criteria for closure moot. At the present time, all children born with spina bifida undergo closure shortly after birth. About 80% of these children will survive their first year, and approximately 60% will survive to reach adulthood.

INITIAL ASSESSMENT

Following neurosurgical closure of the defect, an attempt is frequently made to identify the neurologic level. This is often very difficult in the newborn because spontaneous leg motion can be reflex rather than voluntary. Frequently, it is difficult to be absolutely certain of the neurologic level until the child is a bit older. The classification as to the level of the lesion is, however, important. Probably no other feature will assist the physician in anticipating prognosis, complications, and planning for the orthopaedic management than the neurologic level. Ultimately, approximately one third of these children will be wheelchair-bound, approximately one third will ambulate with minimal gait disturbance, and the remaining third will ambulate intermittently with the use of braces and external ambulatory aids. Ambulatory effort is frequently identified in one of four categories. Community ambulators are those children who walk regularly in their community. Household

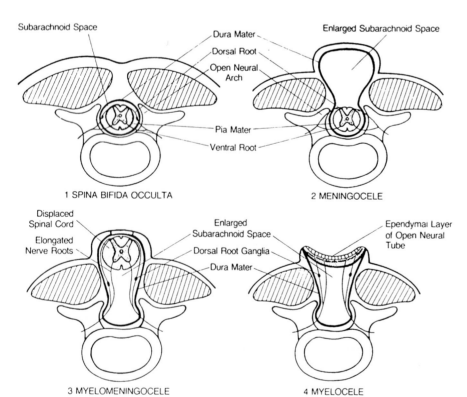

Figure 15–36. Types of spina bifida (based on Patten, 1952). (From Broughton NS: A Textbook of Paediatric Orthopaedics. London, WB Saunders, 1997.)

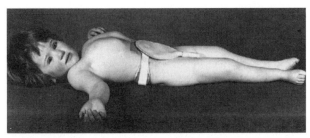

Figure 15–37. Paralysis below the twelfth thoracic roots. This child is aged 6 years and the legs lie, as they did at birth, in a position dictated by the effect of gravity. (From Broughton NS: A Textbook of Paediatric Orthopaedics. London, WB Saunders, 1997.)

ambulators use a wheelchair in the community and at school but are able to ambulate at home or for short distances. Physical therapy ambulators are those children who are able to be upright only with the assistance of the physical therapist in addition to their ambulatory aids. Last are the nonambulators. Frequently, as children get older and heavier, their ambulatory category decreases.

Identification of neurologic level then becomes important in all aspects of patient management. John Sharrard, a British orthopaedic surgeon, developed many of the surgical approaches for these children. His classification of neurologic level is used at the present time. Sharrard class I (Fig. 15–37) is a thoracic level spina bifida with virtually no lower extremity function. Sharrard class II (Fig. 15–38) includes motor levels L1 and L2 and is best identified by a functioning iliopsoas muscle. Sharrard class III (Fig. 15–39) identifies motor levels L3 and L4 and is characterized by the presence of an active quadriceps muscle. Sharrard class IV (Fig. 15–40) identifies motor level L5 and is indicated by posterior tibial and medial hamstring activity.

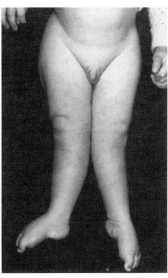

Figure 15–39. Paralysis below the third lumbar roots. The hips lie in flexion and adduction and the knees in extension or hyperextension. There is no muscle power in the feet. (From Broughton NS: A Textbook of Paediatric Orthopaedics. London, WB Saunders, 1997.)

Sharrard class V indicates motor level S1 and is identified by active gastrocnemius function. Finally, Sharrard class VI identifies motor levels S2 and S3, which extend function to the foot intrinsics. In general, Sharrard class I and II patients ultimately resort to wheelchair use. Those in Sharrard class III will usually be household ambulators as children and adolescents, with 50% entering a wheelchair as adults. Sharrard class IV typically are community ambulators in their youth, with 50% becoming household ambulators as adults, and Sharrard class V and VI patients remain as community ambulators.

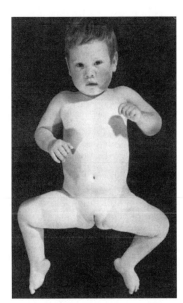

Figure 15–38. Paralysis below the first lumbar roots. Flexion and external rotation of the hips lead to an abducted posture, and a fixed abduction contracture may result. (From Broughton NS: A Textbook of Paediatric Orthopaedics. London, WB Saunders, 1997.)

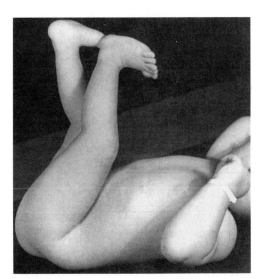

Figure 15–40. Paralysis below the fifth lumbar roots. There is flexion at the hip, some flexion of the knee, and a calcaneus posture of the feet. (From Broughton NS: A Textbook of Paediatric Orthopaedics. London, WB Saunders, 1997.)

TYPES OF DEFORMITIES

Foot deformities are present in three quarters of these patients. They can include severe rigid clubfoot (Fig. 15–41), vertical talus deformity, and calcaneal valgus. The goal of any treatment is to achieve a plantigrade foot which, if nothing else, is braceable. It is absolutely critical to remember that the foot is, for all intents and purposes, anesthetic. This will markedly limit its overall function. Frequently, one is placed in the unfortunate position of dealing with a rigid deformed foot and having to accept, as the end result of treatment, a rigid plantigrade foot. The management of this type of clubfoot is very different than that recommended for a congenital clubfoot. Although early manipulation and casting may stretch the soft tissues, most authors prefer not to cast these children for fear of skin breakdown. Rather, early soft tissue release or talectomy, after 1 year of age, have both been recommended.

Deformities of the knee are likewise varied. Extension contracture, flexion contracture, and valgus deformity (due to iliotibial band contracture) have all been reported. The fixed flexion contracture of the knee is a severe impediment to sitting and walking. As with the clubfoot, manipulation and casting are dangerous, not only because of the skin problems but also due to secondary adaptive changes that will occur in the condyles. It is generally better to release the contracture or, if necessary, perform a distal femoral osteotomy. Obviously, the best treatment would be to prevent the contracture from occurring in the first place. An Ober-Yount release of the iliotibial band will tend to minimize progressive valgus deformity.

Deformities of the hip joint create some of the most complex issues in the management of the myelodysplastic patient. As seen in cerebral palsy, subluxation and dislocation can ultimately result from pelvic obliquity and muscle imbalance. Intrauterine position and habitual postnatal postures complicate the deformities. The pelvic obliquity itself may result from superincumbent spinal anomalies and spinal deformities. Thoracic level patients rarely dislocate their hips because they lack any muscle activity about the hip. The joint therefore is spared deforming forces. Hip flexion contractures will make it extremely difficult for the child to stand upright, whether in a parapodium or in long leg braces. Therefore, early surgical management of hip flexion contractures is recommended. Surgical procedures designed to relocate a subluxed or dislocated hip in a spina bifida patient are similar to those recommended for cerebral palsy. However, unlike the CP child, muscle balancing procedures must be added. In addition, postoperative stiffness is a significant complication. Therefore, careful selection, as well as carefully planned and executed surgery, is required, lest the child be made worse. In addition, the natural history of hip dislocation is different than that seen in cerebral palsy. These hips, left dislocated, do not become painful. However, children with deformities at the L3 level and below tend to lose an ambulatory level if the dislocated hip is not relocated. Therefore, the current recommendation is to relocate hips in children at or below the L3 level. In general, above the L3 level, should both hips be dislocated, most authors would recommend no surgical treatment. The most problematic situation is seen when one hip is located and the other is dislocated in the child above the L3 level. This imbalance only aggravates pelvic obliquity, increases spinal deformity, and alters sitting balance. It is appropriate to wait a reasonable period of time in hopes that the located hip will dislocate. Should this not happen, then the dislocated hip requires reduction.

Two bony complications are noteworthy. Pathologic fractures are not uncommon in these children because of their osteoporotic bone. Usually, these fractures are low velocity in nature and can be managed conservatively with lightweight immobilizing devices. Charcot's arthropathy may be seen in adults. Ambulation on the insensate extremities may initiate neuropathic changes much like those seen in the diabetic. This is especially true for the knee, which is frequently subjected to unprotected varus and valgus stresses. Even the consistent use of an orthosis does not preclude this complication. The cause of death in these patients is usually chronic renal failure or sepsis that follows severe skin ulceration.

Muscular Dystrophies

Most of the muscular dystrophies are hereditary (Table 15–3). Therefore, a careful family history is important when evaluating these children. Frequently, the familial nature of the disease is well known before the child is even referred. When examining children with muscular dystrophies, it is always appropriate to look for such things as abnormal movement, posturing, aberrations of gait, strength, the ability to get up from the floor (Gowers' sign), the facies of the child, and the distribution of weakness. Clearly, a neurologic examination is appropriate in these children. The creatine phosphokinase (CPK) is the most sensitive laboratory test for striated muscle, and the measured levels parallel the rate and amount of muscle necrosis. Electromyography (EMG) and nerve conduction study can be used to differentiate myopathic disease from neuropathic disease; however, this will rarely establish a specific

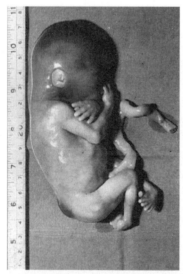

Figure 15–41. A 16-week fetus with a lumbosacral myelomeningocele and rigid equinovarus deformity of both feet at this early stage of development (photograph kindly provided by Dr. Gordon Stark of Edinburgh). (From Broughton NS: A Textbook of Paediatric Orthopaedics. London, WB Saunders, 1997.)

Table 15–3. Etiology and inheritance of neuromuscular disorders

Diagnosis	Inheritance	CPK	Electromyographic Finding	Nerve Conduction	Muscle Biopsy	Orthopaedic Deformity
I. Anterior horn cell						
Spinal muscular atrophy	Autosomal recessive, rarely dominant	Normal to slight elevation	Neuropathic	Normal	Neuropathic	Scoliosis Hip dislocation Flexion contractures
A. Werdnig-Hoffman						
B. Chronic infantile						
C. Kugelberg-Welander						
II. Nerve fiber						
Charcot-Marie-Tooth (HMSN)						
Type I	Autosomal dominant (usually)	Normal	Neuropathic	Decreased	Neuropathic	Cavovarus feet Scoliosis Hip dysplasia
Type II	Autosomal dominant			Can be normal		
Type III	Autosomal recessive			Decreased		
Type IV	Autosomal recessive			Normal		
Type V	Autosomal dominant			Can be normal		
III. Muscle						
A. Dystrophies						
Duchenne's	Sex-linked	Very elevated	Myopathic	Normal	Myopathic	Equinovarus feet Scoliosis Contractures Heart*; intellectual*
Becker's	Sex-linked	Very elevated	Myopathic	Normal	Myopathic	None
Facioscapulohumeral	Autosomal recessive	Normal to slightly high	Myopathic	Normal	Myopathic	Winged scapulae
Limb-girdle	Autosomal recessive	Elevated	Myopathic	Normal	Myopathic	Late contractures
B. Myopathies						
Central core	Autosomal dominant	Normal	Myopathic	Normal	Characteristic	Hip dislocations Scoliosis Pes valgus
Nemaline	Autosomal dominant	Normal	Myopathic	Normal	Characteristic	Scoliosis
Myotubular	Autosomal dominant or recessive, or sex-linked	Normal	Myopathic	Normal	Characteristic	Scoliosis
Fiber type	Autosomal dominant	Normal	Myopathic	Normal	Characteristic	Foot
Minicore	Autosomal dominant	Normal	Myopathic	Normal	Characteristic	Scoliosis
Mitochondrial	Unknown; maybe familial	Normal	Myopathic	Normal	Characteristic	Rare None reported Risk*: heart block
C. Myotonia						
Myotonia congenita	Autosomal dominant and recessive	Normal	Typical	Normal	Muscle hypertrophy	None
Myotonic muscular dystrophy (myotonia atrophica)	Autosomal dominant	Normal	Typical	Normal	Muscle atrophy; motor end-plate changes Cataracts* Cardiac conduction defects*	None
Congenital myotonic	Autosomal dominant	Normal	Typical	Normal	Atrophy type I fibers	None
D. Polymyositis/dermatomyositis	No inheritance	Increased or normal	Myopathic	Normal	Characteristic	None
E. Myasthenia gravis	Variable	Normal	Repetitive nerve stimulus response	Normal	—	None

*Other significant organ involvement.
From Benson MKD, Fixsen JA, MacNicol MF: Children's Orthopaedics and Fractures. Edinburgh, Churchill Livingstone, 1994.

diagnosis. Muscle biopsy is the gold standard for establishing the diagnosis. Although the quadriceps is the most frequently sampled muscle, it is probably best to biopsy the muscle most severely involved. The biopsy can show both myopathic and neuropathic changes. Further electron microscopic studies may allow differentiation between certain dystrophic states. The progressive muscular dystrophies are all noninflammatory, inherited disorders of muscle. They are subdivided based on clinical distribution, the severity of muscle weakness, and the pattern of genetic inheritance.

DUCHENNE'S DYSTROPHY

Duchenne's dystrophy is the most common and most classic of the progressive muscular dystrophies. A sex-linked recessive trait, it is currently under active investigation in the field of molecular genetics. The finding of a single gene defect on the short arm of the X chromosome has been a landmark in diagnosis. The single gene, which is defective, normally codes for dystrophin. This substance is absent in the muscle cells of Duchenne patients. At present it is thought that dystrophin is associated with the triadic junction in skeletal muscle and is important in the calcium-regulated depolarization of these cells.

Characteristically, Duchenne patients are noted to have initiation of their disease between 2 and 7 years of age. Frequently, the child is referred for the evaluation of clumsiness. The classic Gower sign (Fig. 15–42) is usually seen at the time of presentation. The child finds it extremely difficult to arise from the floor and does so by climbing up his or her legs. This is due to weakness of quadriceps and hip extensors. Delayed motor milestones, clumsiness, and the inability to climb stairs are all early findings in this disease. The extent of cardiac involvement is variable and, if severe, may be the ultimate cause of demise.

Management efforts are directed to assist children in maintaining their center of gravity. Therefore, as their hip flexion deformities worsen and lordosis increases, bracing may become more important. Heel cord contractures fre-

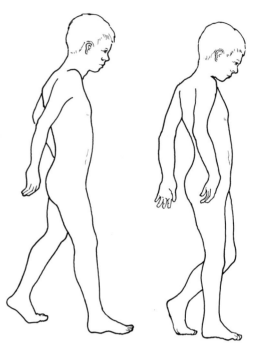

Figure 15–43. Typical gait of a child who has muscular dystrophy. (From Benson MKD, Fixsen JA, MacNicol MF: Children's Orthopaedics and Fractures. Edinburgh, Churchill Livingstone, 1994.)

quently cause knee flexion and truncal hyperextension deformities (Fig. 15–43). In an effort to maintain independent ambulation as long as possible, the clinician may find it necessary to release contractures, particularly at the knee and the heel cord. Once released, bracing will be required. Even with surgical efforts, most children cease independent ambulation by about 11 years of age. Although scoliosis is a frequent problem in the Duchenne child, surgery to correct it should be forestalled as long as possible; once corrected and instrumented, these children will lose the ability to ambulate. Most Duchenne children survive into their early teen years before ultimately succumbing to respiratory failure.

LIMB GIRDLE DYSTROPHY

Autosomal recessive muscular dystrophy is frequently referred to as limb girdle dystrophy. This type is more benign and less common than Duchenne's dystrophy and has a variable age of onset. Typically, the weakness involves the pelvic or shoulder girdle and the progression of this disease is quite slow. However, these patients do not have a normal life expectancy, and death is expected by their mid-40s.

FACIOSCAPULOHUMERAL DYSTROPHY

This type is inherited as an autosomal dominant trait. It has a highly variable age of onset and severity. As the name implies, weakness involves the shoulder girdle and facies. Life expectancy approaches normal levels.

MYOTONIA

A number of myotonic disorders have been identified and are characterized by the inability of skeletal muscle to relax. Most myotonic disorders are autosomal dominant in

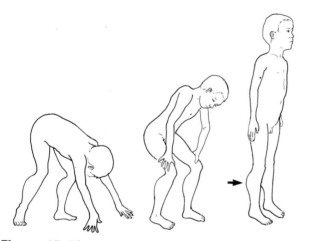

Figure 15–42. Gower's sign: the child arises from the floor by "walking up" the thighs with his hands—a functional test for quadriceps muscle weakness. Note the bulky calf *(arrow)*. (From Benson MKD, Fixsen JA, MacNicol MF: Children's Orthopaedics and Fractures. Edinburgh, Churchill Livingstone, 1994.)

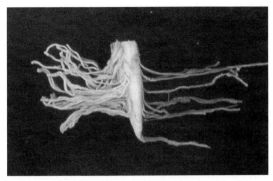

Figure 15–44. Spinal muscular atrophy: section of the spinal cord demonstrating atrophy of the ventral roots resulting from degeneration of the anterior horn cell. In contrast, the dorsal roots are normal. (From Broughton NS: A Textbook of Paediatric Orthopaedics. London, WB Saunders, 1997.)

transmission. Myotonia congenita and myotonia dystrophica are two examples of this group.

CONGENITAL MYOPATHIES

Recently, several congenital myopathies have been characterized. The use of the electron microscope in evaluating the myopathic lesions has permitted diagnosis. The identification of specific and unique intracellular structures has provided the basis for differentiation within the group, including central core disease, nemaline dystrophy, and myotubular myopathy.

Spinal Muscle Atrophy

Spinal muscle atrophy (SMA) is an autosomal recessive disorder with an incidence of 1 in 20,000 live births. Like poliomyelitis, there is destruction of anterior horn cells of the spinal cord with the resulting end-organ changes (Fig. 15–44). Unlike poliomyelitis, however, SMA is associated with systemic involvement. As one would anticipate, the end-organ reflects the pathology: therefore, hypotonia, areflexia, and muscle weakness are characteristic of these syndromes. Sensation, as is the case in poliomyelitis, remains intact.

Historically, eponyms were used to define the subtypes within this group. However, at the present time, three types are identified based on the severity of clinical findings. Type I SMA (acute Werdnig-Hoffmann disease) has its onset at birth and is usually fatal within the first year of life. Type II disease has its onset between 6 months and 2 years of age and has a rather severe course. This type is frequently referred to as chronic Werdnig-Hoffmann disease. Finally, the most benign form, type III, onsets in children older than 2 years of age. The type III disease is frequently referred to as Kugelberg-Welander disease.

The orthopaedic problems encountered by these children are similar to those seen in other neuromuscular diseases. Typically, the hips tend to sublux and dislocate, especially in the type II patients. These are best managed by maintaining the hips in the reduced position. Scoliosis is perhaps the most common orthopaedic problem requiring treatment. Both type II and type III patients have a demonstrated

incidence of 100%, and most of these curves are significant. The scoliosis can be so severe that it actually precludes normal ambulation. Aggressive surgical treatment of the spine in these children will usually keep them ambulatory for a protracted period. In addition, appropriate curve care assists in maintaining appropriate sitting balance.

Arthrogryposis

At the present time, this syndrome is frequently referred to as multiple congenital contractures. In point of fact, arthrogryposis multiplex congenita is not a single disease but rather the final end point for a number of conditions that are associated with intrauterine paralysis. The syndrome is characterized by its congenital nature and the finding of multiple, persistent joint contractures (Fig. 15–45). Both muscle and soft tissue contractures are present at birth. Notably, sensation is normal. There appears to be no specific sex predilection, and there are approximately 500 new cases per year reported in the United States. When the mother is questioned, there is frequently a history of decreased fetal movement and associated oligo- or polyhydramnios.

Opinions vary widely as to whether the syndrome is

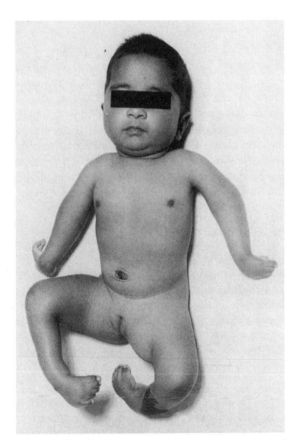

Figure 15–45. Typical appearance of a child with arthrogryposis in all four limbs. Note adduction and internal rotation at the shoulders, extension at the elbows and flexion of the wrist, severe fixed flexion of the knees, and equinovarus deformity of the feet. (From Benson MKD, Fixsen JA, MacNicol MF: Children's Orthopaedics and Fractures. Edinburgh, Churchill Livingstone, 1994.)

primarily neuropathic or myopathic. Most believe that the lesions seen in the muscle are characteristic of neurogenically induced muscle atrophy. Similar changes have been reported in children with myelodysplasia. In general, the concept of genetic transmission has been rejected. At birth, these children present with curved, featureless extremities. The absence of normal skin creases accentuates the spindle shape of the extremities. Joint rigidity is characteristic. The skin tends to be smooth and stretched, with normal sensation. Typically, all four extremities are involved, and the spine is usually spared. One pathognomonic finding is reported to be the thumb-in-palm deformity noted in these children. In addition, the rigid clubfeet in these children have been referred to by some as "resistant" clubfeet to emphasize their nonresponsiveness to standard treatment protocols.

Treatment goals are simply to maintain mobility in the upper extremities and to maintain alignment in the lower extremities for ambulation. Early manipulation and stretching with serial bracing and casting have shown some promise. Ultimately, surgical intervention is required. Because multiple joints are typically affected, the timing of surgical procedures can be tricky. Usually, most authors begin at the hip and work distally, although others choose to approach these deformities in exactly the reverse order.

The hip deformities are similar to those seen in cerebral palsy, with flexion and adduction preceding subluxation and dislocation. Typically, the hip is rigid, whether dislocated or located. For this reason, many believe it is useless to attempt reduction, because no significant motion has been reportedly achieved. In addition, surgical assault may cause avascular necrosis and, ultimately, a painful hip. The knees frequently are contracted, either in hyperextension or flexion. The hyperextended configuration is the more common and is associated with a severe quadriceps contracture. Following a short period of serial casting, quadricepsplasty is the recommended procedure.

The severe talipes equinovarus (clubfoot) is similar to that seen in myelodysplasia. It is a rigid, immobile, deformed foot. The best one can expect from surgery is to convert it to a rigid, plantigrade foot. These "resistant" clubfeet are best managed by early comprehensive releases. Prolonged postoperative immobilization is frequently required to prevent recurrence of deformity.

Upper extremity surgery should be considered only for specific functional goals. Should both elbows be fixed in extension, a posterior capsulotomy will allow one elbow to be placed in flexion. It is generally best to achieve a flexed elbow on one side and an extended one on the other.

Prognostically, about 15% of these children die in the neonatal intensive care unit. Of the remainder, 40% will walk without external aids, another 15% will walk with those aids, and the remainder will be bedridden or wheelchair-bound. The fact that these children have a normal intellect only complicates their already difficult life.

Hereditary Motor Sensory Neuropathy

This term describes a large heterogeneous group of inherited neuropathies. Type I disease is an autosomal dominant condition frequently called *Charcot-Marie-Tooth disease* (hypertrophic form). Type II disease is Charcot-Marie-Tooth disease of the neuronal type. Additional hereditary motor sensory neuropathies have been described but they are primarily adult diseases without orthopaedic implications; thus, they are not included in this chapter.

Charcot-Marie-Tooth (CMT) disease is important in the history of foot deformities. The cavovarus foot is characteristic of this syndrome. The hallmark of the disease is muscle weakness, which is primarily seen in the hands and the feet (peroneal muscles) and associated with areflexia and decreased sensation, especially to light touch. Biopsy of the involved muscle will typically show a neuropathic pattern. It has recently been shown that type I CMT disease results from a DNA duplication of a portion of the short arm of chromosome 17 at loci p11.2 to p12.

These children are frequently seen by the orthopaedist due to gait disturbance and foot deformity (Fig. 15–46). Frequently, the family history is well known at the time of presentation. Although occasional hip and spine deformity has been reported, the greatest focus of the literature has been on the management of the cavus foot. Many diseases can produce a pathologically high arched foot and include spinal cord tumors, Friedreich's ataxia, diastematomyelia, and syringomyelia, to name a few. It is most important to recognize that the cavus foot is never normal. Most of the CMT children will have weakness in their peroneal muscle group. This favors inversion of the foot. Subsequently, there is the development of forefoot adduction and hindfoot varus. The surgical management of these feet presents a challenge. The specific procedures are determined based on the degree of deformity and the flexibility of the foot. Early soft tissue releases and tendon transfers may be adequate to control and delay the cavus deformity. Later, however, bony procedures, whether they be calcaneal and first metatarsal osteotomies or triple arthrodeses, are indicated to maintain a plantigrade foot. Late in the disease, the upper extremity weakness is seen, usually involving the ulnar-innervated intrinsics of the hand. The prognosis for a normal life expectancy is excellent.

CONGENITAL AND HEREDITARY SYNDROMES

A number of orthopaedic abnormalities are the result of congenital limb defects or genetic disease. Obviously, congenital defects may or may not be genetic in nature, and conversely, genetic syndromes may or may not be congenital in nature. In this section an example of each type will be discussed, specifically the prototype chromosomal abnormality that produces musculoskeletal disease in Down's syndrome. Many other chromosomal aberrations are associated with musculoskeletal manifestations, and many of those are very similar to the ones seen in Down's syndrome. Congenital limb deficiency syndromes, on the other hand, are congenital but not hereditary. Proximal femoral focal deficiency and the hypoplastic syndromes of the leg will be presented as examples of this group.

Down's Syndrome

Described in 1866 by Langdon Down, this syndrome has become the prototype for all diseases resulting from a

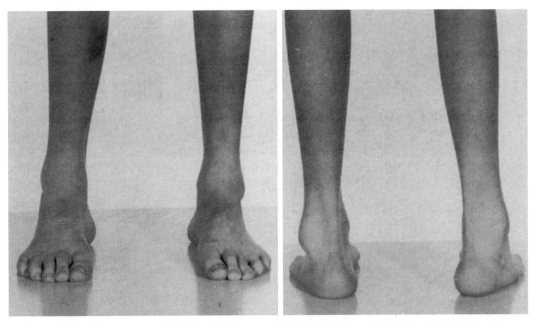

Figure 15–46. Charcot-Marie-Tooth disease. Moderate varus and slight equinus deformities of both feet result from atrophy of peroneal, anterior tibial, and toe extensor muscles. (From Tachdjian MO: Pediatric Orthopedics, 2nd ed. Philadelphia, WB Saunders, 1990.)

chromosomal abnormality. The triplication of genetic material (trisomy 21) was identified be Le Jeune in 1959. A very small percentage (3%) of these children actually has a translocation of genetic material with a normal number of chromosomes. The male-female incidence is equal and the overall incidence is approximately 1.5 children per 1000 live births. The major associated finding is increased maternal age.

The general clinical manifestations seen in these children vary somewhat. Specifically, intelligence levels vary widely. Most children are functioning at a low-normal level and are able to participate in self-care skills, to perform activities of daily living, and to work as adults, usually in sheltered environments. The child's life expectancy is also somewhat variable, depending on associated defects, especially those involving the cardiorespiratory system.

The orthopaedic manifestations of the syndrome are best understood if one appreciates the common thread of the pathology: ligamentous laxity. The orthopaedic abnormalities seen in these children reflect this fact. Patellar subluxation, pes planovalgus, C1–C2 subluxation, scoliosis, and hip subluxation have all been reported in increased incidence in these children. These phenomena are related to a relative alteration in the ratio of collagen fibers to elastic fibers in the ligaments.

The foot abnormalities are typical. Due to severe ligamentous laxity, one sees *severe pes planovalgus*. These flatfeet typically demonstrate prominent heel eversion with depression of the talar head and loss of the longitudinal arch. The foot itself is quite supple, and the findings are similar to those seen in congenital hypermobile flatfeet. Many children also have a prominent metatarsus primus varus and coincident bunion deformity. The feet are best managed conservatively in the young child, using inserts to control the arch. In the older child, if more rigorous control is required, subtalar arthrodesis is an acceptable

option. The bunions usually respond favorably to metatarsal osteotomy and soft tissue realignment procedures.

The problem of patellar instability and subluxation is a direct result of ligamentous laxity. Because the retinaculum is believed to be a major restraint keeping the patella in the intercondylar groove, retinacular insufficiency allows subluxation. In addition, many of these children have modest valgus deformity at the knee, which may also play a role in the patellar instability. Because the patella tends to sublux, these children walk with a stiff-kneed gait. They recognize that, if they do not bend their knee, the patella will not sublux. Unfortunately, nonsurgical management is invariably not helpful to control this problem. Frequently, this leads the physician to select an operative approach. Problems such as hypoplastic intercondylar grooves, fixed dislocations, hypoplastic patellae, angular deformity, and ever-present ligamentous laxity make surgical treatment problematic as well. Soft tissue balancing procedures have been used with resultant redislocation. Bony procedures may show a bit more promise; nevertheless, the redislocation rate remains very high.

Spinal deformity is seen in approximately 50% of institutionalized Down's syndrome patients. Typically, they have a significant scoliosis in the thoracolumbar region. Usually, the scoliotic curves are quite supple and do not require treatment. The spinal pathology of greater significance is C1–C2 subluxation (Fig. 15–47). As seen in juvenile rheumatoid disease and spondyloepiphyseal dysplasia, these children likewise sublux C1 on C2 as a result of the ligamentous laxity. However, unlike the child with juvenile rheumatoid arthritis who stretches the ligament over time, these children have deficient ligaments at the onset. This phenomenon is seen in approximately 25% of Down's children, despite the fact that few, if any, of these children are symptomatic. Routine screening of Down's syndrome children with a lateral flexion/extension view of the cervi-

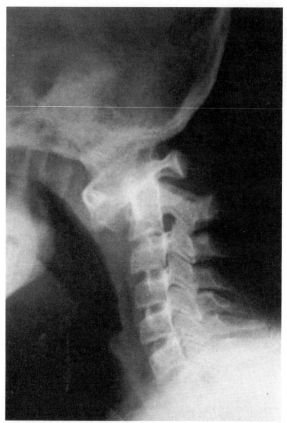

Figure 15–47. Eleven-year-old child with Down's syndrome and gross atlantoaxial instability. The gait was clumsy, and physical examination revealed poor coordination of the extremities. There was no other evidence of motor or sensory impairment or of pathologic reflexes. The patient has no symptoms referable to the cervical spine 2 years after surgical stabilization. (From Benson MKD, Fixsen JA, MacNicol MF: Children's Orthopaedics and Fractures. Edinburgh, Churchill Livingstone, 1994.)

cal spine is recommended. There is still some debate as to appropriate guidelines for activity modification and fusion. Most would agree that under 6 mm of anterior displacement in an asymptomatic child warrants restriction from only very active types of sports. Over 7 mm of ADI (atlantodens interval) on flexion frequently is associated with neurologic deficits; therefore, fusion is frequently required. Early surgical fusion is recommended before the neurologic deficit can progress. Usually, it is necessary to extend the fusion from the occiput to C2, because the arch of C1 is frequently hypoplastic. As one would expect in these children, the incidence of pseudarthrosis after fusion is high.

Hip subluxation and dislocation is also a major problem, occurring in 10% of children. Because many of these patients are living longer, osteoarthritis of the hip is more often seen. The severely involved institutionalized patients are best left untreated should their hips dislocate, because the vast majority do not have pain. Acetabular augmentation procedures with or without capsular procedures are fraught with high complication rates, especially redislocation. Currently, there is increasing enthusiasm for the use of total hip arthroplasty in a highly selected group of ambulatory patients with symptomatic hips. These patients

are at greater risk for implant dislocation and loosening, as well as an increase in the infection rate due to T-cell dysfunction.

Despite the relatively high incidence of complications and recurrence, these children still tend to benefit from many of these surgical procedures, and most can expect functional improvement; therefore, surgical intervention is often appropriate. Many other chromosomal syndromes reflect in part the manifestations classic in Down's syndrome. Because many of the other syndromes are quite rare, it is reasonable to apply some of the principles learned from the management of these children when caring for children with other unique syndromes.

Limb Deficiency Syndromes

Children born with dysplastic bones in the lower extremities present a significant challenge in management (Fig. 15–48). Often, when a child is born with one of these unusual and striking deformities, the guilt-stricken parents want to know the cause. At the present time, few if any hereditary or genetic markers have been identified in relation to these syndromes. Most are considered to be the result of "lightning striking." Other than the use of thalidomide by the pregnant mother in the 1950s and early 1960s, no toxins or drugs have been closely associated with the origin of these defects. It is best to recognize these defects as isolated findings and to make an effort to alleviate the guilt of the parents.

The femur, the fibula, and the tibia have all been reported to be affected by hypoplastic conditions. In the case of the femur, three variations have been identified: proximal femoral focal deficiency, congenital short femur, and hypoplastic femur. Fibular hypoplasia or hemimelia is the most common of the deficiency states in the lower extremity, whereas tibial deficiency syndromes are the rarest.

Proximal femoral focal deficiency (PFFD) is classified using the Aitken grouping (Fig. 15–49). All these children have shortening of the femur, a variable degree of hip dysplasia, hypoplasia of the patella, and a knee flexion contracture. In general, the management of PFFD by lengthening procedures has been less than gratifying. Complications frequently make the use of circular fixators problematic at best. Many authors believe that lengthening protocols are contraindicated in the more severe types of PFFD. Most still favor early knee fusion and amputation surgery in order to fit the child prosthetically, thereby minimizing the number of operative procedures and restoring the child to an active life as quickly as possible.

Fibular hemimelia, as mentioned, is the most common of the lower extremity limb deficiency syndromes. In the absence of the fibula, the foot tends to displace laterally, relative to the tibia, resulting in variable degrees of ankle and hindfoot valgus (Fig. 15–50). The extent of the foot abnormality will parallel the degree of hypoplasia of the fibula. Occasionally, the lateral rays of the foot may be absent. Some tibial bowing and ankle equinus are not unusual. In patients with fibular hemimelia, stabilization of the foot in a plantigrade position and subsequent lengthening procedures have shown favorable results. Despite fairly significant leg length discrepancies, current limb lengthen-

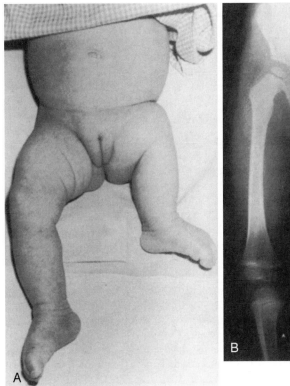
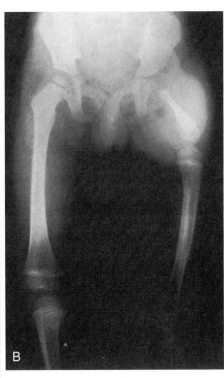

Figure 15–48. *A,* Clinical photograph of a child aged 1 year with proximal femoral focal deficiency. Note the very short femoral segment, which is held flexed and externally rotated. The foot is almost at the level of the opposite knee. *B,* Anteroposterior x-ray of a patient with a similar condition. Note again the very short femoral segment and abnormality below the knee with hypoplasia of the fibula. (From Benson MKD, Fixsen JA, MacNicol MF: Children's Orthopaedics and Fractures. Edinburgh, Churchill Livingstone, 1994.)

ing technology has been successful in achieving a satisfactory functional extremity.

Tibial hemimelia is reported to be extremely rare. Some suggest the incidence to be a low as 1 per 1,000,000 live births. Tibial hypoplasia may be partial or complete. In either event, an "apparent clubfoot" is frequently seen. The severity of the foot deformity parallels the degree of tibial deficiency. Unlike the other limb deficiency syndromes, some cases of tibial hypoplasia have been reported to have a hereditary basis. The Brown procedure has been used to manage this condition by centralizing the foot under the fibula. Long-term results have been marginal at best; therefore, most of the current literature suggests that the best treatment for tibial hemimelia is knee disarticulation surgery. This procedure offers the child the most rapid return to a functional childhood using a prosthesis.

Many unique limb deficiencies, other than those men-

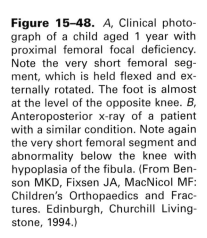

Figure 15–49. The classification of proximal femoral focal deficiency described by Aitken in 1969. Reproduced with permission. (From Benson MKD, Fixsen JA, MacNicol MF: Children's Orthopaedics and Fractures. Edinburgh, Churchill Livingstone, 1994.)

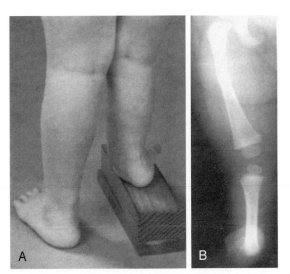

Figure 15–50. *A,* Congenital deficiency of the fibula type II. The heel lies in valgus and the tibia is short. *B,* Radiograph of congenital deficiency of the fibula showing the foot in valgus with deficiency of the lateral ray of the foot. (From Broughton NS: A Textbook of Paediatric Orthopaedics. London, WB Saunders, 1997.)

tioned, have been reported. The classic article of Franz and O'Railly attempted to classify this very heterogenous group of limb deficiency syndromes. They are credited with the introduction of descriptive terms such as *terminal versus intercalary* defects and *transverse versus paraxial* defects. Fortunately, these deficiency syndromes are rare, which has of course made it difficult to collect any series large enough to make treatment recommendations anything more than anecdotal.

REGIONAL ORTHOPAEDIC PROBLEMS

Shoulder and Arm

SPRENGEL'S DEFORMITY

This condition is characterized by a failure of the scapula to descend from its normal embryologic level at C4 to the thoracic region. Typically, the scapula develops adjacent to the cervical somites and completes its descent to the thoracic region by 3 months of fetal life. In Sprengel's deformity the scapula is retained in its cervical position by either a fibrous, cartilaginous, or osteocartilaginous bar. The condition is more common in females than males and more likely to involve the left shoulder for no apparent reason.

The clinical features include a hypoplastic high-riding scapula (Fig. 15–51) with some generalized muscular atrophy of the entire shoulder girdle. In approximately one third of cases, an omovertebral bone can be identified. Despite some loss in range of motion, most of the complaints are primarily cosmetic in nature. It is essential for the physician to recognize that Sprengel's deformity can be associated with other congenital anomalies, including scoliosis, Klippel-Feil anomaly, congenital muscular torticollis, and renal and facial deformities.

The treatment of this condition varies with the severity of the deformity. For the vast majority of patients, in whom the cosmetic deformity is mild and motion is adequate, only observation is required. Surgical correction of the deformity is typically carried out using one of two classic operative procedures. The *Green procedure* is an extraperiosteal release of all the musculature attached to the vertebral border of the scapula. Conversely, the *Woodward procedure*, which is more frequently employed, is executed by releasing the trapezii, rhomboids, and levator musculature from the spinal attachments, resecting the omovertebral bone, and advancing the scapula distally.

The younger the child at the age of surgical correction, the more likely it is to achieve a satisfactory result. After age 7, it is usually necessary to resect and morselize the

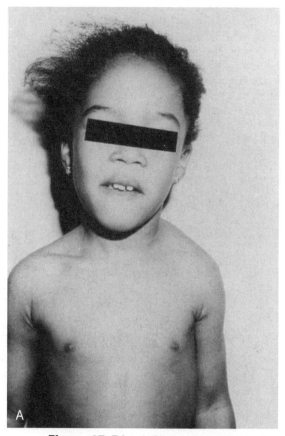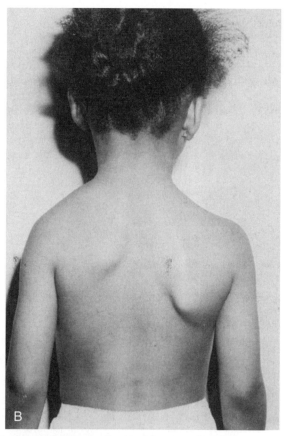

Figure 15–51. *A*, Clinical photograph of a child with a left Sprengel's shoulder, anterior view. *B*, Clinical photograph of a child with a left Sprengel's shoulder, posterior view. Note the elevation and rotation of the scapula. (From Benson MKD, Fixsen JA, MacNicol MF: Children's Orthopaedics and Fractures. Edinburgh, Churchill Livingstone, 1994.)

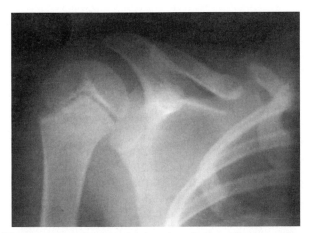

Figure 15–52. Pseudarthrosis of the clavicle. (From Broughton NS: A Textbook of Paediatric Orthopaedics. London, WB Saunders, 1997.)

midportion of the clavicle; otherwise, a traction palsy of the brachial plexus will likely be encountered as the scapula is moved distally. Finally, it is occasionally recommended to simply resect the superior border of the scapula in an effort to improve the appearance of the child's shoulder.

CONGENITAL PSEUDARTHROSIS OF THE CLAVICLE

The clavicle normally ossifies from both medial and lateral centers. Failure of these ossification centers to fuse may result in a central defect in the bone (Fig. 15–52). Typically, children with this defect are born with a mass in the center of the clavicle. Classically, it has been taught that this lesion occurs on the right side, except in the presence of sinus inversus. Recently, however, questions have been raised about this fact. Occasionally, congenital pseudarthrosis is confused with birth fractures of the clavicle. The most reliable method of differentiation between the two is to realize that the birth fracture will heal. Cleidocranial dysostosis, as was discussed in the section on skeletal dysplasias, is another clavicular abnormality that may occasionally be confused with this lesion.

Treatment of this lesion remains controversial. Most authors recommend no surgical intervention because of problems related to skin breakdown and persistent nonunion. Others report good results with excision of the pseudarthrosis and bone grafting with fixation. All authors generally agree that the condition is usually painless and causes virtually no functional deficit.

OBSTETRIC BRACHIAL PLEXUS PALSY

These disorders are the most common types of birth palsies and occur in approximately 1 per 1000 live births. Reportedly, high birth weight, traumatic delivery, lengthy labor, and shoulder dystocia are all risk factors associated with these palsies. Most injuries occur at the level of the neural foramen, with one of three typical patterns being seen. The upper root injuries are referred to as Erb-Duchenne palsy (levels C5 and C6) and are the most common type. Lower root injury has been referred to as Klumpke's paralysis (levels C8 and T1). The third type is paralysis of the entire arm, due to involvement of the entire plexus.

Erb's palsy, which is the most common type, typically involves the roots of C5 and C6, thereby causing paralysis in the deltoid, lateral rotators of the shoulder, biceps brachii, and brachioradialis. The internally rotated and adducted shoulder is characteristic of the syndrome. Hand function is only mildly impaired. The lower root injuries, on the other hand, affect primarily the wrist flexors, the long finger flexors, and hand intrinsics. Therefore, the function of the hand is most prominently affected; the sensation is normal. Diagnosis is usually apparent at birth, when the child demonstrates paralysis of all or part of the upper extremity (Fig. 15–53). Although difficult to identify, the presence of Horner's syndrome should be sought, because it indicates a poor prognosis.

The management of these birth palsies is somewhat controversial. General agreement exists as to the use of physical modalities for stretching and splinting. The greatest improvement should be anticipated within the first 3

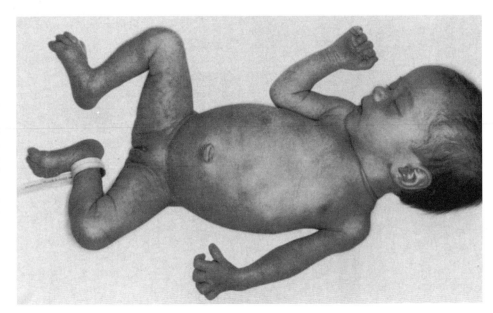

Figure 15–53. Clinical appearance of obstetric brachial plexus palsy paralysis on the left in a newborn infant. The left upper limb lies at the side of the trunk with the elbow in extension. (From Tachdjian MO: Pediatric Orthopedics, 2nd ed. Philadelphia, WB Saunders, 1990.)

months of life. The researchers in Europe have recently reported encouraging results employing brachial plexus exploration at 6 months of age. In children who have achieved no recovery by that time, exploration of the plexus with nerve grafting has reportedly improved function in a significant number of children. In the United States, these techniques have not been completely accepted. Hand function, when poor, is rarely improved in these children.

Children with persistent late deformity are frequently improved by various techniques to improve shoulder rotation. The fixed internal rotation position markedly inhibits hand function. Therefore, anything that will increase the ability of the child to externally rotate the extremity should improve the function of the upper limb. To this end, the Sever release of the pectoralis major and subscapularis muscles has been reported to improve external rotation. The L'Episcopo procedure, which is a transfer of the teres major to a lateral position with the latissimus dorsi, produces a similar effect. Last, in the older child, a rotational osteotomy of the humerus is favored by many as a more reliable procedure. Care must be taken prior to executing any of these procedures to be sure that the humeral head is located in the glenoid, because a number of children have shown posterior dislocation resulting from the internal rotational contracture. Although most of the late sequelae are the result of the contractures, a small number of children are afflicted by a pure flaccid paralysis. In this situation the only options are shoulder arthrodesis and elbow flexorplasty.

Elbow and Forearm

CONGENITAL DISLOCATION OF THE RADIAL HEAD

Perhaps the major significance of this rare condition is in the differentiation between it and an acquired dislocation of the radial head, which unfortunately can occur after an unrecognized Monteggia's fracture dislocation. The congenitally dislocated radial head, typically, is shaped differently than the normal. The head is convex or flattened as opposed to the normal radial head with a central depressed area (Fig. 15–54). The child with a congenital dislocation of the radial head presents when the parents notice a

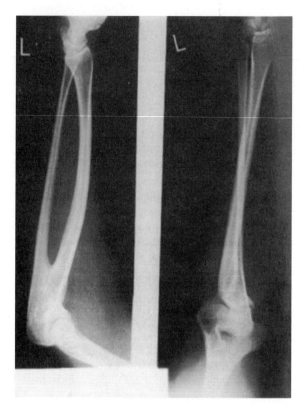

Figure 15–55. Radiograph of congenital radioulnar synostosis, showing cross-fusion in its typical proximal site. (From Benson MKD, Fixsen JA, MacNicol MF: Children's Orthopaedics and Fractures. Edinburgh, Churchill Livingstone, 1994.)

prominent "bump" on the lateral side of the elbow. Some restriction in the pronation and supination range may prompt the initial visit. Rarely is this condition a functional impairment for the child; the vast majority adapt very well.

Treatment of congenital dislocation of the radial head is usually benign neglect. Attempts at surgical reduction of the dislocated radial head are fraught with complications. The vast majority redislocate, frequently leaving the elbow stiffer than it otherwise would have been. Excision of the radial head *after physeal closure* reportedly will improve the appearance of the extremity. The physician must, however, remember the classic admonition: never remove the radial head in a growing child.

CONGENITAL RADIOULNAR SYNOSTOSIS

This abnormal fusion between the ulna and the radius may occur proximally, distally, or in both locations (Fig. 15–55). It is often bilateral and inherited as an autosomal dominant condition. Typically, it is identified in the older child when some mild functional impairment, especially in throwing sports, is recognized. Most children adapt well to the limited motion in the forearm. They are able to compensate with the shoulder and the wrist; therefore, surgery is frequently unnecessary. The physician should not be tempted to try surgical takedown of the synostosis. Procedures designed to resect the synostosis have notoriously poor results. Usually no increase in pronation or supination can be achieved; in fact, should myositis ossificans develop, further loss of function will occur. Attempts at radial head

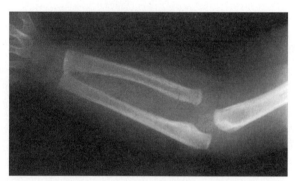

Figure 15–54. Congenital dislocation of the radial head. If a line is drawn along the axis of the radius, it does not pass through the capitellum but passes anteriorly. (From Broughton NS: A Textbook of Paediatric Orthopaedics. London, WB Saunders, 1997.)

resection with or without implants have similarly faced poor results. The only option worthy of consideration is osteotomy, used to place the hand in a more functional position. For example, slight pronation is most desirable for writing or using a keyboard; therefore, the supinated forearm may be osteotomized and placed in pronation, thereby improving the functional position.

NURSEMAID'S ELBOW

This common affliction of the elbow joint is often discussed in chapters on trauma. However, because the basic problem is the hypoplastic radial head or a somewhat attenuated annular ligament, many believe that the "trauma" required to dislocate the radial head is nothing more than normal use of the extremity. Typically, as the child begins to fall with a parent holding his or her hand, a "pop" or "snap," followed by immediate pain, will be appreciated at the elbow. When seen in the emergency facility, the child has pseudoparalysis of the extremity and tenderness diffusely about the elbow. X-rays are always negative. This common syndrome is thought to be a subluxation of the radial head axially through the annular ligament; it is most commonly seen in children under the age of 4 years. By that time, the girth of the radial head has increased so that it is no longer able to slide through the encapsulating annular ligament.

Treatment of the acute nursemaid's elbow need not be excessive. Reduction is usually accomplished by the x-ray technician, who supinates the forearm in order to get the AP exposure. Short-term use of a splint or sling, allowing mobilization as the pain subsides, is all that it is necessary. Parents need to be aware that this elbow is vulnerable and at risk for recurrent subluxation.

RADIAL CLUBHAND

Axial deficiencies on the radial side of the forearm are the most common limb deficiencies in the upper extremity. This particular congenital longitudinal deficiency is reportedly transmitted as an autosomal dominant trait. There is partial or complete absence of the radius, with rare involvement of the ulnar ray being seen (Fig. 15–56). The hand typically is radially deviated and may be lacking the thumb ray. The incidence is 1 in 100,000 live births, with about one half of the cases being bilateral.

It is of the utmost importance for the physician to recognize that radial deficiencies may be associated with other syndromes in approximately 50% of cases (Table 15–4). TAR syndrome (thrombocytopenia and absent radius) is one of the more common. In this group, the thumb is normal. VATER syndrome is the other clustering of anomalies worthy of mention. Here the child is afflicted with vertebral, anal, tracheoesophageal, renal, and radial anomalies.

Despite the deformity, hand function is frequently surprisingly good. As with many of these anomalies in young children, adaptive techniques develop rapidly. Therefore, it is important not to sacrifice a competent functioning hand in an effort to correct what the physician may feel is an unacceptable position. Stretching and splinting have no place in the definitive management of this syndrome. However, they are helpful preoperatively to stretch the soft tissues. Surgically, several different centralization procedures have been described. All involve a soft tissue release and centralization of the carpus onto the distal ulna. Internal fixation techniques and the use of fixators have both been employed.

MADELUNG'S DEFORMITY

True Madelung's deformity is a congenital anomaly. It results from the arrest of the ulnar and volar portions of the distal radial growth plate. As a result, a unique carpal deformity results, referred to as a triangulation defect (Fig. 15–57) of the distal radius. The distal radius and ulna appear V-shaped with the carpus having migrated somewhat centrally. The condition is transmitted as an autoso-

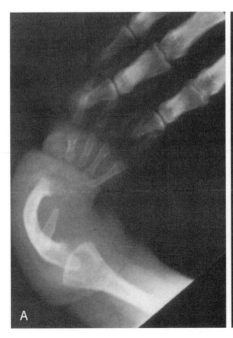
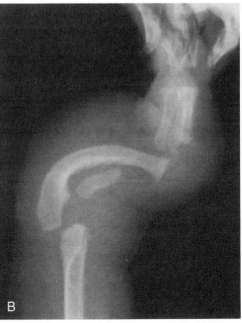

Figure 15–56. Type B congenital longitudinal deficiency of the radius. Anteroposterior (A) and lateral (B) radiographs. Note the partial absence of the distal and middle parts of the radius and the deficiency of the proximal radius with abnormality of the elbow. The ulna is markedly bowed. (From Tachdjian MO: Pediatric Orthopedics, 2nd ed. Philadelphia, WB Saunders, 1990.)

Table 15–4. Congenital malformations associated with congenital longitudinal radial deficiency

Hand	Skeleton, Cardiac anomalies *(Continued)*
Thumb	Coarctation of aorta
Absent	Patent ductus arteriosus
Floating	Dextrocardia
Hypoplastic	Tetralogy of Fallot
Digits	Pulmonary stenosis
Syndactyly	Genitourinary anomalies
Polydactyly	Renal agenesis
Symphalangism	Hypoplasia of kidney
Triphalangism	Horseshoe kidney
Carpus	Pelvic kidney
Deficient radial side—absence of scaphoid and trapezium	Hydronephrosis
Carpal coalition	Urethral valve
Metacarpal joints (MP)	Neurogenic bladder
Excessive hyperextension with limited flexion	Gastrointestinal anomalies
Proximal interphalangeal joints (PIP)	Esophageal atresia
Fixed flexion deformity	Tracheoesophageal fistula
Spine	Rectovaginal fistula
Congenital scoliosis	Imperforate anus
Hemivertebrae	Inguinal hernia
Klippel-Feil syndrome	Pulmonary anomalies
Sacral agenesis	Agenesis of upper lobe of lung
Idiopathic scoliosis	Head anomalies
Skeleton	Cleft lip and palate
Hip dislocation	Craniosynostosis
Congenital high scapula (Sprengel's deformity)	Hydrocephalus
Bowed and short ulna	Cataracts
Radioulnar synostosis (in partial absence of distal radius)	Coloboma
Clubfoot	Ear anomalies
Sternal anomalies	Chromosomal abnormalities
Pectus excavatum	Trisomy 18
Pectus carinatum	
Cardiac anomalies	
Atrial septal defect (Holt-Oram syndrome)	
Ventricular septal defect	

From Broughton NS: A Textbook of Paediatric Orthopaedics. London, WB Saunders, 1997.

mal dominant trait, more common in females and frequently bilateral.

When the anomaly is primarily cosmetic, little or no treatment is required. If it is more severe, surgical options are available and include epiphysiodesis of the distal radial plate to minimize progression, osteotomy of the distal radius to correct deformity, resection of the distal ulna, and ultimately wrist fusion. An acquired type of Madelung's deformity can be seen following damage to the distal radial growth plate that is due to metaphyseal osteomyelitis or trauma.

Hand

CONGENITAL TRIGGER THUMB

Congenital trigger thumb is one of the more common hand problems in the child. Typically, the child presents with "locking" of the interphalangeal joint of the thumb. Usually the deformity is fixed and the "clicking," typical of the adult, is rarely seen in the child. Approximately one third of cases are bilateral; depending on the age of presentation, many will resolve spontaneously. Despite the concern of the parents, it is best to simply observe the child throughout the first year of life because most authors report

spontaneous correction rates as high as 50%. This certainly makes it wise to watch and wait. Those who remain locked are best treated by tenolysis through the A1 pulley. Complications are few and results are excellent.

SYNDACTYLY

Webbing or fusion of two or more fingers is the most common congenital anomaly of the hand. It results from a failure of differentiation between adjacent fingers. The most common web occurs between the long and ring fingers (Fig. 15–58). Males are affected twice as often as females, with a familial incidence of 25%. It is important to determine the extent of soft tissue as well as bony involvement. Those involving only a skin and soft tissue fusion are referred to as a simple syndactyly, whereas those with bony fusions are referred to as a complex syndactyly. As with radial deficiency syndromes, it is important to be sure that these are isolated phenomena. Numerous syndromes and anomalies have been associated with manual and pedal syndactyly; Apert's syndrome and Poland's syndrome are two.

Surgical separation typically will improve finger and therefore hand function. If not separated at an early age, the syndactyly will cause the longer of the two fingers to

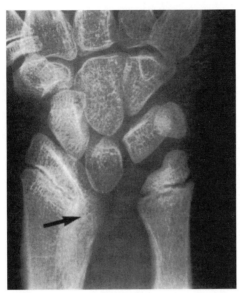

Figure 15–57. Madelung's deformity of the right wrist. (From Tachdjian MO: Pediatric Orthopedics, 2nd ed. Philadelphia, WB Saunders, 1990.)

whites. Blacks commonly manifest a duplicated little finger, being present in 1 in 300 live births. Whites and Asians typically have duplicated thumbs. Little finger duplication is rarely associated with other anomalies or syndromes and is inherited as an autosomal dominant trait. The duplicated thumb, however, is more likely to have associated anomalies. Removal of a duplicated little finger is easily accomplished in the hospital nursery. However, removal of a duplicated thumb is a more complex procedure, since maintenance of ligamentous balance about the MP joint requires a more formal procedure.

The Hip

NORMAL DEVELOPMENT OF THE HIP

For one to understand and appreciate the problems of the immature hip, it is critical to have an understanding of the development of the hip. The bulk of the neonatal hip is cartilaginous (Fig. 15–59). Large portions of the acetabulum and femoral head are not visible by standard radiographic technique because they are still largely cartilage. As one can expect, these cartilaginous portions are ex-

deviate; therefore, surgical intervention is generally recommended within the first year of life.

POLYDACTYLY

An extra digit is usually obvious at birth. Fortunately, the anxiety that it causes the parents is usually unfounded. The supernumerary digit may be postaxial (on the little finger side of the hand) or preaxial (on the thumb side of the hand). Again, it is important to confirm whether or not the extra digit is soft tissue or bony and, if bony, whether it contains only phalanges or in fact its own metacarpal.

Polydactyly is 10 times more common in blacks than

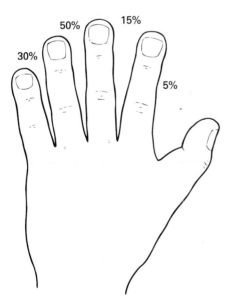

Figure 15–58. The frequency of syndactyly of digital clefts. (From Benson MKD, Fixsen JA, MacNicol MF: Children's Orthopaedics and Fractures. Edinburgh, Churchill Livingstone, 1994.)

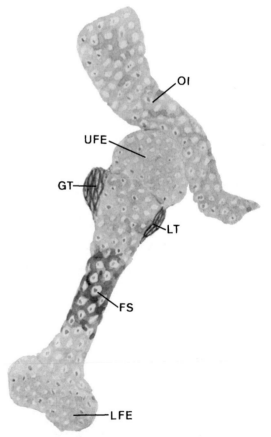

Figure 15–59. Three stages of cell differentiation in the femur: the central portion of the shaft is formed by differentiated cartilage cells, the epiphyses are formed by precartilage cells, and the trochanteric projections are formed by undifferentiated blastemal cells. OI = os innominatum; UFE = upper femoral epiphysis; LFE = lower femoral epiphysis; GT = greater trochanter; LT = lesser trochanter; FS = femoral shaft. (From Tachdjian M: Congenital Dislocation of the Hip. New York, Churchill Livingstone, 1982, p 8.)

tremely labile. They are easily damaged by abnormal mechanical loading and the effect of this damage is usually permanent and irreversible. The acetabulum is constructed of four different cartilage types. The articular surface is covered by hyaline articular cartilage, whereas the triradiate cartilage represents a physeal component of the acetabulum. It is this structure that permits the acetabulum and the pelvis to grow in height. The margin of the acetabulum is surrounded by a fibrocartilaginous labrum, which is critical for circumferential acetabular growth. Last, epiphyseal cartilage can be seen adjacent to the acetabulum, and represents the secondary ossification centers. For normal acetabular growth to occur, it is critical that the femoral head be concentrically located within the acetabulum (Fig. 15–60). Otherwise, should the femoral head lateralize, abnormal joint reaction forces can be expected to alter enchondral ossification and cause variable degrees of acetabular dysplasia.

Similarly, there is an intricate relationship between the acetabulum and the triradiate cartilage. This cartilage is absolutely critical for normal acetabular development and symmetry. Any premature closure of the triradiate will significantly alter acetabular shape. Finally, the marginal labrum, or as it is frequently referred to in the young child, the limbus, contains numerous germinal cells, which are integral for normal progressive acetabular deepening. Damage to this limbus will dramatically alter ultimate acetabular shape as well.

The proximal femur is essentially a composite chondroepiphysis. It is a singular mass of cartilage, which will ultimately develop into not only the capital femoral epiphysis but also the trochanteric apophysis. These two secondary centers develop within the single cartilaginous anlage. In the newborn, cartilage canals can be identified within this chondroepiphysis, suggesting the presence of a blood supply. The ossification center of the femoral head typically appears between the fourth and sixth months of postnatal life. Initially, this center is spherical; subsequently, it expands in a centrifugal fashion. Obviously, the growth and development of the capital femoral epiphysis (CFE) are dependent upon an intact blood supply. At this point in development, the relationship between the CFE and that of the trochanter is such that they are both at the same level in the coronal plane. This relationship, the articulotrochanteric distance (ATD), is therefore said to be neutral. With differential growth, as the femoral neck elongates, the femoral head will ultimately be well above the trochanter (Fig. 15–61), thereby creating a positive ATD. The relationship between the femoral head and the trochanter is critical for normal hip mechanics. By 1 year of age, the initial spherical CFE has adaptively become hemispherical in shape. In addition, with elongation of the femoral neck, the ATD is now obviously positive.

From this point forward, progressive maturation during childhood does not accomplish dramatic configuration changes in the proximal femur. Progressive sophistication of the trabecular pattern, responding to mechanical loading, is prominent at this time. By age 6 years, the calcar is thickening and the trabeculae are becoming more and more stress oriented. All centers are clearly present and continuing to mature. The greater trochanter initially ossifies, as a secondary center, between 5 and 7 years of age. Fusion is generally complete by age 18. The lesser trochanter, on the other hand, does not ossify until adolescence and closes approximately at the time of the greater trochanter. As one can see from this brief discussion of hip embryology, the acetabulum and proximal femur are the most vulnerable in the neonatal and early childhood stages. It is at this time, when large portions of the hip are cartilaginous, that they are very subject to damage by eccentric mechanical loading.

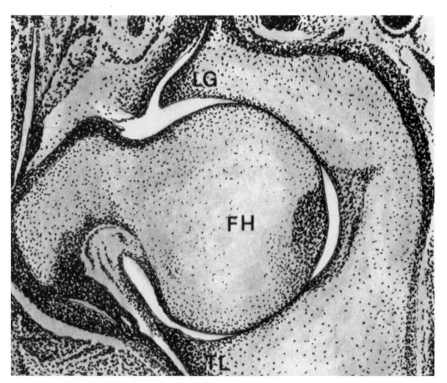

Figure 15–60. Fetus with 70- to 90-mm crown-rump length at the twelfth week of gestation. The femoral head (FH) is almost completely enclosed by the acetabular cavity. The labrum glenoidale (LG) is a well-defined structure contributing to the depth of the cavity. The transverse ligament (TL) remains a fibrous band across the inferior portion of the joint. (From Ralis Z, McKibbin B: Changes in the shape of the human hip joint during its development and their relation to its stability. J Bone Joint Surg 1973;55B:780.)

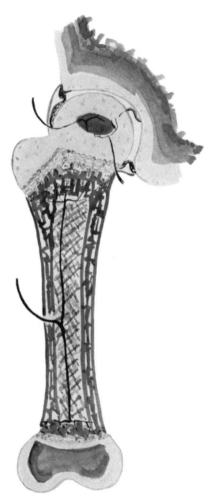

Figure 15–61. Hip joint at about 6 months after birth. Tubulization of the femoral diaphysis with a well-developed inferior ossification center. The superior epiphyseal ossification center is of recent appearance. (From Tachdjian M: Congenital Dislocation of the Hip. New York, Churchill Livingstone, 1982, p 14.)

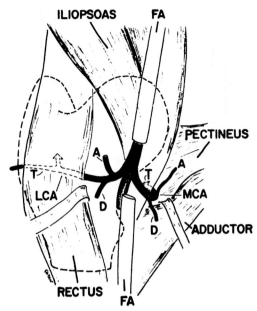

Figure 15–62. Initial course of hip circulation from the femoral artery (FA), which first divides into the profunda femoris. From this latter vessel are derived the medial (MCA) and lateral (LCA) circumflex arteries. Each of these arteries divides into ascending (A), transverse (T), and descending (D) branches. The LCA goes beneath the rectus femoris muscle to reach the proximal femur. The MCA goes between the iliopsoas and the adductor-pectineus muscle group. (From Tachdjian M: Congenital Dislocation of the Hip. New York, Churchill Livingstone, 1982.)

The blood supply of the hip joint is critical to its normal development. In general, the blood supply to the hip is divided into the extracapsular circulation and the intracapsular circulation. The *extracapsular blood supply* (Fig. 15–62) of the proximal femur is predominantly from the profunda femoris artery via its two major branches: the lateral circumflex artery (LCA) and the medial circumflex artery (MCA). This is true for all stages of development. The LCA (Fig. 15–63) sends a small transverse branch to the greater trochanter and prominent branches to the anterior portion of the capital femoral epiphysis. With progressive growth, the significance of the lateral circumflex contribution to the anterior portion of the epiphyseal nucleus recedes, and it largely provides blood to the anterior portion of the femoral neck. The MCA (Fig. 15–64), on the other hand, crosses behind the intertrochanteric notch, where it recurs anterosuperiorly, anastomosing with some of the terminal branches of the LCA (Fig. 15–65). Consequently, a vascular ring is created around the trochanteric and basilar neck regions. This extracapsular ring is a constant finding, although its size and configuration are variable.

The *intracapsular circulation* is highly variable. At birth, both the lateral and medial circumflex vessels provide equal amounts of flow to the capital femoral epiphysis. However, with progressive differential growth and elongation of the femoral neck, the flow from the LCA recedes from the head and predominantly supplies the anterior neck and metaphysis. By 3 to 4 years of age, the MCA exerts

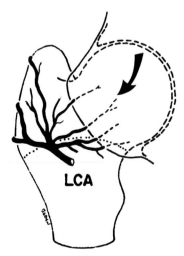

Figure 15–63. Course of lateral circumflex artery (LCA) in the infant stage. The primary distribution is to the greater trochanter. However, small branches penetrate the anterior capsule *(arrow)* to supply a portion of the capital femoral chondroepiphysis. The dotted line shows the course of the common physis, which is primarily extra-articular at this stage. (From Tachdjian M: Congenital Dislocation of the Hip. New York, Churchill Livingstone, 1982, p 61.)

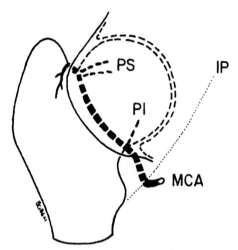

Figure 15–64. Course of medial circumflex artery (MCA) in the infant stage. The vessel wraps around the iliopsoas muscle and tendon (IP) and courses along the posterior intertrochanteric notch, just external to the capsular insertion. The posterosuperior (PS) and posteroinferior (PI) branches are the major vessels penetrating the capital femoral epiphysis. This artery primarily supplies the capital femur, but it also sends some branches to the posterior greater trochanter. (From Tachdjian M: Congenital Dislocation of the Hip. New York, Churchill Livingstone, 1982, p 61.)

its dominance by providing most of the blood to the capital femoral epiphysis. It does so through two systems of vessels. The posteroinferior artery penetrates the capsule in the area of the lesser trochanter, where it lies between the neck and the iliopsoas tendon. In this position, this vessel is relatively mobile and somewhat less vulnerable. On the other hand, the posterosuperior arterial system, which is the more important of the two, enters the capsule posterosuperiorly and proceeds along the superior neck into the capital femoral epiphysis. In this latter location, it tends to

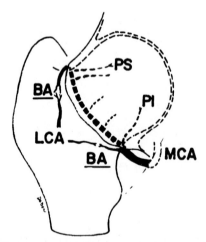

Figure 15–65. The medial circumflex artery (MCA) sends branches around the superior (PS) and inferior (PI) margins of the femoral neck to anastomose with branches of the lateral circumflex artery (LCA). These basal anastomoses (BA) represent the major extracapsular collateral circulation. (From Tachdjian M: Congenital Dislocation of the Hip. New York, Churchill Livingstone, 1982, p 62.)

be partially encased within the articular cartilage. Therefore, it is not mobile and quite vulnerable. These two vessels from the MCA ultimately anastomose, forming a retinacular ring around the femoral neck. Smaller vessels from this ring enter the head through a system of cartilage canals.

Once inside the head, the *intraepiphyseal circulation* (Fig. 15–66) will supply very discrete regions of the capital femoral epiphysis. Prior to ossification within the secondary ossification center, many of these small vessels are essentially end arteries. However, once ossification has occurred, an intraepiphyseal anastomotic network is seen. Therefore, not only does eccentric and aberrant mechanical loading place the cartilage of the hip at risk, but the discrete, and some might say tenuous, vascular supply is also clearly vulnerable. Damage to one or both of these delicate systems of the proximal femur will produce permanent deformity of the hip.

DEVELOPMENTAL DYSPLASIA OF THE HIP

Probably no other abnormality of the immature hip has received as much attention as developmental dysplasia of the hip (DDH). It is important to recognize at the onset, that "developmental," which used to be called "congenital," dysplasia of the hip must be differentiated from hip dislocation seen on a teratogenic basis. Children with neuromuscular disease, arthrogryposis, and other syndromes will frequently demonstrate hip dislocation. These dislocations are essentially different from those in DDH. DDH is a dysplasic condition of the pediatric hip seen at birth or shortly thereafter. It may ultimately lead to subluxation or frank dislocation of the joint. The incidence of this condition is approximately 1 per 1000 live births for true dislocation and approximately 1 per 100 live births for dysplasia and mild subluxation.

The risk factors have similarly been well characterized. First-born females, especially those presenting breech, are at significant risk. A positive family history, ligamentous laxity, and the infamous hip "click" all should signal the examiner to carefully evaluate the infant for this condition. The finding of congenital muscular torticollis has recently been demonstrated to be seen in 20% of children with DDH. Therefore, children who demonstrate this finding should be carefully evaluated for hip dysplasia. At the very onset, one needs to recognize the consequences of inadequate treatment. The natural history of DDH is such that in order to produce a normal hip, three requirements must be met. First, a concentric reduction must be achieved. Second, correction of any residual acetabular dysplasia must be performed, and finally, and perhaps most important, one must avoid the complication of ischemic necrosis of the femoral head; once this occurs, it is impossible to produce a normal hip.

Diagnosis. In the newborn, a careful physical examination of the hip, especially in children with risk factors, is axiomatic. The single best diagnostic tool is the physical examination. It is important that the child be examined on a firm surface to prevent the pelvis from rolling from side to side. Obviously, the child should be completely undressed in order for a complete examination to be performed. In the newborn, ligamentous laxity characterizes the hip examina-

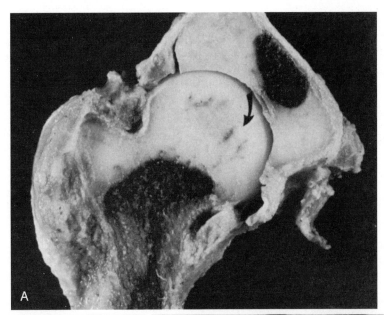

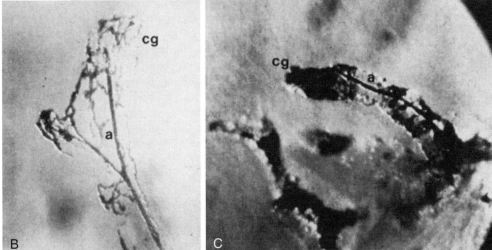

Figure 15–66. *A,* Slab section of infant hip showing terminal branches of cartilage canals *(arrow).* There were no obvious intracartilaginous anastomoses. *B* and *C,* India ink injections of terminal branches showing complexity of these structures. The central artery (a) is surrounded by a capillary glomerulus (cg). (From Tachdjian M: Congenital Dislocation of the Hip. New York, Churchill Livingstone, 1982.)

tion. Inspection may or may not reveal the presence of asymmetric thigh folds. In our current well-fed society, this finding is the norm rather than the exception, and therefore misleading. The classic *Ortolani sign* (Fig. 15–67) is described as the finding of a "click" or "clunk" as the infant's hip is flexed and abducted. This sound essentially occurs when the femoral head reduces over the posterior rim of the acetabulum. Therefore, the Ortolani sign, when positive, indicates that the hip is frankly dislocated. It is the sign of reduction. Conversely, the *Barlow sign* indicates a located hip that is capable of being dislocated. The Barlow sign is performed by flexing and adducting the hip while applying a posteriorly directed force at the knee. With increasing adduction and the anticipated amount of posterior laxity, the femoral head can be dislocated from the socket. This hip is said to be *dislocatable.* The sign is a provocative test for this dislocatability. Frequently, the

experienced examiner will appreciate a subluxable hip. This type of hip cannot be dislocated by a Barlow maneuver, but from a tactile standpoint, the examiner "gets the sense" that with excessive pressure it might be. Essentially, this is a reflection of capsular laxity.

Most children at birth have a hip flexion contracture; this rarely disappears until the fourth to sixth months of life. At approximately 6 weeks postpartum, the signs of instability (Barlow, Ortolani) tend to disappear. This primarily reflects the decrease in ligamentous laxity, with a coincident increase in motion restriction and contracture about the subluxed or dislocated hip. Therefore, by 6 weeks of age, the most important finding is that of limited abduction (Fig. 15–68). Placing the child on a firm surface is essential if subtle changes in hip motion are to be appreciated. If the pelvis is allowed to rotate during the examination, it is common that limited abduction may be masked.

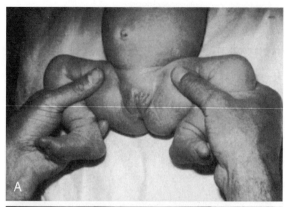

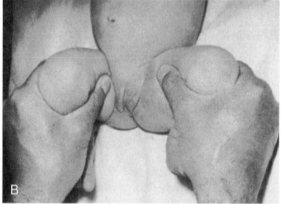

Figure 15-67. *A*, Ortolani's test: when the hip is reduced, full abduction of the flexed hip is possible. *B*, Barlow's test: with the hip flexed and adducted, lateral pressure from the thumb on the proximal femur will demonstrate instability if it is present. (From Benson MKD, Fixsen JA, MacNicol MF: Children's Orthopaedics and Fractures. Edinburgh, Churchill Livingstone, 1994.)

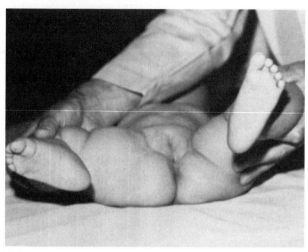

Figure 15-68. Restriction of abduction of the flexed thigh. (From Coleman SS: Congenital Dysplasia and Dislocation of the Hip. CV Mosby, St. Louis, 1978.)

The examiner needs to carefully evaluate one hip in relation to the other in an effort to identify these subtle restrictions in the abduction range.

The *Allis sign (Galeazzi test)* is yet another finding that points to dislocation of the hip (Fig. 15-69). With the child supine on a firm surface, both hips and both knees are flexed. The finding of one knee being lower than the other suggests that the hip is dislocated on the low side. This may be seen any time after birth. The tragedy of bilateral DDH is the frequency of failure to diagnose. Because so many of the classic signs depend on asymmetry, one's diagnostic acumen is markedly altered when both hips are dislocated. Therefore, it is important to carefully examine the thigh folds and to look for a widened perineum. In the older child, typically, the hip flexion deformities persist; in the walking child, these deformities will cause an increased lordotic posture in the lumber region and a waddling gait.

Imaging studies are critically important not only for diagnosis but also for treatment. For many years, the gold standard in the diagnosis of DDH was a standard *AP x-ray of the pelvis* with the hips in the neutral position. In the newborn, this can be extremely misleading for two reasons: first, because of the flexion contracture, the tube is difficult to position; second, and most important, bony markers are absent. In the newborn, as mentioned earlier, the bulk

of the acetabulum and proximal femur are cartilaginous; therefore, relatively little of what one needs to see is truly visible. Unfortunately, what one cannot see is more important than what one can see. By 3 months of age, there has been adequate femoral head ossification as well as ossification about the acetabulum to make the x-ray a very reliable study.

Classic radiographic lines (Fig. 15-70) have been used for many years to assist in the evaluation of the pediatric hip. *Hilgenreiner's line* (Y line) is a horizontal line through the upper margin of the radiolucent triradiate cartilage. *Perkins' line* (vertical line) is drawn from the lateralmost ossified margin of the roof of the acetabulum to intersect, perpendicularly, with the Y line. This creates four quadrants around the hip. In the normal hip, the medial end of the ossified upper femoral metaphysis should lie medial to Perkins' line and below the Y line. In the subluxed hip, it lies lateral to Perkins' line and inferior to the Y line; in the

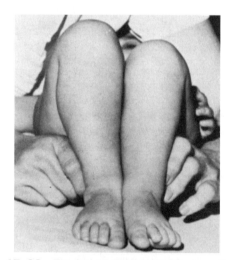

Figure 15-69. The knee level is seen lower on the left, as shown in the Galeazzi test. (From Coleman SS: Congenital Dysplasia and Dislocation of the Hip. CV Mosby, St. Louis, 1978.)

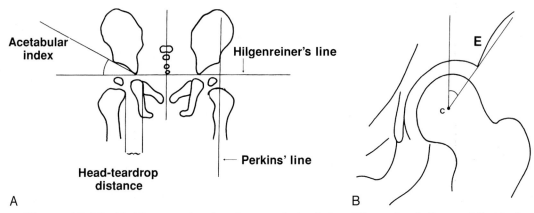

Figure 15–70. *A*, Diagram showing the acetabular index, Hilgenreiner's line and Perkins' line. *B*, The center-edge angle. This becomes useful at about 8 years of age. (From Broughton NS: A Textbook of Paediatric Orthopaedics. London, WB Saunders, 1997.)

case of frank dislocation, the medial end of the ossified metaphysis of the femoral neck lies lateral to Perkins' line and superior to the Y line. *Shenton's line,* between the superior border of the obturator foramen and the medial border of the femoral neck, should form a continuous arc in the normal hip. In the presence of superior and lateral subluxation, this line will be interrupted. For this line to be meaningful, the radiograph must be taken in the true coronal plane with the hips positioned in the neutral position. The acetabular index is the angle formed between the Y line of Hilgenreiner and a line drawn from it to the lateral ossified margin of the acetabular roof. This index may be as high as 35 degrees in the newborn but should rapidly decrease to well below 25 degrees in the older infant. Recently, the teardrop figure (U figure of Koehler), which represents the floor of the acetabulum, has received increased attention. For many years its significance was overlooked. If the teardrop is poorly developed (V-shaped rather than U-shaped), it suggests poor concentric reduction of the hip. For this figure to develop properly there needs to be mechanical interplay between the femoral head and the floor of the acetabulum. The center edge angle (CE angle) is not significant until adequate amounts of cartilage have been replaced by bone. At about age 6 to 8 years, it is a reliable measure of seating of the head in the acetabulum ("docking").

Ultrasound (Fig. 15–71) has become increasingly popular in the evaluation of the pediatric hip. It is most reliable from birth to 3 months of age and becomes decreasingly significant as the child approaches 6 months. Many would say it is the best method to evaluate the hip from infancy to 6 months of age. This study will depict the cartilaginous portions of the acetabulum and the femoral head, which arc those segments not seen on plain x-ray. Two different methods have been popularized, and they are not mutually exclusive. The first method is the static technique described by Graff, and the second is the dynamic stress technique as popularized by Harcke. This latter study is useful not only in diagnosis but also in monitoring treatment. The most common study is done with a direct single coronal image of each hip with the child lying in the lateral position. The study is able to identify the distal portion of the ossified ilium, the ossified medial wall of the acetabulum,

the triradiate cartilage, and the cartilaginous femoral head with the developing ossific nucleus. In addition, the cartilaginous roof of the acetabulum, the labrum, and the capital femoral physis can also be visualized. The alpha angle (Fig. 15–72) is the critical measurement taken. It represents the angle between the reference line and the line across the bony acetabular roof. In the normal hip this angle should be 60 degrees; the smaller the alpha angle, the greater the dysplasia of the hip. The beta angle is used to evaluate the status of the labral margin.

Arthrography is a commonly performed procedure in the follow-up evaluation of these children. It has little role in diagnosis, but for many surgeons, it has an important role in treatment. It allows one to verify the concentricity of the reduction and the depth of docking. The latter term emphasizes the need to deeply seat the femoral head within the acetabulum. Failure to do so has long-standing and sweeping consequences. This procedure, which typically requires a general anesthetic and careful fluoroscopic viewing, will allow the examiner to measure the medial dye pool. Should this dye pool be too wide, one can assume that soft tissue impediments exist, blocking reduction.

Computed tomography (CT) scanning has also been used for the monitoring of treatment. Following closed and open reductions, the CT scan is the most reliable study available to demonstrate the adequacy of the reduction. In addition, the anatomy of the acetabulum can be evaluated further using his technique.

Pathology. The pathologic changes of DDH must be understood in order to effectively manage these hips. Typically, the dysplastic hip has a maldirected, shallow acetabulum. In addition, there are frequently soft tissue impediments, which block the concentric reduction of the femoral head into the acetabulum (Fig. 15–73). There is debate as to which of the soft tissue structures is the most important in blocking this reduction. Nevertheless, there is general agreement that all play a role. The iliopsoas tendon can be demonstrated to create an "hourglass" constriction of the capsule. This capsular constriction in turn creates a stricture, making it impossible for the femoral head to move into the floor of the acetabulum. The acetabular labrum, previously discussed, is critical for normal acetabular de-

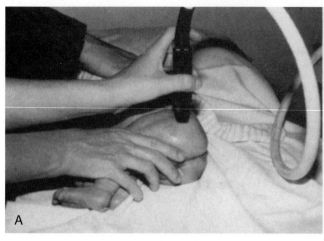

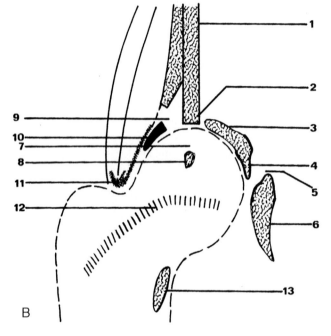

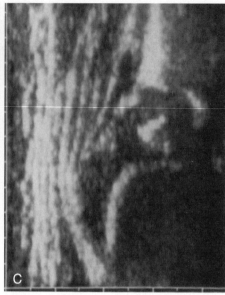

Figure 15–71. Ultrasonography of the hip in congenital hip dislocation. *A*, Lateral decubitus position of the infant for ultrasonographic examination of the hip. *B*, Diagram of structures identified during static nonstress ultrasonography of the hip: 1, iliac bone. 2, the most distal point of the ilium in the roof of the acetabulum. 3, Ossified medial wall of the acetabulum. 4, the inferior end of the iliac bone at the triradiate cartilage. 5, triradiate cartilage. 6, ossified ischium. 7, the cartilaginous femoral head. 8, ossific nucleus of the femoral head. 9, cartilaginous roof of the acetabulum. 10, labrum. 11, intertrochanteric fossa. 12, cartilaginous growth plate of the femoral head. 13, ossified metaphysis of the femoral neck. *C*, Ultrasonogram showing structures. (From Tachdjian MO: Pediatric Orthopedics, 2nd ed. Philadelphia, WB Saunders, 1990.)

velopment. However, in the subluxed and dislocated hip this labrum can become infolded, thereby creating a diaphragm capable of blocking reduction of the head. In addition, in the dislocated hip, the ligamentum teres becomes thickened and redundant, also acting as an anatomic block to reduction. In addition, the normal tissues in the floor of the acetabulum, specifically the pulvinar (haversian gland) and the transverse acetabular ligament, further fill the acetabulum, preventing the femoral head from seating.

Treatment. Treatment of DDH is all too often complex. Frequently, the uninitiated can be easily confused when the discussion of treating DDH is broached. It is very easy to lose sight of the basic goals. It is absolutely critical to recognize the three goals that are key to a successful outcome. Simply stated, the goals of treating DDH at any age are as follows:

1. Reduce the femoral head into the acetabulum.
2. Maintain the reduction of the head in the acetabulum.

3. Do not incur the complications of carrying out these procedures; specifically, avoid avascular necrosis.

If the physician will only focus on these three basic goals, the treatment decisions will frequently be more straightforward. The implementation of these decisions, however, can remain quite vexing.

Birth to 6 Months of Age. The worldwide standard for treating the dysplastic hip in this age group is the *Pavlik harness* (Fig. 15–74). This device can be employed to reduce the dislocated hip and maintain that reduction in the young infant. Because the infant has ligamentous laxity, the Pavlik harness functions as a dynamic splint, allowing active hip flexion and abduction, which are movements that encourage seating of these hips. With reduction comes improved stability, ultimately leading to the goal of a stable concentric reduction. The Pavlik harness, however, is not a panacea. It is critically important in its use that care be exercised in its application and in parental education. The splint must be of appropriate size; otherwise, positioning may be compromised. Its anterior straps are designed to

Figure 15–72. A diagram illustrating visual impression of the position of the femoral head in the acetabulum. 1, Baseline parallel to the ilium. 2, Cartilage roof line from the bony edge of the acetabulum through the labrum. 3, Bony roof line from the bony edge of the acetabulum to the lowest point of the ilium in the center of the joint. Alpha angle is between lines 1 and 3 (the smaller the angle, the more dysplasia present). Beta angle is between lines 1 and 2 (eversion of the labrum and subluxation of the hip indicated by an angle greater than 77 degrees). (From Tachdjian MO: Pediatric Orthopedics, 2nd ed. Philadelphia, WB Saunders, 1990.)

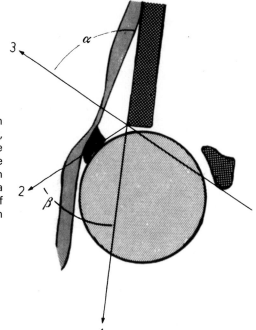

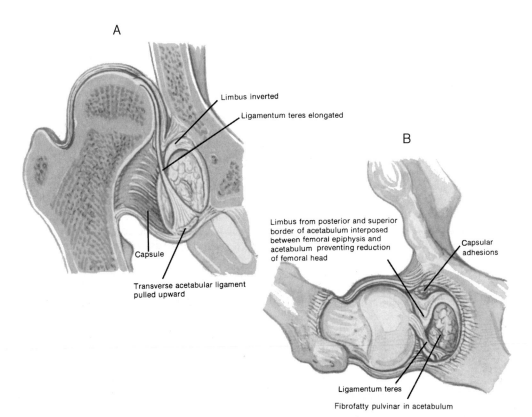

Figure 15–73. Pathology of the dislocated hip that is irreducible owing to intra-articular obstacles. *A,* The hip is dislocated. *B,* It cannot be reduced on flexion, abduction, or lateral rotation. Obstacles to reduction are inverted limbus, ligamentum teres, and fibrofatty pulvinar in the acetabulum. The transverse acetabular ligament is pulled upward with the ligamentum teres. (From Tachdjian MO: Pediatric Orthopedics, 2nd ed. Philadelphia, WB Saunders, 1990.)

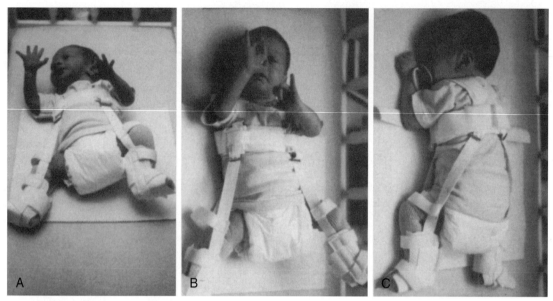

Figure 15–74. The Pavlik harness. (From Tachdjian MO: Pediatric Orthopedics, 2nd ed. Philadelphia, WB Saunders, 1990.)

position the hips at 95 degrees of flexion. The posterior straps are to act as a check, preventing adduction, and do not work as a cinch, pulling the hips into the widely abducted position. The physician should not relegate its maintenance to those untrained in its use. Rather, the child and mother should be seen weekly and the position of the harness carefully checked.

By 3 weeks of age, ultrasound or x-ray must be used to confirm reduction. If the hip is not reduced following 3 weeks of use, other techniques should be employed. This device is not appropriate for children over 6 months of age, for children with muscle imbalance or neuromuscular disease, or for hips that are severely stiff or grossly lax. However, with careful selection and careful maintenance of the device and with ongoing documentation of reduction, one can anticipate 90% success in dysplastic and subluxed hips and 80% success in dislocated hips.

As mentioned previously, the device is not a panacea, and its inappropriate use can result in failure of reduction, femoral nerve palsy (if too flexed), inferior dislocation, and the most severe complication of all, avascular necrosis of the femoral head. Perhaps one of the most difficult decisions to be made by the treating physician is when to discontinue using the Pavlik harness. Certainly one needs to document the stability and adequacy of the reduction prior to considering removal. When employed in a child under 3 months of age, most authors recommend full-time use of the Pavlik harness for 6 to 8 weeks followed by nighttime use for an additional 4 to 8 weeks. Therefore, the total period of wear can range between 2 and 4 months. As a general rule, the older the child at the time of reduction, the longer the Pavlik harness is maintained, again realizing that reduction must be documented. Between 3 and 6 months of age, the Pavlik harness has been documented to be effective; however, as the hip becomes progressively tighter, the use of this harness becomes more problematic. It is difficult to reduce the hip when the hip is contracted. Nevertheless, reduction and maintenance can usually be achieved with the harness up to 6 months of age.

Six to 12 Months of Age. Should diagnosis be delayed or initial treatment in a Pavlik harness fail, then alternative methods are required to relocate the femoral head. Modalities typically used in this age group include traction, with or without the use of an adductor tenotomy, closed reduction under anesthesia, and open reduction.

The use of traction is extremely controversial at the present time. Many believe that it has a role in decreasing the risk of avascular necrosis during treatment. Others believe that it has no efficacy in this mode whatsoever. Frequently, the child who has an extremely narrow safe zone (Fig. 15–75) (in whom the hip is stably reduced within a very narrow range) will be significantly helped by an adductor tenotomy. This simple bedside procedure will frequently widen the safe zone, improve hip stability, and permit reduction and maintenance by closed methods.

Closed reduction has enjoyed somewhat of a checkered past. In the old literature, closed reduction meant the forcible positioning of the femoral head into the acetabulum. This procedure was frequently complicated by relatively high avascular necrosis rates. In addition, the use of extreme positions, such as the Lange or the Lorenz position in the spica cast, only compounded the risk of avascular necrosis. At the present time, closed reduction under anesthesia would better be referred to as "closed positioning" under general anesthesia. No forcible manipulation of the hip should be carried out. Rather, the hip should be placed in the Salter or "human position" with moderate flexion and abduction, and then evaluated for concentric reduction. If the head is adequately reduced as documented by CT scanning, then spica cast immobilization is continued (Fig. 15–76). The time in the cast varies, depending on the instability of the reduction. Most surgeons prefer to change the spica under anesthesia at 4- to 6-week intervals, performing an arthrogram at the time of cast change. Additional documentation with CT scans is also frequently employed.

Open reduction is indicate when the physician is unable to achieve or maintain a concentric reduction. As noted

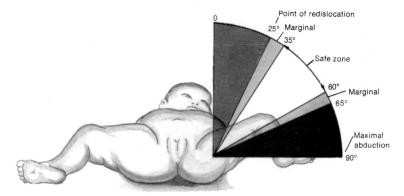

Figure 15–75. Zone of safety. (From Tachdjian MO: Pediatric Orthopedics, 2nd ed. Philadelphia, WB Saunders, 1990.)

earlier, many soft tissue impediments make it difficult to achieve this type of reduction. Should this be the case, then an open reduction is appropriate. The surgical approach, whether it be medial (Ludloff) or anterior (Smith-Peterson) is not as important as the ultimate reduction achieved. Each surgical approach has its proponents, but again, it is important to focus on the goals (achieve a concentric reduction, maintain that reduction, and avoid complications) rather than on the surgical technique. Following open reduction, the patient is immobilized in a hip spica cast for variable periods, based on the stability of the reduction.

Age of Walking. Treatment in this age group is far more complex. It is virtually impossible to achieve a satisfactory reduction without surgical treatment. Depending on the age of the child, various techniques will be employed. These are chosen based on the pathologic deformity to be corrected.

Open reduction is virtually always required. In addition, because of the risk of avascular necrosis in the older child, many authors recommend *femoral shortening*. This procedure, which is usually employed for children over 3 years of age, is said to decrease intra-articular pressure and thereby decrease the risk of avascular necrosis. At the time of femoral shortening, *derotational osteotomy* for persistent anteversion can be carried out. Whether or not one chooses to place the proximal femur in varus depends upon the neck-shaft angle of the femur. Critical analysis following

reduction is important. Arthrographic analysis, as well as radiographic analysis, may help in determining the concentricity of the reduction. In the face of persistent acetabular dysplasia, procedures must be executed to deepen the socket and provide adequate coverage. These procedures can be performed at the time of open reduction or later, as a staged procedure. As mentioned at the onset, persistent acetabular dysplasia condemns the hip to a poor result. Most of the acetabular growth has been achieved by age 4 to 5 years, making it reasonable to follow the hip to that age. If no improvement is seen or the child has reached the age at which no improvement can be anticipated, various pelvic osteotomies are available to correct the dysplasia.

Pelvic Osteotomy. Pelvic osteotomies are an extremely complex group of surgical procedures. It is simplistic to say that the goal is to provide adequate coverage for the femoral head. Nevertheless, that is their major accomplishment. In general, these procedures can be grouped according to what they accomplish.

The first group of pelvic osteotomies is considered to be reconstructive procedures. In that light, the goal is to increase coverage for the femoral head by moving the native acetabulum into a more horizontal position. When accomplished, cartilage-on-cartilage weight bearing is still retained. The *Salter* procedure, described for dysplastic hips in children over 18 months of age, simply moves the acetabulum anteriorly and laterally, improving coverage.

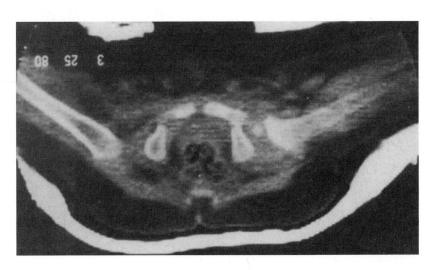

Figure 15–76. Computed tomographic scan showing hip dislocated posteriorly in cast. (From Tachdjian MO: Pediatric Orthopedics, 2nd ed. Philadelphia, WB Saunders, 1990.)

The *Pemberton* procedure (Fig. 15–77) and *Dega* procedure are similar in that they also improve anterior and lateral coverage, with the Dega method adding posterior coverage as well. In addition, they decrease the volume of the acetabulum, which may be a desired result for these shallow sockets. These three osteotomies are best performed in children up to the preadolescent years, when the pelvis still retains some flexibility.

In the older adolescent and in adults, the *Steel* and *Sutherland* osteotomies are used to achieve coverage. Again, these are reconstructive procedures that simply reorient the acetabulum into a more horizontal position. These two procedures require osteotomies through the ilium, the pubis, and, in the case of the Steel osteotomy, the ischium to release the segment of bone containing the acetabulum.

The second group of acetabular procedures is those considered salvage procedures. In this case, one *does not* achieve cartilage-on-cartilage apposition; rather, bone is placed over the femoral head to provide coverage. There is a hope that the interposed capsular structures may go through a process of metaplasia, producing a "cartilaginous-like" tissue. The *Chiari* procedure is the classic salvage osteotomy (Fig. 15–78). Following an osteotomy of the ilium, the proximal fragment is translated over the femoral head to achieve coverage. The *Staheli shelf* procedure uses outer table iliac crest bone as an autograft placed in the supra-acetabular region.

The indications and contraindications for these osteotomies are complex and varied. Specific procedure selection is frequently determined by the experience and prejudice of the surgeon.

Complications. Errors in judgment, errors in the timing of procedures, or errors in execution of those procedures frequently complicate the management of DDH. Redislocation after reduction and avascular necrosis are two of the

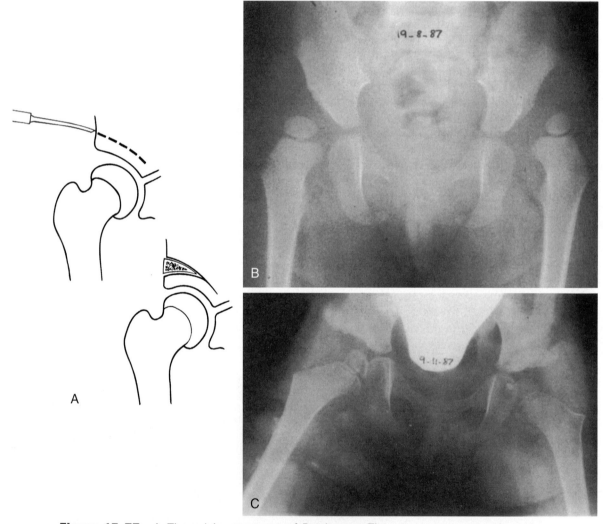

Figure 15–77. *A*, The pelvic osteotomy of Pemberton. The osteotomy curves about 1 cm from the acetabular margin into the triradiate cartilage. Hinging is through the triradiate cartilage as the roof of the acetabulum is brought down and held with a bone graft. *B*, Right hip subluxation and left hip dislocation in a 2¼-year-old girl. *C*, The same child after open reduction of the left hip and bilateral Pemberton's acetabuloplasty. (From Benson MKD, Fixsen JA, MacNicol MF: Children's Orthopaedics and Fractures. Edinburgh, Churchill Livingstone, 1994.)

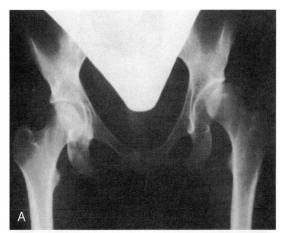

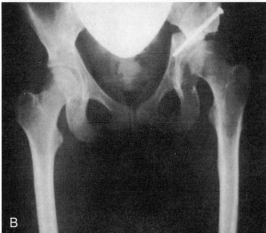

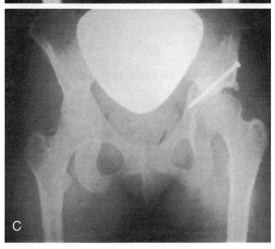

Figure 15–78. The Chiari osteotomy. When, as here *(A)*, subluxation is marked and secondary acetabular changes are beginning to develop, the Chiari osteotomy allows me-dialization of the femoral head and provides a superior bony buttress *(B* and *C)*. (From Benson MKD, Fixsen JA, MacNicol MF: Children's Orthopaedics and Fractures. Edin-burgh, Churchill Livingstone, 1994.)

complications due to these errors. Unfortunately, they can also occur even in the face of appropriate management. Accepting reductions that are less than concentric is a frequent cause of late sequelae. When all is said and done, it must be remembered that DDH is a disease of abnormal

growth. Therefore, even if the management is appropriate, complications, such as acetabular dysplasia, may reflect this aberrant growth.

As mentioned earlier, avascular necrosis (AVN) is the most dreaded of all complications. Salter described the early signs of AVN as seen on the plain x-ray (Table 15–5). Once it occurs, the battle to achieve any functional normalcy is lost. Despite many advances in the manage-ment of DDH, approximately 10% of treated cases will still demonstrate some degree on AVN. Mild cases gener-ally require no treatment, and severe cases generally are not helped by treatment. Night splinting and bracing have been attempted. In addition, acetabuloplasties, trochanteric transfer, and femoral osteotomy have been all suggested in selected cases. Unfortunately, the prognosis for the hip is poor. Recognition of avascular necrosis is generally not difficult. Failure of the ossified nucleus to appear, failure of the ossified nucleus to grow, broadening of the femoral neck, increasing density of the femoral head, and deformity after ossification may all herald this unfortunate event.

Summary. Successful management of the dysplastic hip requires early diagnosis and careful management. There is no place for the frivolous use of the Pavlik harness or other abduction devices. Careful monitoring and follow-up are required if success is to be achieved. It has been said by many individuals that the first person to treat the dysplastic hip is the last person with a chance to produce a normal hip. This only emphasizes the disastrous consequences of inappropriate management.

LEGG-CALVÉ-PERTHES DISEASE

This condition was described in the literature in 1910. Articles by Legg in the United States, Calvé in France, and Perthes in Germany all described a syndrome of idiopathic avascular necrosis of the femoral head in a child. Occasion-ally, Waldenström in Sweden is given credit for pre-empting the other three authors, producing a description of this syndrome in 1909. Unfortunately, he interpreted the condition to be a mild form of tuberculosis; therefore, his name is not frequently associated with the disease. The incidence of Perthes disease is approximately 1 per 1000 in the United States, but it is significantly higher in the United Kingdom. The male-female ratio is about 4:1. Bilat-erality is frequently reported to be approximately 20%.

Etiology. The etiology of this condition remains obscure. Most agree that ischemia is the final common pathway,

Table 15–5. Salter's signs for the early recognition of avascular necrosis

Mottling or fragmentation of the ossific nucleus
Delay in ossification of the ossific nucleus for at least 12 months
Areas of rarefaction, cyst formation, or cupping of the metaphysis
Localized sclerosis of the growth plate
Abnormal growth arrest

From Broughton NS: A Textbook of Paediatric Orthopaedics. London, WB Saunders, 1997.

producing the skeletal changes. The etiology of this ischemic event is clearly debatable. Salter and others have suggested that at least two periods of ischemia are required to produce similar changes in the animal model. In addition, elevated intraosseous venous pressure has been suggested to play a role. Other theories relate to abnormalities in hormones and growth factors, as well as some suggesting that Perthes' disease is a localized chondrodystrophy. These have been not been as well received as the vascular theories. The only other consistent finding is the relative delay in bone age in the affected child. The meaning of this finding remains obscure.

Pathology. The early changes in the femoral head are consistent with ischemia and necrosis; subsequent changes result from repair phenomena. Following the initial necrotic event, enchondral ossification stops in the epiphyseal nucleus; the cartilage overlying it, however, continues to grow. Subchondral collapse due to *bony necrosis* will certainly follow. During this period, the ossification center itself is mechanically labile, and it is not uncommon to see a fracture through this weakened bone. This fracture is seen radiographically as the "crescent sign" (Salter's sign) (Fig. 15–79). Following this necrotic period, *revascularization* occurs. This reparative process is characterized by resorption of dead trabeculae and formation of new bone. As the femoral head heals and remodels, *residual changes* are seen. The process of creeping substitution, whereby new bone replaces the resorbing old necrotic bone, is similar to that seen in areas of fracture callus.

The pathologic changes frequently parallel the stages of the disease: synovitis, necrosis, fragmentation (regeneration), and residua. The *stage of synovitis* lasts approximately 2 weeks. It is characterized by irritability of the hip and a limp; soft tissue swelling and a widened joint space may be seen on the x-ray.

The *avascular stage* lasts approximately 2 months. During that time, the necrotic events are occurring. The capital femoral epiphysis is homogeneously opacified on the x-ray. Some flattening of the head may be seen. It is during this period that the crescent sign is seen.

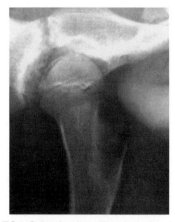

Figure 15–79. Salter's sign. The length of the subchondral fracture line indicates the extent of the involvement of the underlying femoral head. Here the anterior one third of the head is involved. (From Broughton NS: A Textbook of Paediatric Orthopaedics. London, WB Saunders, 1997.)

The *stage of fragmentation or regeneration* is characterized by the repair process. The duration of this stage is approximately 2 years, which is the time required for healing. It takes this long for the dead bone of the necrotic head to be replaced with new viable bone. During this time, rarefaction of the capital femoral epiphysis with irregular ossification of the chondroepiphysis is seen. Also, secondary changes in the femoral neck and physis, as well as teardrop widening, may be noted.

The *stage of residua* is characterized by remaining deformity, once the process has run its course. During healing the femoral head is soft. Eccentric loading can easily deform this pliable growth center, causing late resultant deformity. The active process has resolved. The disease is now static and residual deformity such as coxa plana (flattening of the head), coxa breva (shortening of the neck), and coxa magna (overgrowth of the head), as well as overgrowth of the greater trochanter, may be seen.

Clinical Findings. Typically, these children present with hip pain or a limp. They are usually between 4 and 9 years of age, although an adolescent onset pattern has been described. As mentioned, it is far more common in males than females, and these males typically are small in stature with a delayed bone age. More often than not, their limp is antalgic (caused by pain) in nature, characterized by a shortened stance phase on the involved side. Frequently, hip motion is limited, especially internal rotation. Adductor spasm is commonly seen due to the synovitis of the joint.

Radiologic Findings. Standard x-rays include AP and frog-leg lateral views of the pelvis to include the hips. The radiographic changes parallel the pathologic phenomena. Initially, soft tissue swelling and joint space widening are seen. These changes are rapidly followed by opacification of the necrotic portion of the head. As revascularization begins, rarefaction is the hallmark of this neovascularization. The fragmentation changes of the head actually represent irregular ossification in the capital femoral epiphysis (ossification from multiple centers). Alterations in the height and width of the head are a function of the degree of necrosis. As noted earlier, irregularity of the physis and the metaphysis, occasionally with cystic changes, are often seen as secondary manifestations.

Differential Diagnosis. Most important to consider in the child presenting with a limp and hip irritability is *transient synovitis* of the hip. This will be discussed in the following section. *Multiple epiphyseal dysplasia*, as mentioned earlier, may be confused with this disease. In addition, *tuberculosis* of the child's hip can appear much like Perthes' disease; indeed, this was Waldenström's initial interpretation of the condition. Lastly, *cretinism* must be considered in children with bilateral disease.

Classification. At the present time, three schemes have been proposed to classify Perthes' disease. These methods are all based on radiographic assessment of the involved hip. By far and away, the most widely used is the Catterall classification system. Four groups have been described based upon the percentage of the head involved in the disease process and the degree of collapse seen in those heads (Fig. 15–80). Catterall group I includes those with 25% head involvement, which is largely anterocentral. Group II defines hips with 50% head involvement, being primarily anterolateral. In addition, the medial and lateral columns are intact. Group III extends involvement to 75% of the head, with loss of the medial column, and finally, group IV defines total head involvement. The major problem with the Catterall grouping is interobserver and intraobserver variability.

The *Salter-Thompson classification* is again based on the percentage of subchondral collapse. Two groups are defined: those in group A have less than 50% of the head involved, and those in group B have over 50% of the head involved. Typically, Catterall groups I and II represent hips in Salter group A and Catterall groups III and IV represent hips in Salter group B.

Most recently, the *lateral pillar classification*, as described by Anthony Herring, has gained popularity. In an effort to identify an easily reproducible classification, and eliminate interobserver error, this descriptive grouping was put forth. In addition, these groups can be used prognostically to anticipate probable end results. Group A hips show no lateral pillar (lateral column) involvement. Group B hips demonstrate over 50% lateral pillar height maintained, whereas group C hips show over 50% collapse of the lateral pillar.

In addition to radiographic grouping, a number of classic radiographic signs have been put forward to emphasize the "head at risk" (Fig. 15–81). Pathologically, the head at risk is one that has begun to sublux laterally. This occurs when the head is soft (during the repair phase). If ignored, this lateral subluxation can lead to irreversible changes. These findings suggest a poor prognosis and may indicate a different treatment protocol. Calcification lateral to the epiphysis, subluxation of the hip, horizontal growth plate, and metaphyseal cysts are some of these radiographic signs. Perhaps none is more classic than the finding of Gage's sign. Gage's sign indicates a poor prognosis and, as originally described, is a horizontal V-shaped defect at the junction of the growth plate and the lateral aspect of the neck. In addition to radiographic signs of the head at risk, a number of clinical signs have been described (Table 15–6). Most important among them are the overweight child, progressive loss of motion, and an adduction contracture. In summary, prognostic indicators are centered around the age of onset, the percentage of head involvement, and the radiographic and clinical findings of the head at risk.

Treatment. Despite long-standing recognition of this syndrome, the treatment approaches have changed very little over the past 80 years. It is probably fair to say that as

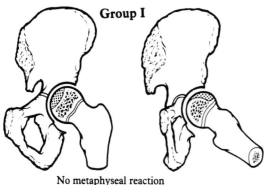

Group I

No metaphyseal reaction
No sequestrum
No subchondral fracture line

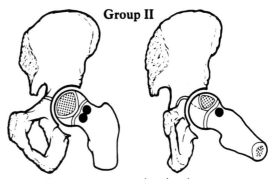

Group II

Sequestrum present—junction clear
Metaphyseal reaction—antero/lateral
Subchondral fracture line—anterior half

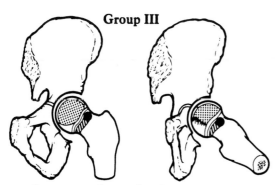

Group III

Sequestrum — large — junction sclerotic
Metaphyseal reaction — diffuse antero/lateral area
Subchondral fracture line — posterior half

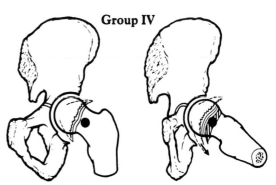

Group IV

Whole head involvement
Metaphyseal reaction — central or diffuse
Posterior remodelling

Figure 15–80. Groups I to IV in Catterall's classification of Perthes' disease. (From Catterall A: The natural history of Perthes' disease. J Bone Joint Surg 1971;53B:37–53.)

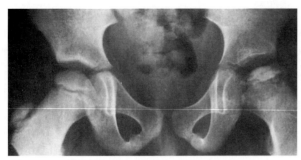

Figure 15–81. Perthes' disease of the left hip in a boy with a chronologic age of 5 years and a bone age of 4½ years. According to the lateral column classification, he is in group C (over 50% loss of lateral column height, although this is somewhat masked by some recent lateral ossification, which also indicates a poor prognosis). A large central area has undergone avascular neurosis. There is a horizontal V-shaped defect at the junction of the growth plate and the lateral aspect of the neck. This is Gage's sign and indicates a poor prognosis, as does the broad band of metaphyseal rarefaction and uncovering of the head. (From Broughton NS: A Textbook of Paediatric Orthopaedics. London, WB Saunders, 1997.)

Table 15–6. Signs of the "head at risk"

Clinical	Progressive loss of movement
	Adduction contracture
	Flexion with abduction
	The heavy child
Radiologic	Gage's sign
	Calcification lateral to the epiphysis
	A diffuse metaphyseal reaction
	Lateral subluxation
	Horizontal growth plate

From Benson MKD, Fixsen JA, MacNicol MF: Children's Orthopaedics and Fractures. Edinburgh, Churchill Livingstone, 1994.

much confusion exists now in the planning of treatment for these children as it did 50 years ago. Several principles, however, have emerged as important in the management of these children. Clearly, the most important measure of success or failure is the development of osteoarthritis of the hip and, if it occurs, the age at which it is seen. Some authors have used age at the time of total hip replacement as a way of assessing outcomes.

The treatment principles, which have been generally accepted as important to successful results, consist of improving and maintaining the range of motion and containment. Emphasis on the concept of containment has remained a consistent treatment principle over the past 30 years. The principle is predicated upon the fact that while the femoral head is in its softened condition it is best to contain it entirely within the acetabulum; by doing so, the femoral head will remodel, assuming the shape superimposed by the acetabulum. Conversely, failure to contain the head permits it to deform, with resulting impingement on the edge of the acetabulum (hinge abduction) (Fig. 15–82). Essentially the implication of the containment theory is that the acetabulum will act as a mold for the regenerating femoral head. If containment is successful, the end result will be a congruous hip joint.

At the time of presentation, the initial goal should be to regain the range of motion. This can be accomplished by

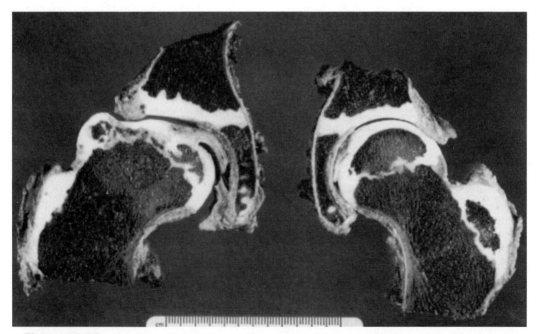

Figure 15–82. Photograph of transverse slab sections taken through the center of the femoral heads in a child of 8 years who died from lymphocytic lymphoma but was also known to have Perthes' disease. On the involved side there is obvious femoral head deformity with impingement between the lateral aspect of the acetabulum and the femoral head, producing a dent. On the opposite normal side there is abnormal thickening of the articular cartilage, particularly on the medial and lateral aspects. (From Benson MKD, Fixsen JA, MacNicol MF: Children's Orthopaedics and Fractures. Edinburgh, Churchill Livingstone, 1994.)

a short period of bed rest, perhaps with the application of longitudinal traction, flexing the knee over a pillow. Nonsteroidal anti-inflammatory drugs (NSAIDs) have been shown to be helpful in this process. Should the child demonstrate a persistent adduction contracture, then adductor tenotomy has been shown to be helpful in regaining range of motion. During this initial period, restricted weight bearing, using crutches or a walker, has proved beneficial. Referral to a physical therapist can be fraught with problems. Typically, in an effort to rapidly achieve motion, the synovitis can actually be worsened. Once range of motion has been improved, then the options for containment should be discussed with the family.

Nonsurgical containment techniques employ devices, whether they be casts or orthoses, to position the hips in abduction and internal rotation. In this position, the femoral head is solely contained within the acetabulum. Gordon Petrie, a Canadian, reported success using two long leg casts, connected with a bar. The legs were placed in 90+ degrees of abduction with internal rotation. These children were admitted to the hospital for cast changes every 6 to 8 weeks, at which time emphasis was placed on range of motion programs. Orthotic devices (Fig. 15–83), such as the Scottish Rite (Atlanta) brace and the Toronto brace, continue to be used to achieve the same effect. Whatever method is chosen, it is important to document that the device is actually containing the femoral head within the acetabulum. Frequently, active boys are able to circumvent the device. Similarly, compliance may become a major issue thwarting the use of nonsurgical approaches.

Surgical containment can be accomplished in several different ways. Proximal femoral *varus derotation osteotomy* has been a popular approach for many years. Its proponents believe that one can provide a legitimate alternative to nonsurgical containment by performing a simple osteotomy of the upper femur. Its critics argue that many of these children are left with a Trendelenburg lurch and a cosmetic asymmetry of the femora. *Pelvic osteotomies* (Fig. 15–84), specifically as described by Salter, have also achieved some popularity. Theoretically, by redirecting the acetabulum, one can improve coverage of the head and thereby improve containment. The Staheli shelf is also currently popular, in some centers, for its relative simplicity in achieving lateral coverage of the head.

Prognosis. The major problem is that few long-term results are available to demonstrate that containment methods are overall effective. The Iowa series, which presents over 40 years of follow-up, indicates that relatively few of these patients have symptoms before the age of 30; even then, their symptoms are relatively modest until the age of 45. Only 8% of patients prior to age 45 had undergone total hip replacement. However, the next decade, between ages 45 and 55, appears to be critical in the deterioration of these hips. By age 56, a full 50% of patients had either undergone total hip replacement or needed total hip replacement. Most of the patients in the Iowa series had been treated by noncontainment methods. Unfortunately, there is no data of this duration to suggest that containment methods dramatically improve outcome. It is clear, however, that once the head has extruded, and especially once hinge abduction occurs, prognosis is generally poor.

At present, some general agreement exists regarding specific treatment protocols based on age of onset. In children aged 5 and under, most authors would recommend simply regaining and maintaining range of motion, without the use of braces, casts, or surgery. The prognosis in this group is excellent.

Between 5 and 8 years of age, treatment protocols again emphasize maintenance of range of motion and the use of some containment method. It is important to remember that surgical containment is not sequentially used with nonsurgical methods. Surgical and nonsurgical methods should be considered as alternatives to one another. If one waits until nonsurgical containment has clearly failed, then surgical containment applied at that point is likewise destined to failure. The decision should be made in conjunction with the family to elect either a nonsurgical or surgical approach. At present, the data are somewhat conflicting regarding the prognosis in this age group.

In children 8 years of age and older, the prognosis is generally considered to be poor, despite the treatment modality chosen. Therefore, most authors recommend only range of motion treatment. Some have suggested the addition of a Staheli shelf in the face of lateral extrusion or hinge abduction. The results of this approach are largely unproved.

Despite the pessimism frequently associated with the diagnosis of Perthes' disease, the vast majority of these children lead a very normal life until their late 20s or early 30s. At that time, hip symptoms develop, and the hip tends to deteriorate over a 10-year period.

Evaluation of Results. The use of *Mose's concentric circles* is one mechanism to evaluate the radiographic result. Typi-

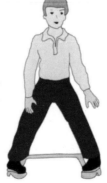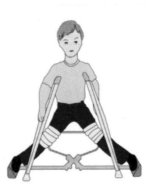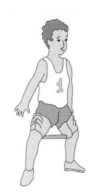

Figure 15–83. Various braces for Legg-Calvé-Perthes disease. Brace management has become less restrictive. Currently, the Atlanta brace *(right)* is most commonly used. (From Broughton NS: A Textbook of Paediatric Orthopaedics. London, WB Saunders, 1997.)

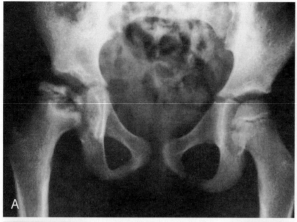
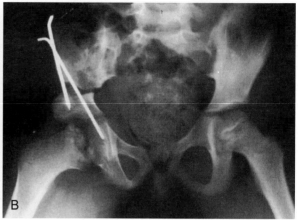
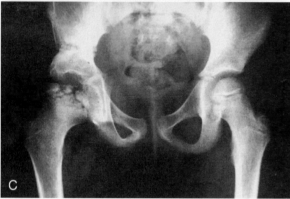

Figure 15–84. *A*, Girl with a bone age of 6 years with less than 50% loss of lateral column height (group B). *B*, Immediately following innominate osteotomy. Note the lateral displacement of the inferior quadrant of the pelvis and the asymmetry of the obturator foramina, indicating forward rotation of the distal pelvis. *C*, Appearance 1 year later. Note the improved containment of the femoral head. (From Broughton NS: A Textbook of Paediatric Orthopaedics. London, WB Saunders, 1997.)

cally, if all the radii of the femoral head fall within 2 mm, one can anticipate a good result. If the radii exhibit between 2 and 4 mm of discrepancy, a fair result is anticipated. Over 4 mm of variation portends a poor prognosis. The *CE angle* of Wiberg, which essentially is a measure of lateral acetabular coverage, is another quantitative measure of prognosis.

Summary. Perthes' disease has been recognized as a specific entity for over 80 years. Despite technologic advances, the treatment of Perthes' disease remains as controversial now as it did when first recognized. Unfortunately, because it is a relatively rare phenomenon, natural history data remains somewhat sparse. Clearly, long-term follow-up data for noncontainment methods exist and overall demonstrate their futility; as yet, containment approaches have yet to show their worth.

TRANSIENT SYNOVITIS OF THE HIP

Transient synovitis of the hip is the most common cause of hip pain and limp in the 5- to 9-year-old age group. It is, however, a diagnosis of exclusion. Other causes of limp must be ruled out before one settles on the diagnosis of transient synovitis.

Characteristically, the child is between ages 4 and 8 and presents with a history of limp of 3 to 4 days in duration. Typically, no systemic findings are reported. With careful history taking, one can frequently uncover a history of an upper respiratory tract infection or ear infection several weeks prior to onset of the limp. Most believe that this represents a nonspecific inflammatory condition of the hip.

Some suggest a postviral allergic synovitis. Nevertheless, the onset tends to be acute, with antalgic limp being the hallmark. The course of this condition is self-limited, and most of the symptoms disappear within 2 weeks. Examining the child demonstrates some restricted motion, particularly in internal rotation and extension. Some local tenderness may be elicited, but systemic symptoms are notably absent.

Imaging techniques are generally not necessary; however, the use of ultrasound is gaining popularity. Some joint effusion and capsular distention are frequently seen. Unfortunately, the first stage of Perthes disease (stage of synovitis) may frequently be confused with transient synovitis of the hip and ultrasound is not able to differentiate between the two. Bone scanning, CT, and MRI scans are not indicated in the evaluation of this disease.

Laboratory studies may be performed to rule out other causes of synovitis. One needs to consider juvenile rheumatoid disease, acute granulomatous septic arthritis, and Lyme disease when evaluating these children. Rarely is sepsis a concern; therefore, aspiration of the hip joint is rarely indicated in these children. However, if sepsis is a genuine consideration, there should be no excuse to defer aspiration. Treatment simply consists of short-term bed rest and activity modification in addition to protected weight bearing. The use of NSAIDs has also proved to be helpful. Recurrence of the acute synovitis does occur and frequently can be associated with a recurrent upper respiratory infection or ear infection. Physical examination and the classic history are usually adequate to diagnose this syndrome and to recommend appropriate treatment modalities.

SLIPPED CAPITAL FEMORAL EPIPHYSIS

In 1888 Mueller, in the German literature, described a condition that he referred to as "bending of the femoral neck in adolescence." This article is considered by most as the initial description of what is now known as slipped capital femoral epiphysis (SCFE). What occurs is a progressive posterior and inferior displacement of the femoral head in relation to the femoral neck. In fact, the femoral head remains relatively stationary within the acetabulum, while the neck displaces anteriorly and superolaterally.

This condition typically presents between 10 and 16 years of age, and 80% of involved patients are obese. Males are 2½ times more likely to be affected than females and there is a higher incidence in blacks. More cases are seen in the summer months for no known reason. The bilaterality incidence is approximately 50%. It has been reported that the left hip is more commonly involved than the right hip, although this fact is debatable. It is critical to be wary of the younger child who presents with a slipped capital femoral epiphysis; in this case, a metabolic etiology should be sought.

Etiology. Most SCFEs are idiopathic without any underlying cause. Because most of the boys are significantly overweight, with delayed pubertal onset, an imbalance between growth hormone and gonadal hormones has frequently been suggested. Endocrine screening of these patients rarely yields any positive findings. There are, however, some specific identifiable etiologies associated with SCFE. Especially when evaluating the younger child, hypothyroidism and hypopituitarism must be considered. In addition, renal osteodystrophy, Marfan's syndrome, and Down's syndrome have all been associated with an increased incidence of SCFEs. Last, although the physical theory seems reasonable based on the size of these children, it has never been proved. Obviously, traumatic separation of the proximal femoral growth plate can occur, but this is best considered to be a Salter I fracture rather than SCFE.

Pathology. Most authors agree that the pathologic portion of the growth plate in SCFE is the zone of hypertrophy (Fig. 15–85). Disorganization of the chondrocyte cell columns occurs with normal alteration in the horizontal and vertical septa. The normal homogeneous matrix in these areas is markedly disoriented and irregular. These changes may cause the physis to be wider than normal. As one would expect, some synovial inflammation and thickening is a common secondary finding. As mentioned earlier, the displacement of the femoral head is posterior and inferior to the femoral neck. As a result, one frequently sees remodeling changes of the posterior femoral neck due to this chronic displacement.

Classification. This is most typically done on the basis of chronology. Acute SCFEs follow a sudden onset of hip pain and have persisted for less than 3 weeks. These are frequently Salter I fractures. A chronic SCFE, on the other hand, is one in which symptoms have lasted longer than 3 weeks and often for many months prior to presentation. Obviously, there are some children who defy classification into these two groups. The child who presents with a prior history of some hip pain complicated by a sudden increase

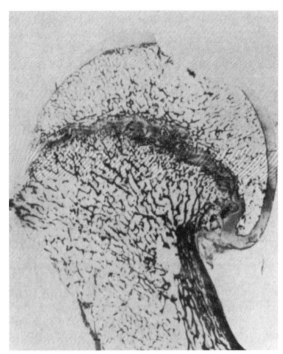

Figure 15–85. Photomicrograph of a specimen of slipped capital femoral epiphysis shows the entire specimen of the femoral head and neck. Note the slipping has occurred through the hypertrophied zone of the physis. (H & E, ×2.) (From Mickelson MR, Ponseti IV, Cooper RR, Maynard JA: The ultrastructure of the growth plate in slipped capital femoral epiphysis. J Bone Joint Surg., 59B:1076, 1977. Reprinted by permission.)

in this pain following an injury is classified as an acute on chronic SCFE.

The extent of the SCFE can also be used to classify these lesions. The pre-SCFE is one in which the child manifests with all the clinical characteristics of the syndrome, but the x-ray for all intents and purposes shows no movement of the femoral head. A mild SCFE has less than one third displacement of the head on the neck. A moderate SCFE has one third to two thirds of displacement of the head on the neck, and the severe SCFE has greater than two thirds displacement of the head on the neck. Last, current literature refers to stable versus unstable SCFEs emphasizing the mobility, which is present between the femoral head and the femoral neck. The hallmark of an unstable slip is the inability of the child to bear weight on the extremity. As is typically seen with chronic SCFEs, most children will walk or limp into the office.

Clinical Presentation. The child with a slipped capital femoral epiphysis that is chronic frequently presents with a history of limp or pain for several weeks to several months. The pain may be localized to the hip (groin) or more typically the knee. The pain in the knee is often attributed to referred pain along the course of the obturator nerve. As mentioned earlier, the child with an acute SCFE is unable to bear weight on the extremity. On physical examination, the body habitus is usually characteristic. The child, when examined in the supine position, will characteristically keep the involved extremity externally rotated. Attempts to range

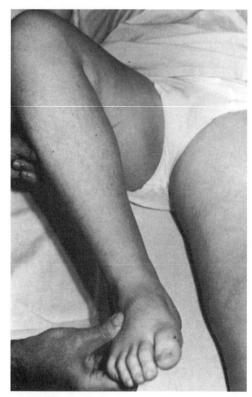

Figure 15–86. Clinical findings in slipped capital femoral epiphysis of the right hip. Hip flexion is limited, and on flexion the hip rotates laterally. (From Tachdjian MO: Pediatric Orthopedics, 2nd ed. Philadelphia, WB Saunders, 1990.)

the hip will usually show significant restriction in flexion and internal rotation. When one attempts to flex the hip, it typically goes into abduction and external rotation (Fig. 15–86).

Imaging Studies. *Plain x-rays* should be obtained in the AP and frog-leg lateral positions. Both hips should be imaged on the same radiograph. It is not unusual that the SCFE not be seen in the AP projection. The use of Klein's line to demonstrate the lesion is important (Fig. 15–87).

This line is drawn along the superior neck and should intersect a small portion of the capital femoral epiphysis in both projections. If it fails to do so, this indicates migration of the head. The extent of the SCFE can also be evaluated on standard x-rays. In addition, remodeling changes of the neck and angular changes of the growth plate can also be appreciated.

Ultrasound has recently been reported to be helpful in the evaluation of these patients. Typically, one can see the presence or absence of joint effusion, evidence of metaphyseal remodeling, and occasionally the degree of the SCFE. In high-grade SCFEs it is occasionally helpful to obtain a *CT scan* to give the treating physician a far better concept of the location of the head in relation to the neck.

Treatment. Again, one must focus on the goals of treatment, if one is to achieve a satisfactory result. Simply stated, the treatment goals for SCFE are as follows:

1. Prevent further displacement of the head.
2. Ensure physeal closure.
3. Avoid complications when doing the first two.

Once the diagnosis is made, the child should be placed on crutches and should avoid weight bearing while hospital admission is planned for the immediate future. The definitive treatment for chronic SCFE is pinning in situ. No attempt should be made to reduce the femoral head by manipulating it onto the neck prior to fixation. The high risks of avascular necrosis and chondrolysis complicating this maneuver make it unwise. Even high-grade SCFEs are best pinned in situ with an osteotomy performed later to correct fixed deformity.

In the case of acute SCFEs or fractures, no remodeling changes have occurred in the femoral neck; therefore, one may consider the use of traction, applied longitudinally with an internal rotation strap, in an effort to restore a more anatomic relation between the head and the neck. Once reduced in this fashion, pinning can then be accomplished with a greater level of safety.

In situ pinning has become the gold standard in the management of this disease. In the past, a number of

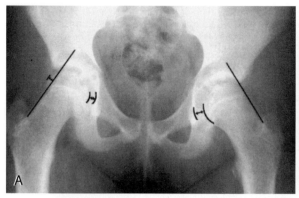
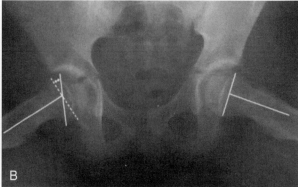

Figure 15–87. *A*, Mild slipped capital femoral epiphyses can be difficult to diagnose radiologically. Comparison with the opposite hip on this anteroposterior radiograph of the pelvis shows the abnormality in the Klein (or Trethowan) line as well as the increased joint space in this patient with a mild right slipped epiphysis. *B*, Frog-leg lateral view of the pelvis confirms the posterior displacement of the head relative to the neck.

devices were used, such as Knowles pins and Hagie pins. At present, the use of a single, large cannulated screw is preferred by most surgeons for the definitive treatment of chronic SCFE. Because of the physeal instability in acute SCFEs, most recommend the use of two screws. Careful radiographic monitoring is required during pin insertion. The screw should cross the growth place in the center and be perpendicular to it in both planes. Care must be taken to ensure that the screw has not entered the joint. Geometrically, it must be remembered that the femoral head is posterior and inferior. Therefore, the initial entry point for screw placement is in the anterior neck (Fig. 15–88). In fact, in high-grade slips it may be necessary for the screw to penetrate the neck anteriorly, exit the neck posteriorly, and then enter the epiphysis.

Postoperatively, most patients are maintained on restricted weight bearing until their synovitis and associated muscle spasm have resolved. Although removal of the screw was popular for many years, at the present time many surgeons elect not to remove the screw, believing that the complications of removal are greater than those associated with leaving it in. In any event, if screw removal is elected, it is critical to be sure that the physis is closed prior to doing so.

Prophylactic routine pinning of the opposite uninvolved side is generally not recommended. However, it should be considered in the young child in whom concerns over significant leg length inequality exist. In addition, any SCFE with an associated endocrine or nutritional syndrome should have both hips pinned, because the bilaterality rate in these conditions approaches 100%.

Complications. *Chondrolysis* describes the global loss of the articular cartilage within the hip joint. Its incidence has been reported to be as high as 10%, and most strikingly, it can occur without surgery. Because of the marked predisposition of blacks to this condition, it has been suggested

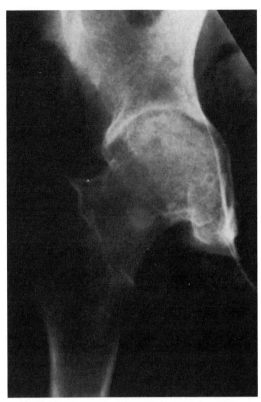

Figure 15–89. Narrowing of the articular cartilage space in chondrolysis of the hip with intrapelvic protrusion of the acetabulum (Otto's pelvis). (From Tachdjian MO: Pediatric Orthopedics, 2nd ed. Philadelphia, WB Saunders, 1990.)

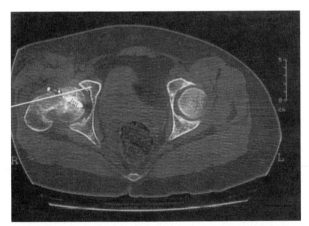

Figure 15–88. Computerized tomography (CT) scan of a chronic severe slipped capital femoral epiphysis with a marked posterior displacement of the epiphysis. It is essential to place the screw through an anterior entry site on the neck. If the screw is placed along the axis of the neck, as shown, the epiphysis is missed or poorly held. CT scans can be used to confirm the position when plain radiographs are difficult to interpret. (From Broughton NS: A Textbook of Paediatric Orthopaedics. London, WB Saunders, 1997.)

that it may actually be an immunologic phenomenon. The concept of an immunologic response to a "sequestered protein" (in this case the proteins of the cartilage) has been put forward by some. Because there appears to be an increased risk of chondrolysis with pin penetration, it has been thought that this supports the immunologic concept. Once the articular cartilage has been breached by the pin, the hip joint becomes vascularized. With vascularization, immunoglobulins now have access to the hip joint, making rejection of the articular cartilage possible. In any event, the syndrome of chondrolysis is characterized by severe loss of joint space (Fig. 15–89) and severe loss of motion. Once it occurs, there is no credible treatment. Symptomatic management including rest, gentle range of motion exercises, and NSAIDs can be helpful in the short term; however, most of these hips go to unsatisfactory results with severe degenerative arthritis and joint contractures. Arthrodesis and arthroplasty are the ultimate treatment for this complication. Because it can occur in the untreated patient, it is considered a complication of the disease.

Avascular necrosis, on the other hand, is a complication of the treatment of SCFE. Most authors agree that it is not part of the natural history of the disease when left untreated. The incidence of avascularity varies with the chronology and severity of the SCFE. It is reported in approximately 5% of chronic slips and approximately 20% of acute slips, especially if manipulation has been performed. Overzealous reduction, poor pin placement, penetration of the head by the pin, and femoral neck osteotomies have all been associated with increased risks of avascular necrosis. Much like chondrolysis, treatment options are limited and generally unsatisfactory. Periods of non–weight bearing with crutches, NSAIDs, and physical therapy have all shown short-term benefits. Although AVN and chondrolysis can coexist, it is important to remember that chondrolysis is a complication of the disease, whereas AVN is a complication of the treatment. Some series have reported AVN in untreated high-grade SCFEs.

Leg length inequality does occur following unilateral slips. If one recalls that approximately 16% of limb length results from the upper femoral plate, it is apparent that premature surgical closure of the plate may cause some discrepancy in limb length. Fortunately, this lesion occurs in adolescence with relatively little time left to grow. Therefore, the inequality rarely exceeds 1 inch.

Deformity of the proximal femur is expected following SCFE. The femoral head will remain in the posterior and inferior position relative to the neck once it has been pinned. This results in some neck varus and external rotational deformity of the limb. Many patients find this cosmetically problematic, if not functionally impairing, in adulthood. Should that be the case, the overall alignment of the proximal femur can be improved using a biplanar intertrochanteric osteotomy as described by Southwick. Although his original osteotomy was performed in the subtrochanteric region, current modifications have placed it in the intertrochanteric position. In this location less proximal femoral deformity is seen, making later arthroplasty a far easier procedure.

Prognosis. As with the other diseases of the immature hip, prognosis is best measured in terms of outcomes. The development of osteoarthritis and the need for joint replacement surgery is probably the best measure of treatment modalities for SCFE. Unfortunately, many long-term studies, such as the one from Iowa, reveal a relatively high incidence of osteoarthritis, even in SCFEs that were well treated without complications. A 10 to 15% incidence of avascular necrosis and a 15% chondrolysis incidence is consistent in many series. As previously mentioned, these two complications often coexist, thereby overlapping the statistics.

Similarly, most long-term series demonstrate the best results with in situ pinning of all SCFEs. The more severe the SCFE and the more acute it is, the more likely that deterioration will be seen early. Arthrodesis or arthroplasty can be utilized to salvage these bad hips.

Knee and Tibia

OSGOOD-SCHLATTER DISEASE

The term "disease" is obviously a misnomer for this entity. Many believe that Osgood-Schlatter disease is better referred to as a condition. This condition was described in 1903 by Osgood in the United States and Schlatter in Switzerland. This condition is the most common of the osteochondroses and is a traction apophysitis. An apophysis is a secondary ossification center, which ultimately develops into a point for muscular attachment. Unlike epiphyses, which are typically loaded in compression, apophyses are loaded in tension. The pull of extremely powerful muscle groups, such as the quadriceps, causes a traction apophysitis. The implication is that low-grade inflammation resulting from chronic mechanical overload, with its resultant swelling and pain, is the source of symptoms in these children.

The typical child presents in the preadolescent years complaining of anterior knee pain. These children will always localize their pain to the tibial tubercle. Characteristically, their pain is made worse with strenuous physical activity and stair climbing. Although the diagnosis is rarely in question based on the clinical evaluation alone, most physicians will obtain x-rays of the knee. The finding of irregular ossification in the area of the tibial tuberosity is not felt to be pathologic.

The treatment of the condition involves both the parents and the child. The parents must be advised that, despite the symptoms, the child is not damaging the knee in any permanent way. The child must understand that the symptoms are primarily activity related. Moderation of activity and the selection of one sport versus many is usually the most help. Adjunctive therapy with icing after activity, lightweight knee straps or braces, and intermittent NSAID administration are all of value. Although some authors have suggested the injection of Xylocaine (lidocaine), this approach has not gained wide acceptance.

OSTEOCHONDRITIS DISSECANS

This condition of the pediatric knee was named by Koenig in the German literature in 1888. It is also considered to be one of the osteochondroses, which are idiopathic self-limited conditions. These conditions result in aberrant enchondral ossification in a local area. Osteochondritis dissecans was recognized by Sir James Paget as a "quiet necrosis." Although the exact etiology of osteochondritis remains uncertain, there has always been the sense that a vascular insult was at its root. Whether this loss of blood flow results from local direct trauma or from a distant mechanism is unclear. The lateral face of the medial femoral condyle is the most frequent location of these lesions (Fig. 15–90). Occasionally, extremely large defects can be seen, giving support to the concept that these lesions may actually represent a partially penetrated skeletal dysplasia.

Most of these patients present in their preadolescent years, complaining of knee pain associated with catching or locking. The physical examination may show a low-grade effusion and direct tenderness over the medial femoral condyle. The plain x-rays, including an AP, lateral, and tunnel view, are usually adequate to make the diagnosis. In recent years, MRI scans have been extremely helpful in documenting the extent of the lesion as well as determining its position.

The treatment is based on the age at presentation and the position of the osteochondritic fragment. In the younger child (8 to 11 years old), one may elect a conservative approach of restricted weight bearing, if the lesion is in situ. In older children (11 to 15 years old), and especially those with unstable lesions, arthroscopic pinning is currently recommended. If the base of the lesion is found to be sclerotic and by inference avascular, drilling, grafting,

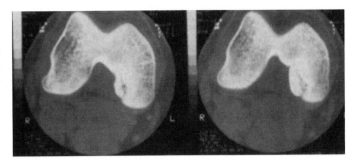

Figure 15–90. Osteochondritis dissecans. Computed tomographic scan of the knee showing osteochondritis dissecans of the medial femoral condyle. Note the clear delineation of the extent of the lesion; the fragment is partially detached. (From Tachdjian MO: Pediatric Orthopedics, 2nd ed. Philadelphia, WB Saunders, 1990.)

or screw fixation have been proposed. Last, the lesion that has displaced into the joint is usually best treated by removal of the fragment. If this fragment constitutes a large portion of the femoral condyle, newer cartilage grafting techniques have been described.

POPLITEAL CYSTS

Baker described the popliteal cyst in 1877. These cysts are essentially synovial cysts located behind the knee. Many communicate directly with the synovial lining of the knee joint, whereas others do not. Most of these cysts tend to be located near the semimembranosus tendon insertion and are typically filled with a gelatinous material. Whereas in adults most popliteal cysts are secondary to intra-articular disease, in children they are believed to be a primary phenomenon.

The parents typically present with the child reporting a mass behind the knee. As one would expect, parental anxiety is high in association with this finding. The child is typically between the ages of 3 and 6 years and has no complaints whatsoever in relation to this mass. Most physicians will obtain an x-ray to exclude other diagnostic possibilities and also to reassure the parents. The use of transillumination and ultrasound have both been reported as helpful, although their value is questionable.

Based on the clinical evaluation and the negative x-ray, the parents can be assured of the diagnosis and advised that the vast majority of these cysts will resolve in a 6-month period. Most authors report about 70% spontaneous regression of these cystic lesions. Surgical excision should be put off until it is clear spontaneous resolution is not likely to occur.

DISCOID MENISCUS

The child who presents with a click or pop in the knee at a relatively young age is almost certain to have pathologic involvement of the meniscus. The meniscus develops from the cells of the interzone as an intra-articular structure. The theory of embryologic delay has been popular for many years. Simply stated, this proposes that the normal C-shaped cartilaginous meniscus is the result of differential changes occurring in an initial "hockey puck"–shaped structure (Fig. 15–91). Current literature, however, suggests that this is not likely to be the cause, leaving the subject of etiology controversial at this point in time.

The vast majority of discoid menisci occur in the lateral compartment and in children between 3 and 7 years of age. Examination shows that most children have no tenderness; however, a loud "clunk" can usually be elicited with flexion and rotational motion of the knee. Persistent clunk-

ing can cause some low-grade effusion and knee pain; in fact, tearing of a discoid meniscus has been reported. MRI scans are certainly more than adequate to confirm the diagnosis, but many take issue with their need. Because this is generally a straightforward clinical diagnosis, the cost of an MRI may make it unnecessary for some. Arthroscopic treatment is usually recommended. Reshaping of the meniscus using arthroscopic techniques has been shown to produce satisfactory results.

BLOUNT'S DISEASE

As discussed earlier, genu varum is a common finding in children. The vast majority of cases are physiologic with correction anticipated with normal growth and development. Blount's disease, on the other hand, is a condition causing progressive varus deformity with an abnormality seen in the medial aspect of the upper tibial growth plate. The condition is very rare in whites but common in blacks, especially in the West Indies. Because many of the children are significantly overweight, excessive loading of the proximal medial tibia has frequently been indicated as the cause of Blount's disease. The infantile onset (1 to 3 years of age), the juvenile onset (4 to 10 years of age), and the adolescent or late onset (after 11 years of age) are the three clinical groups that have been observed. Infantile and juvenile Blount's disease are typically bilateral in distribution, whereas the adolescent form is almost always unilateral.

Clinical findings include obesity, genu varum, and frequently gait disturbances. When observing these children walk, attention should be paid to any translatory motion of the knee. As the varus worsens, not only is angular defor-

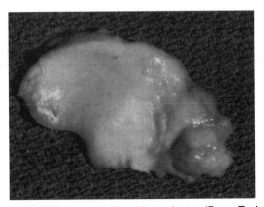

Figure 15–91. Lateral discoid meniscus. (From Tachdjian MO: Pediatric Orthopedics, 2nd ed. Philadelphia, WB Saunders, 1990.)

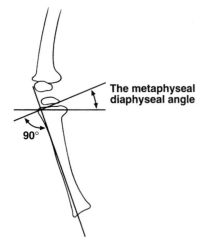

Figure 15–92. Radiologic measurement of the metaphyseal-diaphyseal angle. (From Broughton NS: A Textbook of Paediatric Orthopaedics. London, WB Saunders, 1997.)

mity seen but translation of the tibia laterally under the femur can also be noted. Uncorrected "lateral thrusting" will damage the knee rapidly if allowed to persist.

Radiographic evaluation includes standing APs of both tibias. The metaphyseal-diaphyseal angle of Drennan (Fig. 15–92) is used by many in an effort to differentiate Blount's disease from severe physiologic genu varum. Unfortunately, the debate rages as to the cutoff angle between these two entities. The originally reported 11 degrees is still a somewhat moving target. Most authors feel that an angle of 13 or 14 degrees is more typical of Blount's disease.

The *Langenskiöld classification* has been used for a number of years to grade the severity of Blount's disease. The classification is based upon the radiographic appearance of the proximal tibia (Fig. 15–93). The condition of the growth plate, the extent of the medial beaking, changes in the medial tibial metaphysis, and evidence of premature fusion of the plate medially are all factors in differentiating the grades.

The treatment of Blount's disease depends on the age of the child and the severity of the deformity. The initial use of orthotics in the young child is frequently employed. In concept, the knee-ankle-foot orthosis (KAFO) is designed to protect the extremity in weight bearing and

thereby limit the rate of progression of deformity. Many authors are pessimistic about the true benefits of orthotic management. It is probably best utilized to permit time to pass in order to confirm the diagnosis of Blount's disease rather than mistaking it for severe physiologic tibia vara. If the child clearly is within the high-risk group (an obese, early ambulator who typically is a black female), one should be more aggressive in moving toward a surgical option.

Osteotomy of the proximal tibia to correct the varus and in fact produce valgus in the limb is the definitive surgical treatment. Wedge and dome osteotomies of the tibia both seem to be effective ways to correct the deformity. It is important to osteotomize the fibula at the time of tibial osteotomy. Otherwise, the risk of postoperative compartment syndrome is increased. The use of lateral epiphyseal stapling, although reported, is generally not employed alone except in the older age group. The family should be warned that repeat osteotomies may be required if they are performed at an early age.

CONGENITAL PSEUDARTHROSIS OF THE TIBIA

This poorly understood dysplastic condition of the tibia has puzzled orthopaedists for many years. Not only is the etiology obscure, but the treatment remains controversial. The defect is reportedly confined to the lower half of the tibia, where the bone is clearly abnormal. The diseased bone in this region permits anterolateral angulation. In addition, stenosis of the medullary canal and the ultimate pathologic fracture are the anticipated sequelae. Following fracture, pseudarthrosis is the natural result; the treatment of this pseudarthrosis is characterized by poor results. Many have described the abnormal tissue as hamartomatous in nature. In addition, a relation of this condition to neurofibromatosis has been suggested for many years. Although neurofibromatosis can cause pseudarthroses in numerous bones, this condition often appears as an isolated defect in the tibia. This syndrome is rare, occurring in 1 per 100,000 live births, and is unilateral in the vast majority of cases. It is important to differentiate this condition from congenital posteromedial angulation of the tibia and fibula (Fig. 15–94). This latter condition is obvious at birth, due to the apparent calcaneovalgus foot. The prognosis for posteromedial angulation is far better than that for congenital pseudarthrosis (anterolateral bow).

Clinically, the initial diagnosis is usually made prior to

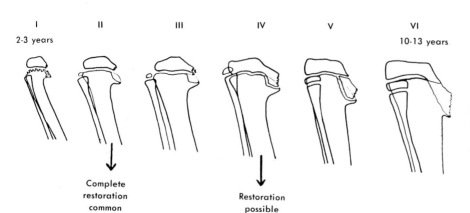

| I | II | III | IV | V | VI |
| 2-3 years | | | | | 10-13 years |

Complete restoration common

Restoration possible

Figure 15–93. Infantile type of tibia vara—the six progressive stages develop with increasing age. (From Langenskiöld A: Tibia vara. Acta Chir 1952;103:9.)

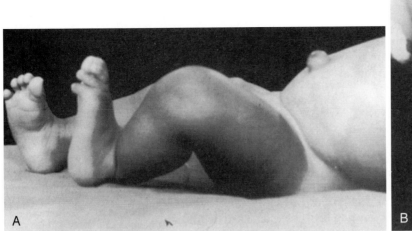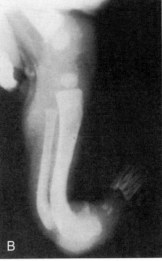

Figure 15–94. *A,* Clinical photograph of a child aged 5 months with tibia recurvatum. Note the calcaneus position of the foot. *B,* Lateral radiograph of the same patient. Note the marked posterior bowing of both the tibia and fibula. (From Benson MKD, Fixsen JA, MacNicol MF: Children's Orthopaedics and Fractures. Edinburgh, Churchill Livingstone, 1994.)

fracture. This phase has frequently been referred to as the prepseudarthrosis stage. Many recommend orthotic protection at this time in an effort to forestall pathologic fracture. Unfortunately, many of these children are exceedingly active, making the ultimate fracture inevitable. The fracture in turn always fails to unite and results in a pseudarthrosis.

Once the pseudarthrosis occurs, the complexity of treatment increases. Despite the operative approach chosen, the extremity typically remains dysplastic, short, and functionally impaired. Most parents are unwilling to accept amputation surgery despite the fact that many still believe it offers the best chance of rapid mobilization for the child.

Current surgical techniques include onlay bone grafting procedures with intermedullary fixation, Ilizarov's bone transport techniques, or the use of a free vascularized fibular transplant. At present, it is fair to say that bone transport surgery is the initial procedure chosen by most physicians. The free fibular transplant is usually reserved as a second-line procedure, when others have failed. After multiple procedures, amputation may remain as the best surgical option.

Foot and Ankle

The child's foot and its normal variations can provide a source of significant anxiety for parents and grandparents alike. Recalling what was mentioned earlier, that 50% of pediatric orthopaedic referrals are for "nondisease," the foot is the source of many of these consultations. The parents and more particularly the grandparents are frequently unhappy with the shape or configuration of the young child's foot. However, relatively few of these feet are pathologic. It is therefore important to recognize which feet are normal and which are abnormal. All children are flatfooted at birth; the arch does not develop until 2 years of age. When children start to walk, they do so with a "toddler gait," which is a flatfooted pattern with a wide base. Heel-toe gait does not develop until after age 2.

Many of the odd shapes of the infant's foot are the result of "uterine-cramming" syndromes and are by no means pathologic. Probably the single most important thing that the physician can do when examining the child's foot is to "feel the foot." In general, feet that are supple and easily correctable with gentle pressure are benign. Conversely, feet that are rigid and stiff are usually pathologic.

CALCANEOVALGUS

The calcaneovalgus foot (Fig. 15–95) will be seen in 1 in 1000 neonates. Typically, the forefoot is dorsiflexed and everted as well as abducted. As a result, the anterodorsal soft tissues tend to be tight. Despite these changes, the foot is usually flexible enough to be gently manipulated into a normal position. This suggests that 99% of these feet are the result of intrauterine positioning, and therefore do not

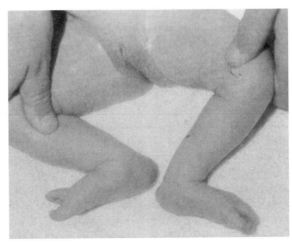

Figure 15–95. Clinical photograph of typical calcaneovalgus feet in the newborn infant. (From Benson MKD, Fixsen JA, MacNicol MF: Children's Orthopaedics and Fractures. Edinburgh, Churchill Livingstone, 1994.)

require significant treatment. Perhaps the most important thing to remember is the need to rule out congenital vertical talus, which can look very similar to this benign foot. The latter is a pathologic, fixed deformity, which prohibits manipulation into a normal position. If confusion exists, a simple x-ray is adequate to make the differential diagnosis. In addition to congenital vertical talus, spinal anomalies and congenital posteromedial bowed tibia may also be associated with the calcaneovalgus foot. If treatment is warranted, stretching exercises, serial casting, or light-weight braces may be helpful.

HYPERMOBILE FLATFEET

Although the hypermobile flatfoot was thought to be pathologic for many years, at the present time it is considered a variation of normal and not a pathologic entity. Typically, this is a genetic trait and frequently is manifest in the parents or grandparents. When the child is standing, the arch is flattened (Fig. 15–96). However, on examination the foot is noted to be very flexible, and if the child is asked to sit down (hence, non–weight-bearing) or stand on their toes, the arch reconstitutes itself. The heel is in modest valgus.

Many of these feet actually improve as the child gets older, with a more definite arch appearing after puberty. Despite the configuration of the foot, this condition is a much bigger problem for the parents than it is for the child. The vast majority of children are asymptomatic during their childhood. Some will develop mild arch symptoms as they get heavier, and others may have some mild calf pain due to heel cord contractures.

Treatment is usually not necessary. However, if for whatever reason one wishes to treat these children, the use of a commercially available arch support is usually more than adequate. If calf pain is present, it is easily remedied with an aggressive heel cord stretching program. The prescription for custom-made inserts in the small child is absolutely unnecessary and outrageously expensive.

The one variation of the hypermobile flatfoot that may require surgery is the associated accessory navicular syndrome. Approximately 25% of these children will have an extra ossicle adjacent to the medial side of the navicular. Typically, this ossicle is contained within the insertion of the posterior tibial tendon. Should the child have pressure

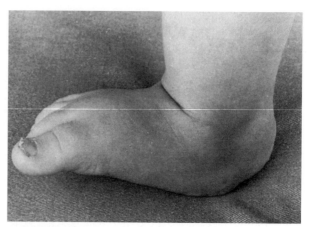

Figure 15–97. Clinical appearance of congenital vertical talus with a rocker bottom foot. (From Broughton NS: A Textbook of Paediatric Orthopaedics. London, WB Saunders, 1997.)

symptoms or develop a painful bursa over this ossicle, the Kidner procedure is recommended. Excision of the ossicle with advancement of the posterior tibial tendon produces predictably good results.

CONGENITAL VERTICAL TALUS

The congenital vertical talus is a true congenital abnormality of the foot. It is one of the causes of a rigid flatfoot—that is, one that does not improve with toe standing or non–weight bearing. Typically, the talus is in a vertical position, causing the navicular to be dislocated onto the dorsum of the neck of the talus. Typically, in the newborn, the foot is described as "serpentine," "Persian slipper," or "congenital rocker bottom" foot (Fig. 15–97). The head of the talus is palpable on the plantar surface of the foot. As a result of the midfoot breach, the posterior capsule and the heel cord tend to be contracted. The forefoot is dorsiflexed and abducted. Approximately 50% of these feet are isolated abnormalities, whereas the others are associated with syndromes, especially myelodysplasia. Examination of these feet shows them to be rigid and not correctable with gentle passive stretch. X-rays, specifically a *forced plantarflexion lateral* view, will confirm vertical position of the talus and the dorsal dislocation of the navicular.

Treatment of congenital vertical talus is best accomplished before the age of walking. Early serial casting is essential preoperatively. The goal is to stretch the skin and tendinous structures as a prelude to surgical correction. Originally, Sherman Coleman had proposed a two-stage surgical corrective procedure. Currently, however, most authors recommend a one-stage procedure, performed much like a comprehensive clubfoot release. Pinning of the deformed osseous structures is critical to maintain the corrected position of the foot. Some also recommend postoperative splinting or bracing, until the child is ambulating, to guard against recurrence.

PERONEAL SPASTIC FLATFOOT

Many articles were written describing a rigid type of flatfoot associated with peroneal muscle spasm. In the early

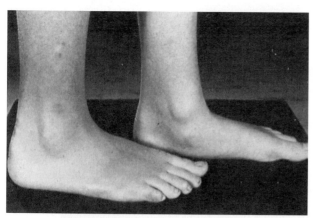

Figure 15–96. Physiologic flatfeet.

literature, the cause and effect became confused. Initially, it was proposed that the rigid flatfoot was the result of, rather than the cause of, the peroneal muscle spasm. Harris and Beath and others pointed out that, indeed, the primary cause of the rigid foot is frequently a tarsal coalition or other hindfoot pathologic condition. Although these feet appear similar to hypermobile flatfoot, simply feeling the foot allows the examiner immediately to appreciate the rigidity characteristic of this condition (Table 15–7).

Tarsal coalitions result from a failure of segmentation during development (Fig. 15–98). Partial or complete fibrous, cartilaginous, or osseous bars persist between two or more adjacent tarsal bones. The calcaneonavicular bar and the talocalcaneal bar are the two most frequently seen. The literature is somewhat controversial regarding which is the most common; however, most authors seem to believe that the calcaneonavicular bar is most often seen. The typical patient is a preadolescent or adolescent, who presents with increasing arch pain or ankle pain following activity. When the foot is evaluated, it is noted to be flat and does not correct with toe standing. Feeling the foot reveals it to be quite rigid and uncorrectable. The heel lies in excessive valgus, and peroneal muscle spasm can usually be appreciated.

Imaging studies are initiated with AP, lateral, and Sloman views of the foot. The calcaneonavicular bar is best

Table 15–7. Classification of flatfeet

Physiologic
Nonphysiologic
Congenital
    Congenital talipes calcaneovalgus
    Congenital vertical talus
Painless
    Flatfoot associated with ligamentous laxity
    Flatfoot associated with tightness of Achilles tendon
    Paralytic flatfoot (cerebral palsy, spina bifida)
Painful or peroneal spasmodic flatfoot
    Tarsal coalition
    Subtalar irritability (idiopathic, septic arthritis, osteoid
      osteoma, juvenile chronic arthritis, traumatic subtalar
      degenerative changes)

From Broughton NS: A Textbook of Paediatric Orthopaedics. London, WB Saunders, 1997.

visualized on the Sloman oblique view. On the other hand, subtalar bars are frequently not apparent on these plain films unless one also requests a Harris "ski jump" view. The finding of a talar beak on the superior aspect of the talar head (Fig. 15–99) is a signal that hindfoot rigidity exists. This beak essentially is a traction spur representing increased talonavicular motion. This increased motion is the result of restricted subtalar or calcaneonavicular motion. The talar beak itself should not be misconstrued as an osteoarthritic change.

The calcaneonavicular bar is, by most reports, the most common. It may be fibrous, cartilaginous, or bony and it may be complete or incomplete. Initial conservative management with commercial arch supports and stretching exercises may be helpful in the younger child. However, in the older child, excision of the bar and extensor brevis

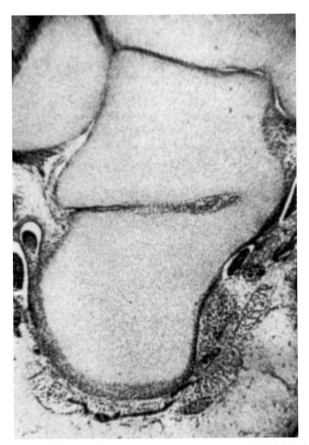

Figure 15–98. Complete medial talocalcaneal bridge in the foot of a 72.3-mm fetus (coronal section). (Courtesy of Barbara Anne Harris Monie; from Harris RI: Retrospect—peroneal spastic flat foot. J Bone Joint Surg 1965; 47A:1658. Reprinted by permission.)

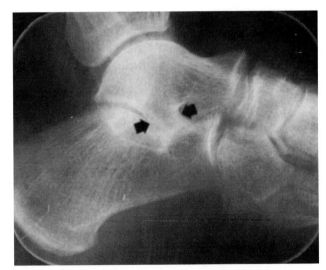

Figure 15–99. Secondary signs of calcaneonavicular coalition as seen in the lateral radiograph of the foot. Note the beaking of the head of the talus, the broadening of the lateral process of the talus, and the narrowing of the cartilage space of the posterior subtalar joint. (From Tachdjian MO: Pediatric Orthopedics, 2nd ed. Philadelphia, WB Saunders, 1990.)

arthroplasty as described by Cowell is recommended. The results of this procedure are generally excellent in relieving pain. The configuration of the foot is not changed by surgery.

The talocalcaneal bar is more problematic. Recall that the subtalar joint has three individual facets (Fig. 15–100): a small anterior facet, a middle facet, and a large posterior facet. The most common coalition is seen involving the medial subtalar facet. Because standard radiographs are usually not helpful in bar localization, a CT scan is a far better study. Not only can it aid in diagnosis, but it can also assist in evaluating extent (Fig. 15–101). Treatment is frequently initiated with a short leg cast to decrease inflammation and pain. Once conservative management has failed, however, bar excision is a reasonable next step. Unfortunately, the prognosis for the resected talocalcaneal bar is not as good as the calcaneonavicular bar. Occasionally, excision will relieve the pain, but it never changes the shape of the foot. Some talocalcaneal bars are so large that resection is not an option. Should the bar be too large or resection fail, the best surgical option is subtalar arthrodesis or triple arthrodesis, depending on secondary changes in adjacent joints.

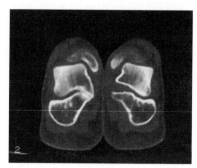

Figure 15–101. Computerized tomographic appearance of talocalcaneal bar in the left foot. The right foot shows the appearance following surgical excision of a similar bar. (From Broughton NS: A Textbook of Paediatric Orthopaedics. London, WB Saunders, 1997.)

METATARSUS ADDUCTUS

Commonly, a small child presents with the complaint of toeing-in. On examination, the entire forefoot is adducted at the tarsometatarsal joint. Frequently, the great toe lies in varus with prominent overactivity of the foot invertors. The foot typically can be manipulated into a neutral position with minimal difficulty. There is no rigidity and no crease is found on the medial plantar aspect of the foot. These findings easily differentiate postural metatarsus adductus from congenital metatarsus varus, the latter being a rigid deformity that is not passively correctable. Some authors have suggested an association between metatarsus adductus and DDH, making careful hip screening important. Others believe that the stated association is artificial. The vast majority of children with metatarsus adductus can be treated by observation. Many classify this condition into three types. Type I will correct with only peroneal stimulation (stroking the bottom of the foot on the lateral border). Type II metatarsus adductus is correctable to neutral with gentle manual pressure. Last, type III metatarsus adductus is not correctable with passive stretch, and many would suggest that this foot actually represents congenital metatarsus varus (Fig. 15–102).

The treatment dilemma is to determine which feet will correct untreated. Unfortunately, the initial severity usually is not related to outcome, and most series suggest that about 10% require treatment. In general, the type I foot requires no treatment whatsoever. The type II foot might best be treated with straight last shoes, stretching, or a lightweight polypropylene brace. The type III foot, which many believe is actually a pathologic congenital metatarsus varus, is best treated by early abductor hallucis and medial capsular release followed by casting and maintenance bracing.

ADOLESCENT BUNION DEFORMITY

Like the adult bunion deformity, that seen in an adolescent characteristically has the same three features: hallux valgus, metatarsus primus varus, and exostosis. The adolescent usually will manifest a significant degree of metatarsus primus varus, which many believe is the hereditary component of the bunion deformity. This deformity in young patients is frequently progressive and considered to be an

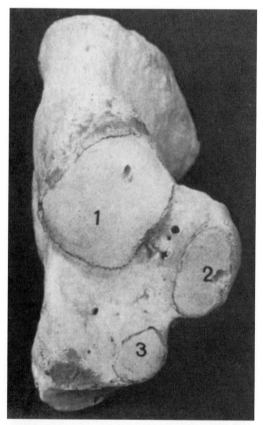

Figure 15–100. The dorsal surface of the calcaneus. Note the three facets of the subtalar joint. The posterior facet (1) is in the posterior compartment. The middle facet (2) and the anterior facet (3) are in the anterior compartment. (Courtesy of Dr. H. Cowell.) (From Tachdjian MO: Pediatric Orthopedics, 2nd ed. Philadelphia, WB Saunders, 1990.)

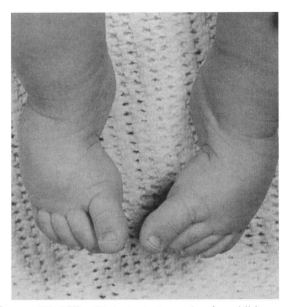

Figure 15–102. Clinical photograph of a child aged 9 months with the severe type of metatarsus varus showing a significant medial crease. This deformity was rigid and not passively correctable. (From Benson MKD, Fixsen JA, MacNicol MF: Children's Orthopaedics and Fractures. Edinburgh, Churchill Livingstone, 1994.)

autosomal dominant condition. There is relatively little place for the conservative treatment of these bunions. Most of these children simply require a widened shoe until such time as correction is required. Most authors still recommend waiting until skeletal maturity prior to surgical treatment of bunions in adolescents. When done early, many series still report only 50 to 60% good results. The surgical treatment should obviously include first metatarsal osteotomy to correct the metatarsus primus varus. Distal soft tissue procedures alone will be woefully inadequate to treat the deformity in this age group.

PES CAVUS

The patient with an elevated arch is frequently said to have a cavus foot. The abnormal elevation of the longitudinal arch is the primary determinant of this anatomic abnormality. The most critical issue is to determine whether the elevated arch is pathologic or physiologic. Unlike flatfoot, a true cavus foot is of significant clinical importance. The vast majority of patients with a true, pathologically elevated arch have a specific neuromuscular disease, which has caused this distal effect. The cavovarus foot is usually rigid. Because of the deformity, secondary changes are frequently seen and include plantar callosities over the metatarsal heads, clawing of the toes, and instability of the hindfoot. This unstable hindfoot typically assumes a varus position.

Most cavus feet are classified based on the apex of the arch deformity. Anterior or forefoot cavus typically shows an apex at the metatarsocuneiform joints. Midfoot cavus usually has as its apex the anterior tuberosity of the calcaneus, and hindfoot cavus (calcaneocavus) is characterized by the vertical position of the os calcis. Frequently the calcaneal pitch angle is greater than 30 degrees.

The true pathogenesis of the cavus deformity is complex and controversial. Weak triceps surae muscles have been associated with calcaneocavus, whereas midfoot cavus has been said to result from overactive long extensors. Whatever the mechanism, once the cavus occurs the first metatarsal typical plantarflexes and the plantar fascia contracts. As previously noted, the overactive long extensors frequently produce secondary clawtoe deformities. With progressive plantarflexion of the first metatarsal the forefoot tends to pronate, which in turn causes the hindfoot to supinate in order to get the foot plantigrade (Fig. 15–103). Initially these deformities are flexible, but as they persist over time, they become rigid.

The evaluation of the patient with a cavus foot must include an aggressive search for neurologic cause. Failure to do so and simply manage the foot deformity is clearly an error both in diagnosis and treatment. The *Coleman lateral block test* (Fig. 15–104) is the classic way in which flexibility of the cavus foot is determined. A 1-inch block is placed under the heel and the lateral border of the foot. This allows the first three metatarsals to fall free of the block and fall into pronation. If the hindfoot supination or varus corrects, the hindfoot is flexible and the deformity requires only forefoot surgery. Conversely, if the hindfoot varus does not correct, then it is rigid and forefoot and hindfoot surgery will be required for correction. Radiographic evaluation includes AP and lateral standing films of the foot. Meary's angle can be used to assess the degree of pes cavus (Fig. 15–105).

The treatment of this deformity is complex. Nonsurgical management is not usually adequate to relieve symptoms or to control the deformity. Therefore, surgical treatment is usually required. Depending on the extent of deformity and the rigidity of the deformity, soft tissue procedures or bony procedures may be required. Plantar fascia release and

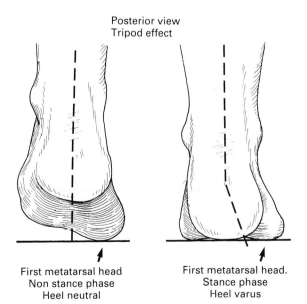

Posterior view
Tripod effect

First metatarsal head
Non stance phase
Heel neutral

First metatarsal head.
Stance phase
Heel varus

Figure 15–103. Drawing to illustrate the tripod effect responsible for producing heel varus as a result of a rigid plantarflexed first metatarsal. (From Benson MKD, Fixsen JA, MacNicol MF: Children's Orthopaedics and Fractures. Edinburgh, Churchill Livingstone, 1994.)

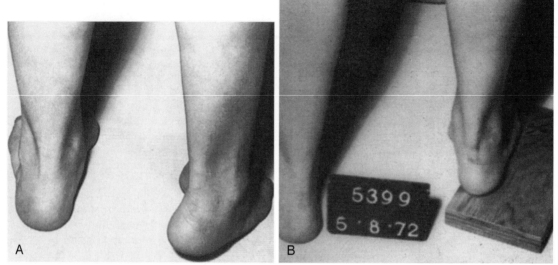

Figure 15–104. Illustration of a method of documenting hindfoot flexibility in a cavovarus foot; posterior view of the foot of a 9-year-old boy with Charcot-Marie-Tooth disease. Note heel varus *(A)*. By placing the heel on a 3-cm block, eliminating the effect of the first metatarsal, the heel assumes a normal position *(B)*. (From Benson MKD, Fixsen JA, MacNicol MF: Children's Orthopaedics and Fractures. Edinburgh, Churchill Livingstone, 1994.)

dorsal wedge osteotomy of the first metatarsal are the mainstays of treatment. If significant inversion is seen, a split anterior tibial tendon transfer may be helpful. With fixed hindfoot deformity, calcaneal osteotomy will be required to correct the hindfoot varus. In the presence of a high-arched midfoot that has been of long standing, a Cole dorsal midfoot osteotomy may be required. If all else fails, triple arthrodesis is the definitive salvage procedure. Because many long-term series show overall patient dissatisfaction with the triple arthrodesis, one should tailor the procedures to the individual patient. Certain neuromuscular diseases seem to have better outcomes with specific procedures. For example, paralytic cavovarus with weak musculature is best treated with a triple arthrodesis. The cavovarus seen in Charcot-Marie-Tooth disease seems to be best managed with plantar release, tendon transfers, and calcaneal osteotomies rather than resorting to a triple arthrodesis.

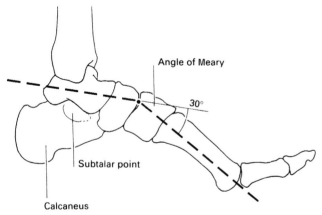

Figure 15–105. Meary's angle. (From Benson MKD, Fixsen JA, MacNicol MF: Children's Orthopaedics and Fractures. Edinburgh, Churchill Livingstone, 1994.)

FOOT PAIN IN CHILDREN

Foot pain is an extremely common complaint and is almost always benign. The child who presents with a painful foot is easily evaluated with a physical examination and standard x-rays. Some of the common causes of pain in the foot of a child are the osteochondroses (local disorder of enchondral growth).

Köhler's disease is osteonecrosis of the tarsal navicular. Typically, this is seen in a 4- to 6-year old child, who presents with pain and swelling around the arch of the foot. The etiology of the syndrome complex is believed to be primarily repetitive trauma. The radiograph will demonstrate generalized opacification and sclerosis of the tarsal navicular. Occasionally, the bone will appear flattened in the lateral projection.

Treatment should be conservative. Many believe that even untreated, this is a self-limited process. During the symptomatic phase, short leg casting followed by a longitudinal arch support is usually adequate to control symptoms. Within 1 year of onset, the x-ray usually demonstrates normalization of the tarsal navicular.

Avascular necrosis of the second metatarsal head (Freiberg's infraction) is a cause of pain typically in the adolescent. The increased incidence in females suggests that the frequent discrepancy in length between the first and second metatarsals may be a factor. Again, repetitive microtrauma has been indicated in many cases. The radiograph will demonstrate flattening of the involved metatarsal head. Additional imaging studies are felt to be overkill.

Conservative treatment is best, with short-term immobilization and appropriate orthotic management. Unfortunately, jumping sports and contact sports will need to be avoided in the short term. Despite conservative treatment, some of these cases do not resolve spontaneously and surgery may be indicated. Various techniques include excision of the necrotic bone with grafting or simple shortening of the metatarsal to relieve the weight bearing on the plantar surface.

Sever's disease is the most common cause of heel pain in children. It also has been described as an avascular necrosis (osteochondrosis) of the calcaneal apophysis. It is better compared to Osgood-Schlatter disease in that it is likely a traction apophysitis. Typically, the patient is 5 to 10 years of age and presents with heel pain during or after activity. Physical findings are generally limited to tenderness over the tuberosity of the os calcis, and x-rays typically show fragmentation changes of the calcaneal apophysis, which are misinterpreted as pathologic. These latter changes reflect only the normal irregular ossification in that secondary ossification center.

Treatment consists of activity modification, intermittent NSAIDs, heel padding, and heel cord stretching exercises. Injection with lidocaine or cortisone should be discouraged.

Miscellaneous causes of foot pain in children have been previously mentioned in the text. Such things as accessory naviculars in association with flatfoot deformity can cause pain on the medial side of the foot. Juvenile rheumatoid arthritis can frequently present with hindfoot pain and subtalar stiffness. Skin changes on the plantar surface of the foot may also cause the child to have pain and limp. Plantar warts frequently will produce plantar pain in the child. Haglund's deformity in the adolescent female is a classic cause of heel pain and is caused by friction from the tight counter of the shoe against the calcaneal tuberosity. Initially a bursa develops, followed by an exostosis. Stress fractures of the calcaneus and the metatarsals have been reported in children and may produce symptoms.

TOE DEFORMITIES

Congenital deformities of the toes are relatively common. Syndactyly can occur and can be partial or complete. A standard x-ray will differentiate between simple (skin involvement only) and complex (skin and bony involvement) syndactylies. The technique chosen for separating the toes depends on the type of deformity seen. Congenital curly toe is a common finding. Frequently, this condition is bilateral and usually affects the second or third toe. Curly toe has a high familial incidence and causes a great deal of parental concern. Unfortunately, it does not correct spontaneously and tends to worsen with growth. Initially, taping and stretching can be used but when symptoms develop, flexor tendon reconstruction is appropriate.

CONGENITAL CLUBFOOT

Referred to as talipes equinovarus, congenital clubfoot is seen in 1 per 1000 live births. It is more common in males than females and occurs bilaterally in 30 to 40% of children. A multifactorial inheritance pattern has been ascribed to this condition. The clinical spectrum is very wide, ranging from severe fixed contractures, in which even surgical intervention is occasionally inadequate to achieve a satisfactory correction, to relatively mild deformities, which may be adequately corrected nonoperatively with serial casting.

Etiology. Numerous theories have been put forward over the years to suggest the cause of this deformity. Clearly, it is not an intrauterine cramming syndrome. Although abnormal uterine forces have been emphasized, the rigidity seen in these feet speaks against the postural nature of these abnormalities. Arrested limb bud development is often cited as a potential etiology. Some authors have demonstrated abnormal muscle fibers in extremities when a clubfoot is seen. Whether or not there is a myopathic basis for clubfoot remains to be seen. Certainly, there is a genetic component to the etiology, because there is an increased incidence in families with affected individuals. It is important, when evaluating the child with a clubfoot, to be sure that the clubfoot is not simply one manifestation of a syndrome. Many dysmorphic and neuromuscular syndromes are characterized in part by talipes equinovarus. Diastrophic dwarfism, arthrogryposis, and chromosomal diseases may all show this condition. In addition, myelodysplasia, spinal muscle atrophy, muscular dystrophy, and occasionally cerebral palsy may likewise present with this foot deformity.

Pathologic Anatomy. Carroll and others believe that the basic pathology is found in the talus. Changes in soft tissues, other bones, and adjacent articulations tend to be secondary to the talar disease and together these changes produce the overall malformation. The neck of the talus is deviated medially and plantarward, causing the subjacent calcaneus to rotate into varus (Fig. 15–106). In turn, the calcaneus dislocates from the calcaneocuboid articulation, and as the forefoot medially subluxes, the navicular is carried dorsally and medially onto the neck of the talus. This can be so extreme that the navicular will articulate with the medial malleolus. It is important to recognize that not only is the talus deviated in an abnormal direction, but the shape of the bone itself is abnormal. The body of the talus is directed laterally within the ankle mortise, but the neck of the talus is angulated medially. Associated with these osseous deformities are contractures of the capsules and ligaments of the ankle and subtalar joints. The tendons of the tibialis posterior, flexor hallucis longus, and flexor digitorum longus are contracted. In addition, intrinsic muscles of the foot, such as the flexor digitorum brevis and abductor hallucis brevis, are contracted. Other associated findings include relative atrophy of the calf and internal tibial torsion.

Clinical Presentation. The foot is typically fixed in equinus with hindfoot varus and forefoot adductus, hence the name *talipes equinovarus* (Fig. 15–107). It is important to note the presence or absence of a crease along the medial column (medial border) of the foot. The entire hindfoot appears to be supinated, carrying much of the midfoot and forefoot with it. "Feeling" the foot is critical in the evaluation. The relative rigidity will be important in determining the extent of treatment required. Obviously, the more rigid the foot, the more likely that surgical intervention will be necessary. Unfortunately, despite the appearance and feel at presentation, it is extremely difficult to predict outcome. The extreme variation in the pathologic anatomy makes the evaluation of long-term results difficult at best.

Radiology. Standard x-rays are the technique used to evaluate the clubfoot. In addition to AP views, a forced dorsiflexion lateral view (Fig. 15–108) is important. On the AP view, one can measure the longitudinal talocalcaneal angle or Kite's angle (Fig. 15–109). Normally, this is 20 to 40 degrees. If less than 20 degrees, hindfoot varus is indicated. The forced dorsiflexion lateral film also allows one to measure the lateral talocalcaneal angle, frequently referred to as the lateral Kite's angle. If this is less than 25 degrees, a parallel relationship between the talus and the calcaneus is suggested. Another feature to be sought on the lateral view is any evidence of superimposition of the ossification centers of the talus and calcaneus. In the absence of this finding, parallelism or "locking" of the subtalar joint is suggested.

Treatment. For many years, nonsurgical treatment was the norm for all clubfeet. Hiram Kite, in his classic text, emphasized protracted, long-term serial casting for the correction of these feet. Unfortunately, this period of casting was frequently extended for several years after the age of walking. Not only was this labor intensive for the physi-

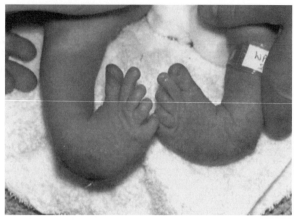

Figure 15–107. Severe clubfeet at birth. (From Broughton NS: A Textbook of Paediatric Orthopedics. London, WB Saunders, 1997.)

cian, it was also problematic for the family. The major problem with protracted casting is the deformation that it may cause to soft osseous and cartilaginous structures within the foot. The finding of the "flat-topped talus" was directly the result of forcible dorsiflexion against a tight heel cord, which occurred during manipulation. One must recognize the limitations of manipulative treatment. It is currently used in an effort to correct the deformity early, recognizing that if the deformity does not respond to a reasonable period of casting, then surgical intervention is required.

Nonoperative treatment includes not only serial casting but taping and bracing. Many orthopaedic surgeons combine these modalities. They use taping for a short period of time after birth in order to stretch the soft tissues gently, and follow this with serial casting for a period of 4 to 6 months. In general, the foot should show clinical and radiographic evidence of correction by 4 to 6 months of age. If casting has been successful, retentive splinting or bracing is then required. If unsuccessful, then surgery is required to complete the correction.

Taping is designed to pull the medial column toward the lateral side. Those who favor taping prepare the skin with tincture of benzoin. The tape is applied to the medial side of the foot, onto the plantar surface and extending up the lateral side of the lower leg. The tape is usually changed weekly and, as one would expect, the major problem is skin breakdown.

Serial casting is the most popular nonsurgical approach in the management of clubfoot. The foot should be manipulated gently for a period of time prior to application of the cast. Emphasis should be placed on gentle molding of the cast following application of the plaster. Ponseti and others have emphasized the importance of meticulous casting technique. Not only is it important in achieving correction, but also in avoiding complications. The casting (Fig. 15–110) should aim at correcting the forefoot adduction and supination and the hindfoot varus initially. Slow gentle stretching of the heel cord is important; otherwise, forcible dorsiflexion against the tight heel cord can cause a midfoot breach and a rocker bottom deformity. Most surgeons prefer long leg casts in order to control foot position and

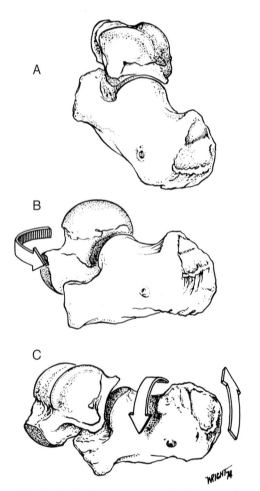

Figure 15–106. Pathomechanics of talipes equinovarus. *A*, Posterolateral view of the calcaneus and talus of a normal foot. *B*, Lateral rotation of the talus. *C*, The anterior part of the calcaneus is pressed by the head of the talus and forced into plantarflexion, rotation, and varus position. (From Carroll N, Murphy R, Leete SF: The pathoanatomy of congenital clubfoot. Orthop Clin North Am 1978; 9:227. Reprinted by permission.)

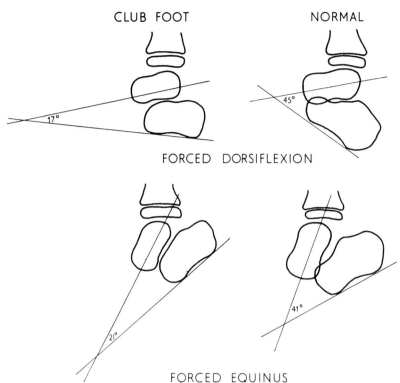

Figure 15–108. The talocalcaneal angle in the normal foot and in talipes equinovarus. The axis of the talus is the line joining the midpoints of the head and body of the talus. The axis of the calcaneus is the line joining the calcaneal tubercles and the anterior plantar convexity of the calcaneus. The normal talocalcaneal angle is between 35 and 50 degrees, and it increases in forced dorsiflexion, whereas in talipes equinovarus, it is less than 35 degrees and is often decreased further by forced dorsiflexion. (From Heywood AWB: The mechanics of the hindfoot in clubfoot as demonstrated radiographically. J Bone Joint Surg 1964; 46B:105.)

prevent the child from removing it. Between birth and 6 weeks, the casts are generally changed weekly. Following that time, cast changes every 2 weeks are usually adequate. Plaster is preferred over fiberglass, because it is more malleable, allowing molding. In addition, the parents can soak the casts off in advance of their next visit. Should correction be achieved using serial casts as determined by clinical examination and radiographic evaluation, then retentive splinting for at least 6 months to 1 year is required. As mentioned, casting complications include dermatitis, skin ulceration, rocker bottom deformity, stiffness, and damage to the distal tibial physis.

Surgical treatment of clubfoot has gained immense popularity. Not only are the long-term consequences of pro-tracted casting avoided, but the problem of the undercorrected clubfoot has been more or less resolved. Currently, the problem is more likely to be overcorrection. Indications for surgical treatment include failure of conservative management, the presence of a severe midfoot crease, a keel-shaped heel, rigid adduction, and the finding of an "atavistic" big toe (dynamic varus). Various surgical approaches have been recommended. In Europe, the tendency is to treat these children surgically within the first 3 months of age. In the United States, most authors prefer to perform surgery when the child is between 6 and 9 months of age. Obviously, the specific surgical technique depends upon the deformity present. Two surgical approaches are popular at this time: (1) the Cincinnati incision (Fig. 15–111) was popularized by Crawford in 1982, and (2) double-incision techniques have been described by Carroll and Eilert. De-

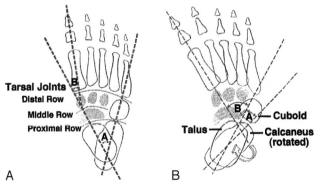

Figure 15–109. *A*, Anteroposterior diagram of the normal foot showing a talocalcaneal angle (A) of 20 to 30 degrees. The angle between the axis of the talus and the first metatarsal (B) is small. *B*, In a clubfoot the talocalcaneal angle is less than 20 degrees (A). The angle between the talus and the first metatarsal is increased (B).

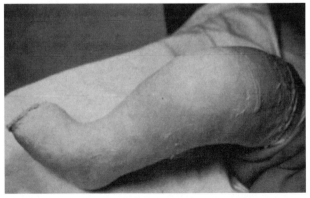

Figure 15–110. Technique of plaster of Paris cast application in talipes equinovarus. (From Tachdjian MO: Pediatric Orthopedics, 2nd ed. Philadelphia, WB Saunders, 1990.)

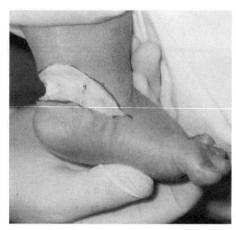

Figure 15–111. The Cincinnati incision for posteromedial release of clubfoot. (From Broughton NS: A Textbook of Paediatric Orthopaedics. London, WB Saunders, 1997.)

spite the skin incision, the technical issues are similar. Most feet require a posteromedial release of the tight structures in order to correct the malpositioned talus and the associated osseous abnormalities. Lateral release is also needed in order to derotate the talus in the ankle mortise. Once corrected, most surgeons use pins to hold the corrected position. Some surgeons favor the use of intraoperative x-ray, whereas others are comfortable without it. Postoperative casting periods vary from 2 to 4 months, with retentive splints being used once the cast is discontinued. Surgical complications include wound infection, distal metaphyseal tibial fractures, flat-topped talus, dorsal talonavicular dislocation, residual calcaneus deformity, and as previously mentioned, overcorrection. Those particularly at risk for overcorrection are children of diabetic mothers, floppy babies, children who have associated eye problems suggesting ligamentous laxity, and those who have had previous surgical intervention. In the overcorrected foot, the calcaneus is in excessive valgus. Extensive interosseous ligament release and inadvertent damage to the deltoid ligament complex are often cited as proximate causes of overcorrection.

Procedures are described both for the undercorrected and overcorrected clubfoot. The undercorrected foot typically has residual forefoot adductus, hindfoot varus, and residual equinus. Depending on the age of the child, various procedures are available to deal with these late deformities. The Heyman-Herndon midfoot capsulotomy or metatarsal osteotomies will correct residual forefoot adductus. Hindfoot varus can be corrected with a laterally based closing wedge Dwyer's osteotomy of the calcaneus or a calcaneal translocation osteotomy. Simple heel cord tenotomy may be all that is required to correct residual equinus.

The overcorrected hindfoot is treated with a calcaneal translocation. Forefoot adduction is generally uncommon. Calcaneus deformity due to an overlengthened Achilles tendon is far more difficult to treat than residual equinus.

Summary. Many questions still remain relative to the management of clubfeet. Because clubfeet are so different in their degree of rigidity and deformity, long-term studies are unable to generalize as to treatment and prognosis. All authors agree as to the importance of recognizing and ruling out associated syndromes. In addition, the physician must make an attempt to quantify and assess the level of deformity so that the surgical treatment can be focused on the areas of particular involvement.

The recognized prognostic indices of a poor result include a failure to respond to treatment, recurrence following surgical treatment, associated anomalies, teratogenic etiology, and a delay in treatment. In addition, the recently described short, fat, rigid foot with a deep medial crease has been clearly shown to resist treatment and have a poor prognosis. It is important to convey to the parents at the initial visit that this a true congenital deformity and that their goals need to be tempered with reality. It is, however, realistic to expect a functional plantigrade foot. The mobility of that foot, however, may be somewhat variable.

MISCELLANEOUS CONDITIONS

Limp

The limping child is a relatively common problem and yet this is difficult to evaluate. Multiple etiologies, the child's difficulty in localizing pain, and a vague history make it essential that the physician have a systematic approach to this problem. Rather than order multiple unpleasant and expensive diagnostic studies, it is usually more valuable to carefully observe and examine the child, especially in a sequential fashion. Generically, a limp is any uneven or laborious gait, or for that matter, any alteration in normal gait sequence. Normal gait classically occurs in two phases—stance and swing. The stance phase is initiated at heel strike for a given limb and terminated with toe-off of that extremity. Stance accounts for approximately 60% of the gait cycle, normally leaving 40% of that cycle for swing. Swing begins when the foot leaves the ground and terminates at heel strike. Three classic aberrations of the gait cycle are important to consider in the evaluation of the child's limp.

Antalgic Gait. Pain is the cause of this gait aberration. Because of pain in the extremity at the time of ground contact, the stance phase is shortened, causing the patient to unload the affected extremity more quickly. Multiple etiologies will cause an antalgic limp, including a fracture in the extremity, toxic synovitis of the hip, and Perthes' disease.

Trendelenburg's Gait. Often referred to as a gluteus medius lurch or abductor lurch, this pattern is due to the incompetence of the abductor lever arm needed to stabilize the pelvis. If one remembers that moment is created by a force acting over a distance ($M = F \times d$), it can be appreciated that altering either factor, the force or the distance (lever arm), will cause a Trendelenburg limp (Fig. 15–112):

- Force alteration (F): muscle weakness as seen in poliomyelitis
- Distance alteration (d): a shortened lever arm as seen in developmental dysplasia of the hip (DDH) or malunited femoral neck fractures

Static examination of the child with a Trendelenburg limp will usually demonstrate a positive Trendelenburg sign on the involved side.

Figure 15–112. Trendelenburg's test. *B,* In single-limb stance, the abductor muscles on the weight-bearing side contract to raise the pelvis on the opposite side *(arrow). C,* If the abductor muscles are weak, the pelvis will drop on the non–weight-bearing side *(arrow).* This drop is compensated by shifting body weight to the opposite side, placing the center of gravity over the limb bearing weight. (From Staheli LT: Fundamentals of Pediatric Orthopedics. New York, Raven Press, 1992.)

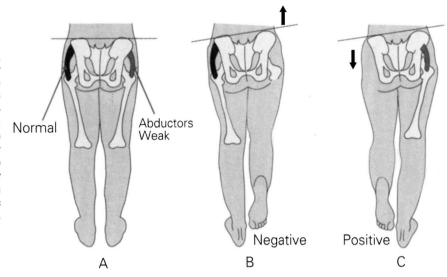

Short Leg Limp. Leg length discrepancy of significance will be manifested as an apparent limp with the pelvis dropping on the short side at the time of ground contact. The Trendelenburg sign, however, is normal because there is usually no pathology of the abductor lever arm.

A careful history should investigate any past traumatic event, systemic symptoms, and the effect on activity. Physical findings such as fever, focal findings of swelling, limitation of motion, and muscle spasm should be sought. Age itself may be a clue to the etiology, because each group seems particularly prone to certain maladies (Fig. 15–113). As shown in Figure 15–113, the very young child (1 to 3 years old) should be suspected of having DDH, trauma, or septic arthritis. The middle age group (4 to 8 years) should be studied for Perthes, toxic synovitis, or juvenile rheumatoid arthritis. In the preadolescent, SCFE and trauma are the likely causes.

The diagnostic workup is frequently initiated with standard x-rays, especially of the hips. It has been said that, if only one x-ray of the limping child can be obtained, it should first and foremost show the hips. A routine hemogram is frequently beneficial, especially in the face of systemic symptoms. A three-phase bone scan is a good second-line study, especially if localization is necessary. Unfortunately, it is not possible to specifically outline all the studies to be routinely obtained. Reaching the correct diagnosis is all too often the result of coinciding historical data, physical findings, laboratory data, and a "gut sense." Several diagnostic algorithms have been proposed that emphasize the basic factors in evaluating pediatric limp. The one put forth by Dr. Staheli is one such example (Fig. 15–114); it is based on the characterization of the type of limp. Others, however, are based more on the clinical features: a history of trauma, the presence or absence of systemic symptoms, and the anatomic localization of findings.

In the presence of a trauma history, appropriate radiographs will frequently disclose the diagnosis. Additional studies, such as a bone scan or MRI scan, will augment the diagnostic algorithm. One should recognize that children can sustain soft tissue trauma without bony injury, frequently accounting for negative imaging studies. Should the trauma history be negative, then the workup will take another turn. In that setting, radiographs are frequently helpful if there are localized findings, but early laboratory data should be sought: complete blood count (CBC), eryth-

Figure 15–113. Causes of limp by age. The causes of limp are related to the age of the child. The fine line shows the range, and the heavy line shows the most common age range of involvement. dys., dystrophy. (From Staheli LT: Fundamentals of Pediatric Orthopedics. New York, Raven Press, 1992.)

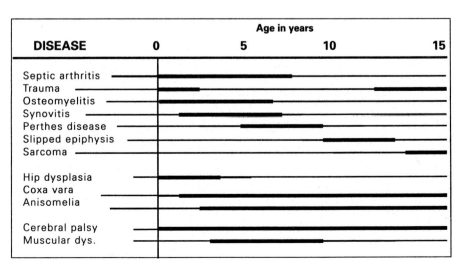

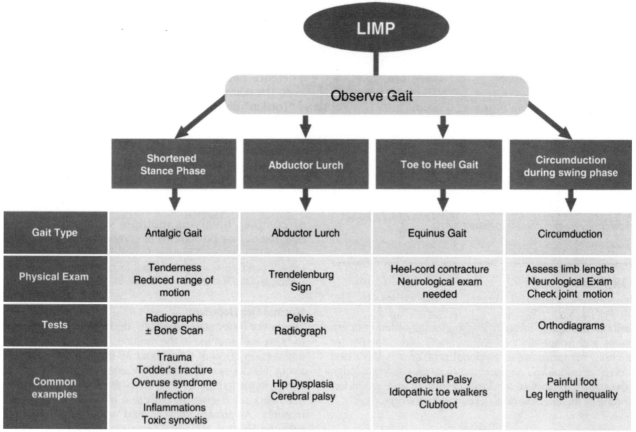

Figure 15–114. Algorithm for evaluation of limping. The major causes of limping are shown. A general categorization is first possible by observation. The exact causes are established by the physical examination and laboratory studies. (From Staheli LT: Fundamentals of Pediatric Orthopedics. New York, Raven Press, 1992.)

rocyte sedimentation rate, C-reactive protein, and in the black child, hemoglobin electrophoresis is worthwhile. In addition, should the child have localized findings, pursuit of the workup for that region is also necessary. The finding of systemic symptoms, especially fever, forces the algorithm to include sepsis, specifically osteomyelitis and septic arthritis. In addition, the inflammatory arthritides in these children must be considered.

Recall that the most common cause of limp in the child 5 to 9 years of age is toxic synovitis. As discussed, this condition is common and self-limited. It is characterized by the absence of systemic findings and the presence of normal laboratory and radiographic studies. Frequently, this diagnosis is obvious; however, should there be any question, further workup is essential because it should be considered a diagnosis of exclusion. Careful history, physical examination, laboratory tests, and radiographic evaluation will usually lead to the correct diagnosis. At the time of initial evaluation, should the diagnosis be elusive, sequential evaluation is a must.

Evaluation of Limb Length Inequality

Frequently, the physician is asked to evaluate the child with a short leg. There are numerous congenital and acquired causes for this, and the treatment will need to be individualized based on the cause and extent of the inequality. Minimal discrepancies can be well tolerated by the individual and require essentially no treatment. On the other hand, extensive discrepancies may require significant procedures to overcome the otherwise anticipated disability.

ETIOLOGY

Many different conditions can cause leg length inequality. Congenital causes such as PFFD and congenital short femur were mentioned earlier in this chapter. DDH with a high dislocation similarly can cause a leg length inequality. Acquired conditions such as the residua of juvenile rheumatoid disease, damage to the growth plate following trauma or infection, and obscure etiologies, such as radiation and burns, are all capable of producing unequal limb lengths. The neuromuscular causes referred to earlier, such as cerebral palsy and poliomyelitis, have been reported to produce limb length inequality.

The evaluation of these children is often difficult and time-consuming. The history should be extensive in order to encompass both congenital and acquired defects. Physical examination should determine not only the extent of the leg length inequality but also the type. Absolute leg length inequality is determined by comparing the length of the two legs from the anterior superior iliac spine to the medial malleolus. Relative leg length inequality, measured from the umbilicus to the medial malleolus, should be excluded at this point. Pelvic obliquity can frequently be the cause of a relative leg length inequality. It would be rare to consider procedures, typically described for true leg length discrepancy, for the management of a relative defect.

Radiographs used in the evaluation of leg length inequality are the scanogram and the orthoroentgenogram (Fig. 15–115). Both of these employ a radiopaque ruler placed under the limbs. The scanogram is used less frequently, because the radiographic technique is very sensitive to patient movement. The orthoroentgenogram is performed using multiple exposures. The hips, the knees, and the ankles are viewed using an orthogonal beam directed at each level. Once performed, both will allow accurate measurement of leg length discrepancy. Most treatment protocols require serial evaluation of leg length inequality. Therefore, most children should be seen at intervals and the radiographic studies obtained. This sequential evaluation allows the physician to judge the degree of inhibition. For example, in the case of many congenital deformities, the discrepancy will worsen with growth; therefore, the growth of the limb is said to be inhibited. On the other hand, discrepancies secondary to trauma tend to remain constant with growth; therefore, no growth inhibition is seen.

Three classic techniques are used for predicting limb length inequality. The first is the growth remaining chart of Green-Anderson. Using this chart and basing the assessment on skeletal age as determined from standard tables, one can assess the amount of growth remaining in a given limb. The second is the Mosely straight line graph, which is based on a logarithmic function. Although significantly more complex to use, many believe it gives a more accurate assessment of limb length inequality and growth remaining for planning purposes. Last, the Menelaus method, which has now been repopularized, is certainly the simplest. It is predicated on the premise that males complete their growth by age 16 and females by age 14. It employs only chronologic age in the calculations. Generalizations are based on the assumption that the distal femoral physis contributes 1 cm per year, the proximal tibial and proximal femoral physes contribute 0.6 cm per year, and the distal tibial plate adds 0.4 cm per year. This method allows the most rapid assessment of growth remaining. Many authors are skeptical as to its reliability, preferring one of the more complex techniques.

MANAGEMENT

Once information is available regarding the current discrepancy and the projected discrepancy at growth cessation, a treatment plan can be devised. In general, several approaches are available. Options include shortening the long leg, lengthening the short leg, lengthening one and shortening the other, or stopping growth in the long leg at a time appropriate to allow the short leg to catch up. Historically, the techniques employed for the management of leg length inequality have been extremely varied and some would say bizarre. The use of ivory pegs to stimulate the growth plate is but one of these unusual historical methods.

At the present time, most authors believe that discrepancies at growth cessation of under 2 cm require no treatment or at most a modest heel lift. Discrepancies between 2 and 5 cm are best managed by a lift, shortening, lengthening, or physeal arrest if the individual is still growing. Discrepancies between 5 and 15 cm are probably best managed with limb lengthening procedures. Last, discrepancies projected to be over 15 cm will probably require prosthetic treatment approaches (Fig. 15–116). The treatment decision must be individualized and other factors must be considered. The age of the patient and the sex of the patient, as well as the height of other family members, must be reviewed. In addition, the desire of the patient or the parents needs to be considered. It is critically important, when projecting discrepancy, to keep in mind whether or not this discrepancy is inhibited. If the pattern is such that the discrepancy will get worse with ongoing growth, it makes planning far more problematic.

If one is satisfied that the projected discrepancy can be legitimately determined while the individual is still growing, then epiphysiodesis (surgical growth plate closure) presents an attractive option. The procedures are simple and safe; in large part, they are predictable within a certain range. Although originally suggested by Blount, his technique of closing the plate with staples is rarely performed at this time. Presently, percutaneous epiphysiodesis, using C-arm control, is a popular, minimally invasive technique. For this procedure to be successful, a relatively accurate projection of discrepancy must be made. The timing of physeal arrest must allow adequate time for the short side to catch up.

Once physeal closure has occurred, then the options of management become more limited. Currently, lengthening techniques for the short limb have been gaining popularity. For discrepancies over 5 cm in the child 8 to 12 years of age, lengthening techniques are of value. It is imperative

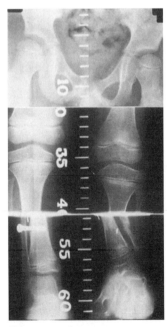

Figure 15–115. An orthoroentgenogram of a short left leg, demonstrating that the shortening is in the tibia. Measurements can be taken against the metal ruler. (From Broughton NS: A Textbook of Paediatric Orthopaedics. London, WB Saunders, 1997.)

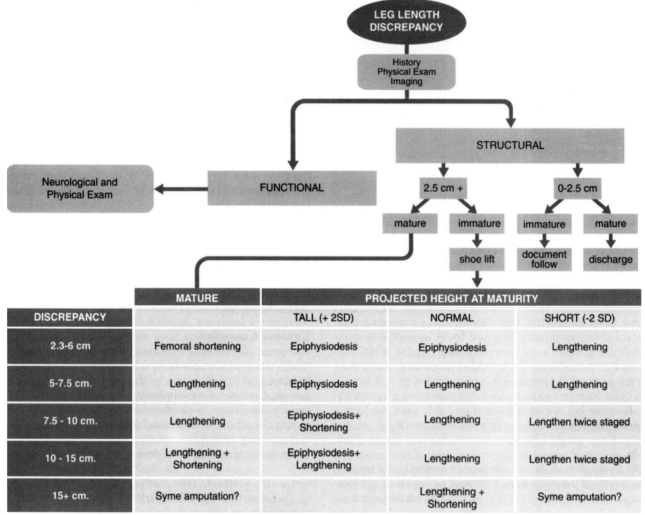

Figure 15–116. Algorithm for management of leg length discrepancy. First, determine or estimate the discrepancy at maturity. If the adolescent is skeletally mature, refer to the column at the left. For children, plan management based on projected height at maturity. (From Staheli LT: Fundamentals of Pediatric Orthopedics. New York, Raven Press, 1992.)

that the child and the parents be fully advised of the rigors of lengthening techniques. Many complications have been reported with the use of distraction osteogenesis techniques. In principle, the short bone is osteotomized in a subperiosteal fashion. An external fixator is applied. The Orthofix (Fig. 15–117) and Ilizarov frames are both popular for this application. Once applied, the device is used to distract the bone over time. With slow distraction of 1 mm per day, time is allowed for the periosteum to make new bone (Fig. 15–118). Essentially, a new tube of diaphyseal bone is formed as the proximal and distal fragments are distracted. For example, if the discrepancy is 7 cm, it will take approximately 70 days to achieve that correction. Once the goal length has been achieved, the fixator is left on for a period of time to allow for solidification of the new diaphyseal cylinder.

Complications of these techniques include equinus deformity, peroneal nerve palsy, systemic hyperemia, and pin track infections. In addition, premature union of the fibula and nonunion of the tibia can complicate lengthening of the leg. Perhaps one of the most common complications of

femoral lengthening is the stiff knee, which must be carefully evaluated and aggressively treated.

The most important question is, "Should anything be done?" It is important to remember that the vast majority of patients with 2 cm of discrepancy have no functional deficit. In addition, over 15 cm of discrepancy cannot be resolved with one single procedure. Despite the current enthusiasm for many of these techniques, one must carefully prepare the family for anticipated complications and be comfortable dealing with those complications when they occur.

SUMMARY

After discussing the many afflictions of the pediatric musculoskeletal system, one can certainly appreciate the veracity of the fact that children are different from adults. The very thing that makes them a child complicates the management of their pathology. That unique factor is growth. Frequently, it benefits them in the resolution of

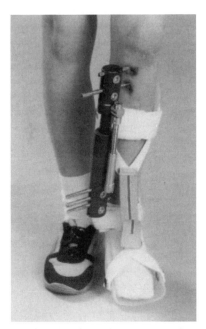

Figure 15–117. The Orthofix uniplanar frame for tibial lengthening. (From Menelaus M: The Management of Limb Inequality. Edinburgh, Churchill Livingstone, 1982.)

Table 15–8. Prevalence of orthopaedic problems in children

Disorder	Prevalence*
Marfan's syndrome	66,000
Achondroplasia	50,000
Idiopathic scoliosis requiring surgery	9000
Neurofibromatosis	3000
Slipped epiphysis	2000 (males), 3000 (females)
Accidental death under 15 years	3000
Perthes' disease	800 (males), 4000 (females)
Clubfoot	700
Spina bifida	700
Cerebral palsy	500
Congenital dysplasia of hip	700
Newborn hip instability	100
Positive screening for scoliosis	30
Spondylolysis	20
Forefoot adduction in newborn	33
Accessory navicular	20
Toeing-in	8
Infant death in Malawi	7
Flatfeet	5
Childhood fracture	2

*Prevalence: The number of children affected during childhood—expressed as the number of normal children for every affected case.

From Wenger DR, Rang M: Art and Practice of Children's Orthopaedics. New York, Raven Press, 1992.

deformity and disease; however, there are times when it only accentuates the process.

Systemic diseases, such as dysplasias, metabolic aberrations, nutritional defects, and hematologic abnormalities, can have wide-reaching impact on the musculoskeletal system. Local phenomena that are neoplastic, infectious, or traumatic in origin can dramatically alter the shape and length of a child's limb. It is frequently difficult to get a perspective on the relative frequency of these conditions. Therefore, Table 15–8 was prepared by Mercer Rang to assist in anticipating the prevalence of many of the diseases

and syndromes discussed here. In addition, an awareness of the child's biologic and mechanical differences can only assist the orthopaedic surgeon in appropriately managing these pathologic states. Despite early diagnosis, appropriate management, and excellent surgical technique, many of these conditions result in less than adequate outcomes. Fortunately for the physician and the child, the converse is usually the case. Despite delay in diagnosis, errors in decision making, and technical misadventures, satisfactory results can be achieved, again proving the astounding reparative ability of the child.

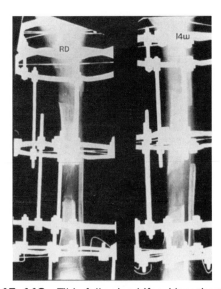

Figure 15–118. Tibia following bifocal lengthening using the Ilizarov frame. (From Menelaus M: The Management of Limb Inequality. Edinburgh, Churchill Livingstone, 1982.)

Bibliography

Benson MKD, Fixsen JA, MacNicol MF: Children's Orthopaedics and Fractures. Edinburgh, Churchill Livingstone, 1994.

Bleck E: Orthopaedic Management of Cerebral Palsy. Saunders Monograph in Clinical Orthopaedics. Vol 2. Philadelphia, WB Saunders, 1979.

Boyer DW, et al: SCFE, long term follow up study of 121 patients. J Bone Joint Surg 1981;63A:85–95.

Broughton N: A Textbook of Paediatric Orthopaedics. London, WB Saunders, 1997.

Carroll N: The pathoanatomy of congenital clubfoot. Orthop Clin North Am 1978;9:225.

Catterall A: The natural history of Perthes disease. J Bone Joint Surg 1971;53B:37–53.

Graf R: New possibilities for the diagnosis of CDH by ultrasonography. J Pediatr Ortho 1983;3:354–360.

Harcke H: Performing dynamic sonography of the infant hip. Am J Radio 1990;155:837–844.

Harris R, Beath T: Hypermobile flatfoot with short Achilles' tendon. J Bone Joint Surg 1948;30A:116.

Kite JH: Nonoperative treatment of congenital clubfoot. Clin Orthop 1972;84:29.

Morrissey R, Weiinstein S; Lovell & Winter's Pediatric Orthopaedics. Philadelphia, JB Lippincott, 1996.

Petrie JG: The abduction weight bearing treatment of Legg Perthes disease. J Bone Joint Surg 1971;53B:54–62.

Ponsetti IV: Observations on pathogenesis and treatment of congenital clubfoot. Clin Orthop 1972;84:50.

Rubin P: The Dynamic Classification of Bone Dysplasias. Chicago, Year Book Medical Publishers, 1964.

Salter R, Thompson G: LCP disease, two group classification. J Bone Joint Surg 1984;66A:479–489.

Southwich W: Osteotomy through the lesser trochanter for SCFE. J Bone Joint Surg 1967;49:807–835.

Staheli L: Fundamentals of Pediatric Orthopaedics. New York, Raven Press, 1992.

Tachdjian M: Pediatric Orthopaedics, 2nd ed. Philadelphia, WB Saunders, 1990.

Tachdjian M: Clinical Pediatric Orthopaedics. Norwalk, CT, Appleton & Lange, 1996.

Wenger D, Rang M: Art and Practice of Pediatric Orthopaedics. New York, Raven Press, 1993.

Chapter 16

Pediatric Spine

William C. Lauerman, M.D.

SPINAL DEFORMITY

Classification

Scoliosis refers to coronal or frontal plane curvature of the spine. It is a complex 3-dimensional deformity including the obvious abnormality seen in the frontal plane, but also involving alteration in sagittal plane balance and rotation in the transverse plane. This combination of abnormalities in the three planes leads to the cosmetically apparent aspects of the deformity including shoulder and pelvis asymmetry, hypokyphosis, apparent junctional kyphosis, and rotational prominence of the rib or flank.

Scoliosis and associated spinal deformities have been classified by the Scoliosis Research Society.[67] Etiologically, scoliosis can be broken down into structural and nonstructural causes. Nonstructural causes of scoliosis include postural curves, hysterical scoliosis, and scoliosis secondary to a leg length discrepancy or contracture about the hips. In addition, nerve root irritation from a herniated nucleus pulposus or from a tumor can cause a nonstructural scoliosis. Nonstructural curves have normal flexibility when the inciting cause is removed, and can be seen radiographically to correct or even overcorrect on bending films.

Most cases of scoliosis are structural, and the assumption should certainly be made that any significant spinal deformity is structural until proven otherwise. The three most common types of scoliosis are idiopathic, in which no known cause has been identified; neuromuscular, in which there is either an underlying neuropathic or myopathic cause; and congenital, consisting of failure of formation or failure of segmentation of an area of the spinal column.

Other conditions in which scoliosis is seen include neurofibromatosis, in which a characteristic curve pattern may constitute one of the essential components of diagnosis. Short, sharp curves with vertebral scalloping, enlargement of the neural foramina, and penciling of the ribs are the hallmarks of neurofibromatous scoliosis, and excessive kyphosis is often seen. When progressive, this type of dystrophic scoliosis in neurofibromatosis can lead to the development of a neurologic deficit often associated with dural ectasia. Also seen in neurofibromatosis is a nondystrophic deformity very similar to idiopathic scoliosis.[8] A variety of estimates have been given as to the incidence of spinal deformity in neurofibromatosis type 1, with estimates ranging from 10 to 60% of affected individuals having either dystrophic or nondystrophic curves.[1]

Collagen disorders such as Marfan's syndrome or Ehlers-Danlos syndrome are also associated with scoliosis. The evaluation of a patient with scoliosis should always include assessment for generalized ligamentous laxity. The child with suspected Marfan's syndrome should be referred for appropriate evaluation including slit lamp examination of the eyes, cardiac evaluation, and pulmonary function testing.[54] Treatment of scoliosis in these patients is similar to that for idiopathic deformity, although the surgeon should be aware of the predilection for complex sagittal plane abnormalities, which must be addressed when surgery is elected; an attempt to save fusion levels such as is common in idiopathic curves may lead to progressive deformity proximal or distal to the fusion or to the development of junctional kyphosis.[59] Other conditions in which scoliosis is seen (Table 16–1) include juvenile rheumatoid arthritis; the osteochondrodystrophies, particularly diastrophic dwarfism; and metabolic disorders such as osteogenesis imperfecta. Scoliosis can also develop following irradiation to either the spine or chest, following burns, or

Table 16–1. Etiology of scoliosis

Idiopathic
Congenital
Neuromuscular
    Polio
    Cerebral palsy
    Posttraumatic (spinal cord injury)
    Spinal muscular atrophy
    Muscular dystrophy
    Friedreich's ataxia
    Charcot-Marie-Tooth disease
    Syringomyelia
    Myelomeningocele
    Arthrogryposis
Neurofibromatosis
Marfan's syndrome
Ehlers-Danlos syndrome
Juvenile rheumatoid arthritis
Spine or spinal cord tumor
Postlaminectomy
Thoracic cage defect/deficiency
Osteochondrodystrophy (dwarfism)
Osteogenesis imperfecta

From Wiesel SW, Delahay JN: Essentials of Orthopaedic Surgery, 2nd ed. Philadelphia, WB Saunders, 1997.

385

following laminectomy for intraspinal conditions, and is seen in almost 100% of individuals sustaining spinal cord injury during childhood.[46]

Kyphosis refers to forward bending of the spine with posterior convex angulation, normally seen between T1 and T10 and ranging, in normal individuals, from 20 to 50 degrees. Mildly increased kyphosis is most commonly postural. Scheuermann's kyphosis is discussed below. Congenital failures of formation, segmentation, or mixed anomalies can lead to excessive kyphosis, as can a variety of neuromuscular conditions including myelomeningocele. Other causes of hyperkyphosis include metabolic bone disease, skeletal dysplasias, and rheumatologic disorders such as ankylosing spondylitis. Progressive hyperkyphosis can also be seen following spine trauma, either with or without injury to the spinal cord, and following laminectomy or irradiation.

Evaluation

A thorough history and physical examination are mandatory when evaluating the patient with a potential spinal deformity. While it is essential to completely define the nature and extent of the spinal deformity, the most important task facing the physician is to ensure, prior to arriving at a diagnosis of idiopathic scoliosis or Scheuermann's kyphosis, that no more serious underlying condition is present. As such, the history should concentrate on the patient's presenting complaint. Is this an asymptomatic deformity, or have pain or neurologic symptoms been present? How was the condition first detected? Pain should be thoroughly investigated. It is not uncommon, particularly once the diagnosis of scoliosis has been made, for individuals with idiopathic scoliosis to complain of pain, which is usually mild and related to activity.[58] On the other hand, the history that an adolescent has begun to limit his or her activities including missing school, refraining from participation in sports or other preferred activities, or regularly taking medication for back pain should be considered out of the ordinary. Such a history, or the history of any neurologic symptoms including pain or paresthesias in the legs, weakness, stumbling or clumsiness, or bowel or bladder dysfunction, merits further investigation. Other important aspects of the history include any family history of spinal deformity, the patient's overall medical condition and history, and the patient's physiologic maturity including a history of menarche. A history of cardiopulmonary dysfunction, while rare, should also be sought.

Lonstein advocates pursuing three areas in the physical examination: the deformity, its cause, and its complications.[42] All patients should be examined in their underwear wearing an examining gown. The socks and shoes must be removed. Examination from the back allows inspection of the entire trunk and axillae as well as inspection of the buttocks to evaluate for any skin abnormalities such as café-au-lait spots. Symmetry of the shoulders, scapula, and pelvis is assessed, as is coronal and sagittal plane balance. The Adams forward bending test brings the rotational rib prominence into relief and is helpful in detecting subtle cases of scoliosis; we find use of the Scoliometer useful in quantifying the rib prominence, and symmetry of greater than 5 degrees suggests a significant likelihood of scoliosis

of more than 20 degrees. The lower extremities should be carefully evaluated for hamstring contractures or contractures about the hips, knees, or ankles. Calf and foot sizes should be compared; any asymmetry may be evidence of an underlying intraspinal abnormality. Thorough neurologic testing should be carried out including testing of light touch sensation, motor strength, tone in the lower extremities, and deep tendon reflexes including testing for ankle clonus. Babinski's sign should be sought and the superficial abdominal reflexes routinely tested. Any evidence of upper motor neuron pathology, or asymmetry in findings from one leg to the other, merits consideration of further radiographic workup.

Routine radiographic evaluation of the patient with spinal deformity consists of a standing frontal and lateral view on a single cassette. It is important on both views to be able to assess the relationship of the head and cervical spine to the pelvis, and the iliac crests must be visualized to assess for Risser's sign of skeletal maturation (Fig. 16–1). All scoliosis patients undergo a lateral radiograph on first presentation, which is only repeated immediately prior to surgery, where indicated. Similarly, bending films are reserved, in almost all cases, for preoperative use to select fusion levels.

Special studies that may be obtained include tomography, computed tomography, bone scan, and magnetic resonance imaging (MRI). Tomography is helpful in defining congenital anomalies such as failures of segmentation or formation, although its use and availability have diminished in recent years. These anomalies are also visualized well on MRI scanning,[13] which, in addition, will also demonstrate almost all intraspinal anomalies, spinal cord tumors, and neoplasms of the vertebral column. In our practice, MRI of the full spine is obtained in patients who are particularly young (below age 8 to 10), or in patients with rapidly

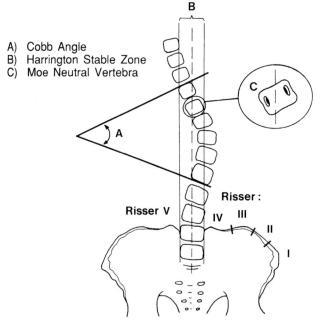

A) Cobb Angle
B) Harrington Stable Zone
C) Moe Neutral Vertebra

Figure 16–1. Measurements for scoliosis. (From Miller MD: Review of Orthopaedics, 2nd ed. Philadelphia, WB Saunders, 1996.)

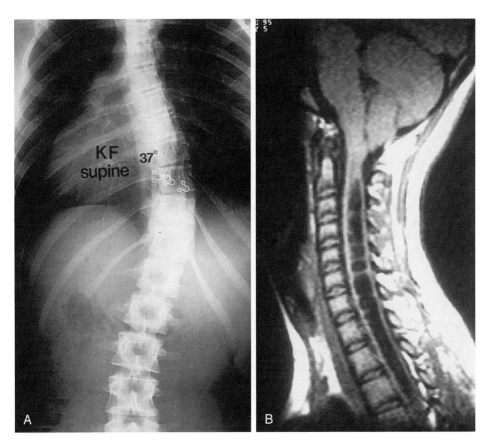

Figure 16–2. *A,* A 12-year-old girl with presumed idiopathic scoliosis. On physical examination, she had asymmetrical superficial abdominal reflexes; all other neurologic findings were normal. *B,* MRI demonstrates a large syrinx in association with an Arnold-Chiari malformation.

progressive curves, with a significant history of pain, or with evidence of neurologic dysfunction such as sensory or motor deficit, deep tendon reflex (DTR) asymmetry or hyperreflexia, clonus, Babinski's sign, or asymmetry of the superficial abdominal reflexes (Fig. 16–2).

Idiopathic Scoliosis

Idiopathic scoliosis can be divided into infantile (before 3 years of age), juvenile (ages 3 to 10 years), and adolescent. The most common form of frontal plane deformity, idiopathic scoliosis remains a diagnosis of exclusion. While no known cause for idiopathic scoliosis has been proven, investigation continues into abnormalities of platelet function, muscle function, collagen structure, and central nervous system, in particular brain stem structure and function. It is known that a history of idiopathic scoliosis in a first-degree relative significantly increases the individual's risk.

The quoted prevalence for idiopathic scoliosis varies depending on the curve magnitude utilized as threshold as well as the technique of detection and age at screening. Estimates have been published that range from 0.3 to 15.3%. When adolescent populations are considered, curves over 10 degrees are found in 0.2 to 0.3%, whereas only 0.02 to 0.03% of individuals are found to have curves over 30 degrees.[73]

The natural history of idiopathic scoliosis has been studied extensively. The factors that have been assessed include the long-term effects of untreated scoliosis on pain, pulmonary dysfunction, and social functioning. Most authors have been unable to define a statistically significant correlation between the presence of scoliosis, no matter the curve type or magnitude, and back pain. A similarly benign natural history in terms of the risk of significant pulmonary dysfunction has also been elaborated, with pulmonary function testing (PFT) changes usually seen only in thoracic curves greater than 60 or 70 degrees and alterations in life expectancy rare with curves less than 100 degrees.[20] The PFT changes of restrictive and constrictive nature seem to be more severe when scoliosis is detected before the age of 8 years.

The risk of curve progression has been extensively studied. Depending on curve magnitude, age, and skeletal maturity, the risk of progression reported varies from 5.2 to 56%. Lonstein and Carlson (Table 16–2), assessing a number of suggested risk factors, found that the most important predictive factors were curve magnitude and skeletal maturity.[44] Double curves are more likely to progress than single

Table 16–2. Incidence of progression as related to the magnitude of the curve and the Risser sign

	Percent of Curves That Progressed	
Risser Sign	*5–19° Curves*	*20–29° Curves*
0, I	22	68
II, III, IV	1.6	23

From Lonstein JE, Carlson JM: The prediction of curve progression in untreated idiopathic scoliosis during growth. J Bone Joint Surg Am 66:1061, 1984; reprinted by permission.

curves, but the most striking finding is that, in skeletally immature patients (Risser 0 to I), curves greater than 20 degrees have a two in three chance of progressing significantly. On the other hand, curves less than 20 degrees, particularly in skeletally mature (Risser II to IV) individuals, are at much less risk. These findings serve as the basis for current recommendations for the institution of treatment in children and adolescents.

Infantile Idiopathic Scoliosis

Defined as idiopathic scoliosis first diagnosed in individuals under 3 years of age, this condition is most common in Europe, particularly in Great Britain, and is rare in the United States. The rarity is such that, in our practice, any infant or toddler diagnosed with scoliosis is assumed to have an underlying neuromuscular disorder or intraspinal anomaly until this can be excluded by a thorough radiographic and medical workup.

It has been established that infantile idiopathic scoliosis consists of two distinct subtypes: resolving and progressive deformities. Progression varies from 8 to 64% among authors and may be related to the presence of developmental anomalies. Mehta in 1972 defined the rib-vertebral angle difference (RVAD) at the apical vertebral.[48] She found that an RVAD of less than 20 degrees was strongly predictive of curve resolution, with the mean RVAD in the resolving group being 11.7 degrees, while in the progressive group the mean RVAD was 25.5 degrees. She also noted that overlapping of the rib head with the vertebral body was a poor prognostic sign.

Treatment depends on differentiating progressive from resolving curves. Curves with an RVAD of less than 20 degrees are typically observed, although treatment will be instituted if progression beyond 30 degrees is noted. Progressive curves are treated initially with the application, under anesthesia, of a well-molded body cast. These growing children frequently require cast changes every 3 months. When the curve has been corrected and maintained at less than 10 degrees, full-time Milwaukee brace wearing is instituted. Surgery is undertaken when the curve cannot be corrected, or at least controlled, with casting or bracing. In the very young child (under age 6 years), instrumentation without fusion is typically elected, while over the age of 6 to 8 instrumentation and fusion are performed. Because of the risk of continued anterior growth and continued rotation of the spine around a posterior fusion mass, the "crankshaft effect," combined anterior and posterior fusion should be considered in patients with open triradiate cartilages.[26]

Juvenile Idiopathic Scoliosis

Diagnosis of idiopathic scoliosis in the patient between 4 and 10 years of age is defined as juvenile idiopathic scoliosis and has been reported in between 12 and 16% of scoliosis patients.[41] It is our experience that the relative proportion of patients being diagnosed at this earlier age appears to be increasing and may represent 25% of the patients in our practice. Treatment principles are similar to those for adolescent idiopathic scoliosis as defined below.

It has been well documented that these patients are at increased risk for curve progression, probably owing not to any difference in the biology of the curve, but to the skeletal immaturity of the patient. We have found that small curves, usually less than 20 degrees, are occasionally seen in these patients, which completely or partially resolve without any treatment. This resolution should be carefully followed, however, to ensure that there is no recurrence of the deformity during the adolescent growth spurt.

Adolescent Idiopathic Scoliosis

Most cases of idiopathic scoliosis are detected during adolescence. Once the adolescent is diagnosed with idiopathic scoliosis, appropriate treatment must be selected. The most important factors in determining treatment are the curve magnitude, the risk of progression, and any history of progression. For a variety of poorly understood reasons, the risk of progression is greatest at the time of this adolescent growth spurt and the need for treatment is highlighted. In many cases, active treatment should be deferred until documented progression is identified or such a high risk or progression is seen that waiting is contraindicated.

A variety of treatment options have been offered and continue to be offered for adolescent idiopathic scoliosis with no evidence of efficacy. These include exercise regimens, physical therapy, chiropractic manipulation, and electrical stimulation. The economic, emotional, and time costs of these interventions, as well as their propensity to distract from more effective intervention, suggest that they should be discouraged. Although decision making can be quite complex in adolescents with idiopathic scoliosis, the viable options for treatment are only three: (1) observation; (2) bracing; (3) surgery.

OBSERVATION

Observation is indicated for patients in whom bracing or surgery is not yet necessary because the curve is either not yet big enough, has not been documented to progress, or is not at significant risk of progression. Observation is also elected for adolescents with a significant curve who may have gone beyond the suitable range for bracing but are not yet candidates for surgical treatment. This would include curves over 40 or 45 degrees in skeletally mature adolescents (Risser III or IV), curves that have not been documented to progress, or well-balanced double major curves of 40 to 50 degrees that are cosmetically unobjectionable in a patient who is near the end of growth.

Observation consists of routine radiographic evaluation and physical examination. Serial assessment of the cosmetic appearance of the curve, shoulder and pelvic balance, coronal and sagittal plane balance, and neurologic status is as important as routine radiographs. Radiographic assessment should be repeated every 4 months at first, and, if the curve is stable, extended to 6-month intervals followed by yearly intervals. The Risser sign is assessed each time until the patient is a Risser V or is 2 to 3 years postmenarchal. Progression of 6 degrees or greater, if the child is still growing, or beyond 45 or 50 degrees if surgery is being contemplated, moves the child up to the next stage of treatment.

BRACING

A number of authors have reported on the results of a variety of orthoses for the control of scoliosis. Relatively few series have concentrated on a single diagnosis and matched treated and untreated patients, and certainly no study exists that has prospectively, in a blinded fashion, compared bracing with observation in patients with adolescent idiopathic scoliosis. Other limitations of previous studies include attempts to brace curves that are either too big or too small to merit treatment, failure to assess patient compliance, and failure to define "failure." Despite these limitations, a review of the literature suggests that, in the appropriate patient, there is an encouraging chance of success with bracing. Lonstein and Winter, in a review of the Milwaukee brace in which they compared 1020 adolescents to previous natural history studies, demonstrated statistically significant success rates for single right thoracic curves of 20 to 39 degrees, particularly for patients with a Risser of 0 or I and curves between 20 and 29 degrees.[45] Nachemson and associates reported on a prospective multicenter study in which patients were randomized by center to observation, electrical stimulation, or thoracolumbosacral orthosis (TLSO) bracing. In addition to demonstrating the failure of electrical stimulation to alter the natural history of these curves, the authors clearly demonstrated a decrease in the failure rate, from 70% to 40%, for bracing when compared with observation or electrical stimulation.[51]

Bracing is indicated for growing children with progressive curves. The factors to be assessed include the magnitude of the curve, whether or not progression has been documented, and the Risser sign (see Fig. 16–1). In our practice, patients with a Risser 0 to II who present with curves between 30 and 40 degrees have bracing recommended, whether or not progression has been documented. Between 25 and 29 degrees, we withhold bracing unless documentation of progression is seen radiographically, although close follow-up is mandatory. We occasionally recommend bracing in the extremely immature patient (Risser 0) with documentation of progression up to 20 to 25 degrees. Finally, factors such as the patient's home situation, ability to pay for one or more orthoses, emotional makeup and response to the concept of brace wear, and reaction to surgery as an eventual possible alternative all must be assessed in recommending bracing.

Virtually all orthoses that we now use for the treatment of idiopathic scoliosis are of the underarm TLSO variety. Reported to be effective in curves with an apex at T8 or below, the TLSO has proven effective for the overwhelming majority of curves treated in our practice. Most right thoracic curves have an apex of T8 or below and left upper thoracic curves, with an apex of T3 or T4, are in our experience unsuitable for bracing. We recommend full-time brace wear for most patients, with the patient allowed to come out of the brace for organized sports activities and for 1 to 2 hours a day for hygiene, etc.[60] It is essential that the patient and parents understand that neither the diagnosis of scoliosis nor the requirement for bracing represents a contraindication to participation in any sort of sports activity and indeed the opposite is true—active participation in sports should be encouraged.

Once the brace is delivered to the patient, a follow-up standing radiograph, in the brace, is obtained 1 month after the institution of brace wear. The prognosis for ultimate success has been demonstrated to be dependent on the initial response to bracing.[2] When good curve correction is seen on the initial x-ray, long-term control of the curve is much more likely (Fig. 16–3). Failure to obtain initial correction in the brace should lead to reevaluation of the adequacy of the brace and possibly alteration or added pad placement. Follow-up radiographs are then obtained, in the brace, every 4 months. When the patient is a Risser IV or is 18 to 24 months post menarchal, weaning ensues and usually takes place over 1 year. It is not uncommon, once weaning is completed, to see a slight increase in curve magnitude over the next year, and it is essential prior to the institution of bracing that the patient and parents understand that the long-term goal of brace treatment is maintenance of the curve. It has been well established that long-term curve correction is rare, and the patient and family should have appropriate expectations going into treatment regarding the eventual outcome of bracing.[41, 60]

SURGERY

The same factors go into the decision for surgical treatment as for bracing: curve magnitude, documented progression, and risk of progression. Surgery is typically elected for immature patients who despite bracing are seen to have curve progression beyond 40 or 45 degrees, skeletally immature patients who present with curves of 45 degrees or greater, or skeletally mature adolescents or young adults presenting with curves of greater than 50 degrees, wherein the risk for curve progression even in adulthood has been clearly documented.[71] These guidelines are modified depending on factors such as curve appearance, overall balance, and patient wishes, but in our practice, 50 degrees represents a fairly rigid cutoff for surgery, since there is such clear evidence that untreated curves beyond 50 degrees will progress through adulthood.

In selecting the appropriate operation for adolescents with idiopathic scoliosis, the options are to approach the spine from an anterior, a posterior, or a combined approach for fusion and/or instrumentation. Selection of fusion area is an important component of surgical decision making, and the underlying principle calls for fusion of all of the involved vertebrae in the curve from a neutrally rotated, balanced (over the sacrum) level cephalad to a neutrally rotated, balanced level caudad (see Fig. 16–1). Exceptions to these rules include King-Moe Type II curves wherein the thoracic curve is larger than the lumbar curve, both curves cross the midline, and the lumbar curve is more flexible (Table 16–3). In this curve pattern, selective fusion of the thoracic curve leads to spontaneous balancing of the lumbar curve and for many surgeons is the preferred approach.[38]

The most common surgical treatment utilized for adolescent idiopathic scoliosis is posterior fusion with posterior instrumentation and iliac crest bone grafting (Fig. 16–4). Once appropriate fusion levels are selected, instrumenta-

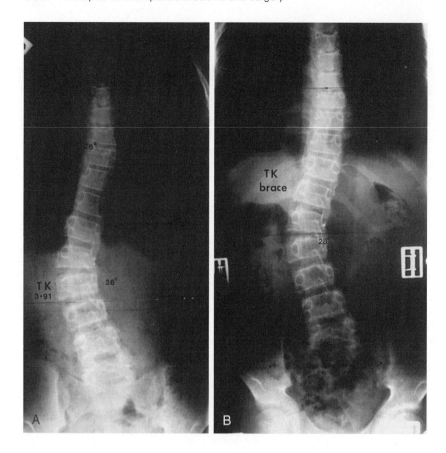

Figure 16–3. *A*, A 14-year-old boy, recently diagnosed with idiopathic scoliosis, with a 36-degree curve. *B*, Initial radiograph in his TLSO demonstrates only 22% curve correction, a poor response. His curve progressed despite bracing, ultimately requiring surgery.

tion, which has evolved from Harrington's original instrumentation to a variety of segmental constructs, spans the entire fusion, usually on both sides of the spine. Correction of 50% or more with a pseudarthrosis rate of 2 to 3% and a risk of neurologic complications of 0.5% or less has been reported. Long-term concerns with posterior fusion and instrumentation include suboptimal three-dimensional correction, the fate of unfused distal levels, and implant-related complications such as dislodgement, loosening, and late infection. In addition, skeletally immature individuals (Risser 0 with open triradiate cartilages) may be at risk for the crankshaft phenomenon and should be observed closely for continued rotation, as manifested by worsening of the rotational rib prominence.

Anterior fusion with anterior instrumentation has been proposed for certain thoracolumbar and lumbar curves as a means of "saving" distal fusion levels. The ability to completely correct and even overcorrect the apical three or four vertebrae of such a curve has been proposed as a means of stopping the instrumentation and fusion construct proximal to the traditionally required neutral, stable level.[33] This approach requires a flexible major curve as well as a flexible fractional curve distally with documented ability of the distal fusion level to approach horizontal on a supine side-bending radiograph (Fig. 16–5). In addition, there is a risk of the creation of kyphosis with the utilization of Zielke's anterior instrumentation and the preoperative lateral radiograph must be scrutinized to ensure that normal sagittal plane contours are present prior to utilizing this technique. It has been suggested that the risk of this type of implant kyphosis is less with newer devices utilizing rigid 1/4 inch rods.[70] Anterior instrumentation and fusion

Table 16–3. **Patterns of idiopathic scoliosis and treatment options (after King-Moe)**

Type	Definition	Flexibility (Flexion-Extension)	Treatment
I	S-Shaped thoracolumbar curve; crosses midline	Lumbar < thoracic (or lumbar curve larger)	Fuse lumbar and thoracic vertebrae
II	S-Shaped thoracolumbar curve; crosses midline	Lumbar > thoracic (and thoracic curve larger)	Fuse thoracic vertebrae*
III	Thoracic curve; lumbar vertebrae do not cross midline	Lumbar vertebrae highly flexible	Fuse thoracic vertebrae
IV	Long thoracic curve	L4 tilts to thoracic curve	Fuse through L4
V	Double thoracic curve	T1 tilts to upper curve	Fuse through T2

*Experience with lumbar curves >50 degrees suggests that large lumbar curves should be included in the fusion for rotational correction.
From Miller MD: Review of Orthopaedics, 2nd ed. Philadelphia, WB Saunders, 1996.

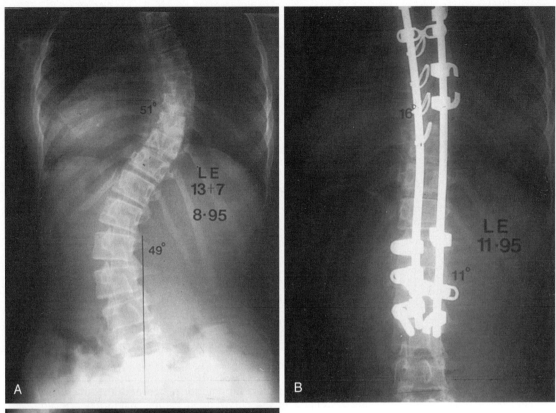

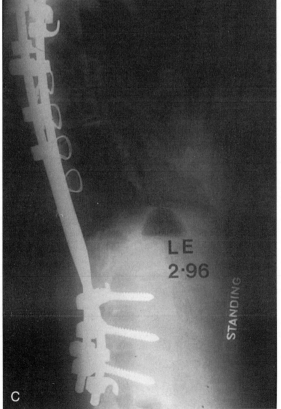

Figure 16–4. A 13-year-old boy recently diagnosed with idiopathic scoliosis. *A,* AP radiograph demonstrates a double-major (King-Moe type I) thoracic and lumbar curve. *B and C,* Posterior fusion with segmental instrumentation yielded excellent curve correction and balance in both planes. The instrumentation was stopped at L3, one level short of the stable L4 vertebra, but good balance of L3 and L4 is seen.

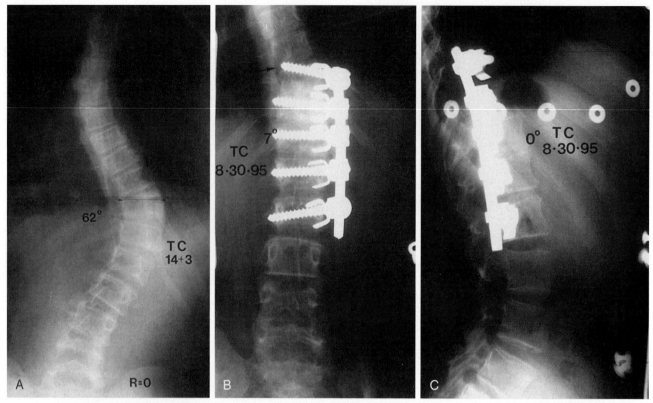

Figure 16–5. *A,* A 14-year-old boy with a 62-degree thoracolumbar curve. Good flexibility of the curve was seen on side-bending, and on reverse side-bending (to left) L2 achieved a horizontal alignment. *B and C,* Following short-segment anterior fusion and instrumentation utilizing a 1/4 inch rod, excellent correction of the curve, good coronal plane balance, and preservation of normal sagittal alignment are seen.

are also being investigated in some centers for use in isolated thoracic curves.

Either a posterior approach with posterior instrumentation or the anterior approach with anterior instrumentation is utilized in the large majority of adolescent curves. A combined approach, consisting of anterior disk excision and interbody fusion followed by posterior fusion with posterior instrumentation, usually performed at the same setting, is undertaken in adolescent idiopathic scoliosis for two main indications: large rigid curves, or to prevent the crankshaft effect in skeletally immature individuals. We consider the combined approach if well-done, physician supervised preoperative bending or traction films fail to show correction of the curve to below 50 degrees. Endoscopic techniques in the thoracic spine have recently been reported with equal degrees of curve correction as are achieved with thoracotomy, although putative cost advantages have not been documented.[53]

Congenital Scoliosis

Congenital anomalous vertebrae may lead to the development of spinal deformities. These deformities range from mild to severe and are among the types of spinal deformity that are most likely to lead to neurologic impairment and even paraplegia. Because of the propensity for certain types of congenital scoliosis to progress rapidly, because of the risk of neurologic impairment and intraspinal anomalies,

and because of the association of congenital spinal deformity with congenital anomalies of other organ systems, all orthopaedic surgeons should be aware of the implications of congenital deformity of the spine when recognized.

CLASSIFICATION

Congenital deformities of the spine are classified by the region of the spine involved, the type of deformity seen (scoliosis, kyphosis, or kyphoscoliosis), and the specific type of vertebral anomaly or anomalies.

The main types of anomalies seen are defects of segmentation and defects of formation. Mixed patterns are quite common and important factors to evaluate in assessing a deformity, and its risk of progression includes whether there is one defect or a combination of defects, as well as the location of abnormality in the frontal, sagittal, and transverse planes. The main types of anomalies (Fig. 16–6) are failures of segmentation, which lead to unilateral unsegmented bar, and failures of formation, which lead to a hemivertebra. Hemivertebrae can be completely segmented, meaning there is disk tissue separating the anomalous vertebra from both vertebra above and below it; semi-segmented, meaning disk tissue is present either above or below the hemivertebra; or non-segmented, meaning it is attached to both vertebra above and below. Hemivertebrae are also described as being incarcerated, meaning that the lateral border of the hemivertebra is in line with or medial to a line drawn from the lateral border of the vertebral body

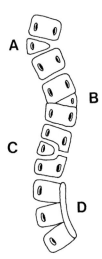

Figure 16–6. Congenital vertebral anomalies leading to scoliosis. *A,* Fully segmented hemivertebra. *B,* Unsegmented hemivertebra. *C,* Incarcerated hemivertebra. *D,* Unilateral unsegmented bar. (From Miller MD: Review of Orthopaedics, 2nd ed. Philadelphia, WB Saunders, 1996.)

above to the vertebral body below. Incarcerated hemivertebrae have a relatively low risk of progression. Hemivertebrae frequently occur in combination with other anomalies. Balanced hemivertebrae on opposite sides of the spine frequently lead to minimal progression and may be benign. On the other hand, a hemivertebra may be combined with a unilateral unsegmented bar on the contralateral side. This combination has the worst prognosis of all congenital scoliosis patterns for relentless progression.

The orthopaedic surgeon should be aware of the association between congenital anomalies of the spine and a number of other congenital birth defects. Other orthopaedic conditions seen include Klippel-Feil syndrome and Sprengel's deformity. The most important association, and the most common, is between congenital deformity of the spine and anomalies of the genitourinary system. Twenty-five to 40% of patients with congenital spine deformity have anomalies of the genitourinary tract, the most common of which is unilateral renal agenesis. This risk is increased in Klippel-Feil syndrome. All patients with congenital spine anomalies should be referred for urologic evaluation and assessed with either renal ultrasound or intravenous pyelography. Six to 10% of patients will be found to have congenital heart disease; the patient's pediatrician should be made aware of this association and the parents encouraged to seek evaluation as indicated.

PROGNOSIS

A number of authors have reviewed the natural history of congenital scoliosis. McMaster and Ohtsuka, in a large review, demonstrated significant progression in 75% of their patients. Both the region of the spine and the type of anomaly impacted on the risk of progression. The worst prognosis was seen in patients with a unilateral unsegmented bar opposite a hemivertebra, with an isolated unilateral unsegmented bar also being at significant risk for progression (Table 16–4). The best prognosis is seen with isolated hemivertebra formation, particularly incarcerated

hemivertebrae that are either semi-segmented or non-segmented. Defects at the thoracolumbar junction had a higher risk of progression than elsewhere; however, because of the impact on shoulder balance, defects in the upper thoracic and cervicothoracic spine resulted in the most readily apparent clinical deformities seen.[47]

TREATMENT

Nonoperative Treatment. Most authors believe that progression in congenital scoliosis is inevitable and the rate is determined by the type of anomaly seen. Knowledge, therefore, of the curve patterns with a high likelihood to progress, such as unilateral unsegmented bars, and curve patterns with a more benign prognosis, such as isolated hemivertebra, is an essential component of selecting appropriate treatment for these patients. Winter and associates have demonstrated that some patients with congenital scoliosis may respond, at least temporarily, to the use of a Milwaukee brace. They suggest that long, flexible curves, particularly at the thoracolumbar junction and in younger children, frequently respond to bracing.[78] The physician must be aware that the overall response of congenital spine deformity to bracing is far less satisfactory than for idiopathic curves and careful comparison of up-to-date radiographs with the patient's pre-bracing films is important to determine when bracing has failed.

Surgery. A number of approaches can be utilized when treating a congenital spinal deformity surgically.[79] The most important elements in decision making include recognizing,

Table 16–4. Progression and treatment options in congenital spinal anomalies

Risk of Progression (Highest to Lowest)	Character of Curve Progression	Treatment Options
Unilateral unsegmented bar with contralateral hemivertebra	Rapid and relentless	Posterior spinal fusion (add anterior fusion for girls <10, boys <12)
Unilateral unsegmented bar	Rapid	Same
Fully segmented hemivertebra	Steady	Anterior spinal fusion Ant/post convex hemiepiphysiodesis (age <5, curve <70°, no kyphosis) Hemivertebra excision
Partially segmented hemivertebra	Less rapid; curve usually <40° at maturity	Observation Hemivertebra excision
Incarcerated hemivertebra	May slowly progress	Observation
Nonsegmented hemivertebra	Little progression	Observation

From Miller MD: Review of Orthopaedics, 2nd ed. Philadelphia, WB Saunders, 1996.

at times in children who are quite young, the need for surgery in patients who have been documented to either have progression or have such a bleak prognosis that surgery should not be delayed, accurately defining the anomaly or anomalies present and appreciating the growth potential of the fused segment of the spine, and assessing the neurologic status of the patient and the risk for neurologic injury associated with surgery. Surgery for congenital deformities of the spine, particularly when instrumentation is utilized, has a greater risk of neurologic injury than almost any other type of deformity surgery. Intraspinal anomalies are seen in as many as 25% of patients with congenital deformity, and the possibility of such a defect should be excluded prior to undertaking surgery. Diastematomyelia, tethered cord, and intraspinal lipoma are all common and can be accurately assessed with MRI scan. MRI is also helpful in defining the congenital vertebral anomalies present.[13]

Prior to selecting the type of surgery to be performed, the surgeon must take into account the age of the patient, the growth potential, the type of deformity and natural history for progression, the area of the spine involved, and the presence of intraspinal anomalies or neurologic deficits. The main types of surgery are (1) posterior fusion, either in situ or with cast or brace correction; (2) posterior fusion and posterior instrumentation; (3) circumferential anterior and posterior fusion in situ or with cast or brace correction; (4) anterior and posterior fusion with instrumentation; (5) anterior and posterior convex hemiepiphysiodesis and arthrodesis; and (6) hemivertebra excision and circumferential fusion. Individualizing appropriate treatment to each patient and spinal deformity is both art and science and is beyond the scope of this chapter. No one operation is right for all types of deformity, but several general principles apply.

Frequently surgery is elected in very young patients with congenital spine deformity and as such the risk of continued growth anteriorly, if posterior fusion alone is selected, must be appreciated. The crankshaft phenomenon is seen in congenital as well as idiopathic deformity and should be considered when selecting appropriate treatment. Patients who are Risser 0 and have open triradiate cartilages should be considered for circumferential fusion unless the anomaly is such that anterior growth is unlikely, such as in a case of congenital kyphoscoliosis.

It has been well documented that surgery utilizing spinal instrumentation in congenital spine deformities poses significant risk for the development of paraplegia. Severe deformity is frequently seen in patients with congenital anomalies, and it is axiomatic that the more complex the surgery, and the more correction that is sought, the greater the risk that entails. The most conservative operation, involving either a posterior or a circumferential fusion and correction with only casting or bracing, frequently results in little if any correction. On the other hand, aggressive attempts at osteotomy, correction through instrumentation, or hemivertebra excision frequently results in remarkable correction but subjects the patient to a greater risk of neurologic catastrophe. These more aggressive procedures are frequently indicated, and in many cases the surgeon, parents, and patient are willing to accept the risks, but each case should be assessed to ensure that the cosmetic,

functional, and physiologic benefits of correction are worth the risks undertaken. In many cases, less aggressive surgery is possible if early recognition of the inevitable need for surgery occurs.

Another consideration in the patient with congenital spine deformity who is undergoing or has undergone surgery is the need for long-term follow-up. Particularly in prepubertal patients, an entirely appropriate operation may be selected and an optimal result achieved, but long-term follow-up may demonstrate curve progression or adding on to the curve many years later. Follow-up through and beyond the period of skeletal maturity is essential, and it is important to warn parents in advance of the significant possibility, when surgery is undertaken for congenital spine deformity, that further surgery may be necessary in the years to come.

Neuromuscular Scoliosis

A number of neuromuscular conditions are seen in which spinal deformity, most commonly scoliosis, is common and contributes significantly to functional deterioration of the patient. Recognition of the risk of spinal deformity, knowledge of the natural history, and integration of these with the patient's overall function and prognosis lead to appropriate decision making.

CLASSIFICATION

Neuromuscular deformity of the spine has been classified by the Scoliosis Research Society as either neuropathic or myopathic.[67] Neuropathic conditions include primary upper motor neuron or lower motor neuron abnormalities. The most common upper motor neuron disorder treated is cerebral palsy; other upper motor neuron conditions include Friedreich's ataxia, Charcot-Marie-Tooth disease, and abnormalities of the spinal cord such as syringomyelia and spinal cord tumors or trauma. Lower motor neuron conditions include poliomyelitis and spinal muscular atrophy. Myopathic conditions include arthrogryposis, congenital hypotonia, and most importantly muscular dystrophy.

PROGNOSIS

The above classification differentiates a number of the neuromuscular conditions and the spinal deformities seen. There are common factors, however, that affect most patients with neuromuscular deformity and that should be appreciated by the orthopaedic surgeon when involved in such a patient's care. Most patients with neuromuscular scoliosis should be considered at relatively high risk for progression, which at times may be astonishingly rapid. The risk of progression is greatest in patients with spastic quadriplegia, particularly those who are nonambulators. The risk is greater once the curve progresses beyond 50 degrees, and the risk of ongoing progression, even after skeletal maturity, must be appreciated.

The physician should be aware of the implication of certain functional landmarks as well, such as the muscular dystrophy patient who becomes a wheelchair ambulator, and the risk of progression signified by this occurrence.[63] Most patients with neuromuscular dysfunction are at risk for, or already have, impaired pulmonary function. This is frequently exacerbated by alterations in the chest cage seen with scoliosis. In some conditions, for example Duchenne's muscular dystrophy, cardiopulmonary compromise is a common cause of death, is very sensitive to worsening scoliosis, and may preclude scoliosis surgery in some cases. In this condition in particular, therefore, it is essential to recognize the development of any significant (greater than 30 degrees) scoliosis, to appreciate the inevitable risk of progression and the implications thereof, and to intervene early in the disease process with surgical stabilization.

The impact of spinal deformity on the overall function of the patient with neuromuscular conditions such as cerebral palsy is frequently the primary determinant in initiating treatment or electing surgery. Progressive scoliosis frequently leads to truncal imbalance, pelvic obliquity, and difficulty sitting. The individual's ability to freely use the upper extremities and ultimately even to sit in a wheelchair may be compromised by worsening scoliosis, and quality of life considerations such as these should not be neglected when considering the appropriateness of treatment. More controversial is the prospect for pain related to severe scoliosis. It has been our experience that parents and caregivers frequently report, following successful surgical treatment, a significant improvement in comfort as well as improved sitting and hygiene.

Evaluation of a patient with neuromuscular spinal deformity includes assessment of the patient's intellectual skills, communications skills, and sitting capabilities. The presence of contractures, particularly about the hips, or pelvic obliquity should be noted. The skin is carefully assessed for turgor and for any areas of skin breakdown. The magnitude of deformity in both the frontal and sagittal plane is evaluated clinically, as is the flexibility of the deformity. The impact of the curve on the patient's ability to sit is assessed, and careful attention must be paid to sagittal plane problems when seated; many patients have poor muscle tone and lack head and trunk control, with a tendency to fall *forward*, which may not be related to the magnitude of scoliosis. It is vital to consider this when planning either surgical or nonsurgical treatment. Standing or sitting radiographs in both the AP and lateral plane, of the entire spine, are performed, and traction views may be used to assess curve flexibility. The extent and direction of pelvic obliquity should be measured.

It is important when considering a patient for surgery for neuromuscular scoliosis to assess the patient's cardiopulmonary function and nutritional status. Formal consultation with a nutritionist, if there is any question about the patient's protein balance and caloric intake, is frequently very helpful. Deferring surgery until positive nitrogen balance has been achieved may help to avoid catastrophic wound complications.

TREATMENT

Nonoperative treatment may include observation, the use of seating support systems, or the use of bracing. Observation is appropriate for mild curves measuring less than 20 to 25 degrees, without functional impairment. Seating support systems are utilized for lesser curves, not requiring bracing, where sitting imbalance or pelvic obliquity is of concern. A well-made seating support system can accommodate pelvic obliquity and minimize the risk of skin complications, can provide assistance in sitting balance, and can be modified to assist in head control.

Bracing is indicated for curves greater than 25 to 30 degrees, particularly if they are documented to progress, in patients with sensate skin. It should be stressed that bracing is *inappropriate* for patients with Duchenne's muscular dystrophy, who should be treated surgically if scoliosis is seen to progress beyond approximately 30 degrees. A total contact TLSO is otherwise employed and is frequently effective in patients with neuropathic conditions. Bracing frequently improves sitting balance and in many cases will provide curve control allowing for continued growth. In most cases, however, surgery is only delayed, but not permanently avoided, with the use of bracing.[14]

Surgery. Surgical treatment is indicated for progressive curves beyond 60 degrees or curves that cannot be controlled with bracing. In very young children (under age 8), we will sometimes observe curves of somewhat greater magnitude as long as control in the brace is possible and sitting balance is maintained. In such cases, careful follow-up is essential, and any evidence that the curve is progressing beyond 80 to 90 degrees or is becoming more rigid warrants surgical intervention no matter the patient's age.

Surgical treatment of neuromuscular scoliosis consists of a posterior spinal fusion with segmental spinal instrumentation. The issues to be addressed by the surgeon include whether or not to extend the fusion to pelvis, the type of segmental instrumentation utilized, and whether or not circumferential fusion, rather than posterior fusion alone, should be employed.

Fusion to the pelvis is employed in neuropathic curves such as cerebral palsy in the presence of fixed pelvic obliquity.[3] Most wheelchair-bound patients who have curves over 60 degrees tend to have subluxated or dislocated hips and frequently have pelvic obliquity and sitting imbalance. Extension of the fusion and instrumentation to the pelvis utilizing the Galveston technique result in significant improvement in sitting balance and pelvic obliquity with better maintenance of correction of both the scoliosis and the pelvic obliquity, when compared with fusion to the lower lumbar spine without extension to the pelvis (Fig. 16–7). Because the deterioration of sitting balance is one of the main indications for surgery in these patients, our preferred technique in most patients who are wheelchair bound with spastic cerebral palsy is segmental sublaminar instrumentation utilizing the Galveston technique with a continuous bilateral rod, inserted bilaterally in the posterior column of the ileum. On the other hand, myopathic conditions such as muscular dystrophy less commonly result in such severe fixed pelvic obliquity that fusion to the pelvis is necessary.

Circumferential anterior and posterior fusion is elected for curves at risk for development of the crankshaft phenomenon, for nonunion, or for curves that are either so large (greater than 90 to 100 degrees), so rigid, or that involve significant kyphosis such that posterior instrumentation alone is unlikely to result in adequate alignment. The crankshaft phenomenon is a concern in the young, skeletally immature patient. Particularly in cerebral palsy, delayed skeletal maturation is common, so simply assessing the patient's age may lead to an underestimation of the

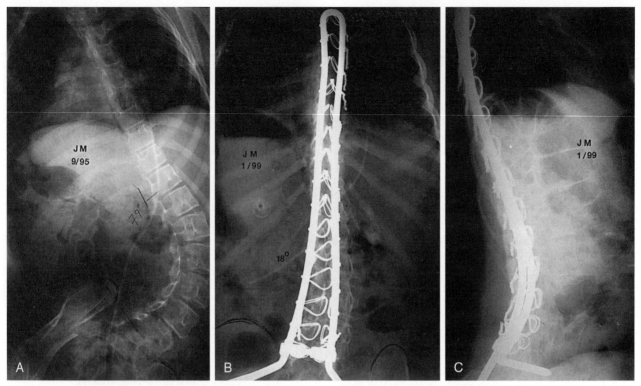

Figure 16–7. A 12-year-old girl with spastic cerebral palsy and total body involvement. She is wheelchair bound and is noted to have progressive scoliosis. *A,* Preoperative AP radiograph demonstrating a 79-degree curve and severe pelvic obliquity. Traction-bending views demonstrated correction to 48 degrees. *B and C,* AP and lateral views 3 years following posterior fusion and segmental instrumentation to the pelvis. Allograft bone was used, and a solid fusion is seen.

potential for continued anterior growth. Assessment of the status of the triradiate cartilages is utilized to help in decision making, and every attempt is made to control curves with bracing long enough to avoid the need for combined anterior and posterior fusion when possible. Conversely, once patients have completed growth, typically after age 20, we frequently see larger curves that tend to be more rigid. These patients are also at greater risk for the development of pseudarthrosis, particularly since banked bone is the predominant type of graft used. In these patients, therefore, circumferential fusion should be considered and the use of femoral ring allografts in the lumbar and lumbosacral region is helpful to protect the posterior instrumentation and preserve lumbar lordosis.

The results of surgery for neuromuscular spinal deformities have varied among authors and are dependent on the underlying disorder. Curve correction of from 50 to 75% is reported for patients with cerebral palsy, and with the use of banked bone a pseudarthrosis rate of 5 to 10% may be anticipated. Fusion to the pelvis utilizing the Galveston technique results in long-lasting improvement in fixed pelvic obliquity and sitting balance in most patients. Complications are not uncommon in these patients, however, and include wound breakdown, deep infection, and nonunion leading at times to instrumentation failure.

Kyphosis

Kyphosis in a growing child and adolescent may be seen secondary to many different conditions. An appreciation of the normal thoracic kyphosis, which ranges from 20 to 50 degrees, is important and will eliminate the need for worry in many cases of mild thoracic roundback. Excessive kyphosis can be seen as a postural phenomenon, secondary to congenital anomalies, in neuromuscular conditions, following trauma, surgery, or irradiation, and in metabolic conditions such as osteogenesis imperfecta. It is also seen associated with various skeletal dysplasias including achondroplasia and neurofibromatosis, in inflammatory disorders, and as a complication of vertebral osteomyelitis, most notably tuberculosis. It should be appreciated that most cases of true scoliosis represent lordoscoliosis, although with greater rotation an apparent kyphotic deformity may ensue. In addition, some scoliosis, such as in neurofibromatosis or Marfan's syndrome, may present as true kyphoscoliosis.

The most common kyphotic disorder seen by the orthopaedist is the adolescent with postural round back. Long-standing complaints of "poor posture" are common and may have been present in other members of the family. An appreciation of the tendency of some adolescents going through puberty to habitually stand with rounded shoulders may explain the perceived increase in kyphosis. Postural roundback may be differentiated from other types of kyphosis such as Scheuermann's disease by the presence of a more generalized hyperkyphosis extending throughout the thoracic spine, which is typically quite flexible.[6] Aching pain in the shoulder girdles and thoracic spinal region is not uncommon with any type of thoracic kyphosis and may be a presenting complaint. In the absence of radiographic evidence of a more serious underlying cause for kyphosis, postural round back is treated with an exercise program involving strengthening of the thoracic extensor musculature and shoulder girdles. Patient compliance is frequently an issue, and the potential for poor compliance should be discussed with the parents. Observation alone may, in many cases, be the most rational approach.

SCHEUERMANN'S KYPHOSIS

In 1920, Scheuermann first described the radiographic manifestations of progressive juvenile kyphosis.[61] In 1964, his son-in-law Sorenson further defined the x-ray definition of juvenile kyphosis and described radiographic criteria that are currently widely accepted: (1) wedging of three adjacent vertebrae of 5 degrees or more, (2) endplate irregularity, and (3) Schmorl's node formation[64] (Fig. 16–8). Bradford has noted that strict adherence to these criteria may exclude certain patients with hyperkyphosis who are at risk for progression and for the development of some of the adverse sequelae associated with Scheuermann's kyphosis. In addition, any such radiographic changes in even a single vertebra in the thoracolumbar or lumbar spine are to be considered abnormal.[6]

The etiology of Scheuermann's disease continues to be debated. Mechanical and metabolic factors have been

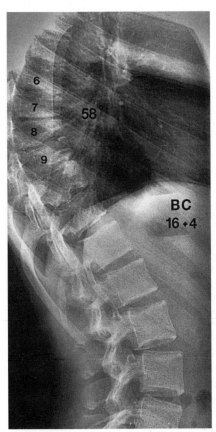

Figure 16–8. A 16-year-old boy with mild thoracic back pain and hyperkyphosis. Radiographic findings diagnostic of Scheuermann's kyphosis are seen in the mid-thoracic region, including endplate irregularities, Schmorl's node formation, and wedging, which is most marked at T8.

suggested, and disruption of the cartilage ring apophysis, abnormalities of the endplates leading to Schmorl's node formation (herniation of disk material through the endplate), and genetic factors have all been implicated. Whether or not these factors are primary or secondary continues to be at issue.

Scheuermann's disease has been described in from 0.4 to 8.3% of the population and appears to be more common in girls than in boys.[8] Unlike scoliosis, juvenile kyphosis is rarely diagnosed prior to age 10 and many times patients are initially seen at or beyond skeletal maturity. Presenting complaints include pain and deformity. Mild to moderate thoracic back pain is more common in more severe deformity, or in deformity at the thoracolumbar junction or the upper lumbar spine. When lower back pain is associated with thoracic kyphosis, spondylolysis needs to be ruled out (investigated).

The radiographic criteria for the diagnosis of Scheuermann's disease have been discussed. Standing x-rays are essential and should include anteroposterior (AP) and lateral views. Mild scoliosis is frequently seen with minimal rotation. We agree with Bradford that Scheuermann's kyphosis is an appropriate diagnosis if Sorenson's x-ray abnormalities are seen with one or more wedged vertebrae in the presence of hyperkyphosis. It should be noted that spontaneous anterior interbody fusion does not occur in Scheuermann's disease, serving to differentiate it from congenital kyphosis.

The natural history of Scheuermann's kyphosis has been assessed by numerous authors but continues to be debated. Progressive hyperkyphosis represents a cosmetic abnormality, and this may be adequate reason to entertain nonoperative or operative treatment. Scheuermann's disease does not, on the other hand, result in pulmonary compromise and has an uncertain relationship to back pain in the adult. Murray and Weinstein, in a long-term follow-up study of patients with untreated Scheuermann's kyphosis, reported an increase in the presence of back pain in affected individuals but did not note significant interference with the ability to hold gainful employment or with long-term function.[50] This is consistent with Sorenson's original report. The risk of progression in Scheuermann's kyphosis must be viewed in light of the gradual increase in kyphosis that is frequently seen through aging. Unlike scoliosis, at this time there is no clear-cut evidence that a certain magnitude of hyperkyphosis results in such a high risk of adult progression as to merit prophylactic treatment in the absence of other indications.

Treatment

Nonoperative. Nonoperative methods of treatment include exercises, casting, and bracing. Casting, while effective, will rarely be tolerated by the adolescent and is typically reserved for use in the infant and toddler. An aggressive exercise regimen is an important adjunct to treatment but will rarely, as an isolated means, result in long-lasting curve correction. It may, however, be effective for generalized well being, hamstring stretching, and relief of mild thoracic back pain.

Bracing was first described by Moe in 1965 for use in juvenile kyphosis.[49] Bradford and coworkers, expanding on Moe's work, reported in 1974 on the results of Milwaukee brace treatment. While improvement is seen, the authors note the importance of at least 1 year of growth remaining as a prerequisite to bracing. Furthermore, more severe kyphoses, greater than 74 degrees, are less likely to improve and are more likely to lose correction when patients are followed for 5 years after cessation of bracing. Long-term maintenance of correction was seen, however, in patients with lesser kyphosis.[8] Underarm orthoses are at a mechanical disadvantage in most cases of Scheuermann's kyphosis but may be utilized for curves with an apex below T9, particularly for Scheuermann's disease occurring at the thoracolumbar junction.[6]

Surgery. Surgery is indicated for adolescent patients who have failed bracing and who have a sufficiently objectionable cosmetic appearance, as perceived by the patient and parents as well as by the surgeon, to merit major spinal surgery. Surgery is occasionally indicated for juvenile kyphosis with ongoing symptomatic complaints of thoracic back pain, but a diligent search for other causes of the pain, both orthopaedic and non-orthopaedic, should be carried out prior to considering surgery for this indication. Finally, surgery is occasionally elected in the adult with curve progression, a cosmetically objectionable appearance, or intractable pain. Pain is seen more frequently with kyphosis greater than 66 degrees and is caused by muscular imbalance owing to hyperkyphosis and/or fixed degenerative changes.

Surgical treatment consists of spinal fusion and almost always includes the use of posterior instrumentation. Combined anterior release of the thickened anterior longitudinal ligament, disk excision, and anterior interbody fusion followed by posterior instrumentation and fusion are frequently employed. The indications for combined anterior and posterior fusion include bigger curves (greater than 70 degrees), and stiffer curves that are unlikely to be correctable to a residual kyphosis of less than 50 or 55 degrees[9] (Fig. 16–9). It is important when undertaking surgery to select the appropriate fusion levels including appreciation of the uppermost kyphotic segment as well as extending the fusion distally, not just to the lowest involved level but to and across the first lordotic disk space. This may require extending the fusion down as low as L2 or even L3, but is necessary to avoid the development of a junctional kyphosis.

Rigid segmental instrumentation is employed. As with fracture constructs, instrumentation can be used to distract, compress, or in a three-point bending mode. Constructs utilizing three-point bending, particularly when sublaminar instrumentation is utilized, have been reported with good initial correction in Scheuermann's but have a significant risk for the development of junctional kyphosis.[21] We prefer utilization of a compression implant in this deformity.

Congenital Kyphosis

Congenital kyphosis is a relatively uncommon type of spinal deformity, but, because of the significant risk of progression and the risk of neurologic compromise, awareness of the manifestations of this condition, the natural history, and appropriate treatment is essential. Congenital kyphosis is seen with failures of formation, failures of

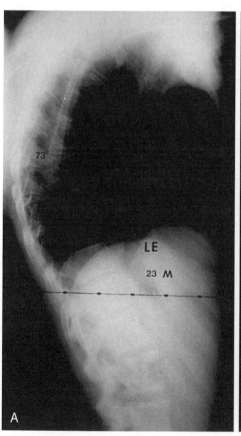
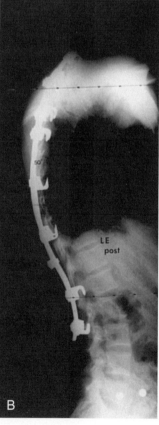

Figure 16–9. A 23-year-old man with persistent, severe thoracic back pain despite 2 years of aggressive exercising and medication usage. *A,* Preoperatively, he has 73 degrees of kyphosis, which corrected to 50 degrees on a hyperextension lateral radiograph. *B,* He was treated with a posterior fusion with posterior instrumentation only, with good correction. Although the kyphosis ends at T12, note that the fusion extends down to L2, into the lordotic part of the spine.

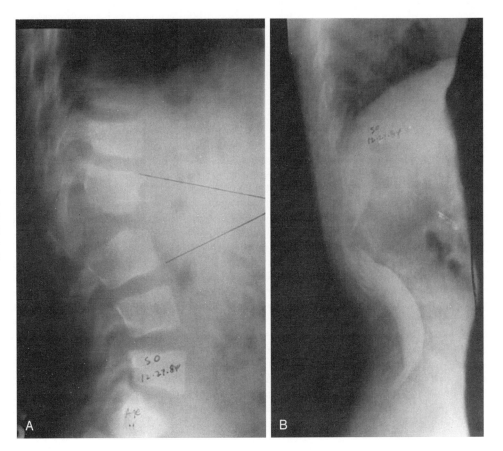

Figure 16–10. *A,* An 11-year-old boy with type I congenital kyphosis (failure of formation) with new onset of enuresis. *B,* Myelography demonstrated a high-grade block.

segmentation, and mixed anomalies. Unlike scoliosis, in congenital kyphosis it is failure of formation, the congenital hemivertebra, that is most ominous.[77] These defects are more common than kyphosis secondary to defective segmentation, and commonly lead to severe deformity. In addition, with the exception of tuberculosis, this deformity poses the greatest risk for the development of neurologic impairment in the absence of surgery (Fig. 16–10).[43]

There is no known nonoperative treatment for congenital kyphosis. Patients with defects of segmentation are at lesser risk for progression but should, upon diagnosis, be treated surgically. The procedure of choice is posterior fusion extending one level above and one level below the anomalous region.

Congenital kyphosis secondary to hemivertebra formation requires prompt intervention, even when seemingly benign. Patients under the age of 5 years and with kyphosis less than 50 to 55 degrees are treated with posterior fusion alone. Instrumentation is not typically required, and immobilization in a hyperextension cast is employed. Consideration should be given to re-exploration and re-grafting at 6 months. Frequently these patients undergo slow gradual improvement in their deformity as a result of continued anterior growth.[77]

For children older than 5 years of age, or with kyphosis greater than 55 degrees, combined anterior and posterior surgery is undertaken. Winter has described thorough release of the anterior tethering structures, resection of disk material back to the posterior anulus bilaterally, and posterior correction utilizing compression instrumentation. Traction, either preoperatively or using distraction instrumenta-

tion at the time of surgery, should be avoided in this condition.[79] The presence of a neurologic deficit may need to be addressed. When an intraspinal anomaly such as diastematomyelia is identified, resection of the "bar" should be considered in the patient with a progressive neurologic deficit. In addition, if significant correction of the spinal deformity is anticipated, the lesion should also be removed. Neurologic deficit is common with progression of the kyphosis and progressive extrusion of the hemivertebra into the spinal canal. In the presence of a mild deficit or an extremely flexible curve, anterior release followed by posterior correction alone may be indicated. Otherwise, formal resection of the hemivertebra with decompression of the dural tube should be undertaken, followed by anterior strut grafting and posterior compression instrumentation and fusion.

CERVICAL SPINE DISORDER

Klippel-Feil Syndrome

In 1912, Klippel and Feil described massive congenital fusion of the cervical spine in a 46-year-old tailor with multiple associated anomalies. Since then, the classic triad of Klippel-Feil syndrome has consisted of a short neck, low posterior hairline, and marked limitation of motion of the neck. Most surgeons now consider any case of congenital fusion of cervical vertebrae to constitute an example of Klippel-Feil syndrome, and to suggest that the patient is at risk for associated anomalies.[56]

The etiology of Klippel-Feil syndrome continues to be disputed. Theories include primary vascular disruption, fetal insult, primary neural tube abnormality, and a primary genetic etiology. The incidence of this condition has never been determined, but reasonable estimates vary from 0.2 to 7 per thousand.

Probably the most important aspect of the Klippel-Feil syndrome is its association with other syndromes and anomalies. Congenital cervical fusion has been reported in fetal alcohol syndrome as well as in Goldenhar's syndrome. Anomalies that are associated with Klippel-Feil syndrome include abnormalities of the musculoskeletal system, craniofacial anomalies, central nervous system anomalies, and anomalies of the genitourinary tract, the cardiovascular system, the gastrointestinal system, and the lungs. The most common musculoskeletal anomaly is scoliosis, which is most often congenital. Sprengel's deformity, cervical ribs, thoracic outlet syndrome, and torticollis are also seen. The most common craniofacial anomaly is hearing loss, reported in 15 to 36% of patients. Synkinesia, involuntary paired movement of the hands and arms, is the most common central nervous system anomaly. It is present in 15 to 20% of young patients with Klippel-Feil syndrome but appears to improve as the individuals get older. The etiology is believed to be failure of adequate decussation of the pyramidal tracts in the upper cervical spine.[32] Several other central nervous system anomalies such as syringomyelia and diastematomyelia have been reported, and an increased incidence of congenital cervical spinal stenosis is a well-known phenomenon; this may be complicated by the development of instability adjacent to the congenital fusion, which is also common in Klippel-Feil.

Genitourinary anomalies are present in 25 to 35% of patients.[9, 19] Distribution is similar to that of congenital scoliosis, and the most common anomaly is unilateral renal agenesis.[35] As with congenital spine deformity, routine screening of the genitourinary tract with ultrasound has been recommended for patients with congenital cervical fusion.[25]

Congenital cervical fusion is, in many individuals, asymptomatic. On the other hand, progressive instability may develop secondary to abnormal stresses on motion segments above or below the areas of congenital fusion and this instability, particularly in individuals with pre-existing stenosis, may lead to clinically significant spinal cord or nerve root compression (Fig. 16–11). Three fusion patterns have been defined[52] that may identify patients with Klippel-Feil syndrome who are at particular risk for neurologic injury. These include two sets of adjacent block vertebrae with one or two intervening open disk spaces, occipitalization of the atlas with a congenital fusion below C2, creating a risk for C1–C2 instability, and congenital fusion with associated cervical stenosis. We have seen several patients with Klippel-Feil syndrome who have developed degenerative changes and instability adjacent to the congenitally fused level with resultant myelopathy.[66]

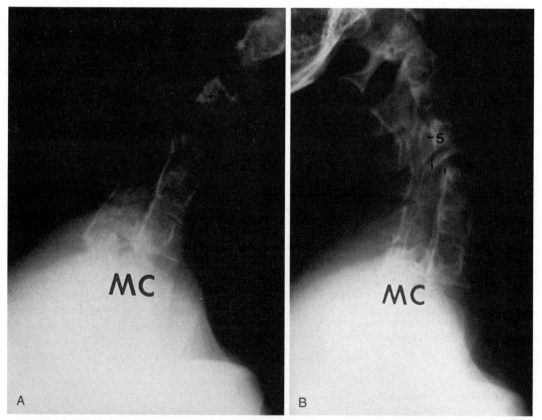

Figure 16–11. A 25-year-old man with neck and arm pain, seen to have congenital cervical fusion from C4 to C6. He was hyperreflexive and had positive Babinski's signs bilaterally. Flexion/extension radiography *(A and B)* demonstrated 8 mm of motion at C3–C4. He was treated with posterior fusion at C3–C4 with complete resolution of his symptoms.

While the literature generally advocates a relatively conservative approach to asymptomatic instability in Klippel-Feil syndrome, we believe that evidence of myelopathy, even mild, in the presence of instability merits surgical stabilization. This minimizes the risk of sudden catastrophic neurologic injury, also seen on occasion in patients with Klippel-Feil syndrome in association with instability adjacent to fused vertebrae.

Os Odontoideum

Os odontoideum refers to a separate ossicle that is unattached to the body of the axis. It is typically located in the region of the normal dens and is believed to originate as part of the ossification center of the dens. The etiology of os odontoideum was originally felt to be failure of fusion of the secondary center of ossification for the dens to the body of the axis. More recent evidence suggests that unrecognized trauma leads to nonunion of fractured dens (Fig. 16–12).[29]

On radiographic evaluation, the os is typically seen as a hypoplastic sclerotic ossicle that may be anterior to, at, or posterior to, the typical location of the dens. Frequently the anterior ring of C1 is enlarged. The os may be fused cephalad to the clivus, a variety referred to as *dystopic os odontoideum*, which has a greater likelihood of neurologic injury.[29]

It has been well documented that os odontoideum can lead to neurologic compromise and even sudden death. Any patient with a history of neurologic impairment or neurologic symptoms who is diagnosed with os odontoideum should undergo surgical stabilization. A more difficult issue is appropriate treatment for the asymptomatic child with os odontoideum. We believe that radiographic evidence of instability (4 mm more of motion at C1–C2 on flexion/extension radiography) is adequate justification for surgical treatment in these children. In the absence of instability, the child is followed with serial dynamic radiography; any evidence of increasing motion, pain, or neurologic sequelae merits surgery.

Atlantoaxial Rotatory Displacement

Atlantoaxial rotatory displacement may be seen following minor trauma, an upper respiratory infection, or head and neck surgery. An acute torticollis is seen, and a classic "cocked robin" appearance has been described. Neck pain is usually present, but in nontraumatic cases neurologic involvement is rare.

The diagnosis of fixed rotatory displacement of C1 on C2 is made radiographically. Plain lateral radiography is obtained to assess for anterior subluxation of the atlas on the axis, which may be absent, mild, or marked. Subtle malalignment of the head or the posterior arch of the C1 may also be seen. The most definitive test is dynamic CT scanning.[28] Axial scanning through the C1–C2 complex with the head rotated 45 degrees to the right and 45 degrees to the left will identify failure of the atlas to rotate normally around the axis, even when the head appears to be turned. This is diagnostic of atlantoaxial rotatory displacement, or fixed rotatory subluxation as it is sometimes called.

Treatment of rotatory subluxation depends on the duration of symptoms and presence of anterior C1–C2 subluxation. Individuals with less than 1 week of symptoms are

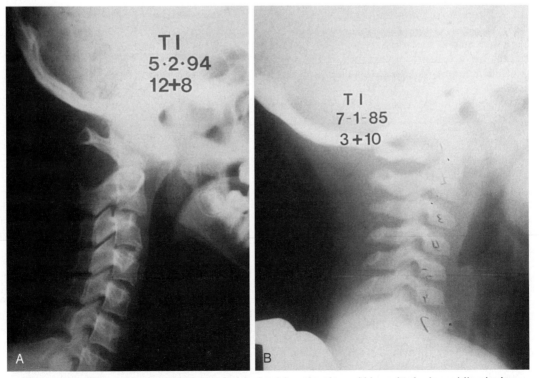

Figure 16–12. A 12-year-old boy who developed neck pain and Lhermitte's sign while playing soccer. *A,* Lateral radiography demonstrates an os odontoideum. History–taking revealed a prior neck injury falling out of a tree at age 3. X-rays at that time *(B)* were normal.

usually treated with a soft cervical collar and rest. In patients who fail to respond or in whom symptoms have persisted for more than 1 week, hospitalization with the use of head halter traction is employed. Muscle relaxants may be employed in this setting. When symptoms have been present for more than 1 month, halo traction is utilized, although a relatively high risk for re-displacement, even after reduction, should be appreciated.[40]

Surgery is elected for atlantoaxial rotatory displacement that has persisted for greater than 3 months, that has recurred following adequate reduction, or in patients in whom neurologic findings are present. In situ C1–C2 fusion is performed. Positioning in a halo vest, with the patient awake following the procedure, is employed to maximize comfort and cosmetic appearance. Residual deformity usually resolves spontaneously over time in the presence of a solid fusion.[40]

Congenital Muscular Torticollis

Congential muscular torticollis is more common in first-born children and in breech deliveries. The etiology is believed to be local compression to the sternocleidomastoid muscle at the time of delivery. A clinical and pathologic picture similar to compartment syndrome has been described.[22] Torticollis is more common on the right side and in children with developmental dysplasia of the hip.

A contracted sternocleidomastoid muscle results in tilting of the head toward the affected side with contralateral rotation of the chin and ill-leveled eyes. If detected early, a mass may be felt in the muscle belly. Deformity of the skull and face may be seen in more severe cases.

Conservative treatment with stretching exercises is the most common form of treatment. In persistent deformity after 1 year of age, surgery is considered. Options include unipolar or bipolar release of the sternocleidomastoid, resection of the muscle, and Z-plasty lengthening. If surgery is delayed later than approximately 3 years of age, the risk of permanent ocular deformity is higher even after torticollis correction.

Down's Syndrome

Upper cervical involvement in Down's syndrome (trisomy 21) has been reported in an alarmingly high proportion of affected children and adults. Both occipitocervical and atlantoaxial instability have been reported, with estimates of occipitocervical instability as high as 60% and C1–C2 instability as high as 20%.[57, 69] An increased incidence of anomalies of the cervical spine, such as os odontoideum, has been identified in individuals with Down's syndrome and C1–C2 instability.

The natural history of atlantoaxial instability in Down's syndrome has not been clearly defined. Burke and coworkers demonstrated a tendency toward gradual progression in some individuals and reported that progressive instability and neurologic impairment were more likely in males and after the age of 10.[16] Most individuals are asymptomatic, however, and screening radiographs taken for the Special Olympics lead in most cases to diagnosis, evaluation, and questions about appropriate treatment.

Most individuals with Down's syndrome and C1–C2 instability are asymptomatic, and the appropriate role for surgical treatment is unclear. An exceedingly high complication rate, including nonunion, infection, neurologic worsening, and even death, has been reported with C1–C2 fusion in these patients, and there is only anecdotal evidence that atlantoaxial instability is associated with neurologic catastrophe (Fig. 16–13).[24, 62] The presence of C1–C2 instability with motion of greater than 4 or 5 mm unfortunately requires restricting high-risk sports participation. Since most surgeons restrict these activities following successful C1–C2 fusion, surgery is not indicated simply to continue Special Olympics participation. Based on the high complication rate reported when surgery is undertaken in this condition, we favor a fairly conservative approach. Certainly, any individual with a clear-cut history of neurologic impairment or evidence of myelopathy on physical examination, and who is documented to have occipitocervical or atlantoaxial instability, should undergo stabilization. When C1–C2 fusion is contemplated, careful scrutiny of the occipitocervical junction should be performed to assess for subtle abnormalities at this level. Otherwise, we favor observation in most cases of atlantoaxial instability in neurologically normal, asymptomatic individuals.[24]

The presence of occipitocervical instability and its significance are less clearly defined. A higher success rate is seen when fusion is extended to the occiput, and we believe that doing so is prudent whenever there is any suggestion of occipitocervical instability. The role of occipitocervical

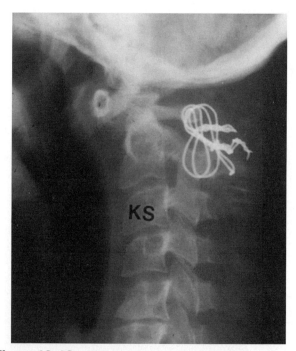

Figure 16–13. A 26-year-old man with Down's syndrome, 6 months following C1–C2 fusion for instability. Lateral radiography demonstrates loss of reduction and nonunion; he had worsening myelopathy and gait disturbance. Two subsequent operations resulted in only partial recovery, and he remained worse neurologically than before his initial operation.

or atlantoaxial stabilization in asymptomatic individuals who are normal neurologically is unclear. We consider surgery for occipitocervical instability of 4 mm or greater (1 mm is normal) or for atlantoaxial instability of 10 mm or greater, although, even in this setting, restriction from high-risk sports such as gymnastics, diving, and soccer and close radiographic follow-up constitute a reasonable approach.[24] This emotionally charged issue should be discussed in detail with the patient and parents. They should be appraised of the uncertain natural history of the disorder and the significant complication rate seen when surgery is elected, and allowed to consider these factors in addition to the risk of neurologic injury.

SPINE INJURY

A relatively small proportion of patients sustaining spinal cord injury (SCI) is made up of children and younger adolescents, but the incidence of SCI in children escalates significantly after 15 years of age. In most series, approximately two thirds of cases of SCI involve cervical spine injury, a slightly greater proportion than the even split between cervical and thoracolumbar injuries seen in adults.[37] Among the possible causes of spine and spinal cord injuries in children are motor vehicle accidents, penetrating injuries, and athletic injuries, but also included are birth injury to the spinal cord and child abuse.

The child's relatively large head size, particularly in young children, figures significantly in the consideration of spine injuries. Because the child's large head will impose a flexed posture on the cervical spine when lying supine, immobilization of the child under age 8 with a potential injury to the neck should be accomplished by placing the torso on a specially elevated pad, or utilizing a customized back board with a recess for the occiput.[36] Large head size also contributes to the pattern of injuries seen under age 8, with the large majority of injuries in younger patients occurring at C2 and above. After age 8, the injury pattern becomes more typical of that seen in teenagers and adults.

Several unique or atypical injury patterns are seen with increased frequency in young children. As noted, a predilection for upper cervical spine injuries is common, most of which heal quite well with nonoperative treatment. Special considerations in immobilization of the young child include modifying the application of the halo. In children under age 4, multiple halo pins, as many as eight in some cases, are utilized, and they should be "finger tight," rather than tightened to the 6 or 8 pounds recommended for adults. Under age 2, a Minerva cast is utilized for upper cervical spine immobilization, in preference to the halo.

A common SCI pattern seen in children is spinal cord injury without radiographic abnormality (SCIWORA).[73] This is more common in younger children and is extremely rare in adults. By definition, these injuries involve neurologic impairment in children who have normal plain radiographs of the spine. The use of MRI and myelography has been described, and MRI may identify physeal injuries or ligamentous disruption where plain films were believed to be nondiagnostic. In addition, cord swelling or disruption may be seen.

The mechanism of injury of SCIWORA is unclear, and it is likely, given the diverse clinical patterns seen, that there is more than one cause for this tragic injury. Mechanisms that have been suggested include physeal injury with subluxation, transient disk herniation, traction injuries to the spinal cord, and infarction of the cord. Pang and Wilberger have suggested that subclinical instability may be present, although the majority of cases reported have not involved any radiographic documentation of instability.[55] The role of immobilization is unclear, but certainly the child with SCI should be immobilized until complete radiographic evaluation of the spine is completed. Normal static radiography does not exclude the possibility of a dislocation or subluxation that has spontaneously reduced, and a pattern of SCIWORA with a stable spine should only be assumed once instability has been excluded. Once this has been done, however, immobilization would appear to be pointless and can interfere with optimal nursing care and rehabilitation.

PSEUDOSUBLUXATION

Cattell and Filtzer first described pseudosubluxation of the cervical spine in children in 1965.[19] They noted the presence of anterior displacement of C2 on C3 in 9% of children; pseudosubluxation has subsequently been reported to occur at C3–C4 as well. It is believed to be facilitated by the more horizontal orientation of the upper cervical facet joints, which become more vertical as the child ages; pseudosubluxation is rarely seen after age 8. Pseudosubluxation of C2 on C3 (Fig. 16–14) may be differentiated from traumatic injury by the absence of a history of sufficient trauma to explain the radiographic injury; by the presence of selective kyphosis throughout the cervical spine, rather than compensatory hyperextension of the segments below C3 seen with a traumatic injury; and by the spontaneous reduction of C2 on C3 when the head is extended. Observation is indicated when pseudosubluxation is diagnosed.

BACK PAIN IN CHILDREN

Back pain in the adult is so common as to be considered a normal variant. Although a bothersome and at times incapacitating condition, most patients and family members accept the fact that backache is a routine occurrence, frequently difficult to diagnose, and often resistant to treatment. When significant back pain occurs in children or adolescents, however, an entirely different approach is seen on the part of family members and referring primary care practitioners.

In our experience, it is important to differentiate between back pain in children and back pain in adolescents. The prevalence of back pain in individuals under age 10 is quite low, with Taimela and coworkers reporting a prevalence of 1% in 7-year-olds, 6% in 10-year-olds, and 18% in 14- to 16-year-olds.[65] This is in keeping with previous reports. It is therefore important to recognize the significance of persistent complaints of back pain in prepubertal children and to very aggressively seek an accurate diagno-

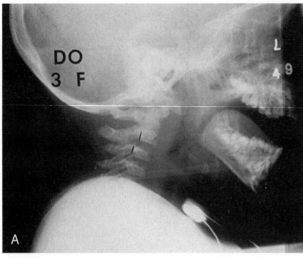

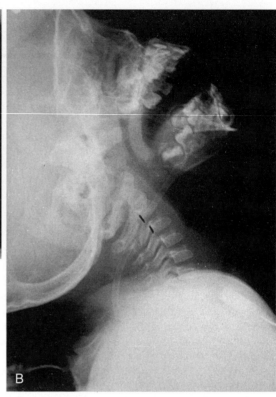

Figure 16–14. *A,* A 3-year-old boy with pseudosubluxation of C2 on C3. Note the horizontal inclination of the facets at the level of subluxation. *B,* In extension, complete reduction is seen.

sis, or at least rule out serious pathology such as infection or tumor.

History

A careful detailed history should be obtained from both the child and parent. The onset of the symptoms should be explored, including any inciting trauma, the location of the pain, and sites of radiation. The occurrence of pain at rest should also be pursued, and explicit questioning about neurologic symptoms such as pain or paresthesias in the legs or recent changes in bowel or bladder habits is important. It is also very helpful to attempt to assess the severity of the symptoms. It is not at all uncommon for adolescents, and even children, to complain of relatively mild back pain with no specific cause; this is particularly true if a diagnosis of scoliosis has recently been made.[18, 58] On the other hand, pain that is of sufficient magnitude to interfere with activities such as attending school or participating in organized sports is much more worrisome, and this sort of activity disturbance should be specifically questioned. Finally, inquiry about the child's general medical status, including a thorough review of systems and questioning about constitutional symptoms, is carried out.

Physical examination is performed with the patient in an examining gown, disrobed down to his or her underwear. The shoes and socks must be removed to adequately evaluate the patient with back pain, either adult or child. An evaluation of gait is carried out, an examination of posture, and palpation for sites of tenderness. Limitation of range of motion or asymmetry of motion is noted. Examination of the back for café-au-lait spots, skin dimples, or hairy patches is performed. Calf or foot asymmetry is sought. Finally, a thorough neurologic evaluation is per-

formed, seeking in particular any upper motor neuron findings or asymmetry of motor or sensory function or of deep tendon reflexes in the lower extremities. The superficial abdominal reflexes are also checked for symmetry.

Imaging Studies

Unlike in the adult, a child or adolescent with significant back pain should almost always be studied radiographically, even on initial evaluation. Plain AP and lateral radiographs of the area in question should be obtained, and dynamic films are helpful if instability is suspected. Standing views of the full spine are utilized for cases of spinal deformity.[68]

Technetium-99 bone scanning is carried out in cases in which the child fails to respond rapidly to nonoperative modalities, where walking or standing are impaired, or when incapacitating symptoms are present. Bone scanning is a sensitive but relatively nonspecific modality that will identify most spinal column and pelvic conditions such as tumors, infections, and spondylolysis. The sensitivity and specificity can be enhanced with single photon emission computed tomography (SPECT) scanning, particularly when the diagnosis of spondylolysis is an issue.[4] MRI is used to supplement the findings on an abnormal bone scan or when an intraspinal lesion is suspected. MRI is more sensitive and more specific in the diagnosis of tumor or infection and is the imaging modality of choice for disk abnormalities including herniation, a cause of back pain in adolescents.

Laboratory testing is occasionally indicated in the child or adolescent with back pain and is more commonly utilized in this setting than in the adult. Urinalysis and complete blood cell count are routine tests obtained, and the sedimentation rate is a good generalized screen for neoplasia or infection. Several blood tests are available to complement the search for underlying rheumatologic disorders, but this testing is usually deferred to the rheumatologist. It is important, however, to bear in mind that, particularly in children, back pain can present with unusual complaints and conversely, back pain can be a symptom of non-orthopaedic intra-abdominal, pelvic, or constitutional conditions.

Differential Diagnosis

Bunnell has suggested dividing back pain in children into four categories: mechanical disorders, developmental disorders, inflammatory disorders, and neoplastic disorders.[15] Some clue as to the underlying nature of the condition may be apparent based on the history and physical examination, but it is the radiographic workup that will ultimately lead to the diagnosis. Since neoplasia and infection are the most ominous conditions associated with back pain, it is important to consider these disorders and rule them out in a timely fashion, prior to assuming that a developmental disorder such as spondylolysis, or a mechanical disorder, is the cause of the patient's symptoms.

Neoplastic disorders are rare but occasionally manifest as spinal pain in the child or adolescent (Fig. 16–15). Pain at rest or atypical spinal deformity is a relatively common presenting complaint in the individual with spinal column tumor. Intraspinal tumors may manifest as back pain or pain in the chest wall, the abdominal wall, or the abdomen as a result of nerve root compression. In addition, lumbar or sacral involvement may lead to leg symptoms, atrophy, or bowel or bladder dysfunction.

Inflammatory disorders include rheumatologic conditions such as juvenile rheumatoid arthritis or aseptic disk space calcification. In addition, vertebral osteomyelitis and discitis may be seen, with a mean age of presentation for spine infection being 6 years of age.[72] Depending on the age of the patient, presenting complaints include back pain, abdominal pain, or refusal to walk, stand, or even sit. When infection of the spine is suspected, the key to prompt diagnosis is early utilization of either bone scanning or MRI. A characteristic MRI picture is seen; findings similar to the adult but typically involving less bony involvement confirm the diagnosis of disk space infection. Biopsy is not mandatory, and we favor the institution of broad-spectrum antibiotics, delivered parenterally for 2 to 3 weeks, followed by oral antibiotics for a total of 6 weeks. Immobilization is accomplished first at bedrest; then, as symptoms allow, activities are increased in a brace or cast. Failure to respond leads to percutaneous biopsy of the affected area, but only rarely is surgical debridement necessary.

Developmental disorders may also lead to back pain in children and adolescents. Scheuermann's kyphosis is one of the more common causes of back pain in adolescents and is typically readily apparent on plain radiographs of the thoracic spine. Scoliosis rarely causes severe pain, but it is not uncommon for the child or adolescent with scoliosis to have relatively mild complaints of pain. We typically do not pursue imaging beyond routine plain radiography unless the pain is so severe as to interfere with school attendance or recreational activities, a neurologic abnormality is seen, or there is particularly rapid curve progression. Spondylolysis and spondylolisthesis are common causes of back pain in children and adolescents and are discussed below.

Mechanical conditions such as disk herniation or overuse syndrome are relatively common causes of back pain, particularly in adolescents. Children and adolescents account for 1 to 2% of patients with disk herniations, and Epstein and colleagues have noted the strong correlation between disk herniation in the adolescent and the presence

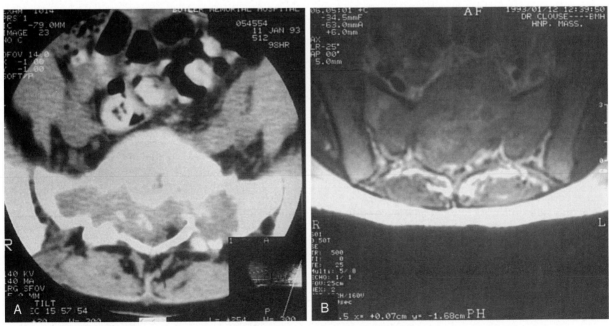

Figure 16–15. CT scan *(A)* and MRI *(B)* of a 16-year-old girl with back and right leg pain, who was found to have a giant cell tumor of the sacrum.

of a straight leg raising sign.[27] MRI is very accurate for the diagnosis of disk herniation and for differentiating true herniated nucleus pulposus from posterior displacement of the apophyseal ring, which also occurs in adolescents.

Overuse syndrome or "lumbar strain" should be considered a diagnosis of exclusion. In our experience, adolescents with back pain frequently are diagnosed with overuse syndrome, but we come to this diagnosis carefully. Plain radiographs are routinely obtained, and in most cases either a bone scan or MRI scan is pursued prior to assuming that there is no abnormality other than a mechanical overuse syndrome. This is particularly true in children under age 10, in whom one can almost always find a specific diagnosis when persistent back pain is present.[39]

Treatment

Neoplastic and inflammatory disorders, when diagnosed as the cause for back pain, are treated as appropriate for the specific condition. Similarly, developmental disorders such as Scheuermann's kyphosis, scoliosis, or spondylolisthesis are treated as described elsewhere in this chapter. It is the treatment of the adolescent with mechanical low back pain that is the most difficult, and this treatment must be individualized.

Depending on the length of the patient's symptoms and the extent of sports-related activities, activity restriction is usually the first approach. If the patient is continuing to participate in his or her full athletic regimen, a cutback of approximately 50% in the level of participation is frequently adequate to allow the mechanical symptoms time to resolve. If this has been tried unsuccessfully, more extensive rest is needed. This frequently requires complete cessation of athletic activity with the exception of walking. Many times this is a source of great consternation on the part of the patient and/or the parents, but if the symptoms are severe enough and of sufficient duration, this is the course we routinely pursue. In addition, we typically prescribe a nonsteroidal anti-inflammatory medication and find the use of moist heat to be helpful.

The patient is reevaluated at 3 to 4 weeks. If the symptoms have improved, gradually increasing activity is instituted. A return to sports can be attempted in 6 to 8 weeks if the patient continues to be sufficiently comfortable. If the child fails to respond, we typically go back to a more strenuous regimen of rest or we consider bracing. Bracing is of uncertain efficacy in the absence of a firm diagnosis such as spondylolysis, but is occasionally utilized in individuals who fail to respond to activity restrictions and nonsteroidal anti-inflammatory medications. Along with treatment, further evaluation is carried out when the pediatric patient does not improve as expected. This may include more sophisticated imaging studies and/or consultation with the patient's pediatrician to investigate whether there are underlying psychosocial circumstances that may contribute to the atypical pain pattern seen.

Spondylolisthesis

Spondylolysis and spondylolisthesis are relatively common conditions, with an overall prevalence of 5 to 6% in adolescents by the end of skeletal growth. Wiltse and colleagues

Table 16–5. Types of spondylolisthesis

Class	Type	Age	Pathology/Other
I	Congenital	Child	Congenital dysplasia of S1 superior facet
II	Isthmic*	5–50	Predisposition leading to elongation/fracture of pars (L5–S1)
III	Degenerative	Older	Facet arthrosis leading to subluxation (L4–L5)
IV	Traumatic	Young	Acute fracture/other than pars
V	Pathologic	Any	Incompetence of bony elements
VI	Postsurgical	Adult	Excessive resection of neural arches/facets

*Most common.
From Miller MD: Review of Orthopaedics, 2nd ed. Philadelphia, WB Saunders, 1996.

have classified spondylolisthesis (Table 16–5), and the most common type seen in children, adolescents, and young adults is type II or isthmic. Isthmic spondylolisthesis occurs secondary to an abnormality of the pars interarticularis. This may either be an acute fracture, which is rare; progressive elongation of the pars; or, most commonly, a stress or fatigue fracture of the pars interarticularis.[74] Fredrickson and coworkers have noted a prevalence of 5.6% for spondylolysis and found that in approximately 75% of cases the defect was bilateral and in about 75% of cases resulted in forward slippage or spondylolisthesis.[30] It is believed that there is a hereditary predisposition to the development of spondylolysis and that the fatigue fracture occurs as the result of repetitive hyperextension stresses in genetically predisposed individuals.[75] It is well accepted that these pars defects are more common in athletes who incur repetitive hyperextension forces in the lower lumbar spine such as gymnasts or interior linemen in football.

Symptomatic isthmic spondylolisthesis is most commonly seen in young and middle-aged adults but may present for evaluation in children and adolescents. Spondylolysis or spondylolisthesis is one of the most common causes of back pain in the pediatric population, and patients present typically with pain in the low back, occasionally radiating into the buttock or posterior thigh. True radicular symptoms are rare. Hamstring spasm is a common complaint, and occasionally, in individuals with high-grade slippage, flattening of the buttocks, a transverse abdominal crease, and a crouched posture and waddling gait—the Phalen-Dickson sign—may be seen.[7] The mechanism of the hamstring spasm is unclear; possible causes include L5 nerve root irritation and an attempt by the body to stabilize the pelvis in the presence of an incompetent posterior arch of L5.

A number of radiographic findings have been described in spondylolysis and spondylolisthesis. Most defects of the pars interarticularis occur at L5, and most can be seen on plain lateral radiography. Further definition of the defect in the pars interarticularis may be seen on the oblique radiograph, where a characteristic "collar" on the neck of the "scotty dog" is seen (Fig. 16–16). On the standing lateral

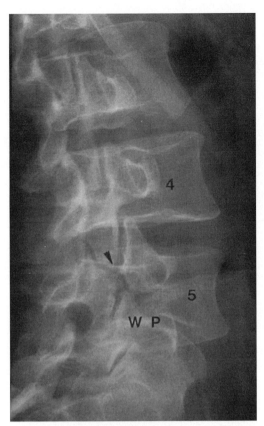

Figure 16–16. Oblique radiograph demonstrating spondylolysis *(arrowhead).*

radiograph, a number of measurements have been suggested to grade the extent of slippage as well as to attempt to assess the risk of further slippage (Fig. 16–17).[76] The three most helpful are the percent slip, graded as I to IV; the slip angle; and the sacral inclination. The percent slip may be related to the propensity for further slippage in the growing child, appears to be related to the development of back pain in adulthood, and is the most commonly used way to define treatment parameters. The slip angle helps to understand the cosmetic deformity present in more severe slips, as the L5 vertebral body rolls into a kyphotic relationship to the sacrum. In addition, the slip angle may also relate to the prognosis for progression. The sacral inclination helps quantify possible deformity. As the L5 vertebral body rolls further into kyphosis, the sacrum, along with the pelvis, rotates backwards, bringing the sacrum into a more vertical alignment with a lesser angle of sacral inclination. This results in flattening of the buttocks, which is the most cosmetically objectionable aspect of severe spondylolisthesis.

TREATMENT

Treatment of spondylolisthesis depends on the grade of the slip as well as the presence or absence of symptoms. Asymptomatic patients who are noted to have spondylolysis alone or a grade I (0 to 25% slippage) spondylolisthesis are typically treated with observation only. No activity restrictions are recommended. Routine radiographic follow-up, measuring the extent of slip on annual standing radiographs, is carried out. Asymptomatic patients with

higher grades of spondylolisthesis are usually restricted from high-risk activities such as gymnastics or contact sports, particularly those such as football or wrestling that result in frequent hyperextension.

The role for prophylactic fusion in isthmic spondylolisthesis, in the absence of symptoms, is somewhat controversial. Because of the risk of further progression or the development of significant back pain in adulthood, most surgeons recommend fusion in the asymptomatic child or adolescent if the percent slippage is greater than 50%. Harris and Weinstein have reported, however, on a series of adults with high-grade spondylolisthesis treated nonoperatively and compared them with individuals who have undergone fusion. Although pain was not uncommon, there was a relatively high level of function in individuals with grades III and IV spondylolisthesis who had not undergone surgery, suggesting that observation may be reasonable in these patients, particularly if they are followed closely for progression.[34]

Symptomatic patients are treated based on the degree of slippage. For grades I or II spondylolisthesis, nonoperative treatment is instituted. This typically constitutes activity restrictions, moist heat, and in some case nonsteroidal anti-inflammatory medications. A brief period of sports restriction, only occasionally requiring bedrest, is frequently helpful in minimizing symptoms, and this is typically followed by a program of hamstring stretching and Williams flexion exercises. If the child continues to be comfortable, gradually increasing activity is instituted as outlined above. Occasionally patients are seen in whom a clear history of trauma suggests an acute etiology for the pars defect. In these patients, some authors suggest casting, although a pantaloon spica is typically required to ade-

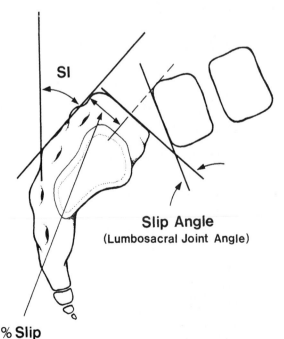

Figure 16–17. Measurement used for evaluation of spondylolisthesis. (From Wiesel SW, Delahay JN: Essentials of Orthopaedic Surgery, 2nd ed. Philadelphia, WB Saunders, 1997.)

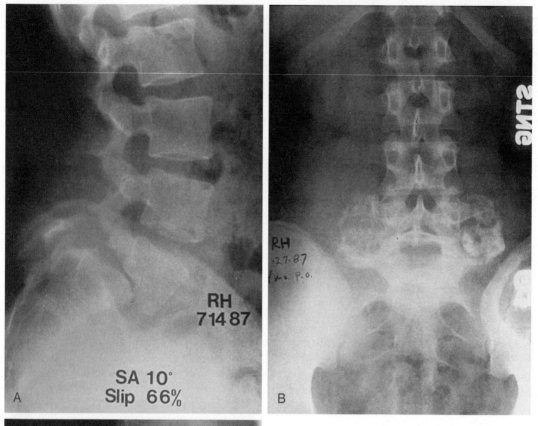

A

RH
714 87

SA 10°
Slip 66%

B

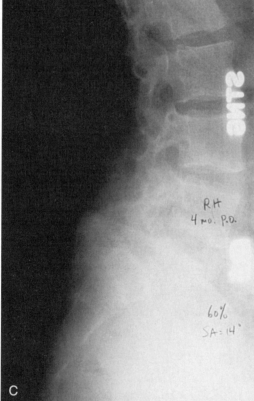

C

Figure 16–18. *A*, A 17-year-old boy with 2 years of back and buttock pain is seen to have a grade III isthmic spondylolisthesis. He was treated with a bilateral intertransverse fusion from L4 to S1, utilizing a muscle-splitting approach, and was immobilized for 4 months in a pantaloon spica. *B* and *C*, taken following cast removal, show good early healing. He experienced complete pain relief and went on to a solid fusion.

quately immobilize the lumbosacral junction. A removable lumbosacral orthosis with a thigh cuff is more commonly utilized in this setting, and bone or SPECT scanning may be helpful in determining whether the pars defect is truly traumatic. In our practice, we almost always treat patients symptomatically rather than in anticipation of healing of the pars defect. We favor activity modification and allow gradually increasing activity depending on the patient's response. We reserve bracing for patients who fail to obtain adequate relief of symptoms with activity modifications or who are unable to resume a reasonable level of activity. Some patients' symptoms are markedly improved when wearing a Boston brace, and we then increase their activity level, in the brace, as tolerated. Some even return to athletic activity while initially wearing the brace.

Surgical treatment is considered for patients who have persistent back pain despite 6 to 12 months of aggressive nonoperative treatment or for patients with spondylolisthesis greater than 50%. The options for surgical treatment include repair of the pars defect, fusion, and reduction. In contrast to the adult, nerve root decompression is rarely indicated in the child or adolescent, even in the presence of significant leg symptoms.

Pars repair may be accomplished through several techniques. Bradford and Iza have described a tension-band wiring technique utilizing autologous bone grafting across the pars defect, with good to excellent results in 80 to 90% of patients. They suggest pars repair for patients younger than age 25, with defects above L5, normal disks and facets, and minimal or no slippage.[10]

Arthrodesis may be accomplished anteriorly or posteriorly, and may utilize instrumentation or dowel grafting. The most common approach in the pediatric population is posterolateral intertransverse fusion (Fig. 16–18). In cases of slippage of greater than 40 to 50%, the fusion is extended to L4. Immobilization with a unilateral spica cast has been demonstrated to result in an increased chance of obtaining a solid fusion.[17] Anterior fusion with or without dowel grafting is indicated for higher degrees of slippage or as part of a revision procedure for a failed fusion.

Reduction of high-grade spondylolisthesis is advocated by some surgeons. The most common indications for reduction include grades III or higher spondylolisthesis including spondyloptosis (complete dislocation of the L5 vertebra into the pelvis), with a cosmetically objectionable appearance sufficient to merit the risks of reduction. In addition, high grades of spondylolisthesis lead to a biomechanical environment in which the intertransverse fusion mass, even if extended up to L4, is under tension and is at significant risk for nonunion or bending and continued progression. In this setting, reduction may be indicated.[7] Techniques of reduction include traction and casting,[5] combined anterior and posterior approaches, posterior instrumentation and reduction,[11, 12] and circumferential L5 vertebral body resection and reduction.[31] Success has been described for all techniques, but all authors have noted a significant risk of complications. Complications of reduction include loss of fixation, loss of correction, and a worrisome rate of neurologic deficits—20 to 30% in some series, although the majority have been transient.[7]

References

1. Akbarnia BA, Gabriel KR, Beckman E, et al: Prevalence of scoliosis in neurofibromatosis. Spine 17(86):S244–S248, 1992.

2. Bassett GS, Bunnell WP, MacEwen GD: Treatment of idiopathic scoliosis with the Wilmington brace. Results in patients with a twenty to thirty-nine degree curve. J Bone Joint Surg 68A:602, 1986.

3. Boachie-Adjei O, Lonstein JE, Winter RB, et al: Management of neuromuscular spinal deformities with Luque segmental instrumentation. J Bone Joint Surg 71A(4):548–562, 1989.

4. Bodner R, Heyman S, Drummond R, Gregg JR: The use of single photon emission computed tomography (SPECT) in the diagnosis of low back pain in young patients. Spine 13:1155, 1988.

5. Bradford DS: Closed reduction of spondylolisthesis: An experience in 22 patients. Spine 13:580, 1988.

6. Bradford DS: Juvenile kyphosis. In Lonstein JE, Bradford DS, Winter RB, Ogilvie JW (eds): Moe's Textbook of Scoliosis and Other Spinal Deformities, 3rd ed. Philadelphia, WB Saunders, 1995.

7. Bradford DS: Spondylolysis and spondylolisthesis. In Lonstein JE, Bradford DS, Winter RB, Ogilvie JW (eds): Moe's Textbook of Scoliosis and Other Spinal Deformities (3rd ed). Philadelphia, WB Saunders, 1995.

8. Bradford DS, Moe JH, Montalvo FJ, Winter RB: Scheuermann's kyphosis and roundback deformity results of Milwaukee brace treatment. J Bone Joint Surg 56A:749, 1974.

9. Bradford DS, Khalid BA, Moe JH, et al: The surgical management of patients with Scheuermann's disease. A review of 24 cases managed by combined anterior and posterior spine fusion. J Bone Joint Surg 62A:705, 1980.

10. Bradford DS, Iza J: Repair of the defect in spondylolysis or minimal degrees of spondylolisthesis by segmental wire fixation and bone grafting. Spine 10:673, 1985.

11. Bradford DS, Gotfried Y: Staged salvage reconstruction of grade IV and V spondylolisthesis. J Bone Joint Surg 69A:191–202, 1987.

12. Bradford DS, Boachie-Adjei O: Treatment of severe spondylolisthesis by anterior and posterior reduction and stabilization. A long-term follow-up study. J Bone Joint Surg 72A:1060–1066, 1990.

13. Bradford DS, Heithoff KB, Cohen M: Intraspinal abnormalities and congenital spine deformities: A radiographic and MRI study. J Pediatric Orthopaedics 11:36–41, 1991.

14. Bradford DS, Hu SS: Neuromuscular spinal deformity. In Lonstein JE, Bradford DS, Winter RB, Ogilvie JW (eds): Moe's Textbook of Scoliosis and Other Spinal Deformities, 3rd ed. Philadelphia, WB Saunders, 1995.

15. Bunnell WA: Back pain in children. Orthop Clin North Am 13:587–604, 1982.

16. Burke SW, French HG, Roberts JM, et al: Chronic atlanto-axial instability in children. J Bone Joint Surg [Am] 67:1356–1360, 1985.

17. Burkus JK, Lonstein JE, Winter RB, Denis F: Long-term evaluation of adolescents treated operatively for spondylolisthesis: A comparison of in situ arthrodesis only with in situ arthrodesis and reduction followed by immobilization in a cast. J Bone Joint Surg 74A:693, 1992.

18. Burton AK, Clarke RD, McClune TD. The natural history of low back pain in adolescents. Spine 21:2323–2328, 1996.

19. Cattell HS, Filtzer DL: Pseudosubluxation and other normal variations in the cervical spine in children. J Bone Joint Surg [Am] 47:1295–1309, 1965.

20. Collis DK, Ponseti IV: Long-term follow-up of patients with idiopathic scoliosis not treated surgically. J Bone Joint Surg 51A:425–445, 1969.

21. Coscia MF, Bradford DS, Ogilvie JW: Scheuermann's kyphosis—results in 19 cases treated by spinal arthrodesis and L-rod instrumentation. Orthop Trans 12:255, 1988.

22. Davids JR, Wenger DR, Mubarak SJ: Congenital muscular torticollis: Sequelae of intrauterine or prenatal compartment syndrome. J Pediatr Orthop 13:141–147, 1993.

23. Dickman CA, Zambranski JM, Hadley MN, et al: Pediatric spinal cord injury without radiographic abnormalities: Report of 26 cases and review of the literature. J Spinal Dis 4:296–305, 1991.

24. Doyle JS, Lauerman WC, et al: Complications and long-term outcome of upper cervical arthrodesis in patients with Down syndrome. Spine 21:1223–1231, 1996.

25. Drvaric DM, Ruderman RJ, Conrad RW, et al: Congenital scoliosis and urinary tract abnormalities: Are intravenous pyelograms necessary? J Pediatr Orthop 7:441–443, 1987.

26. Dubousset J, Herring JA, Shufflebarger H: The crankshaft phenomenon. J Pediatr Orthop 9:541–550, 1989.

27. Epstein JA, Epstein NE, Marc J, et al: Lumbar intervertebral disk herniation in teenage children: Recognition and management of associated anomalies. Spine 9:427, 1984.

28. Fielding JW, Stillwell WT, Chynn KY, Spyropoulos EC: Use of computed tomography for the diagnosis of atlanto-axial rotatory fixation. J Bone Joint Surg [Am] 60:1102–1104, 1978.

29. Fielding JW, Hensinger RN, Hawkins RJ: Os odontoideum. J Bone Joint Surg [Am] 62:376–383, 1980.

30. Fredrickson BE, Baker D, McHolick WJ, et al: The natural history of spondylolysis and spondylolisthesis. J Bone Joint Surg 66A:699, 1984.

31. Gaines RW, Nichols WK: Treatment of spondyloptosis by two-stage L5 vertebrectomy and reduction of L4 onto S1. Spine 10:608–687, 1985.

32. Gunderson CH, Solitare GB: Mirror movements in patients with the Klippel-Feil syndrome. Arch Neurol 18:675–679, 1968.

33. Hall, JE: Anterior surgery in the treatment of idiopathic scoliosis. J Bone Joint Surg [Br] 76B(Suppl I):3, 1994.

34. Harris IE, Weinstein SL: Long-term follow-up of patients with grade III and IV spondylolisthesis. J Bone Joint Surg 69A:960, 1987.

35. Hensinger RN, Lang JE, MacEwen GD: Klippel-Feil syndrome. J Bone Joint Surg [Am] 56:1246–1253j, 1974.

36. Herzenberg JE, et al: Emergency transport and positioning of young children who have an injury to the cervical spine. J Bone Joint Surg [Am] 71:15–22, 1989.

37. Kewalramani LS, Tori JG: Spinal cord trauma in children, neurologic patterns, radiologic features, and pathomechanics of injury. Spine 5:11–18, 1980.

38. King HA, Moe JH, Bradford DS, Winter RB: The selection of fusion levels in thoracic idiopathic scoliosis. J Bone Joint Surg 65A:1302–1313, 1983.

39. King H, Tufel D: Prospective study of back pain in children. Orthop Trans 10:9–10, 1986.

40. Loder RT, Hensinger RN: Developmental abnormalities of the cervical spine. In Weinstein SL (ed): The Pediatric Spine: Principles and Practice. New York, Raven Press, 1994.

41. Lonstein JE: Idiopathic scoliosis. In Lonstein JE, Bradford DS, Winter RB, Ogilvie JW (eds): Moe's Textbook of Scoliosis and Other Spinal Deformities, 3rd ed. Philadelphia, WB Saunders, 1995.

42. Lonstein JE: Patient evaluation. In Lonstein JE, Bradford DS, Winter RB, Ogilvie JW (eds): Moe's Textbook of Scoliosis and Other Spinal Deformities, 3rd ed. Philadelphia, WB Saunders, 1995.

43. Lonstein JE, Winter R, Moe J, et al: Neurologic deficits secondary to spinal deformity: A review of the literature and report of 43 cases. Spine 5:331–355, 1980.

44. Lonstein JE, Carlson JM: The prediction of curve progression in untreated idiopathic scoliosis during growth. J Bone Joint Surg Am 66:1061–1071, 1984.

45. Lonstein JE, Winter RB: Milwaukee brace treatment of adolescent idiopathic scoliosis—review of 1020 patients. J Bone Joint Surg 76A:1207–1221, 1994.

46. Mayfield JK, Erkkila JC, Winter RB: Spine deformity subsequent to acquired childhood spinal cord injury. J Bone Joint Surg 63A(9):1401–1411, 1981.

47. McMaster MJ, Ohtsuka K: The natural history of congenital scoliosis: A study of 251 patients. J Bone Joint Surg 64A:1147, 1982.

48. Mehta MH: The rib-vertebra angle in the early diagnosis between resolving and progressive infantile scoliosis. J Bone Joint Surg 54B:230–243, 1972.

49. Moe JH: Treatment of adolescent kyphosis by nonoperative and operative methods. Manitoba Med Rev 45:481, 1965.

50. Murray PM, Weinstein SL, Spratt KF: The natural history and long-term follow-up of Scheuermann's kyphosis. J Bone Joint Surg 75A:236–248, 1993.

51. Nachemson AL, Peterson LE, et al: Effectiveness of treatment with a brace in girls who have adolescent idiopathic scoliosis. J Bone Joint Surg 77A:815–822, 1995.

52. Nagib MG, Maxwell RE, Chou SN: Identification and management of high-risk patients with Klippel-Feil syndrome. J Neurosurg 61:523–530, 1984.

53. Newton PO, Wenger DR, Mubarak SJ, Meyer RS: Anterior release and fusion in pediatric spinal deformity: A comparison of early outcome and cost of thoracoscopic and open thoracotomy approaches. Spine 22:1398–1406, 1997.

54. Orcutt FV, DeWald RL: The special problems which the Marfan syndrome introduces to scoliosis. J Bone Joint Surg 56A:1763, 1974.

55. Pang D, Wilberger JE: Spinal cord injury without radiographic abnormalities in children. J Neurosurg 57:114–129, 1982.

56. Patel PR, Lauerman WC: Historical perspective. Maurice Kippel. Spine 20:2157–2160, 1995.

57. Peuschel SM, Scola FH: Atlantoaxial instability in individuals with Down syndrome: Epidemiologic, radiographic, and clinical studies. Pediatrics 80:555–560, 1987.

58. Ramierz N, Johnston CE, Browne RH. The prevalence of back pain in children who have idiopathic scoliosis. J Bone Joint Surg 79A:364–368, 1997.

59. Robins PR, Moe JH, Winter RB: Scoliosis in Marfan's syndrome, its characteristics and results of treatment of 35 patients. J Bone Joint Surg 57A:358–368, 1975.

60. Rowe DE, Bernstein SM, et al: A meta-analysis of the efficacy of nonoperative treatments for idiopathic scoliosis. J Bone Joint Surg 79A:664–674, 1997.

61. Scheuermann HW: Kyfosis dorsalis juvenilis. Ugesjr Kaeger 82L:385, 1920.

62. Segal LS, Drummond DS, Zanotti RM, et al: Complications of posterior arthrodesis of the cervical spine in patients who have Down syndrome. J Bone Joint Surg [Am] 73:1547–1554, 1991.

63. Smith AC, Koreska J, Moseley CF: Progression of scoliosis in Duchenne muscular dystrophy. J Bone Joint Surg 71A(7):1066–1074, 1989.

64. Sorenson KH: Scheuermann's Juvenile Kyphosis. Copenhagen, Munksgaard, 1964.

65. Taimela S, Kujala UM, Salminen JJ: The prevalence of low back pain among children and adolescents. A nationwide, cohort-based questionnaire survey in Finland. Spine 22:1132–1136, 1997.

66. Tankersley WS, Lauerman WC, Cain JE: Myelopathy associated with subaxial instability in Klippel-Feil syndrome. Orthop Trans 16(3):824, 1992.

67. Terminology Committee: Scoliosis Research Society: A glossary of scoliosis terms. Spine 1:57–58, 1976.

68. Thompson GH: Back pain in children. J Bone Joint Surg 75A:928–938, 1993.

69. Tredwell SJ, Newman DE, Lockith G: Instability of the upper cervical spine in Down syndrome. J Pediatr Orthop 10:602–606, 1990.

70. Turi M, Johnston CE, Richards BS: Anterior correction of idiopathic scoliosis using TSRH instrumentation. Spine 18:417–422, 1993.

71. Weinstein SL, Ponseti IV: Curve progression in idiopathic scoliosis. J Bone Joint Surg 65A:447–455, 1993.

72. Wenger DR, Bobechko WP, Gilda DL: The spectrum of intervertebral disc-space infections in children. J Bone Joint Surg [Am] 60:100–108, 1979.

73. Wilner S: Prospective prevalence study of scoliosis in southern Sweden. Acta Orthop Scand 53:233, 1982.

74. Wiltse LL, Newman PH, Macnab I: Classification of spondylolysis and spondylolisthesis. Clin Orthop 117:23–29, 1976.

75. Wiltse LL, Widell EH, Jackson DW: Fatigue fracture: The basic lesion in isthmic spondylolisthesis. J Bone Joint Surg 57A:17, 1975.

76. Wiltse LL, Winter RB: Terminology and measurement of spondylolisthesis. J Bone Joint Surg 65A:768, 1983.

77. Winter RB, Moe JH, Wang JF: Congenital kyphosis. J Bone Joint Surg 55A:223–256, 1973.

78. Winter RB, Moe JH, MacEwen GD, Peon-Vidales H: The Milwaukee brace in the nonoperative treatment of congenital scoliosis. Spine 1:85–96, 1976.

79. Winter RB: Congenital spinal deformity. In Lonstein JE, Bradford DS, Winter RB, Ogilvie JW (eds): Moe's Textbook of Scoliosis and Other Spinal Deformities, 3rd ed. Philadelphia, WB Saunders, 1995.

Chapter 17

Musculoskeletal Trauma in Children

John N. Delahay, M.D.

Skeletal injury in the child differs from that of the adult in two principal ways. Significant biologic and mechanical variations make the management and prognosis of these injuries in children unlike care for similar injuries in the adult. In most cases, fractures are easier to manage in children because of the rapidity and certainty of bony union and the ability of the child's bones to remodel. However, certain specific fractures can cause considerable problems that must be understood thoroughly if the surgeon is to obtain optimal results.

Of all the biologic differences, the phenomenon of active skeletal growth is critical and is the fundamental difference between children and adults. Ordinarily, it works in favor of the orthopaedic surgeon, because it is associated with achieving union and active remodeling. Growth is physeal and appositional; both types are key in the remodeling process. Remodeling must be considered in the management of any given fracture. The child has a much greater tolerance for incomplete reduction than the adult. The physician is frequently able to accept a reduction in a child that would be completely inadequate in the adult. A certain amount of displacement, overriding, and angulation will be corrected by this remodeling phenomenon. Unfortunately, residual rotational deformity is not amenable to this type of correction.

The periosteum is the second biologic difference between child and adult. In the adult, the periosteum is a relatively thin fibrous membrane and is not actively osteogenic. In the child, however, this periosteum is extremely thick, highly vascular, and osteogenic. In fact, the periosteum of the child is dual-layered with an outer fibrous layer and an inner osteogenic (cambial) layer. Clearly, this periosteum is important in minimizing fracture displacement and in facilitating fracture healing.

The blood supply to the bone in the child is reportedly richer, leading to more rapid and certain union. However, in certain areas the circulation is as tenuous as in the adult. The femoral head of the child is as vulnerable to avascularity as that of the adult. The lateral condyle of the distal humerus is yet another unique area where blood supply is tenuous, obviously increasing the risk of avascular necrosis and nonunion.

The child may also have pathologic changes of the bone. This is certainly true of the adult as well; however, the lesions seen in the pediatric age group tend to be isolated to an individual bone, whereas in the adult osteoporosis, metastatic disease, and other generalized bone diseases compound fracture healing.

The child's higher activity level is obviously another biologic difference. On one hand, it makes rehabilitation much easier with full functional recovery usually anticipated; on the other, it places the child at risk when the immobilization is discontinued prematurely.

Mechanical differences also exist between the young and aging skeleton. The elasticity of immature bone is impressive. Clearly, the child's bone is able to deform plastically, without necessarily fracturing completely through. Incomplete fractures are typical in this age group. Greenstick and torus fractures reflect this unique ability of the child's bone to plastically deform.

The ultimate mechanical difference in the child is the presence of a "flaw" in the long bone. This flaw, the growth plate, is the weakest segment in a child's bone. Relative to adjacent ligaments and surrounding bone, the physis is the first point of failure with the application of excessive load. Fractures in and around the growth plate typically show crack propagation throughout all four zones. Although many texts suggest that injury is isolated to the hypertrophic zone, this is not the case. Plate failure can occur as a result of all modes of loading: tension, compression, and shear. As a general principle, children will rarely sustain ligamentous injuries because the plate will always fail first. Hence, if suspecting a sprain or dislocation in a child, it is best to think again. Special x-ray views, such as stress films (Fig. 17–1) or more sophisticated imaging studies, may be required to document the injury to the plate. One typical example is observed in the distal fibula. When a young child is suspected of having a "sprained ankle," one should remember that children do not sustain sprains; therefore, assume this to be a physeal injury to the distal fibular growth plate.

These biologic and mechanical differences may potentiate some complications in the child not typically seen in the adult. Growth plate arrest, both partial and complete, can occur following trauma. Should the arrest be complete, the resulting growth slowdown will result in limb length discrepancy. On the other hand, should a portion of the plate prematurely close, angular deformity should be anticipated. Growth stimulation has also been recognized, particularly following fractures of the femoral shaft. As a result, the injured limb is longer than the uninvolved side.

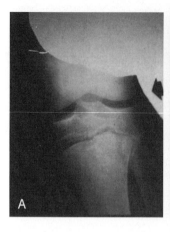
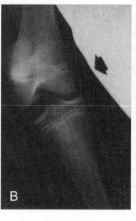
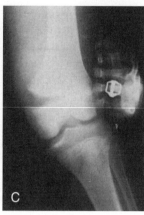

Figure 17–1. Stress films illustrating injury to the proximal tibial physis *(A)*, the medial collateral ligament *(B)*, and the distal femoral physis *(C)* in skeletally immature children. (From Green NE, Swiontkowski MF: Skeletal Trauma in Children, Vol 3. Philadelphia, WB Saunders, 1998.)

A word about remodeling is important. All too often, the uninitiated surgeon presumes that the aggressive remodeling, said to be typical in children, will correct a less than anatomically reduced fracture. More often than not, remodeling will indeed be on the surgeon's side (Fig. 17–2). Unfortunately, there are also numerous instances in which remodeling will not resolve the deformity. Angular deformity in the midshaft of the forearm and varus deformity of the proximal femur are two such examples of this potential pitfall. Similarly, rotational deformity of any long bone cannot be expected to remodel. In addition, one must be careful to assess the age of the child in question. Although true that the biologic and mechanical differences cited here favor the young child, fractures in older children and adolescents behave more like adult injuries. In fact, several specific fractures, such as the triplane and Tillaux fractures of the ankle, are unique in the adolescent. They are referred to as transitional injuries (between child and adult) and are best thought of as adult injuries.

PEDIATRIC POLYTRAUMA

Approximately 10% of all pediatric trauma patients admitted to the hospital are victims of multiple injury. Therefore, an aggressive team approach for these severely injured children is required. In fact, trauma is the leading cause of death in children, accounting for more deaths and disabilities in children older than 1 year of age than all other causes combined. In addition, for every child that dies, four are disabled permanently. The cost in human suffering, not to mention dollars, is overwhelming. It is frightening to realize that the mortality rates for pediatric injury are higher in the United States than in any other Western industrialized nation. It has been reported that motor vehicle accidents and homicides account for the majority of this striking difference. Certainly, motor vehicle accidents are the leading cause of multiple injuries in children (Table 17–1). Tragically, deaths as a result of motor vehicle accidents are most common among adolescents; in this group, alcohol is a significant factor. Even more frightening is the realization that homicide is the second leading cause of death among children; granted, most homicides occur among teenagers, but a startling number occur in children under age 5.

The orthopaedic injuries in the polytrauma patient must be viewed in the context of the child's size and severity of other organ system involvement. Fortunately, children tend to be better able to survive extremely severe injuries and frequently respond better to a given injury than an adult. Care must be taken not to overlook musculoskeletal injuries in the face of what may appear to be more severe trauma.

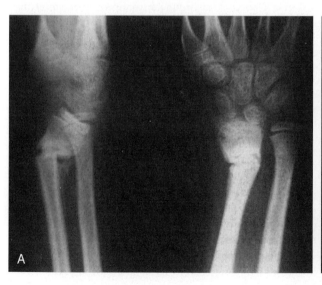
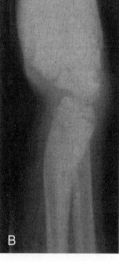

Figure 17–2. Radiograph of the distal radius in an 11-year-old girl at the time of cast removal 6 weeks after injury *(A)*. Lateral radiograph taken 3 months later shows considerable remodeling of the fracture in the plane of the joint *(B)*. (From Green NE, Swiontkowski MF: Skeletal Trauma in Children, Vol 3. Philadelphia, WB Saunders, 1998.)

Table 17–1. Mechanism of injury (from published series)

Mechanism	Marcus et al. (N = 74) (%)	Loder (N = 78) (%)	Kaufmann et al. (N = 376) (%)
Motor vehicle accidents			
Passenger	9	35	18
Pedestrian	76	33	23
Bicycle	3	18	17
Motorcycle	3	5	0
Train	6	1	0
Falls	3	4	24
Other	0	4	19

From Green NE, Swiontkowski MF: Skeletal Trauma in Children, Vol 3. Philadelphia, WB Saunders, 1998.

Spinal trauma, of note, does occur in the pediatric patient, mandating precautions in the transportation of these children. Unique in this age group is the syndrome called SCIWORA (spinal cord injury without radiographic abnormality). Because of the elasticity of the child's spinal cord, it can be damaged, even in the absence of apparent skeletal injury. The use of lap belts also places the child at risk for flexion-distraction injuries of the spine.

The child's pelvis, unlike that of the adult, is extremely plastic and hence deformable. The pelvis may deform under blunt loading without sustaining demonstrable fracture. Unfortunately, the abdominal contents may be severely traumatized in this situation. Injury to the growth plates of the pelvis, specifically the triradiate cartilage and other apophyseal centers, will be reflected later in growth aberrations.

Femoral fractures in the patient with multiple injuries are common; the treatment methods chosen, as well as the timing, significantly affect the outcome. Much like the adult, rapid stabilization of the femoral shaft in the child will markedly decrease time in the intensive care unit and, to a lesser degree, pulmonary complications. Traction treatment in these children is tolerated poorly, especially in the face of head or chest injuries. Internal or external fixation techniques are preferred in order to get the child into the upright position. In addition, it eliminates the need for spica cast immobilization. Although body casts are frequently used in the young child, such casts markedly restrict access to the abdomen and chest.

Upper extremity trauma in the child with multiple injuries may be approached in a fashion similar to that for the isolated injury. Typically, rapid union is the norm and relatively little systemic impact should be anticipated.

Open fractures in the pediatric age group are classified by the Gustilo grouping system, as employed for the adult. The principles of managing open fractures are similar in both age groups. Extensive soft tissue and bone loss will complicate the outcome of the fracture, much as it does in the adult.

Outcomes in this age group can be predicted using the Modified Injury Severity Scale (MISS), as described by Mayer (Table 17–2). This has proved to be useful in predicting morbidity and mortality rates in the pediatric age group. It employs the Glasgow coma scale for grading the neurologic injury; in addition, it reviews damage to individual body areas, such as the face and neck, the chest, the abdomen, and the extremities. Rapid evaluation of the pediatric polytrauma patient can also be assessed using the Pediatric Trauma Score (Table 17–3). Several components such as the size, the airway integrity, the central nervous system integrity, systolic blood pressure, the presence or absence of open wounds, and the amount of skeletal damage can be used to rapidly assess these patients. Total point counts over 8 ensure an excellent prognosis for survival; scores less than 0 indicate a very high risk of death.

INJURIES OF THE UPPER EXTREMITY

Fractures of the Clavicle

The clavicle is the first bone to ossify, and it does so from two primary centers, appearing between the fifth and sixth weeks of fetal life. Ossification, however, is not complete until approximately 25 years of age, when the medial physis of the clavicle closes. Once complete, the clavicle is the only osseous strut between the axial skeleton and the shoulder girdle. The medial third of the clavicle is somewhat round in cross section, whereas the lateral third is flat. The middle third, therefore, is a transition zone, where the overall shape of the clavicle is changing. This anatomic fact is frequently proposed as the rationale for the striking frequency of midshaft fractures.

Fractures of the clavicle span all age groups from neonate to adult. They involve the entire length of the clavicle. In point of fact, birth fractures of the clavicle are the most common fracture in the newborn. These birth injuries correlate with birth weight, the experience of the delivering person, and the use of forceps at the time of delivery. Frequently, the diagnosis is made in the nursery, when the child demonstrates pseudoparalysis of the involved limb and an asymmetric Moro response. It is important to carefully evaluate the child for an associated brachial plexus palsy. These two lesions may coexist, making an obstetric palsy easy to miss when there is pseudoparalysis due to a clavicle fracture. Treatment for these injuries should be simple immobilization of the extremity to the chest wall with a soft wrap of either cast padding or gauze. Healing is rapid and long-term sequelae are virtually nonexistent.

Fractures of the medial end of the clavicle are quite rare, accounting for fewer than 10% of clavicular fractures. More significant is the separation of the medial physis of the clavicle. As noted earlier, this physis does not close until approximately 25 years of age. Therefore, a young adult who presents with a lesion appearing to be a sternoclavicular dislocation should be evaluated carefully for a medial physeal separation. Although some authors prefer a Hobb's view or "serendipity view," most believe that a computed tomography (CT) scan is the most reliable imaging study to diagnose this injury. Fortunately, most of these physeal separations are minimally displaced and can be treated closed. Occasionally, however, posterior displacement can occur, placing the thoracic contents at risk. In this setting, operative reduction and fixation is the preferred method of treatment.

Fractures of the clavicular shaft are one of the more

Table 17-2. The modified injury severity scale (MISS) for multiple-injury children

Body Area	1—Minor	2—Moderate	3—Severe, Not Life-Threatening	4—Severe, Life-Threatening	5—Critical, Survival Uncertain
Neural Face and neck	GSC 13–14 Abrasion or contusions of ocular apparatus or lid Vitreous or conjunctival hemorrhage Fractured teeth	GSC 9–12 Undisplaced facial bone fracture Laceration of eye, disfiguring laceration Retinal detachment	GSC 9–12 Loss of eye, avulsion of optic nerve Displaced facial fracture "Blow-out" fracture of orbit	GSC 5–8 Bone or soft tissue injury with minor destruction	GSC 4 Injuries with airway obstruction
Chest	Muscle ache or chest wall stiffness	Simple rib or sternal fracture	Multiple rib fractures Hemothorax or pneumothorax Diaphragmatic rupture Pulmonary contusion	Open chest wounds Pneumomediastinum Myocardial contusion	Lacerations, tracheal hemomediastinum Aortic laceration Myocardial laceration or rupture
Abdomen	Muscle ache, seatbelt abrasion	Major abdominal wall contusion	Contusion of abdominal organs Retroperitoneal hematoma Extraperitoneal bladder rupture Thoracic or lumbar spine fractures	Minor laceration of abdominal organs Intraperitoneal bladder rupture Spine fractures with paraplegia	Rupture or severe laceration of abdominal vessels or organs
Extremities and pelvic girdle	Minor sprains Simple fractures and dislocations	Open fractures of digits Nondisplaced long bone or pelvic fractures	Displaced long bone or multiple hand or foot fractures Single open long bone fracture Pelvic fractures with displacement Laceration of major nerves or vessels	Multiple closed long bone fractures Amputation of limbs	Multiple open long bone fractures

Note: GSC = Glasgow Coma Scale.
Adapted from Mayer T, Matlak ME, Johnson DG, Walker ML: The Modified Injury Severity Scale in pediatric multiple trauma patients. J Pediatr Surg 1980;15:719; and from Green NE, Swiontkowski MF: Skeletal Trauma in Children, Vol 3. Philadelphia, WB Saunders, 1998.

Table 17–3. Pediatric trauma score (PTS)*

Component	Severity Points		
	+2	+1	−1
Size	>20 kg	10–20 kg	<10 kg
Airway	Normal	Maintainable	Unmaintainable
CNS	Normal	Obtunded	Comatose
Systolic BP	>90 mmHg	90–50 mmHg	<50 mmHg
Open wounds	None	Minor	Major or penetrating
Skeletal	None	Closed fracture	Open or multiple fractures

*PTS ≤ 8 = referral to pediatric trauma center.
Adapted from Tepas JJ III, Ramenofsky ML, Moll HDL, et al: The Pediatric Trauma Score as a predictor of injury severity: An objective assessment. J Trauma 1988;28:425; and from Green NE, Swiontkowski MF: Skeletal Trauma in Children, Vol 3. Philadelphia, WB Saunders, 1998.

common fractures of childhood (Table 17–4). Typically, these fractures result from a fall onto the point of the shoulder, and rarely is diagnosis difficult. Tenderness and swelling along the middle third of the clavicle, associated with pain on motion of the upper extremity, make the diagnosis fairly straightforward. Most of these fractures in the relatively young child are greenstick in nature. Short-term immobilization is adequate treatment. It is best not to apply a figure-of-eight strap immediately upon injury; rather, it is better to wait several days before application of this device. A simple sling and swathe is adequate initial treatment. Perhaps most important in the management of these injuries is to warn the parents about the "bump." The mass of callus that forms around these fractures frequently causes a great deal of parental anxiety; therefore, if warned about it in advance and advised that it should resolve with normal growth, their concerns will be relieved.

Fractures of the distal end of the clavicle are also frequently physeal separations. The distal physis closes at

Table 17–4. The frequency of various fracture types

Type of Fracture	Frequency (%)
Distal forearm	22.7
Hand, phalanges	18.9
Carpal–metacarpal (scaphoid excluded)	8.3
Clavicle	8.1
Ankle	5.5
Tibia, diaphysis	5.0
Tarsal–metatarsal (talus, os calcis excluded)	4.5
Foot, phalanges	3.4
Radius–ulna, diaphysis	3.4
Supracondylar region of the humerus	3.3
Proximal end of the humerus	2.2
Facial skeleton	2.1
Skull	1.8
Femur shaft	1.6
Radial neck	1.2
Vertebrae	1.2

From Benson MKD, Fixsen JA, MacNicol MF: Children's Orthopaedics and Fractures. Edinburgh, Churchill Livingstone, 1994.

approximately age 19. There is a thick periosteal sleeve prominent over the distal portion of the clavicle. This periosteal sleeve and the dense ligaments of the acromioclavicular joint make physeal fracture a more likely event. Once the physis closes, acromioclavicular (AC) separation is the usual injury. Again, the injury typically results from a fall onto the point of the shoulder and simple radiographs are usually adequate to make the diagnosis. Short-term sling and swathe immobilization is adequate treatment for these injuries.

Fractures of the Scapula

The body of the scapula ossifies from a single center appearing approximately in the eighth week of fetal life. In addition, multiple secondary centers of ossification are seen. These secondary centers ultimately develop into processes, such as the acromion and coracoid. Fractures of the scapula are rare in children, and their classification is largely based on their geographic location. For example, fractures of the body, the glenoid, the acromion, and the coracoid are the common ones described. Fractures of the scapular body are stabilized by the bulk muscles around the scapula and respond well to closed treatment. Fractures of the glenoid require operative treatment if the glenohumeral joint is subluxed or dislocated. The other two injuries, acromial and coracoid fractures, are typically avulsion injuries of the secondary growth centers. Depending on the degree of displacement, operative treatment may be required. It is important to remember that os acromiale (Fig. 17–3) may occasionally be confused with an acromial fracture.

Glenohumeral Dislocation

The shoulder interzone is present between the fifth and seventh weeks of embryonic life, with differentiation com-

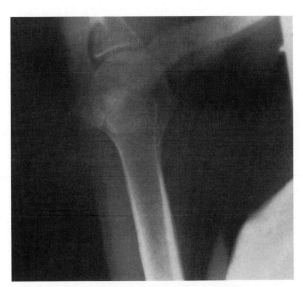

Figure 17–3. This is one of several possible patterns of os acromiale, discovered incidentally on an axillary lateral projection of this patient's glenohumeral joint. (From Green NE, Swiontkowski MF: Skeletal Trauma in Children, Vol 3. Philadelphia, WB Saunders, 1998.)

plete by the ninth week. As in the adult, soft tissue support about the shoulder is critical for glenohumeral stability. As mentioned earlier, dislocation rarely occurs in children because the growth plate will almost always fail prior to ligamentous or soft tissue disruption. Therefore, glenohumeral dislocation is rarely seen in children under 11 years of age. When it does occur, the recurrence rates are high, similar to those seen in young adults. It is also important to be aware of the child who can voluntarily dislocate her or his shoulder. So-called voluntary dislocation is a manifestation of generalized ligamentous laxity, as well as some modest psychological disturbance. It is critically important to recognize this entity and *not* treat it surgically.

Fractures of the Humerus

Fractures of the proximal humerus are again physeal injuries. The proximal humeral physis closes between the ages of 14 and 18 years. It is important to recognize that the geometry of the proximal humeral physis is not planar. Rather, it has been described as "tent-shaped" (Fig. 17–4) with the apex located posteromedially. The other additional anatomic fact of importance is the presence of an attenuated periosteum on the anterolateral surface. Hyperextension with rotation places this area at risk for fracture and is the typical mechanism of injury. Under age 5, these physeal injuries tend to be Salter type I injuries. However, over age 11, they tend to be Salter type II injuries. Between these age groups, there is a mix of lesions seen. In the 5- to 11-year-old age group, both metaphyseal and physeal fractures can be seen. Injuries to this physis have also been reported in newborns; in this age group, the diagnosis is frequently problematic due to the mass of nonossified cartilage making up the proximal humerus. Treatment of proximal humeral physeal injuries is generally nonoperative. The surgeon and child are blessed with huge remodeling potential in this area. An acceptable reduction is said to be angular deformity less than 20 degrees and displacement of less than 50%. Should reduction be required, a general anesthetic is most often employed. Once reduced, immobilization in a shoulder spica or "salute cast" is appropriate

(Fig. 17–5). Occasionally, the arm requires abduction to achieve and maintain the reduction. In this event, adduction of the arm will risk loss of reduction. Should this be the case, percutaneous pinning or open surgery may be deemed a more reasonable option. Sling immobilization for 3 weeks generally completes the treatment, and healing is anticipated in 3 to 4 weeks.

Fractures of the humeral shaft are uncommon in children; when seen, the child is usually over 12 years of age or under 3 years of age. It is critically important to recognize the association between spiral fractures of the humeral shaft and child abuse. In children under 3, acute torsional injury to the upper extremity typically produces this unique spiral lesion. These fractures have also been reported in neonates following difficult delivery and, much like clavicle fractures, are heralded by pseudoparalysis of the upper limb. The vast majority of humeral shaft fractures respond to closed methods of treatment, such as a collar and cuff, a functional brace, or a sling and swathe. Most are "sticky" by 4 weeks, with rapid mobilization thereafter. The polytrauma victim is a good candidate for operative treatment of this fracture.

Injuries About the Child's Elbow

SUPRACONDYLAR FRACTURE

Perhaps no other injury in children produces more physician and parental anxiety than this one. The complications of the injury, as well as the treatment, are legendary in orthopaedic surgery. Satisfactory long-term outcomes are not guaranteed, even with anatomic reduction. However, techniques and practices, which have been advanced over the last decade, have significantly reduced the number of serious complications. The two groups of supracondylar fractures are extension type (95%) and flexion type (5%) injuries based on the mechanism of injury. Supracondylar fractures account for 60% of elbow fractures in children. The incidence of supracondylar fractures is correlated with age. It is almost exclusively an injury of the immature elbow, with the average patient being 6 years old. As one

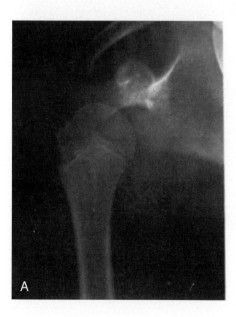

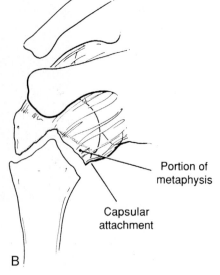

Portion of metaphysis

Capsular attachment

Figure 17–4. *A,* "Tent-shaped" proximal humeral physis. *B,* Glenohumeral capsular attachment site following a fracture. (From Green NE, Swiontkowski MF: Skeletal Trauma in Children, Vol 3. Philadelphia, WB Saunders, 1998.)

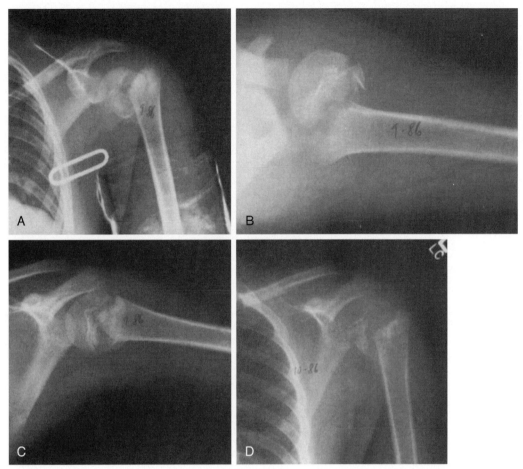

Figure 17–5. *A* and *B,* Type II proximal humerus fracture in a 12-year-old. *C,* Because abduction improved the alignment of the fracture, the patient was treated in abduction. *D,* Three-month x-rays demonstrate more complete healing; the child had a normal shoulder on clinical examination. (From Green NE, Swiontkowski MF: Skeletal Trauma in Children, Vol 3. Philadelphia, WB Saunders, 1998.)

would expect, this injury is twice as common in males as females, simply because of activity level.

The anatomy of the child's elbow differs dramatically from that of the adult. At birth, no epiphyseal structures are present. The first secondary ossification center to appear is that of the capitellum, usually observed at 6 months of age (Fig. 17–6). Following that, in order of appearance, the ossification centers of the radial head, medial epicondyle, trochlea, olecranon, and lateral epicondyle are seen. Initially, these all are part of one large chondroepiphysis. With rapid differential growth, the medial epicondyle forms its own ossification center and the capitellum, trochlea, and lateral epicondyle become one center.

In the supracondylar region, there are two strong columns of bone, one medial and one lateral (Fig. 17–7). Between them is a central "wafer" of bone, which is approximately 1 mm thick. Because of this dramatic decrease in anteroposterior diameter and the acute change in cross-sectional geometry (from cylindric to flattened), the supracondylar region is mechanically vulnerable. With hyperextension loading, which is common in small children, the olecranon tends to lever against the supracondylar region, creating a bending moment. This causes anterior periosteal failure, resulting in the pattern of the hyperexten-

sion failure. In significantly displaced fractures, the anterior periosteal flap can become trapped between the proximal and distal fragments. The fact that hyperextension loading is so common accounts for the preponderance of these injuries. The few flexion injuries seen typically result from a direct fall on the olecranon, thereby bending the supracondylar region in the opposite direction.

The classification most widely accepted is that proposed by Gartland in 1959. Appropriate use of this classification depends on some knowledge of the radiographic anatomy. Important anatomic landmarks and lines seen on the lateral view are reviewed in Figure 17–8. On the anteroposterior view, the most important is Baumann's angle, which is formed between a line perpendicular to the axis of the humerus and a line paralleling the metaphysis on the lateral side of the distal humerus. Baumann's angle normally measures 15 degrees. These lines are important if one is to appropriately use the Gartland classification. The type I fracture is nondisplaced (the anterior humeral line extends through the ossification center of the lateral condyle). Type II injuries show a hinge of intact posterior periosteum and cortex, making them stable in external rotation. The type III injuries are completely displaced and can be further subdivided into those displaced posterolaterally and those

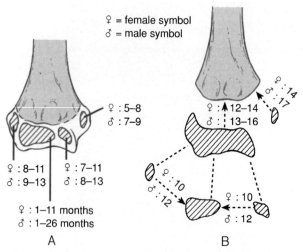

♀ = female symbol
♂ = male symbol

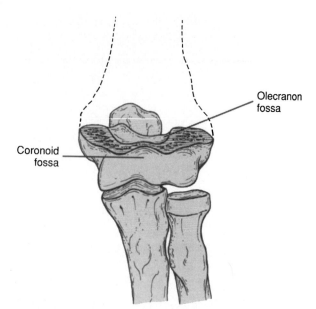

Olecranon
fossa

Coronoid
fossa

Figure 17–6. Ossification and fusion of the growth centers of the distal end of the humerus. *A,* Appearance of the ossification centers of the distal end of the humerus in the early years. If the wear of the ossification center begins before the age of 1 year, the designation is noted with the letter "m," for "months." *B,* Fusion of the ossification centers of the distal humerus. (Adapted from Haraldsson S: On osteochondrosis deformans juvenilis capituli humeri including investigation of intra-osseous vasculature in distal humerus. Acta Orthop Scand [Suppl] 38, 1959. From Green NE, Swiontkowski MF: Skeletal Trauma in Children, Vol 3. Philadelphia, WB Saunders, 1998.)

Figure 17–7. Cross section of the distal humerus through the region of the coronoid fossa. Note that the midportion of the humerus is extremely thin at this level, whereas the medial and lateral sides (columns) are thicker. (From Green NE, Swiontkowski MF: Skeletal Trauma in Children, Vol 3. Philadelphia, WB Saunders, 1998.)

displaced posteromedially; the latter account for about 75% of the total. It is important to note the direction of displacement, because it frequently has an impact on management. Many believe that it may also suggest prognosis.

Complications of supracondylar fractures are the acute

nerve and vascular injuries and the late development of deformity. Nerve palsies have been reported in approximately 10% of patients. Until recently, it had been thought that the posterior interosseous nerve (PIN) was the most common to be damaged. However, in recent years and with careful physical evaluation, many authors are now reporting anterior interosseous nerve (AIN) palsy to be the

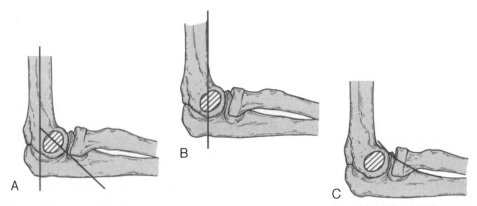

Figure 17–8. Radiographic lines that may be demonstrated on a lateral view of the elbow. *A,* The capitellum of the distal humerus is angulated anteriorly approximately 30 degrees. This angle may be demonstrated by drawing a line parallel to the midpoint of the shaft of the distal humerus; the intersection of that line with a line drawn through the midpoint of the capitellum indicates the anterior inclination of the capitellum. *B,* The anterior humeral line is drawn down the outer edge of the anterior cortex of the distal humerus. As the line is drawn distally through the capitellum the line should pass through the middle of the capitellum. *C,* The anterior coronoid line is drawn along the coronoid fossa of the proximal ulna, which is then continued proximally. It should just touch the capitellum anteriorly. The line will lie posterior to the most anterior portion of the capitellum if the capitellum is angulated anteriorly. If the capitellum is angulated posteriorly, the line will no longer touch the capitellum. (From Green NE, Swiontkowski MF: Skeletal Trauma in Children, Vol 3. Philadelphia, WB Saunders, 1998.)

most common. It is likely that the older literature was flawed because many of these subtle AIN injuries were probably missed. The ulnar nerve is injured approximately one quarter of the time. Prognostically, the vast majority of nerve injuries resolve spontaneously between 3 and 6 months following the injury.

Vascular injury, on the other hand, may be more problematic. There is a rich collateral blood flow in and about the elbow; this circulation is such that even in the face of brachial artery interruption, blood flow to the distal limb is usually adequate. Some authors, however, state that persistent claudication and cold intolerance can complicate healing in such an injury. In the United States today, however, it is rare to see the residua of vascular compromise. Despite the damage to the brachial artery that can result from the anterior spike of the proximal fragment striking the vessel, heightened awareness and improved diagnostic acumen have decreased the long-term morbidity of these injuries. One should not wait for the five Ps of arterial trauma to develop prior to acting. Once pulselessness, paresthesias, paralysis, pallor, and severe pain have developed, irreversible damage almost certainly has been done.

Compartment syndromes can exist in the presence of a pulse, and conversely, the absence of a pulse does not necessarily mandate exploration of the vessel. Recognition of the clinical signs of compartment syndrome is key. Inordinate levels of pain, alterations of skin color, alterations of temperature and hand function, and abnormal capillary refill must all be sought. The use of the Doppler probe to more accurately identify the pulse is also helpful. Currently, digital compartmental monitors are readily available in most facilities and provide a rapid and relatively accurate measurement of intracompartmental pressures. Should these exceed 20 to 30 mmHg (depending on the clinical picture), fasciotomy is indicated. Sending the patient to the radiology department for an arteriogram is generally frowned upon. If the vascular consultant requires such a study, it is best performed on the operating table in order that one can immediately proceed with exploration, if indicated.

There is a significant amount of current literature addressing the problem of the warm pulseless hand. Most of these reports emphasize the fact that excellent peripheral flow can be present while the pulse is absent. Most authors recommend careful observation of the extremity in this setting rather than resorting to invasive studies and surgical exploration. It goes without saying that monitoring of compartmental pressure and capillary refill is required.

Should vascular insufficiency be identified acutely in the emergency room, the most important first step in management is closed reduction of the fracture. Frequently, this will be adequate to return the pulse or improve the appearance of the hand. If not, then further diagnostic studies and possibly exploration will be required. Failure to appropriately treat a compartment syndrome results in irreversible myonecrosis and subsequent contracture. This contracture of the volar musculature of the forearm and the resulting deformity of the hand have been identified for many years as Volkmann's ischemic contracture (Fig. 17–9).

Treatment of these fractures is generally based on the type. The major pitfall surrounding type I injuries is failure to recognize that a given fracture is actually type II. Type

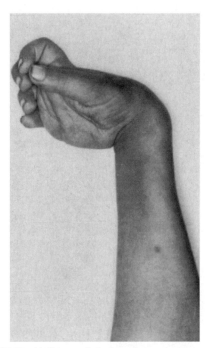

Figure 17–9. Volkmann's ischemic contracture caused by supracondylar fracture of the humerus. (From Tachdjian MO: Pediatric Orthopaedics, 2nd ed. Philadelphia, WB Saunders, 1990.)

I injuries are truly nondisplaced and great care must be taken to document that fact. Occasionally, they will be impacted in varus; if this is the case, it may be necessary to disimpact the fracture. Baumann's angle may be helpful in the evaluation of this deformity. Also, clinical examination with the elbow extended is frequently helpful in the evaluation of the carrying angle. If the injury is truly type I, then application of a long arm cast, after a period of splinting, is usually adequate.

Type II injuries again can suffer from too casual an approach by the physician. Although the posterior cortex is intact by definition, angulation can and frequently does occur. Most authors recommend closed reduction and percutaneous pinning (Fig. 17–10). In any event, a reduction must be achieved and maintained. To do so, it is usually necessary to flex the elbow more than 120 degrees and pronate the forearm. Because this is frequently difficult, due to swelling, many authors choose to pin these fractures.

Type III injuries all require, at least, closed reduction and percutaneous pinning. The initial displacement, whether it be posteromedial or posterolateral, will indicate the location of the intact periosteal hinge (Fig. 17–11). The hinge is typically intact on the side of the displacement. For example, in the more common posteromedially displaced injury, the periosteal hinge is medial. Therefore, pronation, which closes the lateral side and tightens the medial hinge, is generally employed to assist in the reduction of these injuries. Critical x-ray evaluation should be used to document reduction. Rotational and translational residual deformity are less critical than residual varus or valgus tilt. As will be seen, the late deformities, which complicate this injury, result primarily from residual tilt. The tilt, however, usually follows residual rotational defor-

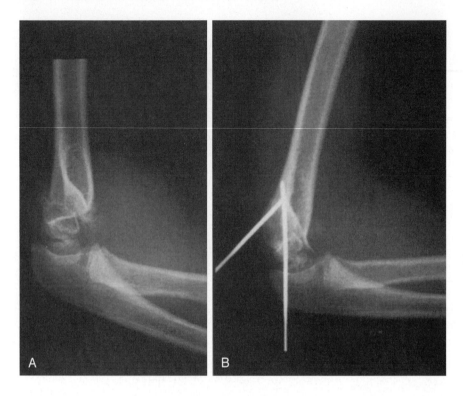

Figure 17–10. Type II supracondylar fracture of the distal humerus. *A,* Lateral radiograph of the distal humerus demonstrating posterior angulation of the distal fragment of the distal humerus. Note that if one drew the anterior humeral line, it would no longer intersect the capitellum, and neither would the coronoid line lie on the anterior aspect of the capitellum. In addition, the capitellum has lost its normal 30 degrees of angulation. *B,* Postreduction radiograph of the distal humerus. (From Green NE, Swiontkowski MF: Skeletal Trauma in Children, Vol 3. Philadelphia, WB Saunders, 1998.)

mity. Therefore, the significance of rotation is that it allows tilt to occur.

Because the amount of flexion required to hold the reduction is frequently greater than 90 degrees (placing the circulation at risk), the currently favored treatment is percutaneous pinning. The number of pins and location of pins are somewhat controversial. Suffice it to say that the strongest mechanical construct is provided by the use of one medial and one lateral pin crossed above the fracture site (Fig. 17–12). Because of the risk of ulnar nerve injury, many surgeons prefer two lateral pins; although not mechanically as strong, this arrangement does protect the nerve. Recently, some authors have suggested using three pins (one medial and two lateral). Should the child demonstrate ulnar nerve symptoms postoperatively, the medial pin can be removed, leaving the child with two pins laterally and negating the need to return to the operating room to insert a second lateral wire. Initially, a splint is applied after surgery, following which a long arm cast is used for a period of 6 weeks. Most surgeons remove the wires at around 4 weeks.

Other techniques have been used for many years in the management of these fractures. Dunlop's traction is a form of skin traction with the arm at the side. Skin breakdown and inordinate amounts of swelling have made it primarily of historic interest. Overhead skeletal traction (Fig. 17–13)

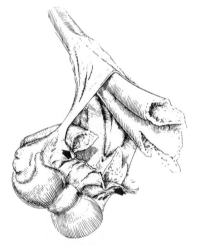

Figure 17–11. The periosteum is completely torn and stripped proximally from the proximal fragment. (From Abraham E, Powers T, Witt P, Ray RD: Experimental hyperextension supracondylar fractures in monkeys. Clin Orthop 171:309–318, 1982.)

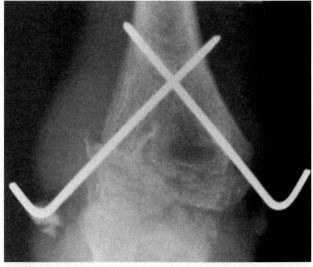

Figure 17–12. Cross pinning of supracondylar fracture.

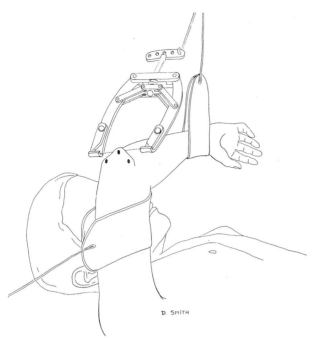

Figure 17–13. Overhead skeletal traction through a pin in the olecranon for treatment of markedly displaced supracondylar fractures of the humerus. (From Smith L: Deformity follow supracondylar fractures of the humerus. J Bone Joint Surg 42A:244, 1960.)

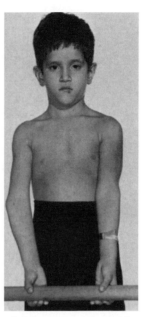

Figure 17–14. Cubitus varus caused by malunion of supracondylar fracture of the humerus. (From Tachdjian MO: Pediatric Orthopaedics, 2nd ed. Philadelphia, WB Saunders, 1990.)

as described by Lyman Smith is still an important technique, especially for observation, should questions arise relative to vascular integrity. This technique allows dependent drainage. It prevents rotation and therefore tilt, and it is a safe alternative should closed reduction and percutaneous pinning not be possible. Open reduction is generally indicated for open fractures, those with serious vascular injury, and those that cannot be reduced and pinned percutaneously. Green and Swiontkowski recommend the use of the medial approach; others prefer the lateral approach, and some use the straight posterior (Campbell) approach. The latter reportedly has an increased incidence of stiffness, and for that reason tends to be employed least often. Current literature suggests that concerns over excessive stiffness with this approach may be unwarranted.

Late deformity, resulting from these fractures, is due to changes in the carrying angle. In turn, these changes result from residual tilt. Cubitus varus (Fig. 17–14) is the more common angular deformity. Classically, this is referred to as the "gunstock" deformity, the incidence of which varies widely in the literature. Most agree that it follows residual medial tilt at the fracture site. Although the gunstock deformity is primarily cosmetic, there is usually a great deal of parental pressure to correct this unsightly deformity. The use of supracondylar osteotomy to correct the deformity is appropriate, but it is best delayed until adolescence; otherwise, it may need to be repeated. Valgus deformity, on the other hand, tends to cause a functional problem. The cosmetic effect is better tolerated. Should valgus deformity result, tardy ulnar nerve palsy is a likely sequel. In this event, early surgical correction is required to minimize the risk of irreversible changes in the ulnar nerve distribution.

LATERAL HUMERAL CONDYLAR FRACTURE

Injuries to this portion of the distal humerus account for about 20% of elbow fractures in children. There is some debate as to whether the mechanism is avulsion or compression, but most authors agree with Green and Swiontkowski that this is a Salter type IV fracture. The location of the fracture line at the articular surface of the humerus is important in determining elbow stability (Fig. 17–15). If

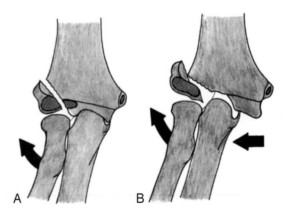

Figure 17–15. Anatomic location of the fracture line in lateral condylar fractures described by Milch. *A,* Type I: The fracture line traverses lateral to the trochlea through the capitulotrochlear groove. The fracture fragment angulates, and the elbow joint is stable; the radial head and olecranon translocate laterally. *B,* Type II: The fracture line courses and exits into the elbow joint at the apex of the trochlea. In this type the elbow joint is unstable. The fracture fragment angulates, and the radial head and olecranon translocate laterally. (Redrawn after Milch HE: Fractures and fracture-dislocations of the humeral condyles. J Trauma 4:592, 1964.)

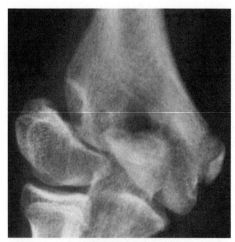

Figure 17–16. Established nonunion of lateral condyle. (From Crawford AH, Wilkins K: Residuals of elbow trauma in children. Orthop Clin North Am 21:273, 1990.)

the fracture line is lateral to the trochlear groove (Milch I) the elbow tends to remain stable. However, should the fracture line go through the trochlear groove or medial to it (Milch II), the elbow tends to sublux laterally.

Great care must be taken in assessment of fracture displacement. There is a tendency to think that many of these fractures are nondisplaced, when indeed there is a slight amount of rotation or translation. Oblique x-rays or arthrograms are useful in determining the degree of displacement. Truly nondisplaced fractures are quite rare. When seen, closed treatment in a long arm cast is appropriate, but it is critical to document the lack of displacement. Many authors elect to surgically pin all these injuries, thereby obviating concerns over the degree of displacement. Many believe that the fragment is bathed in synovial fluid and has an extremely tenuous blood supply, making nonunion (Fig. 17–16) that much more common. Therefore, open reduction and fixation is desirable to rigidly fix the fragment as well as restore the articular surface. Hence, one can anticipate a decreased risk of nonunion and hopefully a decreased risk of growth arrest. Established nonunions are occasionally seen and are exceedingly difficult to treat. Due to the risk of avascular necrosis when explored, many authors recommend leaving them in situ if displacement is minimal. However, should displacement be significant, very cautious open reduction and peg grafting can be attempted to bring about a successful union. Central growth plate arrest has been reported, resulting in the so-called "tent pole" (fishmouth) deformity of the distal humerus (Fig. 17–17).

MEDIAL EPICONDYLAR FRACTURE

Accounting for 10% of elbow fractures and occurring in an older age group, these injuries are frequently associated with elbow dislocations. The application of a valgus stress can avulse the medial epicondyle and subsequently cause the elbow to dislocate. In general, the extent of displacement is the criteria for treatment. Should they be displaced under 5 mm, simple immobilization for 3 weeks is the recommended treatment. Over 5 mm of displacement is an indication for operative treatment. Because of concerns

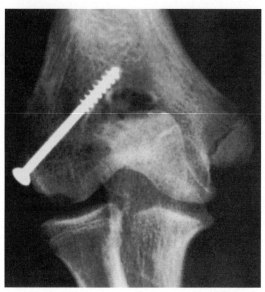

Figure 17–17. This 7-year-old child had a lateral condylar fracture 6 months previously. The small "fish mouth" deformity of the trochlea does not appear to have affected the patient's function. (From Crawford AH, Wilkins K: Residuals of elbow trauma in children. Orthop Clin North Am 21:273, 1990.)

over valgus instability, most authors prefer to pin these fragments in place. It is important to carefully evaluate the location of the fragment because some will be rotated *into* the joint at the time of initial injury.

FRACTURES OF THE PROXIMAL RADIUS

Fractures of the upper end of the radius account for about 10% of fractures about the elbow. Most of these fractures involve the neck or the physis and occur in an older age group. They may occur as isolated injuries or in association with a posterior dislocation. The injuries are graded based on the amount of angulation (Fig. 17–18). Some dispute exists over the amount of angular deformity felt to be acceptable. Salter has reported 15 degrees as the upper limit of acceptability, whereas Mercer Rang has reported 30 degrees. Most authors, however, recommend closed

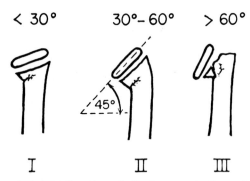

Figure 17–18. Degrees of displacement of proximal radial epiphyses. I. Minimal displacement. II. Moderate displacement. III. Marked displacement. (From O'Brien PI: Injuries involving the proximal radial epiphysis. Clin Orthop 41:52, 1965.)

reduction over 30 degrees of angulation; if the reduction cannot be maintained closed, then consideration should be given to percutaneous pinning. All authors discourage the use of a transcapitellar wire to maintain the reduction, because most wires tend to break in the joint.

FRACTURES OF THE FOREARM

Pediatric forearm fractures account for approximately 45% of fractures in children. Approximately 75% are in the distal third, 20% in the middle third, and 5% in the proximal third. Despite a tradition for closed treatment, there has been increasing enthusiasm for operative treatment, particularly of shaft fractures. This is due, in part, to the fact that remodeling in the 8- to 10-year-old age group is not reliable; also, reports of permanent loss of pronation and supination have encouraged many surgeons to consider surgical treatment. One must temper this enthusiasm with the reality of the satisfactory results reported for 85% of displaced fractures.

Fractures in the middle third of the forearm tend to be deformed by a number of muscle forces (Fig. 17–19). Proximally, the biceps and supinator tend to flex and supinate the proximal segment. The pronator acts in the mid-portion of the forearm, making it necessary to know whether the fracture is proximal or distal to the pronator insertion. Distal fractures frequently are manipulated by the attachment of the brachioradialis muscle. It therefore is easy to appreciate that fractures behave quite differently, based upon their relationship to various muscle attachments. Most forearm fractures in children are the result of a fall on the outstretched hand with a supination force being applied to the pronated forearm. This produces the typical angular and rotational deformity, which tend to be coupled—that is, supination and anterior angular deformity. The more infrequent scenario is for the forearm to be forcibly pronated, thereby producing posterior angular deformity.

In children, the decision making frequently is determined by the physician's evaluation of remodeling potential. The success or failure of the long-term result is often a function of the adequacy of this judgment. Remodeling (Fig. 17–20) depends upon the age of the child, the residual angular deformity, the distance of the fracture from the physis, and the relationship of the angulation to the plane of motion of the adjacent joint. Recognizing that bone tends to resorb on the convexity of deformity and form on the concavity of deformity, there is certainly a reasonable range for satisfactory remodeling. Unfortunately, it is variable and in the preadolescent age group largely unpredictable. In general, one can predict about 10 degrees per year of remodeling in the distal segment. In the middle third of the forearm, the younger the child, the more angular deformity that can be accepted; however, it is probably fair to say that 30 degrees is the maximum amount of angulation acceptable in young children. In addition, if the angular deformity is volar or dorsal, and therefore in the plane of motion of the wrist joint, residual angulation is more likely to remodel than if the angulation is medial or lateral and, hence, out of the plane of motion of the wrist. As stated earlier, rotational deformity will not remodel.

Treatment for the vast majority of forearm fractures is closed reduction and cast application. Long arm casts are

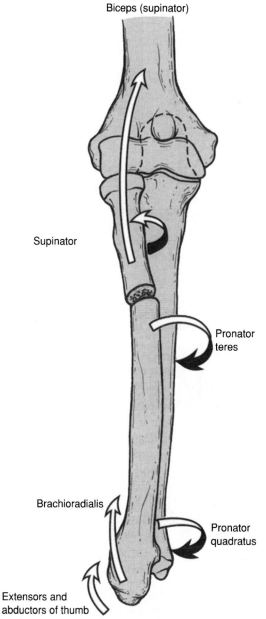

Figure 17–19. Main deforming muscular forces of the forearm. (Redrawn from Cruess RL: The management of forearm injuries. Orthop Clin North Am 4:969, 1973. From Green NE, Swiontkowski MF: Skeletal Trauma in Children, Vol 3. Philadelphia, WB Saunders, 1998.)

the preferred option in most cases. Regular follow-up visits with x-rays are required to document maintenance of reduction. In general, the initial reduction of significantly displaced forearm fractures is best accomplished with adequate sedation or general anesthesia. Although nonunion is rare, malunion does occur. Malunion may be due to the lack of adequate follow-up, improper casting technique, or the improper use of pronation or supination to control fracture maintenance. Malunions are best dealt with early, using manual or drill osteoclasis (refracturing of the callus). However, once the fracture is solidly healed, one may delay an osteotomy for several years.

Refracture rates range from 10 to 15% in most series.

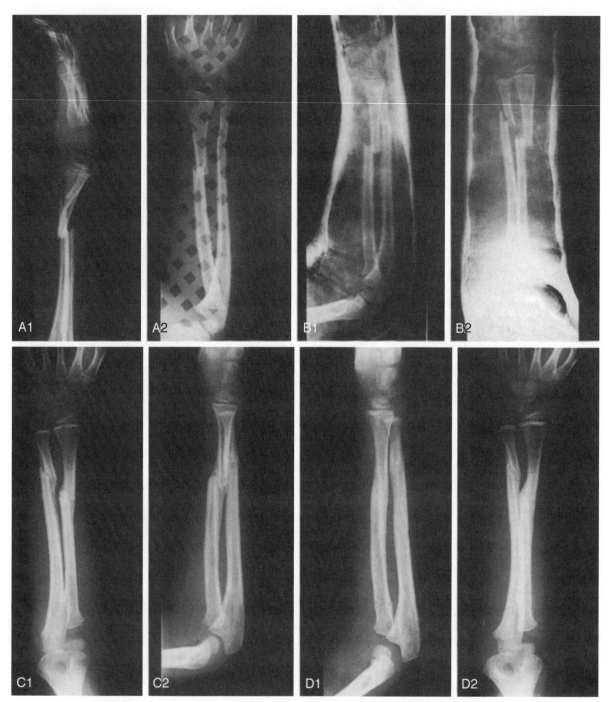

Figure 17–20. Bayonet apposition of the radius and ulna. A 6-year-old boy fell off a swing and sustained a complete fracture of the shaft of the radius *(A1)* and a greenstick fracture of the distal ulna *(A2)*. Note that the distal fragment is volar to the proximal fragment, which differs from the usual dorsal displacement seen with this injury. This appearance is consistent with continued rotation of the forearm after the fracture occurred. The radius was manipulated *(B1)*, with the patient under general anesthesia, so that the distal fragment was dorsal to the proximal fragment, and the usual reduction technique was then attempted. The greenstick fracture of the ulna was completed during the manipulation *(B2)*, increasing the instability of the fracture. An end-to-end reduction could not be obtained, and the fracture was casted in bayonet apposition. Note that the fracture ends of the distal and proximal fragments match in width and shape, indicating correct rotatory alignment. *C1* and *C2*, The cast was removed at 6 weeks. *D1* and *D2*, On follow-up 1 month later, there was full supination and pronation, as in the normal left forearm. (From Green NE, Swiontkowski MF: Skeletal Trauma in Children, Vol 3. Philadelphia, WB Saunders, 1998.)

Because these fractures frequently occur at the previous fracture site, one must assume that such fractures are not entirely new injuries. Persistent angular deformity, osteopenia, and incomplete union should all be considered. Many choose to treat refracture operatively in an effort to obviate the problem in the future. If closed treatment is selected, protracted protection with a forearm orthosis may provide an additional level of protection.

DISTAL RADIAL PHYSEAL FRACTURES

Distal radial physeal fracture is perhaps the most common physeal injury of a major long bone in a child. Approximately 75% occur around the onset of puberty. Most are Salter type II injuries. In the younger child, they are more likely to be Salter type I injuries. The overwhelming majority of these injuries are adequately treated with closed reduction and cast immobilization. The type of cast used is frequently debated, and most authors prefer long arm casts. Complications of this injury are few, with growth plate arrest, either partial or complete, occurring in 7 to 10%.

COMPLEX INJURIES OF THE FOREARM

Children may sustain complex forearm injuries; these injuries are not unique to adults. Specifically, the Monteggia fracture dislocation is seen in children. Dislocation of the radial head, in association with fracture of the proximal ulna, is a well-recognized entity. Interestingly enough, the major problem with this injury in children is failure to recognize the dislocated radial head. For this reason, one should be suspicious of the diagnosis "isolated fracture of the proximal ulna." Monteggia described this injury in 1814 and it was subsequently classified by Bado (Fig. 17–21). When diagnosed early, closed treatment is usually adequate to effect excellent results in children. Late diagnosis of the radial head dislocation presents a much more complex problem. Currently, most authors recommend relocation of the radial head. In order to do this, it is necessary to either shorten the radius or lengthen the ulna. Doing so will allow the radial head to reposition itself opposite to the capitellum without undue pressure. If the length issue is overlooked and the radial head is forced back into position, redislocation will likely result. The Bell-Tawse procedure, which is a reconstruction of the annular ligament, is frequently performed with the relocation procedure.

The Galeazzi fracture dislocation is yet another complex forearm injury. Frequently, disruption of the distal radioulnar joint or a fracture of the ulnar styloid is seen in association with a distal third fracture of the radius. These injuries tend to be very unstable; hence, there is a current wave of enthusiasm for operative fixation of the radius.

HAND INJURIES

Most metacarpal and phalangeal fractures in children are frequently nondisplaced; therefore, they require minimal treatment. Most of the displaced fractures can be adequately reduced closed and immobilized using simple splints. A word of caution: when immobilizing finger fractures, it is important to do so in the *position of function.* Unfortunately, the common practice of immobilizing fingers on tongue blades must be condemned. As a result of this practice, the digit ends up unnecessarily stiff. As is so

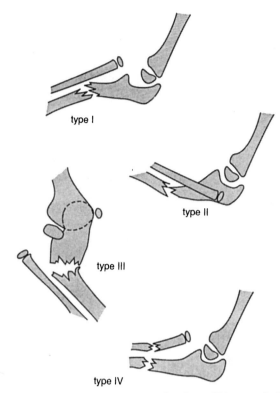

Figure 17–21. The Bado classification of Monteggia fractures. (From Dormans JP, Rang M: The problem of Monteggia fracture dislocations. Orthop Clin North Am 21:252, 1990.)

often the case, when the vast majority of injuries are benign, it is easy to overlook the problem fractures. Therefore, several specific injuries are worthy of note. Condylar fractures (Fig. 17–22), especially if intra-articular, whether they be of the middle or proximal phalanx, require anatomic reduction and fixation. As in adults, degenerative changes and deformity will result if they are not treated appropriately. Physeal fractures occur typically at the base of the proximal phalanx; these are usually Salter type II injuries. Because angulation typically is out of the plane of motion of the joint (usually medial or lateral), remodeling is minimal at best. Therefore, reduction of these injuries is essential; once reduced, they are usually stable with simple buddy taping to the adjacent digit with a small splint. Preadolescents and adolescents will frequently sustain metacarpal fractures and fractures of the thumb as a result of aggressive behavior. These are managed like their adult counterparts.

FRACTURES OF THE PELVIS

As mentioned earlier, the pelvis in the child is far more flexible than that of the adult. Because of the presence of significantly more cartilage, mechanical deformation frequently does not result in fracture; rather, the cartilage allows the pelvis to deform elastically, and recoil, following the removal of load. Unfortunately, the abdominal contents are not necessarily as pliable; thus, with the relative lack of protection provided by the immature pelvis, they are more likely to be damaged.

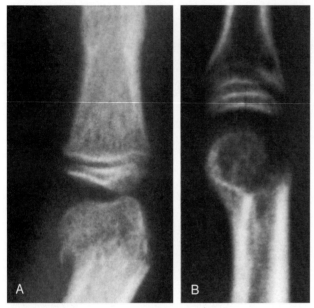

Figure 17–22. *A,* An unstable, angulated phalangeal neck fracture of the proximal phalanx in an 8-year-old child. An oblique radiograph was necessary to show true angulation. *B,* The lateral radiograph suggests rotational deformity, which was confirmed clinically. (From Campbell RM Jr: Fractures and dislocations of the hand and wrist. Orthop Clin North Am 21:228, 1990.)

The triradiate cartilage is a physis, allowing enchondral growth. In point of fact, it is a bilaminar growth plate, producing growth in two directions. Normal triradiate growth is essential for normal acetabular growth and coincidentally normal pelvic height. Reportedly, the ischial segment of the triradiate cartilage contributes the most to pelvic height. In addition to the triradiate, there are a number of secondary ossification centers, most of which fuse to the bony pelvis between 15 and 19 years of age. Avulsion injuries of the secondary centers do occur. Specifically, the iliac apophysis, the anterior inferior iliac spine, and the ischial tuberosity are subject to these types of avulsion injury.

Pelvic trauma in children is primarily the result of pedestrian versus car injuries. These children, as noted earlier, have significant concomitant injuries. Most pelvic injuries are stable, with relatively few unstable pelvic ring fractures being reported. Avulsion injuries of secondary ossification centers usually follow athletic trauma. Despite the pain that they cause, their prognosis is usually excellent.

Treatment of avulsion injuries is usually nonsurgical: rest, activity modification, rehabilitation, and protected weight bearing are adequate to produce satisfactory results. Occasionally, nonunions have been reported. These have occurred primarily following ischial avulsion fractures, although other areas are not immune. In the presence of an established nonunion of an avulsed segment, excision of the fragment and muscle reattachment is usually the best approach. Attempts to reattach the fragment, especially that of the ischium, are complicated by the formation of overabundant callus and heterotopic ossification.

More significant pelvic fractures are classified as they

are in adults. The Tile classification based upon mechanism of injury is most descriptive. Anterior compression, lateral compression, and vertical shear injuries have all been identified in children. As previously mentioned, most pelvic fractures in children, should they occur, are stable. Unstable pelvic fractures usually require fixation to prevent late deformity; their specific management is similar to that for the adult. The more important problem surrounding pelvic trauma in children is the associated visceral injury. Closed head injuries, genitourinary injuries, and gastrointestinal injuries are all unfortunately quite common. Significant retroperitoneal hemorrhage also occurs in this age group. Approximately 20% of children with pelvic fractures will require blood replacement. These are usually the children with unstable pelvic injuries.

Unique in this age group is damage to the triradiate cartilage (Fig. 17–23). Should this occur, the normal height and depth of the acetabulum will not be achieved. The labral growth that occurs at the periphery is usually unaffected. Should premature closure occur, it will result in dysplasia of the acetabulum and possibly subluxation of the hip. Late osteotomies of the pelvis are usually required to treat this unfortunate complication. The vast majority of pelvic fractures in children, however, can be treated with simple bed rest, skeletal traction or a pelvic sling, and protected weight bearing. Early mobilization and activity modification are important in this age group. The key to pelvic trauma in children is to recognize the risks of associated injuries.

FRACTURES OF THE FEMUR

Fractures of the Hip

The head of the femur in the child is at risk for avascular necrosis (AVN), much like in the adult. The tenuous blood supply from the retinacular system is frequently damaged with fractures in and around the proximal femur. The force required to cause this injury in the child is proportionally greater than that required in the adult; thus, children are at greater risk for this dreaded complication than are the elderly. The osteoporotic femoral neck fails at relatively

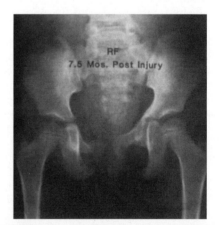

Figure 17–23. A 4-year-old girl, 7½ months after a motor vehicle accident. Triradiate cartilage arrest is seen at left. (From Green NE, Swiontkowski MF: Skeletal Trauma in Children, Vol 3. Philadelphia, WB Saunders, 1998.)

low loads; the normal femoral neck of the child or young adult requires significantly greater load to failure. This, of course, places the blood supply in greater peril, hence increasing the risk of AVN. Fortunately, fractures in this region are relatively uncommon, constituting less than 1% of pediatric fractures. The literature is sparse concerning the treatment and prognosis of these injuries. As would be expected, the vast majority are the result of falls from significant heights and automobile versus pedestrian injuries. In addition, as is the case with pelvic fractures, high energy is required to produce this fracture, making it important to be cognizant of significant associated injuries.

The fractures are still classified using the Delbet grouping (popularized by Colonna), which was first published in 1907 (Fig. 17–24). Four types are described: type I transepiphyseal fractures, type II transcervical fractures, type III cervicotrochanteric fractures, and type IV intertrochanteric fractures.

Despite anecdotal reports over the years referring to the success of closed reduction and spica casting, operative treatment is currently recommended. Concerns regarding the high incidence of AVN have encouraged most authors to recommend immediate reduction and stable fixation. To achieve this, open reduction is frequently required. Following reduction, rigid fixation is accomplished using smooth Steinmann pins or screws. The device used is frequently based on the proximity of the fracture to the growth plate. In an effort not to damage the physis, some would choose smooth pins for more proximal injuries. Most orthopaedic surgeons, however, would prefer to accept the risk of

premature physeal closure and minimize the risk of AVN. The most important goal is to achieve stable, rigid fixation of the fracture. If this results in a physeal arrest, the resulting leg length inequality is easier to treat than AVN of the femoral head. Unfortunately, once AVN develops, the hip is doomed to a poor result. The incidence of AVN varies with the level of the injury. As one would expect, the type I fractures carry a 90% risk of AVN and poor functional results. Types II and III injuries have an incidence of AVN of approximately 50%. Although the type IV fracture is rarely complicated by AVN or premature physeal closure, residual coxa vara (neck/shaft angle less than 135 degrees) deformity frequently requires subsequent treatment. This deformity occasionally results from loss of fixation; therefore, despite the method of internal fixation chosen, most of these children are best managed in a spica cast postoperatively.

Femoral Shaft Fractures

Fractures of the femoral shaft constitute approximately 2% of childhood fractures. In children under 1 year of age, child abuse must be suspected. However, once the child has begun to walk, femoral shaft fractures are not uncommon and are usually accidental. Such things as motor vehicle accidents, falls from heights, and interactions with a sibling have all been reported. The older child usually sustains these injuries during athletic activity or following a fall from a bicycle. The older the child, the more likely that the mechanism of injury will be similar to that seen in the adult. These injuries are more common in males. Although associated injuries are not common, they should be carefully sought, especially in the very young age group. Complex fracture patterns, such as segmental injuries or intra-articular fractures of the knee, are rarely seen in children.

Historically, femoral fractures in children have been treated in a variety of ways. During the nineteenth century, they were managed by various traction modalities and splinting methods. Early in the twentieth century, there was a tendency toward operative correction. The complications incurred during that period brought a return to conservative traction treatment. At present, there is a resurgence of interest in the operative fixation of femoral shaft fractures in children. Clearly, this approach is age-dependent. The management of femoral shaft fractures in infants is nonoperative. Children under 1 year of age who sustained the fracture during delivery or as a result of child abuse can be managed simply in a Pavlik harness or a spica cast. In children between 1 and 2 years of age immediate spica cast application (Fig. 17–25) will usually produce an excellent result. Concerns regarding shortening and angulation are usually unfounded. The dense periosteum around this bone frequently prevents progressive deformity. Despite the popularity of Bryant's traction in the past, most authors recommend against its use because of the high complication rate, especially affecting the noninvolved limb. Both ischemic damage and peroneal nerve palsy have been reported with alarming frequency.

In the young child of 2 to 5 years of age, remodeling is excellent and nonunion is rare. Acceptable angular deformity in the frontal plane is approximately 15 to 20 degrees,

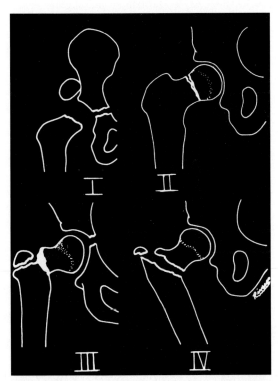

Figure 17–24. Classification of hip fractures in children: I, transepiphyseal, with or without dislocation from the acetabulum; II, transcervical; III, cervicotrochanteric; and IV, trochanteric. (From Canale ST: Fractures of the hip in children and adolescents. Orthop Clin North Am 21:342, 1990.)

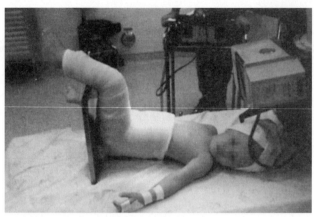

Figure 17–25. Most femoral shaft fractures in infants and young children may be managed in a spica cast at home. The hips are usually positioned in flexion. (From Staheli LT: Fundamentals of Pediatric Orthopedics. New York, Raven Press, 1992.)

with 20 degrees acceptable in the sagittal plane. Traction in the 90-90 position is still the mainstay of treatment in this age group (Fig. 17–26). Typically, the Steinmann pin is placed through the distal femur proximal to the growth plate (from medial to lateral) and traction is applied with the hip in 90 degrees of flexion and the knee in 90 degrees of flexion (90-90 position). Once the fracture site is "sticky," the child may be taken out of traction and placed in a spica cast or cast brace for an additional period of time. Normally, 3 weeks of traction and 3 to 6 weeks of cast immobilization are the recommended course.

The child between 6 and 10 years of age is currently the focus for operative treatment. In an effort to get these children out of the hospital quickly, and mobilize them

rapidly so that they can return to school, various techniques have been described. Some of the more popular ones include open reduction with a small plate and application of a spica cast or cast brace, the use of flexible intramedullary rods such as the Ender nail or rush rod, and the external fixator. All these techniques have their proponents and have shown more than satisfactory results. Stiffness of the hip and knee is avoided and minimal hospital times are recorded.

The management of the preadolescent is somewhat controversial. Many series report excellent results with the use of standard adult nailing techniques. However, a number of case reports of AVN following closed femoral nailing has stimulated a re-evaluation of these techniques. At the present time, most authors do not recommend adult nailing techniques in children under 12. The younger preadolescent is probably better served with the use of an external fixator or flexible intramedullary rod.

Those interested in operative treatment frequently point to the complications of closed treatment, specifically skin breakdown from traction, physeal damage, infection of the pin track, and malunion. Obviously, many complications can result from operative treatment. Nevertheless, the ability to achieve almost anatomic reduction, without marked shortening or angulation, continues to drive the enthusiasm for surgical treatment of these fractures. Short hospital stays, decreased cost, and rapid mobilization of the child also favor these techniques. In addition, parental and physician satisfaction are added benefits.

In general, excellent results have been reported with most methods of managing femoral fractures. Late deformity, such as excessive shortening and angular deformity, usually results from inattention to detail. Nonsurgical treatments mandate more aggressive follow-up. Should excessive shortening be seen, remanipulation of the fracture or

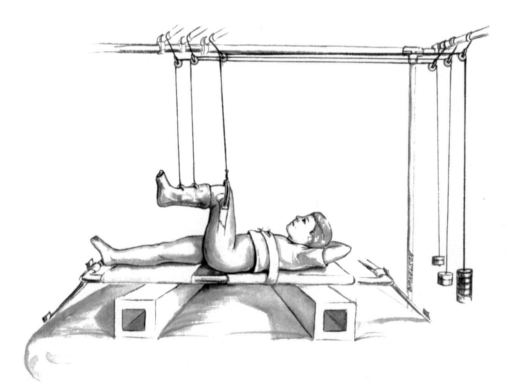

Figure 17–26. The 90-90 skeletal traction with wire through the distal femur is used in children over 2 years of age for treatment of fractures of the femoral shaft. (From Tachdjian MO: Pediatric Orthopaedics, 2nd ed. Philadelphia, WB Saunders, 1990.)

adjustment of the cast may be required. The phenomenon of overgrowth is well documented. The average child's femur, having sustained a fracture, can be expected to overgrow by 1.6 cm. This knowledge should not, however, reassure the surgeon that excessive shortening will be compensated by growth and development.

FRACTURES ABOUT THE KNEE

Fractures about the knee in children comprise a unique group of injuries. A significant amount of lower extremity growth results from the activity of the two growth plates about the knee. The distal femur plate contributes about 1 cm per year, and the proximal tibia plate contributes about 0.6 cm per year. Therefore, injuries about the knee may have far-reaching effects on overall limb length. The distal femoral physis contributes approximately 40% of overall limb length and the proximal tibial plate contributes 25%.

Distal Femoral Fractures

These fractures may occur through the growth plate or purely through the metaphysis. In either event, the gastrocnemius attachments and the attachments of the adductus magnus muscle tend to deform the fracture. In addition, one should remember that the growth plate, like that of the proximal humerus, is not planar; rather, multiple undulations are seen in the distal femoral physis. Also complicating these injuries is the presence of significant neural and vascular structures immediately adjacent.

Distal femoral metaphyseal fractures typically are associated with posterior angular deformity and usually result from motor vehicle accidents or high-energy athletic injuries. The options of treatment include traction followed by casting, cast bracing, open reduction and internal fixation, or external fixation. Surgical treatment is favored in open fractures, older adolescents, polytrauma patients, and in the presence of the floating knee. In addition, if arterial exploration is required, surgical stabilization is appropriate.

The distal femoral physeal fracture is more common. As mentioned earlier, these fracture lines transcend all zones of the growth plate. In addition, due to the undulating nature of the plate, the fracture extends through the "mammillary pegs," which are actually extensions of metaphyseal bone into the undulations of the physis. The fracturing of these pegs, as the physis fails, leads to the high incidence of partial and complete physeal arrest. Rates are reported to be as high as 50%. Salter type II injuries are the most common, with the location (medial or lateral) of the metaphyseal fragment being a function of the mechanism. A varus stress causes a medial "Holland" sign (medial metaphyseal fragment) and, conversely, a valgus stress, fractures the metaphysis laterally.

It is important to remember the principle that ligamentous injury in the presence of an open growth plate is uncommon. Frequently, one is presented with a preadolescent or adolescent who has sustained a knee injury and in whom the initial evaluation suggests ligamentous injury and the x-ray is negative. Keeping in mind the presence of an open growth plate should encourage the physician to seek additional evaluation of this structure. Controversy exists surrounding the use of stress films. Some authors prefer CT scans, and others use classic tomograms. Despite the diagnostic study chosen, most of these injuries will be fractures in the distal femoral physis.

Treatment is based on anatomic reduction. Although 50% of these fractures, treated appropriately, still result in a partial physeal arrest, one should still strive for anatomic restoration. This is usually accomplished under anesthesia with a manipulative reduction and percutaneous pinning (Fig. 17–27). Casting should be used to augment the internal fixation devices. Open treatment with internal fixation devices, such as plates, has been recommended in the older patient, in whom physeal closure is virtually ensured. Recalling that the distal femoral physis grows approximately 1 cm per year, should the plate close in a 14-year-old boy, one can anticipate about 1 inch of leg length inequality. The proximity of the popliteal artery and peroneal nerve should prompt careful evaluation of these patients prior to treatment. Should any question exist regarding vascular integrity, vascular consultation and arteriography should be considered.

Tibial Spine Fractures

This injury is believed to be the pediatric equivalent of an anterior cruciate ligament (ACL) injury in adults. A hyperextension load applied to the immature knee can avulse the anterior tibial eminence. This injury typically occurs in children 8 to 12 years of age. The Meyers and McKeever classification (Fig. 17–28) is the one most often employed. Type I injuries are nondisplaced fractures of the tibial spine. The type II injury suggests the presence of a posterior hinge remaining in the presence of an anteriorly elevated spine. Finally, the type III injury defines a completely displaced and rotated tibial spine.

The treatment of these injuries varies with the degree of displacement. Type I injuries are adequately treated closed with 6 weeks of cast immobilization. The type II injury should be treated by reduction, whether it be closed in hyperextension or arthroscopically. Once reduced, the fracture should be maintained in a cast for a period of 6 weeks. The type III injury always requires operative reduction and fixation. Some authors prefer open surgery, while others favor the use of the arthroscope. If left unreduced, the elevated tibial spine will block extension and ultimately result in a flexion contracture. However, early restoration of anatomy ensures good results in the vast majority of patients.

Proximal Tibial Physeal Fractures

These injuries are similar to those of the distal femoral growth plate. Again, the proximity of the posterior vascular and neural structures must be remembered and evaluated. This injury has been described as the pediatric equivalent of a knee dislocation. That being the case, the physician should have a high index of suspicion of associated vascular injury. Some have suggested a shearing mechanism; others suggest a significant crushing component in the injury. Despite the mechanism, restoration of normal anatomy and maintenance of that reduction are required. Fre-

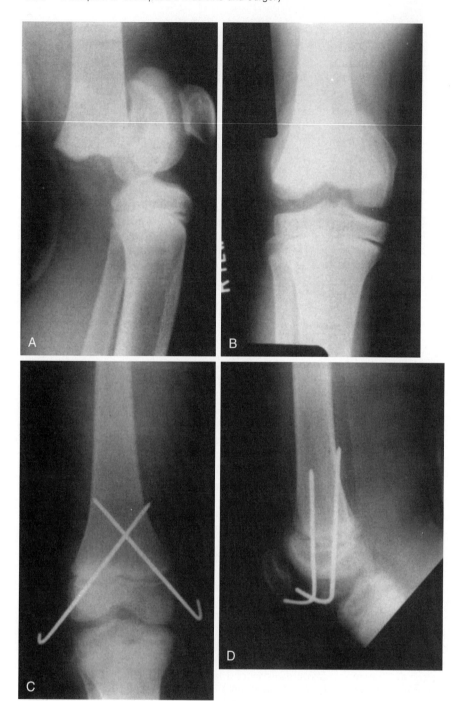

Figure 17–27. Type I fracture of the distal femoral physis of a 13-year-old male. The patient sustained a hyperextension injury of the knee. There was no neurovascular injury. *A*, Lateral radiograph of the knee that shows a completely displaced type I physeal injury of the distal femur with anterior displacement of the femoral condyles. *B*, Anteroposterior radiograph of the same knee demonstrating the displacement of the condyles. *C*, Anteroposterior radiograph after closed reduction and percutaneous pinning showing anatomic restoration of the fracture. Note that the pins are smooth pins that have crossed the physis. *D*, Lateral radiograph of the knee that again shows anatomic reduction of the fracture. (From Green NE, Swiontkowski MF: Skeletal Trauma in Children, Vol 3. Philadelphia, WB Saunders, 1998.)

quently, that is best achieved with a closed reduction and percutaneous pinning. Postoperative augmentation with a cast is usually the best course. As with distal femoral physeal fractures, approximately 40% of these injuries are complicated by partial or complete physeal arrest.

TIBIAL FRACTURES

Proximal Tibial Metaphyseal Fractures

This relatively benign-appearing injury has become a legendary problem for those who manage pediatric trauma. Frequently, it presents in a child under 10 years of age

following modest trauma. The initial evaluation and x-rays suggest a relatively nondisplaced fracture. Careful viewing of the radiograph may show a small fracture gap on the medial side of the proximal tibial metaphysis. Many believe that this injury is actually a greenstick fracture.

Treatment should be aimed at closing this gap. Closure is best accomplished with the child under anesthesia and a C-arm present. The surgeon should apply a varus stress to close the gap. Once closure is accomplished, a well-molded long leg cast with the knee extended should be applied. Following cast application, additional films should be obtained to document reduction. If the gap cannot be closed, it is best to explore the area in search of soft tissue interposition. Occasionally, the pes anserinus has been

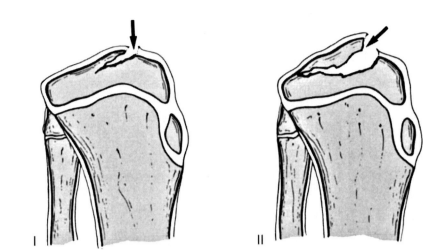
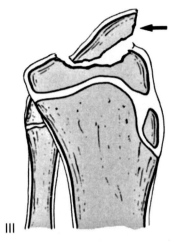

I   II   III

Figure 17–28. Meyers and McKeever classification of fractures of the anterior tibial spine. Type I fracture has no displacement of the fracture. A type II fracture has elevation of the anterior portion of the anterior tibial spine, but with the fracture posteriorly reduced. A type III fracture is totally displaced. (From Green NE, Swiontkowski MF: Skeletal Trauma in Children, Vol 3. Philadelphia, WB Saunders, 1998.)

found in the fracture site. These fractures generally heal within 6 weeks.

The problem, however, comes later. The parents need to be advised prior to initiating treatment to anticipate late valgus deformity (Fig. 17–29). Most authors believe that this deformity results from asymmetrical growth. It is seen even in the face of anatomic reductions with adequate gap closure. This deformity typically develops within 12 to 18 months following fracture. It is most important, however, to recognize that the vast majority of these deformed extremities will spontaneously correct with normal growth and development within 4 years. Therefore, it is important

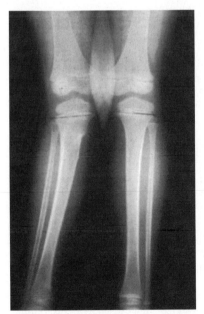

Figure 17–29. Tibia valga following a nondisplaced greenstick fracture of the proximal tibial metaphysis. (From Tachdjian MO: Pediatric Orthopaedics, 2nd ed. Philadelphia, WB Saunders, 1990.)

that the surgeon not embark upon corrective osteotomy until adequate time has been allowed to pass for normal correction to occur. Premature corrective osteotomies are frequently complicated by recurrent deformity. Although it is difficult to resist parental pressure to straighten the "crooked" leg, it is nonetheless in the surgeon's best interest to do so. Zions and other authors have emphasized the spontaneous improvement that can be anticipated following this injury.

Tibial Shaft Fractures

Perhaps the most common tibial fracture in children is the so-called "toddler" fracture. This fracture occurs between 1 and 6 years of age and frequently results from trivial injury. Dunbar applied the name "toddler" fracture in his 1964 article because this injury was most typically seen in younger children. Frequently, the injury can be so subtle that the x-ray may be interpreted as normal. Careful physical examination, however, usually demonstrates localized tenderness over the shaft of the tibia. Some local temperature increase may also be seen. Otherwise, the physical examination is unremarkable. Most of these fractures are spiral in nature and nondisplaced because of the presence of the dense, thick periosteum, which retains it in position. Immobilization in a long leg cast for 3 to 4 weeks is more than adequate treatment.

Fractures of the shaft of the tibia and fibula are quite common in children, constituting 20% of all pediatric fractures. Most result from a direct blow, which typically creates a bending moment in the bone. The resulting transverse fracture is characteristic. As the child gets older, the fracture patterns approximate those of the adult. Obviously, if the mechanism of injury suggests high-speed trauma, associated injuries should be sought.

The treatment is based on the age of the child. Most of these fractures in young children are minimally displaced and can be appropriately managed using nonoperative means. In the adolescent patient with significant deformity, adult treatment options may be considered. External fixators and intramedullary devices are currently being employed by some authors for the management of tibial fractures. Operative techniques are deemed appropriate for open fractures, the floating knee, limbs with neurovascular impairment, and polytrauma.

ANKLE FRACTURES

These injuries primarily involve the physeal plate. Therefore, growth arrest is an important complication. Typically, the arrest is partial and results in angular deformity and joint incongruity; complete physeal arrest has been reported with subsequent leg length discrepancy. Several specific injuries are worthy of note.

The Salter-Harris type III (Fig. 17–30) fracture of the medial malleolus is frequently complicated by premature closure on the medial side of the distal tibial physis. Although unreduced fractures are more likely to demonstrate this complication, it has been reported in well-reduced, well-fixed injuries. The recommended treatment for this injury is accurate reduction of the plate and articular surface with internal fixation using smooth pins or a small cancellous screw. After healing, routine x-rays should be taken at 6-month intervals for 2 years after injury to ensure normal growth. The premature closure and subsequent varus deformity will usually be apparent by that time.

Two unique ankle fractures are seen in the preadolescent and adolescent age group. These fractures frequently have been referred to as "transitional fractures." Such transitional injuries typically occur through the plate that is in the process of closing. In the presence of partial physeal closure of the distal tibia, the application of a deforming force may produce one of these unusual fractures. The juvenile Tillaux fracture is a Salter type III injury of the anterolateral portion of the distal tibial plate. Frequently displaced, these fractures are best managed by open reduction and fixation using small cannulated screws. The complication of concern is articular incongruity and not premature physeal arrest. This growth plate is in the active process of closing; therefore, concerns over premature arrest and angular deformity are unfounded.

The triplane fracture is more complex in its anatomy (Fig. 17–31). The injury is generally thought to be due to external rotation of the supinated foot. The resulting injury is a Salter-Harris type IV fracture occurring in multiple planes. On the x-ray, the fracture will look like a Salter type III injury on the AP view and a Salter type II injury on the lateral projection. The unusual three-dimensional geometry of this fracture makes its treatment difficult. Here, as with the Tillaux injury, the issue is articular congruity, not growth arrest. Triplane fractures require virtually anatomic restoration of the articular surface. Occasionally, this repair can be achieved with a closed reduction and percutaneous pinning. However, should the position be deemed unacceptable and persistent widening of the distal tibial articular surface remain, the surgeon should not hesitate to openly reduce this fracture and fix it with cannulated screws. Postoperative cast immobilization is required. Generally, these are high-energy injuries; therefore, significant swelling should be anticipated.

FRACTURES OF THE FOOT

Fractures of the foot in children are very similar, both in mechanism and management, to those in the adult. Frac-

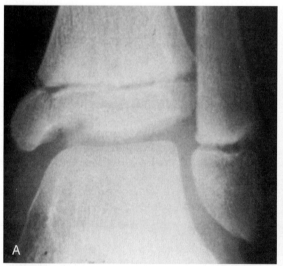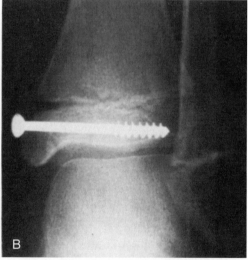

Figure 17–30. *A,* A 10-year-old girl fell off her bike and sustained a supination-inversion injury that caused a Salter-Harris type I fracture of the distal fibular physis and a displaced and laterally rotated type III fracture of the medial distal tibial physis. Closed reduction under general anesthesia did not accurately align the articular surface. *B,* Open reduction through an anterior medial incision was done because closed reduction was not successful. The fragment was secured with a small malleolar screw inserted through a separate medial incision. The screw was placed from the epiphyseal fragment into the remaining epiphysis parallel to the physis. (From Kling TF Jr: Operative treatment of ankle fractures. Orthop Clin North Am 21:385, 1990.)

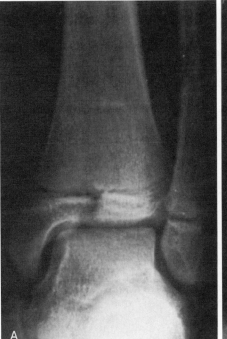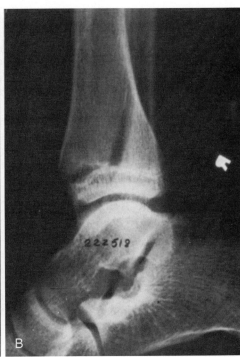

Figure 17–31. Triplane fracture of the ankle—three fragments. The medial and lateral parts of the distal tibial physis are open. *A*, Anteroposterior view showing the Salter-Harris type III physeal injury. *B*, Lateral projection showing the Salter-Harris type II physeal injury. (From Tachdjian MO: Pediatric Orthopaedics, 2nd ed. Philadelphia, WB Saunders, 1990.)

tures of the metatarsals and phalanges are almost ubiquitously managed nonoperatively. Excellent results are usually anticipated. One injury unique in this age group is the stress fracture of the calcaneus. Frequently the child, who presents with heel pain, is diagnosed with Sever's disease. This osteochondrosis of the calcaneal apophysis is common in young children. However, should the tenderness be more distal in the body of the calcaneus and the symptoms be more intense, a stress fracture of the calcaneus should be considered. A bone scan is usually adequate to make the differential diagnosis, because the x-rays are often normal. A short leg cast for 3 to 4 weeks is ordinarily adequate treatment.

COMPLICATIONS OF SKELETAL TRAUMA IN CHILDREN

Myositis ossificans is rare in children. When seen, it typically occurs in the older age group, especially following head trauma and burns. Approximately 10 to 15% of head-injured children will demonstrate some heterotopic ossification.

Cast syndrome was originally recognized following scoliosis surgery with the application of a body jacket. Obstruction of the third portion of the duodenum by the superior mesenteric artery has been recognized as a complication of body casting for many years. Children who are thin seem to be at greatest risk.

Traction-induced hypertension was originally recognized following leg lengthening procedures. It has also been described in children when traction is applied to reduce a long bone fracture. The exact mechanism remains obscure.

Vascular trauma has been discussed in association with several different fractures, specifically those about the knee and those about the elbow. About half of all arterial injuries in children result from penetrating trauma, and about 20% are associated with fractures. Compartment syndrome is of major concern following injury to the limbs. Compartment syndrome in children is somewhat more difficult to diagnose than in adults because the physical findings tend to be more subtle.

Fat embolism, as a clinical syndrome, has been reported in children. Most reports occur in association with femoral and pelvic fractures. Some series suggest that the incidence is ten times greater in adults.

Deep vein thrombosis is fortunately quite uncommon in children. When reported, the findings have been similar to those seen in adults. Usually, this complication occurs in the older child and teenager, particularly in those who are significantly overweight.

Local union problems have been mentioned already. Malunion can complicate many fractures and has a multitude of causes. Nonunion, although rare in the pediatric age group, can occur; one example cited was the lateral humeral condyle.

Synostosis should be differentiated from myositis ossificans. This complication has a poor prognosis. Characteristically, the bone is formed in the interosseous membrane. Usually, synostosis is seen following fractures in the proximal third of the forearm; the extent of the synostosis is directly related to the severity of the initial displacement.

Growth disturbance, secondary to physeal arrest, has been mentioned frequently. Clearly, the degree of deformity will vary with the age and severity of the fracture. Angular deformity is frequently seen secondary to partial physeal arrests, especially when they occur peripherally in the plate. The disastrous central arrest, secondary to a central bony bar, can cause very destructive changes in the plate, as well as significantly impair long bone growth. Techniques to excise physeal bars have been discussed by many authors. CT scans are often used to "map" the extent of the physeal bar. If the physeal bar involves less than 50% of the plate, bar excision can be contemplated. Most techniques involve the insertion of some type of interposition material after excision (fat, silicone, methyl methacrylate). Results from this type of surgery, nevertheless, remain somewhat variable.

Neural injury may occur acutely at the time of fracture or late. Acute injury, such as that seen following supracondylar fractures of the elbow, usually carries a good prognosis. On the other hand, neural trauma due to penetrating injury is less predictable. Late neuropathies, such as the tardy ulnar nerve palsy resulting from progressive elbow valgus, may also be encountered.

Reflex sympathetic dystrophy is rare in children. However, an increasing number of reports suggests that this bizarre syndrome can be seen as early as 8 years of age. Many of these children, as is the case in adults, have psychological overlay issues. Frequently, family problems are readily elicited. Nevertheless, the somatic manifestations are disabling. The course generally is more benign in children, with fewer long-term sequelae.

Because of the resiliency of children and their bones, many physicians are lulled into a false sense of security when treating pediatric fractures. Although it is true that most skeletal injuries in children have an excellent prognosis when treated appropriately, there are, nevertheless, a number of pitfalls in management. It is crucial to be aware of the uniqueness of the child's bone, and the extraordinary potential of the growth plate. The physis is clearly a two-edged sword concerning skeletal trauma. It provides the child with marvelous mechanism for remodeling, and yet injury to it can cause complications unknown in the adult.

BATTERED CHILD SYNDROME

Euphemistically referred to by some as "nonaccidental trauma," this condition was perhaps originally referred to by Caffey in a 1946 report, which linked unexplained intracranial injury and skeletal injury. Kempe, in 1972, introduced the term "battered child syndrome," and a number of articles since that time have made physicians increasingly aware of this horrendous problem. At the present time, there are approximately 1 million victims per year of abuse and neglect. Approximately 25% of these children are physically abused, resulting in 1000 deaths per year. The male-female incidence is roughly equal. Approximately half of the children are under 2 years of age and 40% are between 2 and 5 years of age. The older child is more likely to be the victim of sexual abuse. Multiple articles and news reports have made the general public increasingly aware of this problem. Similarly, it is widely recognized now that early diagnosis is important. Green has stated that should an abused child be returned to his or her home without therapeutic procedures or precautions, approximately 50 to 70% are at risk for further battering and 10% are at risk for death.

Frequently, orthopaedic surgeons are called upon to evaluate injuries in these children. In addition, they are frequently asked to testify as to the likelihood that a given fracture resulted from battery. It has been estimated that approximately one third of battered children sustain musculoskeletal trauma; therefore, orthopaedists are regularly involved in their care. The party responsible for the battering is usually known to the victim. Tragically, the parents (commonly the mother) are at fault. Other members of the household, specifically adult males who are not the biologic father, should be suspected. Many of these children are from lower socioeconomic levels, although child battery is by no means confined to this group.

The diagnosis rests on the finding of a constellation of signs and symptoms that, when viewed collectively, point to battered child syndrome. Most of these children will demonstrate signs of neglect—nutritional, hygienic, and psychological. Most of the children will be withdrawn and extremely anxious while being evaluated by the physician. They will typically avoid eye contact with their parents or caregivers. Sixty percent of physically abused children have only soft tissue injuries. At this stage, the battery has not escalated to the point of skeletal injury. The vast majority of children will demonstrate some cutaneous lesions. Approximately one third will have visceral injuries, and as previously mentioned, approximately one third to one half will have skeletal injuries.

Evaluation of the skin for cutaneous lesions is critical. Certain unique *bruises* may give clues to this syndrome. In very young children, under 1 year of age, a large bruise of the forehead may mean "shaken baby syndrome." Bruises can also be used as an aging technique. Multiple bruises of different colors suggest that they were incurred at different points in time. *Bite marks* should be sought, especially on the upper extremities. The phenomenon of *imprinting* (marks on the skin suggesting impact with a specific object) may be seen. Coat hangers and belt buckles are two commonly employed imprinting devices. *Burns* also are seen in these children. Multiple small burn marks over the body, especially of different ages, may suggest the use of cigarettes or matches to punish the child. When children are dipped in hot water, one will usually see the phenomenon of *popliteal sparing*. When children fall into a bathtub of hot water, they do not have time to bend their knee and therefore the popliteal space is burned. However, if children are purposefully dipped into a tub of hot water, they will flex their knee, thereby protecting their popliteal space from thermal injury. Finally, it is fair to say that burns are never seen in the nonambulatory child unless they are inflicted by an adult.

Eye ground changes, such as multiple *petechial hemorrhages* of the retina, should also be sought. These hemorrhages occur from the shaking of small infants. Bruising of the buccal mucosa and tearing of the *frenulum* under the upper lip can be diagnostic of this syndrome, suggesting that the child's bottle was forcibly pushed into the mouth.

Visceral injury is not uncommon although. Intrathoracic trauma tends to be relatively uncommon because of the presence of the protective rib cage. Usually, all intra-abdominal trauma results from beating with a hand or fist. Occasionally, impact with a thick object, such as a wall, can produce abdominal visceral injury. The most common severe intra-abdominal injury is a fracture of the liver. However, crushed kidneys, torn mesenteries, ruptured in-

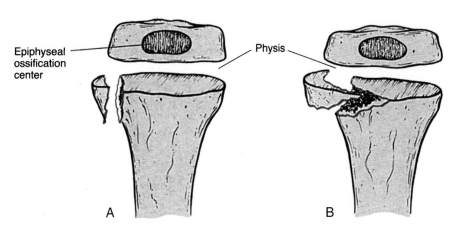

Figure 17–32. The metaphyseal avulsion fractures occurring at the junction of the metaphysis and the physis that are seen in child abuse. The injuries are caused by sudden twisting of the limb. The fracture may be a simple corner fracture *(A)* or a so-called bucket-handle fracture *(B)*. (From Green NE, Swiontkowski MF: Skeletal Trauma in Children, Vol 3. Philadelphia, WB Saunders, 1998.)

testines, fractured pancreas, and rectal perforation, as well as genital injury, have all been reported. One unique visceral injury is the classic esophageal stricture caused by the forced imbibing of caustic liquids.

The skeletal injuries in battered child syndrome have a somewhat unique distribution. They may be seen involving diaphyses of long bones, the metaphyseal/epiphyseal region of long bones, and in the ribs. Certain diaphyseal fractures are indicative of nonaccidental trauma. Perhaps the most pathognomonic long bone fracture is the *spiral fracture of the humerus*, seen in the child under 2 years of age. Most feel that this is virtually diagnostic of battered child syndrome. On the other hand, fracture of the *femoral shaft* in children, once they reach the age of walking, can be quite common and accidental in origin. Battering should be considered in the child under 1 year of age, especially if first-born or neurologically impaired. Additionally bilateral femoral fractures in a child under 1 year of age are almost always nonaccidental; over the age of 4, however, femoral shaft fractures are usually accidental.

Metaphyseal and epiphyseal injuries (Fig. 17–32) are perhaps more indicative of battered child syndrome than those in the diaphysis. The metaphyseal *"corner"* fracture, which is seen in the distal femur, proximal tibia, and distal humerus, and the *bucket-handle fracture*, in which the entire peripheral metaphyseal rim is avulsed, characteristically result from battering. Typically, the small child who is swung by an arm or a leg will suffer repeated varus or valgus stress to the joints. The radiographic finding of periosteal elevation and periosteal new bone suggests failure in this region of the distal long bone. The finding of several of these injuries, especially in different stages of healing, makes battery almost certain.

Rib fractures are common in battered child syndrome. Typically, they result from direct blows to the chest wall. Frequently, they follow a kicking injury. Again, the ribs provide a mirror to age these injuries. Multiple rib fractures, in various stages of healing, again suggest battering.

Last, craniocerebral trauma completes the picture of battered child syndrome. Typically, 25% of battered children under the age of 2 will sustain head injury. In fact, it is the most frequent cause of death. An inadequate explanation for the injury and the presence of multiple associated injuries are two important corroborative facts. It is interesting to note that the pediatric skull can generally withstand a fall from a height of about 3 feet. Therefore, a significant skull fracture that is said to result from falling from a sofa or a changing table should be suspected as potentially nonaccidental. Skull fractures resulting from battering typically involve *multiple sites*. In addition, they manifest *complex configurations*. Depressed fragments are not unusual, and the so-called *growing fracture* suggests that there is ongoing bleeding within the calvarial vault. It is very rare for accidental trauma to produce other than a single narrow fracture line, whereas in battery the single fracture is unusual. The most common bone to be fractured accidentally is the parietal bone. In battery, the parietal remains the most common, but many more fractures are seen in the occipital and temporal bones of the calvarium. This fact should alert the physician to be suspicious of *nonparietal skull fractures*.

The diagnosis of battered child syndrome hinges on the multiple manifestations of the condition. The history taking and physical assessment can glean facts that are important in the overall evaluation of these children. The vague inconsistent history presented by a parent, who somehow seems unusually anxious or nervous, and a child who does not interact well with the parent may raise one's suspicion. A clustering of soft tissue injuries, specific types of fractures, and craniocerebral injury may be confirmatory of one's suspicions. A word of caution, however, is important. There are a number of skeletal manifestations of battered child syndrome that are very characteristic; however, many of them are simply protean and can result from accidental trauma as well. Great care must be exercised by the physician when evaluating these children, as well as when cooperating with state and local agencies in the investigation. Significant harm can be done by errors on both sides of the discussion. Should a child who is truly being battered be returned home inappropriately, the risk of further battery is great. On the other hand, should a simple fracture of the femur be reported as a manifestation of battered child syndrome, irreparable effects on a family can be imparted. Virtually all state and local jurisdictions now have mandatory laws requiring the reporting of suspected cases of battered child syndrome; in fact, the physician may be held liable for failure to do so.

Bibliography

Caffey J: Multiple fractures in the long bones of infants suffering from chronic subdural hematomas. Am J Radiology 56:163–173, 1946.

Dunbar J, et al: Obscure tibial fracture of infants—the toddler's fracture. J Can Assoc Radiol 25:136–144, 1964.

Green FC: Child abuse and neglect. A priority problem for the private physician. Pediatric Clin North Am 22:329–339, 1975.

Green N, Swiontkowski M: Skeletal Trauma in Children. Vol 3. Philadelphia, WB Saunders, 1994.

Kempe C: Helping the battered child and his family. Philadelphia, JB Lippincott, 1972.

MacEwen D, Kasser J, Heinrich S: Pediatric Fractures. Baltimore, Williams & Wilkins, 1993.

Rockwood C, Wilkens K, Beaty J: Fractures in Children, 4th ed. Philadelphia, JB Lippincott, 1996.

Zionts L, et al: Posttraumatic tibia valga. J Pediatr Orthop 7:458–462, 1987.

Section V

Regional Orthopaedic Problems of the Adult

C h a p t e r   18

Adult Spinal Disorders

Sam W. Wiesel, M.D.
William C. Lauerman, M.D.

SPINE TRAUMA

Spinal cord injury (SCI) is without a doubt the most devastating condition encountered by the orthopaedic surgeon. No other injury or condition is as disruptive physically, emotionally, or economically or has the potential for such a high rate of premature death and associated complications. Described originally in the time of Pharaohs, there is a long and almost exclusively pessimistic history of the response of SCI to treatment. Labeled by ancient Egyptian physicians as "an ailment not to be treated," it is only in the latter half of this century, with the evolution of special SCI units, that an improvement in the functional prognosis of SCI patients could be reported. More recent studies demonstrating at least partial efficacy for the pharmacologic management of SCI, and ongoing studies into the utility of newer drugs and drug regimens, hold a promise for continued improvement in the outlook, if not for a "cure," for SCI.

The tragedy of SCI is highlighted by its predilection for young, healthy individuals. Extensive epidemiologic data from model SCI centers in the United States have been compiled, and several trends are apparent.[146] There are approximately 10,000 cases of traumatic SCI annually in the United States. These cases are almost evenly divided between quadriplegia, either incomplete or complete, and paraplegia. The overwhelming majority of the patients are young, with the most common age group, accounting for almost 60% of patients, being individuals between the ages of 16 and 30. SCI occurs most frequently during the summer months of June, July, and August and most commonly on Saturday. It is four times more common in men than in women. It has long been documented that the most common cause of spinal cord injury is motor vehicle accidents, and most estimates have placed this at approximately 50%; falls, civilian violence, and sports have each contributed approximately 15% of injuries. More recent evidence suggests that gunshot wounds (GSW) are contributing increasing numbers of SCI, but a variety of legal and social changes appear to have led to a decrease in motor vehicular injuries.

Several patterns of SCI or neurologic injury following spine trauma may be seen, ranging from complete SCI to isolated nerve root injury. Complete SCI implies complete physiologic, although rarely anatomic, disruption of the spinal cord below the level of injury. With the exception of root sparing, which may be seen for one or even two levels distal to the cord injury, any function further distally is evidence of an *incomplete* SCI. The distinction is important prognostically because of the bleak prognosis with a true complete SCI; recovery of meaningful function distal to the level of injury (with the exception of one to two levels of root recovery) is almost impossible. Incomplete SCI, on the other hand, has significant potential for recovery and this fact may well change the treatment plan. In evaluating the SCI patient the presence of the bulbocavernosus reflex is important when a complete cord injury is apparent. The bulbocavernosus reflex is a normal finding. With the examiner's finger in the rectum, squeezing the glans penis or tugging on the Foley catheter will cause reflexive contraction of the rectal sphincter. If this normal reflex is absent in the acute setting, then the patient is presumed to be in spinal shock. The presence of spinal shock in a patient who otherwise appears to have a complete SCI means that prognostication must be deferred, because the injury may be incomplete but made to appear more severe by the spinal shock. The return of the bulbocavernosus reflex, which should occur within 48 to 72 hours, signifies the end of spinal shock, and appropriate designation of the severity of the injury can at that time be made.

Incomplete SCI syndromes include the anterior cord syndrome in which injury to the anterior horn cells leads to disruption of the corticospinal or motor tract.[19] This disruption most commonly involves the cervical region and has the worst prognosis of all incomplete SCI syndromes. Clinically these patients frequently mimic those with complete injuries, with only patchy distal sparing to differentiate them. Unless rapid recovery of function is seen, a poor outcome is likely. Central cord syndrome is also common and has a somewhat better prognosis. A variable mechanism of injury has been reported, with the original description being of the older patient with pre-existing spondylosis sustaining an extension injury to the cervical spine.[135] On presentation these patients typically have greater involvement of the upper extremities than of the lower extremities and have retained perianal sensation. Lower extremity recovery usually precedes that in the upper extremities. Most patients recover bowel and bladder function and ambulatory capability, although a spastic gait may be seen. Clumsiness of the upper extremities is also a common long-term complication. Brown-Sequard syndrome is common in cases of penetrating trauma. Functional hemisection of the cord leads to ipsilateral paralysis or paresis with contralateral loss of pain and temperature sense, usually two levels below the injury. This syndrome has the best prognosis for recovery with almost all patients regaining the ability to ambulate. Posterior cord syndrome, involving loss of the sensory function of the posterior column, vibratory and position sense, is extremely rare following trauma.[19]

A final mention should be made of neurologic injury in the region of the cauda equina. The spinal cord typically terminates at about the L1–L2 level, and the nerve roots to the lower extremities begin to exit the cord two or three levels proximal to this level. Therefore, neurologic injury at the thoracolumbar junction, and in particular in the lumbar spine, frequently entails injury to the nerve roots of the cauda equina, signifying a lower motor neuron injury. Because these nerve roots are essentially peripheral nerves, the prognosis for recovery is typically better than would be expected for a cord injury and may suggest the need for more aggressive surgical management than would be employed for an equivalent injury at a more proximal level.

EVALUATION

Effective treatment of the patient with spine and spinal cord injury begins with recognition of the injury. In 1979 Bohlman reported on 300 cervical spine injuries, 100 of which were initially missed in the emergency department setting.[15] Although the percentage of missed injuries may now be less than 1 in 3, the most common causes for failure to detect such an injury have not changed. These reasons include the presence of multiple injuries and "an altered level of consciousness" due to the patient sustaining a head injury or being impaired due to alcohol or drug intoxication. Although the patient with a cervical spine or spinal cord injury is frequently medically unstable, this should not distract the trauma team from considering the possibility of injury to the spine. Routine lateral radiography of the cervical spine, with visualization of the superior endplate of T1 as a minimum requirement, is recommended for all polytrauma patients. Discussion of evaluation and treatment of the multiply injured patient is beyond the scope of this chapter, but the stepwise "ABC" approach to such patients should be initiated whenever a spine or spinal cord injury is identified, even if the patient has not been previously identified as a "multiple trauma" patient.

One of the factors to assess is the patient's overall hemodynamic status. Shock in the trauma patient may come about from a variety of causes, the most common of which is hypovolemia. When a spinal cord injury has been identified, however, the possibility of neurogenic shock should be considered. Neurogenic shock occurs due to disruption of sympathetic outflow in the lower cervical and upper thoracic region, leading to decreased peripheral vascular resistance. The hallmarks of neurogenic shock are hypotension and relative bradycardia (rather than the tachycardia that would be expected in hypovolemia). Differentiation between neurogenic and hypovolemic shock may be impossible initially, and an initial presumption of hypovolemic shock leading to fluid resuscitation is reasonable. Failure to respond is best addressed with Swan-Ganz monitoring and the use of pressors as indicated. Ongoing attempts at fluid resuscitation are futile if the underlying cause of the hypotension is neurogenic and may lead to pulmonary edema or worsening of a difficult pulmonary situation later.

When possible, a detailed history should be taken from either the patient or any observers present. Determining the mechanism of injury may contribute to better understanding of the pathoanatomy later seen radiographically. It is important to ask about transient neurologic loss at the scene of injury; a convincing history of temporary loss of motor or sensory function may suggest the occurrence of an incomplete SCI that has resolved rapidly and may affect treatment decision making if a fracture is identified.

Physical examination includes primary and secondary survey of the entire patient and then concentrates on the spine. The entire spine must be inspected and palpated, with the patient log-rolled while maintaining in-line traction of the neck. Ecchymosis, tenderness, or a palpable gap between spinous processes all suggest injury to the posterior elements and supplement information obtained radiographically. Neurologic examination must be detailed, systematic, and documented and should be repeated (along with documentation) at regular intervals. Most SCI centers utilize the American Spinal Injury Association Guidelines for classification and documentation, which is then entered in the patient's chart, facilitating accurate identification of neurologic status, prognostication, and in many cases treatment. The Frankel grading system or a modification of it is also utilized to classify the extent of function following neurologic injury:[2, 58]

- Frankel A: complete SCI
- Frankel B: sensory incomplete
- Frankel C: motor incomplete, motor useless
- Frankel D: motor incomplete, motor useful
    - D1: nonambulatory
    - D2: ambulatory
- Frankel E: normal

In addition to documenting intact or absent levels of sensation, motor function must be clearly defined and graded on a 0 to 5 scale. By convention, the spinal level applied (such as C6 quadriplegic) refers to the lowest level with intact, at least antigravity, strength. It is also important, when performing the neurologic examination, to diligently search for evidence of sacral sparing, such as retained toe flexion, perianal sensation, etc. Rectal examination and evaluation of the bulbocavernosus reflex is routinely carried out as described earlier.

Radiographic assessment begins with a routine lateral cervical spine view and proceeds as indicated. In our center the polytrauma patient who is awake, alert, has no neck pain, is nontender with a normal range of motion, and is neurologically normal undergoes no further radiographic evaluation if the lateral view is negative. The overwhelming majority of cervical spine injuries are apparent on the lateral radiograph,[15, 82] but further views include an AP, supine obliques, and an open mouth odontoid view. The neurologically normal patient with persistent neck tenderness or pain, and who is otherwise medically stable, may be taken for physician supervised (patient performed) flexion/extension lateral radiography.

Computed tomographic (CT) scanning is undertaken when adequate visualization of the entire cervical spine down to the superior endplate of T1 cannot be obtained on plain radiography, or when a fracture or fracture-dislocation is identified. Better definition of bony injury and an accurate assessment of compromise of the spinal canal is obtained with CT. Magnetic resonance imaging (MRI) is utilized to assess for intrinsic cord damage, to evaluate possible cases of posterior ligamentous injury, or to assess for the presence of a herniated disk in a patient with a subluxation or dislocation.[10, 55, 133] The major disadvantage of MRI is logistic, including difficulty introducing an intubated patient or a patient in tongs into the scanner. Injuries to the thoracic and lumbar spine are usually readily apparent on plain radiography. The identification of **any** fracture or dislocation of the spine mandates AP and lateral radiography of the entire spine due to the incidence of associated, noncontiguous injuries, which is as high as 20%. As in the cervical spine, identification of a fracture in the thoracic or lumbar spine is typically followed with CT scanning to better define bony disruption and to determine the presence and extent of spinal canal compromise. MRI scanning is less commonly utilized, but is most helpful for identifying injury to the posterior ligamentous complex.

TREATMENT

Management of the patient with SCI begins with medical stabilization. After initial primary and secondary assessment of the patient, the "ABCs" of treatment include establishment of an airway, breathing, and support of circulation. When intubation is required either nasotracheal intubation or nonmanipulative intubation with continuous in-line traction to the cervical spine is utilized. Hemodynamic evaluation and support, as described earlier, are essential. One component of ongoing neurologic embarrassment in SCI is hypoperfusion of the spinal cord; thus, maintenance of normal blood pressure is mandatory, and appropriate monitoring to differentiate between neurogenic and hypovolemic shock, with treatment as indicated, is vital. Another important step in the overall assessment and management of the patient with SCI is placement of a Foley catheter. Urosepsis was at one time the leading cause of death in SCI patients, but it has diminished significantly in recent years.[12] This is due largely to the importance placed on strict technique for placement of the catheter, as well as early catheter removal and institution of intermittent catheterization for bladder drainage.

Immobilization of the potentially injured cervical spine should be performed at the earliest possible time. Immobilization is routinely accomplished in the field with either a hard collar or sandbags. The use of a spine board for transport contributes to immobilization of the cervical as well as the thoracolumbar spine, but it should be recognized that the spine board is a transportation device and does not represent an ongoing means of immobilization once the patient reaches the hospital.

The most effective and important early step in treating SCI is realignment of the spine. In most cases the application of skeletal traction represents the first step in realignment.[19] We favor the use of Gardner-Wells tongs, which are readily available, inexpensive, and easy to apply. Initial application of 20 lb of traction with increasing weight also serves to immobilize the spine as realignment is accomplished. Certain situations occur, as will be described here, in which traction is either contraindicated or must be applied cautiously, but as a general rule, the application of skeletal traction should be carried out once a skeletal injury is recognized.

Once the spine has been realigned, the presence of ongoing compression on the cord or cauda equina, in the face of a persistent neurologic deficit, suggests that decompression should be considered. Most SCI patients suffer neurologic injury as a result of either malalignment of the spinal canal or anterior compression from retropulsed bone. If a deficit persists after realignment, then a source of ongoing compression should be sought, and is usually easily identified on CT scanning. The role of decompression in incomplete injuries is now reasonably well accepted, with patients who have plateaued neurologically responding well to anterior decompression and stabilization. This is true even in cases of late decompression.[6, 107] The role of decompression in complete injuries is less clear. In the cervical spine there is evidence that decompression may facilitate root recovery and is utilized in selected cases.[8] Little would appear to be gained by decompressing a complete thoracic cord injury but, below T10, injury to nerve roots of the cauda equina may respond favorably to decompression of what otherwise appears to be a complete deficit. We favor an aggressive approach in this setting.

Providing stability to an unstable spine injury, either surgically or nonsurgically, is an essential part of the orthopaedic surgeon's role in managing spine trauma. As will be discussed, the definition of instability varies among different levels of the spine and injury patterns, and therefore, the appropriate means of restabilization vary. Because the modern approach to SCI management includes early participation in rehabilitation, an increasingly aggressive approach to surgical stabilization is undertaken in most SCI centers for patients who are neurologically impaired. Even in the presence of complete SCI, surgical stabilization minimizes or eliminates the need for external immobilization, facilitates early transfer to a rehabilitation center, and may minimize the risk of medical complications such as pneumonia, skin breakdown, and sepsis.

Halo brace immobilization is commonly utilized in the treatment of injuries to the cervical spine, either with or without neurologic deficit. A number of authors have demonstrated the marked increase in rigidity of the halo brace when compared to other external orthoses.[29, 90] The halo is routinely used for immobilization of upper cervical spine injuries such as injuries to the ring of C1 or fractures of C2 and is often applied for unstable injuries of the subaxial spine as well. Limitations of the halo include a well-documented potential for paradoxic motion or "snaking" of the lower cervical spine[156] as well as the risk of pin track complications. Garfin and colleagues have reported on a number of potential complications in the use of the halo.[61] They identified a significant risk of pin loosening and infection when the anterior pins are placed behind the hairline, in the temporalis fossa. They recommend placement anterior to the supraorbital nerve (Fig. 18–1).

In 1990 Bracken and coworkers reported on the results of the use of high-dose methylprednisolone in a multicenter, randomized, double-blind study of patients with com-

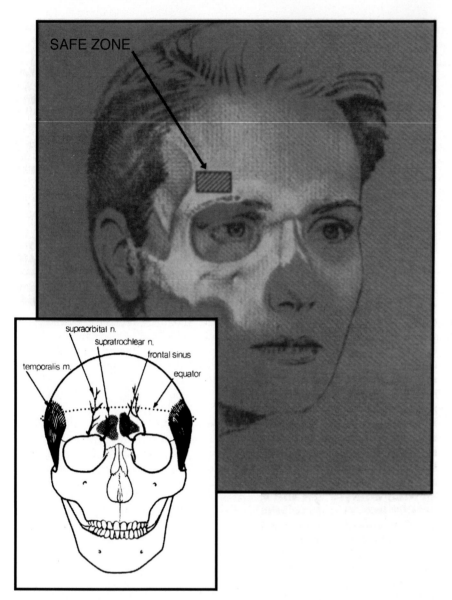

SAFE ZONE

supraorbital n.
supratrochlear n.
frontal sinus
temporalis m.
equator

Figure 18–1. Depiction of the landmarks for anterior halo pin placement and of the "safe zone" as described by Garfin and coworkers. (From Levine AM, Eismont FJ, Garfin SR, Zigler JE: Spine Trauma. Philadelphia, W.B. Saunders, 1998.)

plete and incomplete SCI. Their encouraging results included a significant improvement in motor and sensory function that was particularly dramatic in the patients with incomplete injuries. Although the significance of the functional gains seen, in particular in complete SCI, may be debated, since the publication of this article, the use of this high-dose methylprednisolone protocol has become routine. An initial bolus of 30 mg/kg of body weight followed by infusion of 5.4 mg/kg/hour for 23 hours is administered to any patient who can be treated in the initial 8 hours following the injury and who has a neurologic deficit other than an isolated root injury. Pregnant women and patients under the age of 18 were excluded from the protocol, as were those with penetrating injuries.[20] When this treatment is employed, the risk of complications such as wound infection and gastrointestinal bleeding should be appreciated.

Starting with the Second World War, the final phase of SCI treatment began to develop. Sir Ludwig Guttmann is the best known of a number of individuals who pioneered the concept of specialized rehabilitation centers for the long-term management of SCI patients. The guidelines for these units, as proposed by Guttmann, include the following:[72]

- Transfer to a specialized unit as early as possible following injury
- Management supervised by a physician knowledgeable in and dedicated to SCI care
- A team of allied health professionals trained in the management of SCI complications
- A commitment to vocational rehabilitation
- A commitment to addressing psychosocial and recreational needs
- Provision for lifetime follow-up care of the SCI patient[72]

An ongoing federally sponsored system of SCI rehabilitation centers was begun in this country in 1970. Known as the Model System Centers, these facilities, along with non–federally sponsored centers, address all the above-noted guidelines, paying particular attention to quality of life issues, vocational rehabilitation, and lifetime follow-up. There is now little question that early transfer to such facilities greatly improves the patient's functional and, in particular, emotional outcomes.[9]

Spinal Stability

Stability of the spine has been described as the ability of the spinal motion segment to resist forces, either acutely or chronically, so as to prevent the development of neurologic injury, pain, or spinal deformity.[155] The differences in anatomy, as well as the forces applied, contribute to different concepts of stability for various regions of the spine. Numerous individuals have attempted to define stability, or the lack thereof, for traumatic injuries of the various regions of the spine with varying degrees of success.

White and Panjabi have stressed the importance of considering the concept of "clinical stability" of the spine.[155] This concept takes into account not just radiographic measurements of injury but also the patient's neurologic status and anticipated loads. They and other authors have provided radiographic criteria for the subaxial cervical spine, the thoracic and thoracolumbar spine, and the lumbar spine that includes translation (greater than 3.5 mm or 20% of the subaxial spine,[104] greater than 2.5 mm of the thoracic and thoracolumbar spine,[155] greater than 4.5 mm or 15% of the lumbar spine[121]) and angulation (greater than 11 degrees of the subaxial spine,[154] greater than 5 degrees of the thoracic and thoracolumbar spine,[155] greater than 22 degrees of the lumbar spine[121]). Other authors have suggested that evaluating the injury pattern helps define the presence of instability. Denis has proposed the "three-column theory" of the thoracolumbar spine (Fig. 18–2). He defines the anterior column as consisting of the anterior longitudinal ligament and anterior half of the vertebral body and disk, the middle column as consisting of the posterior longitudinal ligament and posterior half of the vertebral body and disk, and the posterior column as consisting of the posterior bony arch, the facet joints, and the associated ligamentous structures, including the ligamentum flavum, supraspinous, and interspinous ligaments. Disruption of two or more of these three columns is proposed by Denis to suggest instability.[44] McAfee[106] and Ferguson and Allen[56] have also proposed classification systems that help differentiate stable from unstable injuries.

The definition of instability, and its implications, is highly dependent on the patient's overall health and medical status, neurologic status, and the potential healing of the injury. An excellent example, as detailed here, is the Chance or flexion-distraction injury. These three-column injuries are always acutely unstable, but the treatment is dependent on the pathoanatomy; when occurring strictly through bone, a high rate of fracture healing is anticipated and nonoperative treatment is usually employed while, with a soft tissue injury, immobilization will rarely result in adequate healing and long-term instability is anticipated. In this setting operative treatment is preferred. Other factors which may be considered include the patient's body habitus, respiratory status, the presence of intra-abdominal injuries, and neurologic functioning.

CERVICAL SPINE INJURY

Atlanto-Occipital Injury

Fatal craniospinal injuries frequently involve disruption of the occipitocervical junction.[43] Survival following atlanto-

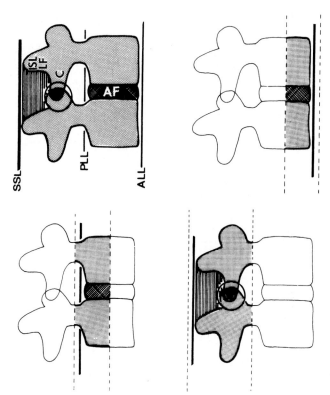

Figure 18–2. Three columns of the thoracolumbar spine, as defined by Denis. AF, annulus fibrosus; ALL, anterior longitudinal ligament; C, facet joint capsule; ISL, interspinous ligament; LF, ligamentum flavum; PLL, posterior longitudinal ligament; SSL, supraspinatus ligament. (From Denis F: The three column spine and its significance in the classification of acute thoracolumbar spinal injuries. Spine 8:817, 1983.)

occipital dislocation, however, is relatively rare due to the high risk of a neurologic injury that is incompatible with life. Surviving patients are usually neurologically intact on presentation, although the potential is great for neurologic worsening if the injury goes unrecognized. Children, particularly those under the age of 8, have a greater predilection for upper cervical spine injury including atlanto-occipital dislocation. Subtle radiographic findings suggest atlanto-occipital dislocation, which may be either anterior (more commonly) or posterior. The most reliable radiographic criterion is the Powers ratio (Fig. 18–3).[122]

Following recognition of this rare injury, aggressive treatment is indicated. Traction is to be avoided, but appropriate positioning of the head in relation to the cervical spine serves to realign the injury. Rigid immobilization is mandatory, and application of a halo vest should be undertaken immediately. Once the patient is medically suitable for surgery, posterior occipitocervical fusion is undertaken, followed by 12 weeks of halo vest immobilization. Because this injury is usually a pure soft tissue injury, nonoperative treatment will almost always result in persistent instability.

C1 Ring Injury

Fracture of the ring of the atlas is a relatively common injury, usually occurring without neurologic sequelae. It is

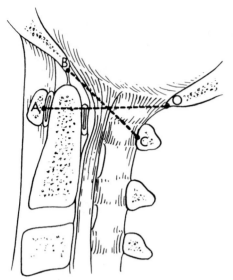

Figure 18–3. The Powers ratio. A, anterior arch of C1; B, basion; O, opisthion; C, posterior arch of C1. The ratio BC:OA should be 1 or less; if it is greater than 1, an anterior occipitocervical dislocation is likely. (From Powers B, Miller MD, Kramer RS, et al: Traumatic anterior atlanto-occipital dislocation. Neurosurgery 4:12–17, 1979.)

important to be aware that, as with all injuries of the upper cervical spine, a particularly high incidence of associated injury to other areas of the cervical spine is to be anticipated. These associated injuries frequently complicate management algorithms and careful scrutiny of high-quality radiographs of the entire neck must be performed.

Fractures of the ring of C1 may occur anteriorly, posteriorly, or laterally and may consist of one to four fractures.[19, 137] A direct blow to the head produces a pure axial loading moment leading, in some cases, to an anterior and posterior fracture on either side of the midline—the "Jefferson fracture."[88] Depending on the degree of force applied, further extrusion laterally at the lateral masses may result in disruption of the transverse atlantal ligament with resultant instability.[143]

Routine radiography may not identify single or even multiple breaks in the ring of the atlas. The open-mouth odontoid view is assessed for lateral spread of the lateral masses; combined extrusion on both sides of 7 mm or more has been reported to be evidence of transverse ligament disruption (Fig. 18–4).[143] When a C1 ring fracture is identified or suspected, CT scanning is helpful in defining the extent of injury and is also useful in assessing fracture healing.

Levine and Edwards recently reported on a series of patients with C1 ring injuries.[99] The most common injury pattern was bilateral fracture of the posterior arch, and only 11 of 34 sustained true Jefferson fractures. Almost all patients can be treated nonsurgically. Patients with three or fewer nondisplaced or minimally displaced fractures are treated with a rigid brace or, when compliance is in question, a halo vest. A halo vest is routinely utilized for Jefferson fractures, which are first reduced by skeletal traction. Associated injuries such as odontoid fracture or transverse ligament rupture complicate management, and

may necessitate a period of halo immobilization to allow for C1 ring fracture healing followed by definitive treatment of C1–2 instability caused by an odontoid nonunion or transverse ligament insufficiency.[99] Management must be individualized in these situations.

Odontoid Fracture

Fractures of the odontoid make up 15 to 20% of all cervical spine injuries. It is interesting that these fractures are particularly common in the very young and the elderly, ages in which failure to recognize the injury, always a common problem, is even more likely. Odontoid fractures are commonly missed on plain radiographs, and undertreatment of these injuries can lead to nonunion, chronic pain, and occasionally neurologic deterioration.

The bony, ligamentous, and vascular anatomy of the dens and surrounding structures is unique and is pertinent in consideration of mechanism of injury, treatment, and complications. The tooth-like projection of the dens provides, along with the cruciate ligamentous complex posterior to it, the intrinsic support of the atlantoaxial complex. Relative thinning of the dens at its base renders this region most susceptible to injury and is the most common site of fracture. Fracture of the dens can also occur, extending into the body of C2 or, rarely, as an avulsion of the tip of the dens. The transverse atlantal ligament forms a sling behind the dens and serves as the primary restraint to anterior translation of C1 on C2. Secondary restraints include the apical and alar ligaments, all of which arise from the skull and insert into the dens itself. Because of the insertion of these ligaments into the dens, prolonged treatment in traction tends to distract the fracture through the waist, and contributes to nonunion.[126] The relatively high nonunion rate seen in type II fractures through the base of the odontoid was at one time felt to be due to a disruption in blood supply to the dens. More recent studies have defined the abundant vascularity to the region around the dens, including contributions from the vertebral and carotid arteries, resulting in a rich anastomosis. This blood supply may be temporarily interrupted in the case of a displaced fracture but is not felt, assuming adequate reduction, to contribute to the risk of nonunion.[119]

In 1974 Anderson and D'Alonzo reported on a series of patients with fractures of the odontoid and suggested a classification system which continues in widespread use today (Fig. 18–5).[5] Type I fractures occur through the tip of the odontoid and are assumed to be avulsion fractures arising from the apical and perhaps the odontoid ligaments. These rare injuries are quite stable, but consideration must be given to the possibility of an associated occipitocervical dislocation. Type II fractures occur through the base of the odontoid and are the most common type seen. Nonunion occurs in 30 to 40% of cases. Risk factors for nonunion that have been reported include increasing patient age, initial displacement of 5 mm or greater, posterior displacement, angulation at the fracture site, and delay in diagnosis.[29] Inability to achieve an anatomic reduction and persistent distraction at the fracture site contribute significantly to the risk of nonunion as well. Type III fractures extend into the body of C2, thereby providing a greater surface area and greater involvement of cancellous bone, promot-

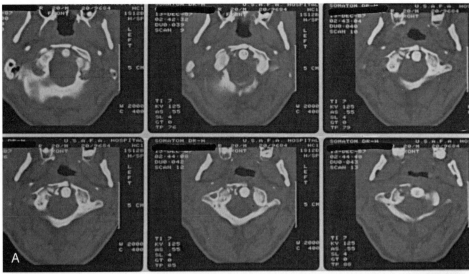

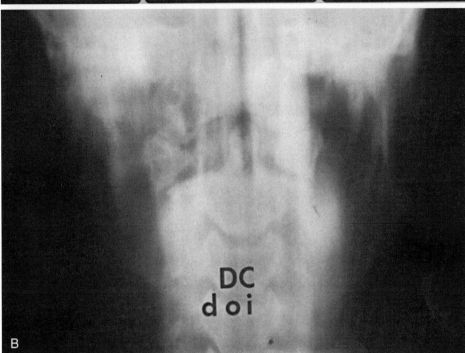

Figure 18–4. CT scan *(A)* and open-mouth tomogram *(B)* of a 37-year-old man with a C1 ring fracture. Spread of lateral masses on open-mouth image is 8 mm, suggesting a transverse ligament rupture.

ing fracture healing. Nonunion and malunion have been reported, however, and the significance of this injury should not be underestimated.[36]

In most cases, fracture of the odontoid is associated with a high-energy injury, particularly motor vehicle accidents, and associated injuries are common. As with other injuries of the upper cervical spine, associated cervical spine injuries are common, and thorough evaluation of the entire spine is mandatory when an odontoid fracture is diagnosed.[74] As mentioned, fracture of the odontoid is a common injury in young children and in the elderly and may, in these cases, be associated with a low-energy injury, including a minor fall. Pre-existent degenerative changes may obscure the radiographic finding of a fracture of the dens in the elderly, and a high index of suspicion is essential. In addition, the authors have seen a number of elderly patients with new onset of neck pain and the radiographic

finding of a chronic nonunion of the odontoid. This represents a difficult therapeutic dilemma, and the degree of instability, anticipated patient demands, and overall health and life expectancy of the patient must be considered when determining appropriate treatment. Patients with fractures of the odontoid typically complain of neck pain, although other injuries, in the emergency department setting, may distract from this complaint. Pain at the base of the skull, occipital neuralgia, and muscle spasm may be seen. Neurologic deficit is relatively rare but has been reported in as many as 10% of patients and is more likely with posterior subluxation.[50]

Failure to recognize a fracture of the odontoid is common and is contributed to by poor quality radiographs, incomplete radiographic evaluation, and distraction of the examiner by the severity of other injuries. Any patient with a blunt injury above the clavicles should be considered at

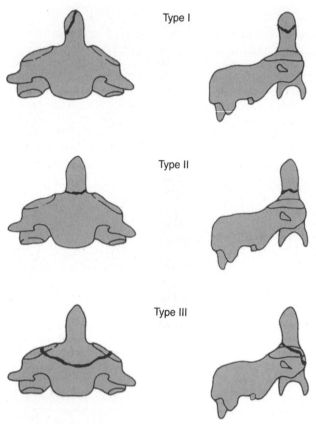

Type I

Type II

Type III

Figure 18–5. Anderson and D'Alonzo's 1974 classification of fractures of the odontoid. (From Anderson LD, D'Alonzo RT: Fractures of the odontoid process of the axis. J Bone Joint Surg Am 56:1664, 1974.)

risk for a cervical spine injury, particularly an injury to the upper cervical spine. Lateral and open-mouth AP radiographs demonstrate the majority of injuries but can be misinterpreted in young children and, in adults, in the presence of significant degenerative changes. CT is commonly used to assess the upper cervical spine but should be interpreted cautiously when a fracture of the odontoid is suspected. If the CT image is obtained in the plane of the fracture, then even with coronal or sagittal reconstructions, the fracture may be missed. Therefore, conventional tomography or MRI is more sensitive for occult fractures of the odontoid.

Treatment of fractures of the odontoid is driven by the classification system of Anderson and D'Alonzo (see Fig. 18–5). Type I fractures, unless seen in conjunction with an occipitocervical dislocation, are stable injuries treated symptomatically only. If an occipitocervical dislocation is seen, then naturally, aggressive craniocervical stabilization is immediately instituted. Type III fractures are generally accepted to be stable and at relatively low risk for nonunion but do necessitate aggressive treatment. The authors favor halo vest immobilization for these injuries; most reported nonunions have occurred when a cervical orthosis, rather than a halo vest, is used.

The treatment of type II fractures, because of their high risk of nonunion, is relatively complex and controversial. Patients who have none of the reported risk factors for nonunion have a favorable prognosis for healing with non-

operative treatment, and halo vest immobilization for a period of 12 weeks is therefore instituted. This treatment would include minimally displaced fractures (4 mm or less of displacement or less than 10 degrees of angulation) that can be anatomically reduced, younger patients, and patients in whom the injury is recognized in the first 7 to 10 days and anatomically reduced. After a period of 12 weeks of halo vest immobilization, the halo is removed, and AP and lateral radiographs are assessed. If a nonunion is present, then flexion/extension lateral radiographs are obtained to see if there is any evidence of motion. A patient with a nonunion and negative flexion/extension radiographs can be followed, but repeat dynamic views should be obtained at 1 month, 3 months, and 1 year to verify that, with increasing neck flexibility when out of the halo, instability has not developed. Patients who have a displaced fracture, a delay in diagnosis, or in whom anatomic reduction cannot be achieved are usually treated surgically, either by C1–2 fusion or direct anterior screw fixation. The age of the patient also affects treatment decision making. An increasing risk of nonunion is seen in patients over the age of 40 years and should be considered when deciding between halo vest immobilization and surgery. In addition, elderly patients (typically 70 years or older) have been documented to tolerate halo vest immobilization particularly poorly with a significant risk of pulmonary complications, emotional distress, and pin loosening. In this setting, therefore, the sometimes difficult decision must be made between either primary surgical treatment or treatment in a cervical orthosis, accepting the relatively high risk of nonunion.

Traditional surgical treatment for a fracture of the odontoid has consisted of posterior C1–2 fusion, which continues to be the "gold standard." Posterior fusion with wiring and iliac crest bone graft in patients with normal bone quality sustaining a traumatic fracture has a high rate of success with minimal complications (Fig. 18–6). Anteriorly displaced fractures occurring through normal bone and with normal lamina of C1 and C2 can be treated in a cervical orthosis following fusion with either Gallie or Brooks wiring techniques. If the fracture is displaced posteriorly or the bone quality is questionable, then halo vest immobilization should be considered.[36, 74] An alternative to fusion with wiring is Magerl's technique of transarticular screw fixation. More technically demanding than wiring, this form of fixation is extremely stable with union reported in as many as 98% of patients, and is appropriate when fusion is selected for patients with associated C1 ring fractures, polytrauma, or in patients who would otherwise require halo vest immobilization and are felt to be at risk for a complication related to use of the halo.[69, 70, 87] The authors favor this technique for most cases of C1–2 fusion in this setting, but it should be noted that a posteriorly displaced fracture that cannot be reduced anatomically may make it technically impossible to direct the screw through the pars of C2 and across the C1–2 facet joint into the body of C1.

A recently described alternative to fusion for fracture of the dens is primary anterior screw fixation. Most authors reserve this technique for acute injuries, and prerequisites for use of the technique include a noncomminuted fracture which is either transverse or angled slightly from anterior to posterior, leaving the fracture line perpendicular to the path of the screw or screws. The fracture must be reducible

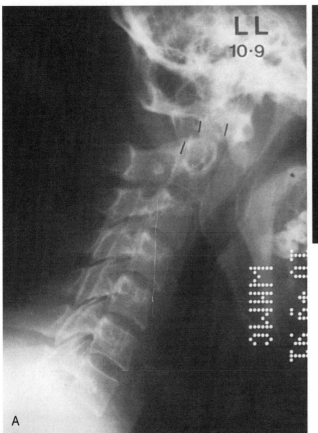

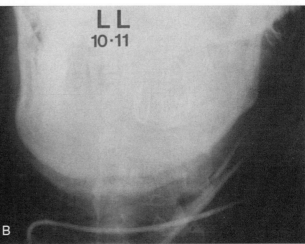

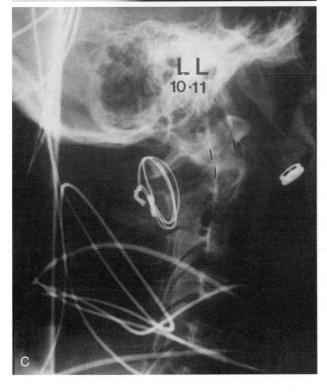

Figure 18–6. A 21-year-old man, noted 2 days post-injury to have an anteriorly displaced type II fracture of the odontoid *(A)*. He was treated with a Brooks and Jenkins fusion *(B and C)*, was immobilized in a hard collar postoperatively, and healed uneventfully.

closed, and care must be taken to assess the patient's neck and chest anatomy to ensure that appropriate drill orientation can be achieved. Familiarity with this technically demanding procedure is essential, and most authors favor the use of two 3.5-mm screws. When successfully performed this technique results in a high rate of fracture healing and an avoidance of the loss of motion seen with C1–2 fusion, which is a significant advantage. The authors make note, however, of the high complication rate, which has been reported in several series.[1]

Hangman's Fracture

Traumatic spondylolisthesis of the axis is a less common injury of the upper cervical spine that, because of its unique historical significance, fascinates physicians of numerous specialties. When judicial hanging was eventually refined sufficiently so that instant death was achieved without avulsing the subject's skull, the submental knot used resulted in a bipedicular fracture of C2 which is now immortalized as the hangman's fracture. The pars interarticularis of the axis represents a zone of transition from the anteriorly placed facet joints of the cervicocranium, from the occiput to C2, to the posteriorly placed facet joints of the subaxial cervical and thoracolumbar spine. The relatively thin pars at this site is therefore susceptible to injury, particularly from a hyperextension force. Subsequent flexion is believed to disrupt the posterior longitudinal ligament (PLL) and the disk, resulting in anterior displacement in more unstable injuries.

Levine and Edwards have classified traumatic spondylolisthesis of the axis based on angulation and translation (Fig. 18–7).[98] Type I fractures involve less than 2 mm of translation with no angulation. Presumed to result primarily from a hyperextension and axial loading injury, these injuries are stable. If physician-supervised flexion/extension radiographs fail to detect motion (implying that the PLL and disk are intact), treatment in a cervical collar is instituted. Close radiographic follow-up is then employed, and a high rate of union anticipated.

Starr and Eismont have described an "atypical" hang-man's fracture, which has also been referred to as type IA. This injury, on at least one side, extends into the vertebral body of C2. It otherwise appears radiographically to be similar to type I injuries, with minimal displacement and no angulation, and should be stable on flexion/extension views. Treatment in a cervical orthosis is appropriate for this type of injury as well.[145]

Type II injuries are divided into type II and type IIA. Displacement and angulation are seen in this group and may, at times, be quite significant. Because of the large size of the spinal canal in relation to the spinal cord at this site, and because anterior displacement of C2 actually enlarges the canal at this level (although the posterior ring of C1 is brought anteriorly and the posterior superior corner of C3 is left in place, posing an eventual risk for cord injury), most displaced hangman's fractures do not result in neurologic injury. Type IIA fractures are differentiated from type II fractures by the radiographic appearance of the fracture line as well as the amount of angulation. A more posterior and oblique fracture line, allowing for marked angulation with a lesser degree of translation, is seen in the type IIA injury (Fig. 18–8). The importance of recognition of this fracture pattern lies in the response to traction; further traction tends to distract through the disk space and should be avoided. Type II fractures are unstable and require an aggressive approach to treatment. Reduction in traction is undertaken. Because of the risk of overdistraction in type IIA injuries, which can occasionally be difficult to differentiate from the far more common type II fracture pattern, initial application of 10 lb of traction is applied and radiographic assessment performed. If distraction at the disk space is seen, then no further traction is applied. If not, then progressive traction is applied, with the neck extended, until the fracture is reduced.[98] Fractures that are displaced more than 5 mm initially have a high risk of redisplacement if immediate mobilization in a halo vest is undertaken. These fractures are typically treated with 4 to 6 weeks of skeletal traction followed by mobilization in a halo vest for a total of 12 weeks of immobilization (Fig. 18–9). It should be noted that even significantly displaced Hangman's fractures will usually heal by virtue of sponta-

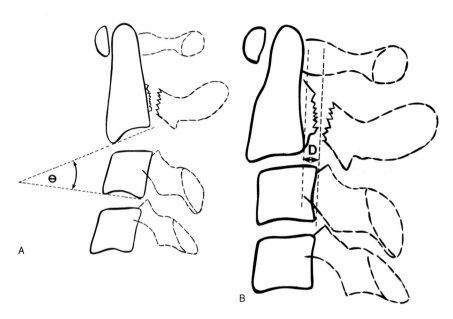

Figure 18–7. Technique described by Levine and Edwards for describing and measuring angulation *(A)* and translation *(B)* in traumatic spondylolisthesis of the axis. (From Levine AM, Edwards CC: Traumatic spondylolisthesis of the axis. J Bone Joint Surg Am 67:217–226, 1985.)

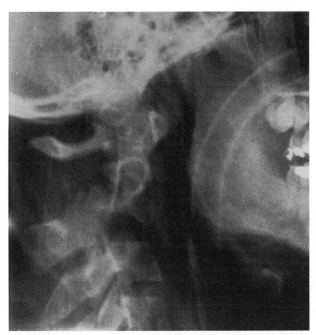

Figure 18–8. Type IIA hangman's fracture. Note the marked angulation.

neous ankylosis at C2–3, underneath the anterior longitudinal ligament which has been stripped off of the body of C3. It is not clear from review of the literature, therefore, exactly what the risk of nonunion is from accepting a fracture that has displaced more than 5 mm. An alternative in treatment of the widely displaced type II fracture is primary osteosynthesis utilizing compression screw fixation across the pars interarticularis.[124] Type IIA fractures are differentiated from type II and are not reduced with the use of skeletal traction. Rather, these injuries are reduced in a halo ring under extension and compression, usually followed by immediate mobilization in a halo vest for 12 weeks.[98]

A type III injury refers to traumatic spondylolisthesis of the axis in conjunction with bilateral dislocation of the C2–3 facet joint. These injuries are not suitable for closed treatment because of the irreducible C2–3 dislocation (Fig. 18–10). Open reduction of the C2–C3 facet dislocation is undertaken and fusion of the C2–3 level performed. The bipedicular fracture of C2 can then be treated either with external immobilization as appropriate, or the operative procedure can include primary osteosynthesis with screw fixation across the fractures or extension of the fusion up to C1.[98]

Vertebral Body Fractures

Vertebral body fractures in the subaxial spine are common injuries whose evaluation and treatment differ significantly from that for injuries to the upper cervical spine. Variables affecting treatment include the fracture pattern seen, associated injuries, and the neurologic status of the patient. Fracture patterns include compression fracture, burst fracture, and a more unstable variant referred to as a "teardrop fracture." In addition, the presence of contiguous fractures at two or more levels further complicates treatment deci-

sion making. Associated injury to the posterior ligamentous structures must also be considered because such damage can render a given fracture significantly more unstable. Finally, the neurologic status of the patient, ranging from normal to an incomplete cord injury to a complete cord injury, has an impact on decisions regarding stabilization as well as the timing of possible surgery.

Fractures of the subaxial vertebral bodies typically occur as a result of an axial load with the extent of the associated flexion force defining the exact injury pattern seen. These injuries can be extremely unstable and, when not recognized, can result in neurologic worsening. Thorough radiographic evaluation down to the superior endplate of T1 is mandatory, and immobilization must be maintained until the possibility of fracture is excluded. Burst fractures at the C7 level are common, and CT scanning, when plain radiographs are inadequate, should demonstrate these injuries.[80]

Treatment of vertebral body fractures depends on all the foregoing factors as well as the patient's general medical status, age, and pre-existing medical conditions. A stable compression fracture, defined as a fracture with less than 40% loss of anterior height and without disruption of the posterior cortex of the body or disruption of the posterior ligamentous complex, in a neurologically normal patient is treated nonoperatively, usually in a cervical orthosis.[97] More severe compression or burst fractures, involving greater than 40% loss of height or disruption of the posterior cortex but without significant retropulsion of fragments or neurologic deficit, are treated with halo vest immobilization. It should be stressed that assessment for a posterior ligamentous injury must be undertaken and the presence of disruption of the posterior ligamentous complex leads to an unacceptably high failure rate with nonoperative treatment. Significant posterior tenderness or ecchymosis, and radiographic findings such as interspinous widening, facet subluxation, or acute kyphotic angulation of greater than 15 degrees, all suggest the possibility of associated posterior soft tissue injury.

Burst fractures of the vertebral body with significant loss of height or with posterior retropulsed fragments causing spinal canal compromise of 20% or more are commonly treated surgically. Again, the presence or absence of posterior ligamentous injury is vital in deciding on appropriate surgical management.[76] If the posterior ligaments are intact, then anterior vertebrectomy and strut graft fusion, usually with tricortical iliac crest, is adequate treatment, and protection of the graft with a cervicothoracic orthosis, such as the Denison brace, achieves an acceptable risk of loss of fixation or nonunion (Fig. 18–11). An alternative would be the use of anterior plate fixation, which appears to lessen the short-term risk of graft dislodgement, although complications related to plate fixation may be seen. In addition, the effect of anterior plate fixation on long-term union is only now being defined. It must be stressed that anterior strut grafting without internal fixation is an acceptable option only in patients with a completely normal posterior column.

The presence of a neurologic deficit has significant impact on the choice and timing of surgical treatment. Persistent neurologic compromise and persistent anterior cord compression from retropulsed bone or disk represents,

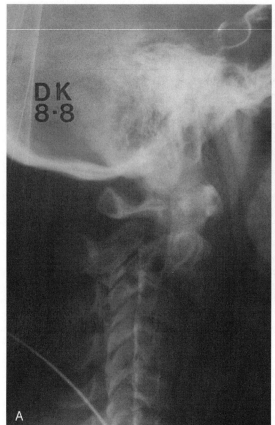

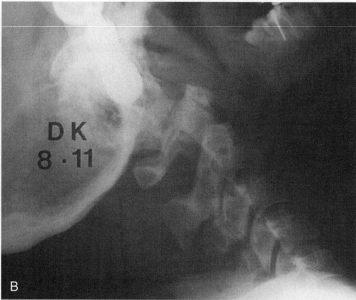

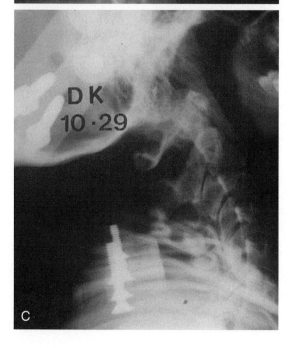

Figure 18–9. Type II hangman's fracture *(A)*. Reduction was obtained in traction *(B)*, which was continued for 6 weeks, then a halo vest was applied for another 6 weeks *(C)*. Anatomic healing resulted.

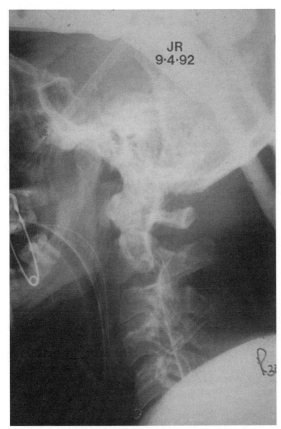

Figure 18–10. Type III hangman's fracture. Halo vest immobilization has not resulted in congruous reduction of C2–3 facets, which require open reduction.

for most authors, an indication for surgical decompression and stabilization. The efficacy of anterior decompression of the spinal cord for neurologic improvement in incomplete SCI is now well accepted.[18] In addition, patients with complete SCI who fail to show evidence of adequate "root recovery" should be considered for anterior decompression. Although the risk-benefit ratio of decompression in these patients is greater than in those with incomplete cord syndromes, facilitation of root recovery is frequently seen, and in patients who are medically stable this approach may be indicated.[8]

The presence of a posterior ligamentous injury significantly affects the treatment of a vertebral body fracture in the cervical spine, as it does elsewhere. Any significant disruption of the posterior stabilizing effect of the posterior column renders a fracture of the vertebral body much more unstable and, in almost all cases, mandates surgical treatment. A commonly seen injury pattern is the so-called "teardrop" fracture. In this injury there is posterior displacement of the posteroinferior corner of the involved vertebral body, acute kyphotic angulation, extrusion anteriorly of a small portion of the anterior cortex of the vertebral body, and loss of parallelism of the facet joint posteriorly (Fig. 18–12). Neurologic injury is common with this injury pattern.[134] Surgical treatment of this injury can consist of anterior or circumferential fusion. Traditionally anterior corpectomy and strut grafting followed by posterior fusion with posterior wiring was recommended. More recent re-

ports have demonstrated the efficacy of anterior strut grafting followed by anterior plating.[2] Although mechanical stability is greater with a combined anterior and posterior approach,[148] a number of authors, including Garvey and coworkers, have reported a high success rate with anterior decompression, structural bone grafting, and stabilization with anterior plating.[63] Although the success of this technique for single-level injuries is well accepted, the presence of two or more contiguous fractures requiring vertebrectomy and plating may be associated with an unacceptably high rate of plate failure, and should merit consideration of a circumferential approach.

Facet Subluxation and Dislocation

Subluxation, dislocation, and fracture-dislocation of the facet joints of the subaxial spine represent a spectrum of injuries. Appropriate treatment of these relatively common injuries requires appreciation of the exact pathologic anatomy as well as the patient's current neurologic status and the expected natural history of the injury. The variation in injury patterns seen includes unilateral and bilateral injuries, subluxation or complete dislocation of one or both facets, and fracture of either the superior facet of the caudad level, which is the most common fracture pattern seen, or fracture of the inferior facet of the cephalad level.[159] An important consideration in assessing the injury is the associated disruption of the ligamentous anatomy of the spine. As with any dislocation, disruption of the joint capsule is seen, but with these injuries, disruption of the ligamentum flavum, interspinous ligament, and the posterior longitudinal ligament may also be present, contributing further to instability. A final consideration is the neurologic status of the patient. Neurologic injury can range from an isolated root deficit to a complete cord injury. It is well accepted that the risk of neurologic injury and the severity of injury seen correlate roughly with the degree of sagittal translation present. Kang and associates have recently demonstrated that the risk of injury is also highly dependent on the pre-existing sagittal canal diameter of the cervical spine.[92] Attention has recently been drawn as well to the potential for creating or worsening a neurologic deficit when reduction of a dislocation is performed in the presence of a disk herniation.[10]

Virtually all facet injuries occur following a flexion injury with the contribution of distraction and/or rotation to the various injury patterns incompletely resolved at this time. C5–6 is the most common injury level seen, but the presence of injuries at C6–7 and even C7–T1 mandates thorough radiographic evaluation down to the superior endplate of T1. In most cases displacement is readily apparent on lateral radiography. The alignment of the facet joints, offset of the spinous processes on the AP view, as well as the presence of subluxation or dislocation on oblique or pillar views of the cervical spine are also helpful in understanding the injury pattern. CT scanning, including reconstructions, provides further information. The role of MRI in the evaluation of these injuries has been debated since Arena, Eismont, and Green first reported on a series of patients with cervical facet subluxation and dislocation, some of whom were made worse neurologically following reduction, with extruded disk herniations.[10, 49] MRI is ex-

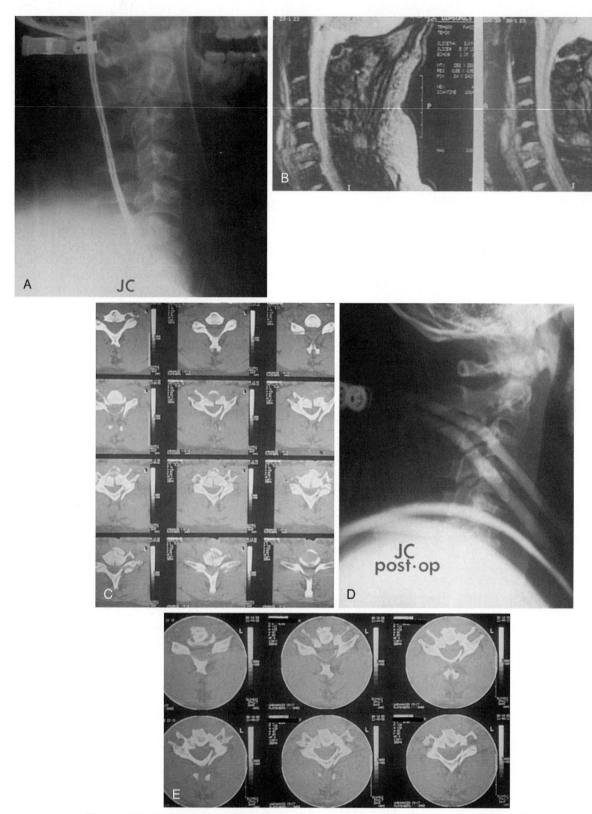

Figure 18–11. A 22-year-old man with a C6 fracture and central cord syndrome. Plain lateral view *(A)* shows relatively mild burst fracture. MRI *(B)* and CT scan *(C)* are preoperative images showing retropulsion into the spinal canal. CT scan demonstrates a laminar fracture, but there is no evidence of ligamentous disruption. *D,* Plain x-ray. *E,* Postoperative CT scan following corpectomy, decompression, and iliac crest strut-grafting. The patient was treated in a cervico-thoracic orthosis for 12 weeks and made a complete neurologic recovery.

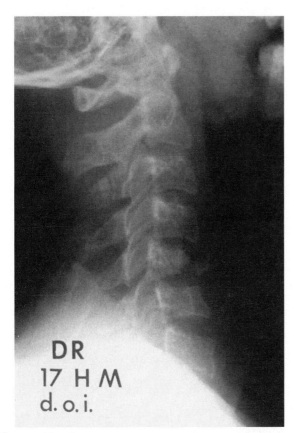

Figure 18–12. Lateral radiograph demonstrating a teardrop fracture in a 17-year-old young man who was a permanent C6 quadriplegic.

tremely sensitive in identifying disk injury, including herniation, but the need for diskectomy is debated and appears to be relatively uncommon. In addition, the logistic difficulty in obtaining an MRI in the emergency department setting, and the timing of urgent reduction versus the need for this test, have not been completely resolved. The authors favor obtaining an MRI prior to closed reduction in any patient who is neurologically normal. Conversely, patients with a complete SCI are reduced closed emergently and, if this is unsuccessful, undergo open reduction and stabilization without imaging unless a delay of less than 1 to 2 hours to obtain a scan is anticipated. Patients with an incomplete cord injury are those who are most likely to benefit from urgent reduction but are also at risk for significant worsening. In these patients we favor, assuming they are awake, alert, and able to provide feedback, the application of skeletal traction and attempted closed reduction. Any evidence of neurologic worsening during this maneuver results in neuroimaging and treatment as indicated. If closed reduction is unsuccessful in a patient with incomplete SCI, then MRI is obtained prior to any attempt at open reduction (Fig. 18–13). If at any point along this algorithm a disk herniation is seen on MRI, then its significance must be assessed. When a clinically significant disk herniation is present, it is suggested by a complete loss of disk height on the plain lateral radiograph. The presence of an extruded disk fragment posterior to the posteroinferior corner of the cephalad vertebral body, a

relatively rare occurrence, is likely to represent a risk following closed reduction, and therefore should be addressed (see Fig. 18–13). Anterior diskectomy is carried out in this setting prior to any reduction, followed by reduction, fusion, and stabilization.

Given the foregoing considerations, the diagnosis of a facet subluxation or dislocation requires reduction and stabilization. In the presence of a neurologic deficit, other than an isolated root injury, reduction is an emergency and is obtained with the application of skeletal traction. In these injuries, once reduction is achieved, stabilization can be carried out electively, usually in the first 48 to 72 hours after injury. Failure to achieve a closed reduction in a patient with a neurologic injury merits urgent open reduction and stabilization.

Neurologic considerations aside, the optimal means of stabilizing these injuries depends on the spectrum of soft tissue and bony injury felt to be present. The most benign injury is a mild subluxation. The presence of mild segmental kyphosis at a given level in a patient presumed to have a neck "sprain" is consistent with this injury. Physician-assisted flexion/extension radiographs are obtained, and if 2 mm or less of translation and 11 degrees or less of angulation is seen, immobilization in a cervical orthosis is instituted.[154] Close radiographic follow-up is mandatory because splinting may result in underappreciation of the extent of injury. Immobilization is usually continued for 10 to 12 weeks, and the authors begin the patients on cervical isometric strengthening exercises, out of the collar, at 3 weeks following the injury. Intractable pain or worsening radiographic instability are treated with posterior fusion and either wiring or plating.

A unilateral or bilateral facet dislocation can be treated either nonoperatively or operatively. Bilateral facet dislocations commonly occur in conjunction with significant disruption of the intraspinous ligament, ligamentum flavum, and often the posterior longitudinal ligament (PLL), and are therefore highly unstable. The pattern of associated ligamentous disruption with a unilateral facet dislocation is typically less severe, and it is certainly less common to see disruption of the PLL. For this reason, nonoperative treatment of a successfully reduced unilateral facet dislocation is a reasonable approach but has a high failure rate for bilateral facet dislocations. Our preference, for either a unilateral or bilateral facet dislocation, is surgical stabilization because of the extremely low risk-benefit ratio of surgical treatment in this setting. The neurologically normal patient is returned much more quickly to normal activity with minimal risk of long-term sequelae, and the neurologically impaired patient is ready to aggressively undergo rehabilitation following surgery without the need for prolonged external immobilization. It should also be noted, when nonoperative treatment of these injuries is considered, that halo vest immobilization has a high risk of redisplacement due to paradoxic motion of the subaxial vertebral bodies, and cannot be assumed to be as reliable as it is in the upper cervical spine.[136, 156]

The presence of a facet fracture changes, at least theoretically, the approach to these injuries. The unilateral facet fracture that is reduced and held anatomically has a high rate of union, which should restore stability. This injury, therefore, represents the most appropriate use of nonopera-

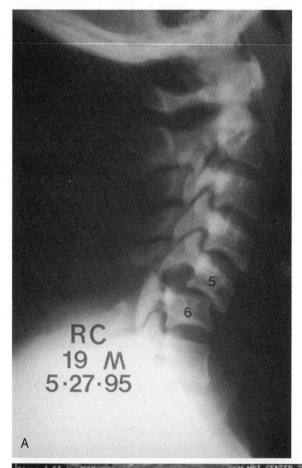

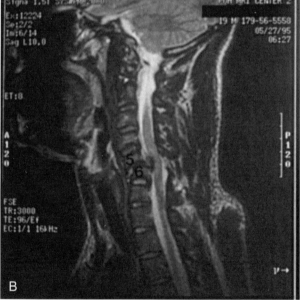

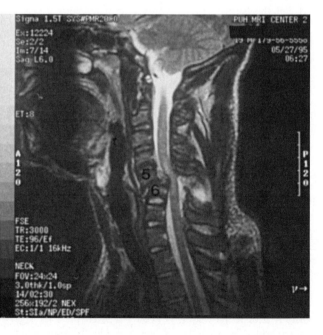

Figure 18–13. A 19-year-old man with a bilateral facet dislocation, demonstrating 50% translation of C5 on C6 on the lateral radiograph *(A)*. Note also the complete loss of disk height seen on the plain radiograph. This is suggestive of the presence of an extruded disk herniation, which was confirmed on the MRI done prior to surgery *(B)*.

tive treatment in the entire spectrum of dislocation and fracture-dislocation of the subaxial cervical spine. There is still, however, a significant risk of redisplacement prior to fracture healing, and many authors favor surgical stabilization of this injury as well.

A final consideration is the patient with a missed injury. This occurs commonly at C6–7 and C7–T1 in unilateral injuries. Radiculopathy may be seen. Successful reduction is unlikely in an injury that is seen more than 4 to 6 weeks after occurrence, and symptomatic treatment should be undertaken. If symptoms persist for greater than 3 months, surgical treatment is indicated. Patients with neck and shoulder pain only are treated with single-level fusion and stabilization; the presence of the disrupted or fractured facet may require modification of standard techniques of wiring or plating. In the presence of nerve root compression resulting in radicular pain, and certainly any objective neurologic deficit, foraminotomy at the involved level is undertaken at the time of fusion.

THORACOLUMBAR INJURY

Compression Fractures

Simple wedge compression fractures make up the majority of traumatic injuries to the thoracic and lumbar spine, even after pathologic fractures through osteoporotic bone are excluded.[117, 161] Axial compression combined with a varying degree of forward flexion produces compressive failure of the anterior aspect of the vertebral body, Denis' anterior column.[44] By definition, a simple wedge compression fracture involves only the anterior column, with preservation of the middle and posterior columns. Other more complex injury patterns may be seen and are increasingly recognized with the advent of more sophisticated imaging modalities and increased awareness on the part of treating physicians. Many fractures that we now define as burst fractures were, prior to the advent of CT, grouped with compression fractures. In addition, an apparent wedge compression fracture of a thoracolumbar vertebral body can be part of a more severe injury complex wherein the posterior ligamentous supports—the interspinous and supraspinous ligaments and ligamentum flavum—fail in tension.[56] This is analogous to the combined vertebral body and ligamentous injury seen in the cervical spine and, as in the cervical spine, radically changes the required treatment.

Most compression fractures of the thoracic and lumbar spine are benign, stable injuries and amenable to nonoperative treatment. It should be borne in mind, however, that in young and middle-aged adults these fractures occur through normal bone and represent relatively high-energy injuries in most cases. The authors therefore feel that benign neglect is inadequate treatment for a compression fracture, at least at the thoracolumbar junction, and an external orthosis is prescribed for 2 to 3 months for most such patients in our practice. Close radiographic follow-up is essential to verify the favorable prognosis and ensure that an unacceptable degree of collapse or angulation is not developing.

Probably the most important aspect of the evaluation of the patient with a wedge compression fracture is to verify the full extent of the injury. Several clues exist on plain radiography to differentiate the wedge compression fracture from its more serious counterpart, the burst fracture. On the lateral view, loss of height of the posterior cortex of the vertebral body or an increase, to greater than 100 degrees, in the angle between the superior endplate and the posterior cortical line at the posterosuperior corner of the vertebral body suggests a burst fracture.[109] On the AP view an increase in the interpedicular distance suggests disruption of the posterior cortex, splaying of the pedicles, and the presence of a burst fracture. Even assessing for these signs, the differentiation may be difficult. Ballock and colleagues reported a misdiagnosis rate of 25% in attempting on plain radiography to differentiate compression from burst fractures. They recommended the routine use of plain CT scanning in the case of all compression fractures to avoid this error.[12] Mistaking a simple wedge compression fracture for a combined vertebral body fracture and ligamentous disruption (referred to by Denis as a flexion-distraction injury or, by Allen and Ferguson, as a compressive-flexion grade III injury[44, 56]) is an even more potentially serious error because the treatment is so different. Flexion-distraction injuries tend to result in greater than 50% loss of vertebral body height anteriorly, in more acute kyphotic angulation, and in interspinous widening that may be seen on either the lateral or AP view (Fig. 18–14).[56] In addition, a patient who on physical examination has marked tenderness in the midline at the fracture level, ecchymosis, or a palpable gap between the spinous processes should be assumed to have sustained tension failure of the posterior column.

Some compression fractures result in neurologic injury, particularly when injuries involve the upper thoracic spine, between levels T2 and T10. Although the rib cage and sternum provide an added degree of stability to fractures in this region, their presence should be understood to imply an even greater degree of energy required to produce such an injury. This factor, in addition to the relatively low spinal canal–spinal cord ratio in the midthoracic spine, as well as the sensitivity of the spinal cord to minor trauma all contribute to a significant risk of injury at this level. Bohlman has reported a high rate of neurologic injury seen with relatively mild fracture-subluxations between T2 and T10, and the possibility of this injury pattern must be considered when evaluating the patient with chest trauma and back pain.[16, 17]

One final consideration is the patient with multiple contiguous wedge compression fractures. A single compression fracture with intact ligaments posteriorly, in a neurologically normal patient, can almost always be treated nonoperatively, but no clear-cut guidelines exist defining appropriate management when two or more contiguous fractures are seen. It has been suggested that the presence of three or more contiguous fractures represents an exceedingly high risk for progressive kyphosis, and in our experience, two adjacent fractures which, when combined constitute the equivalent of 60% loss of vertebral body height, or an acute kyphotic angle of 40 degrees over the expected sagittal contour for that level, should be considered for surgical treatment.[21]

Burst Fractures

Sir Frank Holdsworth was the first to use the term "burst fracture"[86] to describe what is today recognized as one of

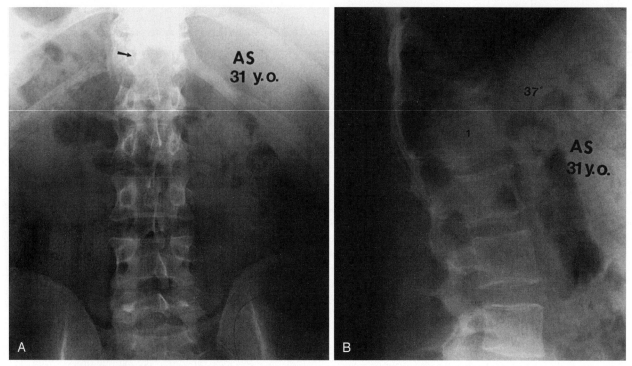

Figure 18–14. AP *(A)* and lateral *(B)* radiographs of a 31-year-old man 6 weeks following an injury to his back, in which he sustained an unrecognized grade III compressive-flexion injury. The AP view shows significant interspinous widening *(arrow),* and the lateral view demonstrates marked anterior compression, preservation of height of the posterior cortex of T12, and significant kyphosis. The patient required surgical stabilization.

the most common injuries to the thoracolumbar spine and one whose treatment continues to be hotly debated. Part of the confusion surrounding treatment of burst fractures stems from differences in definitions among various authors, but most reports are consistent with Holdsworth's original description of a fracture that results from the cephalad disk exploding through the upper endplate into the vertebral body, causing a fracture of both the anterior and posterior cortices. Advances in imaging have enhanced our understanding of the pathoanatomy of this injury, and the retropulsed burst fragment, typically extruded into the canal at the level of the pedicles and causing neural element compression and at times neurologic injury, is now well known (Fig. 18–15). Most surgeons agree with Denis who noted that the posterior column is either intact in a burst fracture or sustains a greenstick type fracture of the lamina or spinous process, but that tension failure of the ligamentous component of the posterior column is not present.[136]

The extent of confusion surrounding this and other injuries is crystallized when an attempt is made to determine whether such a fracture is "stable." Holdsworth originally described the burst fracture and defined it as a stable injury because of the slight risk of progressive deformity or neurologic deficit. Denis on the other hand, utilizing his three-column theory, would define all burst fractures as unstable while McAfee and colleagues in 1982 proposed criteria for an unstable burst fracture, including a progressive neurologic deficit, disruption of the posterior ligamentous complex (which many authors feel would exclude such an injury from classification as a burst fracture), acute kyphosis greater than 20 degrees with a neurologic deficit,

50% loss of vertebral body height in the presence of facet joint subluxation, or the presence of retropulsed bone causing neural element compromise in association with an incomplete neurologic injury.[106] Bradford and McBride have stressed, on the other hand, the importance of a neurologic deficit as a clinical indicator of instability, at

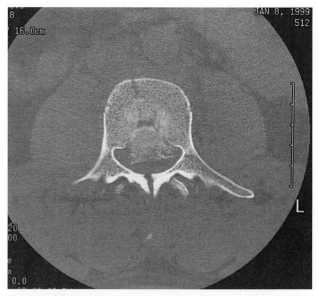

Figure 18–15. CT scan demonstrating characteristic retropulsed bony fragment, occurring at the level of the pedicles in a patient with an L3 burst fracture.

least as it pertains to the appropriateness of surgical stabilization.[21]

Evaluation of the patient with a burst fracture is similar to that described earlier. Radiographic findings commonly seen are described in the previous section. In addition, CT evaluation of a burst fracture is commonly undertaken. The presence of the burst fragment, its exact location in and extent of compromise of the spinal canal, the presence of a laminar fracture, and the integrity of the facet joints are all clearly defined.[108] A percentage estimate of the loss of cross-sectional area of the spinal canal can be made and is suggested by most authors as one of the criteria in determining whether or not surgical treatment is indicated. MRI is less commonly utilized but can be helpful in attempting to determine whether a posterior soft tissue injury has occurred.

Most authors favor surgical treatment for the patient with a burst fracture who is neurologically impaired. In the presence of an incomplete neurologic deficit that has plateaued, decompression, even when performed late, has been reported to yield favorable results by McAfee, Bohlman, and Yuan, who report neurologic improvement in patients decompressed as much as 2 years after injury.[107] Patients with a complete neurologic deficit are commonly treated surgically to facilitate early return to rehabilitation. The authors prefer the anterior approach for decompression of all burst fractures above L4, although posterolateral, transpedicular decompression may be an effective alternative. Laminectomy alone does not contribute to decompression of the cord or cauda equina in the presence of a burst fracture.[22] Decompression performed late requires, by almost all accounts, an anterior approach. Long-term follow-up is lacking, but favorable early results have been seen with the use of anterior fusion and stabilization in conjunction with anterior decompression (Fig. 18–16). Kaneda and colleagues have recently reported remarkable success with a single-stage anterior vertebrectomy and decompression, strut grafting, and stabilization with his anterior instrumentation system. Early examples of instrumentation failure and fusion nonunion have been eliminated with the use of a demanding technique of strut grafting prior to instrumentation.[91]

Posterior instrumentation continues to be widely employed. Acute fractures treated with anterior decompression and strut grafting, without anterior instrumentation, have a significant risk of recurrent deformity unless posterior instrumentation is employed. The significance of this deformity on long-term function is not clear, but following decompression most authors favor either anterior or posterior instrumentation.

Surgery may be elected for patients with a burst fracture who do not require decompression. The precise indications for operating on a neurologically normal patient who sustains a thoracolumbar burst fracture are widely debated.[95] The authors consider surgery in cases in which there is acute kyphotic angulation (greater than 20 degrees more than should be present at that level), greater than 50% compromise of the spinal canal by retropulsed bony fragments, or greater than 50% loss of vertebral body height. We also feel strongly that an apparent burst fracture that includes tension failure of the posterior ligamentous complex should be treated operatively; most such cases fulfill

the preceding criteria for instability due to kyphosis. The neurologically normal patient who undergoes surgery for potential instability is usually treated posteriorly. Traditionally, Harrington rod instrumentation was used and the instrumentation was extended three levels above and two or three levels below the fractured vertebrae. This required an extensive fusion and, with the advent of segmental instrumentation, multiple authors have reported attempts to limit the extent of fusion. The advent of pedicle screw instrumentation led to enthusiasm for single-level fixation above and below the fracture, but unless anterior bone grafting is employed, these constructs are prone to fatigue fracture of one or more screws. We favor the use of a transpedicular instrumentation system extending two levels above and one level below the fracture, supplementing the inferior pedicle screws with infralaminar hooks bilaterally. Another option is the "rod long-fuse short" technique, which saves overall length of fusion but requires a second operation to remove the instrumentation.

One final consideration in the discussion of burst fractures is the management of the patient with a burst fracture of the lower lumbar spine, particularly at levels L4 and L5. These make up a relatively small proportion of the overall numbers of such fractures seen but deserve special consideration. Because of the normal lordosis at this level of the spine, and the passage of the normal center of gravity posterior to the fractured vertebrae, the tendency for these fractures to collapse into progressive kyphosis is less than for injuries at the thoracolumbar junction. In addition, there is relatively more room in the spinal canal for the cauda equina suggesting that the risk of late stenosis is less. For these reasons, several authors have advocated a nonoperative approach for most fractures at L5 and even L4, even when they would appear to fulfill the standard criteria for surgical treatment.[57] We have been satisfied that nonoperative treatment leads to consistently good results in patients with significant collapse, those with retropulsion of up to 60% of the spinal canal, and patients with mild, single nerve root, deficits. When possible a fiberglass body jacket is applied with a single hip pantaloon spica; if the patient's body habitus, other injuries, or other issues preclude the use of a cast, a well-molded, custom-made lumbosacral orthosis (LSO) with a thigh cuff is an acceptable alternative.

Flexion-Distraction Injuries

In 1948 Chance provided the first description of an injury to the lumbar spine involving distraction of the posterior elements, and recommended hyperextension as an optimal means of treatment.[34] His cases predated the use of lap belts, which are now frequently associated with this injury, but many of his other observations remain pertinent. There is a broad spectrum of bony and soft tissue injury seen in both the anterior and posterior columns with flexion-distraction injuries, but all such injuries should raise concern about the possibility of intra-abdominal injury, which is as high as 50%.[7] Although not all patients are wearing a transverse lap belt, or even a seatbelt, a common scenario is the individual wearing a lap belt in a back seat of a car involved in a sudden deceleration injury. Transverse abrasions across the abdominal wall are seen and the spine

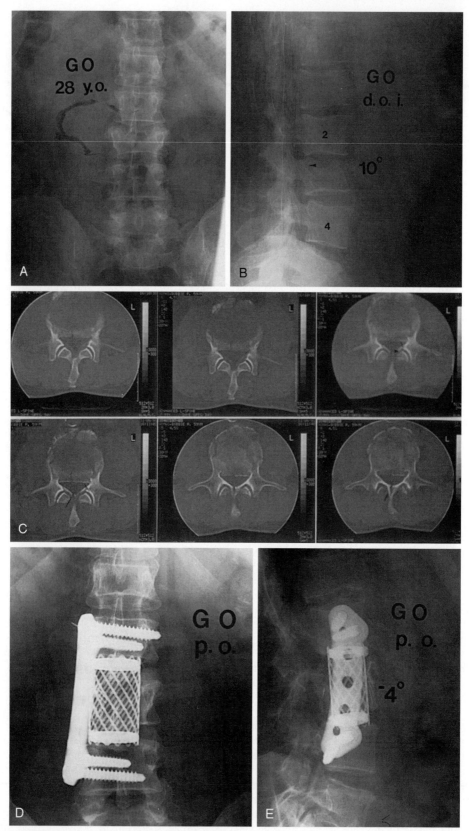

Figure 18–16. A 28-year-old man with a mild neurologic deficit and an L3 burst fracture. The AP view *(A)* demonstrates typical interpedicular widening. The lateral view *(B)* shows collapse with relatively mild kyphotic angulation. Marked angulation and retropulsion at the posterosuperior corner of the body is seen as well *(arrowhead)*. *C,* CT image showing the extent of canal compromise and the presence of a fracture at the spinolaminar junction. *D and E,* AP and lateral views 6 weeks following vertebrectomy through a retroperitoneal approach and reconstruction using a titanium-mesh cage, iliac bone graft, and anterior plating. The patient made a complete neurologic recovery.

rotates around an axis of rotation in the anterior cortex or anterior longitudinal ligament. The lap belt causes blunt trauma to the abdominal viscera in its course toward the spine, where it functions as a fulcrum around which the rotation occurs. The strong correlation between visceral injuries and flexion-distraction injuries of the spine should be remembered by the trauma surgeon when evaluating a patient in whom a lap belt contuses the abdomen resulting in intra-abdominal injury, and by the orthopaedic surgeon evaluating the patient with a flexion-distraction injury.

The standard Chance injury may be pure bone, extending through the spinous process, lamina, pedicle, and vertebral body, pure soft tissue, extending through the interspinous ligament, ligamentum flavum, facet joint capsule, and disk, or mixed, with variable involvement of bone and soft tissue. The common finding among all three is the marked distraction of the posterior elements, moderate distraction of the middle column, and neutral appearance of the far anterior column, reflecting an instantaneous axis of rotation in or about the anterior longitudinal ligament (Fig. 18–17).[64] It is not uncommon to see mild to moderate wedging of the vertebral body reflecting an element of axial loading in addition to pure flexion. Burst-type fractures of the vertebral body may also be seen, reflecting a mechanism of injury that changes from axial loading to sudden flexion, such as in a fall.

Neurologic injury is rare but not unheard of in injuries of this type. As with other areas of the spine, the presence of a neurologic injury is initially treated with realignment, either through an operative or nonoperative approach, followed by stabilization. If there is persistent compression on the cauda equina following reduction, formal decompression is undertaken, usually through a posterior approach. Flexion-distraction injuries are typically highly unstable acutely, and are therefore not amenable to anterior stabilization; if anterior decompression is required, a circumferential approach is typically elected.

The neurologically normal patient may be treated operatively or nonoperatively, depending on associated injuries as well as the pathologic anatomy seen. Pure bony Chance fractures or fractures involving mild wedging of the vertebral body but extending posteriorly through the bony neural arch, are usually treated nonoperatively. The injuries are acutely unstable, but long-term stability is likely if healing occurs; we prefer hyperextension casting because of the potential for losing reduction if a removable orthosis is utilized. On occasion a patient will be deemed unsuitable for casting, and surgery will be elected on that basis alone.

Surgical treatment is elected for Chance injuries that are pure soft tissue or primarily soft tissue and for burst-type fractures with associated tension failure of the posterior ligamentous complex. The instrumentation strategy selected depends on identifying the mechanism of injury and mode of failure of the middle column (see Fig. 18–17).[108] Spinal instrumentation can be utilized to compress, to distract, or to apply a three-point bending force to restore lordosis without distraction. Distraction, in most flexion-distraction injuries, is an inappropriate vector to apply as it will increase the distraction between the posterior elements. Flexion-distraction injuries are either treated with a compression implant for pure three-column distraction injuries, or with a three-point bending type of system to restore

lordosis and only then to distract to restore height, for burst-type fractures of the vertebral body with posterior ligamentous disruption.

Fracture-Dislocation of the Thoracolumbar Spine

The most ominous of all injuries of the thoracolumbar spine is the fracture-dislocation. Several mechanisms have been proposed for the development of a fracture-dislocation, at least one of which includes a severe flexion-distraction injury.[44, 56, 86] The hallmark of fracture-dislocation of the spine, and the essential radiographic finding which should alert the clinician to the high degree of instability involved, is translation. Translation may be seen on either the AP or lateral radiograph and its importance, even when mild, should not be overlooked. In addition, it is important to bear in mind that, as with any dislocation or subluxation, the displacement of the spine may be reduced by the time of radiographic assessment, and may therefore be missed.

Fracture-dislocation of the spine is usually a high-energy injury and is frequently seen in conjunction with a severe neurologic deficit. The exact pathologic anatomy involved depends on the mechanism of injury and the injury severity. Holdsworth first described the "slice fracture," referring to a flexion rotation injury at the thoracolumbar junction with translation in both the AP and lateral planes, and frequently paraplegia (Fig. 18–18).[86] Translation is the most striking finding radiographically and may be associated with fracture of the vertebral body and facet fracture. In this injury the anterior longitudinal ligament (ALL) is typically stripped off of the anterior aspect of the inferior vertebral body, but is usually intact. Another mechanism seen is a severe variant of the flexion-distraction injury. The feature that differentiates this from those discussed in the previous section is translation, typically seen only on the lateral radiograph but which can at times be severe. The ALL is usually intact in this injury as well, but may be stripped off the anterior aspect of the lower vertebral body, although it serves as a valuable aid to reduction. The significance of the translation, in differentiating this from the standard flexion-distraction injury, lies in the greater extent of energy involved in the injury as well as the greater risk for neurologic involvement (Fig. 18–19). A final type of fracture-dislocation involves a pure translational force applied to the spine, typically at the thoracolumbar junction. This rare injury is most commonly the result of hyperextension and shear as has been described, for example, in lumberjacks struck directly on the back by a falling log.[44, 46] These shear-type injuries are the most unstable variant of fracture-dislocation as they typically involve failure of the anterior longitudinal ligament rendering the spine completely unstable.

Assessment of the patient with fracture-dislocation of the spine begins with appreciation of commonly associated injuries. These high-energy injuries may involve trauma to the contents of the thorax, mediastinum, or abdomen, and it is particularly important to consider the possibility of a blunt injury to the aorta. Neurologic injury is common and is typically readily apparent. Complete or near-complete paraplegia is frequently seen, and careful evaluation for sacral sparing should be carried out. Radiographic assessment includes standard AP and lateral views and is fre-

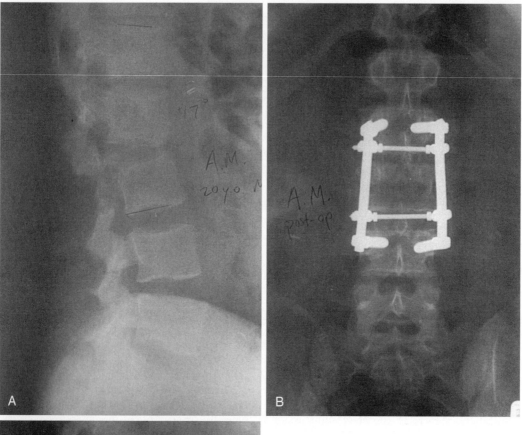

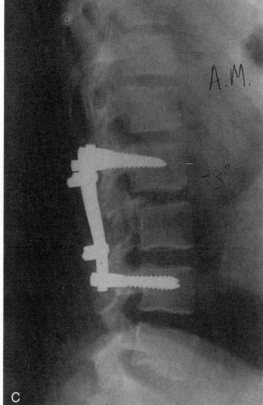

Figure 18–17. This 20-year-old man sustained a "lap belt" injury requiring a colostomy, as well as a mixed soft-tissue and bony Chance injury *(A).* Three weeks following the injury he underwent an open reduction and fusion with a compression implant and transpedicular fixation *(B and C).*

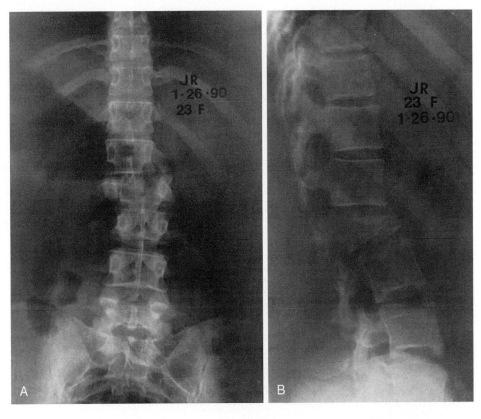

Figure 18–18. AP *(A)* and lateral *(B)* radiographs of a 23-year-old woman with a fracture-dislocation at L1–2 and a severe, near complete neurologic deficit. Following open reduction and stabilization she recovered almost complete neurologic function.

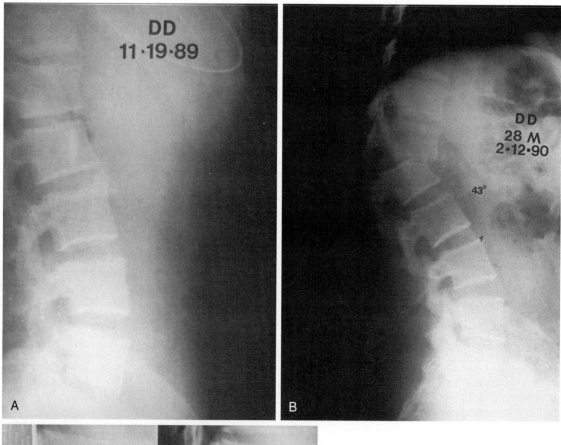

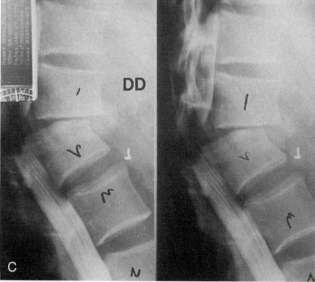

Figure 18–19. This 28-year-old man sustained a seat belt injury requiring laparotomy. The original lumbar spine radiograph was read as normal *(A).* Three months later he had worsening back pain and leg cramping. Plain lateral radiograph *(B)* and myelogram *(C)* demonstrated the extent of the injury, which was a fracture-dislocation that had spontaneously reduced when the patient was supine for the original x-ray.

quently supplemented by CT scanning, with both sagittal and coronal reconstructions being helpful in defining the spectrum of injury seen; understanding the pathologic anatomy and the mechanism of injury greatly facilitates reduction and stabilization. Because the thoracolumbar junction represents a transition zone between the mobile lumbar spine and the relatively stable thoracic spine, as well as a transition from the orientation of the thoracic facet joints to the lumbar facet joints, this is the region of the spine most commonly involved in fracture-dislocation.

Recognition of the presence of a fracture-dislocation stems from recognizing the radiographic hallmark of this injury, which is translation. Once the diagnosis is made, this injury requires surgical stabilization. Because of the inherently unstable nature of the injury, mobilization of the polytrauma patient must be deferred until definitive treatment of the spine is performed, and the orthopaedic surgeon should therefore make every attempt to do so as early as possible, preferably in the first 48 hours following injury. True fracture-dislocation of the spine involves disruption of all three columns, including in some cases the anterior longitudinal ligament, and is the most unstable of all spine injuries. It is, therefore, important to accept that rigid segmental instrumentation should be employed and that strategies designed to minimize the number of levels fused may not be appropriate in these cases. We favor instrumentation extending three levels above and at least two, if not three, levels below the fracture and favor transpedicular instrumentation. If hooks are utilized, then the use of a "claw" construct bilaterally with supplemental hooks or sublaminar wires should be employed. Most patients treated in the first 1 to 2 weeks following injury can be successfully reduced. Even in cases of complete SCI reduction is beneficial. Anatomic or near-anatomic reduction of a fracture-dislocation restores significant stability and lessens the stresses on the surgical implants, may facilitate, however remote, the possibility of neurologic recovery, and may lessen the degree of late pain. In cases of incomplete neurologic injury reduction is the primary means of decompression of the neural elements and should be accomplished expeditiously. Stabilization with segmental instrumentation is carried out and the patient is then reassessed for any persistent canal compromise anteriorly. The presence of persistent bone or disk in the canal is then treated through a separate anterior approach with structural anterior grafting. In general, these highly unstable injuries are not amenable to anterior stabilization alone, and it is therefore our preference to proceed with reduction and rigid fixation through a posterior approach prior to any consideration of anterior surgery.

FRACTURES OF THE SACRUM

The sacrum serves as the junction of the spine with the pelvis. Sacral fractures are relatively common and are usually associated with injury to the pelvic ring. The evaluation and treatment of the sacral fracture, therefore, cannot take place without consideration given to the rest of the pelvis. In some patients, however, the injury to the sacrum is an isolated injury or represents the primary determinant of care.

Denis and associates in 1988 reported on a series of 236 sacral injuries and presented a classification system, which is in widespread use (Fig. 18–20). Although not particularly pertinent when assessing the potential for instability in a sacral fracture, the Denis classification is highly predictive for the risk of neurologic injury.[45] In their series, zone I represents the sacral ala lateral to the neural foramina. Fractures in this region are the most common but have a low (6%) risk of neurologic injury. Zone II describes the region of the neural foramina. Fractures passing through one or more foramina are seen in approximately one third of cases and the risk of neurologic injury increases to 28%. Zone III describes the sacral vertebral bodies. Fractures in this region extend into the sacral canal; although rare (10%), the risk of neurologic deficit is greater than 50%.[45] Sacral fractures can also be classified as vertical, oblique, and transverse.[100] In the absence of significant associated pelvic ring disruption, vertical and oblique fractures are usually stable. Transverse fractures, on the other hand, typically occur through the neural foramina, most commonly at S2–3 or sometimes at S1–2. The high transverse fractures may be sufficiently unstable so as to become painful and will on occasion require operative treatment.

Evaluation of the patient with a sacral injury should include careful evaluation of the perineum, the rectum, and the genitalia. The potential for an open injury should be appreciated. Close neurologic examination of the sacral nerve roots, including assessment of rectal and bladder function, should be carried out. In addition, the L5 nerve

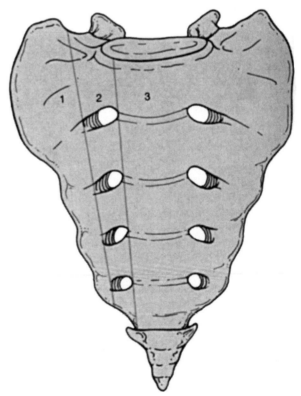

Figure 18–20. Diagrammatic representation of the three zones of sacral fracture described by Denis and coworkers. (Redrawn from Denis F, Davis S, Comfort T: Sacral fractures: An important problem. Clin Orthop 227:67, 1988.)

root, as it passes anteriorly over the sacral ala, is at risk and should be assessed. Radiologic definition of the injury can be difficult on plain radiographs. Inlet and outlet views of the pelvis help define the architecture of the sacrum and should be supplemented with either CT scanning, including sagittal reconstructions, MRI, or both.

Treatment of sacral fractures may include treatment of pelvic ring disruption, treatment of neurologic deficit, or treatment of sacral instability. Evaluation and treatment of pelvic ring disruption is described elsewhere in this book. Neurologic injury in fractures of the sacrum can range from isolated nerve root injury, most commonly L5, as a result of fracture of the anterior and cephalad sacral ala stretching the L5 root as it passes into the pelvis, or S1, as the root enters the S1 neural foramen. The entire cauda equina can be injured in zone III fractures, and a displaced fracture in zone III can result in persistent bony compression on the cauda equina. The role of decompression is not clearly defined. Functional deficit such as rectal atony, loss of bladder function, or L5 or S1 motor deficit, which persists and in which there is clear-cut bony compression, merits consideration for decompression. Understanding of the complex pathoanatomy of fractures in zone I and zone II is essential, and the surgeon must be prepared to follow the affected nerve root much more distally than is typically required for cases of degenerative nerve root compression. Vertical fractures causing neurologic injury are usually stable, and decompression alone is indicated.

On occasion transverse or oblique fractures may result in instability or, by virtue of displacement, persistent distortion of the cauda equina requiring reduction and fixation. The quality of bone found in the sacrum is relatively poor, compared to that seen elsewhere, but the stress on a fracture reduced and fixed with a bilateral plating technique is also relatively low.[101] The need for open reduction and internal fixation of a fracture of the sacrum is, in our experience, exceedingly rare.

One final variant of sacral fracture is the sacral insufficiency fracture. This occurs in middle-aged and elderly patients, typically women, and is a variant of stress fracture. The patient presents with intractable pain over the sacrum, which usually can be clearly differentiated from more characteristic low back pain in the lumbosacral region. The pain is worse with activity and relieved by rest. Plain radiographs and MRI are usually normal or show minimal degenerative changes. The diagnosis is made on technetium bone scan, which shows a characteristic H-pattern on delayed images. Treatment for this condition is supportive with medical management of the patient's osteoporosis, the use of mild analgesics as needed, and gradual activity increases as tolerated.

DEGENERATIVE DISORDERS OF THE SPINE

A major proportion of the adult population is affected by degenerative conditions of the spine. These disorders have a major impact on the cost of health care delivery. Every physician should have a working knowledge of these pathologic conditions and should be able to recognize a serious problem when it arises. In both the cervical spine (myelopathy) and the lumbar spine (cauda equina compression),

disastrous sequelae such as paralysis can occur if these conditions are overlooked.

Spondylosis (osteoarthritis) is the technical term which describes the sequence of degenerative changes that occurs throughout the spine with increasing age. Everyone develops spondylosis, but only a subgroup will complain of symptoms. The physician needs to accurately diagnose the specific etiology for each patient and prescribe the appropriate treatment.

This section will present the degenerative conditions in the cervical, thoracic, and lumbar spine. In each area, the appropriate history, physical findings, and diagnostic studies will be reviewed. By convention, herniated disks are included. For the cervical and lumbar spine a standardized protocol or algorithm will be described.

Cervical Spine

Neck pain is a very common problem that is familiar to most individuals. Most of the conditions can be successfully treated with conservative measures. However, myelopathy, which is compression of the spinal cord, usually requires urgent to emergent invasive methods to prevent poor outcomes. Every clinician should be familiar with the signs and symptoms of the various diagnostic entities that occur in the cervical spine and be able to identify the serious problems that require immediate attention.

HISTORY

The most important information to obtain from a patient's history is the location of the pain. The majority of patients complain of localized symptoms in the neck, with or without referral to pain between the scapulae or shoulders. The pain is described as vague, diffuse, axial, nondermatoma, and poorly localized. The pathogenesis of this type of complaint is attributed to structures innervated by the sinuvertebral nerve or the nerves innervating the paravertebral soft tissues, and it is generally a localized problem.

Another group of patients will complain of neck pain with the addition of arm involvement. This arm pain is secondary to nerve root irritation and is termed radicular pain. The degree of nerve root involvement can vary from a monoradiculopathy to multiple levels of involvement. It is described as a deep aching, burning, or shooting arm pain, often with associated paraesthesias. The pathogenesis of radicular pain can derive from soft tissue (herniated disk), bone (spondylosis), or a combination of the two.

Finally, a third group of patients will complain of symptoms secondary to cervical myelopathy, which is compression of the spinal cord and usually secondary to degenerative changes. The clinical complications vary considerably. The onset of symptoms begin after 50 years of age, and males are more often affected. Onset is usually insidious, although there is occasionally a history of trauma. The natural history is that of initial neurologic deterioration followed by a plateau period lasting several months. The resulting clinical picture is often one of an incomplete spinal lesion with a patchy distribution of the deficits. Disability varies with the number of vertebrae involved and with the degree of involvement at each level.

Common presenting symptoms of cervical myelopathy include numbness and paresthesia in the hands, clumsiness of the fingers, weakness (greatest in the lower extremities), and gait disturbances. Abnormalities of micturition are seen in about one third of cases and indicate more severe cord involvement. Symptoms of radiculopathy can coexist with myelopathy and confuse the clinical picture. Sensory disturbances may show a patchy distribution. Spinothalamic tract (pain and temperature) deficits may be seen in the upper extremities, the thorax, or the lumbar region and may be in a stocking or glove distribution. Posterior column deficits (vibration and proprioception) are more commonly seen in the feet than in the hands. Usually there is no gross sensory impairment but a diminished sense of appreciation of light touch and pinprick. A characteristic broad-based, shuffling gait may be seen, signaling the onset of functionally significant deterioration.

PHYSICAL EXAMINATION

The physical examination should begin with observation of the cervical spine and upper torso unencumbered by clothing. The physical findings are of two different types. One set can be categorized as nonspecific and found in most patients with neck pain, but will not help to localize the type or level of the pathologic process. A decreased range of motion is the most frequent nonspecific finding. It can be secondary to pain or, structurally, to distorted bony and soft tissue elements in the cervical spine. Hyperextension and excessive lateral rotation, however, will usually cause pain, even in a normal individual.

Tenderness is another nonspecific finding that can be quite helpful. Two types of tenderness must be considered. One is diffuse, elicited by compression of the paravertebral muscles, and is found over a wide area of the posterolateral muscle masses. The second type of tenderness is more specific and may help localize the level of the pathology. It can be localized by palpation over each intervertebral foramen and spinous process.

The next part of the physical examination is to isolate the level or levels in the cervical spine responsible for the symptoms. The examination is also important to rule out other sources of pain, which include compressive neuropathies, thoracic outlet syndrome, and chest or shoulder disorders.

The major focus of the examination is directed at finding a neurologic deficit (Table 18–1). A motor deficit (most commonly weak triceps, biceps, or deltoid) or diminished deep tendon reflex is the most likely objective finding in a patient with a radiculopathy. Although less reproducible, manual tests and maneuvers that increase or decrease radicular symptoms may be helpful. In the neck compression test, the patient's head is flexed laterally, slightly rotated toward the symptomatic side, and then compressed to elicit reproduction or aggravation of the radicular symptoms.

Myelopathic physical findings should also be specifically checked. These patients can have a gait disturbance, so they should be observed walking. The extent of motor disability can vary from mild to severe. Pyramidal tract weakness and atrophy are more commonly seen in the lower extremities and are the most common abnormal signs. The usual clinical findings in the lower extremities are spasticity and weakness.

Weakness and wasting of the upper extremities and hands may also be due to combined spondylotic myelopathy and radiculopathy. In this situation the patient usually complains of hand clumsiness. A diminished or absent upper-extremity reflex may be evidence of radiculopathy superimposed on spondylotic myelopathy.

Table 18–1. Cervical radiculopathy symptoms and findings

Disk Level	Nerve Root	Symptoms and Findings
C2–3	C3	*Pain:* Back of neck, mastoid process, pinna of ear *Sensory Change:* Back of neck, mastoid process, pinna of ear *Motor Deficit:* None readily detectable except by EMG *Reflex Change:* None
C3–4	C4	*Pain:* Back of neck, levator scapula, anterior chest *Sensory Change:* Back of neck, levator scapula, anterior chest *Motor Deficit:* None readily detectable except by EMG *Reflex Change:* None
C4–5	C5	*Pain:* Neck, tip of shoulder, anterior arm *Sensory Change:* Deltoid area *Motor Deficit:* Deltoid, biceps *Reflex Change:* Biceps
C5–6	C6	*Pain:* Neck, shoulder, medial border of scapula, lateral arm, dorsal forearm *Sensory Change:* Thumb and index finger *Motor Deficit:* Biceps *Reflex Change:* Biccps
C6–7	C7	*Pain:* Neck, shoulder, medial border of scapula, lateral arm, dorsal forearm *Sensory Change:* Index and middle fingers *Motor Deficit:* Triceps *Reflex Change:* Triceps
C7–T1	C8	*Pain:* Neck, medial border of scapula, medial aspect of arm and forearm *Sensory Change:* Ring and little fingers *Motor Deficit:* Intrinsic muscles of hand *Reflex Change:* None

From Boden S, Wiesel SW, Laws E, et al: The Aging Spine. Philadelphia, W.B. Saunders, 1991, p 46; reprinted by permission.

Sensory deficits in spinothalamic (pain and temperature) and posterior column (vibration and proprioception) function should be documented. Usually there is no gross impairment of sensation; rather, a patchy decrease in light touch and pinprick is seen. Hyperreflexia, clonus, and positive Babinski's signs are seen in the lower extremities. Hoffman's sign and hyperreflexia may be observed in the upper extremities.

DIAGNOSTIC STUDIES

In evaluating any pathologic process one will usually have a choice of several diagnostic tests. The cervical spine is no exception. This section will deal with the most common tests that are routinely used. In general, all these tests play a confirmatory role. In other words, the core of information derived from a thorough history and physical examination should be the basis for a diagnosis; the additional tests are obtained to confirm this clinical impression. Trouble develops when these tests are used for screening purposes because most of them are overly sensitive and relatively unselective. Thus, the studies discussed should never be interpreted in isolation from the overall clinical picture.

Plain Radiographs. Radiographic evaluation of the cervical spine is helpful in assessing patients with neck pain, and the routine study should include anteroposterior, lateral, oblique, and odontoid views. Flexion/extension x-rays are necessary in defining stability. The generally accepted radiographic signs of cervical disk disease are loss of height of the intervertebral disk space, osteophyte formation, secondary encroachment of the intervertebral foramina, and osteoarthritic changes in the apophyseal joints.

It should be stressed that the identification of "some pathology" on plain cervical x-rays does not, per se, indicate the cause of the patient's symptoms. In several series large numbers of asymptomatic patients have shown radiographic evidence of advanced degenerative disk disease. At approximately age 40 some disk degeneration (narrowing) can be expected, particularly at the C5–6 and C6–7 levels. This is considered to represent a normal aging process. The difficult problem with regard to radiographic interpretation is not in the identification of these changes but rather in determining how much significance should be attributed to them.

Radiographic abnormalities of alignment in the cervical spine may also be of clinical significance but they need to be correlated with the whole clinical picture; listhesis or slipping forward or backward (retrolisthesis) of vertebrae upon the vertebrae below it is such a finding.

If "instability" is suspected, dynamic x-rays may be taken. These view the spine from the side, with the head flexed (bent forward) or extended (arched back); the spine normally flexes equally at each spinal level. If one vertebral level is "unstable," that particular vertebra moves more or less and disrupts the symmetry of motion. Again, this finding must be correlated with the whole clinical picture, as its mere presence may be asymptomatic.

Magnetic Resonance Imaging. Magnetic resonance imaging (MRI) is the diagnostic study of choice to identify compression on the neural elements from either soft tissue (herniated disk) or hard tissue (spondylosis). It is also excellent at identifying other entities such as infection or tumor. MRI is a very safe test because it uses neither ionizing radiation nor radioactive contrast agents.

The only caution is that the prevalence rate of abnormalities in asymptomatic patients is very high (19%). Thus, patients with positive findings on the MRI may have no symptoms. This highlights the point that MRI findings should be strictly correlated with the history and physical examination.

Myelography and Computerized Tomography. If the results of the MRI are equivocal or if the patient cannot undergo an MRI, myelography followed by CT may be performed. Myelography and CT do differentiate bone from soft tissue and visualize the spinal cord. Unfortunately, it is an invasive procedure and involves radiation exposure; thus, it is the back-up diagnostic test to an MRI.

Electromyography. Electromyography (EMG) is an electrical test that confirms the interaction of nerve to muscle. The test is performed by placing needles into the muscles to determine if there is an intact nerve supply to that muscle. The EMG is particularly useful in localizing a specific abnormal nerve root. It should be appreciated that it takes 21 days for an EMG to show up as abnormal. After 21 days of pressure on the nerve root, signs of denervation with fibrillation can be observed. Before 21 days, the EMG will be negative in spite of nerve root damage. It should also be noted that there is no qualitative interpretation of this test. Thus, it cannot be said that the EMG is 25 or 75% normal.

The EMG is an electronic extension of the physical examination. Although it is 80 to 90% accurate in establishing cervical radiculopathy as the cause of pain, false negative results do occur. If cervical radiculopathy affects only the sensory root, the EMG will be unable to demonstrate an abnormality. A false-negative examination can occur if the patient with acute symptoms is examined early (4 to 28 days from onset of symptoms). A negative study should be repeated in 2 to 3 weeks if symptoms persist. The accuracy of the EMG increases if both the paraspinal and extremity muscles innervated by the suspected root demonstrate abnormalities.

The EMG is not part of the routine evaluation of the cervical spine. It is indicated to confirm a clinical impression or to rule out other pathologic conditions, such as peripheral neuropathies or compressive neuropathies in the upper extremities.

CLINICAL CONDITIONS

Many conditions may present as neck pain, with or without arm pain, in any particular individual. However, those that are most common will be presented in detail.

Neck Sprain and Neckache. Neck sprain, while a misnomer, describes a clinical condition involving a nonradiating discomfort or pain about the neck area associated with a concomitant loss of neck motion (stiffness). Although the clinical syndrome may present as a headache, most often the pain is located in the middle to lower part of the back of the neck. A history of injury is rarely obtained, but the pain may start after a night's rest or simply on turning the head. The source of the pain is most commonly believed to be the ligaments about the cervical spine or the surrounding muscles. The axial pain may also be produced by small annular tears without disk herniation, or from the facet joints.

The pain associated with a neck sprain is most often a dull aching pain, which is exacerbated by neck motion. The pain is usually abated by rest or immobilization. The pain may be referred to other mesenchymal structures derived from a similar sclerotome during embryogenesis. Common referred pain patterns include the scapular area, the posterior shoulder, the occipital area, or the anterior chest wall (cervical angina pectoris). Those referred pain patterns do not connotate a true radicular pain pattern and are not usually mechanical in origin.

Physical examination of patients with neckache usually reveals nothing more than a locally tender area(s) usually just lateral to the spine. The intensity of the pain is variable, and the loss of cervical motion correlates directly with the pain intensity. The presence of true spasm, defined as a continuous muscle contraction, is rare except in severe cases when the head may be tilted to one side (torticollis).

Because the radiograph in cervical sprain is usually normal, a plain x-ray is usually not warranted on the first visit. If the pain continues for more than 2 weeks or the patient develops other physical findings, then an x-ray should be taken to rule out other more serious causes of the neck pain, such as neoplasia or instability. The prognosis for these individuals is excellent—the natural history is one of complete resolution of the symptoms over several weeks. The mainstay of therapy includes rest and immobilization, usually in a soft cervical orthosis. Although medications such as anti-inflammatory agents or muscle relaxants may aid in the acute management of pain, they do not seem to alter the natural history of the disorder.

Acute Herniated Disk. A herniated disk is defined as the protrusion of the nucleus pulposus through the fibers of the annulus fibrosus (Fig. 18–21). Most acute disk herniations occur posterolaterally and in patients around the fourth decade of life when the nucleus is still gelatinous. The most common areas of disk herniation are C5–6 and C6–7, whereas C7–T1 and C3–4 occur infrequently. Disk herniation of C2–3 is extremely rare. Unlike the lumbar herniated disk, the cervical herniated disk may cause myelopathy in addition to radicular pain owing to the presence of the spinal cord in the cervical region.

The disk herniation usually affects the root numbered lowest for the given disk level; for example, a C3–4 disk affects the C4 root, C4–5 disk affects the fifth cervical root, C5–6 affects the sixth cervical root, C6–7 affects the seventh nerve root, and C7–T1 affects the eighth cervical root. Unlike the lumbar region, the disk herniation does not involve other roots but more commonly presents some evidence of upper motor neuron findings secondary to spinal cord local pressure.

Not every herniated disk is symptomatic. The presence of symptoms depends on the spinal reserve capacity, the presence of inflammation, and the size of the herniation as well as the presence of concomitant disease such as osteophyte formation.

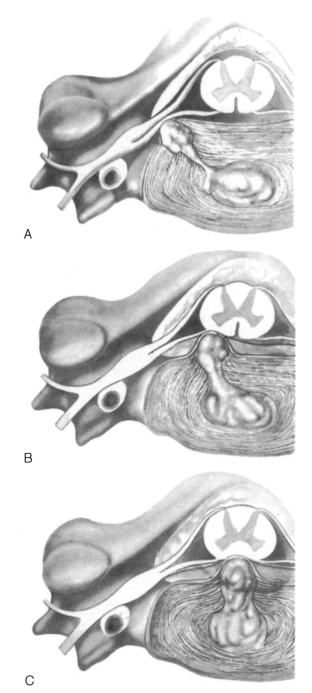

Figure 18–21. Types of soft tissue disk herniation. *A,* lateral, compressing nerve root in the neural foramen. *B,* centrolateral, compressing both the nerve root and spinal cord, and *C,* central, compressing the cord only. (Modified from DePalma AF, Rothman RH: The Intervertebral Disc. Philadelphia, W.B. Saunders Company, 1970, pp 102, 104.)

Clinically, the patient's major complaint is arm pain, not neck pain. The pain is often perceived as starting in the neck area but then radiates from this point down the shoulder, arm, forearm, and usually into the hand, commonly in a dermatomal distribution. The onset of the radicular pain is often gradual, although there can be a sudden onset associated with a tearing or snapping sensation. As time passes, the magnitude of the arm pain will clearly exceed that of the neck or shoulder pain. The arm pain may vary in intensity from severe enough to preclude any use of the arm without severe pain to a dull cramping ache in the arm muscles with use of the arm. The pain is usually severe enough to awaken the patient at night.

Physical examination of the neck usually shows some limitation of motion, and on occasion the patient may tilt the head in a cocked position (torticollis) toward the side of the herniated cervical disk. Extension of the spine will often exacerbate the pain because it further narrows the intervertebral foramina. Axial compression, Valsalva maneuver, and coughing may also exacerbate or re-create the pain pattern.

The presence of a positive neurologic finding is the most helpful aspect of the diagnostic workup, although the neurologic examination may remain normal despite a chronic radicular pattern. Even when a deficit exists, it may not be temporally related to the present symptoms but to a prior attack at a different level. To be significant, the neurologic examination must show objective signs of the reflex diminution, motor weakness, or atrophy. The subjective sensory changes are often difficult to interpret and require a coherent and cooperative patient to be of clinical value. The presence of sensory changes alone are usually not enough to make the diagnosis firm.

Nerve root sensitivity can be elicited by any method that increases the tension of the nerve root. Radicular arm pain is often increased by the Valsalva maneuver or by directly compressing the head. Although these signs are helpful when present, their absence alone does not rule out radicular pain.

The provisional diagnosis of a herniated disk is made by the history and physical examination. The plain x-ray is usually nondiagnostic, although occasionally disk space narrowing at the suspected interspace of foraminal narrowing on the oblique films will be seen. The value of the films is largely to exclude other causes of neck and arm pain. Tests such as an EMG or MRI are confirmatory examinations and should not be used as screening tests because misinformation may ensue (Fig. 18–22).

The treatment for most patients with a herniated disk is nonoperative, and the majority of patients respond to conservative treatment over a period of months. The efficacy of the nonoperative approach depends heavily on the doctor-patient relationship. If a patient is well informed, insightful, and willing to follow instructions, the chances for a successful nonoperative outcome are greatly improved.

The cornerstone to the management of a cervical herniated disk is rest and immobilization. The use of a cervical orthosis greatly increases the likelihood that the patient will rest. Patients should markedly decrease their physical activity for at least 2 weeks and wear the cervical orthosis at all times (especially at night). After the acute pain begins to abate, patients should gradually increase their activity and wean off the orthosis. Most persons will be able to return to work, or at least to light activities, in a month.

Drug therapy is an important adjunct to rest and immobilization. Anti-inflammatory medications, analgesics, and muscle relaxants have historically been used in the acute management of these patients. Because it is commonly believed that the radicular pain is in part inflammatory, the use of aspirin or other nonsteroidal anti-inflammatory medications seems to be appropriate. All these medications have gastrointestinal side effects but are generally well tolerated for brief periods.

Analgesic medication is needed only rarely if the patient is compliant. However, if the pain is severe enough, a brief course of oral codeine may be prescribed. In-hospital intramuscular narcotic injections may be required on rare occasions. Muscle relaxants and the benzodiazepines are truly tranquilizers and central nervous system depressants. As such, they have at best a limited role in the management of the acute herniated disk patient. Although it is true that these medications help patients relax and get their needed rest, the potential for an addictive effect adding to any psychosocial problems patients may have is not, in the majority of patients, worth the long-term risk for the short-term gain.

Surgery is reserved for patients with unremitting radicular symptoms after an adequate period of conservative therapy. The presence of an isolated neurologic finding, such as an absent biceps reflex, is not an indication for surgery. The goal of surgical intervention is to relieve pain. Return of an isolated neurologic deficit is unpredictable. The results of surgery for pain relief are quite good (over 90%) when the history, physical, and diagnostic studies all are confirmatory.

Cervical Spondylosis. Once commonly referred to as "cervical degenerative disk disease," cervical spondylosis is a chronic process defined as the development of osteophytes and other stigmata of degenerative arthritis as a consequence of age-related disk disease. This process may produce a wide range of symptoms. However, it should be stressed that an individual may have significant spondylosis and be asymptomatic.

Cervical spondylosis is believed to be the direct result of age-related changes in the intervertebral disk. These changes include desiccation of the nucleus pulposis, loss of annular elasticity, and narrowing of the disk space with or without disk protrusion or rupture. In turn, secondary changes include overriding of facets, increased motion of the spinal segments, osteophyte formation, inflammation of the synovial joints, and even microfractures. These macro- and microscopic changes can result in various clinical syndromes (spondylosis, ankylosis, central or foraminal spinal stenosis, radiculopathy, myelopathy, or spinal segmental instability).

The typical patient with symptomatic cervical spondylosis is over the age of 40 and complains of neckache. Not infrequently, however, these patients will have very few neck pain symptoms and will present with referred pain patterns: occipital headaches; pain in the shoulder, suboccipital, and intrascapular areas and the anterior chest wall; or other vague symptoms suggestive of anatomic disturbances (e.g., blurring of vision, tinnitus). In patients with predominantly referred pain, a previous history for neck pain is usually obtained.

Physical examination of the patient with cervical spon-

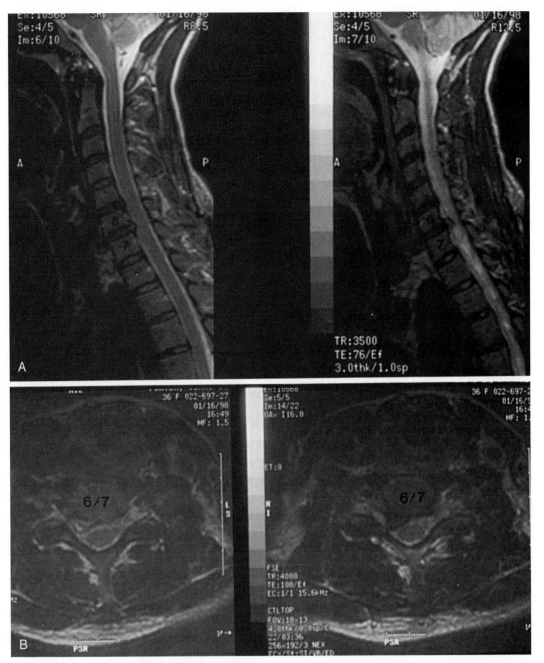

Figure 18–22. MRI of herniated nucleus pulposus.

dylosis is often associated with a dearth of objective find-ings. The patient will usually have some limitation of neck motion associated with midline tenderness. Not infre-quently, palpation of the referred pain areas will also pro-duce local tenderness and should not be confused with local disease. The neurologic examination is normal.

Anteroposterior (AP), lateral, and oblique radiographs of the cervical spine in cervical spondylosis show varying degrees of changes, including disk space narrowing, osteo-phytosis, foraminal narrowing, degenerative changes of the facets, and instability. As previously discussed, these find-ings do not necessarily correlate with symptoms. In large part, the radiograph serves to rule out other more serious

causes of neck and referred pain such as tumors. Further diagnostic testing usually is not warranted.

Cervical spondylosis alone is treated by nonoperative measures. The mainstay of treatment for the acute pain superimposed on the chronic problem is rest and immobili-zation. In addition, oral anti-inflammatory medications like aspirin will be of benefit. Often these medications will need to be administered on a chronic basis or at least intermittently. Trigger-point injections with local anes-thetics (lidocaine) and corticosteroids (triamcinolone) may be therapeutic as well as diagnostic. Once the pain abates the immobilization (usually a soft collar) should be discon-tinued and the patient maintained on a series of cervical isometric exercises. Further counseling with regard to sleeping position, automobile driving, and work is in order. Manipulation and traction are rarely needed and may, in fact, be deleterious to the patient.

Cervical Spondylosis With Myelopathy. When the secondary bony changes of cervical spondylosis encroach on the spinal cord a pathologic process called myelopathy develops. If this involves both the spinal cord and nerve roots, it is called myeloradiculopathy. Radiculopathy, regardless of its etiology, causes shoulder or arm pain.

Myelopathy is the most serious sequela of cervical spondylosis and the most difficult to treat effectively. Less than 5% of patients with cervical spondylosis develop myelopathy, and they are usually between 40 to 60 years of age. The changes of myelopathy are most often gradual and associated with posterior osteophyte formation (called spondylotic bone or hard disk) and spinal canal narrowing (spinal stenosis). Acute myelopathy is most often the result of a central soft disk herniation producing a high-grade block on myelography.

The characteristic stooped, wide-based, and somewhat jerky gait of the aged summarizes the chronic effects of cervical spondylosis with myelopathy. The spinal cord changes may develop from single- or multiple-level disease and as such may not present in a singular or standard manner. A typical clinical presentation of chronic myelopathy begins with the gradual notice of a peculiar sensation in the hands, associated with clumsiness and weakness. The patient will also note lower extremity symptoms that may antedate the upper extremity findings, including difficulty in walking, peculiar sensations, leg weakness, hyperreflexia, spasticity, and clonus. The upper extremity findings start out unilaterally and include hyperreflexia, brisk Hoffman's sign, and muscle atrophy (especially of the hand muscles). Neck pain per se is not a prominent feature of myelopathy. Sensory changes can evolve at these levels and are often a less reliable index of spinal cord disease. The protean nature of the signs and symptoms of cervical myelopathy, along with its potential for severe functional impairment, merit a high index of suspicion in patient evaluation.

Radiographs of the cervical spine in these patients will often reveal advanced degenerative disease including spinal canal narrowing by prominent posterior osteophytosis, variable foraminal narrowing, disk space narrowing, facet joint arthrosis, and instability. Congenital stenosis of the cervical canal is frequently seen, predisposing the patient to the development of myelopathy. The MRI is striking (Fig. 18–23). It will exhibit multiple levels of neural compression, with anterior and posterior defects. The posterior defects are secondary not only to facet arthrosis but to buckling of the ligamentum flavum. For a specific diagnosis as to a patient's complaints the MRI pictures must be correlated with the patient's history and physical examination.

In general, a cervical myelopathy is a surgical disease but is not an absolute indication for surgical decompression. Conservative therapy consisting of immobilization and rest with a soft cervical orthosis offers the myelopathic patient, who is not a good operative risk, a viable option. The goals of surgery in the myelopathic patient are to decompress the spinal cord to prevent further spinal cord compression and vascular compromise. If the myelopathy is progressive despite a trial of conservative treatment, surgery is clearly indicated. These indications may vary slightly from surgeon to surgeon because of the lack of absolute definitive clinical data.

Rheumatoid Arthritis. Rheumatoid arthritis affects 2 to 3% of the population. About 60% of patients with rheumatoid arthritis will exhibit signs and symptoms of cervical spine involvement, whereas up to 86% will have radiographic evidence of cervical disease. Cervical spine involvement secondary to the erosive inflammatory changes of rheumatoid arthritis (synovitis) is divided into three categories: (1) atlantoaxial instability, (2) basilar invagination, and (3) subaxial instability. Atlantoaxial instability is the most common and most senior of the instability patterns affecting 20 to 34% of hospitalized patients. The evaluation of

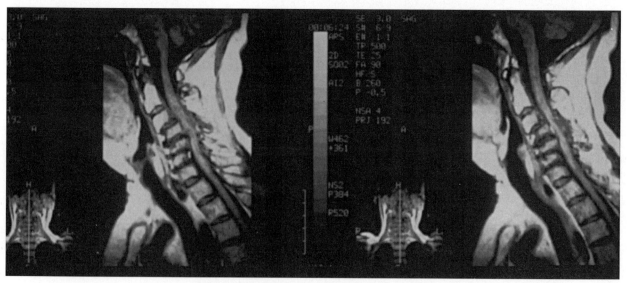

Figure 18–23. MRI of C-spine myelopathy.

a patient with rheumatoid arthritis is difficult because of the multiple system involvement. The physical examination should start with a careful neurologic evaluation to rule out upper motor neuron disease before moving to neck range of motion or other vigorous maneuvers that may harm the patient.

The patient with cervical spine involvement from rheumatoid arthritis most often has neck pain located in the middle posterior neck and occipital area. The range of motion is decreased and crepitus or a feeling of stability may be noted. The neurologic changes can be variable and difficult to elicit in the context of diffuse rheumatoid changes. The evaluation of the patient with cervical rheumatoid arthritis begins with plain radiographs of the neck, which may reveal osteopenia, facet erosion, disk space narrowing, and subluxation of the lower cervical spine (stepladder appearance). To determine whether atlantoaxial disease is present, dynamic flexion/extension views of the lateral upper cervical spine are required.

Basilar invagination is defined as upper migration of the odontoid projecting into the foramen magnum. The addition of a CT scan with or without contrast material in the upper cervical spine can provide valuable information as to the relationship of the bony elements to the spinal cord. Subaxial subluxations are identified by dynamic flexion/extension films.

The majority of these patients, despite rather dramatic disease patterns can be successfully managed nonoperatively. Although the natural history of rheumatoid arthritis predicts a high incidence of involvement of the cervical spine, it is estimated that only a few patients die from medullary compression associated with significant atlantoaxial disease and that, although atlantoaxial disease worsens with time, only 2 to 14% of patients exhibit neurologic progression.

The mainstay in nonoperative therapy is the cervical orthosis (Philadelphia collar). Although this does not fully immobilize the atlantoaxial interval, it does produce symptomatic relief. Some authors have advocated intermittent home traction, but it must be used only with great caution under a physician's direction. Medications have a definite role in the nonoperative management of rheumatoid disease. Initial management includes aspirin in high dosages monitored by serum drug levels. Secondary agents such as methotrexate, chloroquine, or oral steroids are best administered under the direction of a rheumatologist.

CERVICAL SPINE EVALUATION ALGORITHM

The task of the physician, when confronted with the cervical spine patient, is to integrate the patient's complaints into an accurate diagnosis and to prescribe appropriate therapy. Achieving this goal depends on the accuracy of the physician's decision-making ability. Although specific information is not available for every aspect of neck pain, there is a large body of data to guide us in handling these patients. Using this knowledge, which has already been presented, an algorithm for neck pain has been designed.

Webster defines an algorithm as "a set of rules for solving a particular problem in a finite number of steps." It is, in effect, an organized pattern of decision making and thought processes. In this instance we present an algorithm for approaching the universe of cervical spine patients. The algorithm can be followed in sequence (Fig. 18–24) and is also presented in tabular format (Table 18–2).

The primary objective for the physician is to return patients to normal function as quickly as possible. In the course of achieving this goal, the physician must be concerned with other circumstances, which include making efficient and precise use of the diagnostic studies, minimizing the use of ineffectual surgery, and making therapy available at a reasonable cost to society. The algorithm follows well-delineated rules, established from the consensus of a broad segment of qualified spine surgeons. It allows the patient to receive the most helpful diagnostic and therapeutic measures at optimal times.

The algorithm begins with the universe of patients who are initially evaluated for neck pain, with or without arm pain. Patients with major trauma, including fractures, are

Table 18–2. Differential diagnosis of neck pain

Evaluation	Neck Strain	Herniated Nucleus Pulposus	Instability	Degenerative Disk Disease	Myelopathy	Tumor	Spondylo-arthropathy	Metabolic	Infection
Predominant pain (arm vs. neck)	Neck	Arm	Neck	Neck	Neck	Neck	Neck	Neck	Neck
Constitutional symptoms						+	+	±	+
Compression test		+							
Neurologic examination		+			+				
Plain radiographs			±	+	±	±	+	+	±
Lateral motion radiographs			+						
CT scan		+		+	±	+			+
Myelogram		+			+				
Bone scan						+	+	±	+
ESR							+		+
Ca/P/alk phos						+		+	

Key: Ca/P/alk phos indicates calcium, phosphate, and alkaline phosphatase; CT, computed tomography; ESR, erythrocyte sedimentation rate.
From Boden S, Wiesel SW, Laws E, et al: The Aging Spine. Philadelphia, W.B. Saunders, 1991, p 46; reprinted by permission.

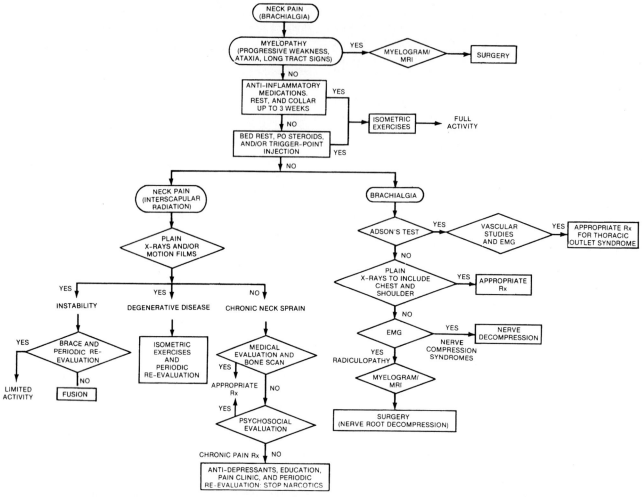

Figure 18–24. Algorithm for evaluation and treatment of cervical spine injury. (From Wiesel SW, et al: Neck Pain. Charlottesville, VA, The Michie Co., 1988; reprinted by permission.)

not included. After an initial medical history and physical examination—and assuming that the patient's symptoms are originating from the cervical spine—the first major decision is to rule out the presence of a cervical myelopathy.

The character and severity of the myelopathy depend on the size, location, and duration of the lesion. Ventrolateral lesions encroach on the nerve roots and lateral aspects of the spinal cord, producing all the manifestations accompanying nerve root compression. The chief radicular signs are weakness, loss of tone and volume of the muscles of the upper extremity, and pressure on the spinal cord may produce pyramidal tract signs and spasticity in the lower extremities.

Midline lesions intrude on the central aspect of the anterior portion of the spinal cord. They produce no signs of nerve root compression. Both lower extremities are primarily involved and the most common problem relates initially to gait disturbance. As the disease progresses, bowel and bladder control may be affected.

Once a diagnosis of cervical myelopathy is made, surgical intervention should be considered without delay. The best results are attained in patients with one or two motor units involved and with myelopathy of a relatively short

duration. The longer pressure has been applied to the neural elements, the poorer the results. A cervical MRI should be obtained in these patients to precisely define the neural compression, and an adequate surgical decompression should be performed as soon as possible to achieve the best results.

After cervical myelopathy has been ruled out, the remaining patients, who constitute an overwhelming majority, should be started on a course of conservative management. At this stage of the patient's course, the specific diagnosis, whether it be a herniated disk or neck strain, is not important because the entire group is treated in the same fashion.

CONSERVATIVE TREATMENT

The primary mode of therapy in both acute and chronic cervical spine disease is immobilization. In the acute neck injuries, immobilization allows for healing of torn and attenuated soft tissues, whereas in chronic conditions immobilization is aimed at reduction of inflammation in the supporting soft tissues and around the nerve roots of the cervical spine.

Immobilization is best achieved by the use of a soft felt collar. It needs to be properly fitted and comfortable on the patient. Initially the collar is worn 24 hours a day. The patient must understand that during sleep the neck is totally unprotected from awkward positions and movements, and therefore the collar is most important.

The other mainstay of the initial treatment is drug therapy. It is directed at reducing inflammation, especially in the soft tissues. A variety of anti-inflammatory medications are available; however, there is no one drug that has proved to be significantly better than all the others. Salicylates have proved to be as effective and safe as the rest and are the least expensive. The dosage must be adequate to achieve a therapeutic blood level. The efficacy of this treatment regimen is predicted on the patient's ability to understand the disease process and the role of each therapeutic modality. The vast majority of patients will respond to this approach in the first 10 days, but a certain percentage will not heal rapidly.

At this juncture a local injection into the area of maximum tenderness should be considered. Localized tender areas in the paravertebral musculature and trapezii will be found in many individuals and are referred to as "trigger points." Marked relief of symptoms is often achieved dramatically by infiltration of these trigger points with a combination of lidocaine (Xylocaine) and 1 mL of a steroid preparation. The object of the injection is to decrease the inflammation in a specific anatomic area. The more localized the trigger point, the more effective this form of therapy.

The patient should be treated conservatively for up to 6 weeks. The majority of cervical spine patients will get better and should be encouraged to gradually increase their activities. The goal is to return to their normal lifestyles. An exercise program should be directed at strengthening the paravertebral musculature, not at increasing the range of motion.

The pathway along this top portion of the algorithm is reversible. Should regression occur—with exacerbation of symptoms—the physician can resort to more stringent conservative measures. These measures may include additional bed rest and stronger anti-inflammatory medication. The majority of patients with neck pain will respond to therapy and return to a normal life pattern within 2 months of the beginning of their problem. If the initial conservative treatment regimen fails, symptomatic patients are divided into two groups. The first group comprises the people who have neck pain as a predominant complaint, with or without interscapular radiation. The second group is made up of those who complain primarily of arm pain (brachialgia).

Neck Pain Predominant. After 6 weeks of conservative therapy with no symptomatic relief, plain roentgenograms with lateral flexion/extension films are carefully examined for abnormalities. One group of patients will have objective evidence of instability. In the lower cervical spine (C3 through C7), instability is identified by horizontal translation of one vertebra on another of more than 3.5 mm, or of an angulatory difference of adjacent vertebrae of more than 11 degrees. The majority of patients with instability will respond well to further nonoperative measures, including a thorough explanation of the problem and some type of bracing. In some cases, these measures will fail and a surgical fusion of the involved spinal segments will be necessary.

Another group of patients complaining of mainly neck pain will be found to have degenerative disease on their plain x-ray films. The roentgenographic signs include loss of height of the intervertebral disk space, osteophyte formation, secondary encroachment of the intervertebral foramina, and osteoarthritic changes in the apophyseal joint. The difficulty is not in identifying these abnormalities on the roentgenogram but in determining their significance.

Degeneration in the cervical spine can be a normal part of the aging process. In a study of matched pairs of asymptomatic and symptomatic patients, it was concluded that large numbers of asymptomatic patients show roentgenographic evidence of advanced degenerative disease. The most significant roentgenographic finding relevant to symptoms was found to be narrowing of the intervertebral disk space, particularly between C5–6 and C6–7. There was no difference between the two groups as far as changes at the apophyseal joints, intervertebral foramina, or posterior articular processes.

These patients should be treated symptomatically with anti-inflammatory medications, support, and trigger point injections as required. In the quiescent stages they should be placed on isometric exercises. Finally, they should be reexamined periodically because some will develop significant pressure on the neurologic elements (myelopathy).

The majority of patients with neck pain will have normal roentgenograms. The diagnosis for this group is neck strain. At this point, with no objective findings, other pathologic conditions must be considered. These patients should undergo bone scan and medical evaluation. The bone scan is an excellent tool, often identifying early spinal tumors or infections not seen on routine roentgenographic examination. A thorough medical search may also reveal problems missed in the early states of neck pain evaluation. If these diagnostic studies are positive, the patient is treated appropriately.

If this workup is negative, the patient should have a thorough psychosocial evaluation. This is predicated on the belief that a patient's disability is related not only to his pathologic anatomy but also to his perception of pain and his stability in relation to his sociologic environment. Drug habituation, alcoholism, depression, and other psychiatric problems are frequently seen in association with neck pain. If the evaluation reveals this type of pathology, proper measures should be instituted to overcome the disability.

Should the outcome of the psychosocial evaluation prove to be normal, the patient can be considered to have chronic neck pain. One must be aware that other outside factors such as compensation or litigation can influence a patient's perception of his subjective pain. Patients with chronic neck pain need encouragement, patience, and education from their physicians. They need to be detoxified from narcotic drugs and placed on an exercise regimen. Many will respond to antidepressant drugs such as amitriptyline (Elavil). All these patients need periodic reevaluation to avoid missing any new or underlying pathology.

Arm Pain Predominant (Brachialgia). Patients who have pain radiating into their arm may be experiencing their symptoms secondary to mechanical pressure and inflammations of the involved nerve roots. This mechanical pressure may arise from a ruptured disk or from bone secondary to degenerative changes. Other pathologic causes of arm pain should be carefully considered. Extrinsic pressure on the vascular structures or on the peripheral nerves are the most likely imitator of brachialgia. Pathologic involvement in the chest and shoulder should also be ruled out.

A careful physical examination should be conducted. If there is any question about these findings, appropriate roentgenograms and an EMG should be obtained. If any of these are positive for peripheral pressure on the nerves or other pathology, the appropriate therapy should be administered.

Should all these studies prove negative and the EMG is consistent, the patient is considered to have brachialgia. One must carefully reevaluate the patient who has a neurologic deficit or a positive EMG; those who have either should undergo an MRI. If the MRI is positive and is consistent with the physical findings, surgical decompression should be considered at this juncture.

It has been repeatedly documented that for surgery to be effective, unequivocal evidence of nerve root compression must be found at surgery. One must have a strong confirmation of mechanical root compression from the neurologic examination and a confirming study before proceeding with any surgery. The indications for surgery are the subjective complaint of arm pain and a neurologic deficit or positive EMG. If the patient does not have these, there is inadequate clinical evidence of root compression to proceed with surgery, regardless of the radiographic findings. For individuals who have met these criteria for cervical decompression, the results will usually be satisfactory: 95% of them can expect good or excellent outcomes.

Thoracic Spine

The thoracic spine differs markedly from both the cervical and lumbar spine because of the support it receives from the rib cage. Although degenerative changes do occur, they very rarely cause symptoms. The only pathologic entity that can result in symptoms is a thoracic disk herniation. It is an uncommon condition but needs to be considered because of the resulting spinal cord compression with its potential serious sequelae.

HISTORY, PHYSICAL EXAMINATION, AND DIAGNOSTIC STUDIES

The clinical presentation is varied. The signs and symptoms depend on the location of the herniation. Three fourths of the cases occur between T8 and L1 with the peak at T11–12. The condition is dynamic with progression of the symptoms. The chronologic progression is pain followed by sensory disturbances, weakness, and finally bowel and bladder dysfunction.

The pain can be midline, unilateral, or bilateral, depending on the location of the herniation. Coughing and sneezing may aggravate the pain. If the herniation is midthoracic, radiation of pain into the chest or abdomen can stimulate cardiac or abdominal disease. Pain from a lower thoracic herniation may radiate to the groin, stimulating urethral calculi or renal disease. Finally, herniated disks at the lowest thoracic levels can impinge on the cauda equina as well as on the distal spinal cord, causing lower extremity pain and simulating a herniated lumbar disk.

The physical examination is most important. A thorough neurologic examination is mandatory and will reveal long tract signs and other evidence of cord compression. Flexion of the neck may induce back or root pain.

Plain spine radiographs are generally not helpful. There is a 70% association of a calcified disk with a symptomatic herniation. Thus, a calcified disk should suggest the diagnosis in the appropriate clinical setting.

The MRI is the diagnostic study of choice. It will demonstrate significant compression of the spinal cord at the involved level. One must correlate the history and physical examination with the MRI findings because there is a significant prevalence rate in asymptomatic individuals.

TREATMENT

If the history, physical examination, and MRI are consistent with a thoracic disk herniation, surgery is generally indicated, not only to relieve symptoms, but to prevent any progression of neurologic deficits. The results of modern surgical techniques are very good to excellent. Diskectomy may be carried out by a costotransversectomy, thoracotomy, or posterolateral technique. The progression is favorable, and early operative intervention is advised.

LUMBAR SPINE

Low back pain occurs much more commonly than neck pain. The lifetime incidence of low back pain is estimated to be 65%. Every physician will be either personally affected (family or friends) or professionally challenged by this problem.

History

A general medical review, especially in the older patient, is imperative. Metabolic, infectious, and malignant disorders may initially present to the physician as low back pain.

The location of the pain is one of the most important historical points. The majority of patients just have back pain with or without referral into the buttocks or posterior thigh. Referred pain is defined as pain in structures that have the same mesodermal origin. These patients have a localized injury, and the referral of pain into the buttocks or thigh does not signify any compression on the neural elements. This type of pain is described as dull, deep, or boring.

Another group of patients complains of pain that originates in the back but travels below the knee into the foot. It is described as sharp and lancinating. It may be accompanied by numbness and tingling. This pain is termed "radicular pain" or a "radiculopathy." A radiculopathy is defined as a mechanical compression of an inflamed nerve root where the pain travels along the anatomic course of the nerve. The compression can be secondary to either soft tissue (disk) or bone. The most common nerve roots affected are L5 and S1—levels that account for pain traveling below the knee.

Finally, one should inquire about changes in bowel or bladder habits. Occasionally, a large midline disk herniation may compress several roots of the cauda equina (Fig. 18–25). This is termed cauda equina compression (CEC)

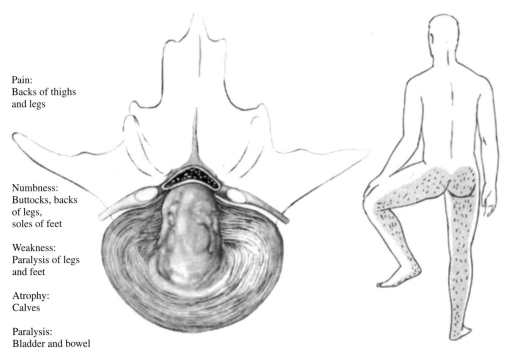

Figure 18–25. Cauda equina compression. (From DePalma, AF, Rothma, RH: The Intervertebral Disc. Philadelphia, W.B. Saunders Company, 1970, p 194; reprinted by permission.)

Pain:
Backs of thighs
and legs

Numbness:
Buttocks, backs
of legs,
soles of feet

Weakness:
Paralysis of legs
and feet

Atrophy:
Calves

Paralysis:
Bladder and bowel

syndrome. Urinary retention or incontinence of bowel and bladder are, along with severe pain, the major symptoms. CEC is a surgical emergency. Spontaneous neurologic recovery has not been observed. Only surgery undertaken promptly can offer any hope of neurologic recovery.

Physical Examination

The physical examination is directed at finding the location of the pain. All patients with low back pain can have some nonspecific findings that vary in degree, depending on the severity of the condition. These findings include a list to one side, tenderness to palpation and percussion, and a decreased range of motion of the lumbar spine and can be present in both radiculopathy and referred pain patients. Their presence denotes that there is a problem but does not identify the etiology or level of the problem.

The neurologic examination may yield objective evidence of nerve root compression. If such evidence is present (Table 18–3), a thorough neurologic evaluation of the lower extremities should be conducted, particularly to check the reflexes and motor findings. Sensory changes may or may not be present, but because of the overlap in the dermatomes of spinal nerves, it is difficult to identify specific root involvement.

In patients with radiculopathies there are several maneuvers that tighten the sciatic nerve, and in so doing, further compress an inflamed lumbar root against a herniated disk or bony spur. These maneuvers are generally termed "tension signs" or a "straight leg raising test (SLRT)." The conventional SLRT is performed with the patient supine. The examiner slowly elevates the leg by the heel with the knee kept straight (Fig. 18–26). This test is positive when the leg pain below the knee is reproduced or intensified; the production of back pain or buttock pain does not

constitute a positive finding. The reliability of the SLRT is age-dependent. In a young patient, a negative test most probably excludes the possibility of a herniated disk. After the age of 30, however, a negative SLRT no longer reliably excludes the diagnosis.

Finally, the physical examination should evaluate some specific problems that can present as low back pain. This

Table 18–3. Clinical features of herniated lumbar disks

L3–4 Disk: L4 Nerve Root

Pain	Lower back, hip, posterolateral thigh, across patella, anteromedial aspect of leg
Numbness	Anteromedial thigh and knee
Weakness	Knee extension
Atrophy	Quadriceps
Reflexes	Knee jerk diminished

L4–5 Disk: L5 Nerve Root

Pain	Sacroiliac region, hip, posterolateral thigh, anterolateral leg
Numbness	Lateral leg, first webspace
Weakness	Dorsiflexion of great toe and foot
Atrophy	Minimal anterior calf
Reflexes	None, or absent posterior tibial tendon reflex

L5–S1 Disk: S1 Nerve Root

Pain	Sacroiliac region, hip, posterolateral thigh/leg
Numbness	Back of calf; lateral heel, foot, and toe
Weakness	Plantar flexion of foot and great toe
Atrophy	Gastrocnemius and soleus
Reflexes	Ankle jerk diminished or absent

From Boden S, Wiesel SW, Laws E, et al: The Aging Spine. Philadelphia, W.B. Saunders, 1991, p 177; reprinted by permission.

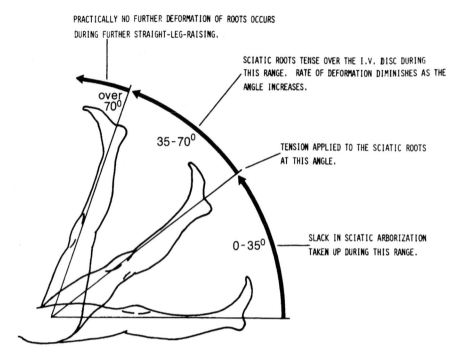

PRACTICALLY NO FURTHER DEFORMATION OF ROOTS OCCURS DURING FURTHER STRAIGHT-LEG-RAISING.

SCIATIC ROOTS TENSE OVER THE I.V. DISC DURING THIS RANGE. RATE OF DEFORMATION DIMINISHES AS THE ANGLE INCREASES.

over 70°

35-70°

TENSION APPLIED TO THE SCIATIC ROOTS AT THIS ANGLE.

0-35°

SLACK IN SCIATIC ARBORIZATION TAKEN UP DURING THIS RANGE.

Figure 18–26. Straight leg raising test. (Modified from Fahrni WH: Observations on straight leg-raising, with special reference to nerve root adhesions. Can J Surg 9:1966; reprinted by permission.)

evaluation includes a peripheral vascular examination, hip joint evaluation, and abdominal examination.

Low back pain can conveniently be divided into three categories: mild, moderate, and severe. Those placed in the mild group have subjective pain without objective findings and should be able to return to customary activity in less than a week. The moderate group is characterized by a limited range of spinal motion and paravertebral muscle spasm as well as pain, and these patients should be able to resume full activity in less than 2 weeks. The severe group includes those patients who are tilted forward or to the side. They have trouble ambulating and can take up to 3 weeks to become functional again.

Because a normal x-ray is a standard finding in a patient complaining of back strain, a radiographic study usually is not necessary on the first visit if the physician feels comfortable with the diagnosis; however, if the response to treatment does not proceed as expected, films should be taken to rule out other more serious problems, such as spondylolisthesis or tumor. The authors' usual recommendation is that if a patient fails to respond to conservative treatment for an acute attack of low back pain after a period of 2 weeks, then a routine lumbosacral spine x-ray series is clinically indicated.

The authors' preferred treatment for low back strain is the functional restorative approach. The mainstay of treatment is controlled physical activity, with the judicious use of trunk flexibility and strengthening exercises as the acute phase subsides. Often, particularly in the obese patient with weak abdominal muscles, a lightweight lumbosacral corset is useful in helping to mobilize those encumbered by low back strain.

Herniated Disk

A herniated disk can be defined as the herniation of the nucleus pulposus through the torn fibers of the annulus

fibrosus. Most disk ruptures occur during the third and fourth decades of life while the nucleus pulposus is still gelatinous. The perforations usually arise through a defect just lateral to the posterior midline where the posterior longitudinal ligament is weakest. The two most common levels for disk herniation are L4–5 and L5–S1. These two disks account for 95% of all lumbar disk herniations; pathology at the L2–3 and L3–4 levels can occur but is relatively uncommon.

Disk herniations at L5–S1 will usually compromise the first sacral nerve root. A lesion at the L4–5 level will most often compress the fifth lumbar root, and a herniation at the L3–4 level more commonly involves the fourth lumbar root. It should be pointed out, however, that variations in root configuration as well as in the position of the herniation itself can modify these relationships. An L4–5 disk rupture can at times affect the first sacral as well as the fifth lumbar root, and in extreme lateral herniations, the nerve exiting at the same level as the disk will be involved.

Not everyone with a disk herniation has significant discomfort. A large herniation in a capacious canal may not be clinically significant because there is no compression of the neural elements, while a minor protrusion in a small canal may be crippling if there is not enough room to accommodate both the disk and the nerve root.

Clinically, the patient's major complaint is pain. Although there may be a prior history of intermittent episodes of localized low back pain, this not always the case. The pain not only is present in the back but also radiates down the leg in the distribution of the affected nerve root. It will usually be described as sharp or lancinating, progressing from the top downward in the involved leg. Its onset may be insidious or sudden and associated with a tearing or snapping sensation in the spine. Occasionally, when sciatica develops, the back pain may resolve because once the annulus has ruptured, it may no longer be under tension. Finally the sciatic pain may vary in intensity; it may be so severe that patients will be unable to ambulate and will feel that their back is "locked." Conversely, the pain may be limited to a dull ache that increases in intensity with ambulation.

On physical examination, there is usually a decreased range of motion in flexion, and patients will tend to drift away from the involved side as they bend. On ambulation, the patients walks with an antalgic gait, holding the involved leg flexed so as to put as little weight as possible on the extremity.

Although neurologic examination may yield objective evidence of nerve root compression, these findings are often undependable because the involved nerve is often still functional. In addition, such deficit may have little temporal relevance if it is related to a prior attack at a different level. To be significant, reflex changes, weakness, atrophy, or sensory loss must conform to the rest of the clinical picture.

When the first sacral root is compressed, the patient may have gastrocnemius-soleus weakness and be unable to repeatedly rise on the toes of that foot. Atrophy of the calf may be apparent, and the ankle (Achilles) reflex is often diminished or absent. Sensory loss, if any, is usually confined to the posterior aspect of the calf and lateral side of the foot.

Involvement of the fifth lumbar nerve root can lead to weakness in extension of the great toe and, less often, to weakness of the everter and dorsiflexors of the foot. An associated sensory deficit can appear over the anterior leg and the dorsomedial aspect of the foot down to the great toe. There are usually no primary reflex changes, but on occasion a diminution in the posterior tibial reflex can be elicited. The absence of this reflex, however, must be symmetric for it to have any clinical significance.

With compression of the fourth lumbar nerve root, the quadriceps muscle is affected. The patient may note weakness in knee extension, and this weakness is often associated with instability. Atrophy of the thigh musculature can be marked. A sensory loss may be apparent over the anteromedial aspect of the thigh, and the patellar tendon reflex is usually diminished.

Nerve root sensitivity can be elicited by any method that creates tension; however, SLRT is most commonly employed. As discussed before, a positive test reproduces the patient's pain down the leg. The reproduction of back pain is not considered positive.

The initial diagnosis of a herniated disk is ordinarily made on the basis of the history and physical examination. Plain x-rays of the lumbosacral spine will rarely add to the diagnosis but should be obtained to help rule out other causes of pain, such as infection or tumor. Other tests such as the EMG, the computerized axial tomography (CAT) scan, and MRI are confirmatory by nature and can be misinformative when used as screening devices.

The treatment for most patients with a herniated disk is nonoperative; 80% of them will respond to conservative therapy when followed over a period of 5 years. The efficacy of nonoperative treatment, however, depends upon a healthy relationship between a capable physician and a well-informed patient. If a patient has insight into the rationale for the prescribed treatment and follows instructions, the chances for success are greatly increased.

One of the most important elements in the nonoperative treatment is controlled physical activity. Patients should markedly decrease their activity. This will sometimes require bed rest and in most cases can be accomplished at home. An acute herniation usually takes at least 2 weeks of significant rest before the pain substantially eases.

Drug therapy is another important part of the treatment, and three categories of pharmacologic agents are commonly used; anti-inflammatory drugs, analgesics, and muscle relaxants or tranquilizers. Inasmuch as the symptoms of low back pain and sciatica result from an inflammatory reaction as well as mechanical compression, the authors feel that anti-inflammatory medication in the form of two aspirin tablets (650 mg) every 4 hours should be taken in conjunction with rest. It should be stressed, however, that no medication can take the place of controlled physical activity. Buffered aspirin can be used by patients with gastrointestinal intolerance. The patient's pain generally will be relieved once the inflammation is brought under control. There may be some numbness or tingling in the involved extremity, but it is usually tolerable. In addition, a large array of NSAIDs are available for the refractory patient.

Analgesic medication is rarely needed if the patient truly rests, because the pain is usually adequately controlled by decreased activity. If the pain is severe enough to require hospitalization, however, then morphine sulfate is the drug of choice; codeine is recommended for use when the patient is home.

There is some question as to whether there actually is a muscle relaxant; all drugs that are designated as such probably act to some degree as tranquilizers. If one is required, though, methocarbamol and carisoprodol are most frequently used, and they can be employed intravenously as well as orally. The use of diazepam (Valium) for this purpose should be discouraged because it is a depressant and often will add to the patient's psychological problems.

Eighty percent of those who follow the above regimen will be markedly improved, but this regimen requires patience because frequently at least 6 weeks will have passed before any additional therapy is indicated. Although the noninvasive treatment of a herniated disk can be quite gratifying, it generally takes a significant period of rest, and the patient must be aware of the time constraints from the beginning in order to understand the rationale behind the measures employed.

The long-term prognosis for the patient with disk herniation is quite good. It has been shown that between 85% and 90% of surgically treated and nonsurgically treated patients were asymptomatic at 4 years. Less than 2% of both groups remained symptomatic at 10 years.

Surgery is indicated for patients with unremitting pain despite an adequate course of conservative therapy (usually 6 weeks). In the properly selected patient who has the appropriate history and physical examination with a confirming diagnostic study, surgery is over 90% successful in relieving leg pain.

Spinal Stenosis

Spinal stenosis can be defined as a narrowing of the spinal canal, and the degree of mechanical pressure on the neural structures within will depend upon the degree of narrowing. Every person's spine, however, becomes narrower with age because of osteoarthritis. Not everyone with a narrowed spinal canal, however, will have symptoms.

For those who do suffer, the discomfort can vary from mild annoyance to an inability to walk. The symptom complex is well documented. Patients of either sex, usually not before their fifth decade, will first complain of vague pains, dysesthesias, and paresthesias with ambulation but will typically have excellent relief of their symptoms when they are sitting or lying supine. The increased lordotic stance assumed with walking, and particularly walking down grades, is most likely the inciting cause. The hyperextension further narrows the spinal canal and increases the symptoms.

With maturation of the syndrome, symptoms may even occur at rest. Muscle weakness, atrophy, and asymmetric reflex changes may then appear; however, as long as the symptoms are only aggravated dynamically, neurologic changes will occur only after the patient is stressed. The following stress test can be used in an outpatient clinic; after a neurologic examination has been performed on the patient, he or she is asked to walk up and down the corridor until symptoms occur or the patient has walked 300 feet. A repeat examination is then done and in many cases the second examination will be positive for a focal neurologic deficit when the first was negative.

Plain x-rays are often helpful in visualizing spinal stenosis, particularly degenerative spinal stenosis. One can see intervertebral disk degeneration, decreased interpedicular distance, a decreased sagittal canal diameter, and facet degeneration. If a patient fails conservative treatment and becomes a surgical candidate, the location and degree of neurologic compression can be assessed with MRI or a CT scan and myelogram.

The majority of patients with spinal stenosis, especially the degenerative and combined variety can be treated non-surgically. Aspirin has been the drug of choice, but the physician must watch for gastric irritation in what is typically an older patient population. Finally, a lumbosacral corset is often helpful in reminding the patient to avoid excessive strain. Symptoms are usually intermittent, and the individual often needs encouragement in getting through the episode without becoming depressed. Nonoperative management is preferable as long as the pain is tolerable.

Lumbar Spine Evaluation Algorithm

As with patients with neck pain, the task of the physician when confronted with low back pain patients is to integrate their complaints into an accurate diagnosis and to prescribe appropriate therapy. This problem (universe of low back pain patients) has been formatted into an algorithm (Fig. 18–27), the aim of which is to select the correct diagnostic category and proper treatment avenues for each patient with low back pain. A specific patient may fall outside the limits of the algorithm and require a different approach, and the physician must constantly be on the alert for exceptions. The algorithm can be followed in sequence and is also presented in a tabular format (Table 18–4).

The information necessary to use the algorithm initially is obtained through the history and physical examination. The key points in the history are differentiation of back pain that is mechanical in nature from nonmechanical pain that is present at rest, detecting changes in bowel or bladder function, and defining the precise location and quality of the pain. The physical examination must be oriented toward ruling out other medical causes of low back pain, assessing neurologic function, and evaluating for the presence of tension signs.

Following the low back pain algorithm, the first major decision is to make a ruling on the presence or absence of CEC syndrome. Mechanical compression of the cauda

Table 18–4. Differential diagnosis of low back pain

Evaluation	Back Strain	Herniated Nucleus Pulposus	Spinal Stenosis	Spondylo-listhesis/ Instability	Spondylo-arthropathy	Infection	Tumor	Metabolic	Hemato-logic	Visceral
Predominant pain (back vs. leg)	Back	Leg (below knee)	Back/leg	Back	Back	Back	Back	Back	Back	Back (buttock, thigh)
Constitutional symptoms					+	+	+	+	+	
Tension sign		+		±						
Neurologic examination		±	± after stress							
Plain x-rays			+	+	+	±	±	+	+	
Lateral motion x-rays				+						
CT/MRI		+	+			+	+			+
Myelogram		+	+							
Bone scan					+	+	+	+	+	
ESR					+	+	+		+	+
Serum chemistries							+	+	+	+

ESR indicates erythrocyte sedimentation rate.
From Borenstein DG, Wiesel SW: Low Back Pain: Medical Diagnosis and Comprehensive Management. Philadelphia, W.B. Saunders, 1989, p 534; reprinted by permission.

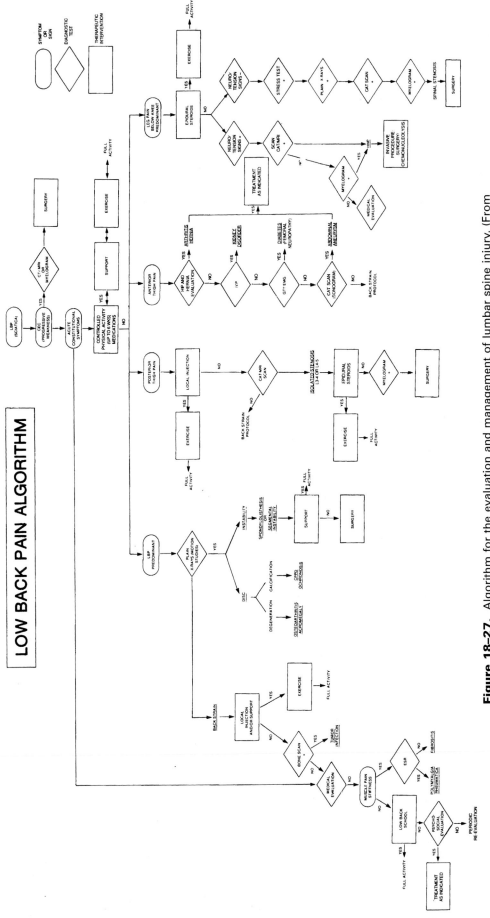

Figure 18–27. Algorithm for the evaluation and management of lumbar spine injury. (From Boden S, Wiesel SW, Laws E, et al: The Aging Spine. Philadelphia, W.B. Saunders Company, 1991, p 156; reprinted by permission.)

equina, with truly progressive motor weakness, is the only surgical emergency in lumbar spine disease. This compression from a massive rupture of the L4–5 disk in the midline is usually due to pressure on the caudal sac, through which pass the nerves to the lower extremities, bowel, and bladder.

The signs and symptoms of CEC are a complex mixture of low back pain, bilateral motor weakness of the lower extremities, bilateral sciatica, saddle anesthesia, and even frank paraplegia with bowel and bladder incontinence or urinary retention. CEC can be caused by either bone or soft tissue damage, the latter generally a ruptured or herniated disk in the midline. These patients should undergo an immediate definitive diagnostic test and, if it is positive, emergency surgical decompression. Historically, the myelogram was the study used in this setting; however, the development of MRI has facilitated the noninvasive diagnosis of CEC. The principal reason for prompt surgical intervention is to arrest the progression of the neuralgic loss; the chance of actual return of lost neurologic function following surgery is small. Although the incidence of CEC syndrome in the entire back pain population is very low, it is the only event that requires immediate operative intervention; if its diagnosis is missed, the consequences can be devastating.

The remaining patients make up the overwhelming majority. They should be started on a course of conservative (nonoperative) therapy, regardless of the diagnosis. At this stage the specific diagnosis, whether a herniated disk or simple back strain, is not important to the therapy because the entire population is treated the same way. A few of these patients will eventually need an invasive procedure (surgery), but at this point there is no way to predict which individuals will respond to conservative therapy and which will not.

Conservative Treatment

The vast majority in this initial group have nonradiating low back pain, termed lumbago or back strain. The etiology of lumbago is not clear. There are several possibilities, including ligamentous or muscular strain, continuous mechanical stress from poor posture, facet joint irritation, or a small tear in the annulus fibrosis. Patients usually complain of pain in the low back, often localized to a single area. On physical examination they demonstrate a decreased range of lumbar spine motion, tenderness to palpation over the involved area, and paraspinal muscle spasm. Their roentgenographic examinations are usually normal, but if therapy is not successful, films should be obtained to rule out other possible etiologic factors. Two exceptions to this rule are patients younger than 20 years of age and patients over age 60; x-rays are important early in the diagnostic process because these patients are more likely to have a diagnosis other than back strain (tumor or infection). Other situations warranting x-rays sooner rather than later include a history of serious trauma, known cancer, unexplained weight loss, or fever.

The early stage of the treatment of low back pain (with or without leg pain) is a waiting game. The passage of time, the use of anti-inflammatory medication, and controlled physical activity are the modalities that have proved safest and most effective. The vast majority of these patients will respond to this approach within the first 10 days, although a small percentage will not. In today's society with its emphasis on quick solutions and "high technology," many patients are pushed too rapidly toward more complex (i.e., invasive) management. This "quick fix" approach has no place in the treatment of low back pain. The physician treats the patient conservatively and waits up to 6 weeks for a response. As already stated, most of these patients will improve within 10 days, a few will take longer.

Once the patients have achieved approximately 80% relief, they should be mobilized with the help of a lightweight, flexible corset. After they become more comfortable and have increased their activity level, they should begin a program of isometric lumbar exercises and return to their normal lifestyles. The pathway along this section of the algorithm is a two-way street; should regression occur with exacerbation of symptoms, the physician can resort to more stringent conservative measures. The patient may require further bed rest. Most acute low back pain patients will proceed along this pathway, returning to a normal life pattern within 2 months of onset of symptoms.

If the initial conservative treatment regimen fails and 6 weeks have passed, symptomatic patients are sorted into four groups. The first group comprises people with low back pain predominating. The second group complains mainly of leg pain, defined as pain radiating below the knee and commonly referred to as sciatica. The third group has anterior thigh pain. Each group follows a separate diagnostic pathway.

REFRACTORY PATIENTS WITH LOW BACK PAIN

Patients who continue to complain predominantly of low back pain for 6 weeks should have plain x-rays carefully examined for abnormalities. Spondylolysis with or without spondylolisthesis is the most common structural abnormality to cause significant low back pain. Approximately 5% of the population has this defect, thought to be caused by a combination of genetics and environmental stress. In spite of this defect most people are able to perform their activities of daily living with little or no discomfort. When symptoms are present, these patients will usually respond to nonoperative measures, including a thorough explanation of the problem, a back support, and exercises. In a small percentage of such cases, conservative treatment fails and a fusion of the involved spinal segments becomes necessary. This is one of the few times primary fusion of the lumbar spine is indicated, and it must be stressed that it is a relatively infrequent occurrence.

The vast majority of patients with pain predominantly in the low back will have normal plain x-rays. The diagnosis at this point is back strain. Before there is any additional workup, a local injection of steroids and lidocaine may be tried at the point of maximum tenderness. This medication can be quite successful, and if there is good response, the patient is begun on exercises, with gradual resumption of normal activity. In some instances, if there are no objective findings, such as a "trigger point," injection can be considered as early as the third week after onset of symptoms.

Should the patient not respond to local injection, other pathology must be seriously sought. A bone scan, along with a general medical evaluation, would be obtained. The bone scan is an excellent tool, often identifying early bone tumors or infections not visible on routine radiographic examinations. It is particularly important to obtain this study in the patient with nonmechanical back pain. If the pain is constant, unremitting, and unrelieved by postural adjustments, more often than not the correct diagnosis will be one of an occult neoplasm or metabolic disorder not readily apparent from other testing.

Approximately 3% of cases of apparent low back pain that present at orthopaedic clinics are attributed to extraspinal causes. A thorough medical search also frequently reveals problems missed earlier such as a posterior penetrating ulcer, pancreatitis, renal disease, or an abdominal aneurysm. If these diagnostic studies are positive, the patient should be transferred into a nonorthopaedic treatment mode and would no longer be in the therapeutic algorithm.

Patients who have no abnormality on their bone scans and do not show other medical disease as a cause for their back pain are then referred for another type of therapy—the low back school. It is believed that many of these patients are suffering from diskogenic pain or facet joint pain syndrome. The low back school concept has as its basis the belief that patients with low back pain, given proper education and understanding of their disease, can often return to a productive and functional life. Ergonomics, the proper and efficient use of the spine in work and recreation, is stressed. Back school need not be an expensive proposition. It can be a one-time classroom session with a review of back problems and a demonstration of exercises with patient participation. This type of educational process has proved to be very effective. It is most important, however, that before they are referred to this type of program, patients are thoroughly screened. One does not want to be in the position of treating a metastatic tumor in a classroom.

If low back school is not successful, the patient should undergo a thorough psychosocial evaluation in an attempt to explain the failure of the previous treatments. This is predicated on the knowledge that a patient's ability is related not only to his or her pathologic anatomy but also to the patient's perception of pain and stability in relation to the social environment. It is quite common to see a stable patient with a frank herniated disk continue working, regarding the disability as only a minor problem, while a hysterical patient takes to bed at the slightest twinge of low back discomfort.

Drug habituation, depression, alcoholism, and other psychiatric problems are seen frequently in association with back pain. If the evaluation suggests any of these problems, proper measures should be instituted to overcome the disability. There are a surprising number of ambulatory patients addicted to commonly prescribed medications using complaints of back pain as an excuse to obtain these drugs. Oxycodone (Percodan) and diazepam, alone or in combination, are the two most popular offenders. Oxycodone is truly addictive; diazepam is both habituating and depressing. Because the complaint of low back pain may be a common manifestation of depression, it is counterproductive to treat such patients with diazepam.

Approximately 2% of patients who initially present with low back pain will fail treatment and elude any diagnosis. There will be no evidence of any structural problem in the back or criteria for an underlying medical disease or psychiatric disorder. This is a very difficult group to manage. The authors' strategy has been to discontinue narcotics, reassure the patients, and periodically reevaluate them. Over time, one third of these patients will be found to have an underlying medical disease; thus, one cannot abandon this group and discontinue treatment. For the remainder, as much physical activity as possible should be encouraged.

REFRACTORY PATIENTS WITH SCIATICA

The next group of patients are those with sciatica, which is pain radiating below the knee. These patients usually experience their symptoms secondary to mechanical pressure and inflammation of the nerve roots that originate in the back and extend down the leg. The etiology of the mechanical pressure can be soft tissue, such as a herniated disk, or bone, or a combination of the two.

At this point in the algorithm, the patient has had up to 6 weeks of controlled physical activity and medication but still has persistent leg pain. The next therapeutic step is an epidural steroid injection, which is performed on an outpatient basis. An epidural injection is worth trying; the chance of success is 40% and the morbidity rate is low, particularly compared with the next treatment step—surgery. The maximum benefit from a single injection is achieved at 2 weeks. The injection may have to be repeated once or twice, and 4 to 6 weeks should pass before its success or failure can be judged.

If epidural steroids are effective in alleviating the patient's leg pain or sciatica, the patient is begun on a program of back exercises and encouraged to return promptly to as normal a lifestyle as possible. Should the epidural steroids prove ineffective, and 3 months have passed since the initial injury without relief of pain, some type of invasive treatment should be considered. The patient group is then divided into those with probable herniated disks and those with symptoms secondary to spinal stenosis.

The physician must now carefully reevaluate the patient for a neurologic deficit and for a positive tension sign or SLRT. For those who have either a neurologic deficit or positive tension signs along with continued leg pain, an MRI scan should be obtained. If the MRI scan is clearly positive and correlates with the clinical findings, there is no need for myelography because it is invasive. If there is any question about the findings, one should proceed with the other noninvasive study not yet done (CT or MRI) or perform a metrizamide myelogram.

As in the cervical spine, there is repeated documentation that for surgery to be effective in the treatment of a herniated disk, the surgeon must find unequivocal operative evidence of a nerve root compression. Accordingly, nerve root compression must be firmly substantiated preoperatively, not only by neurologic examination but also by radiographic data. There is no place for "exploratory" back surgery. Many asymptomatic patients have been found to have abnormal myelograms, EMGs, CT scans, and MRI scans. If the patient has neither a neurologic deficit nor a positive SLRT, then regardless of radiographic findings, there is not enough evidence of root compression to proceed with successful surgery. These patients without objective findings are the ones who have poor results.

If there are no objective findings, the physician should avoid surgery and proceed to psychosocial evaluation. Exceptions should be few and far between. When sympathy for the patient's complaints outweighs the objective evaluation, surgery is fraught with difficulties. For those who meet these specific criteria for lumbar laminectomy, results will be satisfactory; 95% of these patients can expect a good to excellent result.

The second group of patients whose symptoms are based on mechanical pressure on the neural elements are those with spinal stenosis. The diagnosis of spinal stenosis usually can be inferred from the plain x-rays, which will demonstrate facet degeneration, disk degeneration, and decreased interpedicular and sagittal canal diameters. A CT scan or MRI scan can confirm the diagnosis. If symptoms are severe, and there is radiographic evidence of spinal stenosis, surgery is appropriate. Age alone is not a deterrent to surgery; many elderly people who are in good health except for a narrow spinal canal will benefit greatly from adequate decompression of the lumbar spine.

REFRACTORY PATIENTS WITH ANTERIOR THIGH PAIN

A small percentage of patients will have pain that radiates from the back into the anterior thigh. This usually is relieved by rest and anti-inflammatory medication. If the discomfort persists after 6 weeks of treatment, a workup should be initiated to search for an underlying disorder. Although an upper lumbar radiculopathy can cause anterior thigh pain, several other entities must be considered.

A hip problem or hernia can be ruled out with a thorough physical examination. If the hip examination is positive, radiographs should be obtained. An IV pyelogram is useful to evaluate the urinary tract, because kidney stones often may present as anterior thigh pain. Peripheral neuropathy, most commonly secondary to diabetes, also can present initially with anterior thigh pain; a glucose tolerance test as well as an EMG will reveal the underlying problem. Finally, a retroperitoneal tumor can cause symptoms by mechanically pressing on the nerves that innervate the anterior thighs. A CT or MRI scan of the retroperitoneal area will eliminate or confirm this possibility.

If any of the entities reviewed here is diagnosed, the patient is treated accordingly. If no physical cause can be found for the anterior thigh pain, the patient is treated for recalcitrant back strain by the method already outlined.

REFRACTORY PATIENTS WITH POSTERIOR THIGH PAIN

This final group of patients will complain of back pain with radiation into the buttocks and posterior thigh. Most of them will be relieved of their symptoms with 6 weeks of conservative therapy. However, if their pain persists after the initial treatment period, they can be considered to have back strain and given a trigger point injection of steroids and lidocaine in the area of maximum tenderness. If the injection is unsuccessful, it is necessary to distinguish between referred and radicular pain.

As noted earlier, referred pain is pain in mesodermal tissues of the same embryologic origin. The muscles, tendons, and ligaments of the buttocks and posterior thigh have the same embryologic origin as those of the low back. When the low back is injured, pain may be referred to the posterior thigh, where it is perceived by the patient. Referred pain from irritated soft tissues cannot be cured with a surgical procedure.

Radicular pain is caused by compression of an inflamed nerve root along the anatomic course of the nerve. A herniated disk or spinal stenosis in the high lumbar area can cause radiation of pain into the posterior thigh. An MRI or CT scan and an EMG may be used in this situation to differentiate radicular etiology from referred pain or a peripheral nerve lesion. It the studies are within normal limits, the patient is considered to have low back strain and treated according to the algorithm. If a radicular abnormality is found, the patient is diagnosed as having mechanical compression on the neural elements either from a herniated disk or spinal stenosis. Epidural steroids should be tried first; if these drugs do not provide adequate relief, surgery should be contemplated.

This group of patients with unexplained posterior thigh pain is very difficult to treat. The biggest mistake is the performance of surgery on people thought to have radicular pain but who actually have referred pain. Again, referred pain in this setting is not responsive to surgery.

In most instances the treatment of low back pain is no longer a mystery. The algorithm described here presents a series of easy-to-follow and clearly defined decision-making processes. Use of this algorithm provides patients with the most helpful diagnostic and therapeutic measures at the optimal time. It neither denies them helpful surgery nor subjects them to procedures that are useless technical exercises.

Multiple Operations on the Lumbar Spine

Continued pain after low back surgery is a difficult problem. Fifteen percent of all patients who undergo an initial surgical procedure will have significant discomfort and disability. The inherent complexity of these cases necessitates a method of problem solving that is precise and unambiguous.

The best possible solution for preventing recurrent symptoms is to avoid inappropriate initial surgery whenever possible. Again, it must be stressed that proper surgical indication should be strictly adhered to for the first procedure. The idea of "exploring" the low back when the necessary objective criteria are not present is no longer acceptable. In fact, even if there are objective findings but the patient is psychologically unstable or there are compensation litigation factors, the outcome of low back surgery is uncertain. Thus, the initial decision to operate is the most important one. Once the situation of recurrent pain after surgery arises, the potential for a solution is limited at best.

The physician must differentiate the patient with symptoms secondary to a mechanical lesion from one with some other problem. Recurrent herniated disk, spinal instability, and spinal stenosis are the principal mechanical lesions and are amenable to surgical intervention. Scar tissue (arachnoiditis or perineural fibrosis), psychosocial instability, or a systemic medical disease are the nonmechanical problems commonly found in the patient who has undergone multiple low back operations; none of these entities can be relieved by additional surgery.

Successful treatment for these patients is dependent on obtaining an accurate diagnosis. This essential step is often omitted and inappropriate care is rendered.

EVALUATION

The evaluation of the patient who has continuing low back pain following surgery can be quite confusing. The history, physical examination, and roentgenographic studies need to be assessed in a standardized fashion. With accurate information, a diagnosis usually can be obtained.

First, it should be determined if the patient's complaint is based on a medical cause such as pancreatitis or an abdominal aneurysm. Thus, a thorough general medical examination should be routinely performed. In addition, if there is any indication of psychosocial instability, evidenced by alcoholism, drug dependence, or depression, a thorough psychiatric evaluation is necessary. Persons with profound emotional disturbances do not derive any observable benefit from additional surgery. In many cases, once a patient's underlying psychosocial problem has been treated successfully, his somatic back complaints and disability will disappear.

If the lumbar spine is the probable source of the patient's complaints, three specific historical points need clarification. The first is the number of previous lumbar spine operations the patient has undergone. It has been shown that with every subsequent operation, regardless of the diagnosis, the likelihood of a good result decreases. Statistically, the second operation has a 50% chance of success, and beyond two operations, patients are more likely to be made worse than better.

The next important historical point is determination of the pain-free interval following the patient's previous operation. If the patient awoke from surgery with pain still present, the nerve root may not have been properly decompressed or the wrong level may have been explored. If the pain-free interval was longer than 6 months, the patient's recent pain may be due to recurrent disk herniation at the same or a different level. If the pain-free interval was between 1 and 6 months, the diagnosis most often is arachnoiditis or infection.

Finally, the patient's pain pattern must be evaluated. If leg pain predominates, a herniated disk or spinal stenosis is most likely. If back pain is the main complaint, instability, tumor, infection, and arachnoiditis are the major considerations. If both back and leg pain are present, spinal stenosis and arachnoiditis are the possibilities.

Physical examination is the next major step in the evaluation of the patient in whom previous back surgery has failed to relieve pain. The neurologic findings and existence of a tension sign, such as a positive straight leg raising test or sitting root test, are noted. It is most important to have the results of a dependable previous examination so that a comparison can be made between the preoperative and postoperative states. If the preoperative neurologic picture is unchanged and the tension sign is negative, mechanical compression is unlikely. If, however, there is a new neurologic deficit or the tension sign is positive, pressure on the neural elements is possible.

Roentgenographic studies are an important part of the patient's workup. Again, it is most helpful to have a previous set of plain roentgenograms, MRI, CT scans, and myelograms for comparison of the pre- and postoperative situations. The plain roentgenograms are evaluated for the extent and level of previous laminectomy(ies) and for evidence of spinal stenosis. Weight-bearing lateral flexion/extension films of the lumbar spine are examined to see if instability is present. An unstable spine may be the result of the patient's intrinsic disease or secondary to a previous surgical procedure.

Water-soluble myelography and CT play a limited role in evaluating the multiply operated lumbar spine. Although these tests can identify extradural compressions, they cannot distinguish between disk material and epidural scar. The major use of these two tests in combination is for confirmation of arachnoiditis when the diagnosis is otherwise uncertain.

MRI scan is the most valuable diagnostic test in these complicated patients. With the administration of an intravenous paramagnetic contrast material (gadolinium diethylenetriamine penta-acetic acid dimeglumine [Gd-DTPA]), a recurrent disk herniation may be distinguished from epidural scar. A herniated disk is avascular and will not enhance (light up) immediately after the injection of intravenous contrast material; scar tissue, on the other hand is vascular and will enhance with contrast. MRI is also extremely helpful in identifying inflammatory processes such as diskitis, which demonstrates a decreased signal intensity on T_1-weighted images.

MECHANICAL ETIOLOGIES

Three possibilities exist if the patient's pain is caused by a herniated disk. First, the disk that caused the original symptoms may not have been satisfactorily removed. This can happen if the wrong level was decompressed; the laminectomy performed was not adequate to free the neural elements; or a fragment of disk material was left behind. Such patients will continue to have pain because of mechanical pressure on and irritation of the same nerve root that caused the initial symptoms. They will complain predominantly of leg pain, and their neurologic findings, tension signs, and radiographic patterns will remain unchanged from the preoperative state. The distinguishing feature is that they will report no pain-free interval; they will have awakened from the operation complaining of the same preoperative pain. Patients in this group will be aided by a technically correct laminectomy.

A second possibility is that there is a recurrent herniated intervertebral disk at the previously decompressed level. These patients complain of sciatica and have unchanged neurologic findings, tension signs, and radiographic studies. The distinguishing characteristic here is a pain-free interval of greater than 6 months. Another operative procedure is indicated in these patients provided that an MRI scan with gadolinium can demonstrate herniated disk material rather than just scar tissue.

Finally, a herniated disk can occur at a completely different level. Such patients generally will suffer sudden onset of recurrent pain after a pain-free interval of more than 6 months. Sciatica predominates and tension signs are positive. However, a neurologic deficit, if present, and the radiographic signs will be seen at a different level from that on the original studies. A repeat operation for these patients will be beneficial.

Lumbar instability is another condition causing pain on a mechanical basis in the multiply operated back patient. Instability is the abnormal or excessive movement of one vertebra on another, causing pain. The etiology may be the patient's own intrinsic back disease or an excessively wide bilateral laminectomy.[1, 2] Pseudarthrosis resulting from a failed spinal fusion is included in this category because the pain is caused by the instability created by the failed fusion.

Patients with instability will complain predominantly of back pain, and their physical examinations may be negative. Sometimes, the key to diagnosis of these patients is the weight-bearing lateral flexion-extension film; however, it is often difficult to precisely define the anatomic origin of back pain in the presence of radiographic instability. Relative flexion-sagittal plane translation of more than 8% of the anteroposterior diameter of the vertebral body or a relative flexion-sagittal plane rotation of more than 9 degrees between segments is the most commonly cited guideline for instability of the lumbar spine.[3, 4] At the lumbosacral junction the criteria are slightly different; relative translation of more than 6% or rotation of more than 1 degree is significant. These criteria are based on maximum displacements on a single flexion or extension view; however, calculation of relative dynamic translation and rotation from flexion to extension may prove to be a more reliable indication of true instability.

Unfortunately, there is little information to explain why some patients with segmental instability develop back pain while others do not. If there is radiographic evidence of instability in symptomatic patients, spinal fusion (or repair of the pseudarthrosis) may be considered. Additional confirmatory evidence to determine the precise level of origin of the patient's symptoms may be gathered from facet injections and diskography; however, these tests have a substantial rate of false positive results.

Spinal stenosis in the multiply operated back patient can mechanically produce both back and leg pain. The etiology may be secondary to progression of the patient's inherent degenerative spine disease, previous inadequate decompression, or overgrowth of a previous posterior fusion. The physical examination is often inconclusive, although a neurologic deficit may occur following exercise; with reproduction of the patient's symptoms this phenomenon is termed a positive stress test.

The plain films can be suggestive and may display facet degeneration, decreased interpedicular distance, decreased sagittal canal diameter, or disk degeneration. A CT scan will demonstrate bony encroachment upon the neural elements; this is especially helpful in evaluating the lateral recesses and neural foramina. An MRI will show compression of the dural sac at the involved levels. It should be appreciated that spinal stenosis and scar tissue can coexist. Good results can be expected from surgery in at least 70% of properly selected cases, but if there has been a previous laminectomy and spinal fusion, surgery will be less successful. If there is definite evidence of bony compression, a laminectomy is indicated; however, if substantial scar tissue is present, the degree of pain relief the patient can anticipate is uncertain.

Scar tissue (arachnoiditis or epidural fibrosis) and diskitis are nonmechanical causes of recurrent pain in the multiply operated back patient. Although the etiologies and specific locations of these lesions are different, they are discussed in the same section because none of them will respond to another surgical procedure.

Postoperative scar tissue can be divided into two main types based on anatomic location. Scar tissue that occurs beneath the dura is commonly referred to as arachnoiditis. Scar tissue also can form extradurally, either directly on the cauda equina or around a nerve root.

Arachnoiditis is strictly defined as an inflammation of the pia arachnoid membrane surrounding the spinal cord or cauda equina. The condition may be present in varying degrees of severity, from mild thickening of the membranes to solid adhesions. The scarring may be severe enough to obliterate the subarachnoid space and block the flow of contrast agents.

This condition has been attributed to many factors; lumbar spine surgery and previous injections of intrathecal contrast material seem to be the most frequent precipitating factors. This problem is much less common since the advent of water-soluble contrast dyes. Postoperative infection also may play a role in the pathogenesis. The exact mechanics by which arachnoiditis develops from these events is not clear.

There is no uniform clinical presentation for arachnoiditis. Statistically, the history will reveal more than one previous operation and a pain-free interval of between 1 and 6 months. Often these patients will complain of back and leg pain. Physical examination is not conclusive; alterations in neurologic status may be due to a previous operation. As mentioned earlier, myelography, CT, and MRI can be helpful in confirming the diagnosis.

At present there is no effective treatment for arachnoiditis. Surgical intervention has not proved effective in eliminating the scar tissue or significantly reducing the pain. Along with much needed encouragement, there are various nonoperative measures that can be employed. Epidural steroid, transcutaneous nerve stimulation, spinal cord stimulation, operant conditioning, bracing, and patient education have all been tried. None of these will lead to a complete cure, but when used judiciously they can provide symptomatic relief for varying periods of time. Patients should be detoxified from all narcotics, placed on amitriptyline (Elavil), and encouraged to do as much physical activity as possible. Treating these patients is a challenge, and the physician must be willing to devote time and patience to achieve optimal results.

Formation of scar tissue outside the dura on the cauda equina or directly on nerve roots is a relatively common occurrence. This *epidural scar tissue* acts as a constrictive force about the neural elements and frequently can cause postoperative pain. However, although most patients have some epidural scar tissue, only an unpredictable few become symptomatic.

Patients with epidural scarring may present with symptoms from several months to a year or 2 after surgery. They may complain of back pain or leg pain, or both. Commonly there are no new neurologic findings, but there may be positive tension sign purely on the basis of scar formation around a nerve root. Epidural fibrosis is best differentiated from a recurrent herniated disk using gadolinium-enhanced MRI.

As with arachnoiditis, there is no definitive treatment for epidural scar tissue. Prevention may be the best answer, and a free fat graft is sometimes used as an interposition membrane to minimize epidural scar tissue following laminectomy.[12] Use of too thick a fat graft may result in absorption of blood and swelling of the graft; there have been anecdotal reports of postoperative cauda equina syndrome associated with large fat grafts. Once scar has formed, surgery is not successful because scarring will often re-form in greater quantity. The treatment program should be similar to that already described for arachnoiditis.

Diskitis is an uncommon but debilitating complication of lumbar disk surgery. Its pathogenesis is postulated to be direct inoculation of the avascular disk space but is not completely understood.[13] The onset of symptoms usually occurs about 1 month following surgery, and most patients will complain of severe back pain. Physical examination will sometimes reveal fever, a positive tension sign, and occasionally a superficial abscess.

If diskitis is suspected from the history and physical examination, an ESR, blood cultures, and plain radiographs should be obtained. Plain films may not demonstrate the changes of disk space narrowing and endplate erosion in the early stages. MRI should confirm the diagnosis.

Effective treatment has been controversial.[13] The authors recommend placing the patient at bed rest acutely and immobilization of the lumbar spine using a brace or corset. If the patient experiences progressive pain after adequate immobilization or has constitutional symptoms, a needle aspiration biopsy should be performed. If a bacterial organism is identified, 6 weeks of intravenous antibiotics is indicated. There is no need for open disk space biopsy provided the patient responds to conservative therapy. With improvement of symptoms and laboratory findings the patient may ambulate as tolerated.

TUMORS OF THE SPINE

The overwhelming majority of neoplastic afflictions of the spine are metastatic. The skeleton is the third most common site of metastatic deposit, and the spine is the most common skeletal location for metastatic disease. It has been estimated that up to 70% of patients with disseminated cancer will have evidence of skeletal metastasis on autopsy, and symptomatic metastatic disease of the spine is the most frequent clinically significant manifestation.[79] Primary tumors of the spine, on the other hand, are exceedingly rare. Their occurrence, however, extends over the entire age spectrum, and pain, deformity, and paralysis can occur as a result of either benign or malignant primary neoplasms. For this reason, despite their relatively infrequent appearance, these lesions merit review.

Pain is the most common presenting complaint of patients with a tumor of the spine. Back pain almost always precedes neurologic involvement, and a common progression of back pain, followed by radicular pain, followed by cord compression and dysfunction is seen. Other than the age of the patient, very little in history or physical examination serves to differentiate the presence of a primary from a metastatic tumor. Historical points that should serve to alert the physician to the possibility of metastatic disease as the cause for a patient's pain include age over 50; constitutional symptoms such as unexplained weight loss, fever, etc.; night pain; and a history of prior malignancy. Specific questioning about a previous diagnosis of cancer is necessary even though many would assume such infor-

mation to be an obvious point in routine questioning about past medical history, and the treating physician should be aware of the distinct possibility of late presentation of skeletal metastases, particularly in cancer of the breast.

When evaluating the patient with a known primary lesion of the spine, some generalizations can be made regarding the differentiation between benign and malignant disease. Younger patients are more likely to have a benign spinal neoplasm whereas, after the age of 21, over 70% of primary tumors are malignant.[151] As the age group extends into older patients, it becomes apparent that the risk of malignancy, either primary or secondary, is markedly increased in adults in general. The location of the lesion also gives a clue as to its histology. Most lesions of the vertebral body are malignant, including primary and metastatic tumors, whereas disease involving the posterior elements is more likely to be benign.[151]

Evaluation of the patient with a possible spinal tumor begins with the history, concentrating on the points just described. Careful questioning about the location and extent of the pain as well as activities and positions that exacerbate and ameliorate the symptoms is essential. In addition, constitutional symptoms are reviewed, and questioning about bowel and bladder function is carried out; bowel and bladder dysfunction may be seen in cases of cord compression and may, on occasion, precede back pain.[66] On physical examination tenderness, spasm, deformity, and the presence of a mass are sought. Most important, a careful neurologic examination is performed. This assessment must include sensory and motor testing in the extremities as well as sensory pinprick testing along the trunk to determine a subtle sensory pinprick level. The presence or absence of upper motor neuron findings should be ascertained.

Radiographic evaluation includes plain films, scintigraphy, CT scanning, and MRI. Plain radiographs are routinely obtained, although they are relatively insensitive to the presence of either primary or secondary neoplasm. Plain film findings that may be present include pathologic compression fracture, lysis of a vertebral body, or deformity. On AP views, involvement of the pedicle, with destruction of its cortical bone, may lead to the "winking owl sign" (Fig. 18–28). Although most metastatic lesions arise from the vertebral body, it has been well documented that plain radiographic evidence of bony destruction in the vertebral body is not apparent until somewhere between 30 and 50% of the trabecular bone has been destroyed.[51] In many cases, the tumor spreads before this point into the pedicle, where destruction of the mostly cortical bone leads to early radiographic identification of the absent pedicle.

Technetium-99 bone scanning is a highly sensitive test for screening the skeleton for metastatic or any neoplastic disease. Although relatively nonspecific in differentiating tumor from infection or fracture, routine bone scanning is used as a surveillance method, with certain malignancies, to detect early metastases. In addition, the patient with a known pathologic fracture, either secondary to osteopenia or a neoplasm, may benefit from whole body bone scanning to see if there are other lesions that would confirm the presence of widespread metastases and might identify, where necessary, a more suitable source for biopsy.[35, 37]

CT scanning, often in conjunction with myelography,

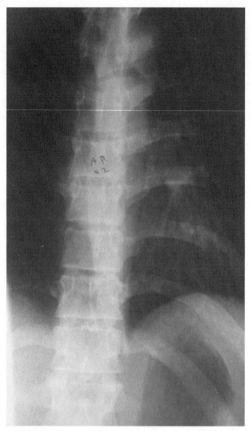

Figure 18–28. A 42-year-old man with a giant cell tumor of the spine. Unilateral absence of the pedicle is seen at T10 on this AP radiograph.

can be used to more clearly delineate the cross-sectional bony anatomy, compression on the cord or cauda equina, and the presence of a soft tissue mass. MRI has largely supplanted CT in the evaluation of most metastatic disease of the spine, but CT can be very helpful in evaluating primary tumors, particularly those involving the posterior elements, and most clearly defines the pathologic anatomy (Fig. 18–29).

MRI has truly evolved as the gold standard for imaging tumors of the spine. Advantages include the lack of ionizing radiation, noninvasiveness, and the ability to identify marrow replacement patterns, soft tissue masses, and neurologic compression.[67] Newer techniques of MRI suggest that it is now the most sensitive means of evaluating neoplastic disease of the spine, and it is certainly the most specific modality for differentiating tumor from infection.[4] This common question is resolved, primarily, by involvement of the disk. Relatively resistant to metastatic spread, the disk is typically spared on plain radiography as well as on MRI in cases of metastatic diseases (Fig. 18–30). On the other hand, infection, which usually arises in the vertebral body, rapidly spreads into the disk, and extensive destruction of the disk is commonly seen on plain radiographic and MRI.

Primary Spine Tumors

Primary tumors of the spine can be differentiated on the basis of tissue origin, location, and age of the patient. Soft

tissue or bony tumors may be seen, and these lesions may arise primarily in the vertebral body or in the posterior elements. In addition, the age of the patient has been demonstrated in several series to provide predictive value as to whether a benign or malignant tumor is present, with adults much more likely to suffer from primary malignancy than are children.[151]

Benign tumors of the spine arise primarily in the posterior elements. Osteoblastoma and osteoid osteoma are benign lesions that commonly arise in the spine, almost always in the posterior elements. These lesions usually occur in adolescence or young adulthood and present as back pain, usually unrelated to activity.[103] Radiographic demonstration, particularly for the smaller osteoid osteoma, may be difficult. When this lesion is suspected, technetium bone scanning enables localization of the lesion which is then better defined on CT scanning. Osteoblastomas are by definition larger than 2 cm and are usually identifiable on plain radiography, although best defined on CT. Either osteoblastoma or osteoid osteoma can result in painful scoliosis and should be considered when pain is the presenting complaint in a patient with spinal deformity.

Excision is the preferred treatment for osteoid osteoma and for osteoblastoma. Intralesional curettage and bone grafting as needed results in excellent pain relief with minimal risk of recurrence.[68, 103] On occasion, an osteoblastoma will destroy enough of the posterior arch and associated facet joint so as to require stabilization, particularly when seen at the thoracolumbar junction, but this is relatively uncommon. Finally, when recognized early, painful scoliosis resulting from the presence of an osteoblastoma or osteoid osteoma will usually resolve. Pettine and Klassen demonstrated that, when the lesion had been symptomatic for 15 months or less, most patients saw resolution of their scoliosis, whereas with symptoms of longer standing improvement was not seen.[120]

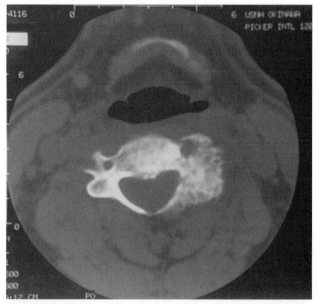

Figure 18–29. CT scan of a chondrosarcoma, clearly illustrating involvement of the lamina, lateral mass, and spread into the vertebral body of C5.

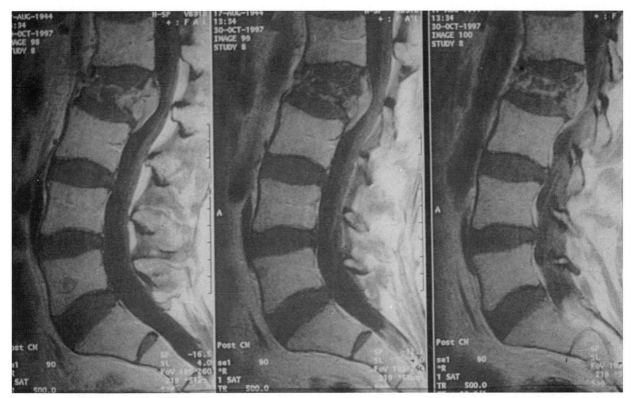

Figure 18–30. Metastatic adenocarcinoma of the colon with L2 pathologic fracture. MRI shows extent of the destruction of L2 but preservation of the disks.

Aneurysmal bone cyst (ABC) is a less common lesion affecting the spine. A lytic, at times fairly extensive lesion is seen radiographically, and the patients typically present with pain. More than one level may be involved. Most lesions arise in the posterior elements, but up to 40% extend into the vertebral body (Fig. 18–31). Treatment involves excision which, in many cases, consists of intralesional curettage. Recurrence is treated with repeat curettage.

At autopsy, approximately 10% of individuals will have evidence of hemangioma somewhere in the spinal column. The correlation between the presence of a hemangioma and back pain is therefore uncertain. The diagnosis of vertebral body hemangioma is typically made on plain radiographs, in which increased trabecular striations and a "jailhouse vertebrae" appearance may be seen. Differentiation from Paget's disease, wherein the vertebral body will actually be enlarged, should be possible on plain radiography. CT and MRI scan will show, on axial images, a punctate appearance to the thickened trabeculae (Fig. 18–32). Occasionally a hemangioma will present with a soft tissue mass, although neurologic impairment is rare. Symptomatic treatment of the patient's back pain usually suffices. In cases in which a hemangioma was believed to be symptomatic we have had success with alcohol sclerotherapy. In addition, radiation treatment has been suggested for refractory pain. Because of the risk of hemorrhage, surgery should be reserved for cases with pathologic fracture and neurologic injury and preoperative embolization considered if possible.

Giant cell tumor is occasionally seen in the spine and typically involves young adults. Usually arising in the vertebral body, extensive destruction and expansion of the bone may be seen.[41] Pain is the most common presenting complaint, but neurologic impairment may ensue. MRI is vital in demonstrating the extent of disease and in helping to guide surgical treatment which, when possible, consists of complete excision and reconstruction, usually through an anterior approach. Savini and associates have reported on the treatment of giant cell tumor of the spine, and although the biologic rationale is unclear they have suggested that this disease behaves more favorably in the spine than in the extremities. Most authors advise against adjuvant radiation following adequate first-time excision.[132]

Primary Malignant Neoplasms of the Spine

Hematogenous malignancies of the spine include multiple myeloma, plasmacytoma, and lymphoma. Multiple myeloma and plasmacytoma represent two ends of a spectrum of B-cell lymphoproliferative disease.[38] Solitary plasmacytoma involves an isolated lesion which commonly occurs in the spine, whereas in multiple myeloma, as the name implies, the disease is disseminated and the prognosis bleak. Anemia is common with multiple myeloma, and the presence of an osteopenic compression fracture in a patient who is anemic should alert the physician to the possibility of myeloma. Although plasmacytoma is considered a precursor to disseminated myeloma, the natural history is significantly better; McLain and Weinstein reported a 5-year survival rate of 60% of patients with solitary plasmacytoma of the spine, whereas the 5-year survival rate in patients with multiple myeloma was only 18%.[111] Local treatment of these lesions consists of radiation in most

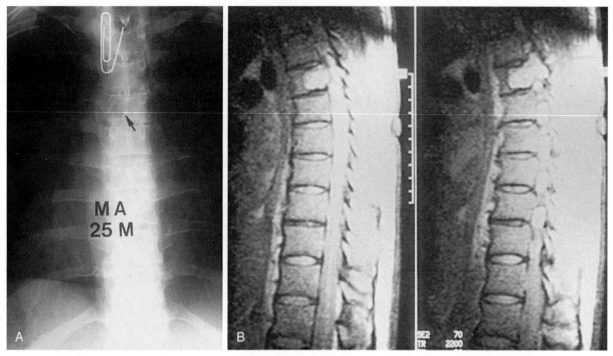

Figure 18–31. A 25-year-old graduate student with thoracic back pain, particularly severe at rest. AP radiograph *(A)* demonstrates the absent pedicle *(arrow)*, and MRI *(B)* shows the involvement of the tumor, and aneurysmal bone cyst, in both the posterior arch and the vertebral body.

cases. The exquisite radiosensitivity of this condition usually renders operative treatment unnecessary, and surgery is reserved for pathologic fracture with spinal instability or neurologic deficit that worsens despite radiation. Mild or moderate degrees of cord compromise due to soft tissue spread of myeloma can usually be treated with radiation.

Lymphoma, either primary or metastatic, can occur as an isolated spinal lesion. Approximately 10% of cases of lymphoma of bone, either primary or secondary, involve the spine with a predilection for the thoracic spine. Local treatment consists of radiotherapy with adjuvant chemo-

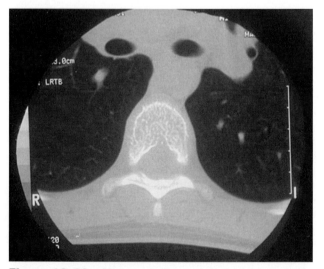

Figure 18–32. CT scan showing typical appearance of a vertebral hemangioma.

therapy if multifocal disease is present. Surgery is reserved for cases of pathologic fracture with instability or neurologic compromise not responding to radiation therapy.

The spine is a rare site for primary osteogenic sarcoma, and treatment of osteosarcoma in this location represents a particularly challenging undertaking. In a review of 27 patients from the Mayo Clinic, Shives and colleagues reported a mean survival of 10 months with only one patient surviving longer than 5 years. Most cases arise in the vertebral body with, at times, extensive soft tissue masses seen. Although the prognosis is poor, an aggressive attempt at en bloc excision and reconstruction, followed by adjuvant therapy, is advocated by the Mayo Clinic group.[138]

As with osteogenic sarcoma, Ewing's sarcoma is occasionally seen in the spine. This disease also demonstrates a predilection for the vertebral body and is most common in the sacrum. The radiosensitivity of Ewing's sarcoma makes high-dose radiotherapy, with adjuvant chemotherapy, the treatment of choice for most lesions. Surgery is undertaken for pathologic fracture with instability or pathologic fracture leading to neurologic impairment. Although better than for osteosarcoma, the prognosis for patients with Ewing's sarcoma of the spine is worse than for extremity disease, and long-term disease-free survival is relatively rare.[125]

Chordoma is a slow-growing malignancy arising from residual notochord in the midline of the spine and skull base. These tumors are most common in the sacrum and the clivus but can be seen in the lumbar, thoracic, or cervical spine also. While the tumor is indolent symptoms develop slowly, and patients frequently have a large paraspinal or presacral mass present at the time of diagnosis. True cure of the patient with chordoma is rare, but long-term survival can be achieved with local disease control. Aggressive surgical excision should be undertaken, even if sacrifice of sacral nerve roots is the price;[115] functional disability related to sacral nerve root resection has been acceptable in most series when compared to the prospect of disease control.

Metastatic Disease of the Spine

The overwhelming majority of spinal tumors represent metastatic lesions, particularly in patients over the age of 40. A history of persistent back pain, unrelieved by rest, particularly in a patient with a known history of cancer should alert the physician to the possibility of a metastatic deposit in the spine. Primary malignancies that most commonly metastasize to bone, and therefore to the spine, include breast, lung, prostate, kidney, and thyroid cancer. Advances in supportive care for patients with these and other types of malignancies, as well as advances in awareness, imaging, and surgical technique have increased greatly the number of patients presenting for surgical treatment of metastatic disease of the spine.

Approximately 90% of metastatic deposits in the spine originate in the vertebral body where the trabecular bone acts as a filter to blood-borne metastases. It is hypothesized that the red marrow of the trabecular bone of the vertebral body provides a favorable environment for deposition and proliferation of tumor. Once deposited, tumor cells are capable of forming a protective fibrin sheath and of secreting osteoclast activating factors and possibly lytic prostaglandins, which furthers their spread.[60] Patients present primarily with pain which, according to Harrington, may be due to cortical expansion with microfracturing and invasion of paravertebral soft tissues, compression of adjacent nerve roots, pathologic fracture with instability, or compression of the spinal cord.[57] The history of pain in a patient with a prior diagnosis of cancer should be viewed as worrisome, even with a remote history of a malignancy presumed to be cured; this is particularly true for carcinoma of the breast.

The diagnosis of metastatic disease of the spine is made radiographically and confirmed by the pathologist. Plain films, as discussed earlier, are relatively insensitive because of the extent of vertebral body destruction that is necessary before a radiographic abnormality is seen.[51] The test of choice is MRI. MRI demonstrates early lesions, accurately defines soft tissue spread, images neural compression, and is extremely specific in differentiating metastatic disease from infection.[4] One common quandary, for which MRI is the most helpful noninvasive modality, is differentiating a pathologic fracture caused by osteopenia from metastatic disease. In our experience most pathologic fractures caused by metastatic deposits are seen with a pattern of diffuse marrow replacement, have involvement at more than one level, or are seen with an associated paraspinal soft tissue mass. The absence of all three of these findings, although not completely reliable in excluding metastatic disease, is reassuring and usually will lead us to recommend against biopsy.

Treatment

Treatment of metastatic disease of the spine may be systemic, local, or both. Systemic treatment consists usually of chemotherapy, as appropriate for the involved tumor. Patients whose disease is amenable to chemotherapy alone rarely come under the treatment of an orthopaedic surgeon, but chemotherapy as the primary mode of treatment should be considered for cancers such as prostate or breast in which metastatic deposit is seen without collapse or neurologic compromise, or for certain hematopoietic malignancies.

Local treatment may consist of radiotherapy, bracing, or surgery. Radiotherapy is the treatment of choice for the large majority of metastatic lesions of the spine. The efficacy of radiotherapy is highly dependent on the radiosensitivity of the tumor present. The most radiosensitive tumors, such as myeloma, lymphoma, Ewing's sarcoma, and to a lesser extent carcinoma of the breast, respond highly favorably to radiotherapy, which should be considered in virtually all such cases unless clear-cut spinal instability is present.[66] On the other hand, radioresistant lesions such as carcinoma of the lung or prostate, GI cancers, or renal cell carcinoma have a much less favorable response to radiotherapy, and surgery should be undertaken, in these diseases, if there is vertebral collapse with pain, borderline instability, or impending neurologic compromise. Obviously, this relatively aggressive surgical approach would be tempered by the overall extent of patient disease, associated medical problems, and the presence of multiple levels of spinal involvement.

Bracing may be used as an adjunct to radiotherapy. Custom-molded thoracolumbosacral or lumbosacral orthoses frequently provide excellent short-term pain relief and may be particularly advantageous in patients with limited life expectancy. Halo vest immobilization should be considered in patients with radiosensitive metastatic lesions in the cervical spine where short-term prophylaxis against neurologic catastrophe is needed, pending disease ablation with either radiotherapy or chemotherapy.

The final method for local treatment is surgery. The indications for surgical intervention in metastatic disease of the spine include (1) the need for tissue for diagnosis; (2) a radioresistant tumor with local collapse or impending neurologic impairment; (3) persistent or recurrent pain or neurologic deficit despite radiotherapy; (4) neurologic deterioration during radiotherapy; (5) neurologic deficit due to bone or disk retropulsion; and (6) spinal instability, either present or impending.[57] All but item 6 are relatively straightforward. The definition of spinal instability in metastatic disease is the source of significant debate.[27, 47, 57] We feel that lesions that result in greater than 50% collapse of the vertebral body, particularly at the thoracolumbar junction, any translational deformity on either AP or lateral radiographs (Fig. 18–33), segmental kyphosis of greater than 20 degrees above that expected at the involved level, and lesions that involve both the anterior and posterior columns should be considered potentially unstable. A highly radiosensitive tumor fulfilling one of those criteria is occasionally treated first with radiotherapy, but otherwise surgery is most likely to preserve neurologic function, relieve pain, and preserve overall function while minimizing the risk of operating through previously radiated tissue.

The surgical approach can be either anterior, posterior, or combined. Because most metastatic lesions arise anteriorly and result in destruction of the anterior column of the

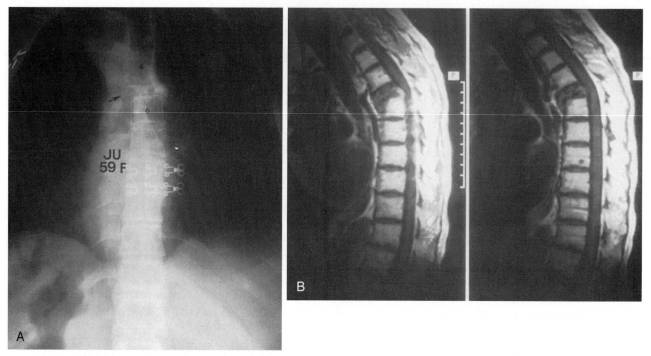

Figure 18–33. A 59-year-old woman with metastatic breast cancer and thoracic back pain. AP radiograph *(A)* demonstrates lateral translation and destruction of T5, which is diagnostic of instability. MRI *(B)* confirms the extent of destruction and collapse in the sagittal plane.

spine, with anterior cord or cauda equina compression, our preferred approach is usually anterior. This approach allows safe and thorough decompression of the spinal canal as well as mechanically sound reconstruction of the anterior column of the spine.[78, 139, 147] Reconstruction can be performed utilizing polymethyl methacrylate (PMMA), bone grafting, or prefabricated cages, such as the Harms cage, which can then be filled with either PMMA or bone. The structural anterior column replacement can be supplemented with anterior instrumentation such as the Kaneda device or specially designed anterior plates. The majority of patients treated in this manner can be managed with an anterior approach alone, eliminating the need for posterior surgery (Fig. 18–34).

Another surgical approach is posterior. Laminectomy alone is relatively inefficient at decompressing the spinal canal and should be avoided in most cases.[75] On the other hand, posterolateral decompression, gaining access to the anterior aspect of the spine by resecting the pedicle, has been reported to have results comparable to the anterior approach in terms of morbidity rate, mortality rate, pain relief, and functional restoration. Bridwell and coworkers have defined the indications for a posterolateral approach, including posterolateral decompression and stabilization with segmental instrumentation, as the presence of translational instability, involvement of more than two vertebral levels, the presence of disease at two separate locations in the spine, and a patient unable to tolerate an anterior procedure.[27] In addition, they advocate the posterolateral approach in cases of circumferential, anterior, and posterior column disease with "napkin ring" constriction of the spinal cord or cauda equina. We believe, however, that clear-cut destruction of both the anterior and posterior

columns with circumferential neural compression is best suited to a combined anterior and posterior approach, allowing thorough decompression and optimal mechanical reconstruction of both the anterior and posterior columns (Fig. 18–35).

Only recently has aggressive surgical treatment of spinal metastases gained wide acceptance. Previous reports of the use of laminectomy for metastatic disease identified an exceedingly high complication rate, including neurologic worsening, with very few patients gaining function or obtaining long-lasting pain relief. Modern techniques of surgery, including either posterolateral or anterior decompression and stabilization, provide clear-cut advantages. Cybulski recently reviewed surgical stabilization for metastatic disease and compared posterolateral to anterior surgery. His meta-analysis of several large series demonstrated 74% neurologic improvement, 85% pain relief, and a combined 7% morbidity and mortality rate for posterolateral decompression and stabilization, but anterior vertebrectomy and reconstruction resulted in 70% neurologic improvement, 84% pain relief, and an 8% morbidity and mortality rate.[40] This reflects our experience that, in the properly selected patient, surgical treatment of metastatic disease of the spine is highly predictable for pain relief, restoration and protection of neurologic function, and an acceptably low complication rate.

SPINE INFECTION

Infections of the spine occupy a perversely important place in the history of orthopaedic surgery in general and spine surgery in particular. Percival Pott's description of spinal

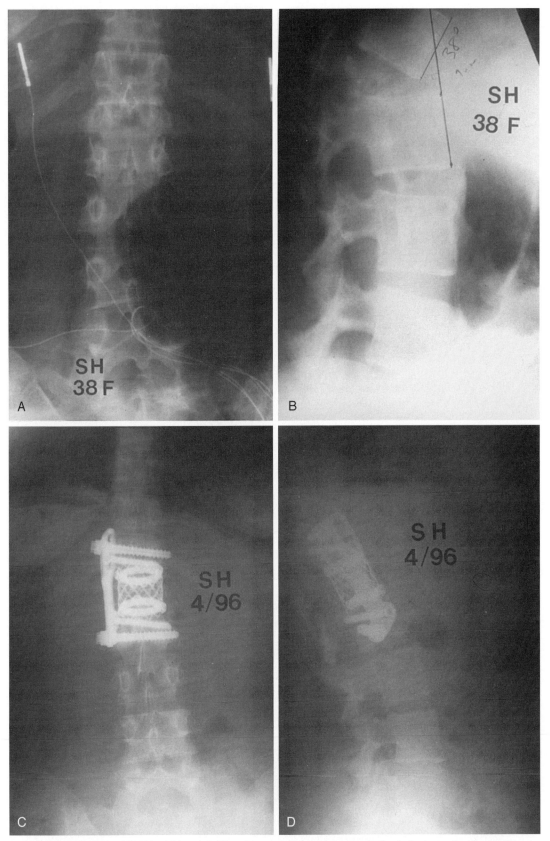

Figure 18–34. AP *(A)* and lateral *(B)* radiographs showing a pathologic fracture and instability in a 38-year-old woman with lymphoma, 2 years after undergoing irradiation. Through a thoracoabdominal exposure, L1 vertebrectomy was performed, and reconstruction was carried out using a titanium-mesh cage with autograft and allograft and supplemented with plate fixation. She had complete relief of her pain and survived for 13 months.

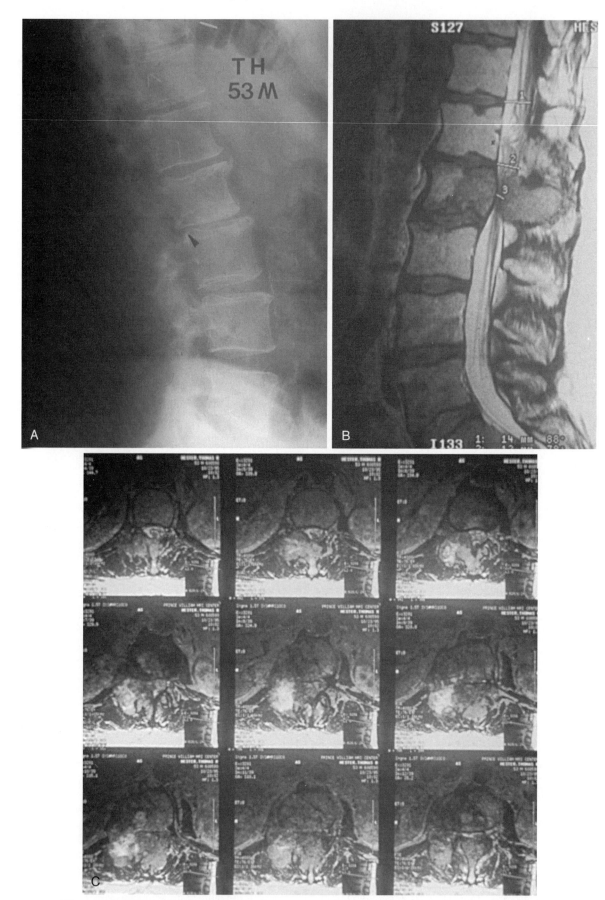

Figure 18–35. Lateral radiograph *(A)* of a 53-year-old man with metastatic hypernephroma. MRI *(B and C)* demonstrate extensive involvement of both the anterior and posterior columns.

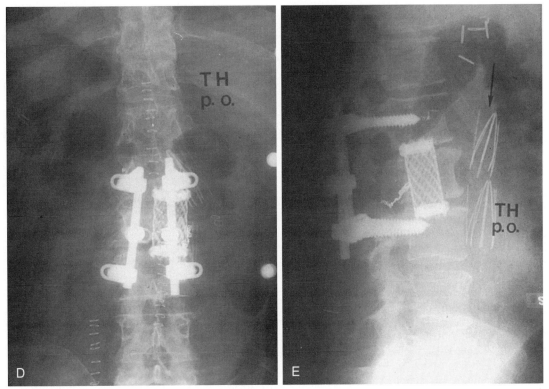

Figure 18–35 *Continued.* He underwent anterior resection and reconstruction followed by posterior decompression and transpedicular stabilization (*D and E*).

tuberculosis and associated paralysis gave rise to the enduring eponym "Pott's paraplegia." Many of this century's seminal advances in spine surgery, including the development of posterior fusion of the spine by Hibbs[83] and Albee[3] related to the treatment of tuberculous spondylitis. Hodgson pioneered anterior surgery of the spine, currently in widespread use for numerous conditions, as treatment for spinal tuberculosis.[85] We now see infections of the spine in numerous settings and caused by a variety of organisms, but despite significant technologic and medical advances in our treatment, the underlying principles of the treatment of infection of the spine are still based largely on the lessons learned from tuberculosis.

Pyogenic Infection

The incidence of pyogenic vertebral osteomyelitis appears to be increasing with an increase in medical and social conditions that lead to immunosuppression. The spine is the site for up to 7% of all cases of osteomyelitis and certainly is the area with the greatest potential for morbidity and, even at this time, death. Although infection of the spine may occur in any age group, there appear to be two peaks; children and adolescents are at risk for a unique form of blood-borne diskitis, and after the age of 50, the risk of infection of the spine again increases. Most, but not all, cases of vertebral osteomyelitis occur in an immunosuppressed patient. Immunosuppressive disorders such as rheumatoid arthritis and diabetes, the use of immunosuppressive medication following transplant surgery, immunosuppressive states such as AIDS, and a history of IV drug abuse are all frequently associated with spine infection.

Approximately 50% of patients with an infection of the spine will give a history of a preceding infection elsewhere; the most common sites of these infections include the genitourinary tract, the skin and soft tissues, and upper respiratory tract.[30, 39, 81] It is not uncommon to obtain a history of a partially treated infection, which further complicates matters. Trauma, once believed to be a predisposing factor, does not play a significant role.

The causative organism seen in most infections of the spine have evolved over time. In the preantibiotic era, *Staphylococcus aureus* predominated. More recently, the incidence of *S. aureus* has dropped significantly, particularly in series involving large numbers of IV drug abusers with an associated increase in gram-negative infections. Of note is the finding of significant numbers of spine infections caused by low virulence organisms such as *Staphylococcus epidermidis* and *Streptococcus* species.[30] Whatever the organism, the overwhelming majority of spinal infections occur via a hematogenous route. The disk itself is avascular in the adult, but a rich arterial anastomotic network in the metaphyseal region of the vertebral body has been demonstrated by Wiley and Trueta.[157] As in the metaphysis of the tibia or other long bones, bacterial deposition in this region of the vertebral body appears to be the first step in infection of the spine. The growing abscess penetrates through the endplate into the avascular disk, which is rapidly destroyed, allowing the infection to then travel into the adjacent vertebral body. The well-known sequelae of disk destruction, collapse, deformity, and paraspinal and epidural abscess formation ensue, with associated morbidity.

The primary manifestations of pyogenic infection of the

spine include pain, neurologic impairment, and signs and symptoms of sepsis. The most common complaint is pain. Carragee recently reviewed a large series of patients and found that over 90% presented with back pain.[30] A number of authors have demonstrated the tendency toward delay in diagnosis; as many as 50% of patients have pain for 3 months or longer prior to the correct diagnosis of spinal sepsis,[128] although greater awareness and improved imaging techniques appear to be lessening this problem. Fever is less common than pain, and is seen only in about one half of patients with osteomyelitis of the spine. From 15 to 20% of patients will present with evidence of neurologic involvement. Eismont and colleagues have identified several factors predisposing to the development of neurologic sequelae, including diabetes, rheumatoid arthritis, increasing age, and a more cephalad level of involvement.[52] Finally, approximately 15% of patients will present with atypical symptoms such as hip pain, abdominal or chest pain, or testicular discomfort. These atypical complaints are more common in infections in the lumbar spine and contribute significantly to prolonged delay in diagnosis.[8]

The importance of recognizing the patient at risk for spinal infection as well as recognizing the common presenting complaints is highlighted by the paucity of specific physical findings suggesting infection. Abscesses are now quite rare in this condition, but are seen more commonly in infections of the cervical or thoracic spine. Significant paraspinal spasm may be seen, and pain on percussion in the midline, at the affected level, is the most specific finding. Laboratory testing should be undertaken whenever infection is suspected but may further confuse the clinical picture. Elevation of the white blood cell count is seen in less than 50% of patients and, when present, is usually mild. The most useful test is the erythrocyte sedimentation rate (ESR).[128] The ESR is elevated in over 90% of patients with documented osteomyelitis of the spine, frequently markedly so. Although the ESR is a nonspecific test, significant elevation in the patient with back pain must be viewed as a potential warning of a serious underlying condition.[33] The C-reactive protein level is also frequently elevated, but its diagnostic use in this condition is not as well documented in the literature as that of the ESR.[149]

Appropriate radiographic evaluation will suggest the presence of infection in most cases. Unfortunately, plain radiographs are relatively insensitive in early infections of the spine, and normal routine x-rays of the back are of limited value. The most common early finding, frequently seen only retrospectively, is soft tissue swelling including loss of the psoas shadow or widening of the retropharyngeal clear space in the neck. Three to four weeks following the establishment of infection, disk space narrowing may be seen.[65] Although disk space narrowing can be due to a number of causes, irregularity and destruction of the bony endplate are not present in degenerative disorders of the spine and should heighten suspicion of infection. Finally, at about 6 weeks, destructive changes in the vertebral body, including collapse and lysis anteriorly, are seen (Fig. 18–36).

Scintigraphy offers a more sensitive way to detect infection of the spine in a timely fashion. Technetium scanning, gallium scanning, or combinations of the two have been advocated.[73] Combined technetium and gallium scanning

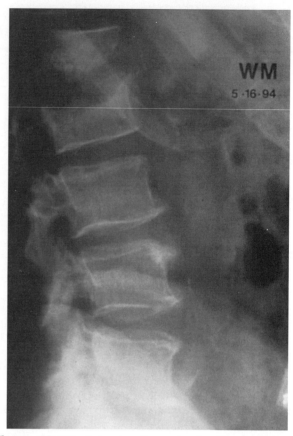

Figure 18–36. Lateral radiograph of a 74-year-old man with a 2-month history of back pain demonstrating endplate destruction and collapse characteristic of vertebral osteomyelitis and diskitis.

has been demonstrated to have an overall accuracy of 94% in diagnosing infection of the spine.[39] Indium-111–labeled leukocyte scanning has been advocated for use in evaluating musculoskeletal sepsis but appears to be less sensitive, in infection of the spine, than more traditional technetium and gallium scanning.[160]

In our practice the imaging modality of choice is MRI. Some of the advantages of MRI have been discussed. MRI may be more sensitive than scintigraphy in the detection of early spine infections and has the advantage of clearly defining associated pathology such as abscess formation, cord or cauda equina compression, etc. Because a positive or even equivocal bone scan will almost always lead to ordering an MRI, our practice is to utilize this test initially when infection of the spine is suspected.[32]

A characteristic MRI picture is seen in vertebral osteomyelitis. We rely most heavily on the T2-weighted images, wherein increased signal is seen in the disk space as well as involved areas of the vertebral bodies. This is more striking following the administration of gadolinium. The most significant finding is the increased signal in the disk space, which clearly differentiates infection from degenerative change. MRI distinctly defines disk and endplate destruction, enabling distinction between infection and tumor of the spine (Fig. 18–37).[4] Overall MRI, although not 100% accurate, is the most sensitive and most specific

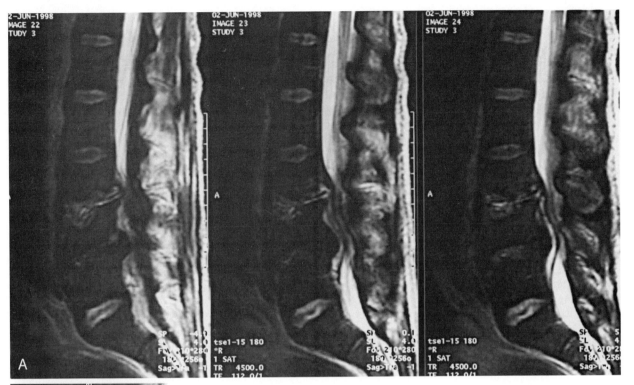

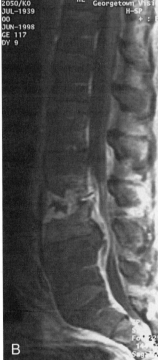

Figure 18–37. A 59-year-old man with end stage renal disease, back pain, and leg pain. *A,* A T2-weighted MRI shows increased signal at the L3–4 disk with destructive changes in the endplates, diagnostic of infection. Questionable changes are seen at L4–5, but *B,* a T1-weighted study after gadolinium injection, shows enhancement at L3–4 but not at L4–5, demonstrating the presence of infection at L3–4 only.

modality in the diagnosis of pyogenic vertebral osteomyelitis.

Before treatment is initiated, laboratory confirmation of the presence of infection and the causative organism should be sought. Confirmation by a positive culture from the spine, the blood, or less desirably the urinary tract is preferable to beginning empiric antibiotic therapy unless systemic sepsis is present. Biopsy of the spine can usually be performed via a percutaneous approach. Fluoroscopy and, when needed, CT guidance allows for minimally invasive access to the entire spine and have been reported to lead to accurate diagnosis in 68 to 86% of cases of vertebral osteomyelitis.[39] When initial percutaneous aspiration does not result in positive culture or histopathologic findings, the decision must then be made about the next step in evaluation and treatment. In our practice, only rarely is empiric medical management undertaken at this stage. We find it helpful to consult with our interventional radiologists to see if they believe that another attempt at biopsy is likely to be more rewarding; if not, we typically proceed with open biopsy and definitive débridement as discussed below.

Treatment of pyogenic vertebral osteomyelitis can be medical or surgical. The type and duration of medical treatment are dictated by the causative organism cultured. Because of the continuous evolution in available antibiotics, we routinely utilize infectious disease consultation to select the agent used. It should be noted that cephalosporin penetration into the nucleus pulposis is less effective than that of bone and, in most cases, the use of an aminoglycoside should be considered.[53] We favor the use of parenteral antibiotics for 6 weeks followed by the use of oral antibiotics, when available, for at least another 6 weeks. When medical management of vertebral osteomyelitis is undertaken, it should be appreciated that a protracted course of treatment is necessary before symptomatic resolution can be expected and we have found that extending treatment for a total of 3 months leads to increased success. Response to treatment can be monitored by response of the ESR.[53, 129] Weekly ESR monitoring for the first 3 to 4 weeks followed by monthly testing until a return to normal is seen will document response of the infection to treatment.

Antibiotic treatment of spinal infections is accompanied by immobilization. The hospitalized patient is usually placed at bed rest for several days and then mobilized, as symptoms allow, in a custom-molded or custom-made orthosis. Ambulatory patients diagnosed in the outpatient setting, now seen with increasing frequency, are not placed at bed rest but are placed into a custom-molded thoracolumbosacral orthosis (TLSO) or cervicothoracic orthosis, depending on the level of involvement.

The indications for surgery include the need for tissue for diagnosis, the presence of significant destruction or deformity, failure of medical management, neurologic deficit caused by spinal cord compression by either abscess, disk, or bone, and the presence of a clinically significant paraspinal or epidural abscess. Each of these indications is somewhat subjective and open to interpretation. As noted, we believe strongly in the need for a bacteriologic diagnosis whenever possible, and when minimally invasive techniques fail we prefer definitive surgical treatment as a means of obtaining tissue, rather than a limited open technique performed under general anesthesia. The extent of bony destruction or deformity leading to the need for surgical treatment has not been clearly defined; it is important when evaluating the patient with a possible neurologic deficit to recognize the extent to which kyphosis can contribute to compression of the spinal cord and cauda equina. Progressive kyphosis with retropulsion of disk or bone will not respond to bracing or antibiotics and should be promptly recognized and treated surgically. Failure of medical management requires the correlation of a number of factors. In the patient with minimal anterior column destruction who is neurologically normal without evidence of abscess formation, we favor a minimum of 4 weeks of antibiotic treatment along with rest followed by bracing. At that time, absence of a significant decrease in the patient's pain as well as the ESR would lead to consideration of either repeat biopsy to ensure that the proper organism is being treated, or definitive surgical treatment.

The significance of the radiographic appearance of abscess formation should be mentioned. The presence of a soft tissue mass in the paraspinal or epidural space is usually not, in our experience, evidence of pus under pressure. Although frequently a large paraspinal or epidural mass is present in a patient with significant destruction or neurologic compromise, in the absence of these more concrete surgical indications we typically prefer to undertake nonoperative treatment and closely follow the patient's clinical course. Awareness of the previously described risk factors for neurologic injury, including increasing age, immunosuppression, and involvement in the cervical spine facilitates appropriate decision making in this setting.[52]

Vertebral osteomyelitis is a disease of the anterior column, involving destruction of vertebral body and disk, kyphotic deformity, and the presence anteriorly of an infected soft tissue mass capable of causing spinal cord injury. It is axiomatic, therefore, that surgical treatment should approach this disease directly. The anterior approach to the spine was pioneered, by Hodgson, for the treatment of tuberculous spondylitis and is still favored in almost all cases of infection.[54, 84] With the exception of limited posterior or posterolateral approaches for biopsy, there is little advantage in an isolated posterior approach for either decompression or stabilization. Laminectomy has been demonstrated to destabilize the infected spine and is in most cases inadequate for decompressing anterior pathology.[52] Thorough débridement of the infection is rarely possible through a posterior approach, even when dissecting anteriorly to gain access to the anterior column. Finally, posterior stabilization of the spine, without mechanically sound reconstruction of the anterior column, is at significant risk for long-term failure in a patient who may well have a normal life expectancy otherwise.

The anterior approach to the cervical, thoracic, or lumbar spine lends itself ideally to thorough surgical débridement, decompression of the spinal cord or cauda equina, and stabilization of the spine. Once débridement of the infection is carried out, and bleeding bone above and below the involved area is seen, autogenous strut grafting has been demonstrated to be safe and effective.[39, 54] Extending this concept to the use of titanium implants, such as mesh cages or plate and screw devices, has been proposed, but there is little in the way of long-term follow-up available.

Anterior stabilization alone, followed by casting or bracing, is usually sufficient for single-level involvement in which the kyphotic deformity can be mostly corrected. The authors reserve posterior stabilization for cases of multilevel disease or cases with residual kyphosis of 20 degrees or greater. This most typically occurs in long-standing infections at the thoracolumbar junction. When posterior stabilization is undertaken, most authors believe that the risk of secondary infection of the orthopaedic implants posteriorly is acceptable, and this has certainly been our experience.

The improvement in outcome seen following medical and surgical management of pyogenic vertebral osteomyelitis, compared to reports from the preantibiotic era, is striking. The risk of neurologic deficit, in the absence of one of the above-described risk factors, is quite low, and patients undergoing anterior débridement and decompression have between a 50 and 100% chance of normal or near-normal function at final follow-up. Nonoperative treatment as outlined previously is successful in the majority of patients, particularly in those who are not immunocompromised, and surgical treatment has a success rate of over 90 to 95% in terms of obtaining solid bony fusion and pain relief.[54] In short, modern surgical and medical techniques have almost completely eliminated the risk of death, in the absence of failure of other organ systems, lead to predictably good rates of healing of the spine with good relief of pain, and lead to predictable improvement in neurologic function when impaired.

Tuberculosis of the Spine

Tuberculosis and tuberculous spondylitis are still common in many developing countries and appear to be increasing again in frequency in the industrialized world, including the United States. In the Western world tuberculosis is primarily a disease of adults, while in Asia and Africa significant numbers of children are affected. It has been estimated that as many as 5% of patients with tuberculosis develop tuberculosis in the spine, with a neurologic deficit reported in 10 to 45% of these patients. The possibility of tuberculous spondylitis should be considered in any individual with persistent unexplained back pain, particularly in patients who have emigrated from, or have recently traveled to, underdeveloped areas of the world, or patients with chronic immunosuppressive disorders such as intravenous drug abuse or human immunodeficiency virus (HIV) infection.[14]

Tuberculous spondylitis usually develops from hematogenous spread, most commonly from the pulmonary system but also on occasion from the genitourinary tract or other sources in the skeleton. Initial inoculation of the spongiosa of the vertebral body leads to local spread of the disease. This spread has been described in several patterns including peridiskal, central, and anterior.[48] Peridiskal spread involves infection of one vertebral body extending out the anterior cortex and under the anterior longitudinal ligament to involve the adjacent body. A distinguishing characteristic of tuberculous spondylitis is the relative resistance of the disk to infection; relative sparing of the disk in the face of significant bony destruction may be seen, unlike pyogenic vertebral osteomyelitis, in which the epicenter of involvement is invariably at the disk space. Other less common patterns of involvement include central involvement, in which significant destruction of the vertebral body occurs without extension anteriorly or into either disk space. Vertebral collapse may occur, and these cases are radiographically similar to metastatic disease. Anterior "skip" lesions may also be seen where spread underneath the anterior longitudinal ligament extends over several segments. Anterior scalloping of each vertebral body is seen radiographically.[48] Only rarely seen are cases consisting of posterior element involvement alone or cases of intraspinal granuloma formation without bony involvement.

Patients with tuberculous spondylitis typically complain of back pain and have evidence of chronic disease, including weight loss and intermittent fever. Local tenderness, muscle spasm, and restricted motion may be seen. Kyphosis, abscess formation, and draining sinuses, while at one time quite common, are now rarely seen in Western countries. Neurologic involvement is more common with more cephalad levels of involvement and has been reported in 10 to 47% of patients with tuberculous spondylitis.[39]

Although many patients with tuberculous spondylitis have been diagnosed previously with tuberculosis, it is certainly not uncommon for spinal involvement to lead to diagnosis. The purified protein derivative (PPD) test is nonspecific for the presence of active disease, but if results are negative, except in the presence of anergy, this finding speaks against tuberculosis. An elevated ESR is commonly seen but is nonspecific. In the authors' experience, an extremely high ESR, sometimes above 100 mm/min, is suggestive of tuberculosis as opposed to other types of vertebral osteomyelitis. Systemic workup of the patient involves chest radiography, which includes apical lordotic views, and culturing of urine, sputum, and gastric washings, and PPD placement.

Radiographic evidence of tuberculosis may be seen on plain films and confirmed on MRI (Fig. 18–38). Because of the relative resistance of the disk space to infection in tuberculosis more extensive bony destruction is commonly seen in this entity, prior to destruction of the disk space, than in pyogenic infection.[141] Vertebral body osteopenia is usually the earliest finding but may not be radiographically apparent until significant destruction has occurred.

As with pyogenic infection, MRI is the imaging modality of choice. MRI findings mirror the above-described pathologic picture, and the differences between pyogenic and tuberculous infection on MRI will therefore reflect the potential for extensive bony destruction before significant disk involvement, multilevel spread under the anterior longitudinal ligament, or central involvement mimicking a tumor. Tuberculous spondylitis is more likely than pyogenic vertebral osteomyelitis to result in extensive abscess formation, either in the paraspinal region or in the psoas (see Fig. 18–38).[141]

Beginning in 1943, chemotherapeutic treatment of tuberculous spondylitis, with the use of streptomycin, was proved to be effective as an adjunct to surgery, with a decline in mortality rate from as high as 72% to under 10% reported.[39] The subsequent introduction of isoniazid, rifampin, and more modern drugs led to attempts to treat this disorder without surgery, utilizing prolonged immobilization. In 1963 the Medical Research Council of Great Britain initiated a comparative study investigating the effi-

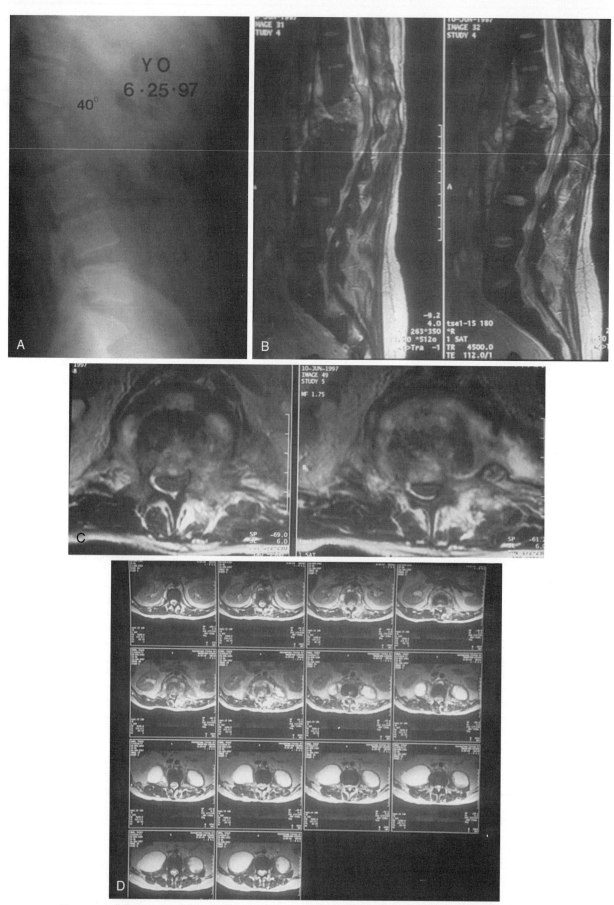

Figure 18–38. *A,* Lateral radiograph showing a pathologic fracture of L1 in a 32-year-old man from Somalia. Marked kyphosis with anterior collapse of L1, but relative preservation of the disks, is seen. *B and C* are MRIs, and a more distal MRI *(D)* shows massive psoas abscesses bilaterally.

498

cacy of various forms of treatment for spinal tuberculosis. This prospective series of trials, relying essentially on randomization by country, has been instrumental in leading to the widespread use of safer, more effective, and less invasive types of treatment, particularly in underdeveloped countries where any sort of spinal surgery entails significant risk. The utility of immobilization, surgery, and chemotherapy, including 6- and 9-month regimens, has been compared. To summarize this extensive and ground-breaking work, ambulant chemotherapy has been shown to be as effective as chemotherapy combined with surgery or with immobilization, in the treatment of most cases of spinal tuberculosis. Nine-month or even 6-month regimens of isoniazid, rifampin, and pyrazinamide are now widely used for most cases of drug-sensitive infection. For most cases surgery was not found to be beneficial, although when surgery was employed, radical resection and bone grafting lead to earlier fusion and less long-term deformity when compared to débridement alone.[112–114] Remarkably, at final follow-up medical management compared favorably to surgery, even in patients with neurologic deficit, although most surgeons favor operation in cases of neurologic impairment.[102, 104, 123, 150]

Based on our experience and these reported results, we favor a 9-month course of medical management for most cases. Surgery is reserved for patients with a neurologic deficit who have failed to respond to 3 months of nonoperative treatment by manifesting pain relief and radiographic findings of healing, or cases involving such extensive multilevel destruction, or deformity, that long-term instability is deemed to be likely.[150] Because of the results documented by the Medical Research Council we are *less likely* to favor surgical treatment, for a given degree of destruction or deformity, in tuberculosis than in pyogenic infection.

When surgical treatment is required, our preferred approach is very similar to the standard Hong Kong procedure originally described by Hodgson.[85] An anterior transthoracic, thoracoabdominal, or retroperitoneal approach is utilized and radical débridement of infected bone and soft tissue is carried out. Thorough exposure across the midline anteriorly is performed, and débridement of paraspinal and psoas abscesses is carried out. Bleeding bone must be seen proximally and distally, and decompression should extend as far back as the posterior longitudinal ligament. Strut grafting consisting of iliac crest, rib, or fibula is undertaken. Our preference is to immobilize the patient in a fiberglass body jacket to protect the strut graft following surgery. In cases of multilevel involvement, potential instability, particularly at the thoracolumbar junction, or a particularly unreliable patient, posterior stabilization is performed, usually under the same anesthetic (Fig. 18–39).

Outcomes following the modern treatment of tuberculous spondylitis have improved with improved chemotherapy, surgical techniques, and quality of inpatient hospital care. The presence of a neurologic deficit increases the risk of perioperative mortality, although modern treatment utilizing appropriate antibiotic coverage at the time of surgery leads to a mortality rate of less than 5%.[14] Recurrent disease following adequate antibiotic treatment was once thought to be quite rare but appears to be increasing in frequency. A highly favorable prognosis can be stated for neurologic impairment, with many patients improving

with or without surgery. Surgery appears to improve the overall recovery rate, and certainly a faster recovery of neurologic function is seen following surgical decompression. Finally, progressive kyphosis must be evaluated. One of the advantages of surgical treatment is lessening the risk of severe spinal deformity, which is greater in cases involving extensive destruction of the vertebral bodies, three or more vertebral bodies, the thoracic spine, and not surprisingly, in patients presenting with marked kyphosis.[123]

Epidural Abscess

Abscess formation in the epidural space occurs almost exclusively in adults and, with increasing numbers of elderly and immunosuppressed patients, appears to be increasing in frequency. Although epidural abscess can occur secondary to spread from a focus of vertebral osteomyelitis, a distinct entity of epidural abscess arising from hematogenous spread from a remote source of infection, or from direct inoculation such as following lumbar puncture, epidural steroid injection, or surgery, is also seen.[42, 105] It is important to distinguish primary epidural abscess from a secondary abscess associated with vertebral osteomyelitis; primary infection of the epidural space is not associated with destruction or instability of the spine, is frequently seen posterior to the cord and cauda equina, and therefore has significantly different treatment implications. It is by all accounts a medical and surgical emergency.

A high index of suspicion is mandatory when approaching the patient with a potential epidural abscess. The initial diagnosis is frequently missed, in approximately 50% of cases, and there are various modes of presentation. Symptoms may be short-lived, of less than 1 to 2 weeks' duration, or chronic extending over several months. The most common findings with acute epidural abscess are fever, back pain, and localized tenderness, but one or all of these may be absent with a more chronic presentation. An ominous progression of the disease has been described.[39] Pain in the midline of the back or neck persists for a variable period of time, followed by radicular pain, possibly weakness, and finally paraparesis and paralysis. The timing of this progression varies, and deterioration to the next neurologic stage may be gradual or sudden.

Diagnosis requires bacteriologic confirmation. Laboratory findings suggestive of epidural abscess include elevation of the ESR, reported by Gardner and associates as a mean of 86.3 mm/hour, and elevation of the white blood cell count, averaging 22,000 cells/mm^3 in the same study.[62] Patients with more long-standing disease typically have less dramatic leukocytosis. Radiographic evaluation is undertaken, but plain radiographic findings are frequently minimal. Myelography historically has been utilized for diagnosis and may require injection above and below the involved level to adequately define the extent of disease. A high-grade block is frequently seen. As with other infections, MRI has evolved as the imaging modality of choice. It provides visualization of the abscess and the extent of neural element compression, and is highly accurate in identifying concurrent vertebral osteomyelitis when present. The sensitivity of MRI is enhanced with the use of gadolinium.[127]

Prompt intervention is required once an epidural abscess

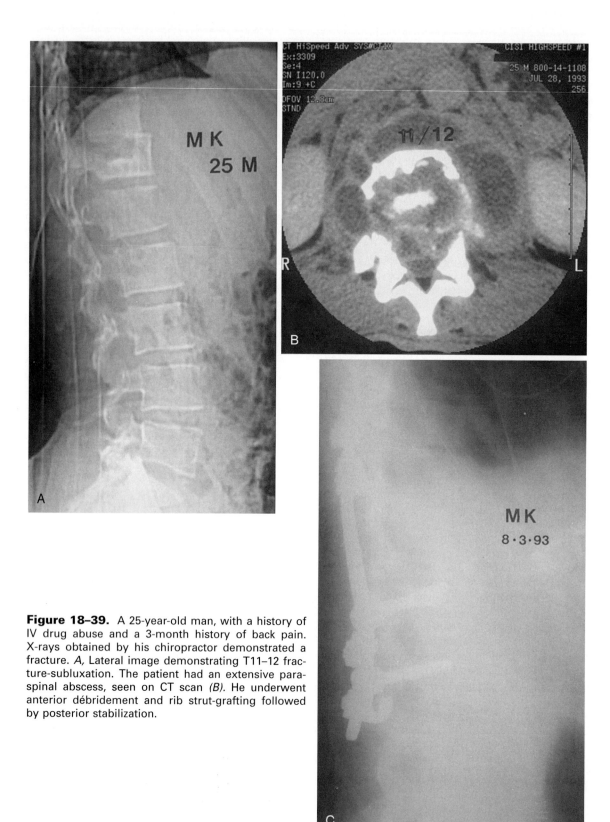

Figure 18–39. A 25-year-old man, with a history of IV drug abuse and a 3-month history of back pain. X-rays obtained by his chiropractor demonstrated a fracture. *A,* Lateral image demonstrating T11–12 fracture-subluxation. The patient had an extensive paraspinal abscess, seen on CT scan *(B).* He underwent anterior débridement and rib strut-grafting followed by posterior stabilization.

is diagnosed. Most authors consider epidural abscess a surgical emergency and we would concur. Certainly all patients, once a bacteriologic diagnosis is achieved or biopsy taken, should be begun on high-dose intravenous antibiotics. Surgery is indicated unless the patient is such a poor surgical candidate, or the disease so extensive, as to render an extremely unfavorable risk-benefit ratio to surgery.[105, 118] Nonsurgical treatment for some neurologically normal patients has been suggested, although this is controversial.[153]

Unlike epidural abscess secondary to vertebral osteomyelitis, primary epidural abscess is routinely treated surgically by laminectomy. Spinal stability can usually be preserved while still thoroughly unroofing and débriding the epidural space. It is imperative to prove intraoperatively that the cephalocaudad extent of decompression is adequate; performing a multilevel laminectomy in an area of the spine with pre-existing kyphosis may lead to progressive deformity and requires close observation.[105]

Aggressive medical and surgical management of epidural abscess has radically improved the historically bleak results. Perioperative death is exceedingly rare, and depending on the duration and extent of neurologic deficit, significant improvement is frequently seen. Poor prognostic factors include dense or long-standing neurologic deficit, diabetes, and advanced age.[62]

ADULT SCOLIOSIS

Scoliosis is a coronal plane curvature occurring most commonly in the thoracic, thoracolumbar, and lumbar spine. Although the frontal curve is the most commonly recognized aspect of the deformity, scoliosis is a three-dimensional abnormality with alterations in the sagittal and axial planes contributing significantly to the cosmetic deformity, as well as to the morbidity seen with this condition. Adult scoliosis refers to scoliosis in the skeletally mature individual, in most series beyond age 20.

The prevalence of spinal deformities in the adult has only recently been elucidated. The prevalence of scoliosis, as well as the severity of the curves identified, increases with increasing age. Kostuik and Bentivoglio reported on 5000 patients undergoing intravenous pyelography, noting 3.9% of these individuals to have thoracolumbar or lumbar curves greater than 10 degrees. They also noted that the overall prevalence of scoliosis was probably somewhat higher, but chest radiographs were not included.[94] Many authors have noted the potential for the de novo development of scoliosis in middle-aged and older patients, as well as the tendency for mild to moderate curves to progress slowly during adulthood, leading to increasing prevalence and severity as older patients are surveyed.[71]

When treating an adult patient with scoliosis, the etiology of the curve is frequently related to the age of the patient. Young and middle-aged adults frequently present with idiopathic scoliosis which may have been diagnosed in adolescence or may be newly identified. Patients' presenting complaints will vary. Some patients present for routine follow-up or because scoliosis has been identified as an incidental finding, for example, following a chest x-ray. The most common presenting complaint is back pain,

and it is incumbent on the physician to clearly identify the location of the pain, in particular whether it is related to the curve or is the more typical low back pain. It is important to recognize that there is no clear-cut correlation between the presence of idiopathic scoliosis and back pain; a certain percentage of adults with scoliosis will develop persistent, at times worsening pain that is clearly related to their curve and are good candidates for either nonsurgical or surgical treatment. On the other hand, many patients with scoliosis present with nonspecific low back pain. In these individuals treatment directed at the scoliosis, particularly surgical treatment, is unlikely to be effective. Curve progression may occur even in adulthood, and is more likely in curves that are greater than 50 degrees at the time of skeletal maturity, particularly right thoracic curves. Slow progression is seen, so it is important to compare curve measurements over a period of 5 or even 10 years to accurately identify possible curve progression.[152] Although pulmonary symptoms, and even respiratory failure, have been reported in scoliosis, the incidence of objective respiratory insufficiency in idiopathic scoliosis is really quite low. An early report by Nachemson on the risk of cardiopulmonary disease in scoliosis included many patients who did not have idiopathic deformity and thus were at greater risk of respiratory failure.[116] Idiopathic scoliosis rarely results in respiratory failure or an increased risk of premature death in curves measuring less than 100 degrees. Finally, cosmesis is a significant concern of many patients with idiopathic scoliosis. This is particularly true in the adult, although many patients are reluctant to identify this to the physician as a reason for seeking treatment.[144]

A second group of patients is seen who have degenerative scoliosis. These patients are typically older and have only recently been diagnosed with scoliosis. The etiology of degenerative scoliosis is uncertain but it is probably related to pre-existing small curves that progress as a response to asymmetric degeneration and collapse in the disks and facets. Significant spondylotic changes are seen with associated rotation, coronal plane curvature, and frequently loss of lumbar lordosis.[71] Central lateral recess, and foraminal stenosis are common, and nerve root compression in the concavity of either the primary lumbar or the lumbosacral fractional curve (opposite the primary curve) is seen. Patients with degenerative scoliosis will typically present with a long history of gradually worsening low back pain and the newer onset of symptoms typical of spinal stenosis (Fig. 18–40).

Evaluation

Evaluation of the patient with scoliosis includes history, physical examination, and radiographic studies. As noted above, the history should begin with a clear definition of why the patient is seeking treatment. If pain is the presenting complaint, then a very detailed description of the exact location of the pain as well as sites of radiation should be sought. Evidence of curve progression, such as loss of height or a notable change, over the last few years, in the fit of clothing, is important. It is also important to ask about the patient's subjective sense of balance, particularly sagittal plane imbalance when previous surgery has been done, suggestive of lumbar flatback syndrome.

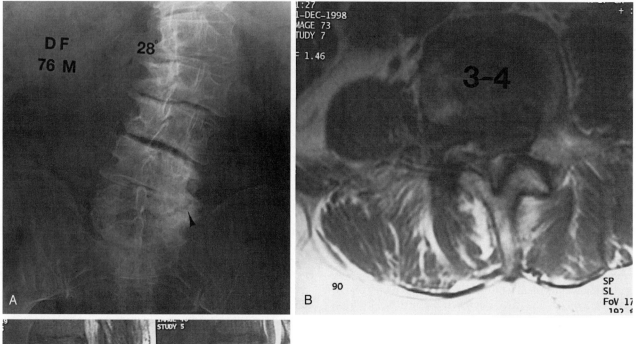

Figure 18–40. A 76-year-old man with progressively worsening back and right leg pain. His AP radiograph shows a right thoracolumbar curve but a left LS fractional curve (concave on the right) with marked collapse at L4–5 *(A)*. Axial MRI *(B)* shows central and right lateral recess stenosis at L3–4. The parasagittal image *(C)* demonstrates severe foraminal stenosis at L4–5 *(arrow)*.

Physical examination includes evaluation of gait, frontal and sagittal plane balance, and range of motion. The presence of a rotational rib or flank deformity is noted. Neurologic testing seeking both upper and lower motor neuron findings is carried out; idiopathic scoliosis never results in spinal cord compression or paraplegia, and the presence of upper motor neuron findings such as clonus or a positive Babinski sign should trigger a search for intraspinal pathology.

Radiographic evaluation includes standing PA and lateral radiographs of the full spine, bending films when surgery is contemplated, and may include supine views of the lumbar and lumbosacral spine to better define degenerative changes in this region. MRI should be obtained in cases of rapid progression, when any upper motor neuron findings are identified, or when lumbar stenosis is suggested by history. It should be noted that the abnormal three-dimensional anatomy seen in degenerative scoliosis, superimposed on the spondylotic changes frequently pres-

ent, may make accurate identification of the site and severity of stenosis difficult on MRI. Postmyelographic CT scanning is frequently utilized in this setting.

Treatment

Many patients with scoliosis present for evaluation and treatment of their backs, but only rarely is surgical treatment necessary. Accurate identification of the patient's major source of concern will in many cases lead to observation as the appropriate form of management. When treatment is indicated many patients either have low back pain, leading to nonoperative management in most cases, or have mild to moderate curve-related pain, which will frequently respond to nonoperative treatment as well.

Nonoperative treatment for low back pain associated with scoliosis is similar to that described earlier. Usually a program of weight reduction, aerobic exercise, and back stretching and strengthening exercises will relieve symptoms. Other nonoperative options that are occasionally utilized include injections, such as epidural steroids or facet joint injections, transcutaneous electrical nerve stimulation (TENS), and medical management of any metabolic abnormalities such as osteoporosis. Occasionally a custom-molded TLSO is utilized in an individual who is a poor surgical candidate.[24]

Operative treatment is reserved for patients with documented curve progression, intractable pain clearly related to the curve itself, or a persistent unacceptable pain pattern secondary to stenosis in a patient with degenerative scoliosis. Cosmesis is rarely identified as the primary indication for surgical treatment, although many patients will attest to its importance if questioned following the surgery.[144]

The surgical treatment of scoliosis consists of spinal fusion. Virtually all modern scoliosis surgery includes fusion and instrumentation, and some form of segmental instrumentation, utilizing pedicle screws, multiple hooks, sublaminar wires, or combinations thereof, is in common use today. As of this writing no widely available alternative to autologous bone grafting is available, so the harvesting of graft from the iliac crest remains common. Alternatives in surgical treatment include posterior fusion with posterior instrumentation, anterior fusion with anterior instrumentation, and combined anterior fusion with posterior fusion and posterior instrumentation. In cases of circumferential anterior and posterior fusion the addition of anterior instrumentation appears to add little to curve correction or to the chance of obtaining a solid fusion.[28]

Posterior fusion with instrumentation is indicated for moderately severe curves, particularly flexible curves, and is most often employed in isolated thoracic curves or when selective thoracic fusion is undertaken (Fig. 18–41). When a curve exceeds 60 to 70 degrees, is particularly rigid, or extends into the thoracolumbar and certainly into the lumbar spine, isolated posterior fusion with instrumentation frequently results in inadequate curve correction or an unacceptable risk of pseudarthrosis.[23] In these cases, a combined anterior approach employing rib bone graft from the convexity of the curve and generous removal of the disks down to the lowest anticipated level of fusion is employed as a first stage. Either under the same anesthetic or several days later, posterior fusion utilizing segmental instrumentation, iliac crest bone grafting, and extending over the entire span of the deformity is performed. We prefer to use a custom-molded TLSO postoperatively in most adults over the age of 30 if there is any question about the adequacy of fixation (Fig. 18–42).

Anterior fusion and anterior instrumentation, without posterior surgery, is more commonly applied in adolescents for flexible thoracolumbar or lumbar curves in an attempt to save a distal fusion level. Although it has been advocated for use in adults, our experience has been that in the adult, the stiffness of the curve, the extent of degenerative changes, and the alterations in sagittal plane contour are such that a combined anterior and posterior approach is more successful.

An even greater challenge is seen when a long scoliosis fusion needs to extend to the sacrum. This is indicated either in patients in whom the L5–S1 level is felt to be the source of their pain or has been shown (on MRI in our practice) to have significant degenerative changes. In addi-

Figure 18–41. A 40-year-old woman with documented progression of her right thoracic scoliosis *(A),* treated with a posterior fusion and segmental instrumentation *(B).*

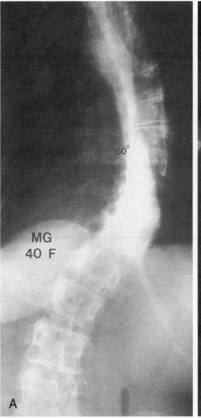
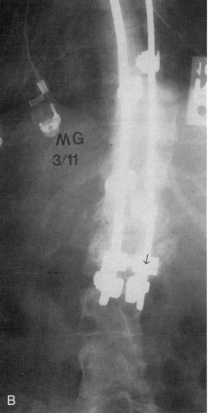

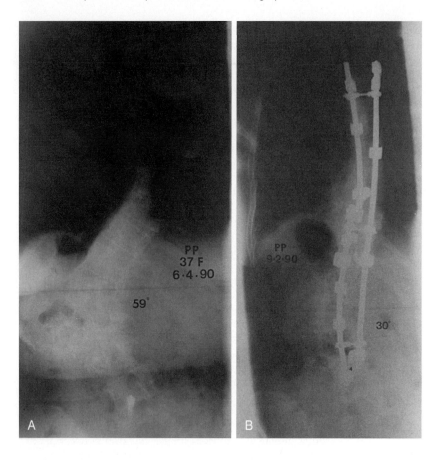

Figure 18–42. A 37-year-old woman with severe midlumbar back pain and lumbar scoliosis *(A)*. She underwent a single-stage anterior spinal fusion from T10 to L4 and posterior spinal fusion with segmental instrumentation *(B)*. She had excellent relief of her back pain.

tion, some surgeons feel that any time a long fusion has to extend to L5, the risk of degenerative change at L5–S1 is such that automatic extension to the sacrum should be undertaken. The risks of implant loosening or failure, loss of lordosis, and nonunion have been shown by several authors to be excessive, leading to a number of potential solutions.[11, 13] The most commonly employed alternative at this time is a combined anterior and posterior approach utilizing structural reconstruction, such as a femoral ring allograft or titanium mesh cage, in the lowest disk spaces (Fig. 18–43). The advantages of this include better preservation of lordosis as well as a decrease in stress on the posterior implant.[35]

The results of surgery for scoliosis in the adult depend on a number of factors including curve etiology, severity, patient age, and the patient's presenting complaint. Pain is the most common indication for surgery in adult scoliosis, but pain relief is frequently inadequate. Careful correlation of the patient's pain complaints with their spinal deformity, as well as establishing realistic goals for the surgery, offers the best hope for minimizing this problem. Curve correction is certainly less in adults than in adolescents, although this can be improved utilizing a combined anterior and posterior approach, in which case curve correction of 40 to 50% is routinely reported.[23, 25, 28] Implant-related complications and loss of correction are also seen; these problems are less common when segmental instrumentation is utilized, and we have found transpedicular fixation to be quite effective in optimizing correction while minimizing implant loosening or dislodgement. Finally, cosmesis is a frequent secondary concern of the patient. Sponseller and

associates reported on the results of the surgical treatment of adults with scoliosis and noted, in addition to significant dissatisfaction in terms of pain relief, very high overall satisfaction with the extent of cosmetic improvement seen.[144]

SPONDYLOLISTHESIS

Spondylolisthesis refers to the forward displacement of one vertebra on another. This common condition has a variety of causes, the most frequent of which are spondylolysis, resulting in isthmic spondylolisthesis, and degenerative changes at the disk and facet joint, resulting in degenerative spondylolisthesis.[158] Degenerative spondylolisthesis is most common at the L4–5 level and is frequently seen in patients with symptoms of spinal stenosis. It has been discussed earlier in this chapter. Isthmic spondylolisthesis most commonly occurs at L5–S1, followed by L4–5, and L3–4. Spondylolysis is present in 5 to 6% of the normal adult population, and most of these defects in the pars interarticularis, which are believed to be fatigue-type fractures, develop in childhood.[59] Symptoms, however, frequently do not occur until adulthood when the onset of disk degeneration leads to narrowing of the neural foramen and the development of back pain, leg pain, and the need for treatment.

Spondylolysis is present in 5 to 6% of the adult population and, approximately 75% of the time, leads to the development of spondylolisthesis.[59] The correlation between spondylolysis or spondylolisthesis and back pain is

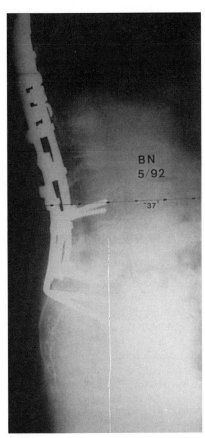

Figure 18–43. Reconstruction construct for long fusion to the sacrum employing fresh-frozen femoral ring allograft anteriorly, bilateral S1 pedicle screws, and Galveston intra-iliac rod placement.

foramen from the proximal stump of the pars all contribute to foraminal stenosis and compression of the exiting nerve root, resulting in radicular symptoms.[96]

Evaluation

History taking in the patient with spondylolisthesis is directed at clearly identifying the location and radiation of the patient's pain, the relative contribution of back pain and leg pain, and the extent of the patient's disability. Physical examination may reveal mild L5 findings in the patient with L5–S1 spondylolisthesis, although the neurologic examination is frequently normal. Straight leg raising test is rarely positive. Limited extension with a painful catch on forced extension of the spine is probably the most common physical finding in patients with isthmic spondylolisthesis, and there is usually a full range of forward flexion.

Radiographic evaluation begins with plain radiography and proceeds to special testing as needed. Plain AP and lateral radiographs, taken in the standing position, provide most of the clinically relevant information needed (Fig. 18–44). Eighty percent of pars defects can be visualized on plain lateral radiographs, and the presence and extent of forward slippage is best defined on this view. Flexion/extension lateral radiography will demonstrate instability when present, which is most common with L4–5 or L3–4 lesions.[131]

Myelography, CT scanning, and MRI have all been utilized in evaluating the patient with isthmic spondylolisthesis. At this time MRI represents the modality of choice for evaluating patients who are being considered

not clear, and there are conflicting findings in the literature. Saraste and coworkers found symptoms to be more common in a group of 255 persons with lumbar spondylolysis or spondylolisthesis than in a control group. They further found that radiographic evidence of disk degeneration and a slip of greater than 10 mm correlated positively with symptoms, as did a low lumbar index, increased lumbar lordosis, and spondylolysis at L4.[130] It is important to be aware when evaluating the patient with back pain and radiographic evidence of spondylolisthesis, however, that this condition may be nonpainful and that there are many other potential sources of pain. Leaping to the conclusion that spondylolisthesis, as seen on plain x-ray, is the source of a patient's pain may lead to unsuccessful treatment. Pain in the adult patient with spondylolisthesis has several potential sources. It is absolutely essential to consider the possibility that there is some other source of the patient's symptoms, rather than the slip. Why spondylolisthesis is painful is not clear, and suggested sources of pain include segmental instability and disk degeneration.[96] Disk degeneration is more common in individuals with isthmic spondylolisthesis, at the level of the slip, and is associated with the presence of low back pain in these patients.[130, 131] Leg pain is frequently present in the adult patient with isthmic spondylolisthesis. Narrowing of the intervertebral foramen due to disk bulging, hypertrophy of the fibrous reparative tissue at the lysis, and a bony beak extending into the

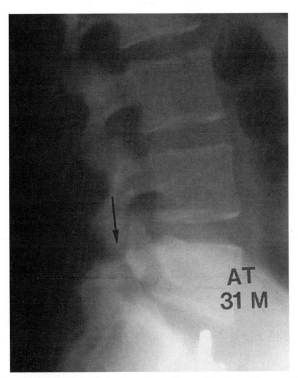

Figure 18–44. Plain lateral radiograph of a 31-year-old man with a grade I L5–S1 isthmic spondylolisthesis. The L5 pars defect *(arrow)* is easily seen.

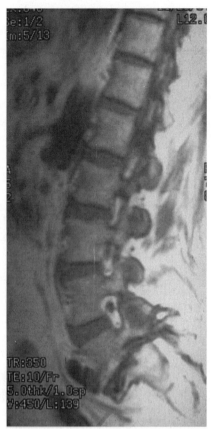

Figure 18–45. Parasagittal MRI of an elderly woman with isthmic L5–S1 spondylolisthesis. Disk space collapse and severe foraminal stenosis is apparent, as are the normal disks and foramina at the more cephalad levels.

for surgical intervention (Fig. 18–45). In addition to its noninvasive nature, MRI has the ability to accurately define the intervertebral foramen and the nerve root in the foramen, to identify possible conus abnormalities, to assess the hydration status of the disks adjacent to the proposed fusion site or to identify disk herniation, and can identify occult defects in the pars interarticularis.[89] MRI has supplanted the use of myelography or CT scanning in our practice.

Treatment

In almost all adults with isthmic spondylolisthesis, nonoperative care is the initial focus of treatment. A generalized back maintenance program including activity modification, weight reduction, generalized aerobic conditioning, and a supervised program of flexion exercises is undertaken. Sinaki and associates compared the results of nonoperative treatment in two groups, randomized to flexion or extension back strengthening exercises. They found that both short-term and long-term results were significantly better in patients who followed a flexion exercise program, with an overall recovery rate of 62%.[140]

A significant number of patients will respond to a conscientious course of nonoperative treatment, but some will ultimately require surgical intervention. The indications for surgery include persistent and intolerable back or leg pain. Because a fusion is routinely undertaken, we do not usually recommend surgery in patients with less than 6 months of symptoms or who have not been in a supervised treatment program for at least 6 to 12 weeks. Progressive slippage and clear-cut worsening of motor function are rare but occasional indications for more urgent surgical intervention.

The mainstay of surgical treatment for isthmic spondylolisthesis is arthrodesis. This can be performed through either an anterior or a posterior approach and can be supplemented with internal fixation or external immobilization. The most common fusion technique utilized, and that most commonly reported in the literature, is posterolateral intertransverse fusion. Most authors recommend single-level fusion for slippage of less than 40 or 50%. In higher grade slips, which are relatively uncommon, extension of the fusion to the next most cephalad level is recommended to increase the success rate.[26] The use of internal fixation, particularly transpedicular instrumentation, is controversial. Zdeblick, in a prospective randomized study, demonstrated that 97% of patients (many with spondylolisthesis) undergoing rigid pedicle screw fixation went on to solid fusion, a significantly higher rate than that seen in patients who underwent semirigid or no internal fixation at all.[162] On the other hand, McGuire and Amundson, in a prospective randomized series of patients with isthmic spondylolisthesis, found no significant difference in the fusion rate when comparing patients fused with and without pedicle screw fixation.[110] In adults, we favor the routine use of pedicle screw instrumentation in patients with a slip greater than 25% who are undergoing decompression, in all patients with slips greater than 50%, in patients undergoing revision fusion, and in patients with radiographically documented instability prior to surgery (Fig. 18–46). The role of instrumentation in patients with grade I spondylolisthesis without preoperative instability remains to be established.[96]

Interbody fusion can be performed through either a posterior or anterior approach. Posterior lumbar interbody fusion has been advocated because of the significant risk of disk space collapse and resultant foraminal narrowing seen in posterolateral fusion alone. Posterior lumbar interbody fusion is typically used as an adjunct to posterolateral fusion and segmental instrumentation; because of the incompetence of the posterior elements, isolated posterior lumbar interbody fusion would appear to have an exceedingly high failure rate. Anterior interbody fusion may be approached through either an anterior transperitoneal or retroperitoneal route. Diskectomy followed by placement of weight-bearing bone graft or fusion cages is undertaken and may be supplemented with posterior stabilization. In addition to these interbody fusion techniques, the use of fibular dowel grafts inserted either from an anterior or a posterior approach has been suggested, again usually as part of a combined procedure along with posterolateral fusion.[142]

The results of fusion are affected by smoking status, degree of slippage, type of fusion selected, and the use of either internal or external immobilization. Kim and associates reported a significantly higher success rate when combined anterior and posterior fusion was performed and when cast immobilization was used following surgery.[93] Improved functional outcome was reported by Hanley and Levy in adults with isthmic spondylolisthesis in noncom-

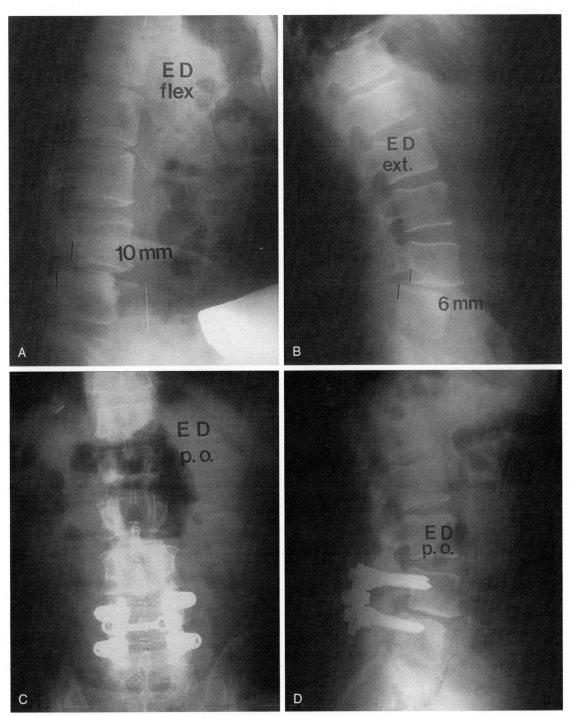

Figure 18–46. A 47-year-old man with isthmic spondylolisthesis at L4–5. As is common at levels above L5–S1, flexion/extension radiography *(A and B)* demonstrate instability. Following posterior fusion and segmental instrumentation, he had complete resolution of his back pain *(C and D).*

pensation cases, women, patients with back pain only, and nonsmokers. They found that the presence of a pseudarthrosis following surgery correlated positively with clinical failure.[77]

The role of decompression continues to be debated. Some authors feel that fusion alone results in stabilization of the motion segment and relieves leg symptoms without the need for formal decompression. Carragee reported on adults with isthmic spondylolisthesis randomized to those undergoing fusion and decompression versus fusion alone. He found a significantly higher success rate, both clinically and radiographically, in patients who underwent fusion without nerve root decompression.[31] Other authors favor routine decompression for patients with clear-cut symptoms of nerve root compression including pain or paresthesias distal to the knee, or objective evidence of nerve root dysfunction such as numbness or weakness.[26, 96] When decompression is undertaken, a thorough foraminotomy is required. We routinely perform removal of the loose posterior arch (Gill procedure) followed by identifying the nerve root medial to the pedicle. The nerve root is followed well out into the foramen with resection of all hypertrophic fibrocartilaginous material from the pars defect, and removal of the proximal stump of the pars. Only rarely is partial resection of the pedicle or ventral osteophyte necessary, and it is extremely uncommon to have to address the disk itself.

In conclusion, isthmic spondylolisthesis or spondylolysis is an extremely common condition, present in 5 to 6% of the adult population, with uncertain clinical implications. Persistent back and leg pain following nonoperative treatment leads to surgical treatment in many cases. Fusion is routinely employed with reported success rates of greater than 90%. Adjunctive internal fixation is gaining widespread acceptance.

References

1. Aebi M, Etter C, Cosica M: Fractures of the dens: Treatment with anterior screw fixation. Spine 1969; 14:1065.
2. Aebi M, Zuber K, Marchesi D: Treatment of cervical spine injuries with interior plating. Indications, techniques, and results. Spine 1991; 16(suppl):538–545.
3. Albee FH: Transplantation of a portion of the tibia into the spine for Pott's disease: A preliminary report. JAMA 1911; 57:885–886.
4. An HS, Vaccare AR, Dolinskas CA, et al: Differentiation between spinal tumors and infections with magnetic resonance imaging. Spine 1991; 16(suppl 8):S334–S338.
5. Anderson LD, D'Alonzo RT: Fractures of the odontoid process of the axis. J Bone Joint. Surg Am 1974; 56:1663.
6. Anderson PA, Bohlman HH: Late anterior decompression of thoracolumbar spine fractures. Semin Spine Surg 1990; 2:54–62.
7. Anderson PA, Rivara FP, Maier R, et al: The epidemiology of seatbelt-associated injuries. J Trauma 1991; 31:60–67.
8. Anderson PA, Bohlman HH: Anterior decompression and arthrodesis of the cervical spine: Long-term motor improvement. Part II. Improvement in complete traumatic quadriplegia. J Bone Joint Surg Am 1992; 74:683–692.
9. Apple DF: Spinal cord injury rehabilitation. In Herkoitz HN, Farfin SR, et al (eds): The Spine, 4th ed. Philadelphia, W.B. Saunders, 1999.
10. Arena MJ, Eismont FJ, Green BA: Intravertebral disc extrusion associated with cervical facet subluxation and dislocation. J Bone Joint Surg Am 1988; 72:43.
11. Balderston RA, Winter RB, Moe JH, et al: Fusion to the sacrum for nonparalytic scoliosis in the adult. Spine 1986; 11:824–829.
12. Ballock RT, Mackersie R, Abitbol J-J, et al: Can burst fractures be predicted from plain radiographs? J Bone Joint Surg Br 1992; 74:147–150.
13. Boachie-Adjei O, Dendrinos GK, Ogilvie JW, Bradford DS: Management of adult spinal deformity with combined anterior-posterior arthrodesis and Luque-Galveston instrumentation. J Spinal Disord 1991; 4:131–141.
14. Boachie-Adjei O, Squillante RG: Tuberculosis of the spine. Orthop Clin North Am 1996; 27:95–103.
15. Bohlman HH: Acute fractures and dislocations of the cervical spine: An analysis of 300 hospitalized patients and review of the literature. J Bone Joint Surg 1979; 61A:1119–1142.
16. Bohlman HH: Treatment of fractures and dislocations of the thoracic and lumbar spine. J Bone Joint Surg Am 1985; 67:165–169.
17. Bohlman H, Freehafer A, Dejak J: The results of treatment of the upper thoracic spine with paralysis. J Bone Joint Surg Am 1985; 67:360–369.
18. Bohlman HH, Anderson PA: Anterior decompression and arthrodesis of the cervical spine: Long-term motor improvement. Part I. Improvement in incomplete traumatic quadriparesis. J Bone Joint Surg Am 1992; 74:671–682.
19. Bohlman HH, Ducker TB: Spine and spinal cord injuries. In Herkowitz HN, Farfin SR, et al (eds): The Spine. Philadelphia, W.B. Saunders, 1999.
20. Bracken MB, Shepard MJ, Collins WF, et al: A randomized, controlled trial of methylprednisolone or naloxone in the treatment of acute spinal injury: Results of the second National Acute Spinal Cord Injury Study. N Engl J Med 1990; 322:1405–1411.
21. Bradford DS, Akbarnia BA, Winter RB, et al: Surgical stabilization of fracture and fracture-dislocations of the thoracic spine. Spine 1977; 2:185–196.
22. Bradford DS, McBride GG: Surgical management of thoracolumbar spine fractures with incomplete neurologic deficits. Clin Orthop 1987; 218:201.
23. Bradford DS: Adult scoliosis: Current concepts of treatment. Clin Orthop 1988; 229:70–87.
24. Bradford DS, Lauerman WC: Fusion techniques for adult spine deformity in spinal fusion—Science and technique. Cotler JM, Cotler HB (eds): Spinal Fusion—Science and Techniques. New York, Springer Verlag, 1990.
25. Bradford DS: Adult scoliosis. In Lonstein JE, Bradford DS, et al (eds): Moe's Textbook of Scoliosis and Other Spinal Deformities, 3rd ed. Philadelphia, W.B. Saunders, 1995.
26. Bradford DS: Spondylolysis and spondylolisthesis. In Lonstein JE, Bradford DS, et al (eds): Moe's Textbook of Scoliosis and Other Spinal Deformities, 3rd ed. Philadelphia, W.B. Saunders, 1995.
27. Bridwell KH, Jenny AB, Saul T, et al: Posterior segmental spinal instrumentation (PSSI) with posterolateral decompression and diskectomy for metastatic thoracic and lumbar spine disease. Spine 1988; 13:1383–1394.
28. Byrd JA, Scoles PV, Winter RB, et al: Adult idiopathic scoliosis treated by anterior and posterior spinal fusion. J Bone Joint Surg 1987; 69A:843–850.
29. Carlson GD, Heller JG, Abitbol JJ, Garfin SR: Odontoid fracture. In Levine AM, Eismont FJ, et al (eds): Spine Trauma. Philadelphia, W.B. Saunders, 1998.
30. Carragee EJ: Biogenic vertebral osteomyelitis. J Bone Joint Surg Am 1997; 79:874.
31. Carragee EJ: Singel level posterolateral arthrodesis, with or without posterior decompression, for the treatment of isthmic spondylolisthesis in adults. A prospective, randomized study. J Bone Joint Surg Am 1997; 79:1175.
32. Carragee EJ: The clinical use of the magnetic resonance imaging in pyogenic vertebral osteomyelitis, Spine 1997; 22:780–785.
33. Carragee EJ, Kim D, van der Vlugt T, Vittum D: The clinical use of erythrocyte sedimentation rate in pyogenic vertebral osteomyelitis. Spine 1997; 22:2089–2093.
34. Chance GQ: Note on a type of flexion fracture of the spine. Br J Radiol 1948; 21:452–453.
35. Citrin DL, Bessent RG, Greig WR: A comparison of sensitivity and accuracy of the ^{99m}Tc phosphate bone scan and skeletal radiograph in the diagnosis of bone metastases. Clin Radiol 1997; 28:107–111.
36. Clark CR, White AA: Fractures of the dens. J Bone Joint Surg Am 1985; 67:1340.
37. Corcoran RJ, Thrall JH, Kyle RW, et al: Solitary abnormalities in

bone scans of patients with extraosseous malignancies. Radiology 1976; 121:663–667.

38. Corwin J, Lindberg RD: Solitary plasmacytoma of bone vs. extramedullary plasmacytoma and their relationship to multiple myeloma. Cancer 1979; 43:1007–1013.

39. Currier BL, Eismont FJ: Infections of the spine. *In* Herkowitz HN, Garfin SR, et al (eds): The Spine, 3rd ed. Philadelphia, W.B. Saunders, 1999.

40. Cybulski GR: Methods of surgical stabilization or metastatic disease of the spine. Neurosurgery 1989; 25:240–252.

41. Dahlin DC: Giant-cell tumor of vertebrae above the sacrum. Cancer 1977; 39:1350–1356.

42. Danner RL, Hartman BJ: Update on spinal epidural abscess: 35 cases and review of the literature. Rev Infect Dis 1987; 9:265–274.

43. Davis D, Bohlman HH, Walker AE, et al: The pathological findings in fatal craniospinal injuries. J. Neurosurg 1971; 34:603–613.

44. Denis F: The three column spine and its significance in the classification of acute thoracolumbar spinal injuries. Spine 1983; 8:817–831.

45. Denis F, Davis S, Comfort T: Sacral fractures: An important problem. Clin Orthop 1988; 227:67.

46. De Oliveira J: A new type of fracture-dislocation of the thoracolumbar spine. J Bone Joint Surg Am 1987; 60:481–488.

47. DeWald RL, Bridwell KH, Prodromas C, Rodts MF: Reconstructive spinal surgery as palliation for metastatic malignancies of the spine. Spine 1985; 10:21–26.

48. Dobson J: Tuberculosis of the spine. An analysis of the results of conservative treatment and of the factors influencing the prognosis. J Bone Joint Surg 1951; 33B:517–531.

49. Doran SE, Papadopoulos SM, Ducker TB, et al: Magnetic resonance imaging documentation of coexistent traumatic locked facets of the cervical spine and disk herniation. J Neurosurg 1993; 79:341–345.

50. Dunn ME, Seljeskog EL: Experience in the management of odontoid process injuries: An analysis of 128 cases. Neurosurgery 1986; 18:306.

51. Edelstyn GA, Gillespie PJ, Grebell ES: The radiologic demonstration of osseous metastases: Experimental observations. Clin Radiol 1967; 18:158–164.

52. Eismont FJ, Bohlman HH, Soni PL, et al: Pyogenic and fungal vertebral osteomyelitis with paralysis. J Bone Joint Surg 1983; 65A:19–29.

53. Eismont FJ, Wiesel SW, Brighton CT, Rothman RH: Antibiotic penetration into rabbit nucleus pulposus. Spine 1987; 12:254–256.

54. Emery SE, Chan DP, Woodwar HR: Treatment of hematogenous pyogenic vertebral osteomyelitis with anterior debridement and primary bone grafting. Spine 1989; 14:284–291.

55. Emery SE, Pathria MN, Wilber RG, et al: Magnetic resonance imaging of post-traumatic spinal ligament injury. J Spinal Disord 1989; 2:229–233.

56. Ferguson RL, Allen BL Jr: A mechanistic classification of thoracolumbar spine fractures. Clin Orthop 1984; 189:77–88.

57. Finn CA, Stauffer ES: Burst fracture of the fifth lumbar vertebra. J Bone Joint Surg Am 1992; 74:398.

58. Frankel HL, Hancock DO, Hyslop G, et al: The value of postural reduction in the initial management of closed injuries of the spine with paraplegia and tetraplegia. Paraplegia 1969; 7:179.

59. Fredrickson BE, Baker D, McHollick WJ, et al: The natural history of spondylolysis and spondylolisthesis. J Bone Joint Surg 1984; 66A:699.

60. Galasko CSB, Bennett A: Relationship of bone destruction in skeletal metastases to osteoclast production and prostaglandins. Nature 1976; 263:508–520.

61. Garfin SR, Botte MJ, Nickel VL, et al: Complications in the use of the halo fixation device. J Bone Joint Surg Am 1986; 68:320–325.

62. Gardner RD, Cammisa FP, Eismont FJ, Green B: Nongranulomatous spinal epidural abscesses. Orthop Trans 1989; 13:562–563.

63. Garvey TA, Eismont FJ, Roberti LJ: Anterior decompression, structural bon grafting, and Caspar plate stabilization for unstable cervical spine fractures and/or dislocations. Spine 1992; 17(suppl):S431–435.

64. Gertzbein SD, Court-Brown CM: Flexion-distraction injuries of the lumbar spine. Mechanisms of injury and classification. Clin Orthop 1988; 227:52–60.

65. Ghormley RK, Bickel WH, Dickson DD: A study of acute infectious lesions of the intervertebral discs. South Med J 1940; 33:347–352.

66. Gilbert RW, Kim JH, Posner JB: Epidural spinal cord compression from metastatic tumor: Diagnosis and treatment. Ann Neurol 1978; 3:40–51.

67. Godersky JC, Smoker WRK, Knutzon R: Use of magnetic resonance imaging in the evaluation of metastatic spinal disease. Neurosurgery 1987; 21:676–680.

68. Griffin JB: Benign osteoblastoma of the thoracic spine. J Bone Joint Surg 1978; 60A:833–835.

69. Grob D, Jeanneret B, Aebi M, et al: Atlanto-axial fusion with transarticular screw fixation. J Bone Joint Surg Br 1991; 73:972.

70. Grob D, Crisco JJ III, Panjabi MM, et al: Biomechanical evaluation of four different posterior atlantoaxial fixation techniques. Spine 1992; 17:480.

71. Grubb SA, Lipscomb HJ, Coorad RW: Degenerative adult onset scoliosis. Spine 1988; 13:241–245.

72. Guttmann L: History of the National Spinal Injuries Centre, Stoke Mandeville Hospital, Aylesbury. Paraplega 1967; 5:115–126.

73. Haase D, Martin R, Marrie T: Radionuclide imaging in pyogenic vertebral osteomyelitis. Clin Nucl Med 1980; 5:533–537.

74. Madley MN, Browner C, Sonntag VK: Axis fracture: A comprehensive review of management and treatment of 107 cases. Neurosurgery 1995; 17:281.

75. Hall AJ, MacKay NNS: The results of laminectomy for compression of the cord or cauda equina by extradural malignant tumor. J Bone Joint Surg 1973; 55B:497–505.

76. Hamilton A, Webb JK: The role of anterior surgery for vertebral fractures with and without cord compression. Clin Orthop 1994; 300:79–89.

77. Hanley EN Jr, Levy JA: Surgical treatment of isthmic lumbosacral spondylolisthesis: Analysis of variables influencing results. Spine 1989; 14:48–50.

78. Harrington KD: The use of methylmethacrylate for vertebral body replacement and anterior stabilization of pathological fracture-dislocations of the spine due to metastatic malignant disease. J Bone Joint Surg 1981; 63:36–46.

79. Harrington KD: Current concepts review: Metastatic disease of the spine. J Bone Joint Surg 1986; 68A:1110–1115.

80. Harris JH Jr: Radiographic evaluation of spinal trauma. Orthop Clin North Am 1986; 17:75–86.

81. Henriques CO: Osteomyelitis as a complication in urology; with special reference to the paravertebral venous plexus. Br J Surg 1958; 46:19–28.

82. Herkowitz HN, Rothman RH: Subacute instability of the cervical spine. Spine 1984; 9:348–357.

83. Hibbs RA: An operation for progressive spinal deformities. NY State Med J 1911; 93:1013–1016.

84. Hodgson AR, Stock FE: Anterior spine fusion for the treatment of tuberculosis of the spine: The operative findings and results of treatment in the first one hundred cases. J Bone Joint Surg 1960; 42A:295–310.

85. Hodgson AR: Report on the findings and results in 300 cases of Pott's disease treated by anterior fusion of the spine. J West Pacific Orthop Assoc J 1964; 1:3.

86. Holdsworth R: Fractures, dislocations, and fracture-dislocations of the spine. J Bone Joint Surg Am 1970; 52:1534.

87. Jeanneret B, Magerl F: Primary posterior fusion C1–2 odontoid fractures: Indications, technique, and results of transarticular screw fixation. J Spinal Disord 1992; 5:464.

88. Jefferson G: Fracture of the atlas vertebra. Br J Surg 1920; 7:407.

89. Jinkins JR, Rauch A: Magnetic resonance imaging of entrapment of lumbar nerve roots in spondylolytic spondylolisthesis. J Bone Joint Surg Am 1994; 76:1643–1648.

90. Johnson RM, Hart DL, Simmons EF, et al: Cervical orthoses: A study comparing their effectiveness in restricting cervical motion in normal subjects. J Bone Joint Surg 1977; 59:332–329.

91. Kaneda K, Taneichi H, Abumi K, et al: Anterior decompression and stabilization with the Kaneda device for thoracolumbar burst fractures associated with neurological deficits. J Bone Joint Surg Am 1997; 79:69.

92. Kang JD, Figgie MP, Bohlman HH: Sagittal measurements of the cervical spine in subaxial fractures and dislocations. An analysis of 288 patients with and without neurologic deficits. J Bone Joint Surg 1994; 76A:1617–1627.

93. Kim SS, Denis F, Lonstein JE, et al: Factors affecting fusion rate in adult spondylolisthesis. Spine 1990; 15:979–984.

94. Kostuik JP, Bentivoglio J: The incidence of low back pain in adult scoliosis. Spine 1981; 6:268–273.

95. Krompinger WJ, Fredrickson BE, Mino DE, et al: Conservative treatment of fractures of the thoracic and lumbar spine. Orthop Clin North Am 1986; 17:161.

96. Lauerman WC, Cain SE: Isthmic spondylolisthesis in the adult. J Am Acad Orthop Surg 1996; 4:201.

97. Lemons VR, Wagner FC Jr: Stabilization of subaxial cervical spina injuries. Surg Neurol 1993; 39:511–518.

98. Levine AM, Edwards CC: The management of traumatic spondylolisthesis of the axis. J Bone Joint Surg Am 1985; 67:217–226.

99. Levine AM, Edward CC: Fractures of the atlas. J Bone Joint Surg Am 1991; 73:680–791.

100. Levine AM: Lumbar and sacral spine trauma. In Browner BD, Jupiter JB, Levine AM, et al (eds): Skeletal Trauma. Philadelphia, W.B. Saunders, 1992.

101. Levine AM, Curria A: Fractures of the sacrum. In Levine AM, Eismont FJ, Garfin SR, Zigler JE (eds): Spine Trauma. Philadelphia, W.B. Saunders, 1998.

102. Lifeso RM, Weaver P, Harder EH: Tuberculous spondylitis in adults. J Bone Joint Surg 1985; 67A:1405–1413.

103. Marsh BW, Bonfiglio M, Brady LP, Enneking WF: Benign osteoblastoma; range of manifestations. J Bone Joint Surg 1975; 57A:1–9.

104. Martin NS: Pott's paraplegia: A report of 120 cases. J Bone Joint Surg 1971; 53B:596–608.

105. Martin RJ, Yuan HA: Neurosurgical care of spinal epidural, subdural, and intramedullary abscesses and arachnoiditis. Orthop Clin North Am 1996; 27:125–136.

106. McAfee PC, Yuan HA, Lasda NA: The unstable burst fracture. Spine 1982; 7:365.

107. McAfee PC, Bohlman HH, Yuan HA: Anterior decompression of traumatic thoracolumbar fractures with incomplete neurological deficit using a retroperitoneal approach. J Bone Joint Surg Am 1985; 67:89.

108. McAfee PC, Yuan HA, Fredrickson BE, et al: The value of computed tomography in thoracolumbar fractures: An analysis of one hundred consecutive cases and a new classification. J Bone Joint Surg Am 1983; 65:461.

109. McGroy BJ, Vanderwilde RS, Currier BL, et al: Diagnosis of subtle thoracolumbar burst fractures: A new radiographic sign. Spine 1993; 19:2282–2285.

110. McGuire RA, Amundson GM: The use of primary fixation in spondylolisthesis with radiculopathy. Orthop Trans 1990; 14:550.

111. McLain RF, Weinstein JN: Solitary plasmacytomas of the spine: A review of 84 cases. J Spinal Disord 1989; 2:69–74.

112. Medical Research Council Working Party on Tuberculosis of the Spine: A controlled trial of six month and nine month regimens of chemotherapy in patients undergoing radical surgery for tuberculosis of the spine in Hong Kong. Tubercle 1986; 67:243–259.

113. Medical Research Council Working Party on Tuberculosis of the Spine: A controlled trial of anterior spinal fusion and debridement in the surgical management of tuberculosis of the spine in patients on standard chemotherapy: A study in Hong Kong. Br J Surg 1974; 61:853–866.

114. Medical Research Council Working Party on Tuberculosis of the Spine: A 10 year assessment of a controlled trial comparing debridement and anterior spinal fusion in the management of tuberculosis of the spine in patients on standard chemotherapy in Hong Kong. J Bone Joint Surg 1982; 64B:393–398.

115. Mindel ER: Current concepts review: Chordoma. J Bone Joint Surg 1981; 63A:501–505.

116. Nachemson A: A long term follow-up study of non-treated scoliosis. J Bone Joint Surg 1969; 50A:203.

117. Nicoll EA: Fractures of the dorso-lumbar spine. J Bone Joint Surg Br 1949; 31:376–394.

118. Nussbaum ES, Rigamonti D, Standiford H, et al: Spinal epidural abscess: A report of 40 cases and review. Surg Neurol 1992; 38:225–231.

119. Parke WW: The vascular relations of the upper cervical vertebrae. Orthop Clin North Am 1978; 9:879.

120. Pettine KA, and Klassen RA: Osteoid-osteoma and osteoblastoma of the spine. J Bone Joint Surg 1986; 68A:354–361.

121. Posner I, White AA, Edwards WT, Hayes WC: A biomechanical analysis of clinical stability of the lumbar lumbosacral spine. Spine 1982; 7:374.

122. Powers B, Miller MD, Kramer RS, et al: Traumatic anterior atlantooccipital dislocation. Neurosurgery 1979; 4:12.

123. Rajasckaran S, Soundarapandian S: Progression of kyphosis in tuberculosis of the spine treated by anterior arthrodesis. J Bone Joint Surg 1989; 71A:1314–1323.

124. Roy-Camille R, Saillant G, Bouchet T: Technique du vissage despedicules de C2. In Roy-Camille R (ed): Cinquiemes Journees d'Orthopedic de la Pitie, Rachis Cervical Superieur. Paris, Masson, 1986, pp 41–43.

125. Russin LA, Robinson MJ, Engle HA, Sonni A: Ewing's sarcoma of the lumbar spine. Clin Orthop 1982; 164:126–129.

126. Ryan MD, Taylor TKF: Odontoid fractures. A rational approach to treatment. J Bone Joint Surg Br 1982; 64:416.

127. Sadato N, Numaguchi Y, Rigamonti D, et al: Spinal epidural abscess with gadolinium-enhanced MRI: Serial follow-up studies and clinical correlations. Neuroradiology 194; 36:44–48.

128. Sapico FL, Montgomerie JZ: Pyogenic vertebral osteomyelitis: Report of nine cases and review of the literature. Rev Infect Dis 1979; I:754–776.

129. Sapico FL: Microbiology and antimicrobial therapy of spinal infections. Orthop Clin North Am 1996; 27:9–13.

130. Saraste H, Nilsson B, Brostrom LA, et al: Relationship between radiological and clinical variables in spondylolysis. Int Orthop 1984; 8:163–174.

131. Saraste H: Long-term clinical and radiological follow-up of spondylolysis and spondylolisthesis. J Pediatr Orthop 1987; 7:631–638.

132. Savini R, Gherlinzoni F, Morandi M, et al: Surgical treatment of giant-cell tumor of the spine. J Bone Joint Surg 1983; 65A:1283–1289.

133. Schaefer DM, Flanders A, Northrup BE, et al: Magnetic resonance imaging of acute cervical spine trauma. Correlation with severity of neurologic injury. Spine 1989; 14:1090–1095.

134. Schneider RC, Kahn EA: Chronic neurological sequelae of acute trauma to the spine and spinal cord. Part I: The significance of the acute-flexion or "tear-drop" fracture-dislocation of the cervical spine. J Bone Joint Surg Am 1956; 38:985–997.

135. Schneider RC, Knighton R: Chronic neurological sequelae of acute trauma to the spine and spinal cord. III: The syndrome of chronic injury to the cervical spinal cord in the region of the central canal. J Bone Joint Surg 1959; 41A:905–919.

136. Sears W, Fazi M: Prediction of stability of cervical spine fracture managed in the halo vest and indications for surgical intervention. J Neurosurg 1990; 72:426–432.

137. Sherk HH: Fractures of the atlas and odontoid. Orthop Clin North Am 1987; 9:973.

138. Shives TC, Dahlin DC, Sim FH, et al: Osteosarcoma of the spine. J Bone Joint Surg 1986; 68A:660–668.

139. Siegal T, Siegal T: Vertebral body resection for epidural compression by malignant tumors. Results of forty-seven consecutive operative procedures. J Bone Joint Surg 1985; 66A:375–382.

140. Sinaki M, Lutness MP, Ilstrup DM, et al: Lumbar spondylolisthesis: Retrospective comparison and three-year follow-up of two conservative treatment programs. Arch Phys Med Rehabil 1989; 70:594–598.

141. Smith AS, Weinstein MA, Mizushima A, et al: MR imaging characteristics of tuberculous spondylitis vs vertebral osteomyelitis. AJR 1989; 153:399–405.

142. Smith MD, Bohlman HH: Spondylolisthesis treated by a single-stage operation combining decompression with in situ posterolateral and anterior fusion: An analysis of eleven patients who had long-term follow-up. J Bone Joint Surg Am 1990; 72:415–421.

143. Spence KF, Decker S, Sell KW: Bursting atlantal fracture associated with rupture of the transverse ligament. J Bone Joint Surg Am 1970; 52:543–549.

144. Sponseller PD, Cohen MS, Nachemson AL, et al: Results of surgical treatment of adults with idiopathic scoliosis. J Bone Joint Surg 1987; 69A:667–675.

145. Starr JK, Eismont FJ: Atypical hangman's fractures. Spine 1993; 18:1954–1957.

146. Stover SL, Fine PR: Spinal Cord Injury, The Facts and Figures. Birmingham, University of Alabama Press, 1986, pp 22, 32.

147. Sundaresan N, Galicich JH, Lane JM, et al: Treatment of neoplastic epidural cord compression by vertebral body resection and stabilization. J Neurosurg 1985; 63:676–684.

148. Sutterlin CE, McAfee PC, Warden KE, et al: A biomechanical evaluation of cervical spinal stabilization methods in a bovine model. Static and cyclical loading. Spine 1988; 13:795–802.

149. Thelander U, Larsson S: Quantitation of C-reactive protein levels

and erythrocyte sedimentation rate after spinal surgery. Spine 1992; 17:400–404.

150. Fuli SM: Results of treatment of spinal tuberculosis by "middle path" regime. J Bone Joint Surg 1975; 57B:13–23.

151. Weinstein JN, McLain RF: Primary tumors of the spine. Spine 1987; 12:843–851.

152. Weinstein SL, Ponseti IV: Curve progression in the idiopathic scoliosis. J Bone Joint Surg 1983; 65A:447–455.

153. Wheeler D, Keiser P, Rigamonti D, Keay S: Medical management of spinal epidural abscesses: Case report and review. Clin Infect Dis 1992; 15:22–27.

154. White AA, Johnson RM, Panjabi MM, et al: Biomechanical analysis of clinical stability of the cervical spine. Clin Orthop 1975; 109:85–96.

155. White AA III, Panjabi MM: Clinical Biomechanics of the Spine, 2nd ed. Philadelphia, J.B. Lippincott, 1990.

156. Whiehill R, Richmann JA, Glaser JA: Failure of immobilization of the cervical spine by halo vest. J Bone Joint Surg Am 1986; 68:326.

157. Wiley AM, Trueta J: The vascular anatomy of the spine and its relationship to pyogenic vertebral osteomyelitis. J Bone Joint Surg 1959; 41B:796–808.

158. Wiltse LL, Newman PH, MacNab I: Classification of spondylolysis and spondylolisthesis. Clin Orthop 1976; 117:23–29.

159. Woodring JH, Goldstein SF: Fractures of the articular processes of the cervical spine. AJR 1982; 139:341–344.

160. Wukich DK, Van Dam BE, Abreu SH: Preoperative indium-labeled white blood cell scintigraphy in suspected osteomyelitis of the axial skeleton. Spine 1988; 13:1168–1170.

161. Young MH: Long-term consequences of stable fractures of the thoracic and lumbar vertebral bodies. J Bone Joint Surg Br 1973; 55:295–300.

162. Zdeblick TA: A prospective, randomized study of lumbar fusion: Preliminary results. Spine 1993; 18:983–991.

Chapter 19

The Shoulder and Arm

Benjamin Shaffer, M.D.

Few joints match the shoulder in its sophistication and versatility. This joint in fact consists of 16 different muscle-tendon units, four bones, three diarthrodial joints, and two soft tissue articulations, all working in synchrony. Whether allowing us to effortlessly place our hand into nearly any position, accurately throw a baseball at 100 miles per hour (or hit 70 home runs in a season!) or power lift, the shoulder is by all accounts an extraordinarily versatile complex. Unfortunately, there is a price for such versatility, and the payment is the frequency with which the shoulder's normal function is compromised by a number of traumatic and atraumatic conditions. This chapter will explore the shoulder's normal functional anatomy, present an overview of evaluation techniques, and review the evaluation and management of common traumatic and atraumatic conditions affecting the shoulder and arm.

FUNCTIONAL ANATOMY

The shoulder complex consists of five articulations working in synchrony (Fig. 19–1). The central articulation in the shoulder is the glenohumeral joint, in which the round humeral head articulates with the oval glenoid. But four other articulations also contribute significantly to shoulder function, both "in sickness and in health," and include the sternoclavicular joint, the acromioclavicular joint, the scapulothoracic articulation, and the subacromial space. Only the glenohumeral, sternoclavicular, and acromioclavicular articulations are true diarthrodial joints (synovial joint with opposing articular surfaces).

The clavicle is an S-shaped bone that serves as a strut to maintain the normal relationship of the shoulder girdle to the body (Fig. 19–2). The medial articulation of this strut is the sternoclavicular (SC) joint, supported by very strong reinforcing ligaments, which account for the infrequency of SC joint injury (Fig. 19–3). Laterally, the clavicle articulates with the scapula through the acromion at the acromioclavicular (AC) joint (Fig. 19–4). Composed of the somewhat weak AC joint capsular fibers, the connection between the lateral clavicle and scapula is additionally reinforced by ligaments connecting the coracoid process of the scapula to the undersurface of the distal clavicle, the coracoclavicular ligaments (conoid and trapezoid). With these exceptions, the scapula (and therefore the attached humerus) has no other skeletal attachments and essentially rests freely against the posterior thoracic wall, with which it "articulates." Occasionally a source of symptoms, this interface is known as the scapulothoracic articulation. Between the anterior aspect of the scapula and the posterior thoracic wall is a bursal lining (a synovial-lined potential sac), the scapulothoracic bursa, which serves as a lubricated frictionless interface for smooth motion (Fig. 19–5).

The last articulation is the subacromial space, which lies between the undersurface of the acromion and superior aspect of the rotator cuff. Like the scapulothoracic articulation, this space provides a frictionless interface between moving structures (the cuff against the acromial undersurface) and is therefore lined by a bursal sac, the subacromial bursa (Fig. 19–6).

The shoulder is not merely a "ball and socket" configuration. Each of these articulations contributes to normal shoulder motion. Most motion occurs at the glenohumeral joint and the scapulothoracic articulation. Two thirds of normal shoulder elevation occurs at the glenohumeral joint, and one third at the scapulothoracic articulation.

The contribution of the scapulothoracic articulation to motion in other planes (such as internal and external rotation) is less substantial. Some joint motion also occurs at the SC and AC joints. The exact amounts are variable, but

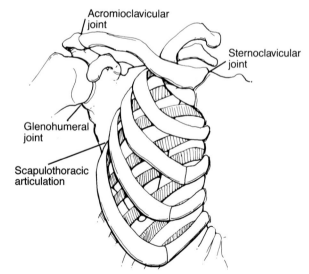

Shoulder

Figure 19–1. The shoulder is composed of four articulations: the glenohumeral, acromioclavicular, sternoclavicular, and scapulothoracic. The subacromial space, between the superior rotator cuff and the acromial undersurface, is sometimes considered a fifth articulation. (From DeLee JC, Drez D: Orthopaedic Sports Medicine: Principles and Practice. Philadelphia, WB Saunders, 1994.)

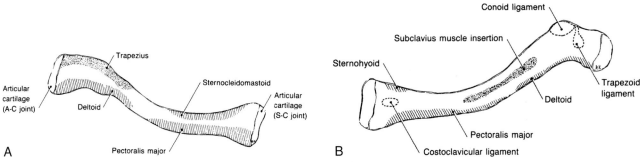

Figure 19–2. The clavicle is an S-shaped strut maintaining the normal relationship between the axial skeleton (spine) and appendicular skeleton (extremity). The superior view *(A)* shows the origins of the deltoid, trapezius, sternocleidomastoid, and pectoralis major. *B,* The inferior surface demonstrates the major ligament insertions and deltoid, pectoralis major, and sternohyoid muscle origins. (From Rockwood CA Jr, Matsen FA III: The Shoulder, 2nd ed. Philadelphia, WB Saunders, 1998.)

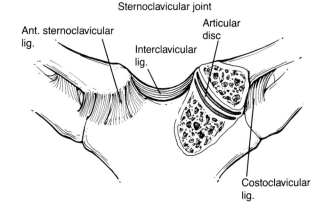

Figure 19–3. Anatomy of the sternoclavicular joint. (From DeLee JC, Drez D: Orthopaedic Sports Medicine: Principles and Practice. Philadelphia, WB Saunders, 1994.)

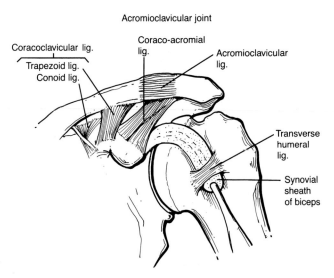

Figure 19–4. Articulation of the acromioclavicular (AC) joint, including the AC capsule and the coracoclavicular ligaments (conoid and trapezoid). (From DeLee JC, Drez D: Orthopaedic Sports Medicine: Principles and Practice. Philadelphia, WB Saunders, 1994.)

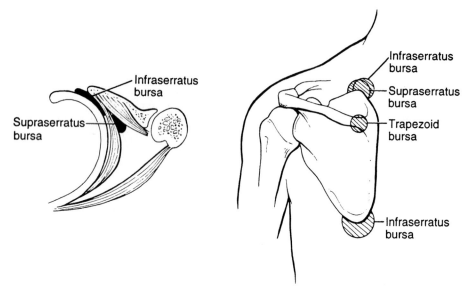

Figure 19–5. Anatomy of the bursae of the scapulothoracic articulation. (From Warner JJP, Ianotti JP, Gerber C [eds]: Complex and Revision Problems in Shoulder Surgery. Philadelphia, Lippincott-Raven, 1997.)

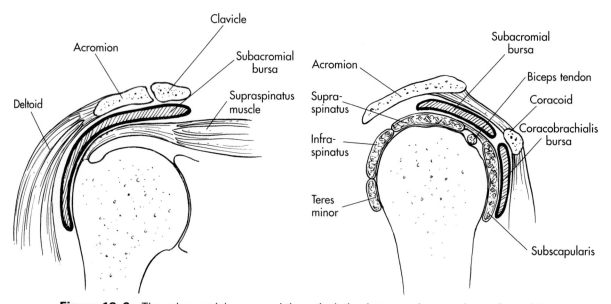

Figure 19–6. The subacromial space and the articulation between the superior surface of the rotator cuff and the acromial undersurface. (From Jobe FW: Operative Techniques in Upper Extremity Sports Injuries. St. Louis, CV Mosby, 1996.)

Figure 19–7. *A*, The labrum, composed of the thickening of the glenohumeral ligament's glenoid insertion, effectively enhances the depth of the otherwise shallow glenoid, improving articulation with the humeral head. *B*, This cadaveric specimen demonstrates the improved congruency afforded the joint by the labrum's presence. (From Rockwood CA Jr, Matsen FA III: The Shoulder, 2nd ed. Philadelphia, WB Saunders, 1998.)

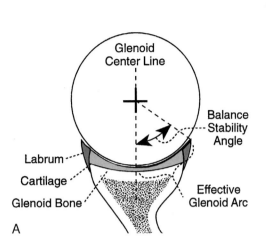
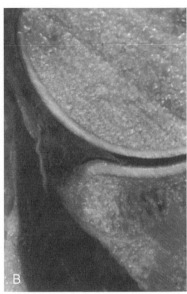

it is important to recognize that these joints are not fixed, and disease or injury can interfere with normal shoulder function, even in the face of a "normal" glenohumeral joint. Likewise, processes affecting the normally smooth frictionless subacromial and scapulothoracic interfaces aversely affect normal shoulder function.

The Glenohumeral Joint

The glenohumeral joint enjoys the dual distinction of being the most mobile and not coincidentally the most frequently dislocated joint in the body. These qualities are due to its shallow ball-and-socket configuration. The skeletal architecture, consisting of a large spherical humeral head articulating with a smaller flat, comma-shaped glenoid is in and of itself insufficient to maintain stability. Stability is enhanced by the presence of the labrum (Fig. 19–7), a rim of fibrous tissue ringing the glenoid rim and enhancing its depth by up to 50%. Although similar in appearance to the knee's meniscus, the labrum is made of fibrous tissue rather than fibrocartilage. It is variable in thickness and occasionally serves as the site of capsular (glenohumeral ligament) attachment.

The most significant constraint providing glenohumeral stability is the surrounding soft tissue envelope or capsule. When viewed from its external surface (during dissection or open surgery), this capsule appears to be a bland fibrous structure similar to that seen surrounding other joints. Yet when viewed from its internal surface (via arthroscopy or histologic examination) the capsule is seen to actually consist of a number of discretely identifiable collagen bundles, each with a specific strategic function. The anterior aspect of the shoulder capsule consists of three distinct ligaments, whose names are derived from their glenoid origin: the superior (SGHL), middle (MGHL), and anterior inferior glenohumeral ligament (AIGHL) complex (Fig. 19–8).

The AIGHL complex is the most important static restraint to anterior instability. This capsular restraint acts like a hammock to support the humeral head. Placing the arm in abduction and external rotation (the "throwing" position) causes the hammock to "tighten up," cradling and thereby stabilizing the humeral head (Fig. 19–9). Failure of this ligament complex to tighten up due to inherent laxity (looseness of the capsular tissue) or detachment along the glenoid rim (known as a "Bankart" lesion) accounts for most cases of anterior shoulder instability (Fig. 19–10). The other glenohumeral ligaments contribute variably in different positions of shoulder function, but to a lesser degree than the AIGHL complex in normal shoulder stability.

A number of muscle groups contribute to normal shoulder function. These muscles can be divided into groups that function to (1) dynamically stabilize the glenohumeral joint, (2) move the glenohumeral joint, (3) move the scapula, and (4) generate shoulder power.

Dynamic Stabilizers

The static stabilizers of the shoulder, which passively contribute to normal stability, include the skeletal architecture of the bone's geometry, the labrum, and the capsuloligamentous restraints. The dynamic stabilizers are those muscles that contribute to normal stability, and include the muscles of the rotator cuff. This important structure is composed of four muscles that originate on the scapula and coalesce as a tendinous cuff to insert on the lesser and greater tuberosities of the proximal humerus (Fig. 19–11). The most well recognized cuff muscle, considered clinically synonymous with most rotator cuff problems, is the supraspinatus. Arising from the suprascapular fossa, the supraspinatus tendon lies directly superior to the glenohumeral joint, attaching to the superior aspect of the greater tuberosity. It is most commonly involved in rotator cuff impingement. Posteriorly lie the infraspinatus and teres minor, the external rotators of the shoulder. The infraspinatus lies directly posterior to the supraspinatus, arising from the infraspinatus fossa to attach to the posterior greater tuberosity, and provides the majority (80%) of external rotation strength. The infraspinatus is the second

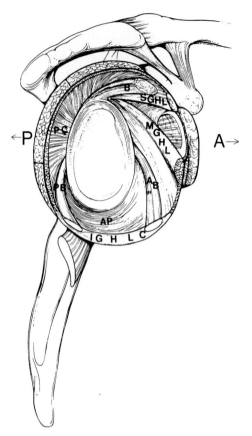

Figure 19–8. In the glenohumeral joint the discrete structures that compose the shoulder capsule include the superior (SGHL), middle (MGHL), and inferior (IGHL) glenohumeral ligaments. Inferiorly, this glenohumeral ligament complex (GHLC) consists of an anterior band (AB), an axillary pouch (AP) and a posterior band (PB). The biceps tendon (B) and posterior capsule (PC) are shown for orientation. (From Wiesel SW, Delahay JN: Essentials of Orthopaedic Surgery, 2nd ed. Philadelphia, WB Saunders, 1997.)

possible with either muscle group alone. For example, if shoulder elevation were to rely only on the deltoid, then upon deltoid contraction the humeral head would simply ride superiorly. If, however, a force in the opposite direction holds the humeral head within the glenoid, then contraction of the deltoid leads to *rotation* of the head and elevation of the arm. Familiarity with this force couple concept is important in understanding how the cuff maintains humeral head centering on the glenoid during normal activity, and how it may fail to do so when diseased or injured.

Although not considered a cuff muscle per se, the long head of the biceps is often considered functionally with the rotator cuff tendons. It arises from the supraglenoid tubercle within the glenohumeral joint and travels distally within the bicipital groove to meet the short head of the biceps (Fig. 19–13). Problems of the biceps tendon around the shoulder are often considered along with cuff problems because of their proximity. The biceps tendon is thought to functionally contribute to humeral head depression during normal function.

Glenohumeral Movers

Although the muscles of the rotator cuff do indeed move the glenohumeral joint, their predominant function is

most commonly involved tendon in rotator cuff disease. Both the supraspinatus and infraspinatus are innervated by the suprascapular nerve.

The teres minor, arising inferiorly to the infraspinatus and attaching along the inferior aspect of the greater tuberosity, is innervated by the axillary nerve.

The fourth and last cuff muscle is the subscapularis, uncommonly involved in the syndrome of cuff impingement. Arising from the subscapular fossa on the anterior aspect of the scapula, innervated by the upper and lower subscapular nerves, this muscle inserts through its tendinous attachment laterally to the lesser tuberosity. It contributes to internal rotation of the arm.

The cuff provides several functions, one of which is to dynamically stabilize the glenohumeral joint. Contraction of cuff muscles in a coordinated fashion applies tension to the underlying ligamentous attachments, thereby reinforcing these constraints and contributing to shoulder stability. Conversely, when disease or fatigue interferes with effective cuff function, appropriate capsule-ligament tightening may fail to occur, leading to symptoms of instability or pain. The cuff also participates with other shoulder muscles as a force couple (Fig. 19–12). A force couple is a paired set of coordinated muscle contractions that together achieve function not

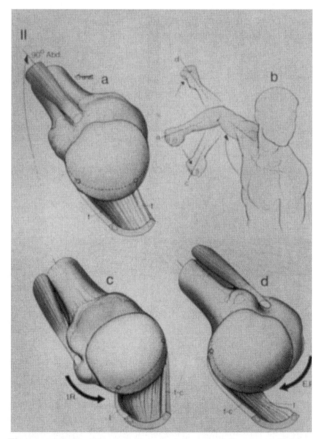

Figure 19–9. The inferior glenohumeral ligament tightens up as the arm is placed in the "throwing" position of abduction and external rotation (a, b). The ligament fans out, supporting the humeral head and preventing anterior inferior translation. c, In internal rotation, the posterior component of the inferior glenohumeral ligament becomes taut. d, In external rotation, the anterior component of the glenohumeral ligament becomes taut. (From Rockwood CA Jr, Matsen FA III: The Shoulder, 2nd ed. Philadelphia, WB Saunders, 1998.)

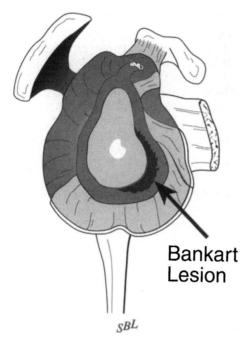

Figure 19–10. A "Bankart" lesion, in which the inferior glenohumeral ligament has been avulsed or detached from the anterior inferior glenoid rim accounts for most cases of traumatic shoulder instability. (From Rockwood CA Jr, Matsen FA III: The Shoulder, 2nd ed. Philadelphia, WB Saunders, 1998.)

thought to be joint stabilization. The muscles directly responsible for generating motion include the deltoid (anterior, middle, and posterior heads), the pectoralis major, latissimus dorsi, and teres major (Fig. 19–14). The deltoid is the largest muscle of the shoulder girdle, a tripennate structure arising from the mid to lateral clavicle, the entire acromion, and scapular spine. The three parts—anterior, middle, and posterior heads—attach to the deltoid tuberosity of the proximal humerus. Innervation is by the axillary nerve emerging posteriorly in the quadrangular space and traveling laterally toward the anterior aspect of the shoulder approximately 5 cm below the acromial edge.

The pectoralis major arises from the manubrium sternum, the first six ribs and the medial two thirds of the clavicle. This powerful internal rotator attaches to the lateral lip of the bicipital tuberosity and is innervated by the medial and lateral pectoral nerves.

The latissimus dorsi arises from a large and broad aponeurosis from T7–L5 as well as the sacrum, ilium, and occasionally the lower three or four ribs and inferior scapular angle to attach to the medial crest of the bicipital tuberosity. The muscle is even more important than the pectoralis major in internal rotation and also contributes to normal shoulder adduction and extension. The thoracodorsal nerve (C6, C7) provides innervation.

The teres major arises from the posterior scapula's inferior lateral border and attaches along with the latissimus dorsi along the medial lip of the bicipital groove, providing internal rotation, adduction, and extension of the arm. Innervation is by the lower subscapular nerve (C5, C6).

Scapular Movers

Normal shoulder movement requires motion at both the glenohumeral joint and the scapulothoracic articulation.

The scapula is in essence a mobile platform from which glenohumeral motion can occur. Normal scapular motion requires orchestrated muscle contraction. The muscles that control scapular movement are known as the scapular rotators and include the trapezius, levator scapulae, rhomboids, and the serratus anterior (Fig. 19–15).

The trapezius is the largest of the scapulothoracic muscles arising from the spinous processes of C7 through T12 and inserting along the scapular spine, acromion, and distal third of the clavicle. Innervated by the spinal accessory nerve, the trapezius acts to retract the scapula.

The levator scapula lies deep to the trapezius and arises from the transverse processes of C1 through C3, inserting on the superior angle of the scapula. As its name implies, it functions to elevate the superior angle of the scapula. Innervation is via deep branches of C3 and C4 as well as the dorsal scapular nerve.

The rhomboids also lay deep to and function similarly to the midportion of the trapezius. Originating from the ligamentum nuchae from C7 through T1 (rhomboid minor) and T2 through T5 (rhomboid major), they insert along the posterior aspect of the medial base of the scapular spine to its inferior angle. Innervated by the dorsal scapular nerve, the rhomboids retract and contribute to elevation of the scapula.

The serratus anterior originates from fleshy slips along

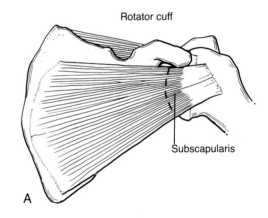

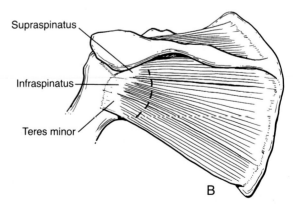

Figure 19–11. The four rotator cuff muscles are shown. The supraspinatus is the cuff muscle most commonly involved in injury. (From DeLee JC, Drez D: Orthopaedic Sports Medicine: Principles and Practice. Philadelphia, WB Saunders, 1994.)

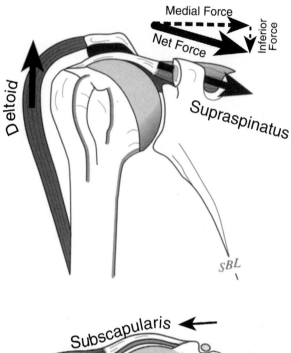

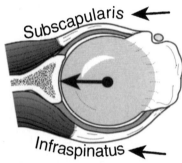

Figure 19–12. The rotator cuff acts as a "force couple" to balance and center the humeral head within the glenoid upon contraction of other shoulder muscles (such as the deltoid). This stabilization phenomenon provided by the cuff is critical to normal shoulder function. (From Rockwood CA Jr, Matsen FA III: The Shoulder, 2nd ed. Philadelphia, WB Saunders, 1998.)

the anterolateral first through ninth ribs and inserts along the anterior surface of the scapula's medial border. Innervated by the long thoracic nerve (C5–C7), the serratus protracts and contributes to upward rotation of the scapula. Serratus dysfunction causes injury of the scapula during forward flexion.

Injury or disease affecting any of these muscle groups or their nerves may lead to scapular dysfunction, improper elevation, and secondary shoulder dysfunction.

Power Generators

Muscles responsible for power generation include the deltoid, pectoralis major, and latissimus dorsi.

Subacromial Space and Bursa

The subacromial space is located between the superior aspect of the anterior rotator cuff and the coracoacromial (CA) arch (consisting of the anterior acromial undersurface,

AC joint, and the CA ligament) (Fig. 19–16). The CA ligament spans the space between the coracoid process and the anterior inferior acromion. Within the subacromial space is a bursa, a sac-like structure whose inner single-cell synovial-lined surface generates synovial fluid. This bursa facilitates frictionless motion between the cuff and the coracoacromial arch. Inflammation, thickening, hypertrophy, and disease can all lead to symptoms at this clinically important interface.

Scapulothoracic Articulation and Bursa

The anterior aspect of the scapula articulates with the posterior thoracic cage. A scapulothoracic bursa provides frictionless motion at this interface (see Fig. 19–5). Pathology within this bursa can occasionally cause posterior shoulder symptoms.

Acromioclavicular Joint

This diarthrodial joint contains a fibrocartilaginous meniscus disk interposed between the distal clavicle and the proximal acromion. Degenerative changes within the disk are age-related. A reinforcing fibrous capsule stabilizes the joint circumferentially. The coracoclavicular (CC) liga-

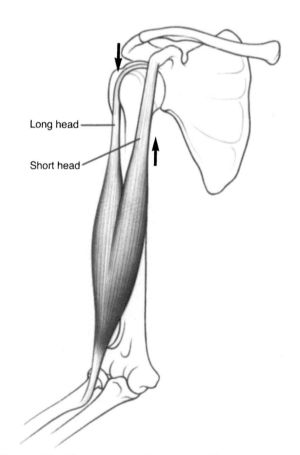

Figure 19–13. The long head of the biceps tendon and its origin within the shoulder at the supraglenoid tubercle of the glenoid. Joined distally by the short head of the biceps, they combine to make the biceps muscle. (From Neer CS II: Shoulder Reconstruction. Philadelphia, WB Saunders, 1990.)

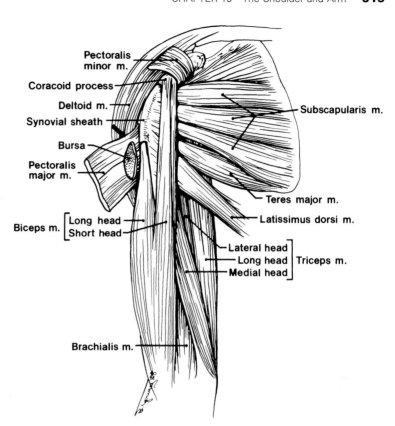

Figure 19–14. The glenohumeral movers include the deltoid, pectoralis major, latissimus dorsi, and teres major muscles. (From Rockwood CA Jr, Matsen FA III: The Shoulder, 2nd ed. Philadelphia, WB Saunders, 1998.)

ments (conoid and trapezoid) provide further stability to this construct (Fig. 19–17).

Sternoclavicular Joint

The medial clavicle articulates with the manubrium sternum at the sternoclavicular joint. The strength of the surrounding fibrous capsular structure as well as ligamentous contributions from the adjacent first rib makes instability of this complex rare (see Fig. 19–3). As a diarthrodial joint, however, this joint is vulnerable to the same processes afflicting synovial joints, including arthritis.

Neurovascular Structures

The brachial plexus, composed of the anterior nerve roots of C5 through T1, provides motor and sensory function to the upper extremity. Familiarity with the roots, trunks, divisions, cords, and individual branches is crucial to understanding peripheral nerve disorders and other common

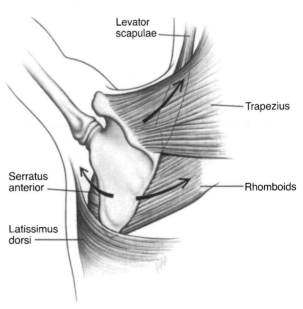

Figure 19–15. Illustration of the scapular "rotators," including the serratus anterior, trapezius, rhomboids, and levator scapulae, responsible for maintaining normal scapular position and contributing to shoulder function. (From Neer CS II: Shoulder Reconstruction. Philadelphia, WB Saunders, 1990.)

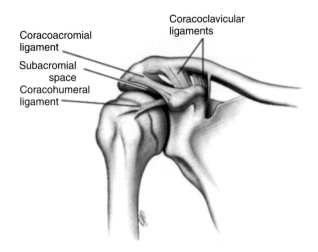

Coracoacromial ligament

Subacromial space

Coracohumeral ligament

Coracoclavicular ligaments

Figure 19–16. The subacromial space lies between the superior aspect of the supraspinatus (rotator cuff) tendon and the acromial undersurface and AC joint. The bursa lining the space serves as a frictionless interface for normal smooth gliding between the tissue planes. (From Neer CS II: Shoulder Reconstruction. Philadelphia, WB Saunders, 1990.)

shoulder disorders (Fig. 19–18). The subclavian artery supplies the upper extremity, becoming the axillary artery as it passes over the first rib. At the inferior border of the latissimus dorsi it becomes the brachial artery.

Arm Musculature

Other important muscles affecting the upper arm include the coracobrachialis, biceps, and triceps (Fig. 19–19). The coracobrachialis has a tendinous origin on the coracoid process and travels distally to attach along the anteromedial surface of the midhumerus. Innervated by the musculocuta-

neous nerve (C5–C6) it contributes to shoulder flexion and adduction.

The biceps is composed of both short and long heads. The short head arises from the coracoid process just lateral to the coracobrachialis and travels immediately parallel to it, including the conjoint tendon seen along anterior shoulder surgery and dissection. In the midhumerus the short head, innervated by the musculocutaneous nerve, combines with the long head (traveling from its intra-articular origin) to become the biceps muscle, terminating in its attachment distal to the elbow in the bicipital tuberosity of the radius. The biceps' main action is at the elbow, where it contrib-

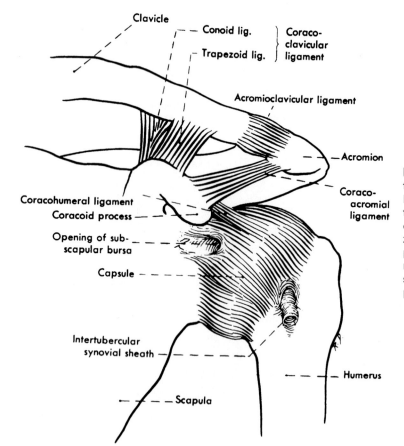

Clavicle

Conoid lig.
Trapezoid lig. } Coraco-clavicular ligament

Acromioclavicular ligament

Acromion

Coraco-acromial ligament

Coracohumeral ligament

Coracoid process

Opening of sub-scapular bursa

Capsule

Intertubercular synovial sheath

Humerus

Scapula

Figure 19–17. The AC joint consists of the distal clavicle, the proximal acromion, a fibrocartilage disk (not seen) between the two ends, and the surrounding joint capsule. Note the presence of the coracoclavicular ligaments (conoid, trapezoid), whose attachment to the distal clavicle provides important support to this otherwise vulnerable joint. (From Wiesel SW, Delahay JN: Essentials of Orthopaedic Surgery, 2nd ed. Philadelphia, WB Saunders, 1997.)

of the proximal arm almost always reflects rotator cuff impingement. Pain radiation is also a key factor; most problems intrinsic to the shoulder do not radiate below the elbow. Because the scapular rotators attach to the base of the cervical spine, pain referral to the neck is not uncommon.

The nature or character of the pain must be determined. Pain that is burning in quality suggests neurologic causes, such as cervical stenosis or disk and brachial neuritis. A dull ache over the anterior shoulder, on the other hand, might indicate rotator cuff pathology. Is the pain caused by certain maneuvers? Pain during overhead activity suggests cuff pathology. Pain when reaching across the body (such as to wash under the opposite axilla) may indicate problems in the AC joint. Conversely, pain in the shoulder of a young, throwing athlete may suggest underlying instability. In the patient whose pain is present only at the extremes of motion, adhesive capsulitis (frozen shoulder) may be responsible. Several conditions, such as rotator cuff impingement and frozen shoulder, cause pain at night, with nocturnal awakening, often from lying on the affected shoulder. Of course, pain at rest may be due to a more serious underlying problem, such as tumor or infection.

Because the shoulder is a common area for referred pain from visceral afferent sources, a careful review of systems must be part of the history. Problems of the cervical spine (stenosis, herniated disk), gastrointestinal tract (gallstones,

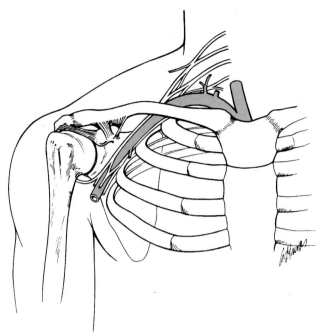

Figure 19–18. The brachial plexus and subclavian artery are seen here, entering the upper extremity underneath the clavicle. (From DeLee JC, Drez D: Orthopaedic Sports Medicine: Principles and Practice. Philadelphia, WB Saunders, 1994.)

utes to supination and flexion. It is thought to contribute to humeral head depression via the long head.

The triceps arises from the shoulder girdle and although it acts mostly at the elbow, can be involved in shoulder problems. A tripennate muscle, the long head arises from the infraglenoid tubercle of the glenoid and the posteroinferior shoulder capsule and inserts posteriorly along the olecranon tip. Innervated by the radial nerve (C6–C8), the long head serves as the medial border of the quadrilateral space, at times of clinical significance. Although involved during throwing activities, its most significant contribution is at the elbow.

EVALUATION OF SHOULDER PROBLEMS

The most common shoulder and arm complaints are pain, stiffness, instability, and/or weakness. Despite advances in sophisticated imaging studies, a thorough history and physical examination remain the benchmark of diagnostic success in evaluating shoulder and arm problems.

History Taking

PAIN

Pain is the most common shoulder problem. It is important to determine when and how it began, whether it is acute or insidious, and where the pain is located. Pain over the top of the shoulder is often due to problems of the AC joint. Pain over the posterior shoulder usually reflects referred pain from the cervical spine, periscapular spasm due to some other intrinsic shoulder disorder, brachial neuritis, or scapulothoracic bursitis. Pain over the lateral aspect

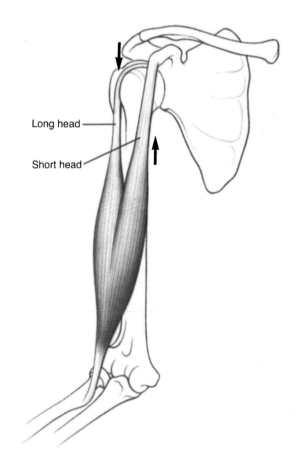

Figure 19–19. Note the dual origin of the biceps muscle with a long and a short head. (From Neer CS II: Shoulder Reconstruction. Philadelphia, WB Saunders, 1990.)

peptic ulcer disease), and cardiopulmonary system can all refer pain to the shoulder or arm.

STIFFNESS

Stiffness is a common shoulder/arm complaint, occurring after trauma, surgery, or any period of immobilization. Sometimes, as in the case of adhesive capsulitis (frozen shoulder), stiffness may occur in the absence of any identifiable cause. Identifying the cause of stiffness is important because of differences in response to treatment.

INSTABILITY

Instability is usually a straightforward complaint, with patients volunteering that they felt their shoulder go "out of place," usually at the time of a traumatic event. The majority of instability episodes occurs with the humeral head dislocating anteriorly. Because these episodes are not always documented (spontaneous reduction or reduction may occur prior to x-ray confirmation), the direction in which the shoulder dislocated, and the position in which their arm was positioned, is important to ascertain. Determine what treatment, if any, was rendered at the time of the first incident, and with any subsequent episodes. Have there been recurrent instability episodes? If so, with what provocation, if any? Recurrent episodes may occur with provocation, such as when rolling over in bed.

Shoulder instability can also present with subluxation, or incomplete separation of the joint surfaces, rather than a full dislocation. For example, anterior subluxation, in which the humeral head translates abnormally anteriorly relative to its normal position within the glenoid, may cause the sense of the shoulder "going out" or "going dead." The unique nature of this particular condition has earned it the name "dead arm syndrome"; patients describe a feeling of the arm going limp or "dead" when placing the arm in the vulnerable cocking position of throwing.

WEAKNESS

Weakness is a less common shoulder complaint, usually occurring in association with pain, stiffness, or instability. Inquire about the onset and severity of weakness, and the presence of associated symptoms, such as numbness or tingling. Common causes of weakness include rotator cuff tear, atrophy from disuse or following trauma, and neurologic disorders.

Functional Assessment

Determine the relationship, if any, pursuits, and the symptoms. This information may be helpful in identifying the potential cause of onset, and instrumental in influencing treatment alternatives. Can the patient perform daily activities, such as washing under the opposite arm, reaching the perineum, reaching overhead, and sleeping on the affected shoulder? Does the patient's occupation require use of the shoulder? The hand dominance may likewise have considerable impact.

Physical Examination

A comprehensive and accurate physical examination of the shoulder includes inspection, palpation, range of motion assessment, strength testing, and neurovascular examination. Familiarity with additional "special" tests useful in the evaluation of specific shoulder conditions is helpful in making the diagnosis.

INSPECTION

The patient must be appropriately gowned to allow inspection of both shoulders and neck. Examination begins with passive inspection of shoulder for asymmetry, mass, swelling, erythema, ecchymoses, and muscular atrophy. Comparison of the two symmetric sides is helpful. Ecchymoses may be present in a number of traumatic shoulder conditions, including fracture, dislocations, muscle ruptures, and acute cuff tears. A globular appearance of the biceps muscle indicates a probable tear of the long head of the biceps (Fig. 19–20). Common abnormalities include the AC joint prominence seen following traumatic AC separation or osteophyte formation. Following anterior shoulder dislocation, the normally round lateral shoulder contour may be flat, accompanied by an abnormal-appearing anterior fullness. Long-standing rotator cuff tears or brachial neuritis may present with mild atrophy or actual hollowing of the normally full supraspinatus or infraspinatus fossa.

Remember that inspection is not just static, but is also dynamic. The examiner should stand in front of the patient and have the patient raise both arms overhead, observing for pain during elevation. Although pain may be present throughout motion, pain during the arc from approximately 90 to 120 degrees suggests rotator cuff impingement, and is known as the painful arc sign. Viewing from behind, while the patient raises both arms overhead, inspect for scapulohumeral rhythm, normally smooth and symmetric. Asymmetry can include abnormal motion, due to scapulothoracic bursitis or scapula restriction, or actual "winging" due to weakness of the scapular rotators (Fig. 19–21). Scapular winging may be better elicited in some patients by having them do a wall push-up or having the patient hold the arm in forward flexion against resistance. Both tests dynamically examine for the integrity of the strength of the serratus anterior (innervated by the long thoracic nerve) (Fig. 19–22).

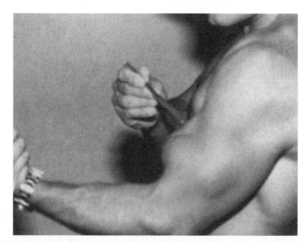

Figure 19–20. Note the globular appearance to this patient who suffered a proximal biceps tendon rupture. (From Neer CS II: Shoulder Reconstruction. Philadelphia, WB Saunders, 1990.)

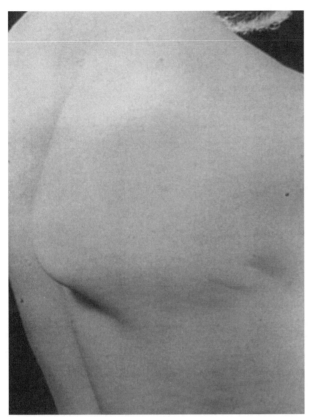

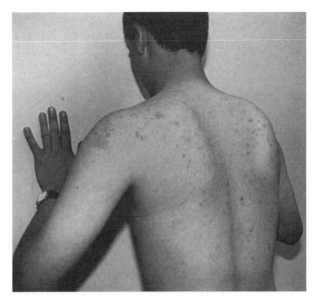

Figure 19–22. Note "winging" of the scapula elicited by asking the patient to do a push-up off the wall, demonstrating serratus anterior weakness. (From Rockwood CA Jr, Matsen FA III: The Shoulder, 2nd ed. Philadelphia, WB Saunders, 1998.)

Figure 19–21. Scapular winging, caused by weakness of the serratus anterior. (From Rockwood CA Jr, Matsen FA III: The Shoulder, 2nd ed. Philadelphia, WB Saunders, 1998, p 172.)

PALPATION

Palpate the shoulder for tenderness, masses, warmth, and crepitus. Begin medially at the sternoclavicular joint and continue laterally along the clavicle, including the AC joint, coracoid, acromion, and scapular spine. Palpate over the trapezius, deltoid, supraspinatus, and infraspinatus. In acute SC or AC joint sprains, focal tenderness is present. In chronic conditions, tenderness may be more generalized, with nonspecific "trigger points" in the surrounding muscles.

During active elevation, palpate directly over the acromion and subacromial space for crepitus. Asymptomatic clicking and/or popping may be normal, but if crepitus is painful and reproduces symptoms, localized to either the AC joint or subacromial bursa, it may reflect significant AC joint, rotator cuff, or glenohumeral joint disease. Crepitus localized to the scapulothoracic bursa may indicate scapulothoracic bursitis, a condition seen in throwing athletes. Although not diagnostic, increased warmth or erythema of the shoulder may suggest infection.

RANGE OF MOTION

In the traumatized or obviously fractured or dislocated shoulder, motion assessment should be considered only after obtaining x-rays. In the nontraumatized patient, in whom fracture or dislocation has been ruled out, determine the patient's active range of motion in forward elevation, external rotation, and internal rotation. With the patient seated, forward elevation is determined by having the patient lift the arm overhead. By definition, elevation is motion that takes place in the plane of the scapula (midway between the coronal and sagittal planes) (Fig. 19–23). External rotation is next checked with the patient's elbow at the side, rotating the arms out as far as possible (Fig. 19–24). Internal rotation is assessed by having the patient put the hand behind the back to touch as high as possible, noting the relationship of the thumb tip to the spinal column. As a reference, the spine of the scapula is considered approximately at the T2 level and the tip at T7 (Fig. 19–25).

If there is any discrepancy compared to the opposite side, more careful measurements of motion are made passively. With the patient supine, compensatory spine and trunk motion is eliminated, and true restriction can be identified. Mild restriction is common in a number of conditions, such as stiffness following immobilization, trauma, surgery, cuff injury, or arthritis. Moderate or severe restriction, particularly in the absence of trauma, suggests adhesive capsulitis as a probable cause.

STRENGTH TESTING

Examine the shoulder girdle for muscular integrity, including the scapula rotators (wall push-up for serratus anterior and shoulder shrug for trapezius) and the primary shoulder movers (pectoralis major and deltoid). The rotator cuff muscles are assessed individually. The supraspinatus (the most commonly affected cuff tendon) is thought to be best isolated with the supraspinatus test (Fig. 19–26). The patient is asked to elevate and hold the arm in the plane of the scapula, with the thumb pointing downward. Inability to maintain this position against gravity or resistance may indicate cuff injury. The "drop arm" sign has been described as specific for rotator cuff tears, but in fact can occur with a number of other painful shoulder conditions

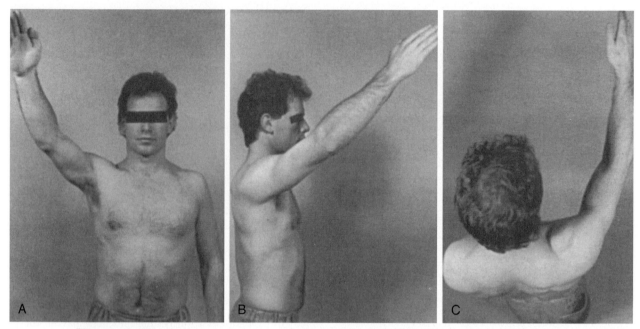

Figure 19–23. Forward elevation occurs with raising of the arm in the plane of the scapula, midway between the sagittal plane and the coronal plane. *(A)* Anterior view, *(B)* lateral view, *(C)* superior view. (From Rockwood CA Jr, Matsen FA III: The Shoulder, 2nd ed. Philadelphia, WB Saunders, 1998.)

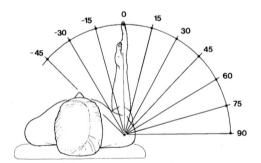 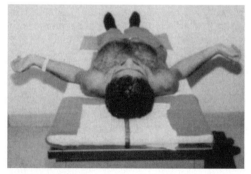

Figure 19–24. External rotation is measured by determining the amount of rotation with the elbow at the patient's side. Having the patient supine prevents the torso from rotating. (From Neer CS II: Shoulder Reconstruction. Philadelphia, WB Saunders, 1990.)

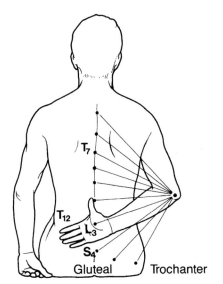
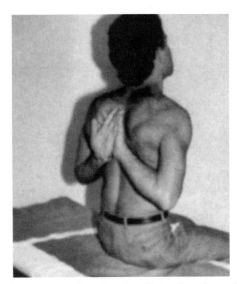

Figure 19–25. Internal rotation is determined by comparing the tip of the thumb to the spinal level, using the top and bottom of the scapula as T2 and T7, respectively. (From Neer CS II: Shoulder Reconstruction. Philadelphia, WB Saunders, 1990.)

Figure 19–26. Supraspinatus integrity/strength is thought to be best determined by having the patient maintain elevation of the arm with the thumb pointing downward against resistance, the so-called "empty a can" position. (From Rockwood CA Jr, Matsen FA III: The Shoulder, 2nd ed. Philadelphia, WB Saunders, 1998.)

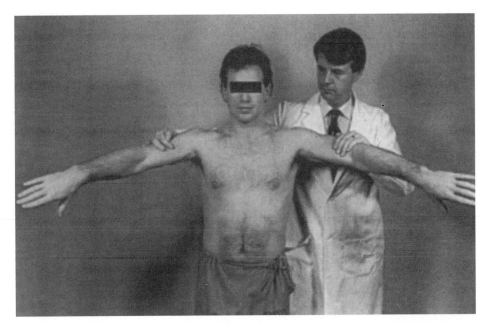

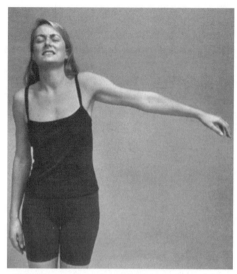

Figure 19–27. In the drop arm test, the arm is placed in elevation and the patient is asked to hold it in this position. Inability to do so constitutes a positive drop arm test, although this is not necessarily specific for rotator cuff tear. (From Reider B: The Orthopaedic Physical Examination. Philadelphia, WB Saunders, 1999.)

(Fig. 19–27). Despite the presence of a full-thickness cuff tear, some patients may still demonstrate very good strength during this maneuver.

The posterior cuff (infraspinatus and teres minor) is examined by having the patient externally rotate against resistance with the elbow at the side (Fig. 19–28). The subscapularis is tested by having the patient try to "lift off" the hand away from the low back. This "lift off" test is positive when the patient is unable to lift the hand away or keep it away, and indicates structural compromise of the uncommonly torn subscapularis tendon (Fig. 19–29).

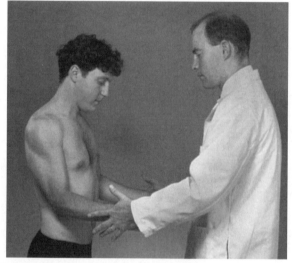

Figure 19–28. Posterior cuff strength and integrity are examined by having the patient maintain the arm against the examiner's efforts at internal rotation with the arm at the side. (From Reider B: The Orthopaedic Physical Examination. Philadelphia, WB Saunders, 1999.)

Neurovascular Assessment

Neurologic examination has already been indirectly initiated through examination of the muscular strength of some specific muscle groups. A thorough examination includes the remaining muscle groups as well as sensory and reflex testing. Sensory evaluation relies on the detection of light touch over the lateral deltoid (axillary nerve), the thumb web space (radial nerve), the radial aspect of the index finger (median nerve), and the ulnar aspect of the little finger (ulnar nerve). Reflex testing involves the biceps (C5), brachioradialis (C6), and triceps (C7). Vascular compromise of the upper extremity is uncommon but can occur following trauma. Examination should include radial and ulnar pulses and, when necessary, the Allen test. In the Allen test, the fist is clenched and both radial and ulnar arteries are compressed. As the hand is opened, pressure is released from the radial or ulnar artery and the hand inspected to determine adequacy of blood flow.

Specific Examinations

Additional physical examination techniques are necessary for the evaluation for specific shoulder conditions, including tests for rotator cuff impingement, glenohumeral instability, and AC joint arthritis. Impingement signs are used to identify the presence of subacromial cuff injury. Several tests have been described, the most common of which are known by the name of the examiner whose descriptions popularized them. They include the Neer and the Hawkins signs, and both rely on reproducing the patient's symptoms by manipulating the shoulder in a way that is thought to mechanically irritate the rotator cuff, which when involved, provokes symptoms. In Neer's impingement sign, the affected arm is elevated in the sagittal plane against the scapula, compressing the cuff against the unyielding coracoacromial arch (Fig. 19–30). Hawkins emphasized forcibly internally rotating the shoulder as a more specific technique (Fig. 19–31). Some have focused on the detection of biceps tendonitis, elicited by having the patient elevate the arm against resistance with the elbow extended and forearm supinated, the Speeds' sign (Fig. 19–32). Frequently positive in the presence of biceps tendonitis, it is also commonly present during impingement due to the proximity of the biceps tendon to the cuff, and therefore is usually considered a nonspecific finding.

Other common shoulder examination techniques involve tests for detecting and quantifying instability. In general, these tests attempt to elicit apprehension, pain, or both, through provocative shoulder positioning. The most common test is for recurrent anterior instability. While the examiner stands behind the seated patient, or with the patient supine, the arm is gently grasped and placed in the position of abduction and progressive external rotation. Known as the apprehension sign, the appearance of apprehension on the patient's countenance (and commonly accompanied by a verbal reaction) indicates impending glenohumeral instability (Fig. 19–33). Posterior instability is detected by adducting the forward flexed and slightly internally rotated arm and applying an axial load posteriorly (Fig. 19–34). Apprehension or the appreciation of symptomatic posterior translation suggests posterior instability.

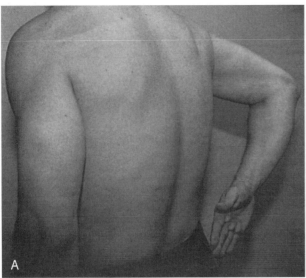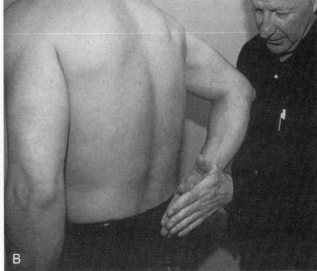

Figure 19–29. The "lift off" test assesses integrity and strength of the subscapularis and is performed by having the patient try to lift the internally rotated (behind the back) positioned hand *(A)* away from the back against examiner resistance *(B)*. (From Rockwood CA Jr, Matsen FA III: The Shoulder, 2nd ed. Philadelphia, WB Saunders, 1998.)

Finally, inferior laxity is assessed by applying longitudinal traction to the adducted arm. The scapula should be fixed with the opposite hand, and attention is placed on the amount of inferior translation compared to the opposite shoulder. Visual indication of laxity occurs with the appearance of a sulcus between the acromion and the humeral head, and this test for inferior laxity is thus known as the sulcus sign (Fig. 19–35). Somewhat nonspecific, this sign may be present in patients with generalized ligament laxity and no history of inferior subluxation.

Examination for ligamentous laxity is helpful, particularly in the young athletic population, and in patients with suspected instability. Laxity can be assessed by examination of the elbows for recurvatum, the metacarpophalangeal joint of the little finger for hyperextension, and the thumb-to-the-forearm sign (Fig. 19–36). Collectively, their presence suggests a generalized laxity pattern that may contribute or predispose to instability.

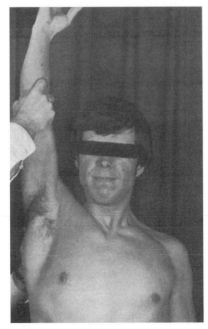

Figure 19–30. The Neer impingement test, performed by elevating the shoulder against the fixed scapula, reproduces pain in terminal elevation. (From Wiesel SW, Delahay JN: Essentials of Orthopaedic Surgery, 2nd ed. Philadelphia, WB Saunders, 1997.)

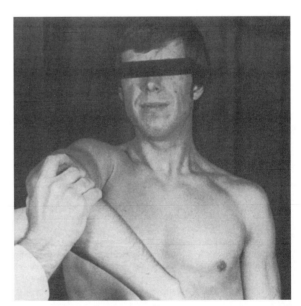

Figure 19–31. In the Hawkins modification of the impingement sign, the elevated arm is internally rotated, reproducing symptoms due to cuff impingement against the acromial and CA ligament undersurface. (From Wiesel SW, Delahay JN: Essentials of Orthopaedic Surgery, 2nd ed. Philadelphia, WB Saunders, 1997.)

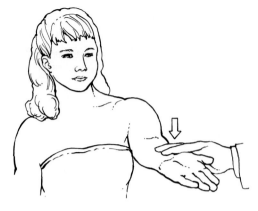

Figure 19–32. In Speeds' sign, patients are asked to maintain their forward flexed supinated forearm against the examiner's resistance. Reproduction of symptoms in the anterior shoulder biceps area suggests possible biceps tendon involvement. (From Jobe FW: Operative Techniques in Upper Extremity Sports Injuries. St. Louis, CV Mosby, 1996.)

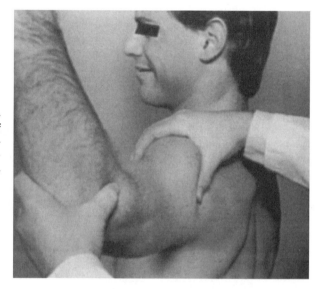

Figure 19–33. The apprehension sign is most commonly elicited for recurrent anterior instability, and involves placement of the shoulder in the abducted externally rotated position, observing the sense of apprehension on the patient's face. (From Rockwood CA Jr, Matsen FA III: The Shoulder, 2nd ed. Philadelphia, WB Saunders, 1998.)

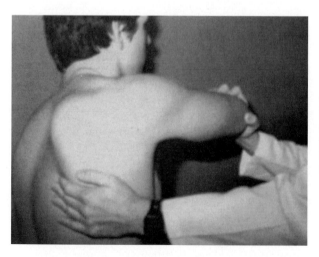

Figure 19–34. Posterior apprehension or translation is tested by axially loading the forward flexed and slightly adducted shoulder, observing for apprehension, discomfort, and translation greater than the opposite shoulder. (From Rockwood CA Jr, Matsen FA III: The Shoulder, 2nd ed. Philadelphia, WB Saunders, 1998.)

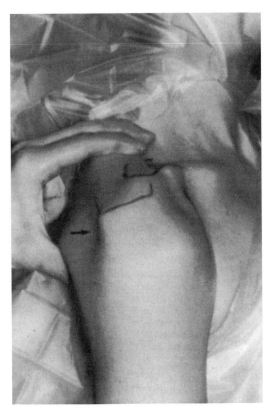

Figure 19–35. The sulcus sign is elicited by attempting to inferiorly translate the humeral head by application of longitudinal traction, observing the sulcus between the lateral acromion and the glenohumeral joint. (From Reider B: Common Sports Injuries. Part II. Sports Medicine: The School-Aged Athletes. Philadelphia, WB Saunders, 1991.)

EXAMINATION FOR REFERRED SYMPTOMS

Shoulder symptoms do not always arise in the shoulder but can be referred from other sources, particularly in the middle-aged and older population, in whom cervical spine problems are common. Remember to evaluate the cervical spine in patients with referred symptoms, stiffness, or pain. Examine for restriction in motion and neurologic findings.

RADIOGRAPHIC EXAMINATION

Standard radiographs include a true AP view (an AP view of the scapula, not the thorax) (Fig. 19–37) and an axillary lateral view (Fig. 19–38A and B). Look for soft tissue abnormality, joint space distance, and bone irregularities. Additional views may be helpful to identify specific problems and are ordered based on history and physical examination findings. For example, suspected calcific tendonitis, or visualization of a faint calcific deposit on the AP view warrants further AP views taken in internal and external rotation.

The acromioclavicular (AC) joint is best visualized with a Zanca view, taken by tilting the x-ray beam 10 degrees cephalad and decreasing the kV by about half (Fig. 19–39). Patients with impingement should be evaluated with the

"Y outlet" view, obtained by shooting the x-ray parallel to the scapular spine, thereby revealing acromial structure (Fig. 19–40).

ARTHROGRAM

Arthrography involves the injection of radiopaque contrast dye into the glenohumeral joint and examining the pattern of dye distribution. It is most useful in the evaluation of rotator cuff tears, in which the dye is no longer contained within the glenohumeral joint but instead leaks through the cuff tear into the subacromial space. The presence of dye in this subacromial location confirms a cuff tear (Fig. 19–41). A second diagnostic entity in which arthrography is helpful is in adhesive capsulitis (frozen shoulder). Patients with this condition demonstrate abnormal blunting of the normal axillary pouch, and accommodate very little injection volume (usually less than 10 ml compared to the normal of 40 or 50 ml).

MAGNETIC RESONANCE IMAGING

Magnetic resonance imaging (MRI) is a very accurate noninvasive imaging technique that has more or less supplanted arthrography in the evaluation of shoulder problems. MRI is most commonly used in evaluating possible rotator cuff tears, for which its accuracy is better than 95% (Fig. 19–42). It is also very helpful in identifying avascular necrosis and tumors. However, the expense and the inordinate sensitivity of this test make it unnecessary in the routine evaluation of most shoulder problems. Even when interpreted by dedicated radiologists, MRI is unreliable in accurately identifying labral injury or disease; it is not the test of choice in evaluating suspected labral tear or instability.

BONE SCAN

Nuclear medicine scans are useful in detecting physiologic increase in blood flow. Because tumors, infections, fractures, and arthritis can all lead to increased blood flow, bone scans in which certain areas "light up" are not specific. However, when analyzed in the context of the patient's history, physical examination, and x-ray findings, bone scan may be very useful. Its greatest utility in the

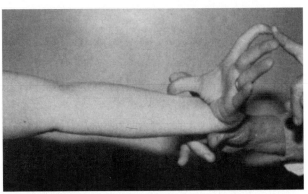

Figure 19–36. Generalized laxity is shown here with both "thumb to the forearm" opposition and finger distal interphalangeal hyperextension. (From Neer CS II: Shoulder Reconstruction. Philadelphia, WB Saunders, 1990.)

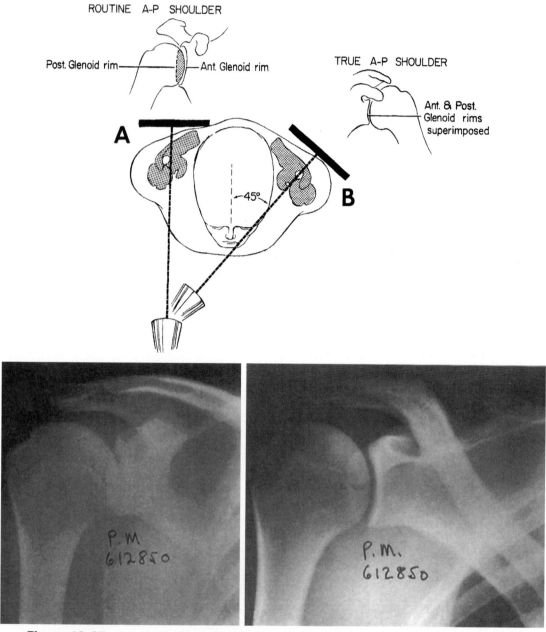

Figure 19–37. A true AP view is obtained by angling the beam about 45 degrees from the coronal plane of the body so that the image is truly perpendicular to the glenohumeral joint. Right radiograph shows the true glenohumeral joint view. (From Wiesel SW, Delahay JN: Essentials of Orthopaedic Surgery, 2nd ed. Philadelphia, WB Saunders, 1997.)

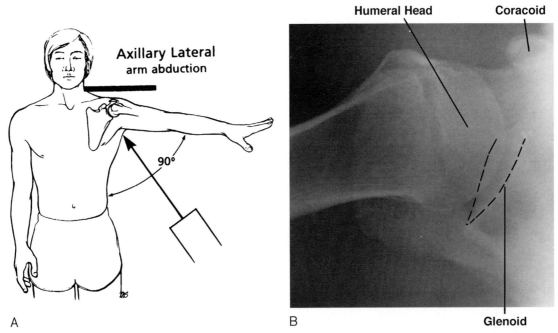

Figure 19–38. An axillary lateral view is obtained by aiming the x-ray beam into the axilla with the plate superiorly. *A* illustrates the technique, and *B* shows the typical axillary lateral appearance. (From Rockwood CA Jr, Matsen FA III: The Shoulder, 2nd ed. Philadelphia, WB Saunders, 1998.)

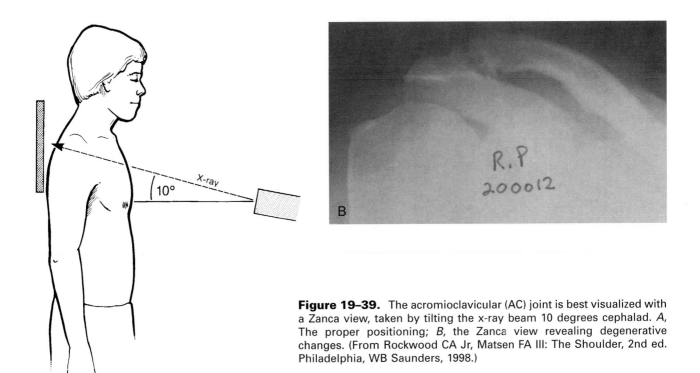

Figure 19–39. The acromioclavicular (AC) joint is best visualized with a Zanca view, taken by tilting the x-ray beam 10 degrees cephalad. *A,* The proper positioning; *B,* the Zanca view revealing degenerative changes. (From Rockwood CA Jr, Matsen FA III: The Shoulder, 2nd ed. Philadelphia, WB Saunders, 1998.)

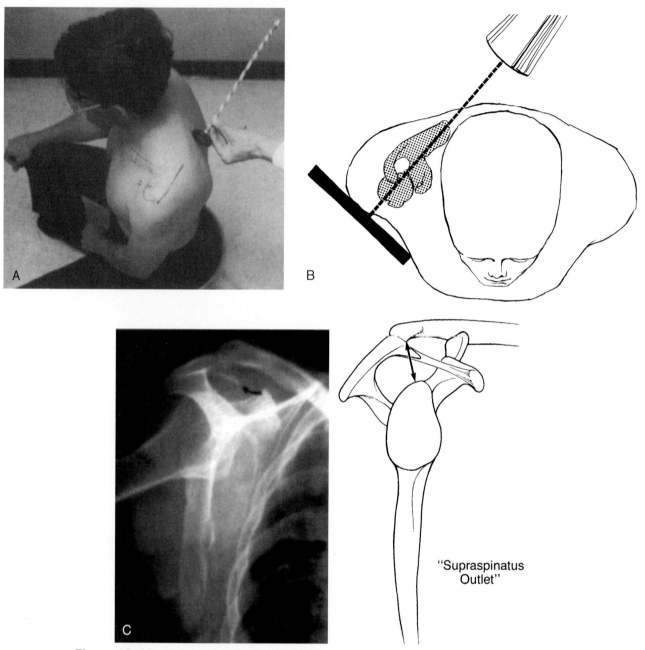

"Supraspinatus
Outlet"

Figure 19–40. The outlet Y view is obtained by shooting the x-ray beam parallel to the base of the spine *(A, B)*, which yields information about the structure of the acromion and injury within the subacromial space. Note the presence of a calcified anterior acromial spur on the outlet view in *C* due to traction of the CA ligament on the acromial attachment. (*C* from Neer CS II: Shoulder Reconstruction. Philadelphia, WB Saunders, 1990.)

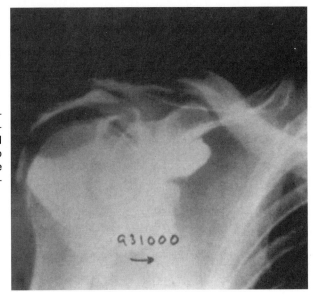

Figure 19–41. An arthrogram is performed by injecting radiopaque contrast material within the glenohumeral joint, observing for the abnormal presence of dye in the subacromial space. A tear of the rotator cuff is indicated by dye leaking into the subacromial space and outlining the superior (bursal) side of the cuff. (From Rockwood CA Jr, Matsen FA III: The Shoulder, 2nd ed. Philadelphia, WB Saunders, 1998.)

shoulder is in evaluating a suspected tumor or AC problems, such as osteolysis of the distal clavicle (Fig. 19–43).

ELECTRODIAGNOSTIC TESTING

Electrodiagnostic tests assess the neurologic status of the upper velocity (NCV) testing. In EMG testing, fine wire electrodes are inserted into upper extremity and paraspinal muscles and record their resting potential and firing patterns. NCV testing examines the speed with which an electrical impulse is conducted through a specific nerve.

ARTHROSCOPY

Diagnostic arthroscopy is the gold standard for evaluation of the shoulder joint. However, it is invasive, expensive, and unnecessary in evaluating most shoulder problems. Diagnostic arthroscopy is reserved for the patient's refractory response to conventional diagnostic evaluation or the patient in whom nonoperative treatment has been ineffective.

TREATMENT OF SHOULDER PROBLEMS

An algorithmic approach is effective in the diagnosis and treatment of most problems. With respect to traumatic injuries, the mnemonic RICE, meaning rest, ice, compression, and elevation, is usually applicable. Rehabilitation, with or without surgery, is effective in the treatment of

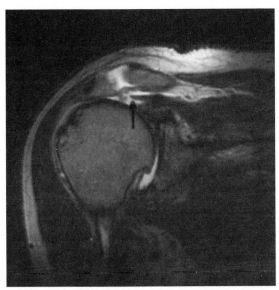

Figure 19–42. MRI is very accurate in demonstrating full-thickness rotator cuff tears, as shown here, although this imaging technology has limitations in distinguishing lesser degrees of partial-thickness cuff injury. The arrow points to the retracted end of the supraspinatus tendon. The white signal reflects fluid present in the region that is normally occupied by tendon whose signal is black. (From Miller MD, Osborne JR, Warner JP, Fu FH: MRI-Arthroscopy Correlative Atlas. Philadelphia, WB Saunders, 1997.)

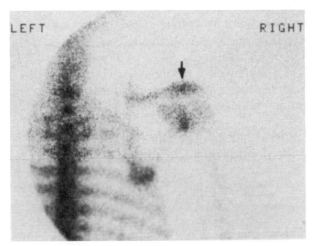

Figure 19–43. A bone scan is helpful in demonstrating osseous defects, in this case showing involvement of the distal AC joint in a case in which plain x-rays were unhelpful in the suspected diagnosis of AC arthritis. The *arrow* points to the site of intensive uptake at the AC joint. (From Neer CS II: Shoulder Reconstruction. Philadelphia, WB Saunders, 1990.)

most shoulder conditions, emphasizing restoration of motion, strength, rhythm, endurance, and function.

This section reviews the evaluation and management of some common traumatic and atraumatic problems affecting the shoulder.

Traumatic Shoulder Conditions

CLAVICLE FRACTURES

The clavicle is the bone most commonly fractured in children, and accounts for roughly two thirds of all adult shoulder fractures.

Anatomy. The clavicle is an S-shaped bone that serves as a "strut" between the axial spine and the appendicular skeleton (see Fig. 19–2). The clavicle suspends the shoulder girdle through its connection to the scapula at the acromioclavicular (AC) joint and through the coracoclavicular ligaments (conoid, trapezoid). Medially, the clavicle is secured to the sternum through strong fibrous capsular attachments and reinforcing costoclavicular ligaments. Laterally, the distal clavicle articulates with the acromial process of the scapula, reinforced by capsular ligaments and the coracoclavicular ligaments. Fractures most commonly occur along the vulnerable middle clavicle, where no reinforcing ligaments are present and muscular attachments are few.

Classification. Fractures are classified according to their anatomic location into medial, middle, and lateral thirds. Eighty percent of clavicle fractures are located in the middle third, made vulnerable by the smaller shaft diameter, absence of soft tissue attachments, and less protected location. Fifteen percent of fractures occur at the lateral end, where fractures are further subdivided according to the

relationship of the fracture pattern to the coracoclavicular ligaments and AC joint (Fig. 19–44). A type I distal clavicle fracture occurs between the coracoclavicular attachments to the clavicular undersurface and the AC joint. The fracture is minimally displaced. Type II fractures occur medial to the attachments of the conoid and trapezoid, resulting in proximal displacement of the clavicle and the appearance clinically of a grade III AC separation. Type III fractures are distal clavicle fractures that extend into the AC joint. Approximately 5% of clavicle fractures occur in the medial one third of the clavicle.

Mechanism of Injury. The most common cause of injury is indirect, by a fall on the outstretched hand. Force is transmitted axially along the shaft of the clavicle, leading to a fracture, usually in the midshaft. Direct injury due to a forceful blow to the clavicle is common in motor vehicle accidents and contact sports.

Presentation. Patients present with pain, swelling, and deformity over the clavicle follow a traumatic injury. Neurologic complaints such as numbness, tingling, or weakness are uncommon. When they do occur, they are usually in association with medial third fractures, where the brachial plexus is in sufficient proximity to the clavicle undersurface to be at risk.

Physical Findings. Visible deformity over the fracture site is common, occasionally with an open injury or "tenting" of the skin directly over a sharp or prominent fracture fragment. Ecchymosis is common as well. In multiple trauma patients, there may be associated injuries to the cervical spine, remaining shoulder girdle, ribs, and underlying vital structures, including the lungs (pneumothorax). Neurologic findings are uncommon, but when they do

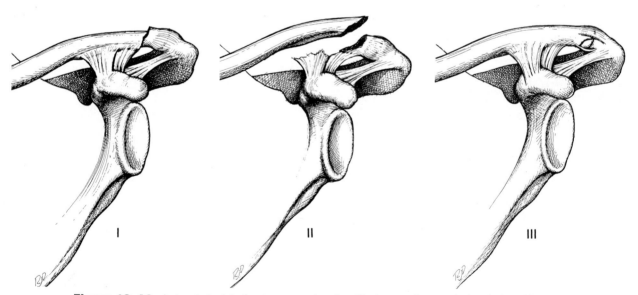

Figure 19–44. Lateral clavicle fractures can be classified according to their relationship with the coracoclavicular (CC) ligaments. In type I, the clavicle is lateral to the CC ligaments, a stable configuration. In type II, the fracture occurs lateral to the CC ligaments, an inherently unstable pattern. Type III involves extension into the AC joint. (From Neer CS II: Shoulder Reconstruction. Philadelphia, WB Saunders, 1990.)

occur, they are usually in the distribution of the ulnar nerve. In the medial third of the clavicle, the medial cord of the plexus lies inferior to the clavicle. Rarely, vascular involvement can occur as a result of injury to the subclavian vein lying beneath the medial third of the clavicle. An expanding hematoma with or without signs of upper extremity ischemia may herald this occurrence.

Radiographic Findings. Two views of the clavicle should be obtained. Medial and middle clavicle fractures require an AP and a 40-degree cephalic tilt view. For lateral clavicle fractures, imaging should be an AP with a 10- to 15-degree cephalic tilt and an axillary lateral view.

Special Tests. Special tests are rarely necessary. Occasionally a CT scan will help image medial third clavicle fractures, particularly in cases in which the sternoclavicular joint may be involved. EMG may be helpful for patients with persistent neurologic deficit following clavicle fracture or in cases of malunion with fracture callus impinging upon the brachial plexus. An arteriogram is indicated to evaluate suspected vascular injury.

Differential Diagnosis. Medial clavicle fractures must be differentiated from sternoclavicular subluxations and dislocations. Because the medial physis (growth plate) is the last in the body to fuse (at age 20 to 25), apparent subluxations or dislocations of the medial sternoclavicular joint

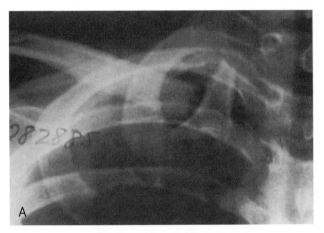

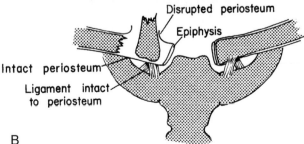

Figure 19–45. Injuries to the medial clavicle in skeletally immature athletes (up to age 25) usually reflect injury to the physis rather than the sternoclavicular joint. This x-ray *(A)* and the accompanying illustration *(B)* show the physeal injury to the medial clavicle, which has displaced to a vertical position. (From Rockwood CA Jr, Matsen FA III: The Shoulder, 2nd ed. Philadelphia. WB Saunders, 1998.)

are considered physeal fractures, rather than actual joint disruptions, until proved otherwise (Fig. 19–45). CT scan is the most helpful diagnostic aid to evaluate this area.

Treatment. The treatment of clavicle fractures is generally nonoperative, involving use of a sling and swathe or figure-of-eight bandage until healing is evident. Nonoperative treatment has been shown to be effective in the vast majority of cases, with fewer than 5% of clavicle fractures proceeding to nonunion. Nonunion is most common in middle third clavicle fractures because it is the location where most clavicle fractures occur. Risk factors for nonunion include the degree of soft tissue injury (amount of trauma) and the amount of displacement. However, few middle third clavicle fractures require operative treatment. Nonunions, when they do occur, are often asymptomatic. Lateral clavicle fractures, particularly type II, are decidedly less common, but statistically are at highest risk of nonunion, occurring in about 20% of these injuries. For this reason, type II distal clavicle fractures are sometimes treated operatively with open reduction and internal fixation. Risk of nonunion of medial third fractures is so low, and the relationship with important neurovascular structures is so high that operative treatment is rarely considered.

Indications for open treatment include the presence of an open fracture, marked displacement with comminution, associated neurovascular injury, fracture in a multiple trauma patient in which upper extremity weight bearing for early mobilization is a priority, and the presence of a type II distal clavicle fracture.

PROXIMAL HUMERUS FRACTURES
Fractures of the proximal humerus account for 5 to 7% of all fractures.

Anatomy. The proximal humerus anatomy consists of the surgical neck dividing the head and shaft, and the articular surface separated from the proximal humerus at the anatomic neck, the lesser and the greater tuberosities, to which the rotator cuff attaches (Fig. 19–46). The biceps tendon courses through the bicipital groove on the anterolateral aspect of the proximal humerus between the lesser and greater tuberosity. Blood supply to the proximal humerus is via several sources, predominantly the anterior and posterior humeral circumflex vessels. The neurovascular structures travel medial to the coracoid and into the upper extremity in the axilla, where they are vulnerable to injury from direct and indirect trauma.

Classification. The most useful proximal humerus classification is the Neer classification, based on the Columbia professor of shoulder surgery whose work helped better understand these injuries (Fig. 19–47). The scheme is simple and involves describing the fracture based on the degree of displacement of the component parts. The four basic parts are the head, the shaft, and the lesser and greater tuberosity. Fractures can be classified on the number of fragments that are displaced. Displacement between two fragments greater than this defined amount makes it a two-part fracture. Displacement of three or more fragments from each other defines a three-part fracture. And the

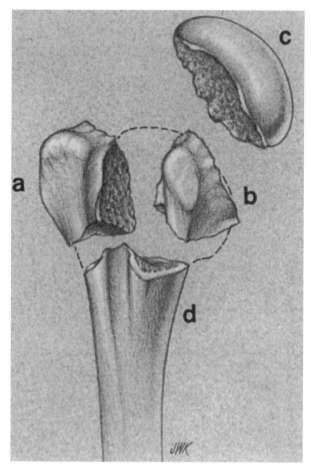

Figure 19–46. The four "parts" inherent to proximal humerus fractures generally separate along the line of their epiphyses. These parts are the humeral head *(c)*, the lesser tuberosity *(b)*, the greater tuberosity *(a)*, and the shaft *(d)*. (From Rockwood CA Jr, Matsen FA III: The Shoulder, 2nd ed. Philadelphia. WB Saunders, 1998.)

falling and landing on one's outstretched hand. The transmitted load often leads to failure of the osteoporotic proximal humerus. The most common fracture is the one-part surgical neck fracture, followed by the two-part, three-part, four-part, and fracture dislocations.

Presentation. The typical presentation is that of pain, swelling and shoulder disability following a fall. The patient usually holds the arm to the side and has often already been placed in a sling.

Physical Findings. The patient is usually in some discomfort on attempting movement. Inspection shows swelling and ecchymoses. The patient is usually reluctant or unable to move the shoulder. Rarely, there may be an expanding hematoma with progressive swelling that suggests an underlying vascular injury. Though uncommon, it may occur in elderly patients whose brittle vessels can be avulsed at the time of the trauma. Distal pulses can remain intact in

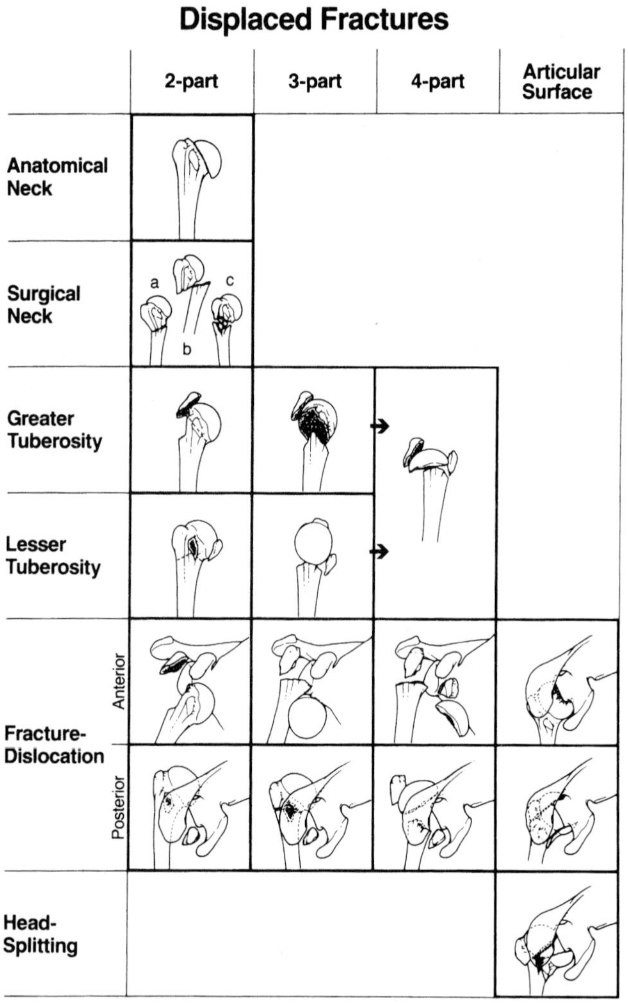

Displaced Fractures

	2-part	3-part	4-part	Articular Surface
Anatomical Neck	◉			
Surgical Neck	a ◉ c / b			
Greater Tuberosity	◉	◉	◉	
Lesser Tuberosity	◉	◉	◉	
Fracture-Dislocation *Anterior*	◉	◉	◉	◉
Fracture-Dislocation *Posterior*	◉	◉	◉	◉
Head-Splitting				◉

Figure 19–47. Fractures of the proximal humerus are best classified according to the scheme of Neer, in which the number of parts were dictated according to their degree of displacement. To be a part, the fragment must be displaced either 1 cm or 45 degrees. (From Rockwood CA Jr, Matsen FA III: The Shoulder, 2nd ed. Philadelphia, WB Saunders, 1998.)

presence of displacement between the head, shaft, and both tuberosities makes up a four-part fracture. To be considered displaced, the fracture fragment must be translated at least 1 cm or rotated 45 degrees. Otherwise, the fracture is considered only a one-part fracture. Under this definition, even a fracture that has multiple planes will be considered a one-part fracture if the criteria for displacement are not met. In addition to the number of parts of the fracture, occasionally a dislocation occurs. Injuries in these cases are described by both the number of parts and the dislocation, such as three-part fracture (Fig. 19–48).

This classification system is useful in communication between clinicians in describing the fracture pattern, as well as in treatment decision making. Eight percent of fractures are one-part fractures involving nondisplaced or minimally displaced fractures of the surgical neck.

Mechanism of Injury. Proximal humerus fractures can occur either by direct or indirect force. In the younger population fractures can occur as a consequence of multiple trauma with direct injury, or on occasion during a violent fall, such as a ski injury. In the older population, diminished bone quality often contributes to indirect injury from

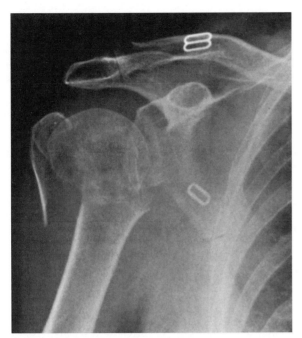

Figure 19–48. This three-part fracture shows displacement of the greater tuberosity, the humeral head, and the shaft from one another, making three distinct parts. (From DeLee JC, Drez D: Orthopaedic Sports Medicine: Principles and Practice. Philadelphia, WB Saunders, 1994.)

about 25% of these cases; diagnosis therefore requires an index of suspicion and evaluation by arteriography when suspected. Neurologic injuries are not uncommon, although they are usually reversible, and should be considered in evaluation. The most common nerves injured in proximal humerus fractures and dislocations include the axillary, suprascapular, radial, and musculocutaneous nerves.

Radiographic Findings. Radiographic evaluation must include a standard true AP view of the glenohumeral joint, a scapular Y view, and an axillary lateral view. Even experienced clinicians vary in interpreting the exact fracture patterns seen in proximal humerus fractures.

Special Tests. Additional tests are rarely necessary, although in some proximal humerus fractures, the pattern can be better elucidated with a CT scan, which may better allow visualization of the fracture fragments and aid in treatment decision making. EMG and NCV testing is reserved for patients with neurologic injury and is usually delayed for about 3 weeks, when denervation can first be detected. Finally, arteriography is helpful in evaluating the uncommon but potentially serious vascular injury.

Differential Diagnosis. The differential diagnosis includes trauma to other upper extremity structures. In the patient who presents with considerable shoulder pain following a fall but with negative x-rays, consider the presence of a nondisplaced proximal humerus fracture or a rotator cuff tear. A nondisplaced fracture or cuff tear can be seen on MRI.

Treatment. Most proximal humerus fractures are treated nonoperatively, with generally good outcomes. The most

common complication following proximal humerus fracture is stiffness. Motion is therefore instituted as early as possible within the limitations of the fracture patterns' stability. For the majority of proximal humerus fractures, the fragments move together as a unit fairly early (within days to weeks of the fracture), and thus emphasis on initiating early motion is encouraged. The degree of displacement, number of fragments, quality of the bone, and compliance and willingness of the patient all influence the decision as to when motion should be started. One-part fractures initially are placed in a sling and swathe for comfort. Early range of motion, usually in the form of "Codman" exercises, is then pursued. These pendulum exercises are carried out by leaning forward and using the "good" arm to gently rotate the injured shoulder in small and progressively larger clockwise and counterclockwise circles (Fig. 19–49).

Displaced fractures are generally treated surgically. This includes two- and three-part fractures and fracture dislocations in most patients, and four-part fractures in some younger patients. The goal of surgery is restoration of anatomy with sufficient fixation to permit early motion. Failure to obtain satisfactory fixation, sufficient to permit early motion, usually leads to a compromised outcome. Patients with head-splitting fractures, four-part fractures, and four-part–fracture dislocations are generally candidates for humeral head replacement using a prosthesis.

In addition to stiffness, other less common complications following proximal humerus fractures include nonunion, malunion, osteonecrosis, and heterotopic ossification.

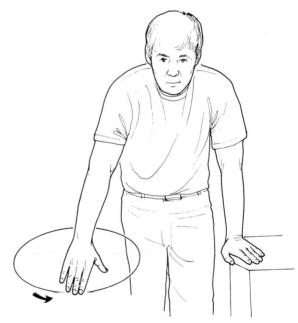

Figure 19–49. Codman pendulum range of motion exercises are performed by having the patient lean forward in a sitting or standing position, and gently allowing passive circular arc of motion to be performed. This allows institution of early motion without subjecting the shoulder to high forces that could disrupt the repair/fixation. (From Neer CS II: Shoulder Reconstruction. Philadelphia, WB Saunders, 1990.)

HUMERAL SHAFT FRACTURE

Fractures of the humeral shaft are common and account for approximately 3% of all shoulder injuries. Most are treatable with nonoperative intervention.

Anatomy. The humerus is bounded by the shoulder joint above and the elbow below, with a surrounding muscular envelope and vulnerable neurovascular structures.

Mechanism of Injury. Both indirect and direct trauma can lead to humeral shaft fractures. A fall on an outstretched hand, direct injury from a motor vehicle accident, or a direct blow to the arm are all common modes of injury.

Classification. Classification generally involves a description of the fracture pattern and its location, such as "an oblique fracture of the middle third of the humerus."

Presentation. Pain in the arm following a traumatic injury is a typical presentation.

Physical Findings. Pain, swelling, ecchymoses, and deformity are commonly present. Inspect for evidence of any open wounds that suggest the presence of an open fracture. The arm may appear shortened, and there may be a grating sensation at the fracture site if the arm is moved. The neurovascular status should be checked, including pulses and motor and sensory testing. Injury to the radial nerve is not uncommon and historically was thought to occur in the distal third of the humerus where spiral fractures are thought to compromise and lacerate the nerve at its emer-gence laterally through the intermuscular septum. Holstein and Lewis described this injury, and this fracture pattern associated with radial nerve injury goes by their name. However, subsequent research and clinical studies have shown that these nerve injuries are usually neuropraxias, which will usually resolve with time. Second, radial nerve injuries are actually most common in the middle shaft of the humerus rather than in the distal third.

Radiographic Findings. X-rays should include AP and lateral views that are 90 degrees to one another. This should be done by having the patient move or moving the x-ray tube rather than attempting to rotate the humerus itself. Films must include the joint above and the joint below. Injury to the proximal or distal humerus must be ruled out.

Special Tests. Special tests are rarely necessary but include the use of electrodiagnostic or vascular studies for the rare occurrence of a neurovascular injury.

Differential Diagnosis. Proximal biceps tendon ruptures can lead to acute upper extremity discomfort, ecchymoses and swelling, along with a globular "Popeye" muscle in the midanterior humerus.

Treatment. Most humeral shaft fractures can be treated nonoperatively with a coaptation splint followed at about 2 weeks with a functional brace (Fig. 19–50). The brace is composed of two polypropylene shells placed on the front and back of the arm and connected by Velcro straps. Muscular contraction actually is thought to enhance frac-

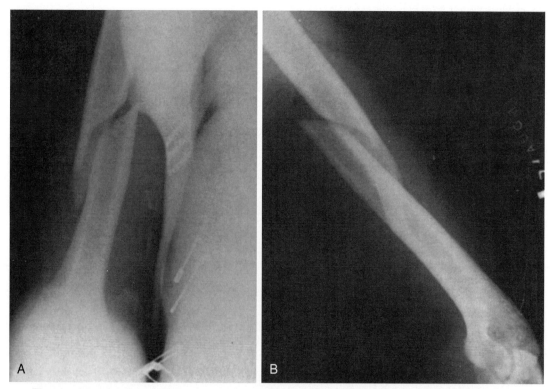

Figure 19–50. This humeral shaft fracture is a spiral configuration and is treated with a functional brace. *A,* The spiral fracture in the anteroposterior radiograph. *B,* The fracture in a lateral view. (From DeLee JC, Drez D: Orthopaedic Sports Medicine: Principles and Practice. Philadelphia, WB Saunders, 1994.)

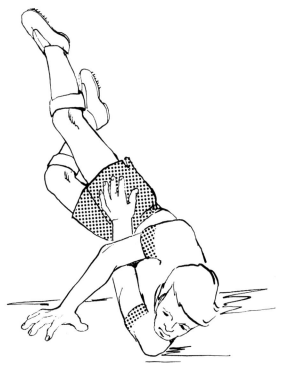

Figure 19–51. The typical mechanism of injury in AC separations involves direct trauma to the point of the shoulder. (From DeLee JC, Drez D: Orthopaedic Sports Medicine: Principles and Practice. Philadelphia, WB Saunders, 1994.)

ture site alignment and stability. Exceptions to closed treatment include most open fractures, segmental fractures, fractures associated with ipsilateral forearm or shoulder girdle trauma (the so-called "floating" humerus fracture), and fractures in multiple-trauma patients (in whom early mobilization is important). Those with neurovascular injury may be surgical candidates, but this requires individual assessment.

ACROMIOCLAVICULAR JOINT SPRAIN (SHOULDER SEPARATION)

Trauma to the acromioclavicular (AC) joint is the most common injury seen in the shoulder. Because the tissue injury is often sufficient to cause joint disruption and "separation" of the acromion from the clavicle, this entity is also known as AC separation.

Relevant Anatomy. The shoulder girdle is suspended from the body via the clavicle, which serves as a supportive strut. Without the clavicle, the shoulder girdle would simply hang down at the side, appearing drooped. The suspension is via two specific structures: (1) the capsule of the AC joint, a thick fibrous envelope that connects the distal clavicle with the acromion, and (2) the coracoclavicular (CC) ligaments (conoid and trapezoid), stout ligaments connecting the undersurface of the clavicle to the coracoid (see Fig. 19–4).

Mechanism of Injury. AC joint injury results from direct trauma to the point of the shoulder, usually from landing directly on it (Fig. 19–51). It is commonly seen in collision sports such as football, rugby, lacrosse, and skiing. The traumatic load applies an inferiorly directed force on the

acromion relative to the clavicle. The degree of injury depends on the severity of this force, with mild injury limited to the AC joint capsule, and more severe injury leading to sprain and ultimate disruption of the supporting CC ligaments.

Classification. In the most commonly used classification scheme, there are three types of sprains, based on the degree of injury to the AC joint and the CC ligaments (Fig. 19–52). In a type I sprain there is a sprain (partial tearing)

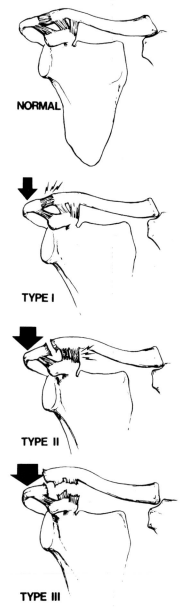

NORMAL

TYPE I

TYPE II

TYPE III

Figure 19–52. AC joint injuries (AC separations) are classified according to the degree of injury to the supporting structures. In type I, there is capsular sprain to the AC joint capsule. In type II, there is sufficient force to disrupt the AC joint capsule and impart some strain to the coracoclavicular (CC) ligaments, with some relative displacement at the AC joint. In type III, the force has been sufficient to disrupt both the AC capsule and the CC ligaments, leading to a complete AC separation. Other types have been described but are less common, and therefore are not included here. (From Rockwood CA Jr, Matsen FA III: The Shoulder, 2nd ed. Philadelphia, WB Saunders, 1998.)

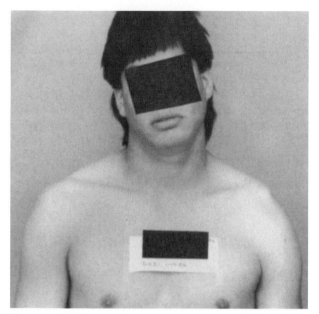

Figure 19–53. This close-up of the left shoulder demonstrates the typical deformity seen in patients with complete (type III) separations, with relative drooping of the shoulder girdle relative to the proximally displaced distal clavicle, creating a "step-off." (From DeLee JC, Drez D: Orthopaedic Sports Medicine: Principles and Practice. Philadelphia, WB Saunders, 1994.)

of the AC joint but no injury to the CC ligaments. Type II describes a complete disruption of the AC joint and a partial sprain of the CC ligaments. In a type III AC separation, there is complete disruption of the AC joint and of the CC ligaments. In essence, a type III AC separation means complete disruption of the normal attachments between the acromion and clavicle. This classification is easy to establish on the basis of the physical and x-ray examinations, and is clinically useful in determining prognosis and treatment. More complex classification schemes include three more types of AC joint injury, but these injuries are uncommon.

Physical Examination. Findings depend upon injury severity. Type I sprains may demonstrate mild swelling and focal tenderness to palpation directly over the AC joint. Most patients are able to elevate the shoulder reasonably comfortably. There is no asymmetry on inspection. Type II sprains are more significant, usually demonstrating a greater amount of focal tenderness, ecchymoses, and desire to avoid moving the shoulder. There may be a small "step-off" of the joint from the relative inferior displacement of the acromion from the relatively superiorly prominent clavicle. In a type III AC separation, the physical findings are even more substantial, including greater degree of swelling, asymmetry, visible "step-off," drooping of the shoulder girdle, and pain on attempted motion (Fig. 19–53).

Radiographic Findings. Proper evaluation of the AC joint requires an AP view and an axillary lateral view. Tilting the AP beam superiorly at about a 10-degree angle and decreasing the kV by half enhances visualization of the AC joint. This view is known as a Zanca view, named by

the clinician that described this finding (see Fig. 19–39). The axillary lateral view allows appreciation of any fracture into the joint and any anterior or posterior displacement. X-rays of a type I AC separation are normal. In a type II, there may be up to 50% displacement, with the clavicle somewhat superior in relation to the acromion. In a type III separation there may be up to 100% displacement (Fig. 19–54).

Special Tests. No special tests are usually necessary. Occasionally, a type III sprain will masquerade as a type I or II and appear minimally displaced or nondisplaced. For this reason, some clinicians have advocated obtaining stress views to ensure that type III separations are not missed. Stress views are obtained by securing weights (5 to 10 lb) to the patient's wrists, and obtaining x-rays of both AC joints (on the same film if possible) (Fig. 19–55). In a type III AC separation, this additional stress will cause the acromion to be inferiorly displaced, thereby "opening up" the AC joint. This test is rarely necessary in clinical practice for two reasons. First, most grade III separations are evident without requiring stress views. Second, making the distinction between grades II and III is usually irrelevant because treatment is usually the same.

Differential Diagnosis. The differential diagnosis includes distal clavicle fracture, which can be seen on x-ray, and osteolysis of the distal clavicle (DCO). In DCO repetitive stresses lead to breakdown of the distal clavicle and progressive activity-related pain in the vicinity of the AC joint. However, the condition is insidious in onset, unrelated to traumatic injury, and unassociated with any "separation" of the AC joint.

Treatment. Temporary activity modification including use of a sling or figure-of-eight bandage is helpful for all AC sprains. In addition, ice for the first 24 hours and use of NSAIDs may be helpful. Definitive treatment is almost always nonoperative. The benefit of the classification sys-

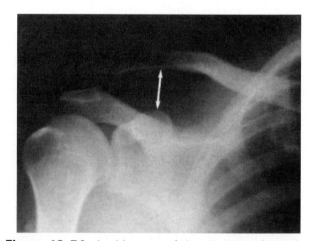

Figure 19–54. In this x-ray of the shoulder of a patient with a type III (complete) AC separation, there is displacement of the distal clavicle in relation to the acromion, appreciated by inspecting the increased coracoclavicular distance *(arrow).* (From Neer CS II: Shoulder Reconstruction. Philadelphia, WB Saunders, 1990.)

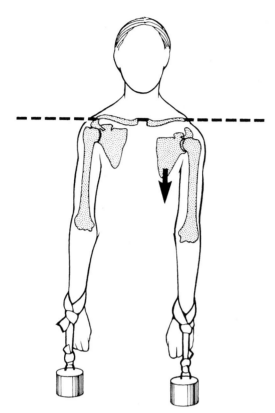

Figure 19–55. This illustration demonstrates the technique of stressing the AC joints in which weights are secured to the patient's forearm or wrist to exaggerate the force and therefore better appreciate any deformity at the AC joint. Note the increased separation of the left AC joint under this stress test. (From Rockwood CA Jr, Matsen FA III: The Shoulder, 2nd ed. Philadelphia, WB Saunders, 1998.)

tem is in recognizing its relationship to prognosis and subsequent problems. Specifically, type I injuries are usually mild and will permit active motion within a few days. Football players with this injury will probably be able to return in time for the next game, though they may be sore. The risk of developing late degenerative changes is on the order of 5%. Type II AC separations are treated identically to type I injuries, with recognition that risk of later degenerative joint changes is slightly higher in type II, perhaps 10%. Time out of competition is usually larger for these moderate sprains, which may require several weeks for substantial improvement. Type III injuries are also treated nonoperatively in most cases. There is no role for use of a special bandage or splint in grade III injuries, because there is no device that will maintain the joint in a "reduced" position. For this reason, the injury is treated for comfort only. A sling is usually just as effective as a figure-of-eight bandage.

Type III sprains usually lead to a longer period of disability, but eventually most people are able to return to their previous level of activity. Problems associated with type III injuries include cosmetic deformity and the risk of late degenerative arthritis or dysfunction. The "bump" will not spontaneously resolve, and patients should be forewarned of this fact. In muscular individuals, deformity may be minimal, whereas in thin patients, the bump may be

quite prominent and noticeable. Nevertheless, most patients learn to tolerate the appearance, and if they can do so, the likelihood of pain or dysfunction is small, estimated at approximately 15%. Surgical intervention is reserved for the small number of patients with type III AC separations who are intolerant of the cosmetic appearance or who cannot afford the "wait and see" approach of nonoperative treatment. Examples of patients sometimes considered surgical candidates include scholarship athletes and heavy laborers whose demands may preclude a delayed hopeful approach, and those who will not tolerate the cosmetic appearance. Symptoms of pain, easy fatigability, or both, occur in about 15% of patients. For this reason, recognition of the potential sequelae after a grade III separation has been described in about 15% of patients. Of symptomatic grade III AC joint–injured patients treated nonoperatively, delayed surgical intervention through a Weaver-Dunn reconstruction is usually successful. This procedure involves reconstruction of the CC ligaments using the CA ligament. Primary surgical intervention is reserved for selected grade III AC joint injuries. Indications for surgery include a dominant arm of an overhead throwing athlete, open injuries, and those with skin compromise (tenting of the overlying skin due to the prominent clavicle).

GLENOHUMERAL INSTABILITY

The shoulder has tremendous *mobility,* but at the expense of stability. Unlike the hip, the shoulder is a loosely constrained joint whose stability is rendered by the surrounding soft tissue capsule. Injury to this vulnerable capsule, particularly in young active individuals, leads to recurrent instability. Anterior dislocation of the glenohumeral joint (in which the humeral head dislocates anterior to the glenoid) is the most common dislocation of any joint, occurring in adolescent and young adult athletes. Posterior dislocation is decidedly less common, accounting for approximately 5% of all cases of shoulder instability.

Presentation. The patient with an anterior shoulder dislocation presents with sudden onset of pain and deformity of the shoulder. Often this follows some traumatic incident in which the shoulder has been felt to "go out of place." When recurrent, the shoulder may dislocate without any significant provocation, such as while sleeping or reaching to pick something up. Posterior dislocations usually occur following a traumatic event as well, and are seen in patients with a sudden load to the posterior shoulder (football linemen), or in those in whom sudden muscle contraction causes the shoulder to dislocate (patients with seizure disorder or following electrocution).

Mechanism of Injury. In anterior dislocation, the arm is usually in a position of abduction and external rotation (the throwing position) at the time of injury. A fall onto the arm, or having the arm forced into further external rotation results in the humeral head being levered out the glenoid anteriorly, resulting in a dislocation. Posterior humeral head dislocations occur when the arm, positioned in front of the body (the push-up position) is loaded directly posteriorly.

Relevant Anatomy. The humeral head surface area is substantially greater than that of the glenoid, comparable to

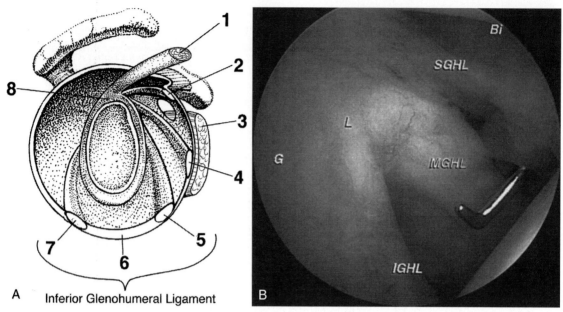

A Inferior Glenohumeral Ligament

Figure 19–56. *A*, The inferior glenohumeral ligament (IGHL), the most important restraint in preventing anterior translation, is shown in this cross section of the glenohumeral joint as one of a number of discrete components appreciated from the inside of the joint. *B*, The arthroscopic view of this complex in relationship to the glenoid (G), including the superior (SGHL), middle (MGHL), and inferior (IGHL) glenohumeral ligaments. Other arthroscopically shown structures are the biceps tendon (Bi) and the labrum (L). (From Rockwood CA Jr, Matsen FA III: The Shoulder, 2nd ed. Philadelphia, WB Saunders, 1998.)

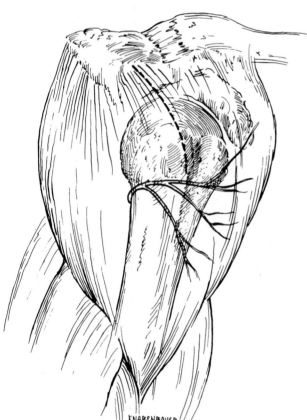

Figure 19–57. This lateral view of the shoulder shows the axillary nerve emerging from the quadrangular space and running anteriorly to provide motor innervation to the entire deltoid. The position relative to the glenohumeral joint renders it vulnerable during shoulder dislocations. (From Rockwood CA Jr, Matsen FA III: The Shoulder, 2nd ed. Philadelphia, WB Saunders, 1998.)

that of a golf ball sitting on a golf tee. Thus, normal shoulder stability is not a consequence of the skeletal design, but by the surrounding soft tissue structures. A fibrous lip of tissue, the labrum, surrounds the glenoid rim, and provides some additional stability by increasing the glenoid socket's depth (see Fig. 19–7). But the surrounding soft tissue envelope, the glenohumeral capsule, renders the greatest stability to the joint. Even more specifically, the anterior and inferior part of the capsular envelope is responsible for preventing anterior instability (in which the humeral head subluxes or dislocates anteriorly to the glenoid). This part of the capsule can be easily seen during arthroscopy, and is known as the anterior inferior glenohumeral ligament complex (Fig. 19–56). When the shoulder dislocates anteriorly, this ligament complex is pulled off or detached from its normal attachment site along the anterior glenoid rim, allowing the humeral head to sublux or dislocate. This detachment is known as a Bankart lesion, named for the physician who in 1903 described its appearance and significance (see Fig. 19–10).

Classification. Shoulder instability can be classified according to direction (anterior, posterior, inferior, or combinations referred to as multidirectional), length of time (acute, chronic), and history (first time, recurrent).

Physical Examination. At the time of presentation following an anterior dislocation, the patient is usually holding the arm at the side, unless at the time of the injury the shoulder either spontaneously or with some manipulation, reduced. When dislocated, the humeral head may be visible anteriorly, and there is noticeable flattening of the normal rounded contour of the lateral aspect of the shoulder (compare to opposite side). The shoulder is tender, and palpation is not specific. Because the axillary nerve travels underneath the surgical neck of the humerus, it is vulnerable to traction stress at the time of the dislocation and is partially stretched and injured up to 30% of the time (Fig. 19–57). Evaluate for possible nerve injury before performing any reduction maneuvers by checking sensation to light touch over the deltoid patch, in comparison with the opposite arm. If there is any question, ask the patient to gently attempt to abduct the shoulder, inspecting and feeling for contraction of the deltoid. Axillary nerve injuries are almost always neuropraxias (self-limiting stretch injuries) and require no specific intervention, but recognizing and documenting its presence prior to manipulation will prevent the implication that the defect was iatrogenic (Fig. 19–58).

Posterior dislocations usually present with the patient holding the arm at the side, avoiding movement. There may be a relative hollowness to the front of the shoulder and a fullness posteriorly. The neurologic examination is usually normal.

Radiographic Findings. A dislocation will be seen on obtaining two views perpendicular to each other prior to and following reduction attempt(s). A true AP view and an axillary lateral view of the glenohumeral joint are standard (Fig. 19–59). Do not be misled and treat on the basis of a single film. Some studies suggest that nearly 80% of posterior dislocations are missed in the emergency room setting because of failure to obtain appropriate films (Fig. 19–60).

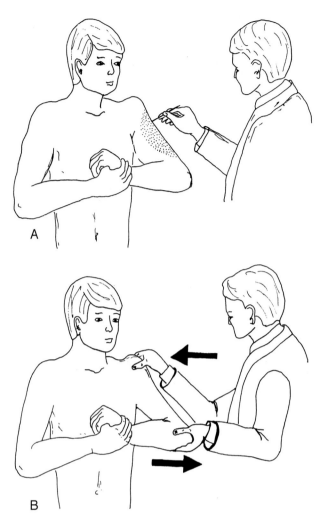

Figure 19–58. Examination for axillary nerve injury is carried out by determining the presence of sensation over the deltoid patch *(A)*. Motor testing can be performed by having the patient try to gently abduct while the examiner holds the patient's elbow *(B)*. (From Stanitski CL, DeLee JC, Drez D Jr: Pediatric and Adolescent Sports Medicine, Vol 3. Philadelphia, WB Saunders, 1994.)

An axillary lateral view can be obtained in nearly every case by careful attentive positioning of the beam. If it cannot be obtained, a CT scan is a reasonable alternative.

A Hill-Sachs lesion has been described as a defect in the posterolateral humeral head as a consequence of impaction upon reduction (Fig. 19–61). This lesion is specific for anterior humeral instability and can best be appreciated with special x-ray views.

Differential Diagnosis. Fractures of the proximal humerus may occur with a dislocation, and x-rays must be obtained to distinguish this entity.

Special Tests. No special tests are necessary in the acute injury. In case of significant axillary nerve injury, electrodiagnostic tests are useful and usually are performed at about 3 weeks after the injury, at which time signs of denervation will usually reliably appear. A CT scan in which air and contrast material have been injected, known as a double-

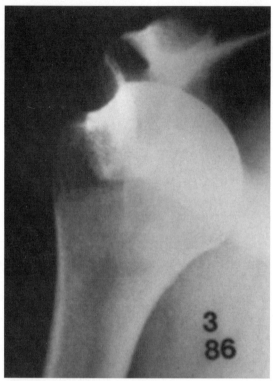

Figure 19–59. Subcoracoid anterior dislocation of the shoulder seen on an AP radiograph. (From DeLee JC, Drez D: Orthopaedic Sports Medicine: Principles and Practice. Philadelphia, WB Saunders, 1994.)

contrast CT of the shoulder, is effective in identifying a Bankart lesion. With the exception of some dedicated and experienced medical centers, MRI has not been as helpful in delineating injury to the labrum and capsular structures.

Definitive Treatment. After clinical and x-ray evaluation, a manipulation should be carried out to achieve reduction. This is usually effected by means of traction-countertraction under some intravenous analgesia and sedation (Fig. 19–62). Typically, a sheet is placed underneath the patient, wrapped around the torso, and used by the assistant to stabilize the body. With gentle longitudinal traction on the arm, reduction usually ensues promptly, with immediate sense of relief to the patient. Alternatively, prone placement with traction on the arm may permit gentle reduction (Fig. 19–63). The neurovascular status is rechecked, followed by application of a sling and postmanipulation films to confirm reduction. The sling is worn for a variable period, depending on the patient's age and history of previous instability. Historically, sling immobilization was recommended for 4 weeks. However, the benefit of immobilization has not been proved and some clinicians question the benefit of more than a few days for comfort. Many studies have demonstrated a direct relationship between risk of instability and age, with those under 20 years of age at highest risk. Some studies cite the risk as high as 85% in this group! In younger patients longer immobilization, up to 4 weeks, is probably reasonable. On the other hand, patients over the age of 30 have only about a 10% recurrence rate, and therefore require less time in a sling. Over

the age of 40, recurrence rate drops substantially. Because of the probability of shoulder stiffness as a complication in this older age group, and the infrequency of recurrent instability, immobilization in this group is only for comfort, with range of motion exercises begun as soon as the patient tolerates movement.

Surgery is reserved for patients with recurrent instability rather than first-time dislocators. In general, after the second episode of instability, the success rate of nonoperative rehabilitation drops dramatically. The goal of surgery is to reattach the usually detached anteroinferior ligament complex (the Bankart lesion) back to its anatomic location along the anterior glenoid rim (Fig. 19–64). Traditionally carried out via open technique, current efforts to achieve stability through arthroscopic techniques are being pursued. Aesthetically and philosophically pleasing, it has not proved as effective as open techniques, but is expected one day to be the definitive treatment of choice for this condition.

PECTORALIS MAJOR TENDON RUPTURES

Tendon injuries of the shoulder girdle are relatively uncommon, but among them, injuries to the pectoralis major are among the most frequent.

Anatomy. The pectoralis major has two origins, a clavicular head and a sternocostal portion. They combine laterally to insert on the proximal humerus. The pectoralis major is one of the major power drivers of the shoulder, and provides strength in shoulder adduction and internal rotation.

Classification. Pectoralis major tears are graded like other sprains according to the degree of injury, from grades I to III. Grade I tears include partial injury, with little hemorrhage, fiber compromise, and usually quick recovery. In a grade II injury, there is substantial tearing of the muscle or

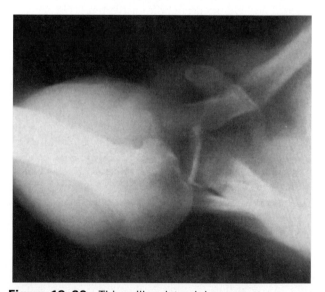

Figure 19–60. This axillary lateral demonstrates an unreduced posterior dislocation, with the humeral head perched on the posterior glenoid. Posterior dislocations are unrecognized in nearly 80% of cases because of failure to obtain this view. (From Neer CS II: Shoulder Reconstruction. Philadelphia, WB Saunders, 1990.)

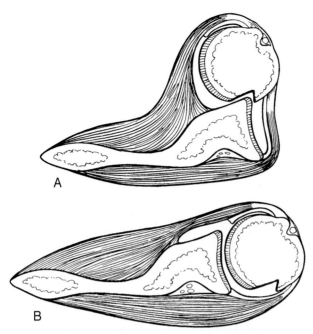

Figure 19–61. A Hill-Sachs lesion is shown in this axial view, in which the anteriorly dislocated humeral head is perched and an impression fracture therefore made on the posterolateral humeral head. (From Wiesel SW, Delahay JN: Essentials of Orthopaedic Surgery, 2nd ed. Philadelphia, WB Saunders, 1997.)

tendon, with partial loss of normal continuity. The amount of swelling, pain, and tenderness is more significant, and there may be detectable deformity at the site of injury. Grade III injuries are complete tears, with loss of normal integrity of the structure. Pectoralis muscle tears can also be classified according to tear location, either within the muscle, at the muscle-tendon junction, or at the tendinous attachment to bone. The most common injury occurs at the muscle-tendon junction.

Mechanism of Injury. The most common presentation is that of a muscular individual performing some feat of

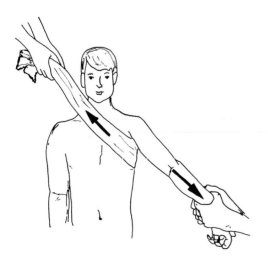

Figure 19–62. Traction-countertraction usually permits relatively gentle reduction of the dislocated shoulder. (From Stanitski CL, DeLee JC, Drez D Jr: Pediatric and Adolescent Sports Medicine, Vol 3. Philadelphia, WB Saunders, 1994.)

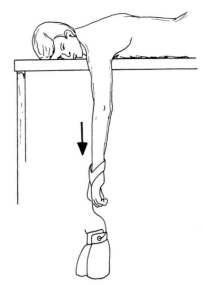

Figure 19–63. Closed reduction of shoulder dislocation may also be achieved by placing the patient prone and applying 10 to 15 lb of weight to the wrist or forearm. (From Stanitski CL, DeLee JC, Drez D Jr: Pediatric and Adolescent Sports Medicine, Vol 3. Philadelphia, WB Saunders, 1994.)

strength, such as trying to lift up the rear end of a car or bench press an inordinate amount of weight. The injury often occurs during an "eccentric" load, such as when doing "negatives" on the down-stroke phase of bench pressing. The force of the contraction exceeds the intrinsic strength of the tissue, leading to acute and overwhelming failure.

Presentation. Sudden pain, swelling, and deformity following an acute injury, usually after lifting something heavy.

Physical Findings. Localized deformity, with asymmetric appearance of the pectoralis fold compared to the opposite side, is seen (Fig. 19–65). There may be swelling and ecchymoses as well. Pain on attempted muscle contraction against resistance both reproduces the pain and may further demonstrate the visible asymmetry.

X-ray. Because this is a soft tissue injury, x-rays are negative.

Special Tests. An MRI is very useful because it enables determination of the site of injury. Although surgical treatment is usually required for restoration of normal muscle integrity, tears of the muscle-tendon junctions are not easily reparable. MRI may help determine the appropriateness of surgical intervention in identifying those with tears near or at the tendinous insertion.

Differential Diagnosis. In the patient with complete detachment, there is little else to consider in the differential. More commonly, patients with a pectoralis injury will go undiagnosed because of clinicians' unfamiliarity with it as a diagnostic entity, and attribute symptoms to a cuff strain.

Treatment. Treatment of grade I and II tears is similar for that of other sprains, namely rest, anti-inflammatory

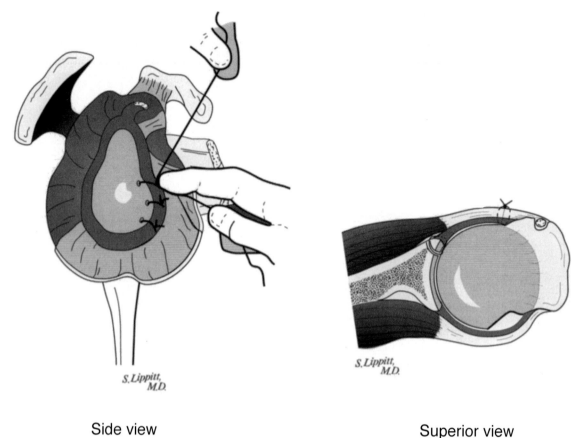

Side view   Superior view

Figure 19–64. In this illustration the detached inferior glenohumeral ligament has been reattached to the anterior glenoid labrum, thereby correcting the "Bankart" lesion. (From Rockwood CA Jr, Matsen FA III: The Shoulder, 2nd ed. Philadelphia, WB Saunders, 1998.)

medication, ice, and local modalities. With time, motion and strength return. For complete tears, surgical intervention with reapproximation of the detached fibers leads to good results in most cases. In patients with muscle-tendon disruptions, surgical repair may not be as effective.

Atraumatic Shoulder Conditions

IMPINGEMENT

The most common atraumatic condition affecting the shoulder is impingement, also known as rotator cuff tendonitis. This condition is responsible for the majority of adult patients presenting with shoulder pain.

Presentation. Anterior shoulder pain is the most common presentation. Symptoms are usually somewhat insidious in onset, and not necessarily related to any specific injury. Alternatively, some patients present with pain after doing something particularly vigorous, such as playing several sets of tennis or falling on the shoulder. The pain is usually a dull ache that radiates laterally to the deltoid insertion. The discomfort is often worse with overhead activity (reaching overhead, serving in tennis, swimming) and may cause nocturnal awakening (especially when lying or rolling onto the affected side).

Pathophysiology. Conventional theories implicate age-related intrinsic degenerative changes in the tendons of the rotator cuff. There may also be some contribution from vascular, traumatic, and mechanical processes.

Relevant Anatomy. The subscapularis, supraspinatus, infraspinatus, and teres minor coalesce as a tendinous cuff to insert on the proximal humerus (see Fig. 19–11). The function of the cuff is primarily that of stabilizing the humeral head, allowing the deltoid to elevate the shoulder (see Fig. 19–12).

The subacromial space, immediately above the cuff, provides a frictionless interface between the cuff and the coracoacromial arch. Normal overhead movements result in smooth frictionless gliding of the rotator cuff's bursal surface within the coracoacromial arch. This arch is composed of the subacromial undersurface, CA ligament, and the AC joint (Fig. 19–66). Any process that interferes with cuff mechanics (failing to maintain the humeral head centered on the glenoid) or compromises the normal outlet through which the otherwise normal cuff passes (abnormal acromial tilt, shape, or spur) can lead to encroachment on the rotator cuff. This mechanical encroachment is termed *impingement* (Fig. 19–67).

Classification. Impingement has been classified clinically by Neer into three stages, which, although somewhat indistinct, offer a way to consider impingement for treatment purposes (Fig. 19–68). In Stage I, symptoms are mild, related to overuse or work with the arm overhead, and are

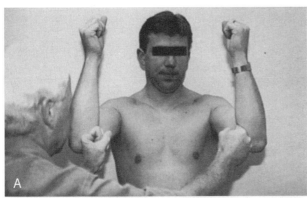
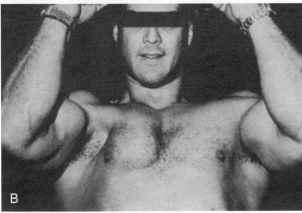

Figure 19–65. Disruption of the pectoralis major muscle is shown here by active adduction of the shoulders against resistance, with obvious asymmetry of this patient's right pectoralis muscle, consistent with a complete tear. (From Rockwood CA Jr, Matsen FA III: The Shoulder, 2nd ed. Philadelphia, WB Saunders, 1998.)

seen in younger individuals (under age 25). Cuff pathology at this early stage is believed due to edema and hemorrhage, and is reversible with rest. Stage II impingement occurs in a slightly older patient, between 25 and 40 years of age. Symptoms are often present for weeks or months at the time of presentation. This stage involves less reversible pathologic cuff changes of tendinitis and fibrosis. In stage III impingement, patients are usually over the age of 45, and symptoms are often chronic. Rotator cuff structural damage is to some degree irreversible, including full-thickness tears. The most common tendon involved is that of the supraspinatus, with the infraspinatus next most common. Tearing of the subscapularis tendon and teres minor are uncommon.

Physical Examination. The patient is observed from the front while raising the arms overhead to notice the "impingement arc sign," which shows discomfort usually seen during elevation between 70 and 120 degrees. Observing from behind, there may be asymmetry in the elevation because of this discomfort. Active and passive range of motion is not actually restricted. The most reliable physical findings are the impingement signs. Best known for the name of the examiner who described them, these signs take advantage of manipulating the shoulder in a way that reproduces the patient's symptoms, suggesting impinge-

ment as a likely cause. In Neer's impingement sign, the affected arm is elevated in the sagittal plane against the scapula, compressing the cuff against the unyielding coracoacromial arch (see Fig. 19–30). Hawkins emphasized adding an internal component to the manipulation to more specifically elicit impingement. While the scapula is held in a fixed position, the arm is elevated and gently internally rotated and adducted, reproducing the pain in the presence of impingement (see Fig. 19–31).

Testing the individual tendons further helps in the assessment of cuff injury. Because involvement of the supraspinatus tendon is most common, testing for impingement relies on examining this muscle. Supraspinatus testing is performed by having the patient place and maintain the arm in the "empty beer can position" with the arm elevated in the plane of the scapula at about 90 degrees and the thumb pointing downward (see Fig. 19–26). Pain during this test, or inability to maintain this position, suggests the possibility of cuff disease. Similarly, involvement of the posterior cuff (infraspinatus) is determined by checking strength in external rotation. With the elbow fixed at the side, the patient is asked to maintain the position of the arm out to the side against the examiner's efforts to internally rotate the arm. Although the "drop arm" sign has been described as specific for rotator cuff tears, neither weakness in supraspinatus nor external rotation strength testing are indicative of cuff tears. Pain, weakness due to disease, nerve injury, and noncompliance can all present with weakness. Conversely, some patients with documented full-thickness cuff tears can still have good strength on manual examination.

Radiographic Findings. X-ray findings are nonspecific. AP views usually show sclerosis of the undersurface of the acromion and greater tuberosity. The presence of a "pseudocyst" of the greater tuberosity due to the presence of localized disuse is not uncommon. Other nonspecific findings include degenerative changes in the AC joint, which may or may not reflect clinical disease. Narrowing of the acromiohumeral interval is an important finding, and indicates long-standing and probably uncorrectable full-thickness (and usually massive) rotator cuff tear (Fig. 19–69).

An axillary lateral view is helpful in evaluating possible abnormal ossification centers, known as os acromiale. This condition is rarely seen (about 2% of the population has this persistent ossification center), but when it exists, it increases the risk of impingement and influences treatment (Fig. 19–70).

The most important x-ray is an outlet view in which the coracoacromial arch outlet is visualized. This view, taken parallel to the plane of the scapula spine, angled 10 to 30 degrees inferiorly, allows direct visualization of the space and particularly the structure of the acromion. The acromion has been classified according to its shape as types I, II, and III (see Fig. 19–40). Type I involves a straight smooth acromion. Type II shows a curved acromion, and type III demonstrates a significant acromial spur (Fig. 19–71). These types are important because they influence treatment strategies.

Special Tests. In the impingement injection test, symptomatic relief following the injection of 3 to 5 ml of 1%

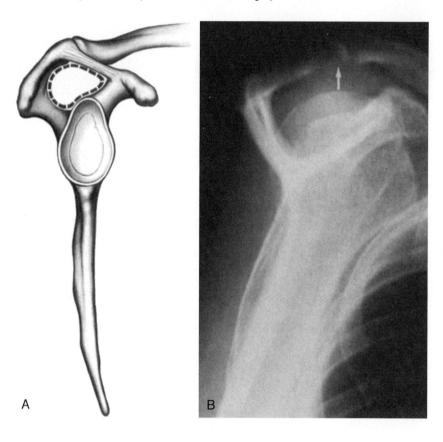

Figure 19–66. The coracoacromial arch consists of the subacromial undersurface, coracoacromial (CA) ligament, and acromioclavicular (AC) joint. (From Neer CS II: Shoulder Reconstruction. Philadelphia, WB Saunders, 1990.)

lidocaine into the subacromial bursa indicates the likelihood that disruption within this space is responsible for the symptoms (Fig. 19–72). More sophisticated imaging tests are appropriate in the patient in whom a cuff tear is suspected or in whom treatment has been ineffective. Imaging of the rotator cuff is achieved through arthrography or MRI. In an arthrogram, dye injected into the glenohumeral joint will normally outline the joint and the undersurface of the rotator cuff. In the presence of a tear, dye leaks through the defect into the subacromial space and can be seen on x-ray (see Fig. 19–41). MRI has by and large superseded use of the arthrogram because of its sensitivity, noninvasiveness, improved accuracy in detecting full-thickness cuff tears, and ability to visualize other structures (see Fig. 19–42).

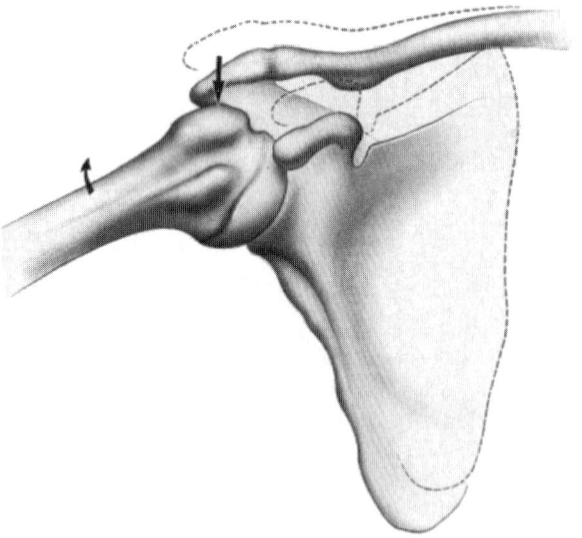

Differential Diagnosis. The differential diagnosis of impingement is that of shoulder pain in general, and includes the early frozen shoulder, arthritis (degenerative, inflammatory), osteonecrosis, infection, traumatic intra-articular injuries, and tumor. AC arthritis can contribute to impingement symptoms because of both its proximity to the cuff and its actual mechanical contribution from inferior AC joint osteophytes. The AC joint must be carefully examined to rule out its involvement in the patient's symptoms. This examination is best performed by the cross body adduction test in which the shoulder is passively adducted across the body, attempting to reproduce the patient's symptoms (Fig. 19–73). Because impingement is generally considered a problem of middle-aged and older adults, younger patients with signs and symptoms of impingement should be examined for occult instability as the most likely etiology.

Treatment. Treatment of impingement depends upon the stage. Stages I and II are usually treatable nonoperatively. The principles of such treatment include (1) elimination of inflammation and pain, (2) restoration of motion, (3) improvement of cuff and scapular rotator strength, (4) restoration of normal scapulohumeral rhythm and coordination, (5) restoration of conditioning, (6) reinitiation of simi-

Figure 19–67. Impingement occurs when the cuff is mechanically compressed on the underside of the acromion or AC joint, resulting in potential wear and damage to the tendon. (From Neer CS II: Shoulder Reconstruction. Philadelphia, WB Saunders, 1990.)

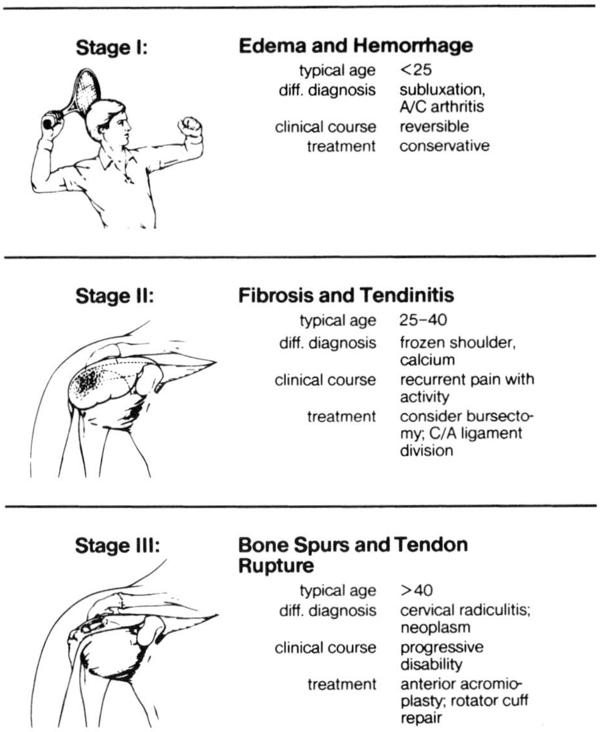

Stage I:	**Edema and Hemorrhage**	
	typical age	<25
	diff. diagnosis	subluxation, A/C arthritis
	clinical course	reversible
	treatment	conservative

Stage II:	**Fibrosis and Tendinitis**	
	typical age	25–40
	diff. diagnosis	frozen shoulder, calcium
	clinical course	recurrent pain with activity
	treatment	consider bursectomy; C/A ligament division

Stage III:	**Bone Spurs and Tendon Rupture**	
	typical age	>40
	diff. diagnosis	cervical radiculitis; neoplasm
	clinical course	progressive disability
	treatment	anterior acromioplasty; rotator cuff repair

Figure 19–68. The most commonly used classification of impingement is by Neer, in which stages are divided into three progressive levels along a continuum. (From Neer CS II: Shoulder Reconstruction. Philadelphia, WB Saunders, 1990.)

lar biomechanical motion and activity, attending to and correcting activity mechanics as necessary, and (7) gradually returning the patient to activity.

In addition to the use of NSAIDs, corticosteroid preparations injected into the subacromial space have been found effective in decreasing pain and inflammation. Because of

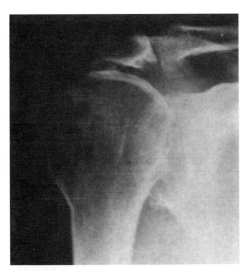

Figure 19–69. Narrowing of the acromiohumeral interval is seen on this AP radiograph, indicating long-standing cuff disease with proximal humeral migration. (From Neer CS II: Shoulder Reconstruction. Philadelphia, WB Saunders, 1990.)

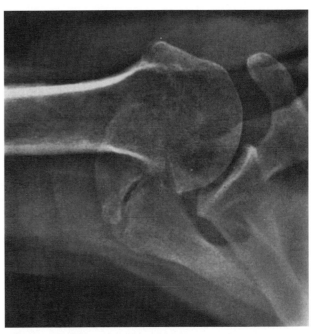

Figure 19–70. An axillary lateral x-ray demonstrates an os acromiale. This relatively uncommon persistent ossification of the acromion contributes to impingement and may require excision or internal fixation. (From Rockwood CA Jr, Matsen FA III: The Shoulder, 2nd ed. Philadelphia, WB Saunders, 1998.)

concern about possible tendon damage, injections are used infrequently, and the number of injections is limited to no more than three in a 1-year period.

Therapy may last only several weeks for the minimally symptomatic athlete who suffers overuse or may require months for the chronically symptomatic older patient. Surgery is reserved for those patients with persistent symptoms despite an adequate trial of therapy and those who have proven symptomatic cuff tears. Of course, the indication for surgical intervention is further influenced by the degree of disability and the patient's goals. Surgery involves either open or arthroscopic decompression of the subacromial space and, when necessary, debridement and repair of the rotator cuff (Fig. 19–74).

CALCIFIC TENDINITIS

Calcific tendinitis is a common disorder in which calcification occurs within the rotator cuff.

Presentation. Calcific tendinitis presents variably. Most commonly, mild impingement symptoms lead to medical evaluation, and x-rays reveal evidence of calcification within the subacromial space. Less commonly, acute shoulder pain may lead the patient in the fourth to fifth decade of life to present for evaluation.

Pathophysiology. The etiology of this condition is unknown, but it is thought to be mediated by the deposition of calcification amid metaplastic chondroid tissue within the tendons of the rotator cuff. Primary degeneration of the cuff initiating deposition of hydroxyapatite crystals and calcification remains an unproven theory.

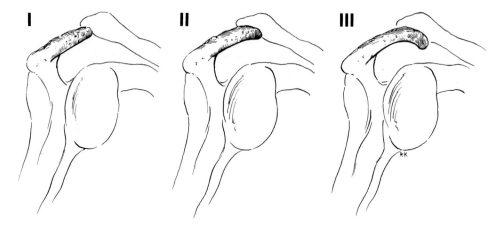

Figure 19–71. Acromial structure has been classified by Bigliani and Morrison on the basis of an "outlet" view, with types I, II, and III. In type I the acromion is relatively flat. Type II shows some rounding or slight compromise of the outlet. Type III shows a hook, with a prominent spur projecting from the anterior inferior acromial undersurface. (From Rockwood CA Jr, Matsen FA III: The Shoulder, 2nd ed. Philadelphia, WB Saunders, 1998.)

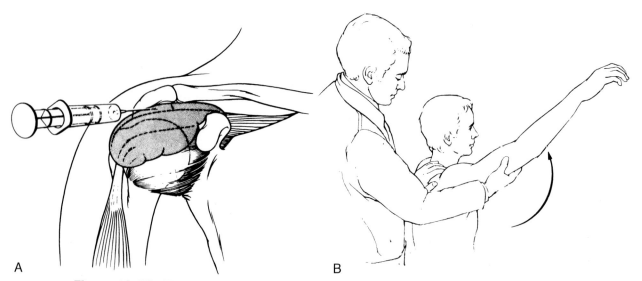

Figure 19–72. The lidocaine impingement test is performed with the injection of lidocaine into the subacromial space (A). If pain is relieved and repeat impingement signs are decreased or eliminated (B), subacromial impingement most likely accounts for the patient's symptoms. (From Neer CS II: Shoulder Reconstruction. Philadelphia, WB Saunders, 1990.)

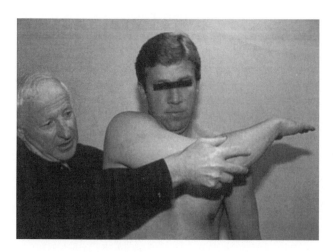

Figure 19–73. Pain in the AC joint on passive adduction of the shoulder suggests AC injury. (From Rockwood CA Jr, Matsen FA III: The Shoulder, 2nd ed. Philadelphia, WB Saunders, 1998.)

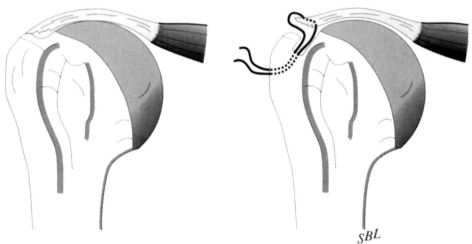

Figure 19–74. This open procedure shows reattachment of the torn edge of the supraspinatus back to its tuberosity insertion, a rather typical approach in rotator cuff repair surgery. (From Rockwood CA Jr, Matsen FA III: The Shoulder, 2nd ed. Philadelphia, WB Saunders, 1998.)

Physical Examination. In the nonacute phase, physical findings are similar to those of impingement, and Neer and Hawkins impingement signs are elicited. Motion is not usually restricted. In the acute painful phase, patients may have marked restriction in both active and passive range of motion.

Radiographic Findings. X-rays establish the diagnosis, with calcific deposits visualized within the tendinous portion of the cuff near its insertion. Because a single AP view may miss the deposit if there are overlying shadows, additional AP views in internal and external rotation help visualize and locate any calcific densities (Fig. 19–75). The supraspinatus is by far the most common location for calcium deposits. Less commonly the salts will localize in the tendon of the infraspinatus. An outlet view allows visualization of the coracoacromial arch and the relationship of the calcium to the arch itself.

Differential Diagnosis. Calcific tendinitis is differentiated from impingement radiographically by the presence of calcific deposits. The patient with acute calcific tendonitis, in which the calcium salts are thought to be undergoing active resorption (also known as the resorptive phase) presents with pain similar to that seen in septic shoulder. The patient is often unwilling to allow any passive shoulder movement. Subacromial lidocaine and corticosteroid injection into the region of the deposit is diagnostic as well as therapeutic. In the patient with suspected septic arthritis, joint aspiration and study of aspirate for cell count, differential blood cell count, Gram stain, and culture are indicated. Dystrophic calcifications seen at the terminal insertion of the cuff in cases of impingement with degenerative change differs from that of calcific tendonitis, in which the deposits are located within the tendon of the cuff.

Special Tests. Radiographs are diagnostic. No further tests are necessary.

Definitive Treatment. Most patients respond to simple nonoperative treatment including analgesics, anti-inflammatory medications, local modalities including ultrasound, and occasionally, corticosteroid injections. Some patients benefit from "needling" the deposit percutaneously. For those with symptoms refractory to nonoperative management, open or arthroscopic surgical excision of the chalk-like calcific deposits is usually effective.

ACROMIOCLAVICULAR JOINT ARTHRITIS

Arthritis of the AC joint is very common and, because of its proximity to the subacromial space, often contributes to symptoms in patients with cuff impingement. Arthritis of this joint can be primary degenerative osteoarthritis or a posttraumatic development.

Presentation. The most common presentation is that of pain over the top of the shoulder, occasionally radiating up

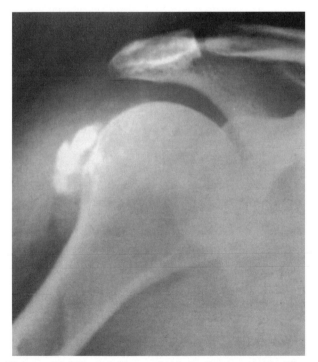

Figure 19–75. Calcific tendinitis is shown on this AP radiograph, occupying the region of insertion of the infraspinatus rotator cuff tendon. (From Rockwood CA Jr, Matsen FA III: The Shoulder, 2nd ed. Philadelphia, WB Saunders, 1998.)

into the trapezius or down the shoulder. The pain is often a mild ache, worsened with specific activities, such as reaching across the body (washing under the opposite axilla) or behind (unfastening their bra, reaching for a wallet). Symptoms are often worse at night, and may awaken the patient, usually when rolling on or lying on the affected shoulder. Usually only one shoulder is affected.

Pathophysiology. AC joint arthritis can occur as a consequence of several disease processes. The three most common entities include primary osteoarthritis, posttraumatic degenerative arthritis, and osteolysis of the distal clavicle. Primary osteoarthritis is similar to that afflicting other synovial joints, namely, progressive thinning and damage to the chondral surfaces leading to narrowing of the joint spaces, the formation of reactive sclerosis, osteophyte formation, and juxta-articular cyst formation. Primary osteoarthritis is very common, with known intrinsic degeneration of the intra-articular meniscal disk in the majority of patients by the fourth decade. Radiographic arthritis is present in the majority of adults over the age of 50. Of course, this doesn't mean these patients are necessarily symptomatic. Most patients, in fact, are not.

Symptomatic posttraumatic arthritis is a common cause of AC symptoms, occurring in approximately 10 to 15% of those with grade I and grade II AC separations. A history of trauma from a previous fall or injury during contact sport (football, rugby, hockey, skiing) commonly precedes symptom onset. Identifying this subset of patients with a history of trauma is important because treatment may differ from that rendered the patient with atraumatic primary arthritis.

The third condition presenting as AC arthritis is osteolysis of the distal clavicle. Patients with this condition are generally younger, and typically are involved in repetitive weight-lifting activities. They complain of pain over the AC joint, particularly worse with bench pressing, dips, flies, and push-ups. The etiology of this condition is thought to be due to stress fractures of the subchondral bone and secondary joint breakdown.

Relevant Anatomy. The AC joint is composed of the distal clavicle and its articulation with the proximal acromion. Both surfaces are covered by articular (hyaline) cartilage. A fibrocartilage disk separates the joint surfaces. Surrounding the joint is a capsular envelope.

Physical Examination. Inspection may reveal prominence due to previous trauma with residual separation or joint hypertrophy. Palpation yields tenderness over the AC joint. The AC joint can be compressed by having the patient place the arm in adduction across the body. This maneuver loads the AC joint and is thought to reproduce symptoms when AC injury is present (see Fig. 19–73). Examination for joint instability can be performed by grasping the distal clavicle and attempting to translate it in an anteroposterior or superoinferior direction.

Radiographic Findings. The AC joint is best imaged in the AP plane by modifying the true AP view by aiming the beam approximately 10 degrees cephalad, and decreasing the kV by about half. This Zanca view best demonstrates the AC joint, and in degenerative arthritis may reveal joint space narrowing, sclerosis, extra-articular cyst formation, and osteophyte formation (Fig. 19–76). An axillary lateral view provides further information regarding joint space and also reveals information about AC alignment. In osteolysis, the distal clavicle is enlarged and appears radiolucent. The joint space in this condition may actually appear to be increased.

Differential Diagnosis. AC joint symptoms may be due to a number of conditions other than arthritis. Possibilities include traumatic injury to the intra-articular meniscal disk, AC sprain, chronic pain following previous AC separation, and less commonly, atraumatic conditions such as inflammatory arthritis.

Special Tests. Rarely, stress tests will be helpful in determining the presence of an instability component to the patient's complaint. A bone scan may prove useful in the patient with convincing symptoms of AC joint pain but negative plain films (see Fig. 19–43). Injection of 1% lidocaine into the AC joint followed by repeat physical examination is helpful in cases of diagnostic uncertainty (Fig. 19–77). Because of variable joint obliquity, an AP x-ray is helpful in ensuring proper targeting of the injection.

Definitive Treatment. Treatment of osteoarthritis, posttraumatic degenerative arthritis, and osteolysis is similar. First, it must be stated that the condition, commonly present on x-ray throughout the adult population, must be symptomatic to warrant treatment. Second, initial treatment involves activity modification and NSAIDs. In the mildly symptomatic patient, this may be sufficient. In the weight-lifting athlete with osteolysis, changing the grip distance or simply eliminating bench pressing or dips from the workout routine may be enough to eliminate symptoms. Persistent symptoms warrant corticosteroid injection directly into the joint, which is often dramatically, if not permanently, effective. Up to three injections are administered before the option of surgical resection is entertained.

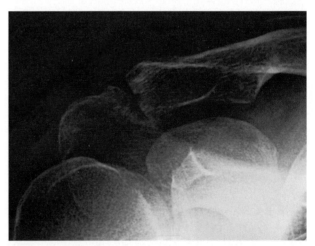

Figure 19–76. This Zanca view demonstrates typical radiographic findings of AC arthritis, including sclerosis, joint space narrowing, and subchondral cyst formation.

Surgical joint debridement and removal of the distal end of the clavicle can be curative in the majority of cases. The only caveat to this is in patients with unrecognized residual AC joint instability, in whom surgical resection may exacerbate symptoms.

FROZEN SHOULDER (ADHESIVE CAPSULITIS)

Occurring in up to 5% of the population, frozen shoulder is a clinical syndrome in which there is restriction in glenohumeral motion for which no specific cause can be determined.

Presentation. The typical presentation is that of a 50-year-old female complaining of progressive pain and stiffness in her nondominant shoulder of several months' duration. The pain is usually generalized or vague over the lateral aspect of the shoulder. Discomfort is often nocturnal, particularly when lying on the affected side, and is accompanied by nocturnal awakening. Stiffness often develops with time. The patient may note difficulty reaching behind, fastening or unfastening the bra, washing hair, and as stiffness progresses, using her arm overhead.

Pathophysiology. Despite familiarity with this condition for more than 50 years, the etiology of frozen shoulder remains unknown. The name "adhesive capsulitis" has been used synonymously with frozen shoulder because of the adhesive and restrictive qualities that have been described affecting the shoulder capsule.

Classification. Frozen shoulder has been divided into three distinct but overlapping clinical phases—painful, stiffening, and thawing. The painful phase is the first phase, with onset usually insidious and progressive. In the next, the stiffening phase, pain resolves, with patients noting stiffness. Finally, the shoulder begins to "thaw" in the third and final phase. The benefit of this classification system is in applying treatment based on the clinical stage of presentation. The disadvantage is the inability to definitively identify the phase the patient may be in at the time of initial presentation or to confidently predict each stage's duration. In general, each stage can last several months, with the entire course of the disorder lasting, in some cases, more than a year. Frozen shoulder is thought to be ultimately a self-limiting disorder in most patients, although a small degree of residual pain or stiffness is not uncommon.

Physical Examination. The hallmark of the physical examination is restriction in both active and passive motion of variable severity. Restriction is present in several planes, including forward elevation and external and internal rotation.

Radiographic Findings. Other than the nonspecific findings of osteopenia (decreased bone density), patients with frozen shoulder have no specific x-ray findings.

Differential Diagnosis. The condition most commonly presenting as a "locked" shoulder is a posterior shoulder dislocation. This entity can be ruled out by obtaining a history of trauma and identifying the dislocated humeral

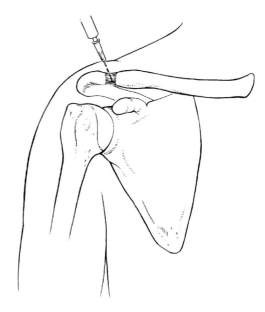

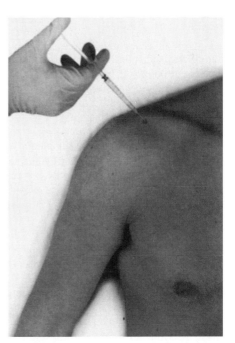

Figure 19–77. Direct injection of the AC joint is performed to determine its contribution to the patient's symptoms. (From Saunders S, Cameron G: Injection Techniques in Orthopaedic and Sports Medicine. Philadelphia, WB Saunders, 1997.)

head on an axillary lateral x-ray. Some shoulders are painful and stiff but not truly "frozen." These include patients with other intrinsic shoulder problems in which stiffness is but one component (arthritis and rotator cuff impingement) and those following trauma or surgery.

Special Tests. The diagnosis of frozen shoulder is made on clinical grounds. There are no laboratory tests specific for this entity. Rather it is a diagnosis of exclusion. The most reliable confirmatory test is an arthrogram, in which contrast agent is injected into the glenohumeral joint. An arthrogram in the typical frozen shoulder demonstrates less than 10 ml of contrast fluid (compared to the normal 15 to 20 ml) accommodated by the shoulder joint capsule, and a blunted (instead of normal) axillary fold.

Treatment. This condition is somewhat frustrating to treat, because resolution of tightness is slow and the recovery timetable is unpredictable. Patients are instructed and supervised in therapy exercises to restore motion. NSAIDs and corticosteroid injections may be effective during the early painful phase. Occasionally, refractory symptoms with persistent motion restriction may warrant operative intervention. At the time of surgery, manipulation under anesthesia and arthroscopic release of extracapsular and capsular adhesions are generally successful.

GLENOHUMERAL ARTHRITIS

Though much less common than arthritis of the weight-bearing hip and knee joints, degenerative arthritis of the glenohumeral joint is still relatively common, thought to occur in up to 20% of adults. Osteoarthritis is considered the most common cause, but other diseases can also lead to degenerative joint breakdown.

Presentation. The exact presentation varies depending on the nature of the problem. In general, pain in the shoulder is the most common presenting complaint, often accompanied by stiffness. Symptoms are typically insidious in onset, progressive, and chronic. Discomfort is worsened with activity and may lead to nocturnal awakening, particularly if they lie on the affected shoulder. Patients will often note a "grating" sensation due to the articular incongruity. Functionally, limitations such as inability to wash under the opposite axilla, reach overhead, or reach their perineal area for daily hygiene are common, especially late in the course.

Pathophysiology and Classification. The pathophysiology of degenerative arthritis is unknown. Degenerative arthritis may be classified as either primary or secondary. Primary degenerative or osteoarthritis is the most common cause of shoulder arthritis and is idiopathic. Whether the inciting problem involves a primary metabolic disturbance within chondrocytes, or is due to disease within the subchondral bone that secondarily affects the vulnerable unsupported chondral surface, is unknown. The pathology is thought to mimic the same processes responsible for osteoarthritis of other synovial joints. Joint changes include progressive loss of normal articular cartilage, increased stress to the subchondral bone, osteophyte, and juxta-articular cyst formation.

Secondary degenerative arthritis is less common, but involves the same end-stage degenerative process following some predisposing injury, surgery, or disease. The most common causes of secondary osteoarthritis include intra-articular fractures (glenohumeral head), recurrent or chronic instability, avascular necrosis, or cuff tear arthropathy.

Fractures that compromise the normal articular congruency of the joint naturally predispose to the development of arthritis. Although uncommon, up to 20% of patients with recurrent instability are thought to be at risk of developing osteoarthritis. Avascular necrosis, in which vascular compromise of the humeral head occurs, can lead to collapse, joint incongruity, and arthritis. Cuff tear arthropathy, in which a massive irreparable cuff defect leads to proximal humeral head migration and articulation with the acromial undersurface, can lead to wearing of the superior humeral head and the development of arthritis.

Physical Examination. The findings to some degree depend upon the etiology of the patient's complaint. In primary osteoarthritis, inspection may reveal modest atrophy from disuse. There is often asynchrony on shoulder elevation with both pain and restriction on active motion. Passive motion is likewise restricted, usually in several planes. There is often nonspecific tenderness about the shoulder, including on palpation over the posterior joint line, and a grating sensation may be felt over the glenohumeral joint during active motion. Patients with a history of previous trauma or surgery may have other visible signs, including scars and/or more specific patterns of restriction (such as the significant loss of normal external rotation following a previous anterior reconstruction for instability).

Radiographic Findings. X-rays should include a true AP view and an axillary lateral view, and will demonstrate the classic features seen in degenerative arthritis (Fig. 19–78). These features include narrowing of the glenohumeral joint space, subchondral sclerosis, osteophyte formation, and juxta-articular cyst formation. Often there are small loose bodies seen in the axillary pouch. The axillary lateral film is very important because it is often the most helpful in identifying eccentric glenoid erosion, a critical development when considering treatment alternatives, particularly arthroplasty.

Differential Diagnosis. The differential diagnosis of glenohumeral osteoarthritis is substantial and includes all conditions that present with a painful, stiff shoulder. The combination of history, physical examination, and radiographic findings should allow the diagnosis to be easily established in most cases. However, a number of conditions can present similarly but must be distinguished. These conditions include inflammatory arthritis, osteonecrosis, rotator cuff arthropathy, neuropathic arthropathy, and septic arthritis.

Inflammatory arthritis is a relatively common disorder affecting the glenohumeral joint. Mediated by an inflammatory enzymatic destructive process in which the synovium and articular cartilage are progressively destroyed, this process is more insidious and rarely occurs in isolation. Most patients have symptoms bilaterally, as well as other joint involvement, which not uncommonly can include other upper extremity joints such as the elbows, wrists, hands, and even acromioclavicular and sternoclavicular joints. A careful history is often helpful in distinguishing this condition from that of osteoarthritis. Radiographic findings differ from those in osteoarthritis, with osteopenia the hallmark rather than sclerosis and osteophyte formation. Weakness on examination commonly reflects the more compromised soft tissues involved along with the joint itself in this process.

Osteonecrosis is a relatively uncommon condition in which some atraumatic process leads to necrosis of the humeral head. Etiologies as disparate as alcoholism,

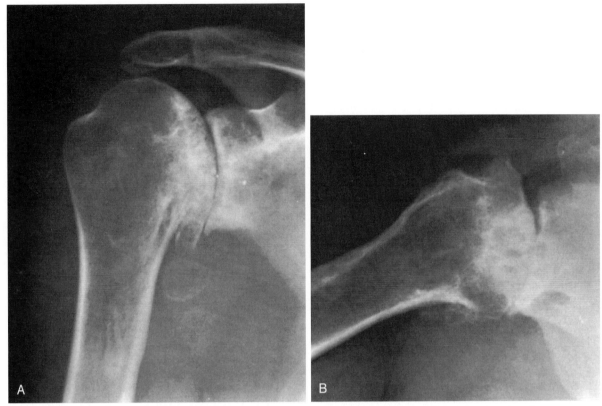

Figure 19–78. Osteoarthritis of the glenohumeral joint is seen on these AP *(A)* and axillary lateral *(B)* radiographs. Note the presence of sclerosis, joint space narrowing, osteophyte formation, and subchondral cysts. The axillary lateral view is particularly valuable in demonstrating the degree of joint space narrowing, which is considerably worse appearing than might be appreciated from merely an AP view. (From Rockwood CA Jr, Matsen FA III: The Shoulder, 2nd ed. Philadelphia, WB Saunders, 1998.)

chronic steroid use, sickle cell disease, hyperuricemia, Gaucher's disease, pancreatitis, hyperlipidemia, lymphoma, and organ transplantation have been implicated in the risk of vascular insult to the humeral head. Symptoms include pain, often at rest and at night. Early radiographs may be negative, requiring bone scan or MRI for detection. Later in the disease course, sclerosis of the head, subchondral fracture, and eventually collapse of the head and end-stage arthritis can be seen (Fig. 19–79). The appropriate patient history accompanied by telling radiographic changes suggests this possible diagnosis.

Rotator cuff arthropathy is an uncommon problem seen in patients with chronic massive irreparable rotator cuff tear. These patients are usually quite disabled and are unable to comfortably elevate the arm. X-rays differ from those of primary osteoarthritis, in that the humeral head has migrated proximally in cuff tear arthropathy. The head is often seen to articulate with the undersurface of the acromion. In fact, some have described this process of the humeral head's articulation as acetabularization of the acromion (Fig. 19–80).

The exact cause of cuff tear arthropathy is unknown, but it is thought to be a mechanical consequence of cuff tear in which muscle dynamics allow the unrestricted head to ride superiorly. Wear from direct mechanical contact leads to chondral degeneration beginning on the superior aspect of the head and leading eventually to the same pain

and limitations as seen with primary degenerative arthritis. Diagnosis is established by x-ray, which shows evidence of the head articulating with the acromial undersurface, in addition to the typical signs of degenerative osteoarthritis.

Neuropathic arthropathy is a distinctly uncommon entity but must be considered within the differential because when missed will create substantial problems. Loss of normal trophic and proprioceptive influence due to neurologic disease causes destructive loss of the normal joint anatomy. The most common causes of this problem include diabetes mellitus and syringomyelia of the cervical spine. Patients will usually present with some shoulder pain and disability, but the most dramatic findings are found on x-ray, which demonstrate significant destructive joint changes. Osseous debris around the joint is a classic finding (Fig. 19–81). Because this condition occurs most commonly due to underlying neurologic disease, workup should include a thorough neurologic examination (electromyography, cervical spine x-rays, and MRI).

Finally, septic arthritis, although relatively uncommon, can present with shoulder pain and restriction. Patients are often somewhat debilitated and may have constitutional signs (i.e., fever, chills, and malaise). The diagnosis is confirmed by joint aspiration with Gram stain, complete blood cell count, differential blood cell count, and culture.

Special Tests. In the straightforward presentation of degenerative arthritis, no special tests are necessary. Because of

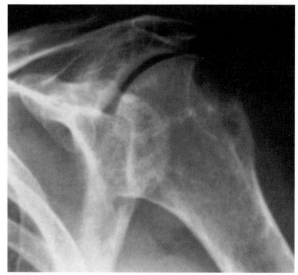

Figure 19–79. This AP view of a left shoulder shows rather typical findings of inflammatory arthritis in its active form, including cartilage loss, periarticular erosions, and hypertrophic synovitis. (From Rockwood CA Jr, Matsen FA III: The Shoulder, 2nd ed. Philadelphia, WB Saunders, 1998.)

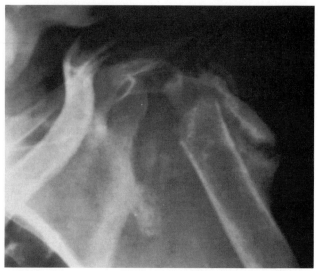

Figure 19–81. Neuropathic joint should be considered in the face of shoulder disability and destructive changes in the absence of a history of significant trauma. Consideration for underlying disease, such as syringomyelia of the cervical spine, and diabetes, must be given. (From Rockwood CA Jr, Matsen FA III: The Shoulder, 2nd ed. Philadelphia, WB Saunders, 1998.)

the tendency for osteoarthritis to lead to posterior glenoid erosion, and because this can pejoratively influence reconstruction efforts, CT scan may be useful in assessing glenoid bone stock. MRI or bone scan may be useful in confirming suspected osteonecrosis. Elecrodiagnostic studies are reserved for the patient with suspected Charcot neuropathy.

Treatment. Treatment of arthritis is variable, depending upon the specific diagnosis. Primary degenerative osteoarthritis is treated symptomatically, including activity modification and use of anti-inflammatory medications. The

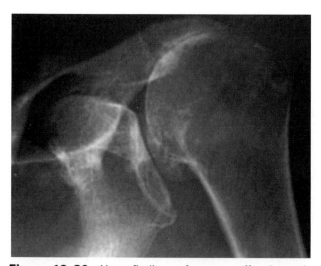

Figure 19–80. X-ray findings of rotator cuff arthropathy in which progressive changes following massive cuff tear include proximal humeral head migration, degenerative arthritis, and acetabularization of the undersurface of the acromion. (From Rockwood CA Jr, Matsen FA III: The Shoulder, 2nd ed. Philadelphia, WB Saunders, 1998.)

judicious use of intra-articular corticosteroid injections may allow comfortable functioning without further intervention for years in the properly selected patient. Definitive treatment for those patients refractory to nonoperative treatment involves prosthetic replacement of the worn proximal humerus and glenoid articular surfaces (Fig. 19–82). Studies have demonstrated remarkable degree of pain relief and restoration of function in patients with uncomplicated primary osteoarthritis. The humeral head is replaced by a metal ball (usually of cobalt chrome) connected to a stem secured within the humeral shaft by press fit or methyl methacrylate (bone cement). The glenoid component, composed of polyethylene, is cemented to the glenoid.

Shoulder replacement is also effective in treating patients with osteoarthritis following previous trauma, surgery, or osteonecrosis. In each of these conditions the surrounding cuff responsible for normal shoulder functioning is usually intact, and helps restore normal function postoperatively. Precise intraoperative surgical technique to accurately position the components and restore soft tissues to normal degree of laxity and careful postoperative therapy are critical for successful outcome following shoulder replacement.

Shoulder replacement is not as effective in treating those with inflammatory arthritis because compromise of the pathologically affected cuff and muscular atrophy prevent restoration of normal function postoperatively. In postoperative rehabilitation, these patients are often managed with recognition of their frequent concomitant disease (other upper or lower extremity joint involvement), and weakened cuff, using limited-goals rehabilitation.

Shoulder replacement should not be considered in treating patients with either a neuropathic shoulder or septic arthritis. Arthrodesis, in which the glenohumeral joint is surgically fused, is a reasonable alternative to arthroplasty

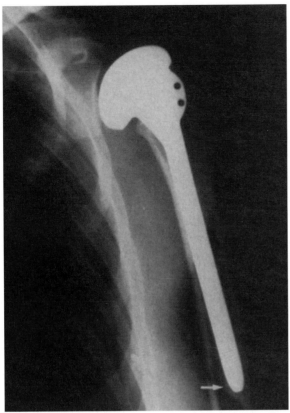

Figure 19–82. This AP view demonstrates the appearance of a total shoulder replacement, in which the worn glenohumeral articular surfaces have been replaced by a metal proximal humeral and polyethylene (plastic) glenoid component. (From Neer CS II: Shoulder Reconstruction. Philadelphia, WB Saunders, 1990.)

in certain patients, including arthritis accompanied by infection, significant motor loss (dysfunctional deltoid or cuff), and failed previous surgery for instability or arthritis.

BRACHIAL NEURITIS

Also known as Parsonage-Turner syndrome, brachial neuritis is an uncommon condition that is responsible for a distinct pattern of shoulder pain. This disorder deserves attention in that only through familiarity as a diagnostic entity can it be recognized and therefore treated.

Presentation. The hallmark of the presentation is usually that of acute onset of a burning type of ache or pain deep within the shoulder. Pain is almost always the most striking part of the patients' complaint, although they may also note weakness. Pain is usually located posteriorly in the vicinity of the scapula, although it can be anywhere, including in the anterior, lateral, or axillary area. Radiation of pain down the arm is not uncommon.

Pathophysiology. The etiology of this condition is not known but is thought by some to be viral-mediated. The pathophysiology involves some sort of neurologic disorder in which the brachial plexus is affected with dysfunction most commonly of the upper trunk. Any of the nerves of the plexus can be involved, although the most common

include the suprascapular and the axillary nerve. Pathologic changes are thought to be self-limited with eventual regeneration of the diseased neural tissue.

Physical Examination. Physical examination findings are most significant for the neurologic manifestations. Specifically, inspection will often reveal atrophy, even in the very early stages (within the first 2 weeks) of the disorder. Atrophy of the supraspinatus or infraspinatus may be substantial. Motor examination yields weakness of muscles affected by the involved nerves. The most common muscles include the deltoid (axillary nerve), supraspinatus, and infraspinatus. The deltoid anterior, middle, and posterior heads are tested gently against resistance while watching and palpating for contraction in each of the individual components. The supraspinatus is tested by having the patient raise and maintain the elevated arm in the plane of the scapula (midway between the coronal and sagittal planes) at 90 degrees with the thumb pointing down. The infraspinatus is tested by having the patient place and hold the elbow against the side while the examiner applies an internal rotation force to the arm. Sensation for the axillary nerve can be tested over the axillary patch of the proximal lateral shoulder. There is no sensory area to correlate with the suprascapular nerve.

Radiographic Findings. X-rays are negative in brachial neuritis.

Differential Diagnosis. The most common differential diagnosis with this condition is radiculopathy from an impinged cervical spine root due to herniated disk or stenosis. Sometimes this differentiation is clinically difficult, because patients with acute brachial neuritis and acute herniated disks can present with significant pain, restricted neck movement, and neurologic findings. In general, however, patients with brachial neuritis usually have normal neck motion. Furthermore, patients with acute cervical disease rarely have atrophy at the time of initial examination.

Also to be considered are other causes of acute shoulder pain, including the early frozen shoulder, calcific tendonitis (the resorptive phase), and septic arthritis. Frozen shoulder in the early phase may be very painful, but rarely is atrophy present, and weakness is very uncommon. Calcific tendonitis may be very painful, particularly in the resorptive phase, but is visible radiographically. A septic shoulder usually hurts to move, and although pain may cause mild weakness, strength is usually reasonable. Diagnostic confirmation is through aspiration and appropriate laboratory studies.

A final consideration, particularly in the younger athlete, and described in volleyball players, is that of suprascapular neuropathy. This entity is due to direct compression of the suprascapular nerve either under the transverse scapular ligament at the scapular notch or at the spinoglenoid notch. Both of these conditions can lead to pain and weakness, but weakness is the most common presenting complaint. Rarely do these patients have considerable pain. MRI evaluation is sometimes helpful in identifying focal ganglion lesions responsible for nerve compression.

Special Tests. Electrodiagnostic (EMG and NCV) tests are confirmatory for this condition and help discriminate between peripheral (brachial plexus) and cervical injury.

Treatment. Pain management is the most important early treatment, including use of a tapering course of oral corticosteroid, supplemented as necessary with strong analgesics. Narcotic pain medicine may be initially necessary in treating this problem. The pain usually subsides within a few weeks of onset, leaving a sometimes weak and dysfunctional shoulder. Instruction in physical therapy is important so that the patient can independently carry out exercises, but recovery takes a long time, and by some accounts may be incomplete. Permanent weakness of a mild degree is the rule rather than the exception. Maximal recovery may take a year or longer. The role of electrical stimulation for trophic influence on muscles has been described but no proven outcome data are available to support its use.

Other Conditions

A number of other, less common conditions afflict the shoulder and should be considered in the differential diagnosis of the patient with shoulder pain. These conditions include other traumatic disorders such as intra-articular injuries to the labrum or articular cartilage, and atraumatic problems including multidirectional instability, reflex sym-

pathetic dystrophy, and thoracic outlet syndrome. In-depth discussion of each of these less common entities is beyond the scope of this chapter, but important in the management of the patient with shoulder complaints.

SUMMARY AND CONCLUSIONS

The shoulder is uniquely designed to provide precision and power through a vastly unconstrained range of motion. Yet the price of such mobility is stability, which is one of the most common clinical problems facing the practitioner. Other common afflictions of the shoulder include degenerative processes involving the soft tissue and articular cartilage about this construct, including impingement, arthritis, and joint sprains. Successful evaluation and treatment of most shoulder conditions require a careful history, physical examination, and radiographic examination. Special tests such as magnetic resonance imaging, electrodiagnostic testing, and bone scan are helpful in certain diagnostic conditions. Nonoperative treatment is effective in the management of most shoulder problems.

Bibliography

Iannotti JP, Williams GR: Disorders of the Shoulder: Diagnosis and Management. Philadelphia, Lippincott Williams & Wilkins, 1999.
Rockwood CA Jr, Matsen FA III: The Shoulder, 2nd ed. Vols. 1 and 2. Philadelphia, WB Saunders, 1998.

C h a p t e r 20

The Elbow and the Forearm

Mustafa A. Haque, M.D.

Although the elbow and forearm are often ignored in training and teaching situations, they play a very important role in the function of the upper extremity. The tremendous range of motion present in the shoulder allows the hand to be positioned on the outer circumference of a sphere. The flexion-extension and pronation-supination of the elbow and forearm allows positioning of the hand within that sphere. This positioning is crucial for our ability to perform our activities of daily living, including such functions as feeding, clothing, and cleaning oneself, and work and recreational activities such as lifting, writing, and throwing. When elbow and forearm function is compromised by pain, injury, or limited motion, significant disability can result. The goals of this chapter are to present the functional anatomy of the elbow and forearm, highlight some of the more common injuries and conditions that can affect this region, and present an approach to their treatment.

FUNCTIONAL ANATOMY

The bony anatomy of the elbow and forearm is well defined. The distal humerus starts at the end of the humeral shaft; as it descends into the elbow region it flattens and flares out to form medial and lateral columns (Fig. 20–1). The medial column is much smaller in diameter than the lateral. It diverges 40 to 45 degrees from the long axis of the humerus, whereas the lateral condyle diverges only about 20 degrees laterally. The two columns are joined at the articular surface by the trochlea to form a triangular construct, which gives the distal humerus a great deal of strength. The lateral epicondyle is a small outcropping from the lateral column; it provides the origin for the lateral collateral ligaments, supinator, extensors, and the anconeus. The medial epicondyle is a more prominent bone outcropping just medial to the medial condyle. It is the origin for the ulnar collateral ligaments, the flexor pronator mass, and it also forms the roof of the cubital tunnel.

The lateral condyle projects distally to become the capitellum (Fig. 20–2). This is a hemispherical structure that projects 30 degrees anteriorly to the axis of the humeral shaft. It has cartilage only on the anterior and anteromedial aspects. The posterior aspect is flat and devoid of an articular surface. This is an important spot for plate fixation. The medial condyle consists mainly of the trochlea, which spans the region between the capitellum and the medial epicondyle. This is a biconcave cylindrical bone formation that has been equated to a spool. It has a medial ridge that has a greater diameter than the lateral and projects more distally. This helps form the carrying angle of

the elbow. The arc of articular cartilage around the trochlea from in the sagittal plane is between 300 and 330 degrees, and this allows for the tremendous flexion and extension at the elbow while maintaining constant stability. A capitellotrochlear sulcus separates the medial and lateral condyles. The bony columns and condyles create two fossae on the front and back of the elbow. These are respectively called the coronoid and olecranon fossa; they allow for the coronoid and olecranon processes to extend below the level of the diameter of the bone in extremes of flexion and extension.

The overall alignment of the distal humerus is such that there is a 30-degree anterior projection of the articular surfaces relative to the axis of the shaft. There are 5 degrees of internal rotation from the epicondylar axis and approximately 6 degrees of valgus to the axis of the shaft. This helps provide a carrying angle of 14 to 18 degrees formed by the trochlea in the sigmoid notch of the proximal ulna (Fig. 20–3).

The proximal ulna is characterized by the olecranon and coronoid processes, which frame the sigmoid notch posteriorly and anteriorly (Fig. 20–4). The sigmoid or semilunar notch forms a deep trough that cradles the trochlea of the distal humerus. This forms a very stable articulation, and approximately 50% of the stability of the elbow is due to this bony configuration alone. The radial aspect of the proximal ulna has a radial or lesser sigmoid notch. This zone provides the articular interface between the proximal ulna and the radial head. Farther distally and radially there is a bony prominence called the crista supinatoris (see Fig. 20–4). This forms one of the insertions of the radial collateral ligament and is part of the origin for the supinator muscle.

The proximal radius has a radial head with a cup-shaped articular surface that interfaces with the capitellum (Fig. 20–5). The sides of the radial head are covered with articular cartilage for an arc of nearly 240 degrees. This region interfaces with the lesser sigmoid notch to provide nearly 180 degrees of pronation and supination. There is then a very short segment of radial neck that extends down to the level of the biceps tuberosity on which the biceps tendon inserts. The bone then continues on as a long tubular shaft with a radially directed bow across the length of the forearm. The radius then begins to flare out distally, and its metaphyseal region becomes the broad-based distal radius that supports the carpus (Fig. 20–6). The ulna rapidly narrows down to a cylindrical shaft going from proximal to distal and stays subcutaneous on the ulnar side. Its distal end has a small flare into an ulnar head that articulates

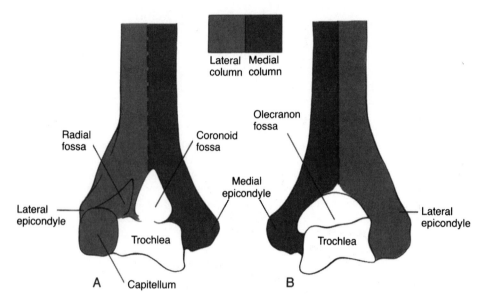

Figure 20–1. Anterior *(A)* and posterior *(B)* views of the medial and lateral columns of the distal humerus. (From Browner BD, Jupiter JB, Levine AM, Trafton PG [eds]: Skeletal Trauma. Philadelphia, WB Saunders, 1992, p 1148.)

Figure 20–2. The bony landmarks of the anterior aspect of the distal humerus. (From Morrey BF [ed]: The Elbow and Its Disorders, 2nd ed. Philadelphia, WB Saunders, 1993, p 20.)

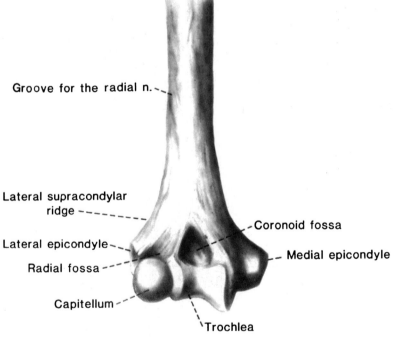

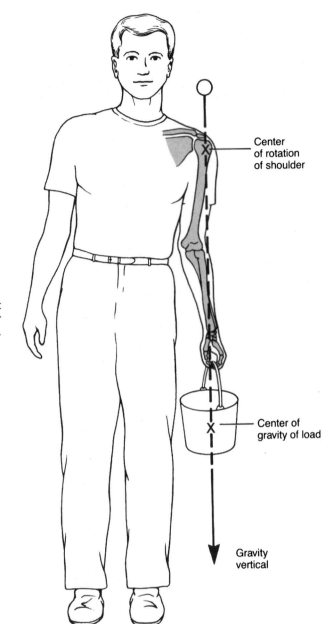

Figure 20–3. With the elbow in full extension, an object held is truly suspended rather than carried. (From Browner BD, Jupiter JB, Levine AM, Trafton PG [eds]: Skeletal Trauma. Philadelphia, WB Saunders, 1992, p 1147.)

Center of rotation of shoulder

Center of gravity of load

Gravity vertical

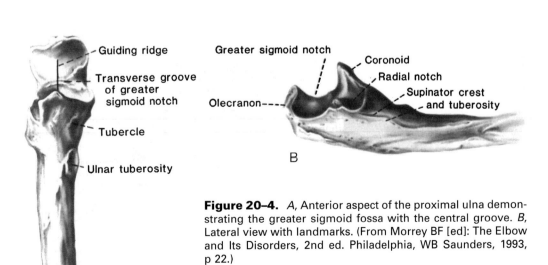

Guiding ridge

Transverse groove of greater sigmoid notch

Tubercle

Ulnar tuberosity

Greater sigmoid notch

Coronoid

Radial notch

Supinator crest and tuberosity

Olecranon

A

B

Figure 20–4. *A*, Anterior aspect of the proximal ulna demonstrating the greater sigmoid fossa with the central groove. *B*, Lateral view with landmarks. (From Morrey BF [ed]: The Elbow and Its Disorders, 2nd ed. Philadelphia, WB Saunders, 1993, p 22.)

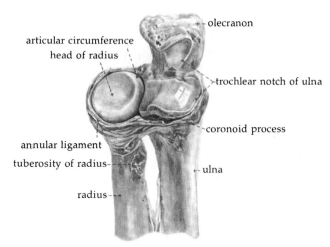

Figure 20–5. Hyaline cartilage covers approximately 240 degrees of the outside circumference of the radial head, allowing its articulation with the proximal ulna at the radial notch of the ulna. (From Langman J, Woerdeman MW: Atlas of Medical Anatomy. Philadelphia, WB Saunders, 1976.)

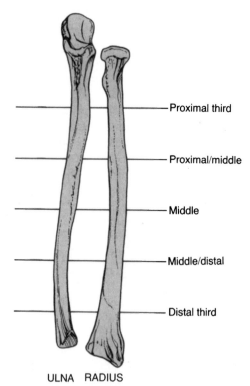

Figure 20–6. Division of the forearm skeleton into thirds for surgical classification. (From Browner BD, Jupiter JB, Levine AM, Trafton PG [eds]: Skeletal Trauma. Philadelphia, WB Saunders, 1992, p 1096.)

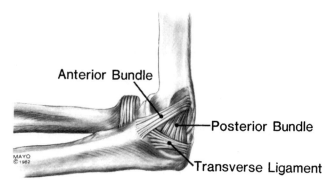

Figure 20–7. The classic orientation of the medial collateral ligament, including the anterior and posterior bundles, and the transverse ligament. This last structure contributes relatively little to elbow stability. (From Morrey BF [ed]: The Elbow and Its Disorders, 2nd ed. Philadelphia, WB Saunders, 1993, p 29.)

with the distal radius at the distal radioulnar joint and with a carpus by means of the triangular fibrocartilage complex. The ulnar styloid on the most ulnar side of this is an anchor point for the triangular fibrocartilage complex and other ligaments from the ulnar aspect of the wrist.

One of the most important stabilizers of the elbow is the medial collateral ligament (Fig. 20–7). This can be broken down into three bundles: the anterior bundle origi-

nates on the medial epicondyle and inserts on the base of the coronoid. It is nearly isometric and is taut throughout the range of motion. This is thought to be the most important restraint to valgus stress. There is a posterior bundle that extends from the medial epicondyle to the edge of the olecranon; it is taut mainly in 90 degrees of flexion. Lastly, there is a transverse segment that extends from the medial tip of the olecranon to the edge of the coronoid. This segment has no known function. The anterior and posterior bundles, with their origin just anterior to the tip of the medial epicondyle, are at risk for injury during medial epicondylectomy.

The lateral collateral ligament complex consists of several structures (Fig. 20–8). The lateral ulnar collateral ligament originates on the lateral epicondyle and extends to the crista supinatoris on the ulna. It is isometric and, therefore, taut in both flexion and extension. It is thought to be the primary restraint to varus stress. The annular ligament extends from the anterior border of the radial notch to the posterior border; it surrounds and stabilizes the radial head. The anterior fibers of this are taut in supination, and the posterior fibers are taut in pronation. The radial collateral ligament extends from the lateral epicondyle to the annular ligament. It is taut in flexion, extension, and part of supination. It forms a mild varus restraint. The accessory collateral ligament originates on the annular ligament and inserts on the crista supinatoris. It stabilizes the annular ligament in varus stress.

The capsule of the elbow consists of thin fibrous tissue structures with discrete thickenings. Anteriorly, the most commonly described thickenings are the transverse and oblique bands. The transverse runs proximal to the medial trochlea and inserts onto the annular ligament. The oblique band runs superior to the capitellum and inserts on the lateral coronoid. These structures are taut in extension. The maximum volume of the elbow capsule is at 80 degrees of flexion and is approximately 25 to 30 mL.

The two main ligamentous structures of the forearm are the interosseus membrane and the triangular fibrocartilage complex. The interosseous membrane is actually a complex of ligamentous bands joining the radius to the ulna; the most important of these is the central band that runs in an oblique fashion proximally from the radius to distally on

Figure 20–8. More detailed representation of the radial collateral ligament complex showing a portion termed the *radial collateral ligament* that extends from the humerus to the annular ligament. This is the portion that is most commonly meant when referring to the radial or lateral collateral ligament. (From Morrey BF [ed]: The Elbow and Its Disorders, 2nd ed. Philadelphia, WB Saunders, 1993, p 30.)

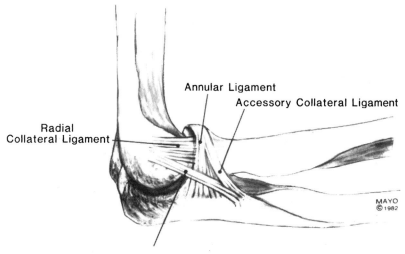

the ulna with an orientation of 21 degrees to the longitudinal axis of the ulna. This structure has important implications in the longitudinal stability of the radius after a radial head fracture or excision. Other main segments of the interosseous membrane include a proximal interosseus band, accessory bands, and membranous segments. These structures are more variable and have less well-defined functional importance (Fig. 20–9).

The triangular fibrocartilage complex is a ligament and fibrocartilage structure that runs from the base of the ulnar styloid to the sigmoid notch of the radius and also has ligamentous attachments to the carpus itself. It plays a very

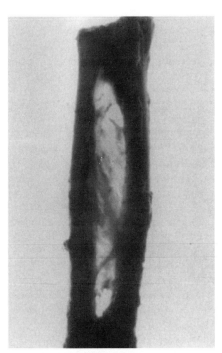

Figure 20–9. Back-lighted specimen of the forearm demonstrating the thickened center portion that comprises the interosseous ligament of the forearm. (From Hotchkiss RN: Injuries to the interosseous ligament of the forearm. Hand Clin 10:394, 1994.)

important role in radioulnar stability and function. This structure is discussed in more detail in Chapter 21.

MUSCLES

The muscles around the elbow and forearm can be broken down into five separate groups based on function. The two groups that originate in the upper arm include the flexor and extensor compartments. The flexor compartment is on the anterior surface and consists of the biceps and the brachialis. The biceps is a powerful elbow flexor and forearm supinator. It becomes tendinous in the distal few centimeters of the upper arm. It has two insertions on the forearm. The most anterior part of the tendon becomes an aponeurotic segment that flares ulnarly over the proximal forearm and inserts onto the fascia of the flexor pronator mass. This segment is called the bicipital aponeurosis or lacertus fibrosus. The remainder of the tendon dives between the pronator teres and the brachioradialis and inserts into the bicipital tuberosity of the radius. Deep to the biceps is the brachialis muscle, which is the main flexor of the forearm. This originates on the distal half of the anterior surface of the humerus and the intermuscular septum and inserts into the coronoid process of the ulnar.

The posterior compartment of the upper arm consists mainly of the triceps muscle. As its name implies, the triceps muscle has three heads. The long head originates on the infraglenoid tubercle of the scapula, the lateral head originates on the posterior surface of the humerus superior to the radial groove, and the medial head originates on the posterior surface of the humerus inferior to the radial groove. These three heads come together and cover the posterior aspect of the humerus. They insert on the proximal end of the olecranon and the deep fascia of the forearm. They are the primary extensors of the elbow.

The three muscle groups of the forearm consist of the mobile wad, the flexor pronator mass, and the extensor mass. The mobile wad is an outcropping of three muscles on the radial aspect of the elbow and forearm. They consist of the brachioradialis, the extensor carpi radialis longus, and the extensor carpi radialis brevis. The brachioradialis takes its origin on the upper two thirds of the supracondylar ridge of the distal humerus. It runs superficial and slightly volar to the radial wrist extensors and inserts on the lateral aspect of the distal radius just proximal to the radial styloid process. It functions as an elbow flexor. The extensor carpi radialis longus and brevis run slightly dorsal and distal to the brachioradialis, and they insert on the index and middle metacarpals of the hand, respectively. They are the strongest extensors of the wrist. The extensor compartment of the forearm has a common origin from the region of the lateral epicondyle and distally. It consists of all of the finger extensors and the extensor carpi ulnaris. In addition, there is a muscle called the anconeus. This relatively small triangular muscle originates on the lateral epicondyle of the humerus and inserts on the lateral aspect of the olecranon and adjacent posterior surface of the proximal humerus. It is thought to assist the triceps with elbow extension.

The flexor pronator mass takes its origin from the medial epicondyle and medial aspect of the proximal arm as well as the interosseous membrane of the middle and distal thirds of the radius. It consists of the muscles that flex the wrists and fingers as well as the pronator teres.

ARTERIES AND VEINS OF THE ELBOW AND FOREARM

The brachial artery, which is the continuation of the axillary artery at the shoulder, runs along with the median nerve just anterior to the medial intermuscular septum and medial to the biceps. As it approaches the elbow, it runs underneath the bicipital aponeurosis just medial to the biceps tendon. At the level of the neck of the radius the brachial artery bifurcates into the radial artery and the ulnar artery (Fig. 20–10). The radial artery, which is the smaller of the two branches, runs underneath the muscle belly of the brachioradialis until it becomes tendinous and the radial artery is superficial and found just adjacent to the flexor carpi radialis tendon all the way to the level of the wrist. Its main branch in the forearm is the radial recurrent branch, which begins just distal to the origin of the radial artery and is sent between the brachioradialis and the brachialis muscles to help form the elbow anastomosis. The radial artery also gives off multiple branches to the muscles on the lateral side of the forearm. From its origin, the ulnar artery passes deep to the pronator teres in a distal and medial direction and continues for a short while with the median nerve between the two heads of the flexor digitorum superficialis. It starts to become posterior at the junction of the proximal and middle thirds of the forearm, where it lies on the flexor digitorum profundus. In the distal two thirds of the forearm, the artery lies just lateral to the ulnar nerve and runs alongside this until it enters Guyon's canal superficial to the flexor retinaculum at the wrist.

The ulnar artery also has multiple branches. One is the anterior ulnar recurrent artery, which arises just inferior to the ulnotrochlear joint and runs between the brachialis and pronator teres muscles. It supplies these muscles and joins in with branches of the brachial artery in the elbow anastomosis. Another branch is the posterior ulnar recurrent ar-

tery, which arises just distal to the anterior ulnar recurrent. It passes deep to the tendon of the flexor carpi ulnaris and posterior to the medial epicondyle to join the elbow anastomosis. In the distal part of the cubital fossa, the ulnar artery gives off the common interosseous artery, which soon divides into the anterior and posterior interosseous arteries. These vessels run anterior and posterior to the interosseous membrane and supply adjacent muscles.

NERVES

The main nerves in the elbow and forearm region are musculocutaneous, radial, ulnar, median, and medial antebrachial cutaneous nerves. They will only be briefly discussed here because they are discussed in more detail in the hand and wrist section.

The musculocutaneous nerve is one of the two terminal branches of the lateral cord of the brachial plexus (Fig. 20–11). It supplies motor innervation to the coracobrachialis, the brachialis, and the biceps muscles, and it runs between the biceps and brachialis until the biceps become tendinous. At this level the nerve continues on as the lateral antebrachial cutaneous nerve, which supplies cutaneous sensation to the lateral aspect of the forearm and thumb.

The radial nerve descends posteriorly in the upper arm until it reaches the junction of the middle and distal thirds of the humerus, then it penetrates the lateral intermuscular septum and continues distally between the brachialis and brachioradialis muscles (Fig. 20–12). At the level of the lateral epicondyle of the humerus, the radial nerve splits into a superficial branch, which runs underneath the brachioradialis and supplies sensation to the dorsum of the hand and fingers, and a deep or posterior interosseous branch that dives underneath the supinator muscle and again becomes a posterior structure. It supplies motor innervation to the wrists and finger extensors. The terminal branch of this runs on the posterior interosseous membrane and supplies some sensory fibers to the wrist itself.

The ulnar nerve is the terminal branch of the medial cord of the brachial plexus (Fig. 20–13). It passes through the medial intermuscular septum at the midhumerus level and then travels medial to the triceps. It enters the cubital tunnel behind the medial epicondyle and passes distally under the ligament of Osborne, a fascial band between the humeral and ulnar head of the flexor carpi ulnaris. It then runs on the volar aspect of the flexor digitorum profundus muscle and at the midway point of the forearm joins up with the ulnar artery and runs ulnar and adjacent to this. It does not give off any innervation in the upper arm, but in the forearm it innervates the flexor carpi ulnaris and the flexor digitorum profundus slips to the ring and small fingers. At the level of the wrist it enters into Guyon's canal along with the ulnar artery to supply sensation and motor function to a significant part of the hand.

The median nerve runs in the upper arm on the lateral aspect of the brachial artery until it reaches the middle of the arm, where it crosses to the medial side and is also adjacent to the brachialis muscle. It enters into the cubital fossa and runs deep to the lacertus fibrosus. It then enters into the interval between the two heads of the pronator teres. At this level it gives off the anterior interosseous

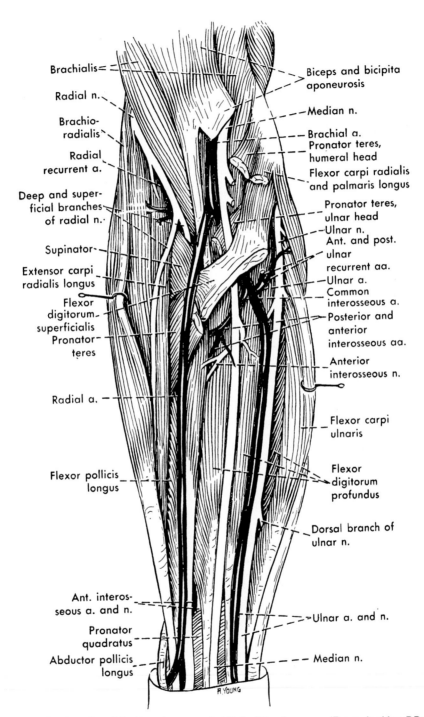

Brachialis

Radial n.

Brachio-
radialis

Radial
recurrent a.

Deep and super-
ficial branches
of radial n.

Supinator

Extensor carpi
radialis longus

Flexor
digitorum
superficialis

Pronator
teres

Radial a.

Flexor pollicis
longus

Ant. interos-
seous a. and n.

Pronator
quadratus

Abductor pollicis
longus

Biceps and bicipita
aponeurosis

Median n.

Brachial a.
Pronator teres,
humeral head

Flexor carpi radialis
and palmaris longus

Pronator teres,
ulnar head

Ulnar n.

Ant. and post.
ulnar
recurrent aa.

Ulnar a.

Common
interosseous a.

Posterior and
anterior
interosseous aa.

Anterior
interosseous n.

Flexor carpi
ulnaris

Flexor
digitorum
profundus

Dorsal branch of
ulnar n.

Ulnar a. and n.

Median n.

R. YOUNG

Figure 20–10. Arteries *(black)* and nerves *(white)* of the forearm. (From Jenkins DB: Hollinshead's Functional Anatomy of the Limbs and Back, 6th ed. Philadelphia, WB Saunders, 1991,
p 131.)

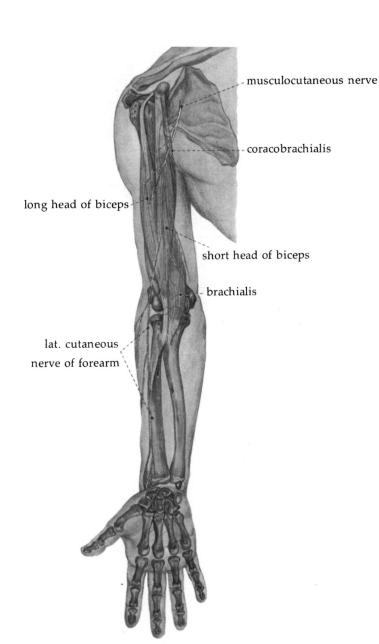

musculocutaneous nerve

coracobrachialis

long head of biceps

short head of biceps

brachialis

lat. cutaneous
nerve of forearm

Figure 20–11. The musculocutaneous nerve innervates the flexors of the elbow and continues distal to the joint as the lateral cutaneous nerve of the forearm. (From Langman J, Woerdeman MW: Atlas of Medical Anatomy. Philadelphia, WB Saunders, 1976.)

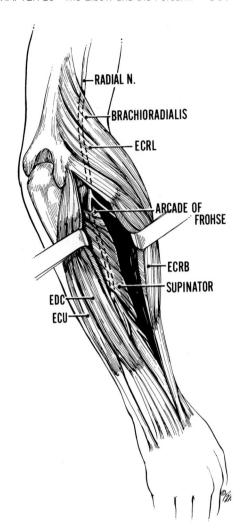

Figure 20–12. Extension of the posterior Thompson approach to the radial tunnel. ECRB, extensor carpi radialis brevis; ECRL, extensor carpi radialis longus; ECU, extensor carpi ulnaris; EDC, extensor digitorum communis. (From Green DP, Hotchkiss RN, Pederson WC: Green's Operative Hand Surgery, 4th ed. Philadelphia, WB Saunders, 1999, p 1436.)

branch, which courses in a radial direction, supplying motor innervation to the flexor pollicis longus, the index and middle finger, flexor digitorum profundus, and the pronator quadratus. The remaining segment of median nerve runs volar to the flexor digitorum profundus and innervates the flexor digitorum superficialis. In the distal third of the forearm it becomes more superficial and gives off the palmar cutaneous branch, which supplies sensory innervation to the thenar eminence. The remainder of the nerve runs along with the flexor digitorum superficialis and profundus tendons into the carpal tunnel.

The medial antebrachial cutaneous nerve arises from the medial cord of the brachial plexus proximal to the origin of the ulnar nerve. It descends through the upper arm medial to the axillary artery and then medial and anterior to the brachial artery. Just proximal to the elbow it passes through an aperture in the brachial fascia and becomes a subcutaneous structure supplying cutaneous innervation to the medial aspect of the forearm.

ELBOW BIOMECHANICS

Motion about the elbow and forearm occurs in two planes: (1) the flexion-extension plane and (2) the pronation-supination plane. Although these tasks seem quite simple, the biomechanics of this motion and the load transfer that can result is quite complex. Motion is also quite constrained with only 3 to 4 degrees of varus and valgus or axial rotation laxity at the elbow. Normal flexion and extension passes through an arch from 0 to 150 degrees, normal pronation is about 75 degrees, and supination can reach 85 to 90 degrees. In classical teaching, the arc required for functional use of the elbow and forearm involves a 30- to 130-degree flexion-extension arch and 50 degrees of pronation and 50 degrees of supination. This has been challenged by some more recent studies, one of which showed that patients could do the majority of their activities of daily living with a 75- to 120-degree arch of flexion and extension.

The axis of rotation for elbow flexion and extension goes through the center of the capitellum and the center of the trochlea (Fig. 20–14). On the lateral side this is identified by the center of the lateral condyle; on the medial side this is marked by the anterior-inferior border of the medial epicondyle. This axis of flexion-extension is 5 degrees internally rotated relative to the epicondylar axis. It is 5 to 8 degrees in valgus from the perpendicular to the long axis of the humeral shaft. Understanding of this flexion-extension axis rotation has allowed for the development of dynamic external fixators about the elbow. The angle between the humeral shaft and the ulnar shaft in full extension

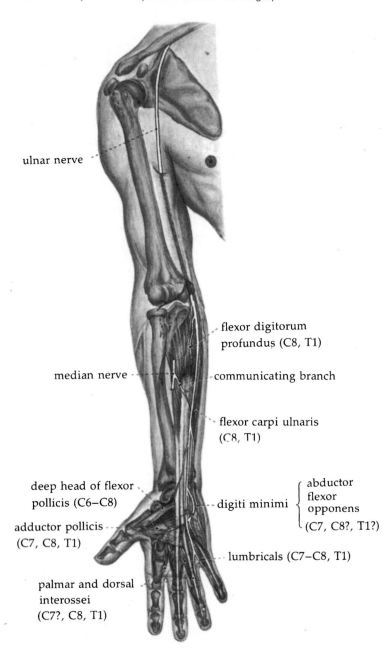

ulnar nerve

flexor digitorum
profundus (C8, T1)

median nerve

communicating branch

flexor carpi ulnaris
(C8, T1)

deep head of flexor
pollicis (C6–C8)

digiti minimi { abductor flexor opponens (C7, C8?, T1?)

adductor pollicis
(C7, C8, T1)

lumbricals (C7–C8, T1)

palmar and dorsal
interossei
(C7?, C8, T1)

Figure 20–13. Muscles innervated by the right ulnar nerve. There are no muscular branches of this nerve above the elbow joint. (From Langman J, Woerdeman MW: Atlas of Medical Anatomy. Philadelphia, WB Saunders, 1976.)

is called a carrying angle of the elbow. It varies between 10 to 15 degrees for men and is slightly greater in women. It allows us to carry objects with the elbow in full extension and clear our hips while ambulating. The axis of rotation for pronation and supination begins at the center of the radiocapitellar joint and extends through the fovea of the distal ulnar. Forearm pronation-supination is highly dependent on the arc of curvature of the radius (radial bow), which allows it to pass about the ulnar. This motion leaves the radius slightly short relative to the ulna in full pronation compared with its position in full supination. Several studies have also shown that there is some slight axial rotation of the ulna relative to the humerus during full arm rotation. In full supination the ulna externally rotates, and in full pronation it internally rotates slightly.

Biomechanical studies in the mid 1980s suggested that force transmission from the hand to the forearm resulted in 82% of load transfer to the distal radius and approximately 18% to the distal ulna. Measurements at the elbow region, however, had shown that load transmission was approximately distributed to 57% at the radiocapitellar joint and 43% at the ulnotrochlear segment. The oblique central band fibers of the interosseous membrane, which run from a proximal radial to a distal ulnar direction, are believed to transfer load from the radius to the ulna. More recent studies have suggested that in a normal valgus position the vast majority of load is transferred from the hand to the arm through the radius with relatively little loading being shifted to the ulnar. In situations with radial head resection, however, all of the load is transferred to the ulnar through the interosseous membrane. This structure is crucial to preventing proximal migration of the radial shaft.

The long lever arm of the forearm leads to very high stresses at the elbow. Loads of over 3000 newtons, or

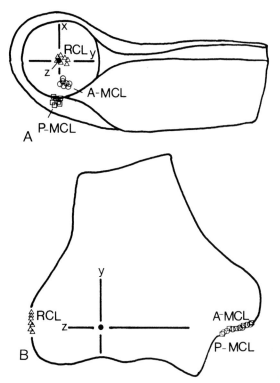

Figure 20–14. *A,* Lateral view of the distal aspect of the humerus demonstrating the locus of the medial and radial collateral ligaments (MCL, RCL) referable to the axis of rotation, Z. *B,* Frontal projection of the distal humerus showing the locus of the original of the radial medial collateral ligaments. Note that of these various components, only the radial collateral ligament lies in the axis of rotation, Z, thereby explaining the length-tension relationship of these ligaments. (From Morrey BF, An KN: Functional anatomy of the elbow ligaments. Clin Orthop 201:84, 1985.)

nearly four times body weight, have been recorded in biomechanical studies, leading some to consider the elbow to be a weight-bearing joint.

The stability of the elbow joint is in great part due to the bony configuration. The deep ulnotrochlear articulation provides more than 50% percent of the stability of the elbow alone. In full flexion, the coronoid process becomes deeply embedded in the coronoid fossa, providing excellent stability. In addition, the radial head is also seated in a radial fossa just proximal to the capitellum, further adding to stability. In full extension, the olecranon tip is deeply locked in the olecranon fossa, constraining the elbow from varus or valgus displacement. The coronoid prevents anterior translation of the distal humerus from the elbow in nearly all positions, and coronoid fractures need to be monitored closely for any resultant instability. The radial head adds to the stability on axial loading of the forearm and is an important secondary stabilizer to valgus stress. Ligamentous stabilizers include the collateral ligaments and the anterior and posterior capsule. The capsule is taut in full extension and provides significant varus-valgus and rotational stability in this position. However, in full flexion it has little additional stabilizing force. The anterior band of the medial collateral ligament is a primary stabilizer to valgus stress; however, when sectioned if the radial head

is intact, only minimal increase in laxity occurs. The lateral collateral ligament is a primary stabilizer to varus stress, and rupture of this ligament can cause instability. Various reconstructions are described for chronic instability due to rupture of this isometric ligament. The posterior capsule adds stability to the joint when it is in full flexion; when the elbow is extended, it is completely lax and adds very little as a stabilizer.

The stability of the radioulnar relationship in the forearm is due mainly to two structures: the interosseous membrane and the triangular fibrocartilage complex. When both of these structures are disrupted, significant instability at the distal radioulnar joint can result. If any injury or resection of the radial head is also present, axial instability can also result. These complex disorders are ones for which we have few adequate treatment options. Recently, attempts at reconstructing the central band of the interosseous membrane have been performed, but the numbers are too small to draw firm conclusions about the results. Radioulnar synostosis, or conversion to a one-bone forearm, remains the only salvage procedure; it can be very debilitating.

EVALUATION OF ELBOW AND FOREARM PROBLEMS

Evaluation of elbow and forearm problems relies on a thorough history and physical examination, radiographic evaluation, and other pertinent tests when necessary.

History

Elbow and forearm problems can be categorized into two major groups: (1) acute traumatic injuries and (2) chronic or insidious onset conditions. In a situation of acute trauma, the detailed history of the event should be obtained. The mechanism of injury, the position of the upper extremity, initial treatment, and subsequent symptoms are all very important toward guiding evaluation and treatment. It is also important to elicit a history of any prior injury or underlying symptoms of the elbow and forearm.

For more chronic conditions, the most common complaint is pain, although stiffness and occasional mechanical symptoms such as throwing or catching may also be involved. It is important to characterize the symptoms very carefully, starting with the exact location. Then one should ask what the nature of the pain is. Is it burning or radiating (nerve), or is it aching related only to activities (tendinitis)? Does it hurt at night or at rest (tumors, infection)? Is it associated with other symptoms such as neck pain (referred pathology from the cervical spine) or wrist pain (distal radioulnar joint problems)?

What is the relationship of the patient's activity to the symptoms? For example, for a throwing athlete, when during the pitch or throw does the pain occur? Medial elbow pain when the arm is in the "cocking" position suggests medial collateral ligament pathology, whereas medial pain during the follow-through suggests involvement of the flexor pronator group. Is there clicking, catching, or other symptoms (particularly at the distal radioulnar joint or with rotational motion)?

What treatments, if any, have helped should be determined. Has the patient had any corticosteroid injections? What types of other treatments (e.g., physical therapy, nonsteroidal anti-inflammatory medications) has the patient had and with what effect? Has the patient had any previous surgery?

The elbow is commonly involved, and sometimes the first joint affected, in inflammatory arthritides. Therefore, it is important to elicit a history of other joint complaints, known arthritis, and family history. Is there a history of skin problems suggesting lupus, dermatitis, or psoriasis or of gastrointestinal problems suggesting colitis? Have there been any systemic symptoms of illness such as malaise or fevers suggesting possible infectious etiology?

Numbness, tingling, and weakness may be obvious clues to neurologic involvement. However, particularly in forearm nerve entrapment syndromes, pain may be the only presenting problem. In addition to questioning about these symptoms, one should ask about new-onset clumsiness or easy fatigability.

Perhaps the most important part of the history is determining how the symptoms interfere with function. Inability to flex the elbow completely is well tolerated by most patients because we generally rely on an arc of 30 to 130 degrees for activities of daily living. However, in patients with compromise of shoulder motion (e.g., patients with rheumatoid arthritis), further restriction of elbow or forearm motion can interfere with their ability to feed or clean themselves. One must ask if the patient is right or left hand dominant. Frequently, patients will demand a more aggressive approach when their dominant arm is affected.

Physical Examination

Physical examination of the elbow and forearm begins with inspection, palpation, range of motion assessment, and evaluation for strength and neurovascular integrity. These can be followed by special tests designed to evaluate specific conditions. A proper physical examination must also include a very directed examination of the shoulder, wrist, and hand and, in some cases, the cervical spine.

Inspection begins from the moment one starts to interact with the patient. One should observe the use patterns of the affected extremity even as the history is being taken. Does the patient offer the hand of the affected side to shake hands with the physician? Are there obvious adaptive motions that the patient uses to avoid pain on that side? A more formal visual examination is then performed to look for swelling, ecchymosis, atrophy, asymmetry, or unusual prominences. In the situations of trauma, one should carefully make sure there is no open wound in the region of a fracture or dislocation. The carrying angle formed between the longitudinal axis of the humerus and forearm, which is normally 10 to 15 degrees, should be evaluated (Fig. 20–15).

With the elbow flexed to 90 degrees, the normal bony prominences of the medial and lateral epicondyles and the olecranon form an equilateral triangle (Fig. 20–16). In dislocations and some fractures, this normal relationship is distorted. One should look for evidence of joint swelling laterally by inspection of the soft tissue triangle bordered by the radial head, the olecranon tip, and the lateral epicondyle.

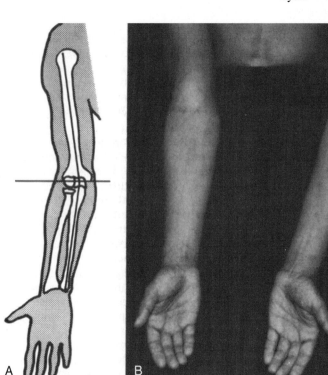
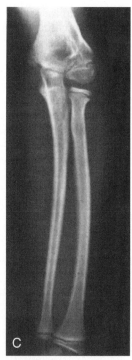

Figure 20–15. *A,* The carrying angle is a clinical measurement of the angle formed by the forearm and the humerus with the elbow extended. *B* and *C,* The normal 10- to 15-degree carrying angle can be altered by injury about the elbow, causing a varus carrying angle or the so-called gunstock deformity. (From Morrey BF [ed]: The Elbow and Its Disorders, 2nd ed. Philadelphia, WB Saunders, 1993, p 74.)

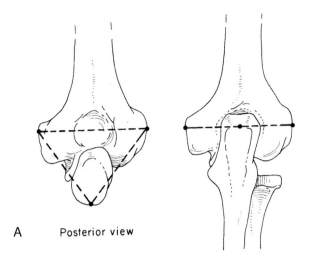

A   Posterior view

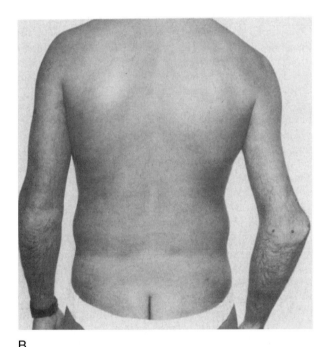

B

Figure 20–16. With the elbow flexed to 90 degrees, the medial and lateral epicondyles and tip of the olecranon form an equilateral triangle when viewed from posterior. When the elbow is extended, this relationship is changed to a straight line connecting these three bony landmarks *(A)*. The relationship is altered with displaced, intra-articular distal humeral fractures *(B)*. (From Morrey BF [ed]: The Elbow and Its Disorders, 2nd ed. Philadelphia, WB Saunders, 1993, p 78.)

The area is palpated for tenderness, soft tissue integrity, and crepitus. The anterior, medial, lateral, and posterior structures are evaluated in an organized systematic fashion in an attempt to pinpoint the area of tenderness to as specific a region as possible. For example, lateral epicondylitis or tennis elbow causes focal tenderness over the lateral epicondyle. Tenderness more distally in the forearm may suggest a posterior interosseous nerve entrapment instead. Medial elbow pain may reflect medial epicondylitis or golfer's elbow if the patient is tender directly over the epicondyle. When it is more distal, it may be due to medial collateral ligament insufficiency; and when it is more posterior, it may indicate ulnar neuropathy. Palpation is done posteriorly over the olecranon fossa as one looks for any presence of a bursa over the olecranon tip occasionally containing fluid, palpable fibrous fragments, or both (olecranon bursitis). Palpation over the antecubital fossa is done to evaluate any defects in the biceps tendon attachment (distal biceps tendon rupture). When the patient complains of forearm pain, both the radius and ulna can be palpated for a significant part of their length in the forearm. Palpation should also be done over the soft tissues, particularly in the common regions for nerve entrapment. Tenderness is checked for around the distal radioulnar joint, particularly in the presence of other elbow trauma.

Both active and passive motion are checked for noting any difference between them. If passive motion is greater than active motion and the patient is relatively free of pain, muscle and/or nerve injury are possible causes. In the absence of trauma, pain on passive elbow motion suggests an infection.

The location and the timing of pain during motion are noted. Discomfort in extension is common in posterior olecranon impingement. Painful crepitus over the radiocapitellar joint during pronation and supination indicates pathology such as degenerative arthritis or radial neck fracture.

The amount of detail devoted to the neurologic examination depends on the patient's symptoms, but one should be familiar with a routine sensory, motor, and reflex examination. Sensation to light touch should be checked in the following areas for specific peripheral nerves: ulnar nerve—ulnar aspect of the small finger; median nerve—radial border of the index finger; radial nerve—dorsal first web space; and musculocutaneous nerve—lateral forearm. When evaluating from a perspective of cervical nerve roots, there is considerable overlap; however, the generally accepted autonomous regions include the lateral deltoid for the C5 dermatome, the lateral dorsal first web space for C6, the middle finger for C7, the ulnar border of the small finger for C8, and the medial elbow for T1.

Strength testing can also be done on both the nerve root and peripheral nerve basis. C5 function is tested with deltoid strength, C6 with wrist extension strength, C7 with triceps, finger extensors, or wrist flexors, C8 with finger flexors, and T1 with finger abduction. With the use of the peripheral nerve basis, the radial nerve is evaluated with wrist extension; its posterior interosseous branch is evaluated with extension or thumb interphalangeal extension or finger metaphalangeal extension. The ulnar nerve is evaluated with abduction of the small finger. The median nerve is evaluated with thumb abduction, and the anterior interosseous branch is evaluated with index finger distal interphalangeal flexion. The axillary nerve is checked with deltoid function, and the musculocutaneous nerve is checked with biceps function. Reflex testing for the biceps evaluates C5 function; that for the brachioradialis, C6 function; and that for the triceps, C7 function.

Vascular assessment of the arm includes palpation of the radial and ulnar arteries at the wrist and the brachial artery at the antecubital fossa.

Additional special physical examination tests can be extremely useful in helping to pinpoint diagnoses. These directed examination points will be addressed in further discussion on the specific conditions. Entrapment neuropathies are discussed in Chapter 21 on hand and wrist surgery.

X-Ray Examination

Anteroposterior (AP) and lateral x-rays are the minimum views necessary to evaluate the elbow joints. One should make sure a true AP view of the distal humerus and proximal ulnar and radius is obtained and the AP elbow film is not taken with the elbow in significant flexion, because this can hide certain traumatic conditions. After trauma, additional views such as oblique and radial head views are often helpful. For forearm injuries, AP and lateral views usually suffice for evaluation, although sometimes oblique views add useful information. One should also consider getting proper wrist films to evaluate the distal radioulnar joint and rule out accompanying wrist injuries.

Stress x-rays may be helpful in evaluating patients with suspected tears of the medial or lateral collateral ligament of the elbow or, in some situations, injury to the distal radioulnar joint. For elbow stress films one can inject lidocaine into the soft spot between the radial head, the olecranon, and the lateral epicondyle to help anesthetize the joint (Fig. 20–17) and then perform manual stress in an effort to open up either the medial or lateral side. A difference between the affected and normal elbow of more than 2 mm is considered significant.

Computed tomographic (CT) scans can be useful in helping evaluate details of fracture fragments, as well as looking for osseous changes. They are also helpful for evaluating loose bodies and osteochondritis dissecans lesions. Magnetic resonance imaging (MRI) can also be very useful at times. MRI is particularly helpful in soft tissue injuries such as distal biceps tendon ruptures in situations in which the results of physical examination are equivocal. It can also be very useful for localizing loose bodies. An MRI evaluation should be obtained in any situation in which soft tissue tumor is present in the forearm or elbow region. Technetium bone scanning is very useful for evaluating degenerative changes and stress fractures of the elbow and forearm region (Fig. 20–18).

Electromyography (EMG) and nerve conduction velocity studies (NCS) should be obtained when one is trying to rule out a neurologic component to the patient's symptoms. They are very helpful in defining nerve injury or entrapment. One must keep in mind there is a wide range of normal values; and in young athletes, in particular, a normal test can be obtained despite nerve compression. Comparison testing with the opposite side or with other uninvolved nerves can be very helpful.

Arthroscopy of the elbow is a relatively new technique that can be useful for both diagnosis and treatment of elbow pathology. Because of the very tight concentration of important nerves, blood vessels, and muscle and tendon structures around the elbow, however, the procedure is quite risky. It should only be performed by surgeons who are very comfortable with the anatomy surrounding the elbow and who have experience in the technique. Its indications are also somewhat limited. Diagnostically, it can be helpful for identifying intra-articular pathology that is represented by pain, snapping, or locking when other imaging studies are negative. Therapeutically, it has been used for removal of loose bodies (Fig. 20–19), treatment of osteochondritis dissecans lesions, debridement of infection, excision of osteophytes, synovectomy and biopsy, and even excision of the radial head and, in some cases, acute fracture care. Many of these indications, however, are debated, and many elbow surgeons would counter they should be done under an open procedure. Contraindications for elbow arthroscopy include severe contracture, previous nerve transposition, and significant body distortion; and a relative contraindication is prior open-elbow surgery.

TREATMENT OF ELBOW AND FOREARM PROBLEMS

The treatment of elbow and forearm problems can be approached with a broad division into traumatic and atraumatic conditions. One general principle of elbow treatment is the avoidance of immobilization for longer than absolutely necessary. The elbow has a high propensity for developing contractures after immobilization, particularly with fractures or dislocations. The resultant loss of motion can be disabling, and the treatment for regaining motion can be prolonged and difficult. When necessary, splinting should be with the elbow in 90 degrees of flexion and neutral pronation and supination to allow for maximal capsular volume and the maintenance of the most useful arc of function.

Anytime a traumatic injury occurs in the elbow and forearm region, after appropriate initial treatment, one should carefully follow the patient's neurovascular examination because the multiple confined fascial planes leave patients at risk for compartment syndromes and other neurovascular compromise.

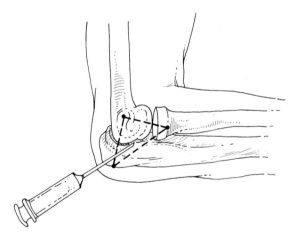

Figure 20–17. Elbow joint aspiration or injection is readily performed by inserting the needle in the midportion of the triangular space formed by the lateral epicondyle, radial head, and tip of the olecranon. This area is coincident with the infracondylar recess, which becomes distended if an effusion is present. (From Morrey BF [ed]: The Elbow and Its Disorders, 2nd ed. Philadelphia, WB Saunders, 1993, p 85.)

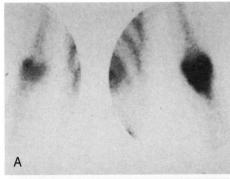
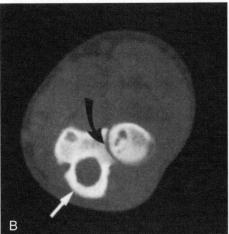
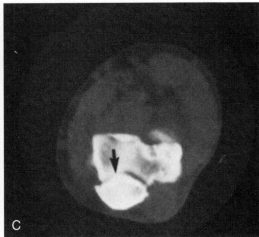

Figure 20–18. *A,* Isotope scan of the elbow in a patient with chronic elbow pain. There is diffusely increased uptake in the elbow region. *B* and *C,* CT scans demonstrate degenerative changes with a degenerative cyst *(white arrow)* and degenerative changes in the radioulnar *(curved black arrow* in *B)* and ulnar-trochlear articulations *(straight arrow* in *C).* (From Morrey BF [ed]: The Elbow and Its Disorders, 2nd ed. Philadelphia, WB Saunders, 1993, p 111.)

Nonoperative Treatment

REHABILITATION

Rehabilitation, either through a patient-guided regimen or through formal occupational physical therapy, plays a large part in treatment of elbow and forearm problems. The goals of this therapy should be directed toward (1) reduction of pain and inflammation; (2) maximizing of range of motion; (3) rebuilding strength; and (4) return to normal function and activity. These rehabilitation issues can often be very difficult. They should be carefully supervised by the treating physician and used in combination with other modalities, including oral anti-inflammatory medications and selective use of corticosteroid injections.

The reduction of pain and inflammation can be a difficult treatment problem. The initial treatment for this follows the RICE principle with *r*est, *i*ce, *c*ompression, and *e*levation. From this one usually starts careful stretching and strengthening exercises, along with ice and heat massage, ultrasound, and iontophoresis as directed by the physician and in conjunction with the therapist. Restoration of motion is done through careful stretching exercises. As noted earlier, one of the best ways to avoid problems with stiffness is to immobilize the elbow for as short a period as possible. When a patient is trying to regain motion it is very important to emphasize the use of active and active-assisted range-of-motion exercises only. In some cases, very gentle passive range of motion can be used, but aggressive passive motion is to be strictly avoided. This is because the elbow and forearm are particularly susceptible to the formation of heterotopic ossification when soft tissue

trauma or bleeding in muscles occurs. This can lead to further loss of motion, such as loss of extension when the brachialis muscle is involved, or even the formation of a radioulnar synostosis preventing pronation and supination in some cases. Continuous passive motion can be useful, particularly immediately after a traumatic situation or after surgery. In the immediate postoperative period, a continous scalene or axillary block can provide several days of pain relief and help the patient begin an early motion program. In other situations, after a plateau is reached with active and active-assisted range-of-motion exercises alone, static and dynamic splinting can be used to help obtain further gains in motion.

ANTI-INFLAMMATORY MEDICATIONS

The use of anti-inflammatory medications can be extremely helpful in elbow and forearm conditions. This can generally be broken down into two sections. The first is the use of non-steroidal anti-inflammatory drugs (NSAIDs). These medications act by blocking the enzyme cyclooxygenase and preventing the production of many inflammatory mediators. They are especially useful for repetitive and microtrauma type pain around the elbow and for arthritic problems. Postsurgically, they can also be used to help prevent heterotopic ossification formation. These are, however, systemic medications with many side effects, primarily gastrointestinal upset and ulcer formation, but also potential liver and kidney problems. If a patient is on these medications chronically, he or she should be carefully monitored.

Another form of anti-inflammatory treatment about the elbow involves the use of corticosteroid injections. This

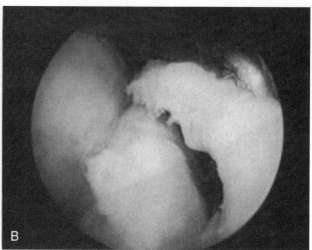

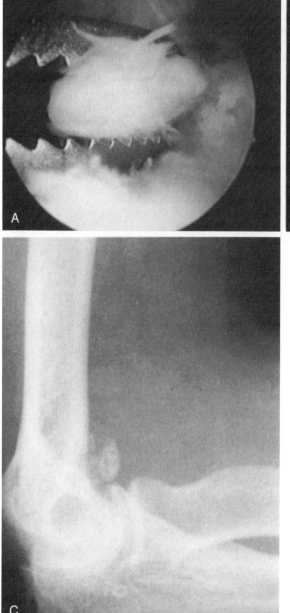

Figure 20–19. *A,* Loose body being grasped and removed from the posterior elbow joint. *B,* Loose body being grasped and removed from the anterior elbow joint. *C,* Radiograph of a patient with synovial chondromatosis and several loose bodies. These can be readily removed arthroscopically and the pathologic synovium excised. (From Morrey BF [ed]: The Elbow and Its Disorders, 2nd ed. Philadelphia, WB Saunders, 1993, p 126.)

involves direct injection of a corticosteroid preparation into the region of pain and inflammation and is one of the most powerful delivery systems to help relieve pain and inflammation. The risks involved include infection, skin discoloration, and tendon rupture, and this procedure should be used very judiciously. The number and frequency of injections that may be given is controversial; however, most would agree no more than three to four injections should be given in a region over the course of a year.

Operative Treatment

Surgical intervention about the elbow is reserved for situations in which nonoperative treatment has failed or is inappropriate, such as traumatic situations requiring debridement or rigid internal fixation. Surgery can be per-

formed by means of open or arthroscopic techniques as described previously.

TRAUMA

Distal Humerus Fractures

Distal humeral fractures constitute approximately 2% of all fractures. There is a high rate of associated injuries; for example, bicondylar fractures have a 50% rate of being open. Distal humeral fractures, in general, have an 18% rate of associated neural injury and a 4% rate of vascular injury. These injuries result from a wide variety of mechanisms.

Initial evaluation should include a careful history, followed by examination of the entire upper extremity with palpation of the elbow and careful neurovascular examination. X-rays should include AP, lateral, and oblique views of the elbow, along with full-length humerus and forearm films. Traction views can be very helpful to define the fracture pattern. If these studies are still inadequate, a CT scan should be obtained.

Treatment goals include fracture healing with pain-free motion and good function. The treatment options include casting, traction, percutaneous pin fixation, rigid internal fixation, and primary total elbow arthroplasty. Casting requires immobilization of the elbow for several weeks; and, in an adult, it leads to a stiff joint and a poor result. Olecranon pin traction involves a long hospital stay and requires that the patient remain bedridden; it allows some motion but eventually it does require casting. It used to be the treatment of choice in displaced fractures before improvement of open reduction and internal fixation techniques. Percutaneous pinning is another option, but the fixation is generally not strong enough to allow early motion, and fractures must be splinted.

Open reduction and internal fixation is now the gold standard of treatment for displaced distal humerus fractures in adults. It allows direct visualization and anatomic reduction of the articular surface, and rigid internal fixation with plates and screws creates enough stability to start early range of motion and reduce stiffness and heterotopic ossification.

For severely comminuted fractures in elderly patients, primary total-elbow replacement has a role as well. It can allow for immediate return to function without trying to achieve bony union, but the implant limitations of most total-elbow replacements require that this be reserved in the trauma situation for low-demand patients.

One of the most useful classification schemes for treatment and prognosis is the AO classification. In this system, type A fractures are extra-articular, type B fractures are unicondylar intra-articular, and type C fractures are bicondylar intra-articular. All of these types are further broken down into two major subtypes.

Type A1 fractures are epicondylar fractures. They occur either through direct trauma or severe varus or valgus force. Treatment usually involves casting unless a large displaced fragment is present (particularly with the medial epicondyle), if there is displacement into the joint, or if there is elbow instability. In these situations, open reduction with internal fixation with screws should be performed.

Type A2 and A3 fractures are transcondylar fractures that are either simple or comminuted, respectively. They usually occur by a fall on an outstretched hand with an axially directed force on the elbow. This extension-type fracture is the most common. It can also occur through anteriorly directed force on the dorsum of a flexed elbow. This is the flexion-type injury. Except for completely nondisplaced fractures or patients with severe osteopenia, these fractures are treated with open reduction and rigid bicolumn fixation, using plates at 90 degrees to each other. One should be a direct posterior plate on the lateral column and the other should be a direct medial plate. In very low transcondylar fractures, one should transpose the ulnar nerve and use the ulnar groove for fixation.

Type B1 and B2 fractures are unicondylar fractures. They usually occur through axial loading with slight varus or valgus positioning. The medial edge of the radial head or the lateral edge of the olecranon impacts the capitellotrochlear sulcus and causes a fracture through a shear mechanism. Treatment of the lateral condylar fractures is through open reduction and internal fixation with lag screws or a plate. Screws alone work fine when the fracture extends proximal to the olecranon fossa. Unicondylar fractures can be treated with lag screw fixation with excellent results.

Type B3 fractures are capitellum fractures (Fig. 20–20). There are three major types of capitellum fractures. Type I fractures are complete fractures of the capitellum, leaving a large fragment with little or no comminution. They can be treated with closed reduction and casting for 3 to 4 weeks, but most authors now advocate an open reduction and rigid compressive fixation with either Herbert screws or standard small fragment screws directly from posterior to anterior. This fixation and early mobilization greatly improve the functional outcome. Type II fractures are shearing injuries of the articular surface, and type III fractures involve fragmentation of the capitellum. Both of these types should be treated with open excision of the fracture fragments.

The C type bicondylar intra-articular fractures are complex injuries that can be very difficult to treat. They usually involve the olecranon driving into the distal humerus as a wedge with the elbow flexed to greater than 90 degrees. The preferred treatment for these injuries involves open reduction and internal fixation followed by early range of motion (Fig. 20–21). Situations in which this is not possible include extensive comminution or severe concomitant medical problems in the patient, making surgical risks unacceptable. In these situations one can try short-term traction followed by casting or a cuff and collar with early motion, the so-called bag of bones treatment. For severely comminuted fractures in patients with low functional demands, primary total arthroplasty has produced good results.

Overall, treatment of all these fractures ranges from 70

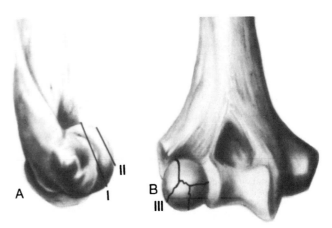

Figure 20–20. The type I capitellar fracture involves a large portion of bone, often the entire structure. Type II is a shear fracture, often with minimal subchondral bone, and may displace posteriorly *(A)*. A type III fracture is a comminuted fracture with varying amounts of displacement of the fracture fragments *(B)*. (From Morrey BF [ed]: The Elbow and Its Disorders, 2nd ed. Philadelphia, WB Saunders, 1993, p 356.)

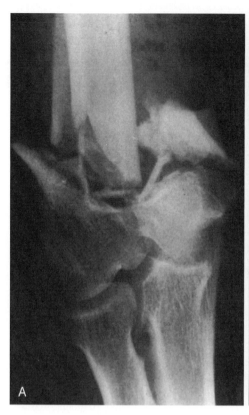
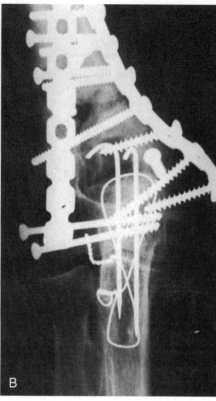

Figure 20–21. An "H" type intra-articular fracture *(A)* represents an exceptionally difficult surgical procedure *(B)*. (From Morrey BF [ed]: The Elbow and Its Disorders, 2nd ed. Philadelphia, WB Saunders, 1993, p 344.)

to 95% good to excellent results, depending on the types. Complications include hardware pain, nerve dysfunction, infection, heterotopic calcification, stiffness, nonunion, and fixation failures.

Radial Head Fractures

Fractures of the radial head or neck are common injuries that make up more than one third of elbow fractures. These injuries usually occur through axial loading of the elbow in full pronation and slight valgus. Suspected injuries to the radial head should be evaluated with AP and lateral x-rays of the elbow, along with a radial head view. Treatment of these injuries is guided by the Mason classification (Fig. 20–22). Type I fractures are non-displaced injuries. They are generally stable fractures and should be treated with approximately a week of immobilization, followed by early range of motion. Type II are displaced fractures involving less than 30% of the articular surface. Treatment of these injuries is controversial. If the elbow is stable and the patient has no block to pronation or supination, non-operative treatment as for type I injuries is indicated. When wide displacement is present, or the fragment reduces motion, surgery is indicated. Options include open reduction and internal fixation, simple fragment excision, and excision of the entire radial head with or without placement of a spacer. For young patients with an injury that can be reduced anatomically, open reduction and internal fixation is the treatment of choice.

Type III radial head injuries are comminuted fractures. There is a consensus that this should be treated with excision of the radial head. When the medial lateral collateral ligament is intact, the elbow will still remain stable to valgus stress. If the axial loading injury did not injure

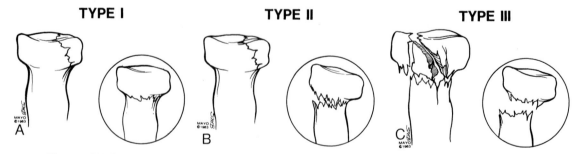

Figure 20–22. Recommended classification of radial head fractures. The exact definition of the type II fracture is often difficult to determine. Type IV is not included because it represents a complicated fracture. (From Morrey BF [ed]: The Elbow and Its Disorders, 2nd ed. Philadelphia, WB Saunders, 1993, p 385.)

the triangular fibrocartilage complex or the interosseous membrane, the radius will not migrate proximally either. If any of the previously mentioned ligaments are ruptured, however, radial head replacement is indicated, rather than simple excision. This can be done either with a silicon spacer or with a titanium radial head. Because of concerns about synovitis and wear, the silicon spacer should be removed at 1 to 2 years. Earlier results with titanium spacers suggest they may be left in long term with no adverse effects.

Type IV injuries of the radial head involve radial head fracture associated with elbow dislocation. These should be treated with reduction of the elbow and treatment of the radial head fracture as described above in types I through III.

Olecranon Fractures

Olecranon fractures are also common elbow injuries. They usually result from a direct blow on the proximal ulna. Evaluation should involve the standard examination and AP and lateral x-rays of the elbow. The Mayo classification is the most useful for determining treatment. It is based on displacement, stability, and comminution.

Type I fractures are non-displaced fractures. These stable injuries should be treated with 1 week of immobilization followed by gentle motion as tolerated. Internal fixation can be used in situations in which patients absolutely cannot risk displacement of their fractures or non-union. However, this treatment is not usually necessary.

Type II fractures are displaced stable fractures, and they are divided into subtypes A and B, which are non-comminuted or comminuted, respectively. Stability is determined by the presence or absence of subluxation of the humerus through the fracture site. Type IIA fractures, the stable non-displaced non-comminuted fractures, should be treated with open reduction and internal fixation, either with Kirschner wires and the tension band technique (Figs. 20–23, 20–24) or with a 6.5-mm cancellous screw and the tension band technique. When comminution is present, as in type IIB, the treatment advocated by Morrey is based on the age of the patient. For patients older than age 50 years, he recommends excision of the fracture fragments and reattachment of the triceps tendon just adjacent to the articular cartilage. In younger patients he recommends open reduction and internal fixation with a contoured 3.5-mm dynamic compression plate. For unstable displaced fractures (type III), the non-comminuted fracture can be treated with open reduction and internal fixation alone. When comminution is present, Morrey recommends addition of a dynamic distraction fixator, which allows for healing of the fracture and early motion without stress on the segments of comminution.

Fracture of the Coronoid

Coronoid fractures are uncommon compared with other elbow fractures, but they have significant implications regarding the stability of the elbow. They have been classified into three types (Fig. 20–25). Type I is a small avulsion injury of the tip of the coronoid. It is sometimes the only indication of an elbow dislocation that spontaneously

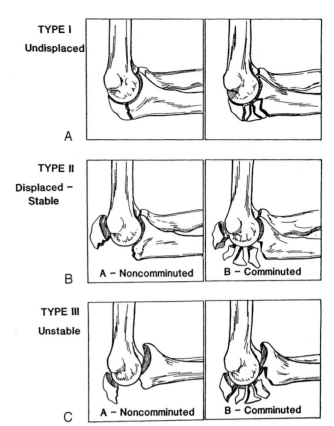

Figure 20–23. *A*, A type II fracture is displaced but stable, with comminuted or non-comminuted fracture. *B*, The Mayo classification is based on three variables: displacement, stability, and comminution. Type I is an undisplaced fracture with minimal or no comminution. *C*, The type III and least common fracture is one that is unstable. This is usually comminuted and with associated radial head fracture but occasionally presents as a non-comminuted fracture. (From Morrey BF [ed]: The Elbow and Its Disorders, 3rd ed. Philadelphia, WB Saunders, 2000, p 368.)

reduced. The treatment is simple early mobilization of the elbow. Type II fractures involve less than 50% of the process. When the elbow is stable, these are treated with early mobilization. Type III injuries involve greater than 50% of the height of the coronoid process. They can often lead to elbow instability because the anterior medial band of the medial collateral ligament attaches at this site. Type III and unstable type II fractures should be treated with open reduction and internal fixation. Morrey advocates the use of a dynamic fixator in addition to allow early range of motion without stressing the repair.

Forearm Fractures

Fractures of the diaphyseal forearm must be treated in a fashion that will allow for full healing in anatomic alignment. If they are allowed to heal with any significant displacement, particularly in the radius, significant loss of motion in pronation and supination can result. Because of this, non-surgical management of forearm fractures is limited to stable isolated ulnar shaft fractures. The criteria for stability here is less than 10 degrees of angulation and less

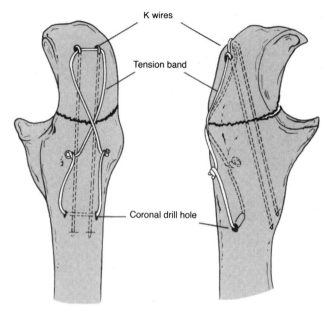

Figure 20–24. A transverse olecranon fracture is optimally treated by a tension band wire technique. Note the placement of the two parallel Kirschner wires from dorsal proximal to anterior distal to engage in the anterior cortex. This minimizes the problem of Kirschner wire migration. (From Browner BD, Jupiter JB, Levine AM, Trafton PG [eds]: Skeletal Trauma. Philadelphia, WB Saunders, 1992, p 1138.)

than 50% of displacement. In rare cases of non-displaced isolated fractures of the radius that cause no alteration of the normal radial bow, one can sometimes consider doing non-operative treatment as well. Non-operative intervention is not considered the standard of care for both bone forearm fractures because of their propensity for shortening and angulation.

Evaluation of forearm fractures should start at the elbow with careful inspection and palpation and extend distally down the shaft of the forearm to the wrist and hand. One

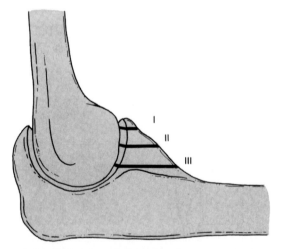

Figure 20–25. The coronoid fracture has been classified into three types by Regan and Morrey. (From Browner BD, Jupiter JB, Levine AM, Trafton PG [eds]: Skeletal Trauma. Philadelphia, WB Saunders, 1992, p 1145.)

should note carefully whether there is any compromise of the skin that could suggest an open fracture, and these fractures should be categorized according to the Gustilo classification. Finger motion should be carefully examined for pain with passive stretch or pain out of proportion to the injury, because compartment syndrome is not uncommon. A careful neurologic examination should be performed, although neurovascular injury is quite uncommon with closed forearm fractures. It becomes much more common with open injuries. One should also carefully check the stability of the distal radial ulnar joint and the elbow. Associated injuries are discussed later.

Surgical treatment options include external fixation, intramedullary fixation, and plate fixation. External fixation is usually reserved for high-grade open injuries and some situations with bone loss. Overall results are fairly good, but there is a high rate of re-displacement and some studies have shown re-reduction is required in up to 10% of patients. Another treatment option is intramedullary nailing. This was previously done mainly with Rush rods or other flexible intramedullary nails; they maintain good axial alignment; however, they provide little rotational stability. Some newer rods have been developed that are more rigid, statically locked intramedullary nails. No long-term results are available yet for these instruments.

The most common fixation technique involves plate fixation. It is recommended one use reasonably stout plates such as the 3.5-mm dynamic compression or LC-DCP plate. Autogenous iliac crest bone grafting is recommended for fractures with comminution involving more than 30% of the diameter of the cortical shaft.

Complications of internal fixation include infection, which is relatively rare; nerve injury, which is usually a traction injury as a result of an approach; hardware failure; and non-union. To avoid the last two problems, bone grafting of comminuted fractures is advocated, and it is recommended at least six cortices of purchase be obtained proximal and distal to the fracture site. Synostosis is another problem that can occur, particularly in both-bone forearm fractures at the same level. The risk factors include situations with high-energy trauma, head injury, and fixation of both bones through the same incision. If synostosis occurs in a position that inhibits function, patients can have resection of this. Results are good in only about 50% of these resections. Plate removal should be discouraged, because re-fracture occurs in 4 to 20% of patients after this. Re-fracture can occur either through the old fracture site or through a screw hole. If, because of severe hardware discomfort, the plate needs to be removed, one should try to wait until less 20 months after the fracture fixation to allow for full remodeling of the fracture site.

Elbow and Forearm Instability

DISLOCATIONS

Dislocations of the elbow are second only to those of the shoulder in frequency. They usually present after a fall on an outstretched arm. This results in either a hyperextension overload, which levers the olecranon tip in the fossa and pushes the ulnar humeral joint out of position, or axial loading in a slightly flexed position, which directly pushes the ulnar humeral joint out of position. There are high rates of associated injuries, including fractures of the radial head in 10 to 50% of dislocations, medial or lateral epicondylar avulsion injuries in 12% of patients, and coronoid fractures in 10%. On physical examination one finds physical deformity of the elbow with loss of the bony equilateral triangle (see Fig. 20–16). Swelling is often severe and can lead to compartment syndrome. There is usually significant loss of motion. A careful neurologic examination is mandated; the ulnar nerve is the most commonly injured nerve.

AP and lateral x-rays are sufficient to make the diagnosis. The radial head should line up with the capitellum on both views. Failure to do so suggests residual subluxation or dislocation.

The classification scheme for elbow dislocations is based on the positioning of the radius and ulna. Posterior dislocations are the most common, followed by anterior dislocation. Medial and lateral dislocations are less common, and a divergent dislocation in which the proximal radioulnar joint is also dislocated is rare.

The goals of treating these injuries include rapid concentric reduction performed in as atraumatic fashion as possible. Intravenous sedation and an intra-articular block with lidocaine should be performed, and in some cases general anesthesia is necessary. For dislocations of long standing, one should perform an open reduction rather than cause further cartilage damage by traumatic manipulation. The most common dislocations are posterior, and they can be usually closed reduced with longitudinal traction and slight flexion. The physician's thumb can be used to exert direct pressure on the olecranon tip and ease the proximal ulna back into position. After reduction, while the patient is still sedated or anesthetized, a careful assessment of stability is performed. The elbow is placed in a well-padded long-arm splint in 90 degrees of flexion and then started on an active motion program with extension blocks or bracing only as defined by the post-reduction examination. It is critical to avoid more than 1 or 2 weeks of immobilization to prevent stiffness and heterotopic ossification.

Chronic elbow instability can be difficult to diagnose and treat. Anterior and posterior instabilities can occur after dislocations. They are usually the result of non-union or malunion of type III coronoid fractures or olecranon fractures. Sometimes there is anterior capsule and brachialis insertion disruption as well. Addressing the source of the pathology usually produces a stable elbow. Other types of instability include varus, valgus, and posterolateral rotatory instabilities. These can all be the result of the injury caused by a dislocation; however, posterolateral rotatory instability is a spectrum of instability that can result from an isolated initial sprain. Valgus instability can also result from chronic overload situations. There are situations in which varus and valgus instability can be produced iatrogenically, particularly after medial epicondylectomy for ulnar neuritis and after excessive debridement for lateral epicondylitis. Varus instability is the result of a complete disruption of the lateral collateral ligament with failure to heal or excessive attenuation. Likewise, in valgus instability, the anterior band of the medial collateral ligament does not heal or has chronic attenuation. This is most common when there is associated radial head fracture or excision. Posterolateral rotatory instability occurs in a progressive

fashion. Stage I instability starts with disruption of the ulnar lateral collateral ligament. Stage II can result in a perched subluxation and also involves rupture of the anterior and/or posterior capsule, and stage III has an associated metacarpophalangeal disruption (Fig. 20–26). The symptoms for posterolateral rotatory instability and varus instability are similar. They include lateral elbow pain and often a flexion contracture. Patients have clicking and recurrent symptoms of popping or subluxation of the elbow.

In valgus instability, patients have a sensation of "giving way" of the medial elbow. They have medial pain and tenderness, especially with throwing. Easy fatigability is a common symptom in throwers and laborers, and ulnar nerve symptoms are also common.

The physical examination for these conditions is best done under block or general anesthesia. A varus stress test is done with the patient prone with shoulder abducted and fully internally rotated. The elbow is flexed to 15 degrees and placed under varus stress. The valgus stress test is done supine or sitting with the shoulder abducted and fully externally rotated. The elbow is flexed at 15 degrees, the forearm is pronated, and valgus stress is placed on the elbow (Fig. 20–27). Posterolateral rotatory instability is tested with a pivot shift test of the elbow (Fig. 20–28). For this, the patient is supine. The shoulder is externally rotated; the elbow is flexed with the forearm fully supinated. The examiner grasps the humerus and forearm and extends the elbow slowly while applying valgus stress, supination, and axial compression. In full extension one sees a posterior prominence and dimpling of the skin just proximal to

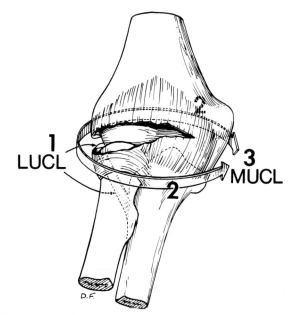

Figure 20–26. Soft tissue injury progresses in a "circle," from lateral to medial, in three stages. In stage 1, the lateral ulnar collateral ligament (LUCL) is disrupted. In stage 2, the other lateral ligamentous structures and the anterior and posterior capsule are disrupted. In stage 3, disruption of the medial ulnar collateral ligament (MUCL) can be partial with disruption of the posterior MUCL only (3A) or complete (3B). (From O'Driscoll SW, Morrey BF, Korinek S, An K-N: Elbow subluxation and dislocation: A spectrum of instability. Clin Orthop 280:186–197, 1992.)

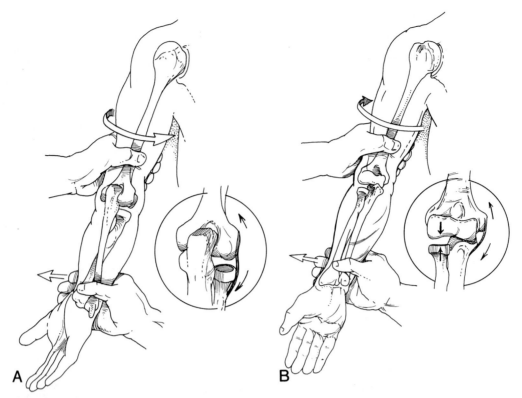

Figure 20–27. *A*, Varus instability of the elbow is measured with the humerus in full internal rotation and a varus stress applied to the slightly flexed joint. *B*, Valgus instability is evaluated with the humerus in full external rotation while a valgus stress is applied to the slightly flexed joint. (From Morrey BF [ed]: The Elbow and Its Disorders, 2nd ed. Philadelphia, WB Saunders, 1993, p 83.)

the radial head. A lateral x-ray shows subluxation of the radius from the capitellum. As the elbow is taken back into flexion, one can produce an audible palpable clunk from the reduction.

X-ray examination shows very few findings on plain x-rays. Arthrography can be good acutely but has a low yield in chronic cases. Stress radiographs under anesthesia are diagnostic. MRI is increasingly being found to be helpful, particularly in diagnosis of incomplete medial ulnar collateral ligament sprains.

Treatment of posterolateral rotatory instability or varus instability involves a reconstruction of lateral ligamentous structures. This is done through a modified Kocher approach. When adequate ligamentous material is available, a direct repair can be performed with reattachment of the avulsed lateral ulnar collateral ligament. One can also plicate the anterior and posterior capsules to supplement this. When inadequate ligament material is available, one should reconstruct the lateral ulnar collateral ligament with a tendinous graft such as palmaris longus or semitendinosus (Fig. 20–29). One must be careful to find the isometric point on the lateral epicondyle for the attachment point.

For chronic valgus instability, a recent rupture in a young patient can sometimes be treated with a mid substance repair or an ulnar-sided reattachment. However, in most cases the preferred treatment for this injury is an anterior transposition of the ulnar nerve and a ligament reconstruction with palmaris longus or other tendon graft. Recent studies have shown up to 74% excellent outcome with reconstructions if there is no history of prior surgery to the elbow.

COMPLEX FRACTURE DISLOCATION OF THE ELBOW AND FOREARM

In addition to the previously mentioned dislocations and instability of the elbow, there are combination injuries that are well described that involve radius or ulna fractures and associated dislocation of the elbow or disruption of the forearm and wrist ligamentous structures. These include the Galeazzi fracture, the Monteggia fractures and their variants, and the Essex-Lopresti fracture-dislocations.

The significance of distal and middle third fractures of the radial shaft with associated distal radioulnar joint disruption was first recognized in 1934 by Galeazzi. He described the severe instability of these injuries and recommended that open reduction and internal fixation be performed. Campbell later termed this fracture the "fracture of necessity," implying the absolute necessity of surgical management for this injury. Other authors have found over 90% failure rates with closed treatment. The diagnosis is made by examination and x-rays. Fractures of the ulnar styloid may or may not be present. Initial treatment is straightforward in that rigid internal fixation of the radial shaft fracture is required. After this is completed, the distal radioulnar joint should be checked for stability. If stable, the patient should be splinted in full supination to allow for healing of the volar and dorsal radioulnar ligaments at the wrist. If there is instability and no ulnar styloid fracture, the triangular fibrocartilage complex should be repaired through drill holes in the fovea of the ulna. If an ulnar styloid fracture is present with instability, open reduction and internal fixation should be done.

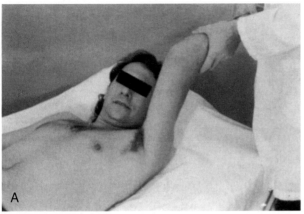

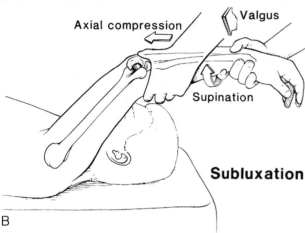

Figure 20–28. *A,* The lateral pivot-shift test of the elbow for posterolateral rotatory instability is performed with the patient supine. A supination valgus moment is applied during flexion. This causes the elbow to subluxate and creates apprehension in the patient. Further flexion produces a palpable, audible clunk as the elbow reduces if the patient is able to relax enough to permit that part of the examination. This usually is not possible and requires a general anesthetic. *B,* Schematic representation of the lateral pivot shift test. (From O'Driscoll SW, Bell DF, Morrey BF: Posterolateral rotatory instability of the elbow. J Bone Joint Surg 73A:440, 1991.)

The eponym given to proximal ulna fractures and associated radial head dislocation is the Monteggia fracture. Four main classes were described by Bado (Fig. 20–30). Type I is an anterior dislocation of the radial head with an apex anterior fracture of the ulnar shaft. Type II is a posterior or posterolateral dislocation of the radial head with an apex posterior angulation of the ulnar shaft. Type III is a lateral or anterolateral dislocation of the radial head and a proximal ulnar metaphyseal fracture. Type IV, a relatively rare injury, involves dislocation of the radial head with a proximal third diaphyseal fracture of both the radius and ulna. There are many variants of these injury patterns. The main value in recognizing them is the understanding that dislocations and soft tissue injuries can also be present in the presence of bony injuries. The constellation of these injuries in adults makes it imperative to perform an open reduction and internal fixation. Delays in treatment can lead to poor outcomes.

The diagnosis is made through physical examination and with AP, lateral, and oblique x-rays of the elbow. One

must be careful to visualize the radiocapitellar joint well with any proximal ulnar fracture. A high index of suspicion should be present for these types of injuries.

Although good results with closed reduction have been found in children, as mentioned earlier, in adults these injury complexes require open reduction and rigid internal fixation of the ulnar fracture with 3.5 mm dynamic compression plates. The radial head usually reduces spontaneously with open reduction of the ulna. If a comminuted fracture of the radial head is present, then excision may be required. We recommend placement of a permanent titanium spacer for this situation. Frequent radiographic examinations in the first few weeks should be obtained to ensure maintenance of reduction of the radial head.

Complications of this injury include posterior interosseous nerve palsy, which is usually a neurapraxia secondary to stretch and usually resolves completely with observation. Non-union can occur if comminution or bone loss is present; therefore, in these situations bone grafting should be performed. Proximal radial ulnar synostosis and/or heterotopic ossification can occur, particularly if surgery is performed late. When extensive comminution or soft tissue stripping is present in these injuries, one should consider prophylactic irradiation with a single dose of 700 cGy.

Essex-Lopresti lesions are the result of a radial head fracture associated with partial or complete rupture of the interosseous membrane and the triangular fibrocartilage complex at the wrist. This results in instability of the distal radioulnar joint.

The diagnosis is made by maintaining a very high index of suspicion for these injuries. At any time a radial head fracture is found, one should carefully examine the wrist for tenderness at the distal radioulnar joint and instability at that site. Radiographic suggestion of distal radioulnar joint instability includes widening of the joint, dorsal displacement of the ulnar head on a true lateral of the wrist, and a fracture of the ulnar styloid base. The treatment involves open reduction and internal fixation of the radial head fracture, if at all possible. When extensive comminution is present, a prosthetic radial head replacement should be used. If gross instability of the distal radial ulnar joint

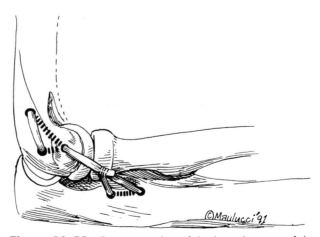

Figure 20–29. Reconstruction of the lateral aspect of the elbow. The function of the lateral ulnar collateral ligament is replicated by the palmaris longus tendon. (From Morrey BF [ed]: The Elbow and Its Disorders, 2nd ed. Philadelphia, WB Saunders, 1993, p 461.)

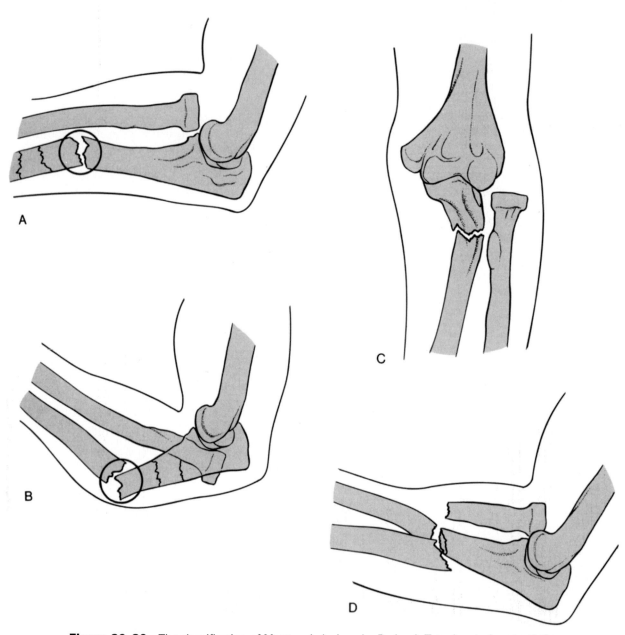

Figure 20–30. The classification of Monteggia lesions by Bado. *A,* Type I: anterior angulation of the ulnar fracture and anterior dislocation of the radial head. *B,* Type II: posterior angulation of the ulnar fracture and posterior dislocation of the radial head. *C,* Type III: fracture of the proximal ulna metaphysis and lateral dislocation of the radial head. *D,* Type IV: anterior dislocation of the radial head and fracture of the radial and ulnar shafts. (From Browner BD, Jupiter JB, Levine AM, Trafton PG [eds]: Skeletal Trauma. Philadelphia, WB Saunders, 1992, p 1117.)

is present, a repair of the triangular fibrocartilage complex should be performed. The radius and ulna should be pinned together for 6 weeks. If gross instability of the distal radioulnar joint is no longer present after radial head fixation and replacement, the forearm can be maintained in a Muenster cast for 6 weeks to allow the triangular fibrocartilage complex to heal.

Soft Tissue Trauma Around the Elbow and Forearm

Soft tissue trauma around the elbow and forearm including injury to the skin, nerves, blood vessels, and muscle and tendon are usually the result of traumatic lacerations or open fractures. When present, these wounds should be addressed by direct exploration in the operating room and repair of all the injured structures. Outcomes are determined by the extent of injury and the number of injured structures. Around the elbow itself, because of the high concentration of neurovascular structures, open injuries can be devastating. For the ulnar nerve in particular, the long distance from the site of injury to the innervated muscles can preclude good return of intrinsic function in the hand. Microvascular reconstruction of arteries in the forearm has mixed results. When an isolated artery is injured, direct repairs have been shown to maintain only a 50% patency rate, even under the best of circumstances. This is probably due to shunting through the excellent collateral flow and stasis at the site of repair.

From the distal third of the forearm to the wrist, lacerations can result in a complex known informally as the "spaghetti wrist," with injury to multiple tendons, nerves, and blood vessels. These injuries should be treated with immediate exploration and repair of all injured structures. Postoperative rehabilitation is critical to return of adequate function.

One significant tendon injury that occurs about the elbow without an open laceration is the distal biceps tendon rupture. This nearly always results from an eccentric loading injury to the biceps tendon in muscular men from the age of 30 to 50. It can occur as a strain to the distal biceps, a partial tear at the tuberosity or at the muscular tendinous junction or most commonly as a complete rupture of the tendon insertion at the tuberosity. The diagnosis for complete ruptures is usually made by history and clinical examination. Patients often feel a pop in their elbow when this happens. They tend to have significant ecchymosis in the antecubital space and tenderness in the region just lateral to the lacertus fibrosus. Patients are weak in flexion and particularly weak in supination with the elbow fully flexed. The condition is also quite painful. If the diagnosis is unclear, an MRI can be helpful, but it is rarely required.

A complete rupture should undergo surgical reattachment to the tuberosity as soon as possible. Exposure can be through a two-incision technique with (1) a small anterior incision to isolate the tendon stump and pass it down toward the tuberosity and (2) a longitudinal dorsal incision for reattachment to the radius (Fig. 20–31). The other option is a long volar incision with a radial approach of Henry to reach the tuberosity. Reattachment to the biceps tuberosity is either by excavating the tuberosity, passing the tendon stump into it, and anchoring it through drill holes, or by using suture anchors.

This immediate reconstruction is easiest when done within 2 weeks of the initial injury. After this, extensive scarring occurs in the region of the tendon stump and retraction of the biceps muscle itself makes it difficult to perform a reattachment. However, successful repairs have been reported up to 3 months out from the initial injury. When significant delay is present and one is unable to perform reattachment, two options are available. The first is tenodesis of the biceps to the brachialis. This helps restore elbow flexion strength but produces no change at all in the deficit in supination strength. When supination strength must be improved, one can attempt an augmentation reconstruction either with tendon autograft or a ligament augmentation device.

The results of immediate, direct reattachment to the tuberosity have shown that in the dominant extremity, flexion and supination strength approach normal. In the non-dominant elbow, patients end up 15 to 25% weaker. When this injury is treated with non-operative management, patients can expect a deficit in flexion strength of 15 to 20%. The supination weakness, however, ranges from 30 to 50% and can be the more problematic loss.

Complications of surgical treatment have included posterior interosseous nerve palsies, particularly with a single anterior approach. With the two-incision technique, reports of up to 5% incidence of heterotopic ossification and even synostosis between the radius and ulna have been reported.

OVERUSE SYNDROMES OF THE ELBOW

Lateral Epicondylitis

Lateral epicondylitis is a painful overuse disorder of the extensor origin at the lateral epicondyle. It is an extremely common condition and usually presents in the fourth to fifth decade of life. It is more common in men than women. There are many occupational and reactional stresses that seem to be associated with it. The condition has the eponym of "tennis elbow," because the classic presentation is from repetitive stresses to the lateral epicondyle from backhand strokes in tennis. However, the condition affects 1 to 2% of the general population, and less than 5% of these people have a history of racquet use. Ten to 20% of patients experience an acute event inciting the onset of this pain.

Differential diagnoses includes radial tunnel syndrome, in which the posterior interosseous nerve is entrapped under the origin of the supinator; radiocapitellar joint arthritis, which is rarely present; and subtle lateral instability of the elbow.

Physical examination should include direct palpation of the lateral epicondyle with the elbow in 90 degrees of flexion; palpation and pressure 3 to 4 cm distally to rule out tenderness over the posterior interosseous nerve; resisted wrist dorsiflexion with the elbow extended; resisted supination, which is more painful with radial tunnel syndrome; palpation over the radiocapitellar joint; and posterolateral pivot shift testing of the elbow.

X-rays can show some epicondylar calcification in 5 to 20% of patients. However, this has very little prognostic value. MRI has very little use in this problem.

When trying to differentiate between this diagnosis and

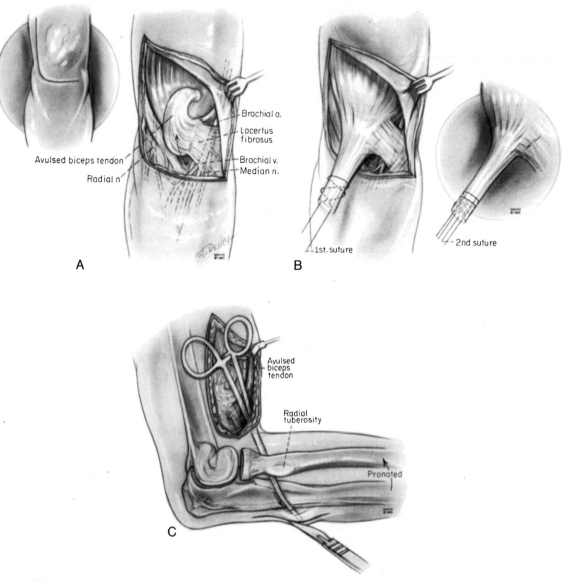

Figure 20–31.   *A,* The proximal portion of a Henry incision is used to expose the antecubital space proximally. The retracted biceps tendon is identified, taking care to avoid injury to the brachial artery and median and radial nerves and their branches. *B,* Two Bunnel sutures are placed in the end of the tendon. *C,* A blunt instrument is introduced in the tract of the biceps tendon, and the skin is indented on the volar aspect of the proximal forearm. An incision is made over this instrument.

posterior interosseous nerve entrapment, which is concurrently present up to 5% of the time, one must rely heavily on physical findings because EMG and nerve conduction studies have little role in radial tunnel syndrome. Selected injection with corticosteroids and local anesthetics can be very helpful in separating the diagnoses and can be curative at times. Analysis of pathologic tissue samples from this condition has shown it is a degenerative process, mainly within the origin of the extensor carpi radialis brevis tendon. The resultant tissue has been called "angiofibroblastic proliferation" by Nirschl and Pettrone.

The mainstay of treatment is non-surgical. Initial management includes activity modification with rest and avoidance of a fully pronated position; anti-inflammatory medications; and counterforce bracing, which helps relieve some

of the strains placed on the common extensor origin by the wrist and finger extensor muscles. Corticosteroid injection in the area of the anterior lateral epicondyle can often be curative. Recent studies have shown even shock-wave lithotripsy may have some role in the treatment of this condition. However, it seems modalities such as ultrasound, massage, and iontophoresis may not have real benefit. Usually 90% of patients respond well to this non-surgical management approach. Surgery is indicated only for the remaining 5 to 10% of patients who have not responded to at least 6 months of non-operative management and have continued moderate to severe pain that limits their ability to perform activities of their choice.

The most commonly performed procedure for this involves a small incision directly over the distal third of the

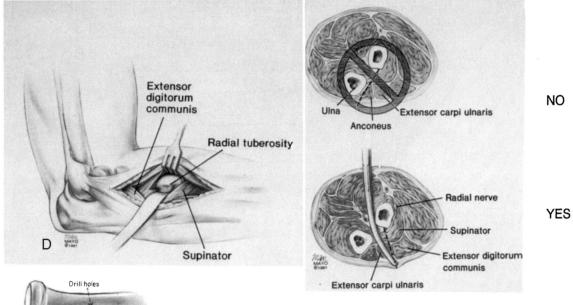

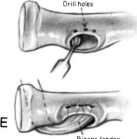

Figure 20–31 *Continued. D*, The common extensor and supinator muscles are then split to expose the radial tuberosity. The ulna is *not* exposed. Full pronation of the forearm brings the tuberosity into the field. *E*, The radial tuberosity is excavated using a high-speed burr. The biceps tendon is then brought through its previous tract and reinserted into the radial tuberosity with two non-absorbable sutures. (From Morrey BF [ed]: The Elbow and Its Disorders, 2nd ed. Philadelphia, WB Saunders, 1993, pp 495–496.)

lateral epicondyle and extending 1 or 2 cm beyond this (Fig. 20–32). The common extensor origin is incised longitudinally at its anterior third, and the underlying extensor carpi radialis brevis origin is explored (see Fig. 20–31). Any degenerative tissue is carefully excised, and the underlying lateral epicondyle is decorticated. The common extensor origin is loosely closed, and patients wear a splint for 2 weeks. After this, gradual increase in range of motion and strengthening is progressed, and the patient is allowed to return to full activity at 3 months. This approach has shown a success rate of greater than 90%. When surgical failure is present, one must be careful to make sure the posterior interosseous nerve is not involved, iatrogenic instability has not been created, and there is no herniation of synovial fluid.

Medial Epicondylitis

Medial epicondylitis has been given the eponym of "golfer's elbow." It is an overuse disorder of the flexor pronator origin along the medial epicondyle that is analogous to that of the extensor origin in lateral epicondylitis. The degenerative changes seem to be mainly within the pronator teres and flexor carpi radialis origins. Differential diagnoses include cubital tunnel syndrome with entrapment of the ulnar nerve. This is frequently a concomitant problem. Other possible diagnoses include medial epicondylar apophysitis in skeletally immature athletes ("Little Leaguer's elbow") and medial collateral ligament injury resulting in valgus stress instability.

Patients are mainly in the fourth to five decades of life

with men outnumbering women in 2:1 ratio. There are many recreational or occupational stress factors for this. Many patients note an acute inciting event. Many patients also have other chronic disorders including carpal tunnel syndrome and rotator cuff tendinitis.

On physical examination patients have direct epicondylar tenderness and provocation of symptoms with resisted forearm pronation and resisted wrist flexion. One must carefully test the ulnar nerve for irritability with direct palpation or percussion (Tinel's test), reproduction of symptoms with prolonged elbow flexion, and painful subluxation of the nerve. The medial collateral ligament should be tested with a valgus stress examination.

X-rays reveal epicondylar calcification in 10%. Gravity valgus x-rays can be helpful to determine mild instability. MRI has little role in this diagnosis. However, EMGs can be very helpful with assessing ulnar nerve irritability.

Again, non-surgical management is the mainstay of therapy and 90 to 95% of patients will respond to measures as described for lateral epicondylitis.

This condition has been classified by Gabel and Morrey into type IA, in which there are no ulnar nerve signs or symptoms; type IB, in which there are minimal or mild ulnar nerve signs and symptoms; and type II, in which moderate or severe associated ulnar nerve symptoms are present.

Surgical management is fairly similar to that of lateral epicondylitis in that a 2- to 3-cm incision can be made just anterior to the medial epicondyle in a longitudinal fashion, the flexor pronator mass is elevated from proximal to distal, and underlying involved degenerative tissue is resected.

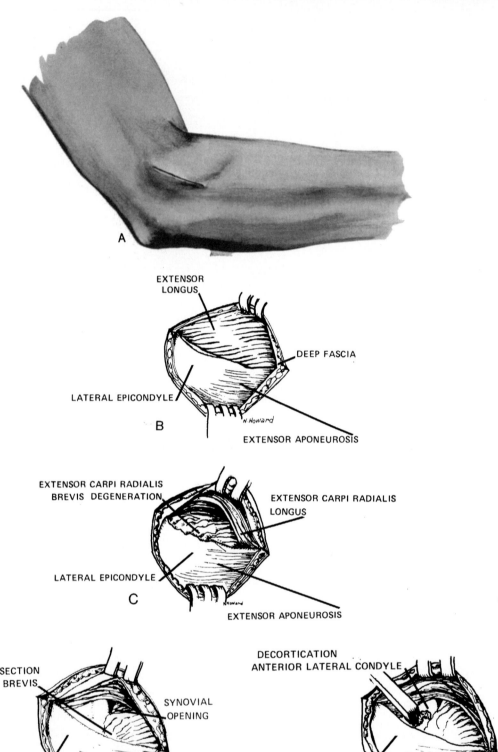

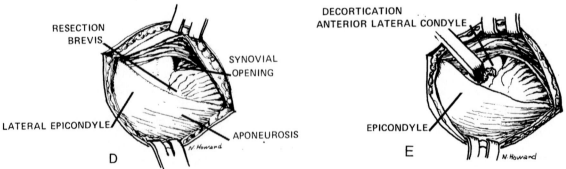

Figure 20–32. *A,* Skin incision. *B,* Incision at interface of extensor longus and aponeurosis. *C,* Anterior retraction of extensor longus, exposing the origin of the extensor brevis. Note that the extensor longus is thin (2 to 3 mm) at this level. A common error is to dissect too deeply, thereby failing to clearly identify the extensor brevis origin. *D,* Excision of pathologic tissue, usually of extensor brevis origin. A small incision may be made through the synovium for visual inspection of the lateral compartment. *E,* Vascular enhancement is accomplished by osteotome decortication as shown, or three to four holes (5/64 inch) are drilled through cortical bone to cancellous areas to enhance the vascular supply. Drilling causes less postoperative pain. (From Nirschl RP, Pettrone F: Tennis elbow. The surgical treatment of lateral epicondylitis. J Bone Joint Surg Am 61:832, 1979.)

One must be careful not to go below the level of the accessory anterior oblique ligament to avoid creation of instability of the elbow. Part of the medial epicondyle is decorticated, and loose closure of the tendon remnants are recommended.

When mild ulnar nerve symptoms are present, releasing of cubital tunnel is indicated and when severe symptoms are present, one should consider an anterior submuscular transposition of the ulnar nerve with elevation of the pronator mass. The results of surgical management have shown a greater than 90% success rate in patients with minimal ulnar nerve involvement, but only 40% good to excellent results when the ulnar nerve is severely involved. The final recovery from surgery can take up to 2 years.

Olecranon Bursitis

Olecranon bursitis is a very common elbow problem as well. This usually presents as a large focal swelling within the olecranon bursa after an episode of overuse or direct trauma. It is also very common in rheumatoid patients. Lateral x-rays of the elbow frequently reveal an olecranon osteophyte.

Treatment is non-surgical initially with a compressive Ace wrap or elbow pad. Oral anti-inflammatory agents are also very helpful in decreasing the swelling and discomfort in the area. Aspiration alone rarely cures this, because the fluid readily reaccumulates. The addition of a corticosteroid injection after aspiration lowers the rate of recurrence but greatly increases the potential complication rate. One can develop a chronic sinus tract or infection when using this treatment.

Septic olecranon bursitis presents in a similar fashion. In an acute setting one should just treat this with oral antibiotics, although some authors have advocated aspiration as well. In more advanced states, where loculations are present, one usually waits until the acute inflammation dies down and then a resection of the bursa can be performed.

ELBOW AND FOREARM STIFFNESS

Stiffness in the elbow and forearm is a fairly common problem and can present one of the more difficult challenges for the surgeon to treat. It is most frequently present after a fracture or direct trauma to the elbow but can also result from burns, head injuries, immobilization after elective surgery, infection, hemophilia, or arthritis. Normal elbow range of motion involves full extension, 140 degrees of flexion, and approximately 80 degrees of both pronation and supination. When there is loss of range of motion, significant disability can develop. Loss of pronation decreases the patient's ability to use a keyboard or write. Loss of supination limits the ability to reach and lift or use a spoon. Loss of flexion inhibits feeding and grooming as well as perineal care. The generally accepted range of motion required for activities of daily living is from 30 to 130 degrees of elbow extension to flexion and 50 degrees of pronation and 50 degrees of supination. Elbow flexion and extension stiffness can be due to intrinsic causes such as adhesions or interarticular stepoffs or bony blocks that restrict joint motion. They can also be due to extrinsic causes such as heterotopic bone or capsular contracture, which almost always becomes a factor with long-standing contracture. O'Driscoll stated that there are four stages of elbow stiffness. Stage I is caused by bleeding and occurs within hours after injury or surgery. Treatment and prevention of further loss is performed by elevation, compression, and keeping the elbow either in a fully extended position to avoid accumulation of blood or moving it through a full range of motion. Stage II is edema that occurs within days of the insult. The treatment is to keep the elbow moving through a full range of motion. Stage III involves early scar tissue formation and takes weeks after the initial injury. Again, treatment is to keep the elbow moving through as full a range of motion as possible and keep increasing this range of motion or use static splints. Stage IV involves the formation of organized scar. This takes months to occur, and the treatment involves splinting for up to a year. Surgical treatment is indicated if splints fail or if the patient presents with a contracture of more than 1 year in duration. Much of this post-surgical stiffness can be prevented by using meticulous surgical technique, achieving excellent hemostasis, and starting range of motion exercises right away. Continuous passive motion is becoming an increasingly useful method for regaining early elbow range of motion. It should be set for full motion so that the elbow is alternatively flexed and extended to tighten tissues and prevent edema. When the patient starts formal occupational or physical therapy, emphasis should be on active and active-assisted range of motion. Overaggressive/passive exercises should be avoided because of the risk of fracture, bleeding, and heterotopic ossification.

In evaluating a patient with a stiff elbow, one should obtain a history about the limitation of the patient's activities of daily living and the direction that the patient would most like to regain motion, either in flexion or extension, and previous treatment protocols, including dynamic splinting. Imaging studies including AP and lateral x-rays should be obtained to evaluate for bony deformity as a cause. For patients with less than 1 year since the onset of the stiffness, we recommend progressive static splinting as well as anti-inflammatory medications. The success of splinting is inversely related to the duration of contracture. The results are quite poor after 12 months. Indications for surgery include failed conservative management for greater than a year and loss of extension of more than 30 degrees or loss of flexion of more than 120 degrees. Surgical management consists of open capsular release, usually done through a posterior skin incision and either a lateral modified Kocher approach or a medial Bryan-Morrey approach. Every effort should be made to leave the triceps intact, and a wide capsular excision should be performed. When marked intrinsic contracture is present and greater than 50 percent of the joint surface is destroyed, the patient may be a candidate for distraction interposition arthroplasty with a fascia lata graft and a dynamic external fixator. Morrey has established excellent results with this technique for regaining the functional range of motion, but he warns that it is a very technically demanding procedure with potentially high rates of complications. Arthroscopic release of capsular contracture has been advocated by some surgeons, but this procedure, too, is very technically demanding. The normal volume of the elbow capsule is 25 to 30 mL, but in a contracted elbow it can be as little as 6 mL. This prevents the normal displacement of the surrounding neurovascular structures and leaves them more susceptible to injury with portal placement. It also makes it difficult to maneuver an arthroscope and shaver within the joint, and any intrinsic scarring or adhesions also makes it difficult to see. It is unsafe to excise large segments of capsule; one should consider this procedure an arthroscopic release rather than capsular excision.

Heterotopic ossification is the formation of normal bone in an abnormal site. The elbow is one of the most common sites for post-traumatic heterotopic bone formation, and it can cause marked loss of motion. Patients usually present with pain and decreased range of motion. It frequently occurs at a point when the patient was otherwise progressing well with their restoration of elbow function. Physical examination may reveal increased warmth, mild erythema, and swelling. X-rays are rarely positive within 3 weeks of surgery or fracture, although soft tissue swelling may be visualized. At this point, overaggressive therapy should be avoided because passive stretching tends to cause

local bleeding, which exacerbates the formation of new bone. Technetium bone scanning can be helpful for detecting early heterotopic ossification and can later help determine when the metabolic activity of the ectopic bone has diminished (Fig. 20–33). Laboratory assays such as serum alkaline phosphatase can be useful, but many authors have questioned their role in decision making regarding resection of heterotopic ossification.

The decision to surgically treat this condition should be made exclusively on the functional limitations. As we know from our experience in the hip, many patients have radiographically significant heterotopic ossification with minimal functional loss. In the elbow, one should specifically note presence or absence of bony compression of the ulnar nerve that can commonly occur, particularly after a brain injury. This would push one to consider resection of the heterotopic bone. Once the decision has been made to resect the heterotopic ossification, the timing is very important. The generally accepted time frame is 1 year after the onset of new bone formation. However, Morrey states that the decision should be based solely on radiographic imaging that shows maturation of the bone with

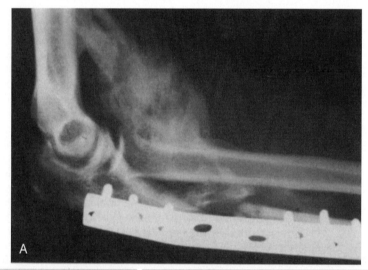

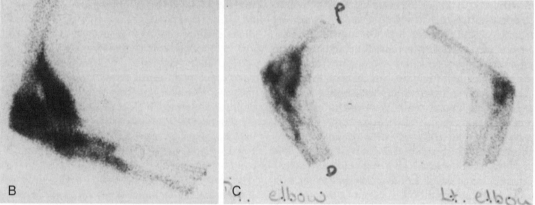

Figure 20–33. A 26-year-old man was involved in a motor vehicle accident and sustained a dislocation of his right elbow with a proximal ulnar fracture. Open reduction and internal fixation of the ulna was done 3 weeks after his injury. He was first seen at the Mayo Clinic 4 months later with extensive (A) ectopic bone. The technetium-99m scan showed marked uptake at 4 months (B), which persisted for 18 months (C). (From Morrey BF [ed]: The Elbow and Its Disorders, 2nd ed. Philadelphia, WB Saunders, 1993, p 507.)

normal trabecular formation. When this is present, earlier resection of the heterotopic ossification may be advantageous to avoid further establishment of contracture and the possibility of long-term cartilage destruction. Several approaches are available for resection of heterotopic ossification about the elbow; the one chosen should provide the most direct access to the bone bridge with a minimal amount of soft tissue trauma. Often several deep approaches are required to allow for full capsular resection at the same time.

Limitations of forearm motion can be due to heterotopic ossification sometimes leading to synostosis. Malunion is also a significant cause of loss of forearm rotation, with loss of the radial bow or closure of the interosseous space, interrupting pronation and supination. Another effect of malunion is shortening or proximal migration of the radius, which results in ulnar impaction at the wrist. There also are congenital causes including radial head dislocation, ulnar bowing, and radioulnar synostosis. In these conditions in particular there is very little hope of restoring functional pronation and supination. When a congenital radioulnar synostosis is present and the forearm is fixed in more than 60 degrees of pronation or any amount of supination, the patient will have marked difficulties with activities of daily living. Simmons and associates have advocated a derotational osteotomy through the synostosis site and placement of the forearm into an individualized position of between 15 to 60 degrees of pronation. When bilateral congenital synostoses are present, the positioning of the forearm is somewhat controversial. Some have advocated 20 to 30 degrees of supination for the non-dominant hand and 30 to 45 degrees of pronation for the dominant hand. Simmons and associates recommended 10 to 20 degrees of pronation for the dominant extremity and neutral positioning for the non-dominant extremity.

The principles of treatment in situations of adult loss of pronation and supination again involve true demonstration of disability, an accurate assessment of the cause as mentioned earlier, and then surgical treatment of the involved segment. When malunion is present, surgical intervention should be geared toward the position of the deformity. When midshaft or both-bone fractures are present, one must correct the angular and rotational deformity with rigid internal fixation to allow for immediate range of motion, and patients tend to improve slowly. With distal radial malunions several options are possible, including osteotomy of the radius for actual correction of the malunion, ulnar shortening osteotomy, distal ulna resection (also called a Darrach procedure), and the Sauvé-Kapandji procedure, which involves leveling and arthrodesis of the distal radioulnar joint and proximal pseudarthrosis formation through the ulna. The procedure of choice should be based on the patient's lifestyle, functional demands, and type of deformity. Proximal malunions can be very difficult to solve. Radial head excision is one option. It carries the risk, however, of proximal migration of the radius and further problems at the distal radioulnar joint if an interosseous ligament injury is present.

Synostosis in the forearm again should be approached based on the position of the bony union. When synostosis is present at the proximal radioulnar joint, resection of the radial head is the procedure of choice. When there is significant heterotopic ossification at the bicipital tuberosity level, it should be resected and either fat or fascia or muscle should be interposed into the region to prevent recurrence of synostosis. At the diaphyseal level, heterotopic ossification or synostosis is directly resected along with the involved regions of the interosseous membrane. The central band of the interosseous membrane can be taken as well unless the radial head has been resected. This would lead to axial instability of the radius with proximal migration. When this problem is present with accompanying angular deformity at the fracture site, the deformity should be corrected as well to maximize the chances for full return of rotation of the forearm. The radial and ulnar shafts in the region where the synostosis is resected should be covered with either fat interposition or silicone rubber sheeting to help prevent recurrence of the synostosis. When distal forearm heterotopic ossification is present, it is frequently within the pronator quadratus musculature itself, leading to synostosis. Although direct resection is possible, it is far easier and results are more predictable when a Sauvé-Kapandji procedure is performed. In the rare instances when heterotopic ossification or synostosis involves the distal radioulnar joint itself, the procedure of choice involves resection of the distal ulna rather than attempt at bony resection and reconstruction of the distal radioulnar joint. In all of these surgical situations one should stick to several general principles: the radius and ulna should be approached through separate incisions, trauma to the interosseous membrane should be avoided, meticulous hemostasis should be obtained, and careful irrigation of any bone dust must be performed. If an osteotomy is required, stable fixation methods should be used to allow for immediate rotational range of motion. One should consider adjunctive therapy as well, including use of indomethacin or low-dose radiation therapy. After long-standing synostosis or stiffness of pronation and supination, contracture of the soft tissues may also be involved. Soft tissue procedures such as resection of the volar or dorsal capsule of the distal radioulnar joint as recently described by Kleinman and Graham may be required.

ELBOW ARTHRITIS

Although relatively uncommon, arthritis of the elbow can create profound disability in upper extremity use. Advances in non-implant and implant arthroplasty techniques over the past few decades have markedly improved our ability to treat various forms of arthritis of the elbow, and this should be kept in mind when evaluating patients with this disease. The three main types of arthritis of the elbow in descending order of frequency are rheumatoid arthritis, post-traumatic arthritis, and osteoarthritis. Treatment options range from basic medical management to total joint replacement. In this section the various types of arthritis and their non-surgical treatment are discussed, followed by surgical options.

Rheumatoid Arthritis

Twenty to 50% of patients with rheumatoid arthritis eventually develop involvement of the elbow. They frequently also have involvement of the shoulder and wrist, further compromising upper extremity function. The process usually begins as a painful synovitis of the joint. When severe enough involvement at the radiocapitellar joint is present, a posterior interosseous nerve palsy can result from the resulting compression. If synovitis persists, there is eventual destruction of the cartilaginous surfaces of the joint and gradual disruption of surrounding ligamentous structures. Finally, the disease progresses to the point of extensive loss of subchondral bone and gross ligamentous instability or a situation where near ankylosis occurs. Physical examination should start with observation to see if there is an olecranon bursitis, obvious rheumatoid nodules, or gross deformity. Range of motion and its limitations should be checked. A careful neurovascular examination with particular focus on the ulnar nerve and the posterior interosseous nerve is done next, then stability testing is performed.

True AP and lateral x-rays of the elbow are usually sufficient for the diagnosis and planning of treatment. These plain x-rays give an accurate staging of rheumatoid arthritis, with grade I disease being active synovitis but no significant radiographic changes with the possible exception of periarticular osteopenia. Grade II has more advanced and unremitting synovitis. The radiographic changes involve symmetrical joint space narrowing but no extensive destruction. Grade III changes result in changes in the subchondral bone. Grade IIIA is a milder type with subchondral cyst formation. Grade IIIB is extensive loss of subchondral bone or ankylosis of the joint. Grade IV shows gross destruction of all the normal articular architecture (Fig. 20–34).

Initial management of the early stages of rheumatoid arthritis of the elbow begins with standard non-surgical treatment. Patients with very low-grade disease are started on aspirin or anti-inflammatory medications. Depending on the staging of other joints and the advancement in the elbow, more powerful systemic medications are tried, including antimalarials, corticosteroids, methotrexate, and so on. Physical therapy is a useful adjunct for maintaining muscle strength and range of motion about the elbow. Splinting can be useful in acute situations to help a synovitic flare resolve. Corticosteroid injections are also very useful in alleviating the inflammatory process in acute flareups.

Post-traumatic Arthritis

Post-traumatic arthritis of the elbow results from extensive articular cartilage loss at the time of injury, articular step-offs, residual instability, and non-union. The resulting pain, stiffness, and/or instability can be disabling to the use of the upper extremity. This patient population is typically younger than those with rheumatoid arthritis or osteoarthritis. Evaluation should include the routine history and physical examination as well as standard AP and lateral x-rays of the elbow.

Results of treatment in this group of patients have not been as encouraging as those in patients with rheumatoid arthritis and osteoarthritis. This is most likely due to the younger age and higher demand nature of these patients. Non-surgical management involves standard activity modification and anti-inflammatory use. Corticosteroid injection

may provide some temporary relief. Beyond this, little can be done non-operatively.

Primary Osteoarthritis of the Elbow

Primary osteoarthritis of the elbow is a relatively uncommon condition that affects mainly middle-aged men, with the peak incidence around age 50 but a range from age 20 to 65. It is primarily present in heavy laborers and patients with chronic elbow overuse. These patients develop a very typical pattern of osteophyte formation of the tip of the olecranon as well as the coronoid process. They also develop osteophytes within the coronoid and olecranon fossas. There is arthritis formation about the radial head in approximately a fourth of the patients and a similar percentage have loose body formations within the joint. Patients present with loss of motion, which they notice most in extension. However, flexion losses are often more severe. Impingement pain with terminal flexion and extension is also a major component and one of the primary reasons for surgical intervention. Catching and locking may be present, and a high percentage of patients have ulnar nerve entrapment symptoms as well.

Surgical Intervention for Elbow Arthritis

Surgical treatment of rheumatoid arthritis, post-traumatic arthritis, or osteoarthritis of the elbow is indicated when non-operative management has failed and when patients are experiencing functional loss due to their symptoms. Treatment options available include debridement, either arthroscopically or open, ulnohumeral arthroplasty, interposition arthroplasty with or without distraction, and total elbow replacement.

Debridement involves resection of synovitis, loose bodies, and other debris, as well as osteophytes within the joint. It is indicated in earlier stages of many types of elbow arthritis. In rheumatoid arthritis the pannus proliferation can be resected to reduce the pain and swelling at the elbow. Many have also advocated resection of the radial head to relieve the painful loss of motion that it can cause. One study has shown a 70% success rate with excellent relief of pain over 6 years after radial head resection and synovectomy with 14% of patients needing re-operation. Little functional gain is obtained, however, in stage IIIB or stage IV rheumatoid arthritis, and most would advocate that a total elbow replacement in these patients is a much more predictable and lasting procedure. Arthroscopic debridement of the early stage rheumatoid elbow can be an effective procedure if one is able to perform an adequate synovectomy. This is a technically difficult procedure and should be done by physicians with significant experience in elbow arthroscopy. Long-term results are not available for this procedure.

Debridement alone has little role in post-traumatic or primary arthritis of the elbow. The one exception is when a loose body is causing a direct mechanical blockage. Arthroscopic or open removal is then indicated.

Ulnohumeral or Outerbridge-Kashiwagi arthroplasty is the procedure of choice for treatment of primary osteoarthritis of the elbow. It involves extensive debridement of the joint and resection of olecranon, coronoid, and fossa

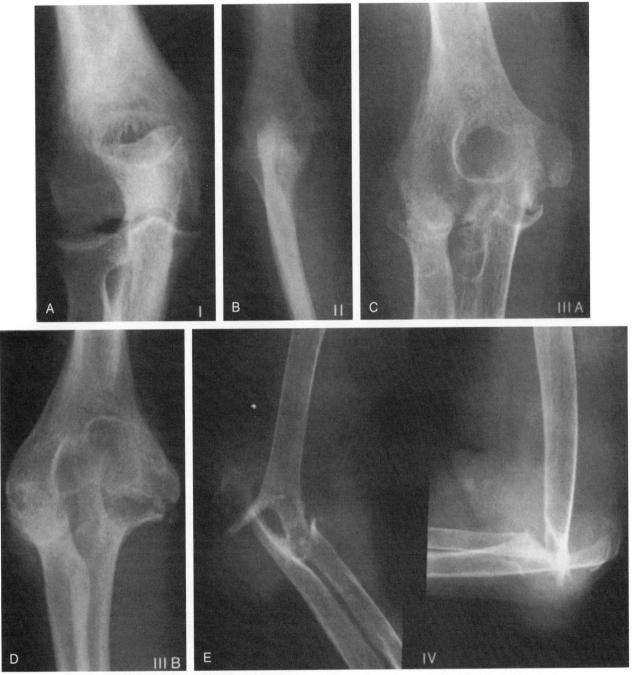

Figure 20–34. Mayo classification of rheumatoid involvement of the elbow. *A*, Synovitis, grade I. *B*, Joint narrowing, grade II. *C*, Architectural changes, moderate, grade IIIA. *D*, Severe, grade IIIB. *E*, Gross destruction, grade IV. (From Morrey BF [ed]: The Elbow and Its Disorders, 2nd ed. Philadelphia, WB Saunders, 1993, p 756.)

osteophytes and decompression of the ulnar nerve when indicated. The elbow is entered through a triceps-splitting or a triceps-reflecting (Bryan-Morrey) approach. An osteotome is used to resect the olecranon tip and its osteophytes. A large trephine on a high-speed drill is then used to create a window through the bone between the olecranon and coronoid fossae, which is often thickened over a centimeter from its normal paper-thin state by osteophytes. Through this window, the anterior joint is debrided and the coronoid osteophyte is resected (Fig. 20–35). This procedure is ex-

cellent for reducing pain, although it does not usually eliminate it completely, and most patients can expect 20- to 30- degree gains in their flexion/extension arc. Complication rates are very low. Radiographic recurrence rates of up to 50% at 5 years have been reported, but the functional decrease from this is unknown.

Interposition arthroplasty for the elbow consists of resection of destroyed joint surfaces and use of interposed material (e.g., fascia lata, cutis, or fat) to provide a stable, gliding surface for motion. It was introduced in the United

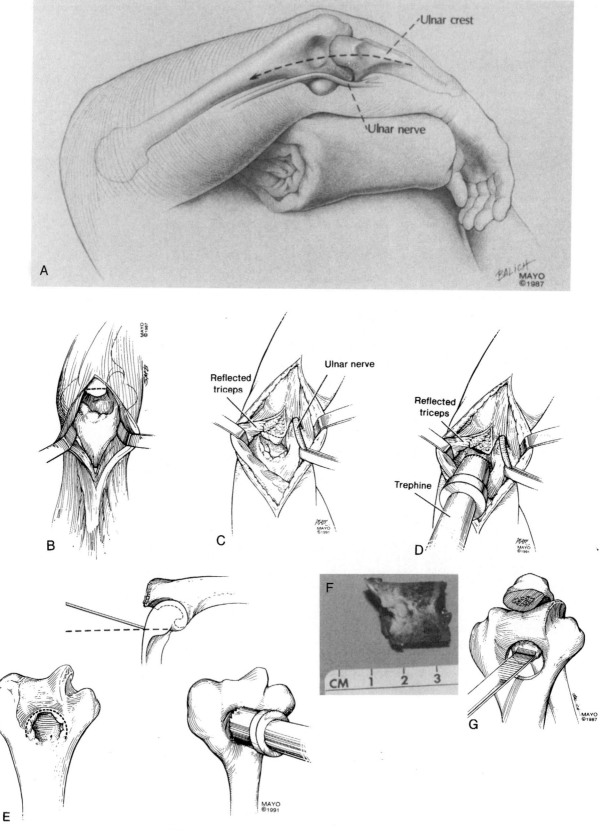

Figure 20–35. *See legend on opposite page*

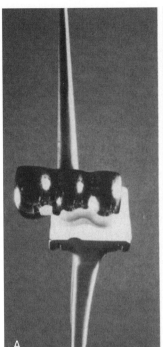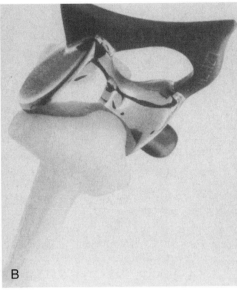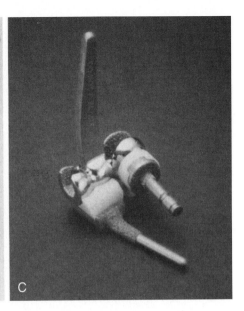

Figure 20–36. *A,* Capitellocondylar unconstrained elbow prosthesis; ulnohumeral resurfacing articular; capitelloradial head articular surface. *B,* Souter-Strathclyde unconstrained elbow prosthesis; ulnohumeral articulation only. *C,* Pritchard unconstrained radioulnohumeral articulation. (From Morrey BF [ed]: The Elbow and Its Disorders, 2nd ed. Philadelphia, WB Saunders, 1993, p 630.)

States in the early 1900s, and until the development of successful implant arthroplasties in the late 1960s, it was one of the only options for pain relief and restoration of motion in arthritic or ankylosed elbows. Today, its use is mainly for post-traumatic arthritis in a young, high-demand patient who cannot comply with the low-weight-bearing restrictions of a total elbow replacement. Morrey advocates that the procedure be performed with the addition of a distraction fixator to allow for early motion with stability while the interposition graft heals. His review of 13 patients with 5-year follow-up showed 78% satisfactory results in patients with no underlying instability. Instability and residual pain are the main problems with this treatment. Recent results in patients with rheumatoid arthritis suggest that pain relief and functional improvement from interposition arthroplasty are inferior to those obtained with total elbow replacement, and they suggest the procedure not be used in this patient population.

Total elbow replacement has evolved into a safe and

highly effective method for treating severe arthritis of this joint. There are two main designs in use today: unconstrained and semiconstrained. The unconstrained designs are unlinked surface replacement prostheses; their main drawback has been instablity when soft tissue balancing is not perfect (Fig. 20–36). The semiconstrained designs consist of ulnar and humeral components linked by a "sloppy hinge" that allows for a few degrees of rotational and varus-valgus motion to decrease stress on the bone-cement interfaces (Fig. 20–37). The primary problem with this design has been stem breakage, and patients with these implants should not lift more than 10 pounds with the affected extremity for the rest of their lives.

The results of total elbow arthroplasty, particularly with those reported for the Mayo-Coonrad semiconstrained system, are now excellent. In patients with rheumatoid arthritis 91% had satisfactory results at an average of 4 years of follow-up. Recent data for post-traumatic arthritis patients show 83% satisfactory results with over 5-year

Figure 20–35. *A,* The surgical technique to perform an ulnohumeral arthroplasty with the patient in the rotated supine position. A straight incision is placed just medial to the olecranon. *B,* The triceps tendon is split and retracted to expose the proximal ulna and distal humerus. *C,* The preferable alternative is to reflect the medial half of the triceps insertion from the olecranon. The tip of the olecranon is removed along with the olecranon osteophyte. *D,* The olecranon fossa is foraminectomized with a trephine. *E,* This crucial maneuver is made by following the contour of the trochlea and the trephine is oriented slightly proximal because the distal articulation of the humerus is anteriorly rotated. *F,* The humeral core is removed. *G,* The humerus is flexed, any anterior loose bodies that may be present are removed, and the osteophyte of the coronoid is removed with an osteotome through the foramen. (Reprinted by permission, Mayo Foundation, 1987.)

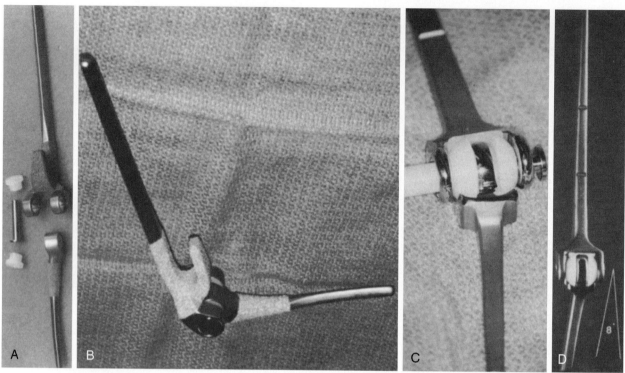

Figure 20–37. *A*, Mayo-Coonrad semiconstrained elbow prosthesis, disarticulated. Polyethylene bearing surface; centered distal humerus and proximal ulna. *B*, Mayo-Coonrad prosthesis, articulated. *C*, Pritchard semiconstrained elbow prosthesis, disarticulated to show polyethylene hinge and ulnohumeral articulation surfaces. *D*, Pritchard-Walker semiconstrained articulated ulnohumeral components with 8 degrees valgus carrying angle and 8 to 10 degrees varus-valgus toggle. (From Morrey BF [ed]: The Elbow and Its Disorders, 2nd ed. Philadelphia, WB Saunders, 1993, p 630.)

follow-up. Patients in these two groups had outstanding pain relief and significant improvement in range of motion. Complications included infection, loosening, ulnar component fracture, ulna fracture, and triceps avulsion.

SUMMARY

The elbow and forearm are involved in a wide range of pathologic processes, from tendinopathies that are sometimes easily treatable to complex post-traumatic disorders. With a firm understanding of the anatomy and these disease processes, one can determine the diagnoses and help patients return to maximum function.

Selected Readings

Browner BD, Jupiter JB, Levine AM, Trafton PG (eds): Skeletal Trauma. Philadelphia, WB Saunders, 1992.

Morrey BF (ed): The Elbow and Its Disorders, 2nd ed. Philadelphia, WB Saunders, 1993.

Morrey BF (ed): The Elbow—Masters Techniques in Orthopaedic Surgery. New York, Raven Press, 1994.

Norris TR (ed): Orthopaedic Knowledge Update: Shoulder and Elbow. Rosemont, IL, American Academy of Orthopaedic Surgeons, 1997.

Weiss A-PC (ed): Difficult disorders of the elbow and forearm. Hand Clin 10(3), 1994.

GWENT HEALTHCARE NHS TRUST
LIBRARY
ROYAL GWENT HOSPITAL
NEWPORT

Chapter 21

Hand and Wrist Surgery

Mustafa A. Haque, M.D.

The role of our hands in our day-to-day activities is so vast and far reaching that few of us can even imagine its extent until we are faced with a hand injury or limitation of our own. Our hands, more than any other organ that an orthopaedic surgeon manages in practice, allow us to interface with the rest of the world. They allow us to touch, hold, gesture, manipulate objects, eat, and defend ourselves. The tactile stereognosis they provide can even let a blind patient read Braille. They are usually open and visible for others to see.

Numerous congenital and acquired conditions affect the hand. The results of these conditions can sometimes be devastating, both to the patient's ability to function and to their self-esteem. Fortunately, great advances in the care of these conditions have developed in the past century, and we can now significantly improve function in many cases. In this chapter a brief introduction is provided to the diagnosis and management of some of these conditions.

ANATOMY

The underlying themes of the anatomy and biomechanics of the hand and wrist are motion and balance. The tremendous motion present in the hand is evidenced by the total active motion present in a finger, which is normally near 260 degrees. For this to occur while maintaining stability at the multiple joints involved, a finally tuned balance must be present between the active muscle and tendon motor units of the hand, the complex bony anatomy, and the static ligamentous stabilizers. Any process that upsets this balance can lead to progressive deformity and loss of function. Conversely, by restoring the balance, even with fusion of selected joints, function can often be greatly improved. Keeping the two themes of motion and balance in mind while studying this anatomy will help with understanding the structures of the hand and wrist and their function.

Bone and Ligament

CARPAL STRUCTURES

The bony anatomy of the wrist is made up of the radius, ulna, eight carpal bones (scaphoid, lunate, triquetrum, pisiform, trapezium, trapezoid, capitate, and hamate), and the metacarpal bases (Fig. 21–1). The articulations between these bones can be grouped into the distal radioulnar joint

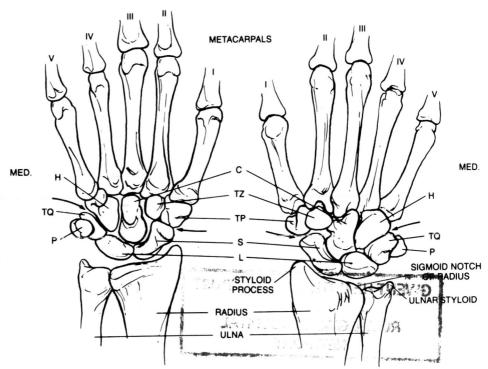

Figure 21–1. The joints of the wrist. Palmar *(left)* and dorsal *(right)* views of the right wrist. H, hamate; C, capitate; TZ, trapezoid; TP, trapezium; TQ, triquetrum; P, pisiform; L, lunate; S, scaphoid. The *arrows* mark the division of the proximal and distal rows at the midcarpal joint. (Illustration by Elizabeth Roselius, © 1985. Reprinted with permission from Taleisnik J: The Wrist. New York, Churchill Livingstone, 1985, p 2.)

(DRUJ), the radiocarpal joint, the midcarpal joints, and the carpometacarpal (CMC) joints. From these joints we obtain wrist flexion/extension, pronation and supination, and radial and ulnar deviation. The biomechanics of the wrist are extremely complex; and in spite of the contributions of countless researchers in the field, it is an area about which we have much to learn.

The carpal bones can be divided into a proximal and distal row with the scaphoid as the link between the two. The distal row consists of the trapezium, trapezoid, capitate, and hamate. The index and middle metacarpals have very tight ligamentous attachments to the distal row, and their CMC joints are essentially immobile. There is much more mobility at the CMC joints of the ring and small fingers to allow for cupping of the hand. The thumb CMC articulation is often described as having a double saddle configuration; it allows full circumduction of the thumb, but it is stable enough to support tremendous force during pinch, grasp, and opposition. The palmar oblique ligament from the trapezoid to the thumb metacarpal base is one of the main stabilizers for this joint.

A key point in the dynamics of the carpal bones is that none has a primary muscle attachment. All of their motion is directed by their articular anatomy and their ligamentous attachments. This is true particularly of the proximal row, because it lacks the rigid capsular structures of the CMC joints of the index and middle finger. The proximal row moves much like a middle link in a chain, and it has been termed the *intercalary segment*. The bones of the proximal row are tightly bound to each other by the scapholunate and lunatotriquetral interosseous ligaments. These ligaments keep their respective bones closely attached while allowing a controlled amount of rotational motion between them. For example, in going from ulnar to radial deviation, the scaphoid bone goes into a palmar-flexed position but the lunate remains relatively neutral (Fig. 21–2). If the scapholunate interosseous ligament is disrupted, an instability pattern can develop and the lunate can become permanently dorsiflexed relative to the scaphoid.

The proximal row is further guided by strong extraosseous ligaments, which are mainly thickenings of the wrist capsule. The most important are thought to be the volar radial ligaments defined by Landsmeer and Berger to be the radioscaphoid-capitate, the long radiolunate, and the short radiolunate (Fig. 21–3). They form the proximal anchor for the proximal row, with the short radiolunate probably being the most important. The radioscapholunate ligament, previously thought to be a key structure, is now thought to be more of a vascular entity than a stabilizer. On the ulnar side of the wrist, the ulnocarpal ligaments, consisting of the ulnolunate, ulnotriquetral, and ulnocapitate ligaments provide a tether for the carpus. When ruptured or attenuated, as in advanced rheumatoid arthritis, an intercarpal supination deformity can result.

Dorsally there are only two ligaments of structural importance: the dorsal transverse intercarpal ligament that runs from the distal pole of the scaphoid to the triquetrum and the dorsal radiocarpal ligament that runs from the radius to the triquetrum (see Fig. 21–3). The V-shaped area between these ligaments is filled with a thin redundant capsule that allows for increased interligamentous distance in going from wrist extension to flexion.

The radiocarpal joint anatomy is defined by the articular surface of the radius. It has a volar tilt of approximately 12 degrees and inclination from the radial styloid to the ulnar border of 22 degrees. Its most proximal point is usually even or distal to the level of the ulna. It has a triangular scaphoid fossa separated from the rectangular lunate fossa by a ridge. These fossae provide highly congruous articulations with the scaphoid and lunate, and articular stepoffs from fractures are poorly tolerated.

The last important articulation in the carpal region is the DRUJ. Although surgical procedures for this articulation have been present for a long time, it is only within the past two decades that we have really started to understand the functional anatomy of this joint. The distal ulna has two articular regions: the ulnar pole, which points to the carpus, and the ulnar seat, which interfaces with the sig-

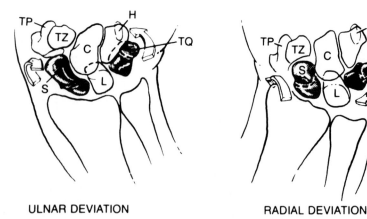

ULNAR DEVIATION   RADIAL DEVIATION

Figure 21–2. In the ulnar deviation, the bones of the proximal row are extended. The scaphoid appears elongated, the shape of the lunate appears trapezoidal, and the triquetrum is distal in relation to the hamate. TP, trapezium; TZ, trapezoid; C, capitate; H, hamate; TQ, triquetrum; L, lunate; S, scaphoid. In radial deviation, the bones of the proximal row are flexed toward the palm. The scaphoid appears foreshortened, the lunate appears triangular, and the triquetrum is proximal in relation to the hamate. (Illustration by Elizabeth Roselius, © 1985. Reprinted with permission from Taleisnik J: The Wrist. New York, Churchill Livingstone, 1985, p 8.)

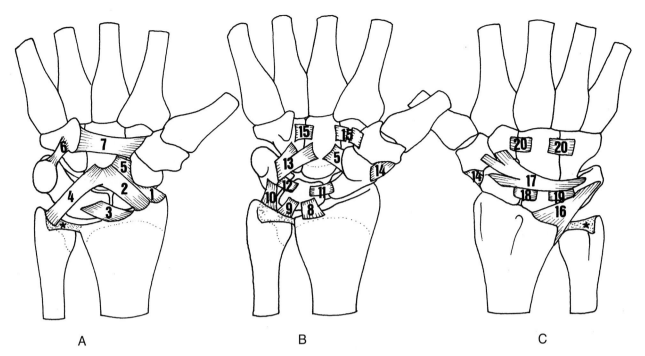

A   B   C

Figure 21–3. Schematic representation of the most consistently present wrist ligaments. These drawings do not aim to replicate the exact shape and dimensions of the actual ligaments, nor their frequent anatomic variation. *A,* Palmar superficial ligaments: (1) radioscaphoid, (2) radiocapitate, (3) long radiolunate, (4) ulnocapitate, (5) scaphocapitate, (6) pisohamate, and (7) flexor retinaculum or transverse carpal ligament. *B,* Palmar deep ligaments: (8) short radiolunate; (9) ulnolunate; (10) ulnotriquetral; (11) palmar scapholunate; (12) palmar lunatotriquetral; (13) triquetral-hamate-capitate, also known as the ulnar limb of the arcuate ligament; (14) dorsolateral scaphotrapezial; and (15) palmar transverse interosseous ligaments of the distal row. *C,* Dorsal ligaments: (16) radiotriquetral; (17) triquetrum-scaphoid-trapezium-trapezoid, also known as the dorsal intercarpal ligament; (18) dorsal scapholunate; (19) dorsal lunatotriquetral; and (20) dorsal transverse interosseous ligaments of the distal row. (From Green DP, Hotchkiss RN, Pederson WC [eds]: Operative Hand Surgery, 4th ed. New York, Churchill Livingstone, 1999, p 867.)

moid notch of the radius. The ulnar seat, which has a 130-degree arc of articular cartilage, has a far smaller radius of curvature than the sigmoid notch. This incongruous joint allows a combination of rotational and translational motion (Fig. 21–4). The joint capsule is very specialized for this. The volar and dorsal aspects are thin and redundant and can accommodate the ulnar head as it slides volarly and dorsally from full supination to full pronation. The inferior aspect is much more stout and has more stabilizing effect. Distally, the DRUJ and the ulnar pole are covered by a structure known as the triangular fibrocartilage complex (TFCC). This structure is a continuous ligament and fibrocartilaginous body with several distinct areas that have been labeled the volar and dorsal radioulnar ligaments, the articular disk, the ulnar collateral ligament, the meniscus homolog, and the ulnotriquetral and ulnolunate ligaments (Fig. 21–5). Its purpose is to transmit force from the carpus to the ulnar pole and to stabilize the DRUJ.

METACARPAL AND PHALANGEAL STRUCTURES
The tubular bones of the hand are uniquely designed for grasp. Their lengths follow Fibonacci's series from the distal phalanx to the metacarpal (i.e., the length of the metacarpal is the sum of the lengths of the proximal and middle phalanges; the length of the proximal phalanx is the sum of the lengths of the middle and distal phalanges).

This allows for full flexion into a fist. The structure of the joints maximize motion and stability. The metacarpal heads are cam/shaped, with greater volar/dorsal diameter than proximal/distal. The radial and ulnar collateral ligaments originate on the dorsal half of the metacarpal and insert onto the volar half of the proximal phalangeal base. They

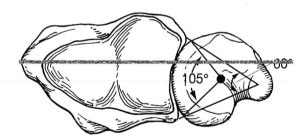

Figure 21–4. The radius of curvature of the seat of the ulna is 10 mm, with the arcs subtending an angle of 105 degrees. The radius of curvature of the sigmoid notch is approximately 15 mm, and the arcs subtend an angle of approximately 60 degrees. Thus, the distal radioulnar joint is not purely congruent. This anatomic feature allows for the translational motion of the ulna within the sigmoid notch during prosupination. (From Lichtman DM, Alexander AH [eds]: The Wrist and its Disorders, 2nd ed. Philadelphia, WB Saunders, 1997, p 387.)

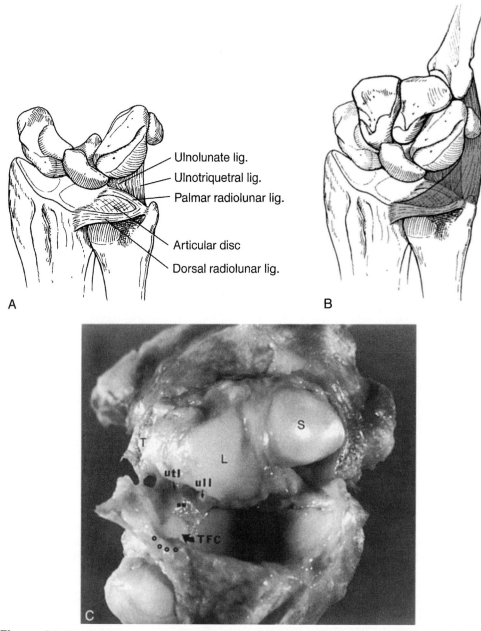

Ulnolunate lig.

Ulnotriquetral lig.

Palmar radiolunar lig.

Articular disc

Dorsal radiolunar lig.

Figure 21–5. *A,* Diagrammatic drawing of the triangular fibrocartilage complex, depicting the triangular fibrocartilage itself with its dorsal and palmar radioulnar ligaments. The ulnolunate and ulnotriquetral ligaments run from the fovea of the ulna to the carpus. *B,* Same view as in *A* with the addition of the meniscal reflection. *C,* Anatomic dissection of the triangular fibrocartilage complex. Of note is that the meniscus homolog, the ulnar collateral ligament, and the subsheath of the extensor carpi ulnaris tendon are not depicted in this anatomic dissection. TFC, articular disk of triangular fibrocartilage; open circles, dorsal radioulnar ligament; squares, palmar radioulnar ligament; utl, ulnotriquetral ligament; ull, ulnolunate ligament; T, triquetrum; L, lunate; S, scaphoid. (From Lichtman DM, Alexander AH [eds]: The Wrist and its Disorders, 2nd ed. Philadelphia, WB Saunders, 1997, p 388.)

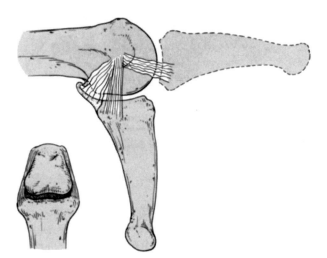

Figure 21–6. Metacarpophalangeal joint. The metacarpal head is wider on its volar projection and has a curve of increasing diameter from dorsal to palmar. Both explain why the collateral ligament is lax in extension and taut in flexion. (From Browner BD, Jupiter JB, Levine AM, Trafton PG: Skeletal Trauma. Philadelphia, WB Saunders, 1992, p 928.)

are taut in flexion and lax in extension (Fig. 21–6). A volar fibrocartilaginous thickening of the joint capsule, the volar plate, provides stability against hyperextension and excess radial and ulnar deviation in full extension. This structure also helps provide a gliding surface over the joint for the overlying flexor tendons.

In the phalanges the heads are more bicondylar, and therefore the interphalangeal (IP) joints have more inherent radioulnar stability. The collateral ligaments are positioned similarly to the metacarpophalangeal (MCP) joints, but the volar plates are better developed. Their origins on the volar phalangeal necks can thicken and form "check reins" in disease states, leading to a flexion contracture.

Muscle and Tendon

EXTRINSIC FLEXORS

The flexors of the hand and wrist originate from the medial epicondyle of the humerus, the proximal ulna, and the interosseous membrane. In the distal third of the forearm, they become tendinous. The wrist flexors, the flexor carpi radialis (FCR), the flexor carpi ulnaris (FCU), and the palmaris longus (PL), stay superficial throughout their course in the forearm. The PL inserts on the palmar aponeurosis; it is a very weak wrist flexor, and it helps to cup the hand. The FCR hugs the carpal bones and goes to insert on the volar aspect of the index metacarpal base, with lesser insertions onto the middle metacarpal base, the trapezium, and the trapezoid. The FCU continues to the pisiform as a sesamoid at the wrist and passes distally to insert on the small finger metacarpal base.

The extrinsic finger flexors include the flexor pollicis longus (FPL), the flexor digitorum superficialis (FDS), and the flexor digitorum profundus (FDP). At the level of the wrist they pass along with the median nerve underneath the transverse carpal ligament. Distal to this they fan out

toward the individual digits. The lumbrical muscles take origin from the FDP tendons at this point. At the level of the MP joints, the flexor tendons enter fibro-osseous tunnels, which promote gliding and prevent bowstringing of the tendons as the finger flexes. The tunnels are commonly called flexor sheaths; their roofs consist of fibrous tissue with specific thickenings called the annular and cruciate pulleys (Fig. 21–7). The annular pulleys are bandlike; the A-1, A-3, and A-5 pulleys are at the levels of the MP, proximal IP (PIP), and distal IP (DIP) joints, respectively. The A-2 and A-4 pulleys are at the bases of the proximal and middle phalanges; they are the most important in prevention of bowstringing of the tendons. The cruciate pulleys, C-1, C-2, and C-3, are between the distal four annular pulleys; they collapse readily during flexion. Within the sheaths, the tendons have a synovial lining that further aids gliding motion and has a role in tendon nutrition. The tendons also have vincula, which provide a modest dorsal blood supply to the tendons.

The flexor tendon anatomy is designed for differential flexion at the PIP and DIP joints. The FDS tendons start volar to the FDP tendons. At the level of the MP joints, they split into radial and ulnar slips and pass dorsal to the FDP tendon (Camper's chiasm) to insert on the middle two thirds of the middle phalanx. The FDP tendons continue centrally to insert on the distal phalanx base (Fig. 21–8).

The thumb, with only one flexor tendon, has a slightly different arrangement. The FPL passes underneath the A-1 pulley just proximal to the MP joint, then the oblique pulley over the proximal phalanx, then the A-2 pulley at the IP joint, before its insertion onto the distal phalanx base.

EXTRINSIC EXTENSORS

The extensors originate on the lateral epicondyle, the radial shaft, and the radial half of the interosseous membrane; they become tendinous in the distal half of the forearm. The tendons become grouped together by similar function and then pass underneath the extensor retinaculum of the wrist in six distinct compartments. The compartments and their contents are shown below in Figure 21–9. The wrist extensors, extensor carpi radialis longus (ECRL), the extensor carpi radialis brevis (ECRB), and the extensor carpi ulnaris (ECU) continue on to insert onto the index, middle, and small metacarpal bases, respectively. They balance each other, with the ECRL, providing a radial deviation moment, the ECU an ulnar deviation moment, and the ECRB a neutral moment. They also balance out the wrist flexors by having a nearly similar total cross-sectional muscle area.

The thumb extensors provide some extension across all three joints. The extensor pollicis longus (EPL) inserts on the distal phalanx base, the extensor pollicis brevis (EPB) inserts on the dorsal base of the proximal phalanx, and the abductor pollicis longus (APL) inserts on the radial aspect of the metacarpal base, providing extension and weak abduction.

The extensor mechanism of the other digits is much more complex, allowing a single tendon to extend three joints. After exiting the fourth and fifth dorsal compartments, the extensor digitorum communis (EDC), the extensor indicis proprius (EIP), and the extensor digiti minimi (EDM) travel up to the dorsum of the palm to the MP

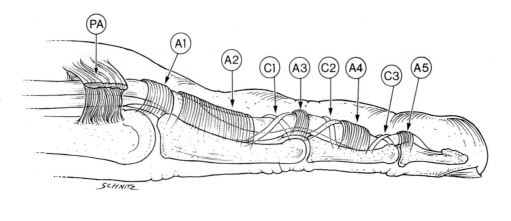

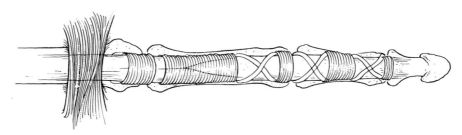

Figure 21–7. Lateral *(top)* and palmar *(bottom)* views of a finger depict the components of the digital flexor sheath. The sturdy annular pulleys (A1, A2, A3, A4, and A5) are important biomechanically in keeping the tendons closely applied to the phalanges. The thin, pliable cruciate pulleys (C1, C2, and C3) collapse to allow full digital flexion. A recently described addition is the palmar aponeurosis pulley (PA), which adds to the biomechanical efficiency of the sheath system. (From Green DP, Hotchkiss RN, Pederson WC [eds]: Operative Hand Surgery, 4th ed. New York, Churchill Livingstone, 1999, p 1853.)

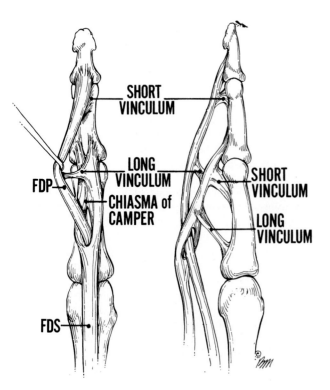

Figure 21–8. The flexor digitorum profundus (FDP) passes through the tails of the flexor digitorum superficialis (FDS) on the way to its insertion into the distal phalanx. (From Green DP, Hotchkiss RN, Pederson WC [eds]: Operative Hand Surgery, 4th ed. New York, Churchill Livingstone, 1999, p 1899.)

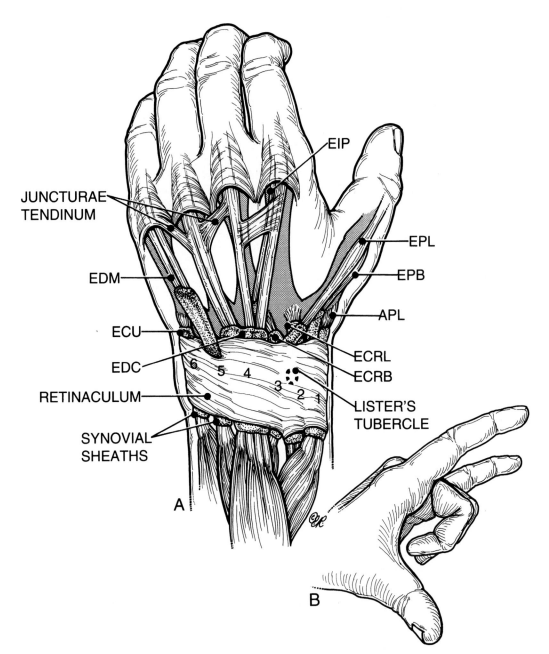

Figure 21–9. *A,* The extensor tendons gain entrance to the hand from the forearm through a series of six canals, five fibro-osseous and one fibrous (the fifth dorsal compartment, which contains the extensor digiti minimi [EDM]). The first compartment contains the abductor pollicis longus (APL) and extensor pollicis brevis (EPB); the second, the radial wrist extensors; the third, the extensor pollicis longus (EPL), which angles around Lister's tubercle; the fourth, the extensor digitorum communis (EDC) to the fingers, as well as the extensor indicis proprius (EIP): the fifth, the EDM; and the sixth, the extensor carpi ulnaris (ECU). The communis tendons are joined distally near the MP joints by fibrous interconnections called juncturae tendinum. These juncturae are found only between the communis tendons and may aid in surgical recognition of the proprius tendon of the index finger. The proprius tendons are usually positioned to the ulnar side of the adjacent communis tendons, but variations may be present that alter this arrangement. Beneath the retinaculum, the extensor tendons are covered with a synovial sheath. *B,* The proprius tendons to the index and little fingers are capable of independent extension, and their function may be evaluated as depicted. With the middle and ring fingers flexed into the palm, the proprius tendons can extend the ring and little fingers. Independent extension of the index, however, is not always lost after transfer of the indicis proprius and is less likely to be lost if the extensor hood is not injured and is probably never lost if the hood is preserved and the junctura tendinum between the index and middle fingers is excised. This finger represents the usual anatomic arrangement found over the wrist and hand, but variations are common. ECRB, extensor carpi radialis brevis; ECRL, extensor carpi radialis longus. (From Green DP, Hotchkiss RN, Pederson WC [eds]: Operative Hand Surgery, 4th ed. New York, Churchill Livingstone, 1999, p 1951.)

joints. The EIP and the EDM are ulnar to their respective EDC tendons. Fibrous connections called juncturae tendinum connect the EDC tendons just proximal to the MP joints (see Fig. 21–8). The tendons are anchored and centralized over the MP joint by the sagittal bands, horizontal fibers that run from the volar plate, and transverse metacarpal ligaments. The sagittal bands also act as a sling to help extend the proximal phalanx base at the MP joint. Just distal to this, the extensor hood (see Fig. 21–9) is joined by the tendons of the lumbricals and the interossei, which come to the sides of the mechanism and form the lateral bands. Proximal to the PIP joint the tendon trifurcates to form a central slip, which inserts on the dorsal base of the middle phalanx, and two other segments adjoin the lateral bands and continue distally to insert on the distal phalanx. The terminal tendon is further joined by the oblique retinacular ligament (ligament of Landsmeer) on the radial side. This ligament originates on the flexor tendon sheath and runs volar to the PIP joint before becoming a dorsal structure. It may allow some independent DIP extension when the PIP joint is flexed.

INTRINSIC HAND MUSCLES

The intrinsic muscles originate and insert in the hand; they include the thenar, hypothenar, interosseous, lumbrical, and abductor pollicis muscles. The thenar muscles are the opponens pollicis, abductor pollicis brevis (APB), and the flexor pollicis brevis (FPB). They bring the thumb out of the plane of the wrist and the hand, pronate the thumb to meet the other fingers, and provide power flexion for both pinch and grip. The APB is the most superficial muscle of the group; it originates on the flexor retinaculum and the tubercles of the scaphoid and trapezium and inserts on the lateral capsule of the thumb MP joint and the lateral aspect of the proximal phalanx base. Its function is abduction and flexion of the metacarpal and slight flexion of the proximal phalanx; it is the most important muscle for opposition. The FPB is deep to the APB and has two heads. The superficial head is innervated by the recurrent motor branch of the median nerve like the other thenar muscles, and the deep head is innervated by the ulnar nerve and can preserve some opposition function in the face of a median nerve palsy. The opponens pollicis inserts along the whole length of the volar radial surface of the thumb metacarpal. Its main function is metacarpal flexion.

The adductor pollicis muscle has two heads: (1) the oblique head originates from the base of the index and middle metacarpals as well as the capitate and (2) the transverse originates from the volar aspect of the middle metacarpal shaft. The two heads converge and insert on the ulnar sesamoid of the thumb MP joint, which is connected to the proximal phalanx by the volar plate. This muscle is a powerful adductor of the thumb and plays an important role in both pinch and power grasp. The hypothenar muscles originate from the pisiform, the hook of the hamate, and the volar carpal ligament. They insert on the small finger metacarpal and proximal phalanx base and flex, adduct, and abduct the small finger to allow cupping of the hand and ease of opposition. They are all ulnarly innervated.

The lumbricals are the only muscles in the body that originate and insert solely on other tendons. They originate

from the index to small finger FDP tendons and pass volar to the transverse metacarpal ligament and axis of rotation of the MP joint. They then progress distally to join the radial lateral band. This allows them to cause flexion at the MP joint and extension at the PIP and DIP joints. They can also radially deviate the digits. The index and middle lumbricals are innervated by the median nerve, and the ring and small finger are innervated by the ulnar nerve. There are four dorsal and three volar interosseous muscles. They originate on the metacarpal shafts and insert on the bases of the proximal phalanx and the dorsal expansions of the extensor mechanism. The dorsal interossei abduct the digits, and the volar ones adduct them. Both groups assist the lumbricals with MP flexion and IP extension. They are all ulnarly innervated.

Vascular Anatomy

The arterial supply to the hands and wrist is through the radial and ulnar arteries. These vessels are the terminal branches of the brachial artery when it bifurcates at the level of the bicipital aponeurosis in the volar proximal forearm. The first branch of the ulnar artery is the common interosseous artery, which quickly branches into anterior and posterior branches that course along the interosseous membrane of the forearm. The anterior interosseous artery has a median branch that runs with the median nerve through the carpal tunnel. This structure involutes with normal fetal development, but in about 5% of people it persists as a median artery and contributes to the superficial arch.

The radial artery is the smaller of the two forearm arteries. It runs in the forearm just radial to the FCR tendon. At the level of radiocarpal joint, it produces a volar branch that runs distally to join the superficial arch. The remainder of the vessel then passes dorsally under the APL and EPB tendons and runs along the floor of the anatomical snuffbox. It passes between the heads of the first dorsal interosseous muscle to enter the palm. There, it gives off the princeps pollicis and the radialis indicis arteries to supply the thumb and the radial side of the index, respectively. The terminal segment of the artery goes on to form the deep palmar arch.

The ulnar artery contributes the dominant supply to the hand. It runs in the forearm deep to the FCU, superficial to the FDP, and just radial to the ulnar nerve. It enters the palm along with the nerve through Guyon's canal with the transverse carpal ligament as the floor and the volar carpal ligament as the roof. It then gives off a deep palmar branch and continues distally and across the hand to form the superficial palmar arch. The deep branch dives through the hypothenar muscles to anastomose with the deep arch (Fig. 21–10).

The deep arch is proximal to the superficial arch. It gives off three palmar metacarpal arteries, which anastomose with three common palmar metacarpal digital arteries from the superficial arch. These common arteries further divide into two proper digital arteries each to supply the fingers.

There is tremendous variability in the superficial arch. The "classic" co-dominant arch with both the radial and ulnar arteries anastomosed is present in only one third of

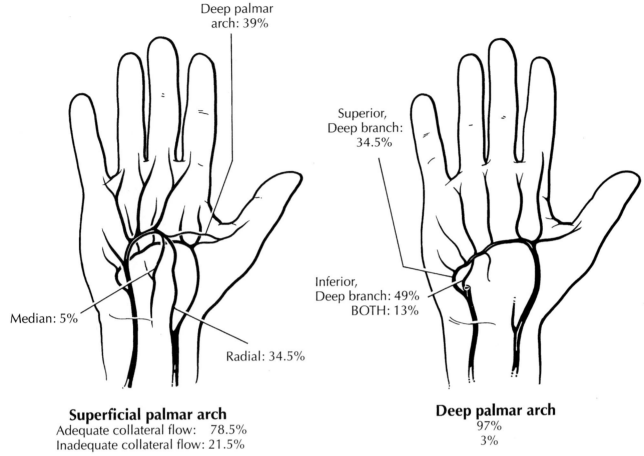

Figure 21–10. The superficial palmar arch is completed by branches from the deep palmar arch, radial artery, or median artery in 78.5% of patients; the remaining 21.5% are "incomplete." The deep palmar arch is completed by the superior branch of the ulnar artery, the inferior branch of the ulnar artery, or both in 98.5% of patients. (Modified from Koman LA, Urbaniak JR: Ulnar artery thrombosis. *In* Brunelli S [ed]: Textbook of Surgery. Milan, Masson, 1988.)

patients. The ulnar artery supplies the arch alone in about 40% of people, and other variants make up the rest. Because of this variability it is important to test blood flow using Allen's test or some other technique before performing procedures such as cannulating the radial artery (Fig. 21–11).

Nerve Anatomy

Three major nerves supply the hand: the median, ulnar, and radial. The radial nerve completes all of its motor innervation by the mid forearm, and only two sensory branches continue distally. The posterior interosseous branch runs along the interosseous membrane, and then enters the radial side of the fourth dorsal compartment to give some sensory fibers to the dorsum of the wrist. The superficial branch of the radial nerve exits between the brachioradialis and ECRL tendons to give sensation to the dorsum of the thumb, the first and second web space, and the dorsum of the index and part of the middle finger.

The median nerve gives off its palmar cutaneous branch several centimeters proximal to the wrist crease (Fig. 21–12). The branch runs along the ulnar border of the FCR

and becomes superficial at the wrist to supply sensation to the thenar eminence. The remaining median nerve passes through the carpal tunnel and then gives off a recurrent motor branch that supplies motor innervation to the thenar muscles. The terminal branches of the median nerve then become the sensory digital nerves to the thumb, index, middle, and the radial half of the ring finger.

The ulnar nerve has dorsal and palmar sensory branches that exit proximal to the wrist, but the bulk of the nerve passes through Guyon's canal. Just distal to this, the nerve divides into superficial and deep branches. The superficial branch travels distally to form the digital nerves into the small finger and the ulnar aspect of the ring finger. The deep branch supplies motor innervation to all of the hand intrinsic muscles except those listed under the median nerve (Fig. 21–13).

The digital nerves run just volar and midline to the digital arteries in the fingers. The neurovascular bundle is surrounded by osteocutaneous ligaments with Grayson's ligaments presenting as bands volarly and Cleland's ligaments forming a continuous sheet dorsally. These ligaments help protect the artery and nerve and allow for their excursion with flexion and extension.

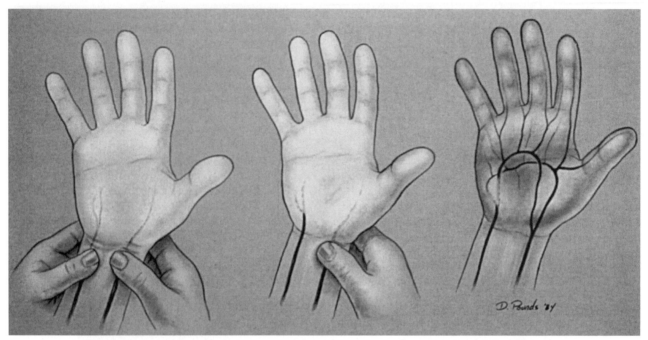

Figure 21–11. The Allen test is represented schematically. Blood is exsanguinated from the hand, and both the radial and ulnar arteries are compressed *(left)*. After release of the ulnar artery *(middle)*, no blood flow passes through the occluded artery and the palm remains pale. With release of the radial artery *(right)*, the entire hand will fill rapidly through the radial artery if the arch is complete. The order of the testing maneuvers can be reversed to test the radial artery in a similar fashion. The test is best described as demonstrating flow or no flow through a specific artery. (From Koman LA: Diagnostic study of vascular lesions. Hand Clin 1:217–231, 1985.)

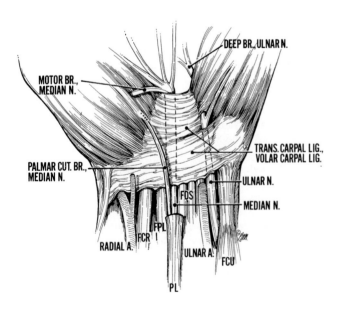

Figure 21–12. The palmar cutaneous branch of the median nerve lies radial to the median nerve and ulnar to the flexor carpi radialis (FCR) tendon. It may pierce either the volar carpal or transverse carpal ligament or the antebrachial fascia before it becomes subcutaneous. FDS, flexor digitorum superficialis; FPL, flexor pollicis longus; FCU, flexor carpi ulnaris; PL, palmaris longus. (From Green DP, Hotchkiss RN, Pederson WC [eds]: Operative Hand Surgery, 4th ed. New York, Churchill Livingstone, 1999, p 1416.)

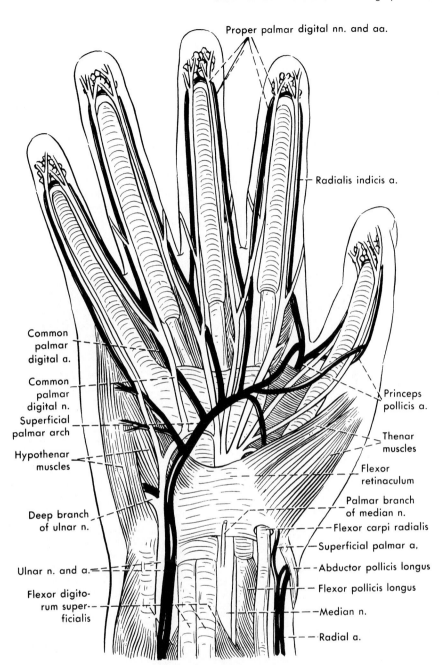

Figure 21–13. Nerves and vessels of the hand. (From Jenkins DB: Hollinshead's Functional Anatomy of the Limbs and Back, 6th ed. Philadelphia, WB Saunders, 1991.)

Proper palmar digital nn. and aa.

Radialis indicis a.

Common palmar digital a.

Common palmar digital n.

Superficial palmar arch

Hypothenar muscles

Deep branch of ulnar n.

Ulnar n. and a.

Flexor digitorum superficialis

Princeps pollicis a.

Thenar muscles

Flexor retinaculum

Palmar branch of median n.

Flexor carpi radialis

Superficial palmar a.

Abductor pollicis longus

Flexor pollicis longus

Median n.

Radial a.

EVALUATION OF THE HAND AND WRIST

In evaluating the hand and wrist, one should always address certain key issues in the history. It is crucial to know which hand is dominant, the patient's occupation, and the patient's hobbies. One should always consider special uses of the hand, such as wheelchair propulsion in a tetraplegic or weight-bearing hand use. The patient's age, systemic health problems, medications, and allergies play an obvious role in guiding diagnosis and treatment, and they need to be asked specifically. Psychosocial issues such as chronic depression or involvement in a workers' compensation claim or a legal action related to the hand condition have an effect on the patient's outcome as well and need to be addressed.

For traumatic hand injuries one should ask the patient the details of how the injury occurred: when did the injury occur and how much time has elapsed? The environment in which it occurred is important: was there exposure to extreme temperatures that could have led to a burn or frostbite? If there is an open wound, was there exposure to gross contamination such as barnyard material? How exactly did the injury happen? Was there a crush component? Did the patient manipulate the hand or have any treatment in the field? Is there any numbness, tingling, or other indication of nerve or vessel compromise? The patient's immune status as well as his or her prior tetanus prophylaxis should be questioned as well.

For nontraumatic conditions, it is important to characterize the symptoms in as much detail as possible. When did the pain or other symptoms start? Where exactly is it located, and is there any radiation to other areas? What is the character of the symptoms: is there sharp or dull pain? Is there tingling, numbness, or altered sensation suggestive of nerve injury? Is there any weakness? Is there a feeling of unstable joint motion or click or giving way? What makes the symptoms better or worse? Does the patient have any involvement of other joints in other areas of the body, suggesting a systemic process? How much functional impairment is present? All of these issues help one to focus on the rest of the evaluation and on diagnosis and treatment.

The physical examination should start with a brief assessment of the patient's general appearance and health. A screening examination including range of motion and palpation for tenderness of the neck, shoulder, elbow, and forearm is indicated, especially after trauma or when the patient has neurologic symptoms. The hand and wrist examination should start out with an inspection of the region, and any deformities, swelling, ecchymosis, or cyanosis should be documented. Then palpation begins. The pulses and the capillary refill are checked. Systematic palpation of the entire hand should be performed to isolate the areas of tenderness or other symptoms. Both the active and passive range of motion are checked of all the involved and surrounding joints. A sensory examination using light touch and two-point discrimination and other modalities as indicated is very useful for detecting nerve compromise and documenting the patient's baseline sensation. Grip and pinch strength, as well as manual muscle testing of radial, ulnar, and median innervated groups, is also useful in assessing the nerve and muscle status of the hand.

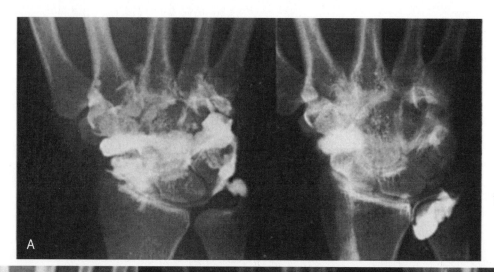

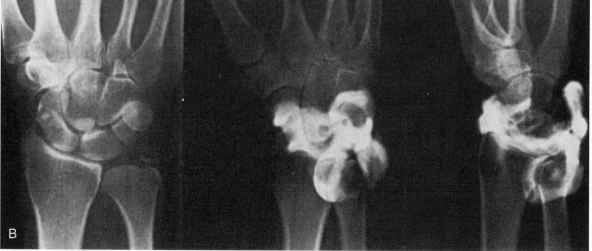

Figure 21–14. *A,* Arthrogram showing the radiocarpal and radioulnar joints in sequential injections. No perforation of the triangular fibrocartilage complex (TFCC) exists, but dye penetration into the intercarpal joints is seen through a surgically demonstrated triquetral lunate disruption. The prestyloid recess is well seen, as well as dye penetration from the midcarpal joints into the flexor carpi radialis tendon sheath. *B,* These x-rays were taken after a single radiocarpal injection in a different patient. They show communication of dye into the distal radioulnar joint through a chronic perforation. The dye collection in the prestyloid area may indicate chronic detachment of the TFCC through an avulsion of the styloid rather than a TFCC perforation. Dye also communicates with the pisotriquetral joint (see far right) but not the midcarpal joints. (From Green DP, Hotchkiss RN, Pederson WC [eds]: Operative Hand Surgery, 4th ed. New York, Churchill Livingstone, 1999, p 1001.)

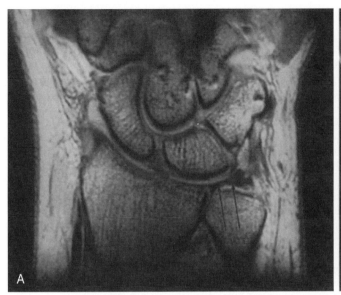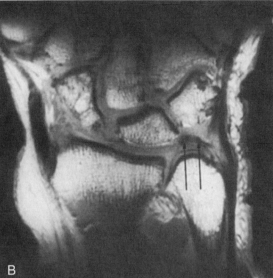

Figure 21–15. T$_1$-weighted imaging of the triangular fibrocartilage complex (TFCC), which appears black *(arrows)*. *A*, Normal TFCC. Note the uniform black image extending from the ulnar aspect of the distal radius ulnarward over the ulnar head. *B*, Abnormal TFCC. Note the bunched appearance of the TFCC over the ulnar head as it appears to have lifted from its origin off the radius. (From Lichtman DM, Alexander AH [eds]: The Wrist and its Disorders, 2nd ed. Philadelphia, WB Saunders, 1997, p 406.)

Detailed evaluation of the patient's symptoms is then indicated. The symptoms should be pinpointed as closely as possible to any anatomic location. The patient is asked to indicate what maneuvers elicit pain. The many provocative tests for the hand and wrist are discussed under the sections for the specific conditions. Comparison examination with an asymptomatic opposite side is an invaluable tool when the patient's findings are at all equivocal. Selective injection with 1 to 2 mL of 1% lidocaine can help with isolating the source of pain, but one must be careful, because diffuse injections can actually cloud the picture even further.

Routine imaging of the hand and wrist begins with anteroposterior (AP), lateral, and oblique x-rays. There are many special views for documenting specific bone and ligament injuries, and some of these, too, are discussed later. Other imaging modalities can be very helpful in making diagnosis in this region as well. Radionuclide scanning has been very helpful in detecting occult fractures, osteonecrosis, infection, and reflex sympathetic dystrophy. Computed tornographic (CT) scanning can help with intra-articular stepoffs of the distal radius and aid with confirming a diagnosis of scaphoid non-unions. Arthrography has been mainly used to detect ligament and TFCC tears (Fig. 21–14). The use of magnetic resonance imaging (MRI) in the hand and wrist is advancing rapidly; it is now the modality of choice for many hand surgeons to detect scapholunate or TFCC tears, occult scaphoid fractures, and occult ganglion cysts (Fig. 21–15). It is largely replacing bone scans for detecting Kienböck's disease (avascular necrosis of the lunate), and it may soon be used to help detect partial tendon ruptures.

Wrist arthroscopy as well is developing rapidly, both for diagnostic and therapeutic purposes. It is one of the only ways to detect isolated chondral lesions within the wrist, and it is the gold standard now for detection of TFCC and

many ligament tears (Fig. 21–16). Many hand surgeons now advocate arthroscopy instead of MRI or other studies for ulnar-sided wrist pain because its sensitivity and specificity are much higher and it allows concurrent treatment of the problem at the time of diagnosis.

TRAUMA

Because of its constant exposure and vulnerable position at the end of the upper extremity, the hand is subject to a wide variety of traumatic conditions. A surgeon who treats these injuries must be familiar with the principles of bony fixation, tendon repair, soft tissue coverage, and, in some cases, microscopic nerve and vessel reconstruction. The treatment also needs to be geared toward rapid return to use and minimal functional loss. The concepts presented here provide a brief overview for treatment.

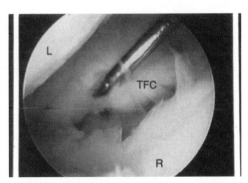

Figure 21–16. Radiocarpal joint, degenerative tear in the triangular fibrocartilage (TFC). Note the ragged edges of the degenerated tear. The lunate (L), which has some minor chondromalacia, can be seen along with the lunate facet of the radius (R). (From Osterman AL [ed]: Basic wrist arthroscopy and endoscopy. Hand Clin 10[4], 1994, Color Fig. 15.)

Fractures and Dislocations

PHALANGEAL INJURIES

Fractures of the phalanges are extremely common. Although union rates are very high, deformity is often poorly accepted in the hand and improper treatment can lead to problems of stiffness and loss of function. Thirty to 50% of these injuries are open, and these tend to have poor treatment results.

Distal phalangeal injuries can be broken down into tuft, shaft, and articular fractures. Tuft fractures are usually caused by crush injuries; they are nearly always stable because of the tough fibrous septa that anchor the skin to the bone. These injuries are often associated with injuries to the overlying nail bed. When there is a subungual hematoma, the nail should be perforated to decompress this area and provide pain relief. Hematomas involving more than 50% of the nail bed indicate large nail bed tears; they should be treated with removal of the nail and repair of the sterile matrix.

Distal phalangeal shaft fractures that are nondisplaced also tend to be stabilized by the surrounding soft tissue and nail plate; they should be treated with splinting of the DIP joint only for 3 weeks or until the area is relatively pain free. Widely displaced fractures of the shaft can be open or cause nail matrix injury. The soft tissue injury should be addressed, and if the fracture is unstable it can be pinned longitudinally. Articular fractures of the distal phalanx can be displaced by the pull of the FDP or extensor tendons. When a large volar fragment is avulsed with the FDP tendon, open reduction and internal fixation (ORIF) is indicated. When a dorsal avulsion is present, hyperextension splinting will often lead to a good result as long as the joint is not subluxed. When subluxation is present, ORIF or, in some instances, a transarticular pinning should be performed.

Proximal and middle phalangeal fractures can be categorized into condyle, neck, shaft, and base fractures. Fractures that can be treated well non-operatively have the following characteristics: little or no displacement, alignment maintained throughout the range of motion, less than 10 degrees of sagittal or coronal plane deformity in the diaphysis, less than 20 degrees of sagittal plane angulation in the metaphysis, and no rotational deformity. Fractures in which one should consider surgical fixation include rotated fractures, comminuted fractures, severely displaced fractures, short oblique fractures, proximal phalanx neck fractures, volar base middle phalanx fractures, and those with extensive soft tissue injury.

The non-operative treatment options for these fractures include buddy taping for truly stable fractures, aluminum-foam splinting, extension block splinting in special situations, and casting. When cast immobilization is used, the hand should be positioned in an intrinsic plus position. The wrist is extended 15 to 20 degrees. The MP joints are flexed to 60 degrees or more, and the IP joints are in full extension (Fig. 21–17). This minimizes the development of stiffness by keeping the MP collaterals and IP volar plates at their maximum length. Phalangeal fractures heal rapidly. One can almost always start a gentle motion program by 3 weeks, and longer periods of immobilization only lead to further stiffness.

Operative fixation options include Kirschner wiring (either crossed or intermedullary), intraosseous wiring, lag screw fixation, plate fixation, external fixation (both dynamic and static), and intermedullary rodding. All have their advantages and disadvantages. If one chooses to use screw fixation, the width of the fragment must be at least three times the diameter of the screw to avoid further comminution or failure of fixation (Fig. 21–18).

Fractures around the PIP joint have special importance, because there are multiple deforming forces and joint sub-

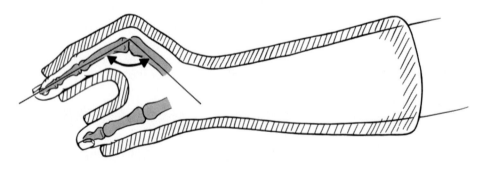

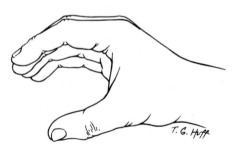

Figure 21–17. The position of immobilization of the hand involves splinting the wrist in 20 degrees of extension, the metacarpophalangeal joints in 60 to 70 degrees of flexion, and the interphalangeal joints in extension. (From Browner BD, Jupiter JB, Levine AM, Trafton PG: Skeletal Trauma. Philadelphia, WB Saunders, 1992, p 933.)

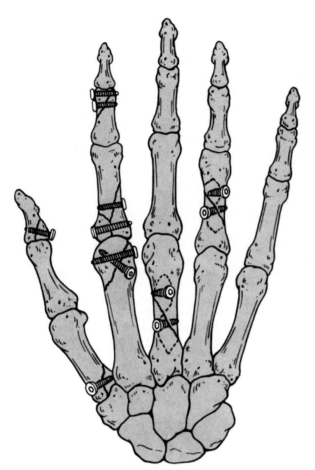

Figure 21–18. Optimal fracture patterns for interfragmentary screw fixation in the hand. (From Browner BD, Jupiter JB, Levine AM, Trafton PG: Skeletal Trauma. Philadelphia, WB Saunders, 1992, p 945.)

luxation is common with displaced fractures. It is also very important to restore motion at this joint; the normal PIP joint has a flexion/extension arc of over 110 degrees, and stiffness in this joint severely limits its use. Newer dynamic external fixators are particularly helpful for treating axial, crush, or "pilon" injuries of the middle phalanx base.

Isolated dislocations of the PIP joint can be dorsal, palmar, and lateral. They are usually easily reduced with digital or wrist block anesthesia followed by longitudinal traction and manipulation. Once the reduction is obtained, stability in flexion and extension should be checked. If stable, the joint should be treated with extension block splinting (Fig. 21–19). If unstable, or if a reduction is not obtained, open reduction may be required to remove interposed soft tissue. Dislocations of the DIP and MP joints are less common. DIP joint dislocations are most often dorsal; they tend to be easily reducible and stable after reduction. MP joint dislocations can be problematic to treat. The volar plate is firmly attached to the proximal phalanx base and often becomes interposed into the joint, thus preventing reduction. For this situation we recommend a dorsal approach to incise and to ease the volar plate back into place, making the reduction easy. Early range of motion must be started to avoid stiffness (Fig. 21–20).

The thumb MP joint is susceptible to an ulnar collateral ligament rupture, which is given the eponyms "gamekeep-

er's" or "skier's" thumb. The stability of the joint should be tested in full extension and 30 degrees of flexion to relax the volar plate. If opening with radial stress is more than 25 degrees greater than that of the contralateral thumb, a complete rupture is present. If an incomplete injury is present, thumb spica casting for 4 to 6 weeks followed by a hand-based orthosis is indicated. Most authors advocate that an immediate open repair should be performed for complete tears. In many cases, the torn ligament becomes displaced behind the adductor pollicis insertion (Stener lesion) and has no hope of healing without open treatment.

Metacarpal fractures make up nearly one third of all hand fractures. Fractures of the metacarpal head are uncommon and usually extend into the joint surface. A simple fracture pattern should be treated with anatomic reduction and pinning or screw fixation. More comminuted patterns are very difficult to treat, and some have even advocated immediate silicone arthroplasty. Stiffness is a common complication for all of these fractures. Metacarpal neck fractures are extremely common. Acceptable alignment for these fractures requires no rotational deformity and less than 15 degrees of apex dorsal angulation for the index and middle fingers. The angulation acceptable for the small finger is widely debated, with some authors recommending reduction and pinning for apex dorsal angulation greater than 30 degrees whereas others accept up to 70 degrees. The Jahss maneuver is the best way to perform a closed reduction. It involves flexion of the joint to 90 degrees, correction of rotational and radial/ulnar deformity, and axial pressure on the proximal phalanx to correct the sagittal plane alignment (Fig. 21–21). It is often difficult, however, to maintain this reduction in plaster alone. Multiple buried intermedullary or "bouquet" pinning as advocated by Foucher is a very useful method for fixing these fractures in patients who cannot tolerate the 4 weeks of cast treatment or those who must bear weight on the hand.

Metacarpal shaft fractures have acceptable alignment when no rotational deformity and no angular deformity is present in the index and middle fingers or when less than 30 degrees of sagittal plane deformity is present in the ring and small fingers. Indications for open reduction include open fractures, unstable or irreducible fractures, and multiple fractures. The techniques available are the same as for phalangeal fractures, with the additional option of pinning the fractured metacarpal to an adjacent intact metacarpal, thus using it as a built-in external fixator.

Metacarpal base fractures and dislocations form another important group of injuries. Bennett's fracture of the thumb metacarpal base is caused by an axially directed force to a flexed thumb. The metacarpal subluxates radially, proximally, and dorsally while a small volar ulnar fragment remains in position, anchored by the volar oblique ligament. The treatment is usually closed reduction and percutaneous pinning (Fig. 21–22). If this is not possible, or if the fragment is large enough, open reduction and screw fixation can be performed. Rolando's fractures involve a comminuted fracture of the thumb metacarpal base. These usually reduce well with longitudinal traction and pronation. If so, they can be treated with percutaneous pinning; if not, ORIF is indicated. The most common fracture-dislocations of the small metacarpal base have been given the eponym "reverse Bennett's" fractures. A small radial fragment remains attached to the ulnar facet of the fourth

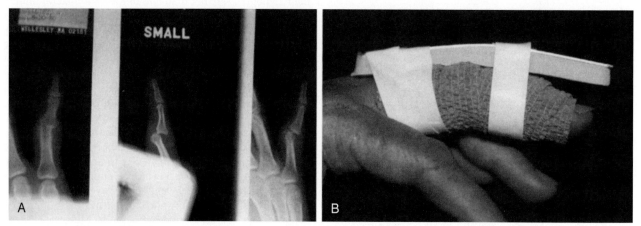

Figure 21–19. A dorsal dislocation of the proximal interphalangeal joint in an 18-year-old man. *A,* Lateral radiographs demonstrate the dorsal displacement of the middle phalanx on the proximal phalanx. *B,* After metacarpal block and closed manipulative reduction, the digit is wrapped with an elastic crepe bandage and a dorsal extension block Alumafoam splint is applied. (From Browner BD, Jupiter JB, Levine AM, Trafton PG: Skeletal Trauma. Philadelphia, WB Saunders, 1992, p 1015.)

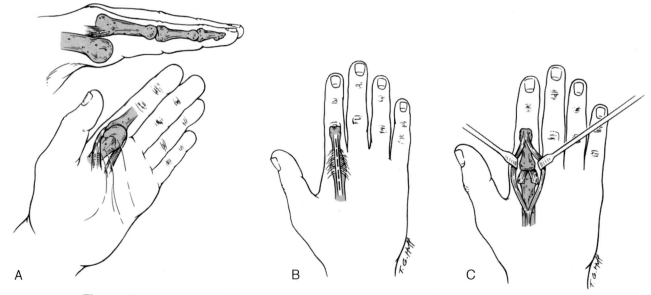

Figure 21–20. A dorsal dislocation of the metacarpophalangeal joint is considered "complex," because a closed reduction is rarely successful because of interposition of the palmar plate. *A,* The palmar plate displaces dorsal to the metacarpal head. In addition, the metacarpal head "buttonholes" between the flexor tendons and lumbrical muscle. *B,* Surgical reduction of the complex dislocation is readily accomplished through a dorsal approach splitting the common extensor. *C,* The palmar plate is splinted longitudinally, followed by atraumatic reduction of the metacarpal. (From Browner BD, Jupiter JB, Levine AM, Trafton PG: Skeletal Trauma. Philadelphia, WB Saunders, 1992, p 1016.)

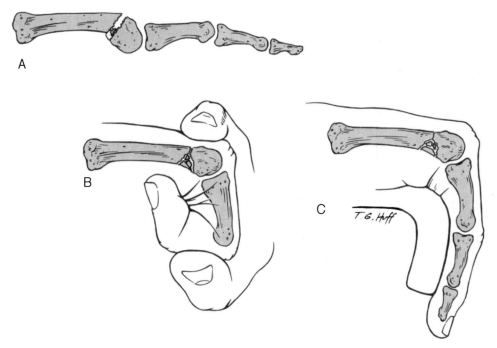

Figure 21–21. A displaced metacarpal neck can be reduced by flexing the metacarpophalangeal joint to 90 degrees and using the proximal phalanx to control rotation and as a lever to push up the metacarpal head. *A*, A displaced neck fracture is generally associated with comminution on the volar surface. *B*, Fracture reduction used the proximal phalanx to push up the metacarpal head. *C*, Immobilization in plaster should place the metacarpophalangeal joint in 70 to 90 degrees of flexion and the proximal interphalangeal joints close to full extension. (From Browner BD, Jupiter JB, Levine AM, Trafton PG: Skeletal Trauma. Philadelphia, WB Saunders, 1992, p 961.)

metacarpal, whereas the ECU insertion pulls the rest of the metacarpal base into dorsal and proximal subluxation. This, too, can be treated with closed reduction and pinning unless a hamate fracture is also present.

CARPAL FRACTURES

The most common carpal fractures are in the scaphoid; they account for up to 60 or 70% of these injuries. The most common mechanism is a fall on an outstretched hand, and the classic physical finding is anatomical snuffbox tenderness. Radiographic evaluation should include posteroanterior (PA) views in both neutral and full ulnar deviation as well as lateral and oblique views of the wrist. The ulnar deviation PA profiles the scaphoid along its entire length, making it the best view for visualization of fractures of the waist or proximal pole. A negative set of x-rays does not always rule out this injury, however, because some non-displaced fractures do not show up on early images. A patient with snuffbox tenderness and normal x-rays should be treated in a thumb spica cast for 3 weeks after which repeat physical examination and radiography should be performed. X-rays at this point may reveal the fracture site as normal resorption occurs. If the patient still has tenderness and negative plain films, further evaluation with an MRI, CT scan, or bone scan is indicated. Although many different classifications are available, Herbert's is one of the best for guiding treatment. He distinguishes them into four major types. Type A includes stable acute fractures, namely fractures of the tubercle and incomplete fractures through the waist. Type B contains unstable

acute fractures including distal oblique fractures, complete fractures through the waist, proximal pole fractures, and trans-scaphoid perilunate fracture-dislocations. Type C includes delayed unions, and type D includes established non-unions.

The problems associated with scaphoid fractures in particular include non-unions, malunions, and osteonecrosis. Non-unions for completely undisplaced fractures are relatively rare, and healing rates of 94 to 98.5% have been reported for cast immobilization of fresh non-displaced fractures. However, these unions may take anywhere from 12 weeks to up to 6 months to occur. When the diagnosis of the fracture and treatment is delayed beyond 3 weeks, or if there is any displacement at all at the fracture site, or if a proximal pole fracture is present, non-union rates increase steadily. Malunions are also a problem because these fractures tend to have volar comminution and can collapse into apex dorsal angulation, often known as a humpback deformity. If severe enough, it can lead to carpal instability patterns and a progressive degenerative change within the wrist. Osteonecrosis often results in these fractures because of the tenuous blood supply, which enters mainly through the dorsal distal ridge of the scaphoid. Proximal pole fractures are at particularly increased risk for avascular necrosis. For these reasons, many hand surgeons advocate that non-displaced fractures may be treated closed in a long-arm thumb spica cast for at least 6 weeks. This can be changed to a short-arm thumb spica cast later, and the cast must be changed often enough to keep it snug. Waist fractures average up to 12 weeks for healing and

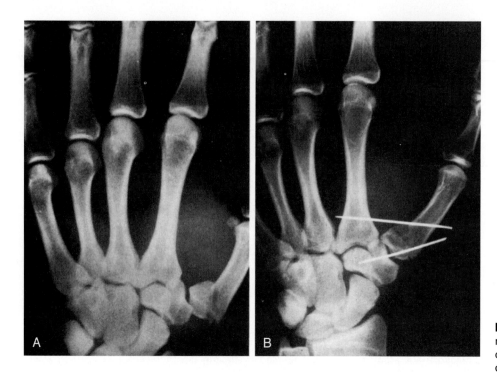

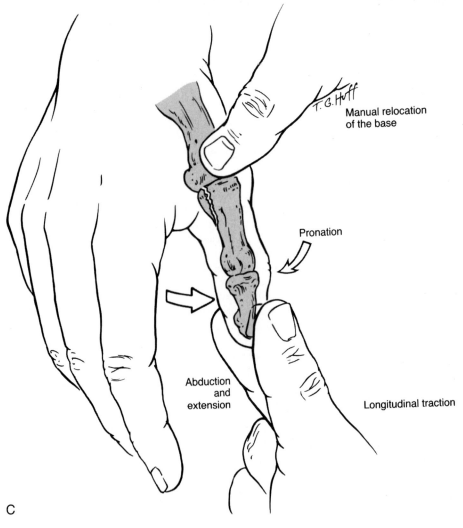

Figure 21–22. A 36-year-old man sustained a displaced oblique epibasal fracture of his dominant thumb metacarpal. *A,* The fracture was reduced with traction and manual pressure on the base of the metacarpal and stabilized with 0.045-inch Kirschner wires placed percutaneously *(B). C,* Reduction of a displaced Bennett fracture-dislocation includes longitudinal traction on the end of the thumb coupled with abduction, extension, and pronation of the metacarpal. Manual pressure on the base will aid in its relocation. (From Browner BD, Jupiter JB, Levine AM, Trafton PG: Skeletal Trauma. Philadelphia, WB Saunders, 1992, p 970.)

may require up to 6 months of immobilization. Proximal pole fractures average 25 weeks of immobilization. Any offset or instability pattern should be considered a displaced fracture and should be treated with ORIF with Kirschner wires or a compression screw such as the Herbert screw or the newer Acutrak screws (Fig. 21–23). Bone grafting should be done if there is any significant comminution to help correct the humpback deformity.

In cases of non-union or delayed union, the fracture pattern should again be evaluated for displacement. In non-displaced fractures, there are some who have advocated electrical stimulation, but evidence of this improving the outcome is equivocal. Russe bone grafting, which uses a corticocancellous "sandwich" of iliac crest graft, has been the standard of care for non-union; however, Greene showed in his study that if the proximal pole was completely avascular the union rate was almost 0%. Internal fixation with a Herbert bone screw and bone grafting seems to have improved the results for non-union and there are much higher union rates even in the face of avascular proximal poles. When there is displacement or humpback type of deformity of the non-union, most would recommend resection of the wedge-shaped defect of the non-union and replacement with a wedge-shaped iliac crest bone graft augmented with an internal fixation including pins or Herbert screw. Several vascularized bone grafts have been developed for use in scaphoid non-unions, the most popular one now being the pedicled distal radius graft described by Zaidemberg. The addition of these vascularized grafts can bring healing rates for non-unions to nearly 100%.

Acute fractures of the lunate have rarely been described, but Kienböck's disease, a pattern of non-displaced fractures and subsequent osteonecrosis, is well known. The lunate blood supply is also a tenuous one due to its extensive articular surface area, which limits blood vessel entry into the bone. Kienböck's disease is thought to be due either to trauma causing a direct interruption of the intraosseous blood supply or stress in an ulnar-negative variance overloading the bone and causing resultant osteonecrosis (Fig.

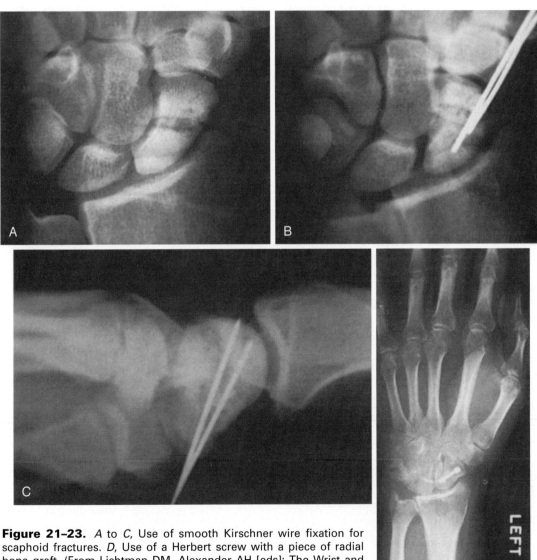

Figure 21–23. *A* to *C,* Use of smooth Kirschner wire fixation for scaphoid fractures. *D,* Use of a Herbert screw with a piece of radial bone graft. (From Lichtman DM, Alexander AH [eds]: The Wrist and its Disorders, 2nd ed. Philadelphia, WB Saunders, 1997, p 195.)

21–24). Patients present with central wrist pain and limitation of motion. The condition can often be difficult to diagnose, and one should maintain a high index of suspicion for it. When plain radiographs are negative, and one suspects this disease, an MRI or bone scan confirms the diagnosis. Lichtman's x-ray classification assigns stage I disease to lunates with no visible changes or a stress fracture detectable on tomography only. Stage 2 shows lunate sclerosis. Stage 3 involves lunate collapse, with subtypes A and B differentiated by the absence or presence of fixed rotatory instability of the scaphoid. Stage 4 disease involves pancarpal arthrosis. Stage 1 can be treated by immobilization only; and, for some patients, the symptoms resolve over time with only mild loss of motion and grip strength. However, when patients have progressive pain in stage I through 3A disease, joint leveling procedures such as radial shortening or ulnar lengthening, limited wrist arthrodesis such as scaphoid-trapezium-trapezoid (STT), capitohamate, or scaphocapitate fusion to unload the lunate; or revascularization procedures such as the one described by Horii should be considered. The option of silicon implant replacement has proved to be largely a failure and should not be used at this point in time. When rotatory subluxation of the scaphoid is present, an intercarpal fusion or proximal row carpectomy (PRC) is the procedure of choice. For stage 4 disease, PRC or total-wrist fusions are the best options.

Triquetral fractures are the third most common fractures of the carpus. They usually present as a dorsal avulsion fracture best seen on lateral x-ray films. This simple fracture pattern can be treated with 4 to 6 weeks of cast immobilization, followed by range of motion exercises. Triquetral body fractures occur uncommonly. If they are displaced or part of a greater fracture-dislocation, they should undergo ORIF.

Fractures of the trapezium can occur at either the trapezial ridge or the body. The ridge fractures usually result from a direct blow to the volar aspect of the wrist. These can be treated very easily by cast immobilization for 3 to 6 weeks. Fractures of the trapezial body require ORIF if there is any displacement.

Capitate fractures are rare in isolation. They can be associated with a scaphoid fracture as part of a greater arc type of injury, which is discussed later. ORIF is usually indicated because the proximal capitate can move out of position, and there are also high risks of osteonecrosis with this fracture.

Fractures of the hamate can occur as either hook or body fractures. The body fractures are relatively uncommon unless associated with a fourth or fifth metacarpal base fracture-dislocation. These can be treated closed if they are non-displaced, but if they are unstable or displaced they should undergo either closed reduction and percutaneous pinning or ORIF when unstable or irreducible. Hook of the hamate fractures are often related to a direct blow to the region. They can be difficult to diagnose. A carpal tunnel view of the wrist or a CT scan can usually confirm the diagnosis. When non-displaced these fractures should be treated with cast immobilization for 4 to 6 weeks. If they are displaced or there is a painful non-union, they should be treated with excision.

Pisiform fractures are also quite uncommon and sometimes difficult to diagnose. AP and true lateral films of the wrist as well as a carpal tunnel view can be helpful. These fractures can usually be treated in a short-arm cast with slight wrist flexion. If painful non-union or pisotriquetral arthritis results, the pisiform can be excised.

Distal radius fractures are the most common of all upper extremity fractures. In spite of this high rate of occurrence and the myriads of clinical and biomechanical studies that have been performed, an inclusive algorithm for treating these injuries and producing a predictably good outcome has yet to be developed. Distal radius fractures can be separated into high- and low-energy injuries. Low-energy injuries typically occur in elderly women who fall on an outstretched wrist. The tendency in the past has been to

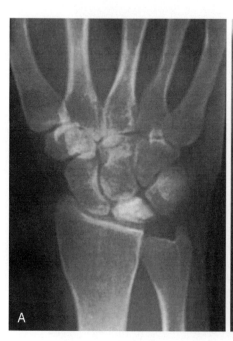
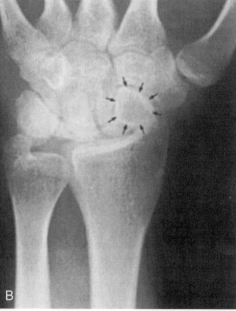

Figure 21–24. *A,* Anteroposterior view of early stage of Kienböck's disease demonstrating a normal relationship of the scaphoid to the remaining carpus. *B,* Late-stage Kienböck's disease, in which scaphoid rotation has led to a characteristic appearance referred to as the "ring sign" on an anteroposterior view. (From Lichtman DM, Alexander AH [eds]: The Wrist and its Disorders, 2nd ed. Philadelphia, WB Saunders, 1997, p 332.)

use closed treatment here owing to perceived low demands, concurrent medical problems, and the usual poor bone stock. This is changing as better surgical techniques have developed. The high-energy injuries tend to occur in younger patients from sports, industrial, or motor vehicle trauma. They usually have more comminution, displacement, and articular involvement. If treated improperly or inadequately, significant disability can develop.

Evaluation should begin with a history of the traumatic incident and the patient's functional goals and medical state. The examination should include evaluation of the shoulder, elbow, wrist, and hand, because the normal mechanisms can cause injury anywhere in the upper extremity. The examination specific to the wrist should address soft tissue injury, deformity, carpal injury, and neurovascular status. AP, lateral, and oblique x-rays usually suffice for planning management, but tomography or CT scans can help evaluate articular stepoffs, and traction views and MRI are helpful for assessing intracarpal pathology. Comparison films of the uninvolved side are very helpful, particularly for assessing the patient's normal ulnar variance. Three other radiographic parameters that should be assessed on the normal side include the radial height (the linear height from the radius at the DRUJ to the styloid tip—usually 12 mm), the radial inclination (the angle between the axis of the radial shaft and the articular surface of the radius—usually 22 degrees), and the radial tilt (the slope from the dorsal to volar lips of the radius on the lateral view—usually 12 degrees) (Fig. 21–25).

There are several classification schemes for these injuries, but none can comprehensively guide treatment. One should formulate a treatment plan based on the following: articular displacement (radiocarpal or DRUJ), loss of radial height, loss of volar tilt, amount of comminution, carpal alignment, and patient factors such as age, bone quality, medical status, and demands for use. Once these factors are determined one needs to decide whether reduction is needed, and if so whether it should be open or closed (Fig. 21–26). Acceptable alignment in an active, healthy patient requires no articular stepoff greater than 2 mm, neutral tilt, minimal shortening, a congruent DRUJ, and no resulting carpal malalignment. If these are not present or cannot be obtained with closed treatment, open reduction is warranted.

PALMAR TILT

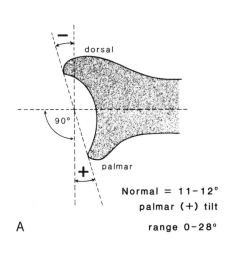

Normal = 11–12°

palmar (+) tilt

range 0–28°

A

RADIAL INCLINATION

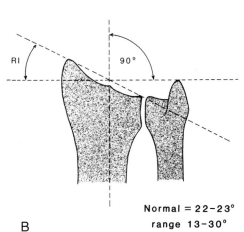

Normal = 22–23°

range 13–30°

B

RADIAL LENGTH

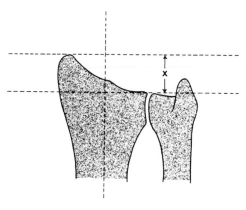

Normal x = 11–12 mm

range 8–18 mm

C

Figure 21–25. The radiographic measurements of the anatomy of the distal radius. *A,* In the sagittal plane, the normal palmar tilt averages 11 to 12 degrees. *B,* In the front plane, the average radial inclination is 22 to 23 degrees. *C,* In the frontal plane, the radial length (height) averages 11 to 12 mm in reference to the distal radioulnar joint. (From Jupiter JB, Masem M: Reconstruction of post-traumatic deformity of the distal radius and ulna. Hand Clin 4:378, 1988.)

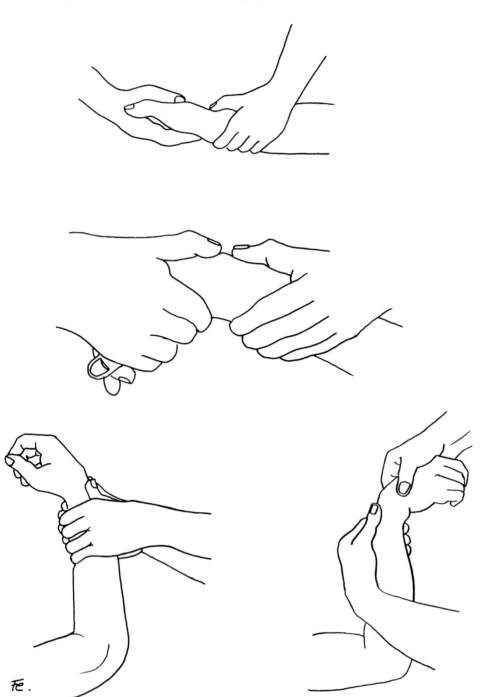

Figure 21–26. Manual reduction of Colles' fracture. *Top,* Disimpaction with traction and extension of the wrist. *Middle*, Reduction with flexion and ulnar deviation. *Bottom*, Stabilization with "double-thumb" pressure on the distal fragment in pronation, flexion, and ulnar deviation. (From Green DP, Hotchkiss RN, Pederson WC [eds]: Operative Hand Surgery, 4th ed. New York, Churchill Livingstone, 1999, p 946.)

The next decision is the type of immobilization to use. Adult distal radius fractures typically require 5 to 8 weeks to heal, and proper immobilization must maintain the reduction for that time period, and sometimes longer. Options include some form of casting, percutaneous pinning, external fixation, or internal fixation. Casting alone works best with fractures that have some inherent stability; they typically have little initial displacement or comminution. If one attempts to use this method after a closed reduction, a proper three-point mold and wrist positioning to maximize ligamentous stabilization of the fracture should be used. Percutaneous pinning is an excellent method for minimally invasive fixation of fractures. Pins can be introduced through reduced fracture fragments or into the fracture site itself as described by Kapandji to aid with fracture reduction (Fig. 21–27). Pinning alone does not work well for fractures with extensive comminution, intra-articular step-offs, or volar displacement. External fixation of distal radius fractures works through the principle of ligamentotaxis: when intact radiocarpal ligaments are placed under traction, they pull fracture fragments into proper alignment, producing an indirect reduction (Fig. 21–28). This method is highly effective for extra-articular fractures, and it can be used as an adjunct to pin or other fixation in intra-articular fractures. Internal fixation with plates and screws is becoming more popular with the advent of new, low-

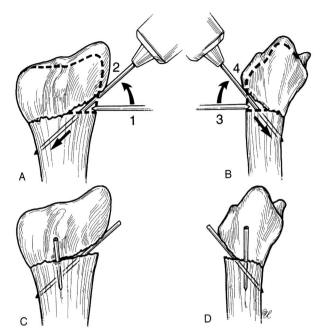

Figure 21-27. Kapandji technique of "double intrafocal wire fixation" to both reduce and maintain distal radial fractures. A 0.045- or 0.0625-inch Kirschner wire is introduced into the fracture in a radial-to-ulnar direction. When the wire reaches the ulnar cortex of the radius, the wire is used to elevate the radial fragment and re-create the radial inclination. This wire is then introduced into the proximal ulnar cortex of the radius for stability. A second wire is introduced at 90 degrees to the first in a similar manner to restore and maintain volar tilt. (From Green DP, Hotchkiss RN, Pederson WC [eds]: Operative Hand Surgery, 4th ed. New York, Churchill Livingstone, 1999, p 951.)

profile plates. This fixation is ideal for intra-articular shear fractures (i.e., volar or dorsal Barton's fractures), comminuted fractures requiring bone graft, and revision situations such as osteotomies for malunions.

TFCC Tears

The anatomy of the TFCC has been described earlier. It is commonly injured with falls on an outstretched wrist, and it is a major cause of ulnar-sided wrist pain (thought by many to be the low back pain of hand surgery). Typical examination findings include tenderness just volar to the ulnar styloid, pain or clicking with an ulnocarpal grind test (pronation and supination of the maximally ulnar-deviated, axially loaded wrist), and, in severe cases, DRUJ instability. X-ray examination is usually negative, but it helps determine ulnar variance and rule out other sources of ulnar pain, such as triquetral or pisiform fracture and lunatotriquetral dissociation. Arthrography was once the best study available for these injuries, but MRI has proved to be more accurate and is now the imaging study of choice. Arthroscopy is advocated by many as the definitive study for staging TFCC tears, and many prominent hand surgeons will go directly to this when the history and physical examination point strongly to this injury. They believe that this approach avoids the wasted time and costs of additional tests, which can be inconclusive and do not allow

immediate treatment of the patient. One should note that deep tears of the volar and dorsal radioulnar ligaments sometimes cannot be detected even with arthroscopy.

Palmer has created a very useful classification scheme for these injuries (Table 21-1). It broadly groups them into traumatic (class 1) (Fig. 21-29) or degenerative (class 2) (Fig. 21-30) lesions, with multiple subtypes. The traumatic lesions can be treated acutely with 4 weeks of immobilization in slight flexion and ulnar deviation if no gross instability or subluxation is present. If symptoms persist, arthroscopic or open treatment is indicated. Class 1A tears involve a central tear of the articular disk, usually 2 to 3 mm ulnar to the radial attachments. These injuries are in an avascular zone (Fig. 21-31) and cannot be repaired. Good results have been obtained with simple arthroscopic debridement of these tears, unless an ulnar positive variance is present (Figs. 21-32 and 21-33). Class 1B lesions are ulnar-sided avulsions, with or without an ulnar styloid fracture. These lesions can destabilize the DRUJ and should be repaired. If an ulnar styloid fracture is present, ORIF with Kirschner wires or a tension band technique is indicated. If the injury is purely ligamentous, it is in a highly vascular segment, and both open and arthroscopically assisted repairs have produced good results. Class 1C injuries involve rupture of the volar ulnocarpal ligaments as they insert on the lunate or triquetrum. These lesions often require arthroscopy for diagnosis, but treatment requires an open repair. Class 1D tears are radial-sided avulsions, with or without a sigmoid notch fracture. Treatment is controversial, but I advocate an open or arthroscopic reattachment.

Class 2, or degenerative, lesions result from chronic wear and have been given the general name of ulnocarpal abutment syndrome. They are frequently the result of overloading secondary to a positive ulnar variance. Class 2A lesions have wear and thinning of the TFCC. Class 2B lesions have TFCC wear plus lunate or ulnar chondroma-

Table 21-1. Classification of TFCC abnormalities

Class 1 Traumatic
  A. Central perforation
  B. Ulnar avulsion
      With distal ulnar fracture
      Without distal ulnar fracture
  C. Distal avulsion
  D. Radial avulsion
      With sigmoid notch fracture
      Without sigmoid notch fracture
Class 2 Degenerative (ulnocarpal abutment syndrome)
  A. TFCC wear
  B. TFCC wear
      Plus lunate and/or ulnar chondromalacia
  C. TFCC perforation
      Plus lunate and/or ulnar chondromalacia
  D. TFCC perforation
      Plus lunate and/or ulnar chondromalacia
      Plus lunatotriquetral ligament perforation
  E. TFCC perforation
      Plus lunate and/or ulnar chondromalacia
      Plus lunatotriquetral ligament perforation
      Plus ulnocarpal arthritis

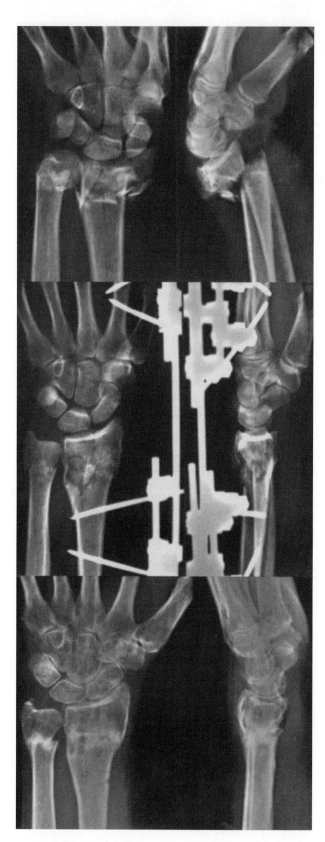

Figure 21–28. Comminuted unstable distal forearm fracture *(top)* treated by external fixation and primary autogenous iliac bone grafting *(middle)*. The frame was removed at 5 weeks and the wrist protected with a removable wrist splint for another 3 weeks. Follow-up x-rays *(bottom)* demonstrate uneventful healing and satisfactory joint alignment. (From Green DP, Hotchkiss RN, Pederson WC [eds]: Operative Hand Surgery, 4th ed. New York, Churchill Livingstone, 1999, p 954.)

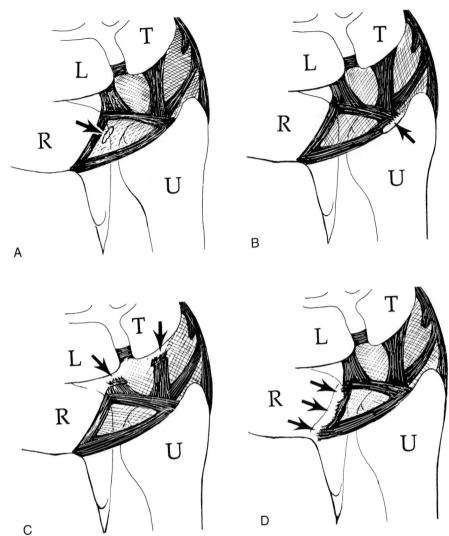

Figure 21–29. Drawing of traumatic, or class 1, abnormalities of the triangular fibrocartilage complex. *A*, Class 1A, central perforation *(arrow)*. *B*, Class 1B, ulnar avulsion *(arrow)*, with or without distal ulnar fracture. *C*, Class 1C, distal avulsion *(arrows)*. *D*, Class 1D, radial avulsion *(arrows)*, with or without sigmoid notch fracture. L, lunate; R, radius; T, triquetrum; U, ulna. (From Palmer AK: Triangular fibrocartilage complex lesions: a classification. J Hand Surg Am 14:594–606, 1989.)

lacia. Class 2C adds perforation of the TFCC, whereas class 2D further adds lunatotriquetral ligament tears. Class 2E injuries have all the features of class 2D plus ulnocarpal arthritis. Initial treatment is conservative with immobilization, activity modification, non-steroidal anti-inflammatory drugs (NSAIDs), and corticosteroid injections. When after 3 months this treatment fails, surgery should be considered. Classes 2A through 2D should be treated with some type of ulnar shortening procedure, either formal shortening with plate fixation or a wafer procedure (open or arthroscopic) that resects just enough ulnar pole to make the wrist ulnar negative in variance. In class 2D lesions this is followed by an assessment of lunatotriquetral instability. If the complex is still unstable, a lunatotriquetral fusion or dorsal capsulorrhaphy is indicated. Class 2E lesions should be treated with a Suave-Kapandji or Darrach procedure.

Carpal Instability

Carpal instability is one of the most difficult problems in hand surgery from every standpoint, including conceptualization, diagnosis, and treatment. The range of injuries represented by this broad term goes from a simple wrist sprain or tear of a single ligament to a complete dislocation of the wrist. Evaluation of these injuries starts with a good history. Frequently they occur during a fall on an outstretched wrist, but they can also be caused by axial loading and other injury patterns. It is helpful to know the exact mechanism. The patient's symptoms are also extremely useful; for example, if the patient has a clunk or instability type sensation with specific motions of the wrist, this can help with the diagnosis. Accurate localization of the pain helps determine which ligaments are injured. Physical examination should start with a basic examination of the wrist, including inspection, palpation, range of motion, and strength and sensory testing. Specific tests regarding instability include the scaphoid shift test and the lunatotriquetral shear test. The scaphoid shift test was described by Watson to test specifically for scapholunate ligament injuries. It involves direct pressure on the scaphoid tubercle starting in a position of ulnar deviation and, while continuing to place pressure on the scaphoid tubercle, bringing the wrist into full radial deviation (Fig. 21–34). Under normal situations the scaphoid palmar flexes in this motion pattern. When the scapholunate ligament is interrupted, the direct pressure placed on the scaphoid tubercle can prevent this palmar flexion, and one can actually subluxate the scaphoid from its normal position. This results in significant pain

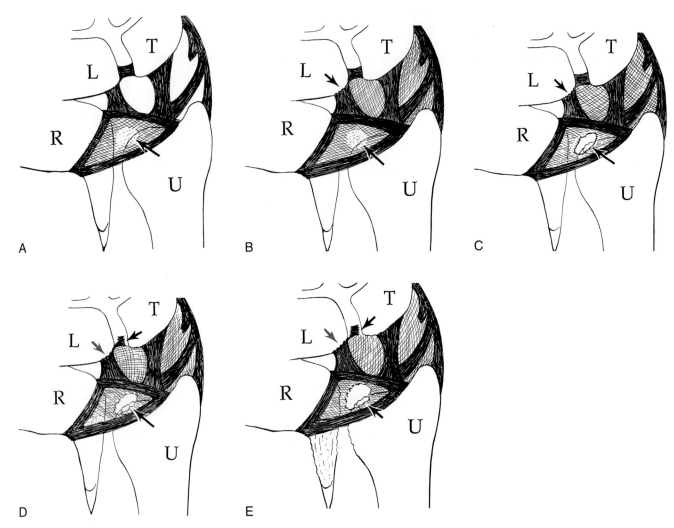

Figure 21–30. Drawing of degenerative, or class 2, abnormalities of the triangular fibrocartilage complex (TFCC), or ulnocarpal abutment syndrome. *A,* Class 2A, TFCC wear *(arrow)*. *B,* Class 2B, TFCC wear with lunate *(small arrow)* and/or ulnar *(large arrow)* chondromalacia. *C,* Class 2C, TFCC perforation with lunate *(small arrow)* and/or ulnar *(large arrow)* chondromalacia. *D,* Class 2D, TFCC perforation with lunate *(arrow)* and/or ulnar *(large arrow)* chondromalacia and lunatotriquetral ligament perforation *(small arrow)*. *E,* Class 2E, TFCC perforation with lunate *(arrow)* and/or ulnar *(large arrow)* chondromalacia, lunatotriquetal ligament perforation *(small arrow)*, and ulnocarpal arthritis. L, lunate; R, radius; T, triquetrum; U, ulna. (From Palmer AK: Triangular fibrocartilage complex lesions: a classification. J Hand Surg Am 14:594–606, 1989.)

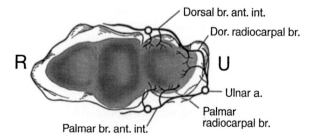

Figure 21–31. Depiction of the vascular supply to the triangular fibrocartilage through the following branches (labeled with abbreviated names): dorsal and palmar radiocarpal branches of the ulnar artery, the palmar branch of the anterior interosseous artery, and the dorsal branch of the anterior interosseous artery. Note the avascularity of the central and radial aspects of the triangular fibrocartilage. R, radius; U, ulna. (From Lichtman DM, Alexander AH [eds]: The Wrist and its Disorders, 2nd ed. Philadelphia, WB Saunders, 1997, p 393.)

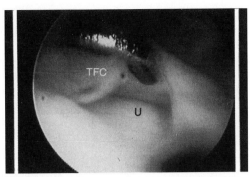

Figure 21–32. Radiocarpal joint, left wrist. Traumatic central tear, triangular fibrocartilage (TFC) with redundant flap. Probe is elevating the tear and shows the laxity of the TFC. The distal ulna (U) is normal and free of chondromalacia in this patient with negative ulnar variance. (From Osterman AL [ed]: Basic wrist arthroscopy and endoscopy. Hand Clin 10[4], 1994, Color Fig. 12.)

and often can cause a clunk. The lunatotriquetral shear test as described by Kleinman is very useful for determining lunatotriquetral instability. The lunate is stabilized in the front and back with the thumb and index fingers of one hand, then the thumb and index of the other hand grasp the triquetrum and are used to create a shear force across the lunatotriquetral interval. Increased translation compared to the opposite side indicates a tear in this region.

The x-ray examination for carpal instability begins with the standard PA, lateral, and 45-degree semipronated oblique views of the wrist. Some additional views can be useful: the clenched-fist AP accentuates scapholunate interval widening; ulnar and radial deviation PA, and flexion and extension lateral views help determine dynamic instability; and a scaphoid view helps identify scaphoid fractures. One should first rule out fractures or static instabilities, including scapholunate widening. Three smooth arcs (Gilula's lines) (Fig. 21–35) can be drawn on the PA view; stepoffs from these lines suggest disruptions of carpal relationships. Carpal bone angles should be carefully evaluated; the most important ones are on the lateral view and they include the scapholunate, the capital lunate, and the radial lunate angles (Fig. 21–36). Carpal height ratios help in determining proximal migration of the carpus (Fig. 21–37).

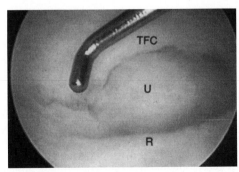

Figure 21–33. Radiocarpal arthroscopy. Postoperative view after debridement of the unstable portion of the flap tear in the triangular fibrocartilage (TFC). The underlying normal distal ulna (U) is noted. Also seen in foreground is the edge of lunate facet of radius (R). The probe shows the smooth ulnar edge of the debrided TFC. (From Osterman AL [ed]: Basic wrist arthroscopy and endoscopy. Hand Clin 10[4], 1994, Color Fig. 13.)

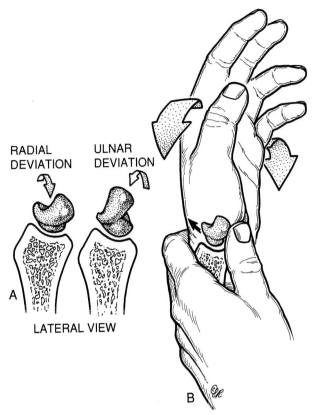

RADIAL DEVIATION ULNAR DEVIATION

LATERAL VIEW

Figure 21–34. Mechanism of scaphoid shift. *A,* When the wrist is in ulnar deviation, the scaphoid dorsiflexes and its long axis approaches alignment with the axis of the radius. In radial deviation, the scaphoid volarflexes. Its long axis lies more perpendicular to the axis of the radius, and its distal pole becomes prominent on the palmar side of the wrist. *B,* During the scaphoid shift maneuver, the examiner's thumb resists the normal volar tilt of the scaphoid. (From Green DP, Hotchkiss RN, Pederson WC [eds]: Operative Hand Surgery, 4th ed. New York, Churchill Livingstone, 1999, p 115.)

One should also look for ulnar translation of the carpus. Fluoroscopy or cineradiography can definitively show relative carpal bone motion, and both are useful for diagnosing the less common midcarpal instabilities. Arthrograms are excellent for diagnosing ligament ruptures, although numerous studies have shown positive arthrograms on the patient's asymptomatic side as well, making it difficult to interpret what is an important finding. As sequencing techniques and resolution improve for MRI, it is becoming the imaging technique of choice for identifying scapholunate ligament tears and occult fractures in the wrist.

The classification developed by the surgeons at the Mayo Clinic is probably the most useful one for addressing these injuries. Their first category is called carpal instability dissociative. The first subgrouping is dorsiflexion intercalated segment instability (DISI), normally the result of a disruption of the scapholunate (SL) interosseous ligament. Classic x-ray findings for this include a widened scapholunate interval on the AP x-ray compared with other intercarpal spacing: a scapholunate gap of greater than 3 mm (the "Terry Thomas sign") is considered diagnostic of this disruption. Other important findings include an increase in the scapholunate angle as well as the capital lunate and radiolunate angles in the true lateral view. On the PA view,

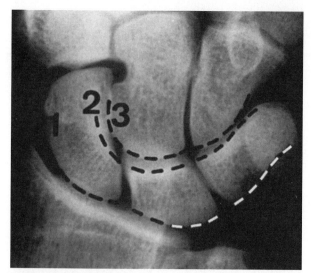

Figure 21–35. Three smooth, curved lines join the proximal and distal cortical surfaces of the carpal bones that help assess normal carpal relationships. A disruption or stepoff in any one of these lines may indicate a major carpal derangement. (From Green DP, Hotchkiss RN, Pederson WC [eds]: Operative Hand Surgery, 4th ed. New York, Churchill Livingstone, 1999, p 876.)

the scaphoid appears foreshortened secondary to its volar flexion and there is a so-called cortical ring sign resulting from an end-on view of the scaphoid tubercle.

The other subgrouping in the dissociative carpal instabilities is the volar flexion intercalated segment instability (VISI); this usually results from a lunatotriquetral dissociation. This injury pattern is much less common than the DISI pattern, and it has been much more difficult to produce under experimental conditions.

The next category of instabilities is the carpal instability nondissociative; this involves injury between the carpal rows of the entire wrist. The first type is radiocarpal instability; this is relatively rare and usually involves disruption of either the volar or the dorsal radiocarpal ligaments with subsequent drift of the carpus. The diagnosis can be very hard to make. The next subgrouping is the midcarpal instabilities. They are caused either by ligament injuries, ligament laxity, or malunion of distal radius fractures causing abnormal orientation of the proximal row. The diagnosis is confirmed by an abnormal capitolunate angle on the true lateral view (Fig. 21–38). The last subgrouping is the ulnar translocation; this is most commonly present in patients with rheumatoid arthritis of the wrist. In post-traumatic situations, it was once thought that injury to the radiolunate ligaments allowed ulnar drift of the wrist; however, now it seems that much more global ligamentous injury is required for this instability pattern.

The third category of carpal instabilities are the complex instabilities. They are the result of perilunate dislocations, which can either be isolated volar/dorsal perilunate dislocations or the somewhat more common transscaphoid perilunate dislocations. These perilunate injuries can go through a greater arc, which usually involves fracture through the scaphoid and then rupture of the perilunate ligamentous structures resulting in dislocation, or they can go through a lesser arc, where the carpal injury is purely ligamentous (Fig. 21–39). This lesser arc injury can sometimes be associated with a radial styloid fracture. For this

reason, displaced radial styloid fractures should be investigated thoroughly to detect any associated intercarpal instability patterns.

The work of Mayfield and colleagues describing a progressive perilunar instability has been very helpful in our understanding of this problem (Fig. 21–40). By using a

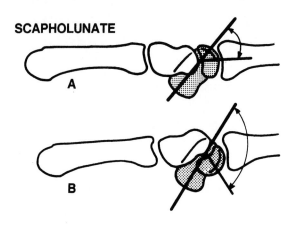

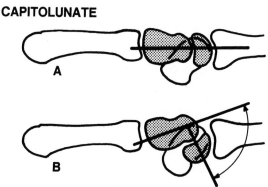

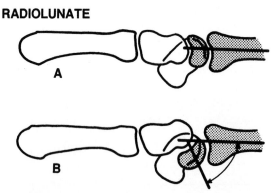

Figure 21–36. The carpal bone angles are of considerable aid in identifying carpal instability patterns. In each illustration the normal angle (A) is shown in comparison with the abnormal angle (B) seen when there is a DISI pattern of carpal instability. The scapholunate angle, when greater than 80 degrees, is definitive evidence of either a scapholunate dissociation or a palmarly displaced scaphoid fracture. The capitolunate angle should theoretically be 0 degrees with the wrist in neutral, but the range of normal probably extends to as much as 15 degrees. The radiolunate angle is abnormal if it exceeds 15 degrees. (From Green DP, Hotchkiss RN, Pederson WC [eds] Operative Hand Surgery, 4th ed. New York, Churchill Livingstone, 1999, p 878.)

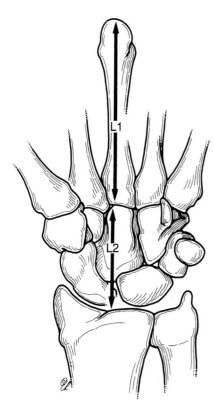

Figure 21–37. The carpal height ratio is calculated by dividing the carpal height (L2) by the length of the third metacarpal (L1). The normal is 0.54 ± 0.03. (From Youm Y, McMurthy RY, Flatt AE, Gillespie TE: Kinematics of the wrist: I. An experimental study of radial-ulnar deviation and flexion-extension. J Bone Joint Surg Am 60:423–431, 1978.)

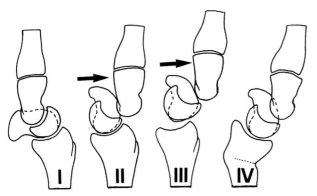

Figure 21–38. Lichtman's classification of midcarpal instabilities (MCIs). Type I (palmar MCI): the whole proximal row appears abnormally flexed in the lateral view. Type II (dorsal MCI): normal alignment in standard x-rays but abnormal midcarpal subluxation when a dorsally directed force *(black arrow)* is applied. Type III (dorsal and palmar MCI): both midcarpal and radiocarpal joints are abnormally subluxable in a palmar and dorsal direction, usually the consequence of increased global laxity. Type IV (extrinsic MCI): the midcarpal dysfunction is the consequence of an extracarpal problem, usually a malunited distal radius as shown here. (From Green DP, Hotchkiss RN, Pederson WC [eds]: Operative Hand Surgery, 4th ed. New York, Churchill Livingstone, 1999, p 905.)

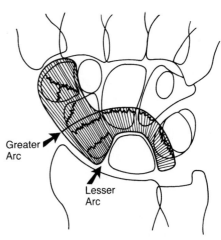

Figure 21–39. The greater arc and lesser arc paths of carpal injury. The greater arc injuries tend to occur with the hand radially deviated, transmitting the force through the scaphoid and creating primarily a bony (perilunate) instability. The lesser arc injuries occur with the hand less radially deviated, creating primarily a ligamentous perilunate instability. (From Weber ER, Chao EV: An experimental approach to the mechanism of scaphoid wrist fractures. J Hand Surg 3:142–148, 1978.)

cadaveric model in forced dorsiflexion, intercarpal supination, and ulnar deviation they were able to come up with four stages of instability. The first stage involved scapholunate and radioscaphoid ligament ruptures. The second stage showed capitolunate instability, the third stage showed lunatotriquetral ligament disruption, and the fourth stage showed lunate dislocation, which is nearly always volar.

The fourth broad category of carpal instability is the longitudinal or axial loading instabilities. This is subgrouped further into axial ulnar, axial radial, and combined (Fig. 21–41). These tend to be high-energy injuries with severe soft tissue damage. The best results have been with open reduction and pin or screw fixation with aggressive treatment of the soft tissue injuries.

The treatment of carpal instabilities is difficult and controversial. For an isolated scapholunate ligament tear that is acute (meaning within the first 6 weeks to 3 months), the consensus now seems to be open reduction and some combination of a primary ligament repair or capsulodesis (Fig. 21–42). For more chronic instabilities, a pattern of degeneration described by Watson as scapholunate advanced collapse (SLAC) can result (Fig. 21–43). There is a progressive cartilage loss starting at the radial styloid and ending with pancarpal arthritis that develops from untreated DISI instabilities or scaphoid malunions. The recommended treatment for chronic instability without SLAC changes would include open reduction and attempted soft tissue reconstructions such as Blatt capsulodesis or other ligamentous procedures (Fig. 21–44). Some have advocated going immediately to limited intercarpal fusion such as the STT fusion or the capitohamate triquetrolunate (CHTL or four-corner) arthrodesis. The use of proximal row carpectomy is becoming increasingly popular, and results in some studies have been excellent, with near full restoration of grip strength and range of motion.

Treatment of lunatotriquetral instabilities is also contro-

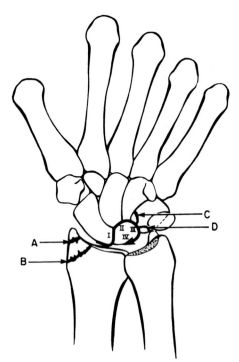

Figure 21–40. The perilunate pattern of injury to the volar ligaments of the wrist is divided into four stages. Stage I is a partial disruption of the scapholunate joint. Stage II is a complete disruption of the scapholuante joint. Stage III is a disruption of the scapholunate, capitolunate, and triquetrolunate joints. Stage IV is a disruption of all the preceding stages and the dorsal radiocarpal ligaments, allowing volar lunate dislocation or dorsal perilunate dislocation. Occasionally, radial styloid (A, B) or triquetrum (C, D) fractures accompany perilunate ligament injuries. Other fracture patterns also occur (see Fig. 12–8). (From Mayfield JK, Johnson RP, Kilcoyne RF: Carpal dislocations: Pathomechanics and progressive perilunar instability. J Hand Surg 5:226–241, 1980.)

Figure 21–41. Schematic representation of the most frequently reported axial fracture-dislocations. In axial-radial dislocations (above) there is an unstable segment displacing in a radial direction, whereas the opposite instability is seen among the axial-ulnar derangements (below). (From Garcia-Elias M, Dobyns JH, Cooney WP III, Linscheid RL: Traumatic axial dislocations of the carpus. J Hand Surg 14A:446–457, 1989.)

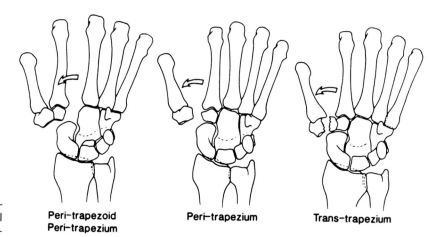

Peri-trapezoid
Peri-trapezium

Peri-trapezium

Trans-trapezium

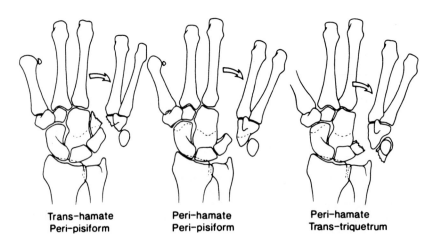

Trans-hamate
Peri-pisiform

Peri-hamate
Peri-pisiform

Peri-hamate
Trans-triquetrum

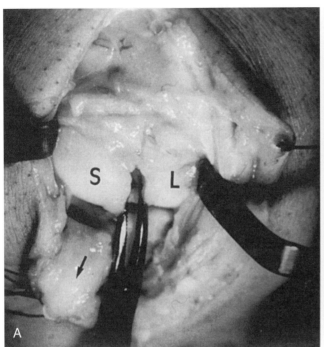

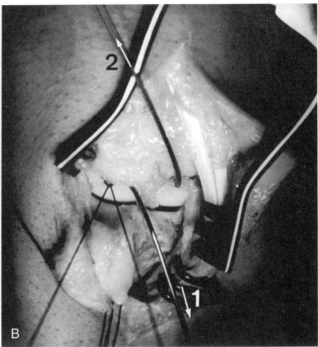

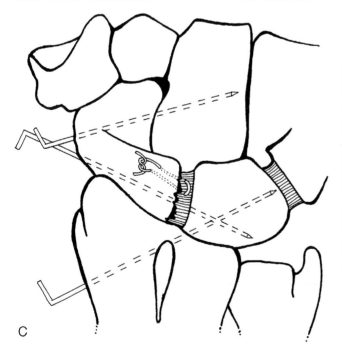

Figure 21–42. Open reduction and scapholunate ligament repair in a 27-year-old man who sustained a scapholunate dissociation 6 weeks before surgery. *A,* Through a dorsal approach, a proximally based capsular flap is created *(black arrow)* for later capsulodesis. With forceps, the scapholunate interval is opened, allowing inspection of the anterior aspect of the joint. *B,* Method of reduction of the joint using two Kirschner wires as joysticks. By pulling the wire inserted into the scaphoid (S) (1) proximally and ulnarly, while the wire in the lunate (L) (2) is held distally and radially, the joint usually becomes anatomically reduced. *C,* At this point, the transosseous sutures previously placed as suggested by Linscheid are tied, and then Kirschner wires securing the reduced carpal bones are inserted. (From Green DP, Hotchkiss RN, Pederson WC [eds]: Operative Hand Surgery, 4th ed. New York, Churchill Livingstone, 1999, p 988.)

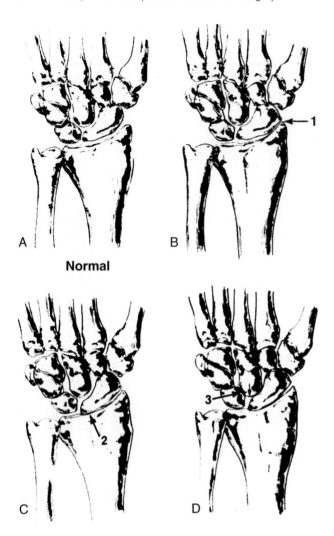

Normal

Figure 21–43. The most common pattern of degenerative arthritis seen in untreated chronic scapholunate instability is termed SLAC wrist, or scapholunate advanced collapse deformity. This predictably progressive sequence of degenerative changes associated with chronic scapholunate injuries is subdivided into three stages according to the location of the secondary arthrosis. *A,* Normal wrist for comparison. *B,* Stage I SLAC wrist manifests as arthrosis limited to the radial styloid-scaphoid articular (1). *C,* In stage II, arthrosis involves the entire radioscaphoid articulation (2). *D,* Stage III is signified by the presence of capitolunate arthrosis (3). (From Watson KH, Ryu J: Degeneration disorders of the carpus. Orthop Clin North Am 15:337–354, 1984.)

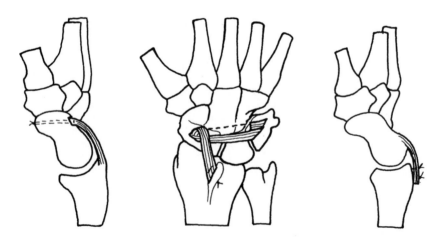

BLATT 1987   LINSCHEID 1992   HERBERT 1996

Figure 21–44. During the surgical approach to treat rotatory subluxation of the scaphoid, a dorsal capsulodesis of the radioscaphoid joint may be created and later used to help prevent recurrence of the scaphoid flexion tendency. The first and most popular method was described by Blatt, which uses a proximally based capsular flap. Linscheid and Dobyns preferred using a strip of the dorsal intercarpal ligament, whereas a distal based capsular flap was suggested by Herbert et al. (From Green DP, Hotchkiss RN, Pederson WC [eds]: Operative Hand Surgery, 4th ed. New York, Churchill Livingstone, 1999, p 889.)

versial. For injuries that are caught very early and seem to be isolated lunatotriquetral sprains, casting for 4 to 6 weeks will usually result in good pain relief. For situations with disassociation of the lunatotriquetral ligament or obvious tear, arthroscopy of the wrist with limited debridement of the tear has produced reasonably good results, as described by Arnold Peter-Weiss. Other options for treatment include lunatotriquetral arthrodesis and four-corner fusion.

SOFT TISSUE

Skin and Nail Trauma

Injury to the skin and the nail region is extremely common. As mentioned earlier, when there is a subungual hematoma that is relatively small, isolated perforation of the nail with release of the fluid can help relieve the pain and soft tissue compression greatly. However, when more than 50% of the nail is involved, the nail should be removed and the larger nail bed laceration should be repaired with fine chromic gut stitches. A stent should be placed under the nail fold to keep it open, and this should be discontinued at approximately 2 weeks.

Fingertip amputations that are very distal can be treated with isolated debridement; and in situations in which the skin laceration is clean, defatting of the amputated part and replacement of the skin as a full-thickness skin graft to the tip of the wound can be done in the emergency department with excellent results. In other situations, with adequate digital block anesthesia, the bone can be ronguered back proximally and the skin primarily closed. It is important not to close the skin in such a way as to volarly angulate the nail bed because this can lead to a nail deformity. Full-thickness skin loss on the fingertip pulp can be treated by a variety of methods. If no bone is exposed, this area can be allowed to granulate over by performing wet to dry dressing changes. Because of the excellent vascularity of the hand, this will usually heal completely; often this tip even becomes sensate. When the area seems too large or the patient cannot tolerate long periods of dressing changes, there are a variety of local advancement flaps available. These include the volar V-Y advancement flap (Atasoy-Kleinert) (Fig. 21–45) and the lateral V-Y advancement flap (Kutler) (Fig. 21–46). For the tip of the thumb, a Moberg slide can be performed. Cross finger flaps are also available. For children, thenar flaps are an option (Fig. 21–47). In adults, however, they cause PIP contractures and should not be used.

Lacerations of the hand should be treated in the emergency department by evaluating the laceration and then covering it with a saline-soaked sterile gauze pad. The wound itself should not be extensively explored in the emergency department setting. Most of the important information can be obtained by examining the digits distal to the wound. Flexor and extensor tendon function can be examined, and vascularity and sensation can also indicate whether or not the wound involves a digital artery or nerve injury. One should avoid trying to clamp any bleeding vessels blindly in this situation, because the digital nerves are directly adjacent to the arteries in the fingers and can be severely damaged by this procedure. Digital vessels nearly always stop bleeding under direct pressure alone. If

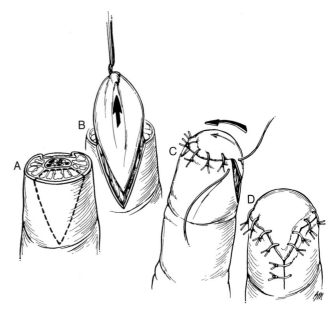

Figure 21–45. The Atasoy-Kleinert volar V-Y technique is applicable to distal tip injuries with bone exposed and when the distal injury is either transverse or oblique and sloping in a volar distal-to-distal proximal direction. In injuries with more volar pad loss, there is usually insufficient skin for this technique to be used. (From Green DP, Hotchkiss RN, Pederson WC [eds]: Operative Hand Surgery, 4th ed. New York, Churchill Livingstone, 1999, p 50.)

the evaluation of the distal digit indicates that no deep structures have been injured, then the wound can be irrigated out locally in the emergency department and closed. For adults, 4–0 or 5–0 nylon simple stitches usually suffice. For children, it is wise to use an absorbable stitch such as

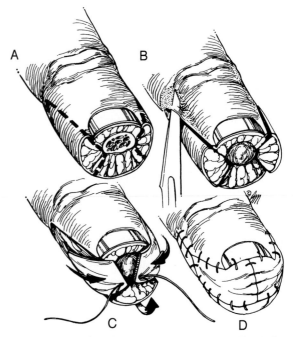

Figure 21–46. Kutler lateral V-Y technique. (From Green DP, Hotchkiss RN, Pederson WC [eds]: Operative Hand Surgery, 4th ed. New York, Churchill Livingstone, 1999, p 52.)

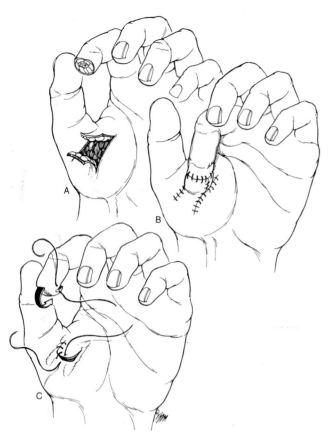

Figure 21–47. The thenar "H-flap" as described by Smith and Albin. (From Green DP, Hotchkiss RN, Pederson WC [eds]: Operative Hand Surgery, 4th ed. New York, Churchill Livingstone, 1999, p 55.)

5–0 chromic gut to avoid the agony of suture removal in a small child.

Tendon Injuries

FLEXOR TENDON INJURIES

Injuries to the flexor and extensor tendons can have devastating effects on the function of the hand. The flexor tendons in particular have been studied very extensively because of the difficulty in obtaining good results with injuries within the flexor tendon sheath. Tendon healing occurs by a combination of intrinsic and extrinsic mechanisms, with fibroblasts from the tendons themselves as well as from the surrounding peritendinous tissue contributing to the process. The complete healing process takes about 8 weeks (Fig. 21–48). The initial or inflammatory phase begins immediately after the injury when the defect is filled with blood clot and inflammatory tissue. As these cells proliferate they promote migration of more fibroblasts into the repair site and begin the healing process. This is followed by a fibroblastic stage. At approximately 1 week from injury, the fibroblasts begin secreting collagen, a process that continues for approximately 4 more weeks. It is supplemented by local factors, particularly fibronectin, which acts as a chemotactic factor for fibroblasts and promotes their adherence to denatured collagen. At about 4 weeks the remodeling phase begins: the fibroblasts begin

to re-orient themselves in line with the tendon, and the collagen fibrils re-align with them. At 6 weeks the repair gap is completely filled with collagen. The maturation process continues; as physiologic loading begins, the tensile strength of the repair increases steadily.

Adhesion formation within the flexor tendon sheath comes from a combination of the initial trauma in the region with subsequent fibrous tissue healing and from immobilization, which leads to fibrosis within the sheath. For these reasons early motion has been crucial in obtaining good results with flexor tendon injuries. To do this, one must obtain a repair that is strong enough to uphold the stress of early motion and prevent gapping at the repair site. Many different suture techniques have been advocated. However, most would now agree that one should try to achieve a repair with at least four core strands of suture and supplement this with a running epitenon stitch. I recommend the technique advocated by Strickland (Fig. 21–49). It uses a 2–0 Ethibond or other nonabsorbable braided suture in a modified Kessler stitch and then a central horizontal mattress stitch to give a total of four core strands crossing the repair site. A running, locked 6–0 nylon or prolene epitenon stitch is used to further supplement the repair.

Flexor tendon injuries are defined by the zone in which the injury occurs (Fig. 21–50). Zone I is the region distal to the FDS insertion. Although it is in the fibro-osseous sheath, the only tendon present is the FDP, and overall results of repair are good. One particular injury pattern here is a rupture of the insertion of the FDP tendon at the distal phalanx base. This can occur with or without an accompanying bony avulsion. Direct repair or reinsertion of the tendon into the distal phalanx base using a pull-out stitch or Mitek suture anchor gives very good results. If the laceration is more proximal and within the tendon substance, one should attempt to perform a direct repair because advancement of the tendon greater than 1 cm can cause a flexion deformity.

Zone II is the region that begins with the fibro-osseous tunnel at the A-pulley and extends to the FDS insertion. This zone has traditionally had the worst results with direct repair; and early in the 20th century, Bunnel stated that direct repair not be done here. However, with our advances in techniques, primary repair of acute flexor tendon injuries is now recommended regardless of the zone in which it occurs. In zone II, atraumatic technique and aggressive postoperative rehabilitation are crucial to obtaining a good result. One should try to repair both the FDS and the FDP tendons when possible.

Zone III is in the palm; it is the zone of lumbrical muscle origin. Repairs in this region can provide good results; however, there is often other serious soft tissue injury including blood vessel and nerve injuries that can sometimes compromise the overall function of the hand. Zone IV is the carpal tunnel; the tight space in which the flexor tendons and the median nerve are contained at this level can lead to injuries involving multiple tendons and sometimes the nerve ("spaghetti wrist"). The resulting adhesions and neurologic deficits frequently compromise outcomes. Zone V is the wrist and forearm. Here, the tendons are subject to their least constraint; therefore, the prognosis for tendon reconstruction is best in this zone.

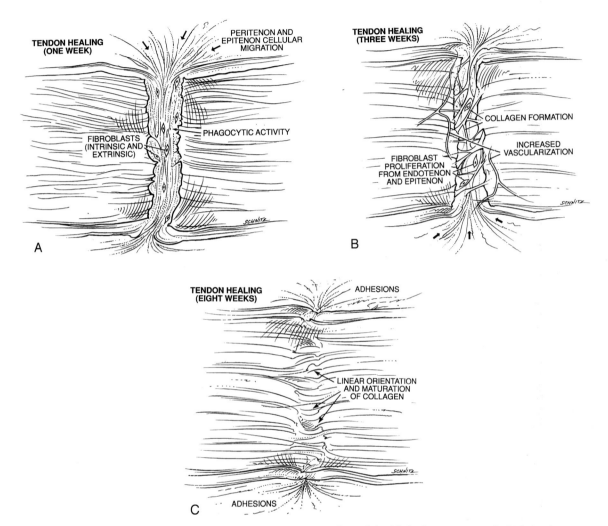

Figure 21–48. Tendon healing. Artist's representation of the biologic sequence. *A,* At 1 week an inflammatory response predominates, and the laceration site is filled with cells that originate from the extrinsic peritendinous tissues and from the epitenon and endotenon. The cells proliferate; their function is largely phagocytosis and also the synthesis of new collagen. *B,* At 3 weeks there is marked fibroblastic proliferation from the endotenon and epitenon, and these fibroblasts participate in both synthesis and resorption of collagen. The fibroblasts and collagen are in a plane perpendicular to the long axis of the tendon, and revascularization increases at the repair site, including penetration of the former "avascular zones" by new vessel. *C,* At 8 weeks the collagen is mature and realigned in linear fashion. Adhesions are stimulated both by the initial trauma to the tendon and sheath and by immobilization. (From Green DP, Hotchkiss RN, Pederson WC [eds]: Operative Hand Surgery, 4th ed. New York, Churchill Livingstone, 1999, p 1856.)

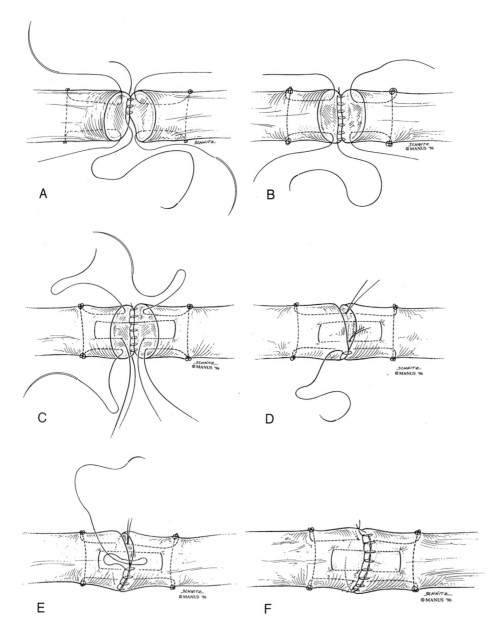

A

B

C

D

E

F

Figure 21–49. *A,* Tajima "core" sutures in place. The back wall (dorsal) running lock peripheral epitendinous stitch is in progress. *B,* Back wall suture completed. *C,* Mattress "core" suture added in the palmar tendon gap. *D,* All "core" sutures tied. *E,* Completion of the running lock peripheral epitendinous suture. *F,* Repair completed.

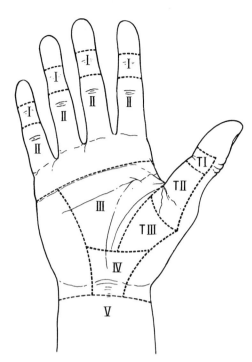

Figure 21–50. Flexor zones of the hand. Note thumb bones (T). (From Tubiana R: The Hand, vol 3. Philadelphia, WB Saunders, 1986, p 172.)

In situations in which diagnosis or treatment of the flexor tendon injury is delayed, the patient is often best served by doing a two-staged reconstruction. This involves placement of a silicon rod, as designed by Hunter within the existing flexor tendon sheath or a reconstructed sheath when excessive scarring is present. The patient is allowed to undergo passive range of motion for approximately 3 months. The immune reaction to the mobile silicon rod creates a synovial sheath. This allows a gliding surface for a tendon graft that is placed at a later procedure.

EXTENSOR TENDON INJURIES

Extensor tendon injuries were once thought to be simple problems that required very little thought in repair or rehabilitation. However, as we understand these problems better, we realize that they are nearly as complex as flexor tendon injuries and often as hard to obtain a good outcome. The zones of injury (Fig. 21–51) are labeled I through IX (Table 21–2). The zone I injuries are given the eponym of a mallet finger because they cause a droop of the distal phalanx at the DIP joint. These are frequently closed injuries, and they can be treated with extension splinting in a Stack or other type of splint. Many bony mallet fractures can also be treated in the same fashion. Untreated mallet fingers can lead to a significant imbalance in the finger, causing a so-called swan-neck deformity with DIP flexion and PIP hyperextension. The lateral bands become dorsally migrated and stuck in that position, and this further accentuates the deformity. Several reconstructions are available for this type of deformity, but early recognition and treatment of mallet deformities can frequently avoid this difficult situation.

Zone II extensor tendon injuries are more often due to

a laceration or crush injury. If they are incomplete they can be treated with active motion in 7 to 10 days. When complete, however, they should be sutured and an appropriate splinting regimen started. Zone III injuries are those directly over the PIP joint; they cause what is called a "boutonniére" deformity. Here, the central slip of the extensor tendon is disrupted and the PIP joint goes into a flexion deformity. These injuries are frequently closed, and when this is the case they can be treated with a splinting regimen that involves maintenance of full extension at the

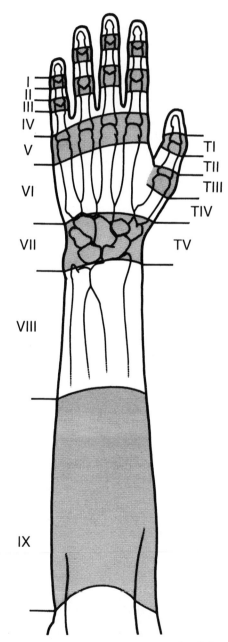

Figure 21–51. Zones of extensor tendon injury. The extensor mechanism can be injured from the fingertip to the mid and proximal forearm. Nine zones (I to IX) have been identified to aid in the classification and discussion of treatment (see Table 21–2). (From Green DP, Hotchkiss RN, Pederson WC [eds]: Operative Hand Surgery, 4th ed. New York, Churchill Livingstone, 1999, p 1956.)

Table 21–2. Zones of injury

Zone	Finger	Thumb
I	DIP joint	Interphalangeal joint
II	Middle phalanx	Proximal phalanx
III	PIP joint	MCP joint
IV	Proximal phalanx	Metacarpal
V	MCP joint	Carpometacarpal joint/radial
VI	Metacarpal	styloid
VII	Dorsal retinaculum	
VIII	Distal forearm	
IX	Mid- and proximal forearm	

DIP = distal interphalangeal; PIP = proximal interphalangeal; MCP = metacarpophalangeal.

PIP joint while allowing flexion at the DIP and MP joints. Open lacerations in this region often enter the PIP joint, and the wound should be thoroughly debrided and the tendon primarily repaired. When these injuries go untreated, the chronic boutonniére deformity results: there is fixed flexion at the PIP joint, the lateral bands become subluxed volar to the axis of rotation of the PIP joint, and they cause a hyperextension deformity at the distal phalanx. This can be a very difficult problem to treat. One option is the Fowler procedure; it involves release of the terminal extensor tendon from the distal phalanx base to allow for correction of the hyperextension deformity at the DIP joint and provide more extensor force at the PIP joint. Another option is repair of the central slip with re-establishment of the lateral bands dorsal to the axis of rotation of the PIP joint. Extensor tendon injuries in the other zones generally require direct repair. Of particular note is injury to the sagittal bands. When the sagittal bands are ruptured at the level of the MP joint, the extensor tendon can subluxate, usually in an ulnar direction. When this is a closed, traumatic acute tear this injury can often be successfully treated by immobilization of the MP joint in full extension for 4 to 6 weeks. In other situations an open repair should be performed (Fig. 21–52).

Nerve Repair

Nerve injury from lacerations or crush injuries to the hand are relatively common, and one should always be careful to examine for loss of sensation or motor function. When a lacerated nerve is found, surgical repair is generally indicated. The key aspects of repair are meticulous microsurgical technique with appropriate equipment, magnification, and suture. One must be very careful to resect all damaged nerve tissue, because the resulting scar tissue will prevent nerve healing. The nerve repair must be tension free. When this is not possible with direct suture, an interposition graft should be used. In general, epineural repair should be performed, because the results of grouped fascicular and other more involved repairs have not proven superior. Postoperative motor and sensory re-education can help maximize the patient's result.

Replantation

Advances in microsurgical techniques and instrumentation in the late 1950s and early 1960s led to the ability to replant detached limbs. The first arm replantation was performed in 1962 by Roger Malt in Boston, and the first thumb replant was performed by Komatsu Tamai in Japan in 1965. Since these early efforts, our ability to perform this procedure has improved steadily. Reports of survival rates for clean digital amputations with no crush or avulsion component are now greater than 90% when replantation is performed in experienced centers. Issues now focus on indications for replantation to optimize patient function and return to work.

Whenever a part of the hand or upper extremity is amputated, the initial care should involve wrapping the part in saline-soaked gauze and placing it inside a plastic bag or sterile container. This should be placed on ice for transport to the definitive care center. The treating physician should perform a routine evaluation of the injury and focus on some specific aspects of the amputation. Which digit is involved is very important; replanted border digits tend not to be used because of secondary stiffness. The type of injury (i.e., a sharp, guillotine-type amputation versus one with extensive crush or avulsion components), the number of digits involved, and the level of injury are all crucial pieces of information. The duration of ischemia is very important; ischemia time of more than 12 hours for the digits or more than 6 hours for areas proximal to the wrist leads to a very poor outcome. Cooling of parts can help allow an ischemia time of 24 hours for digits and 10 to 12 hours for major limbs. The amount of contamination should be assessed, as well as the patient's age, other associated injuries, and ability to cooperate with a prolonged rehabilitation period.

The generally accepted indications for replantation at this time include thumb amputation, multiple digit amputation, amputations that are at the level of the wrist or proximal and transmetacarpal amputations, or any amputation in a child. Contraindications include severe crush injury, multiple level injury in the same digit, degloving injuries, massive contamination, prolonged ischemia time, prolonged warm ischemia time, or a frozen part. Relative contraindications are amputation of a single digit other than the thumb and an amputation distal to the DIP joint.

When replantation is to be attempted, the first step is a thorough debridement of both the proximal and distal parts with careful isolation of the vital structures, including the blood vessels, nerves, tendon, and so on. The bone should be shortened and fixed first to allow for decreased tension on the neurovascular structures. After this, the extensors and then the flexors should be repaired, followed by repair of the arteries, the nerves, and the veins. Obviously, careful microvascular technique should be adhered to. There is significant controversy about postoperative anticoagulation. Several different regimens are available, including the use of aspirin alone, heparin, dextran, or other anticoagulants to prevent early thrombosis of the replanted digits.

As stated earlier, the survival rates for clean amputations that are replanted approach 90%. They are significantly worse for crush- or avulsion-type injuries. The functional results, however, vary greatly. Urbaniak has shown in his study that replantation of digits other than the thumb that are done distal to the FDS insertion have the best results. These had significantly less contracture of the PIP joints than those replanted proximally. Aside from stiffness, lack

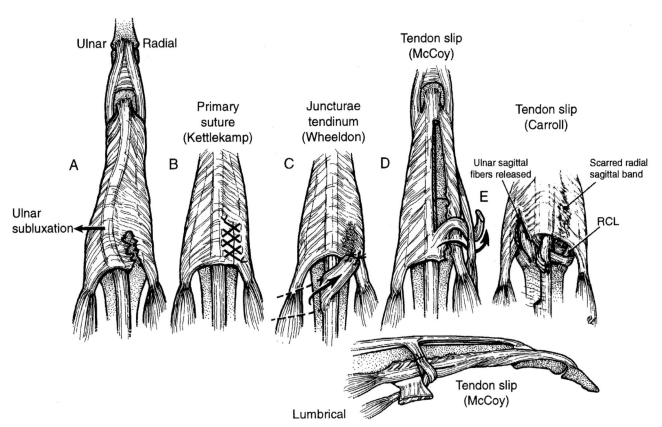

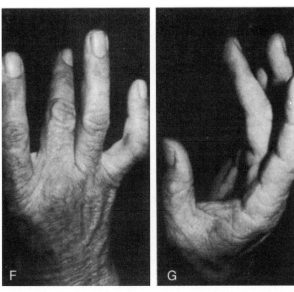

Figure 21–52. Nonrheumatoid subluxation or dislocation of the extensor tendon at the metaphalangeal joint usually occurs after forceful flexion or extension of the finger. The lesion is secondary to a tear of the radial portion of the sagittal band *(A)*, which allows ulnar subluxation of the extensor tendon. Although acute lacerations (relatively rare injuries) or spontaneous ruptures are satisfactorily treated by primary suture of the laceration or rupture using a cross stitch *(B)*, closed sagittal band injuries are best treated by splinting if seen within 2 weeks of injury. Late cases may require additional reconstruction. *(C)*, Wheeldon described a method using a portion of the junctura tendinum to stabilize the tendon over the dorsum of the joint. The junctura is lapped over the extensor tendon and sutured to the joint capsule on the radial side. *D*, McCoy and Winsky also devised a technique for stabilizing the extensor by removing a portion of the extensor tendon on the radial side of the finger, passing it around the lumbrical tendon, and suturing it back to itself. *E*, Carroll and colleagues modified a technique originally described by Kilgore and associates for stabilizing the extensor by forming a distally based slip of tendon from the ulnar side of the extensor digitorum communis, wrapping it around the radial collateral ligament (RCL), and then suturing it back to itself under proper tension. *F* and *G*, The clinical picture of chronic ulnar subluxation of the extensor tendon in the long finger. Note the ulnar deviation and extensor lag. (From Green DP, Hotchkiss RN, Pederson WC [eds]: Operative Hand Surgery, 4th ed. New York, Churchill Livingstone, 1999, p 1979.)

of sensibility, cold sensitivity, and chronic pain can be significant problems. Return of protective sensation often occurs with primary repair or grafting of the digital nerve when the replantation is done.

In summary, replantation is a powerful tool but has many downsides to it. One should use very judicious evaluation of the patient and careful decision making in deciding to perform this major surgery.

APPROACH TO THE MANGLED HAND AND FOREARM

Mangling injuries to the hand and forearm can be some of the most devastating injuries in a person's life. The injuries can occur from industrial, agricultural, or domestic machinery as well as in situations with high-velocity gunshot wounds and motor vehicle accidents. In general, a treating physician should take a careful assessment of the extent of the injury and what parts remain and what has been lost. After this the patient should be taken to the operating room for a very aggressive debridement at the initial stage. The decision of amputation versus limb salvage should be made only after reassessment at this time. In centers where these types of injuries are commonly seen and an aggressive team approach can be performed, it has been advocated that a full reconstruction of bone and soft tissues be performed at the initial setting. This helps prevent further loss of function secondary to immobilization. In most centers, however, this is not an option; therefore, after the initial debridement, stabilization of the bones and any vascular reconstruction should be performed. This should be followed as soon as possible by soft tissue reconstruction for coverage of the wound and a carefully thought out reconstruction protocol to maximize the patient's function. These patients all require an extensive, long-term rehabilitation and support; their ability to cooperate with this situation should be part of the decision-making process for limb salvage versus amputation.

COMPRESSIVE NEUROPATHIES

Compressive neuropathies are due to mechanical compression leading to local nerve ischemia and dysfunction. In the upper extremity, they tend to occur in predictable areas and have a common pathophysiology with various amounts of compression leading to increasing injury to the nerve. Traction is also thought to have a role in this disease process. When diagnosed and released early, nerve recovery is predictably good; however, after long-standing injury, decompression may only halt the progression of disease rather than reverse the symptoms.

The generalized assessment of the patient in whom a compressive neuropathy is suspected should involve careful history and physical examination. One should focus on finding objective signs of sensory or motor changes and trying to isolate the exact level at which the compression is present. The concept of a double crush phenomenon should be carefully kept in mind as well. Patients with cervical radiculopathy can develop decreased axoplasmic transport along the nerve and become more susceptible to distal nerve compression. In these cases both sites may require decompression. Some predisposing factors to compressive neuropathy include systemic or inflammatory processes such as diabetes, hyperthyroidism, rheumatoid arthritis, and infection. Conditions that alter fluid balance, including pregnancy and hemodialysis, sarcoidosis, lipidosis, and abnormal anatomical morphology including supracondylar processes or persistent median arteries, and acute injuries that can cause swelling or hematoma in the region of the nerve should be investigated. Sensory testing should be carefully performed; it should include some measure of vibratory or two-point discrimination. Electromyographic (EMG) and nerve conduction velocity studies are often the only objective tests that can help assess these problems. They are particularly useful in patients who have secondary gain issues, especially workers' compensation patients who may be well versed in the signs and symptoms of common neuropathies such as carpal tunnel or cubital tunnel syndrome.

Carpal tunnel syndrome, or compression of the median nerve as it passes underneath the transverse carpal ligament, is the most common upper extremity compressive neuropathy. Symptoms initially start as numbness, which is mainly in the radial volar distribution of the hand and usually worse at night. This progresses to pain and paresthesias, and it can manifest as motor weakness and wasting in the thenar region after long periods of compression. At times pain will radiate proximally up the arm to the shoulder. On physical examination, provocative testing includes Tinel's test, which involves tapping over the transverse carpal ligament. The test is positive if this elicits paresthesias in the median nerve distribution of the hand. Another commonly used provocative test is Phalen's test, in which the wrist is flexed maximally; if numbness or paresthesias are elicited within 60 seconds the test is considered positive. A carpal tunnel compression test is probably the most sensitive of provocative tests. It involves direct compression of the transverse carpal ligament region with the examiner's thumb, and if paresthesias are elicited within 30 seconds the test is considered positive.

Non-operative treatment includes wrist splinting in a neutral position at night, oral anti-inflammatory medications to decrease synovitis and edema, and management of underlying medical problems. Corticosteroid injections can be performed directly into the carpal tunnel, and for 80% of patients this will provide a transient relief but only 22% have continued symptomatic relief at 12 months. In patients who have less than 1 year of symptoms, normal two-point discrimination, less than 1 to 2 msec of prolongation of their sensory and motor latencies, and no denervation potentials or atrophy, 40% will be symptom-free at 1 year after a corticosteroid injection. Even in patients who do not have lasting relief, an initial transient alleviation of symptoms is a good prognostic factor for surgical release of the transverse carpal ligament.

Indications for release of the carpal ligament include failure of the previously mentioned conservative treatments, the presence of weakness or denervation potentials, or rapidly progressive symptoms. Although carpal tunnel release is the most common procedure performed by hand surgeons, the best method for performing it is still a very controversial issue. Many authors recommend an endoscopic release of the transverse carpal ligament, either through a single- or a double-portal technique. They state that the advantages include shorter return to work and less pillar pain. Recent studies, however, have shown that the difference in outcomes between open and endoscopic carpal tunnel release is minimal and these small benefits must be weighed against significant potential complications. The most common complication after endoscopic carpal tunnel release is incomplete release, but injuries to the superficial arch, the median and ulnar nerves, and the flexor tendons have all been reported. The incidence of pillar pain has not been eliminated by endoscopic carpal tunnel release either. This palmar pain is poorly understood, and some have thought that is due to alteration of the pisotriquetral joint mechanics. Another formerly controversial area is the use of internal neurolysis; studies have shown conclusively that it adds no benefit at all to the simple release of the transverse carpal ligament and it subjects the nerve to considerable potential harm. It should not be performed.

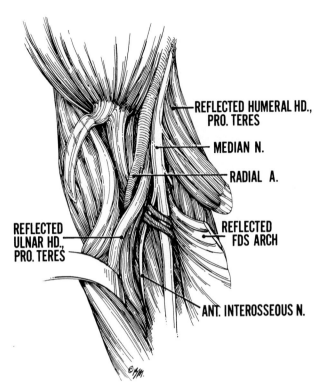

Figure 21–53. The radial origin of the flexor digitorum superficialis muscle is elevated by subperiosteal dissection to expose the deep volar compartment and the anterior interosseous nerve. (From Green DP, Hotchkiss RN, Pederson WC [eds]: Operative Hand Surgery, 4th ed. New York, Churchill Livingstone, 1999, p 1420.)

Pronator syndrome involves median nerve compression at one of several potential proximal sites including a supracondylar process of the humerus with an accompanying ligament of Struthers, the bicipital aponeurosis, the arch of the origin of the pronator teres, and the origin of the flexor digitorum superficialis (Fig. 21–53). Diagnostic features that help distinguish this from carpal tunnel syndrome include the presenting symptom of pain in the volar forearm that increases with activity, numbness in the palmar cutaneous branch distribution, a negative result of Phalen's test, a positive result of Tinel's test in the forearm, pain in the forearm with resisted pronation, or pain with resisted flexion of the PIP joints of the long and ring fingers. X-rays should be obtained to rule out a supracondylar process, and EMG and nerve conduction tests are very helpful in distinguishing this from carpal tunnel syndrome. Initial treatment is conservative with rest and long-arm splinting the elbow in 90 degrees of flexion and slight supination. If the patient fails up to 6 months of nonoperative treatment, then exploration and decompression of the previously mentioned sites should be performed. However, the outcomes are variable after surgical decompression.

A slightly more distal median nerve compression results in an anterior interosseous syndrome. The anterior interosseous nerve divides from the median nerve 4 to 6 cm below the elbow. It innervates the FPL, FDP to the index and middle fingers, and the pronator quadratus. It has absolutely no sensory innervation. This nerve branch can be com-

pressed under tendinous bands from the deep head of the pronator teres, the origin of the FDS, or the origin of the FCR. Symptoms with which a patient presents are forearm pain followed by paresis or paralysis of the previously mentioned muscles. The differential diagnosis includes rupture of the FPL, and sometimes this can be very confusing because patients can present with isolated decreased strength in a single digit. Further differential includes brachial neuritis or partial lesion of the median nerve or the lateral cord. Initial treatment involves splinting of the elbow for 8 to 12 weeks. If the patient fails 3 to 6 months of conservative management, then surgical decompression is recommended.

The ulnar nerve can be compressed in two major regions, the first being the elbow and the second being the wrist. At the elbow there are five general sites of compression (Fig. 21–54). The first and most proximal is in the region of the intramuscular septum; compression here can be caused by an arcade of Struthers (a dorsal fibrous structure), by the medial intramuscular septum itself, by hypertrophy of the medial head of the triceps, or by a snapping medial head of the triceps. The second major site is the region of the medial epicondyle in which compression can be caused by a valgus deformity of a bone or if the nerve actually subluxes outside of the groove. The epicondylar groove itself is another site of compression: any lesion within the groove including bony outcroppings or an anconeus epitrochlearis anomalous muscle can cause neuropathy. Just distal to this, in the cubital tunnel, compression can be caused by a thickened ligament of Osborne,

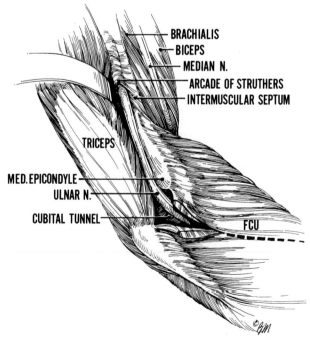

Figure 21–54. Mobilization of the ulnar nerve and any associated vessels necessitates decompression of the cubital tunnel, fasciotomy of the flexor carpi ulnaris, and dissection along the ulnar nerve, at least 8 cm proximal to the medial epicondyle. (From Green DP, Hotchkiss RN, Pederson WC [eds]: Operative Hand Surgery, 4th ed. New York, Churchill Livingstone, 1999, p 1425.)

the fascia of the two heads of FCU. As it exits from underneath the FCU, the nerve can enter the fifth site compression by the deep flexor pronator aponeurosis. These patients present with symptoms varying from mild numbness and paresthesias in the ring and small fingers to severe medial elbow pain, dysesthesias, and hand weakness. Full physical examination of the neck and arm is indicated to rule out cervical or thoracic outlet compression. The two provocative tests in this region include the elbow flexion test in which the elbow is maintained in full flexion with the wrist in full extension for 1 minute. If paresthesias or numbness occurs in an ulnar nerve distribution, this is positive. Tinel's testing in the cubital tunnel region can also be very helpful. When the patient has clear-cut symptoms and physical examination findings, an EMG and nerve conduction test is not required, but it can be helpful in equivocal cases. These tests are also very helpful in determining the site of nerve compression and eliminating polyneuropathy or motor neuron disease from the differential. Initial treatment is conservative with extension splinting at night, rest, and avoidance of provocative activities. If this management fails, surgical options include decompression in situ, medial epicondylectomy, anterior subcutaneous transposition, anterior intramuscular transposition, and submuscular transposition. Decompression in situ is contraindicated in patients with subluxation of the tendon and also for patients with severe neuropathy. The other procedures overall have very similar results. We recommend anterior subcutaneous transposition except for revision situations, when submuscular transposition should be performed.

The ulnar nerve can also be entrapped at Guyon's canal of the wrist, a condition called ulnar tunnel syndrome (Fig. 21–55). This can be caused by stenosis of the canal secondary to a tight volar carpal ligament or compression secondary to ganglions, lipomas, fractures of the hook of the hamate, or thrombosis or aneurysm of the ulnar artery. Tinel's testing and the absence of numbness in the dorsal ulnar cutaneous branch distribution can help with making a diagnosis. EMG and nerve conduction velocities are also quite helpful. Release of the volar carpal ligament and addressing any other pathology can completely relieve the symptoms if caught relatively early.

Compression of the radial nerve in the vicinity of the elbow can produce two different types of syndromes despite compression at the same sites. The nerve bifurcates into a superficial branch and a posterior interosseous branch just proximal to the elbow. The posterior interosseous nerve can become compressed just distal to this by fibrous bands from the radiocapitellar joint, the recurrent radial vessels, the tendinous origin of the ECRB, the tendinous origin of the supinator (the arcade of Frohse), and also at the distal fascial edge of the supinator as it exits from underneath (Fig. 21–56). One syndrome that arises from compression at these sites is called posterior interosseous syndrome. Entrapment is most common at the proximal edge of the supinator, but compression can also occur from rheumatoid synovitis of the radiocapitellar joint or by ganglia in the region. Patients have no sensory deficit. They rarely complain of pain, but they have complete or partial motor paralysis in the posterior interosseous nerve distribution. One way to differentiate this from a more proximal radial nerve palsy is the fact that wrist extension is preserved by

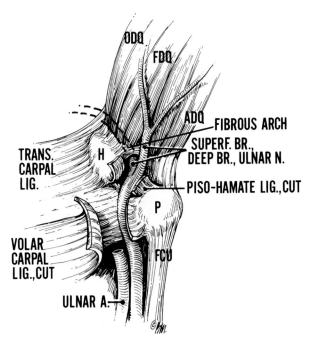

Figure 21–55. The ulnar nerve courses through Guyon's canal between the volar carpal ligament and the transverse carpal ligament. ODQ, opponens digiti quinti (muscle); FDQ, flexor digiti quinti (muscle); ADQ, abductor digiti quinti (muscle); P, pisiform; H, hamate; FCU, flexor carpi ulnaris. (From Green DP, Hotchkiss RN, Pederson WC [eds]: Operative Hand Surgery, 4th ed. New York, Churchill Livingstone, 1999, p 1431.)

the intact innervation of the ECRL. Initial treatment can include up to 12 weeks of rest and observation from the onset of symptoms. However, if there is any failure to improve or if symptoms progress at all during this time period, surgical decompression of the posterior interosseous nerve should be undertaken without further delay. All possible sites of compression should be released, and good to excellent results can be expected in more than 85% of patients, although it may take up to 18 months for full recovery to occur.

Radial tunnel syndrome is a condition that starts with a chief complaint of pain in the proximal radial forearm. The symptoms are often work related, with repetitive elbow extension or supination being two of the possible inciting activities. The pain is usually described as deep and aching. On physical examination, tenderness over the radial nerve approximately four fingerbreaths distal to the lateral epicondyle is one of the hallmark findings. Pain on resisted middle finger extension with the elbow at 45 degrees of flexion and the wrist in neutral as well as pain on resisted supination are the key provocative tests. The main differential diagnosis is lateral epicondylitis, and it is often very difficult to distinguish these two. Selective injection with 1% lidocaine into the region of the posterior interosseous nerve that produces a complete palsy of this nerve is one of the most helpful tests if it causes complete relief of pain. One should note that lateral epicondylitis and radial tunnel syndrome co-exist in up to 5 to 10% of patients, and in some situations release of both of these problems is required. This disease has never been documented to progress to motor loss, and initial treatment for radial tunnel syndrome is always conservative with rest and avoidance distinguishing these various entities. When Wartenberg's syndrome is diagnosed, the initial treatment is non-operative with splinting, NSAIDs, and change in work activities. If this fails, then surgical release is indicated.

The last compressive neuropathy to be discussed here is thoracic outlet syndrome. There are two types of this condition; one is vascular and one is neurogenic. The vascular type is more common and usually involves compression of the subclavian artery. The neurogenic variety is relatively rare, and the diagnosis is generally a clinical one. The compression is due to such structures as cervical ribs, the scalene muscles, abnormal fibrous bands, or a hypertrophic head of the sternocleidomastoid muscle compromising the space available for the brachial plexus (Fig. 21–57). The condition is found most commonly in young or middle-aged females. Symptoms are variable but can include frequent headaches, neck pain, and non-specific pain and weakness in the upper extremity. More classically, it will present in a pattern similar to ulnar nerve compression at the elbow combined with neck pain and neurologic symptoms that are worse with overhead activity. Adson's test, which involves obliteration of the radial pulse with slight abduction of the shoulder in the coronal plane and rotation of the neck to the affected side, as well as Roos' test, which involves numbness or tingling of the ulnar-sided digits with 90 degrees of abduction of the shoulder, 90 degrees of external rotation, and opening and closing the hands rapidly for up to 3 minutes help make the diagnosis. Electrophysiologic testing is sometimes equivocal but can be helpful in making a diagnosis. X-rays of the neck and chest should be performed to help check for cervical ribs,

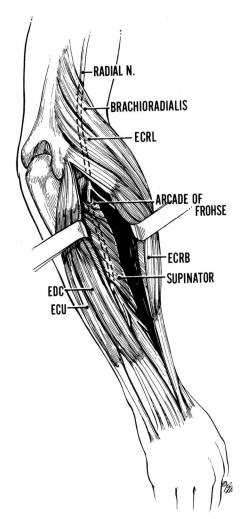

Figure 21–56. Extension of the posterior Thompson approach to the radial tunnel. ECRL, extensor carpi radialis longus; ECRB, extensor carpi radialis brevis; EDC, extensor digitorum communis; ECU, extensor carpi ulnaris. (From Green DP, Hotchkiss RN, Pederson WC [eds] Operative Hand Surgery, 4th ed. New York, Churchill Livingstone, 1999, p 1436.)

of provocative positions. Splinting with the wrist in dorsiflexion and the forearm in slight supination is also useful. If this fails, then surgical exploration and decompression of the nerve can be attempted. Unfortunately, the published results for this procedure show good to excellent outcomes in only 40 to 70% of patients.

The superficial radial nerve is a purely sensory branch that runs in the forearm underneath the brachioradialis and exits dorsally between the tendons of the brachioradialis and the ECRL. It can become compressed between these two tendons, especially with forearm pronation. This condition is known as Wartenberg's syndrome. Patients typically present with pain, numbness, and paresthesias over the dorsoradial aspect of the wrist radiating down to the first web space dorsally. This is made worse with pronation of the wrist or wrist extension. The differential diagnosis includes de Quervain's tenosynovitis, which can usually be distinguished by a good physical examination, as well as lateral antebrachial cutaneous nerve compression. Selective injection with local anesthetics again is very helpful in

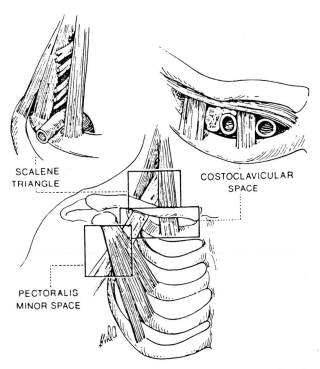

Figure 21–57. Three sites of possible compression for thoracic outlet compression syndrome. (From Berger AC, Kleinert JM: Work-related vascular injuries and diseases. *In* Kasdan ML [ed]: Occupational Hand and Upper Extremity Injuries and Diseases. Philadelphia, Hanley and Belfus, 1991, pp 319–339.)

Pancoast's tumors, and other diseases or anomalies. Cervical stenosis and radiculopathy are among the chief conditions in the differential diagnosis. This condition should be treated non-operatively for a long period of time unless there is an obvious structural abnormality that is found in the evaluation. Initial therapy includes strengthening of the upper extremity, the trapezius, and neck muscles as well as stretching and postural exercises. In addition, weight loss and other modalities can be helpful. If these fail, then surgical treatment options include anterior scalenotomy, exploration and resection of any anomalous fibrous bands, or first rib resection through an axillary approach. Transaxillary first rib resection has reported 90% good-to-excellent results. There is considerable risk in this procedure. Patients should be carefully counseled regarding the potential complications from any of these surgical procedures.

ARTHRITIC CONDITIONS OF THE HAND AND WRIST

Degenerative Arthritis

Degenerative arthritis is a disease that occurs in diarthrodial joints when abnormal cartilage or abnormal loading is present. It tends to be a progressive condition that produces focal erosive lesions, cartilage destruction, subchondral sclerosis, and cyst formation, as well as peripheral osteophyte formation. It can be classified as either primary, which tends to be a disease of older women with no underlying risk factor or injury in a given joint, or secondary, which is due to underlying factors including trauma, osteonecrosis, developmental dyplasia, or metabolic abnormality such as calcium pyrophosphate deposition disease.

Patients present mainly with pain, decreased range of motion, and sometimes progressive deformity. X-rays show characteristic findings of decreased joint space, indicating cartilage loss, subchondral cyst formation, subchondral sclerosis, and peripheral osteophyte formation. Other imaging studies are rarely necessary. The most commonly involved sites in the hand and wrist include the DIP joint, the PIP joint, the trapeziometacarpal joint, the STT joint, and the region around the scaphoid and lunate in post-traumatic SLAC wrist-type problems. Initial treatment is usually non-operative and involves rest, splinting (especially when there is any kind of instability), therapy to maintain supporting muscle strength and range of motion, and non-steroidal anti-inflammatory medications. Intra-articular corticosteroid injections can also provide excellent symptomatic relief.

Surgical intervention should be considered when the patient has deformity or instability that interferes with function or pain refractory to non-operative treatment. Treatment options need to be carefully individualized to the patient and to the affected joint; they include debridement, arthroplasty, and arthrodesis. Our discussion of these treatment options is directed toward the individual joints.

The DIP joint is one of the most frequently involved. Often arthritis at this joint presents as a mucous cyst on the dorsolateral aspect of the joint, which frequently can be painful. When excising the cyst one needs to be sure to debride the underlying osteophyte that caused it. In severe cases, particularly when there is instability resulting in pain or inability to pinch, arthrodesis is indicated. This should be done in 15 degrees of flexion of the index and cascade to 30 degrees for the small finger.

The PIP joint is also frequently involved. Large osteophytes can form, giving characteristic dorsal prominences called Bouchard's nodes. Surgical indications again are severe pain, deformities, and instability. The goals are to create a stable post in the index and sometimes the middle finger for pinch. In the small finger one would prefer to maintain motion to allow for power grip. Debridement is rarely indicated at the PIP joint. Arthroplasty can be done, and the silicon interposition arthroplasties are the best available treatments for this. One can expect a 50- to 60-degree arc of motion with fair radioulnar stability. Patients tend to have improved grasp secondary to painless motion in more useful arc. Another option that is useful for patients who have mainly volar arthritis (sometimes secondary to an older fracture dislocation) is volar plate arthroplasty, in which the volar plate is advanced into the area where there is cartilage and bone loss and allowed to heal in this position. This allows relatively pain free motion at the joint. Arthrodesis is also an option, but it should be reserved for the index and middle fingers unless other finger joints are considered essentially unsalvageable. PIP joints should be fused in 40 degrees of flexion for the index finger and cascade to 55 degrees for the small finger if necessary.

The MP joints are less frequently involved in degenerative arthritis. When they are it is usually post-traumatic in nature. When severe painful arthritis is present, a silicon implant arthroplasty is the procedure of choice, and results are excellent.

The trapeziometacarpal joint is one of the most common sites of hand and wrist arthritis that eventually will require surgical intervention. It starts with mild instability secondary to attenuation of the volar beak ligament and progresses to the loss of the joint space anteriorly and dorsoradial subluxation, leading to a metacarpal adduction deformity. It also leads to progressive MP hyperextension deformity, further impairing the patient's ability to grasp objects or oppose the thumb. In the early stages when subluxation alone is present, ligament reconstruction with local tendons is an excellent option. When a higher stage of the disease is present with volar degeneration and mild sclerotic changes, one can consider a 30-degree closing wedge osteotomy of the metacarpal to shift the load to the dorsal half of the joint. This is a particularly good option for young laborers. Stage III disease of the trapeziometacarpal joint implies end-stage degenerative changes. The treatment options include fusion or arthroplasty. Fusion was quite popular in the past. It produced excellent relief of pain despite high rates of radiographic nonunion. However, the loss of range of motion and the excellent results of arthroplasty have made this procedure less popular. Several implant arthroplasties have been available since the mid 1960s. The Swanson silicon arthroplasty was one of the earliest. It provided excellent pain relief but resulted in many complications including recurrent subluxation and silicon synovitis, so it is rarely used now. Other implants such as metal and polyethylene hemi- and total joint arthroplasties for trapeziometacarpal arthritis have had reasonably good results, with instability being one of the few complications.

Non-implant arthroplasties of the trapeziometacarpal joint have been present for many years as well. Excision arthroplasty was one of the earliest options. It was introduced in the late 1940s and gave excellent results for pain relief. Many hand surgeons, however, thought that this procedure resulted in weakness and excessive proximal migration of the metacarpal base. In 1970, Carroll and Froimson popularized tendon interposition arthroplasty. This procedure involves resection of the trapezium and use of either the PL or a portion of the FCR tendon, which is harvested separately and rolled up and sutured into a "anchovy" interposition. This is placed in the site of the resected trapezium and used as a spacer to allow for scar formation. Results show excellent relief of pain; however, many patients do have proximal migration of their metacarpal base as well as decreased pinch strength. More recently, the concept of ligament reconstruction and tendon interposition arthroplasty was introduced by Burton and Pelligrini (Fig. 21–58). The procedure calls for resection of the trapezium, followed by reconstruction of the volar beak ligament by passing a segment of the FCR tendon through a drill hole in the base of the first metacarpal. Further tendon is rolled up into an interposition graft to help fill the void from the previously present trapezium. The results of this procedure have been outstanding, with reproducible and predictable increases in grip and pinch strength as well as excellent pain relief. Many variations on this procedure have been developed with the use of different local tendons

and different types of weaves. Most have produced similarly excellent results with shorter follow-up available.

The procedure of choice for arthritis at this joint is still quite controversial. Some recent studies have questioned the need for interposition or ligament reconstruction, stating that functional results show no difference when compared with straight excisional arthroplasty. My feeling, however, is that ligament reconstruction and tendon interposition are important adjuncts in maintaining pinch strength.

Isolated STT arthritis is much less common and even more rarely requires surgical intervention. Treatment options include joint debridement, limited resection and tendon interposition arthroplasty, and STT arthrodesis. No clear consensus is present as to which is the best procedure.

The SLAC wrist, as described earlier in the section about trauma, is the result of progressive degeneration from a scapholunate dissociation or a scaphoid fracture nonunion or malunion. This process begins with radial styloid arthritis and progresses to capitolunate and eventually proximal migration of the capitate (Fig. 21–59). The radiolunate joint is usually spared. If the capitolunate joint is minimally involved, an excellent surgical option is proximal row carpectomy, which can maintain range of motion and fairly good grip strength. Another option is scaphoid excision with capitate, hamate, triquetral, and lunate arthrodesis (Fig. 21–60). This is called an SLAC wrist procedure or CHTL fusion; it has had overall excellent results from the standpoint of pain relief; however, patients do lose approximately 50% of their wrist range of motion. In severe cases, wrist fusion is an excellent option but obviously sacrifices motion for pain relief.

DRUJ arthritis is often seen after fractures or instability of this joint. Patients present with painful pronation and supination. Surgical treatment options include resection of the distal ulna as described by Darrach, with or without an added ECU stabilization, hemiresection-interposition arthroplasty as described by Bowers, and synostosis of the distal radioulnar joint with proximal pseudarthrosis formation as described by Sauve and Kapandji.

Rheumatoid Arthritis

Rheumatoid arthritis is a systemic inflammatory autoimmune disease that affects initially the soft tissues and then secondarily bone. It leads to synovial proliferation within joints and around tendons. Progressive destruction of these tissues results in secondary antibody reactions followed by lysozyme release from white blood cells, oxygen free radical formation, and collagenase release from the synovium. Cartilage and ligamentous structures as well as tendons themselves are eventually affected, leading to joint pain, severe loss of motion, instability and resulting deformities, tendon ruptures, and compressive neuropathies. In stage I disease, patients have early tenosynovitis or synovitis and treatment is non-surgical. In stage II, there is persistent tenosynovitis or synovitis lasting beyond 3 to 6 months of non-operative treatment, and the recommended treatment is tenosynovectomy and synovectomy. Stage III involves specific deformities and requires surgical reconstruction. Stage IV involves severe crippling disease and requires

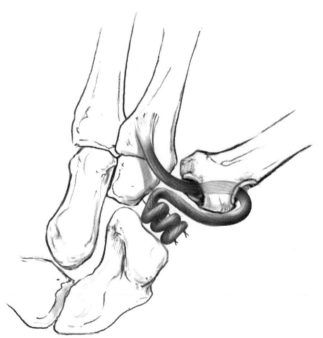

Figure 21–58. The ligament reconstruction tendon interposition (LRTI) as currently performed by Burton. The full thickness of flexor carpi radialis tendon attached only to the second metacarpal base is led through a hole at the first metacarpal base and is sutured back on itself to reconstruct an anterior ulnar ligament. The remainder is sewn accordion-style to make an interposition wad that replaces the completely excised trapezium. (From Lichtman DM, Alexander AH [eds]: The Wrist and its Disorders, 2nd ed. Philadelphia, WB Saunders, 1997, p 453.)

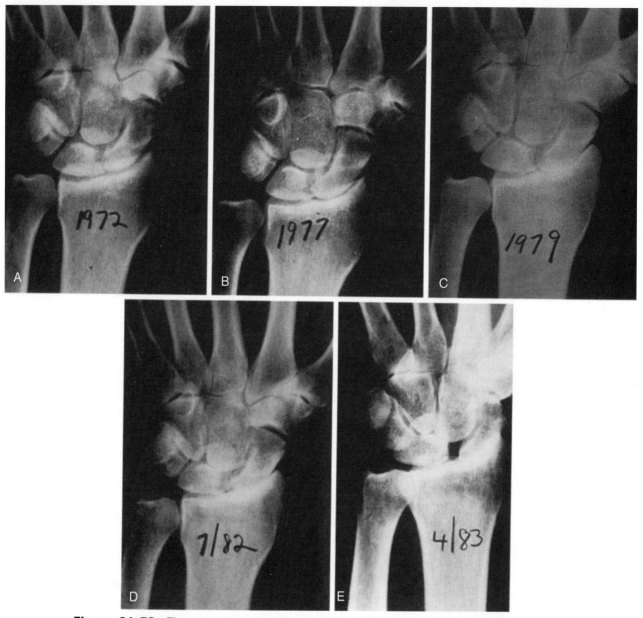

Figure 21–59. The natural progression of SLAC wrist. This 11-year sequence of x-rays demonstrates the progression to SLAC wrist, beginning with symptomatic dorsal wrist syndrome. *A*, In 1972, the patient is symptomatic from scapholunate overload without significant radiographic changes. *B*, The scaphoid is rotating under load, and early narrowing of the radioscaphoid joint is present. *C*, By 1979, complete destruction of the radioscaphoid joint and early narrowing of the capitolunate joint have occurred. *D*, By 1982, there is complete loss of the capitolunate joint space. *E*, By 1983, the scaphoid is now static in its displacement. There is erosion of the scaphoid into the radius, capitolunate joint destruction, hamate-lunate joint narrowing, and proximal migration of the capitate. The radiolunate joint, however, remains normal. (From Green DP, Hotchkiss RN, Pederson WC [eds]: Operative Hand Surgery, 4th ed. New York, Churchill Livingstone, 1999, p 123.)

salvage procedures, which are often fusions or joint replacement.

Non-operative management consists of initial rest and splinting, particularly for acute flare-ups; thereafter, exercise is instituted to maintain muscle mass and help with balance and function. Systemic medications are started, first with non-steroidal anti-inflammatory medications and progressing to corticosteroids, methotrexate, and other op-

tions. Local corticosteroid injections are useful, particularly for synovitis in a localized flare-up. Counseling should be instituted early on, so that patients can understand the course of their disease and what can be done to maintain and assist with their function.

Surgical intervention is directed toward the specific problems of the patient and their stage. For persistent tenosynovitis a tenosynovectomy is indicated. This is an

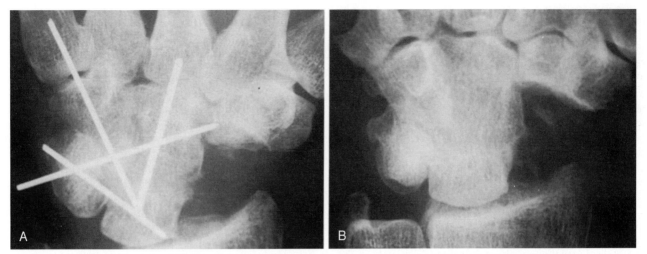

Figure 21–60. SLAC wrist reconstruction. *A,* Postoperative radiographic examination 6 weeks after SLAC reconstruction with limited wrist arthrodesis and scaphoid excision demonstrates typical pin placement and adequate bony consolidation. *B,* Six months after SLAC reconstruction, the arthrodesis is radiographically solid and the radiolunate joint well preserved. Note the ulnar displacement of the capitate on the lunate, which tightens the radioscaphocapitate ligament and prevents ulnar translation. (From Green DP, Hotchkiss RN, Pederson WC [eds]: Operative Hand Surgery, 4th ed. New York, Churchill Livingstone, 1999, p 126.)

excellent procedure with a very good predictable outcome. After tenosynovectomy, extensor tendon ruptures are extremely rare.

Tendon ruptures are caused by synovial infiltration and weakening, attritional wear from osteophytes, and iatrogenic causes such as injection in the region of the tendon. Some common patterns are present. The Vaughn-Jackson lesion is the best known and most common of these. It involves a subluxated, osteophytic, and often razor sharp ulnar head that causes EDM and EDC tendon ruptures. Lister's tubercle can also become osteophytic and razor sharp and cause rupture to the EPL tendon. The Mannerfelt lesion is a scaphotrapezial joint osteophyte that causes FPL rupture. The diagnosis of extensor tendon rupture is made when MP joints are passively correctable to full extension, but the patient cannot actively maintain this. There is also no tenodesis affect; therefore, passive wrist flexion does not result in MP extension. The diagnosis of a solitary EDM rupture is made by holding the index, middle, and ring fingers passively flexed and asking the patient to actively extend the small finger. Rupture of the EDM prevents independent extension of the small finger. The differential diagnosis of extensor tendon ruptures includes subluxation of the extensors at the MP joint, in which patients can maintain but cannot obtain active extension of the MP joint; subluxation of the MP joints, which is visible on x-rays; posterior interosseous nerve compressive neuropathy, in which the tenodesis effect is maintained but the patient has no active MP extension; and locked flexor tendon, in which patients are unable to passively extend the MP joint.

The treatment of extensor tendon ruptures involves resection of bony spikes, tenosynovectomy, and tendon reconstructions. For an isolated EPL rupture, one should transfer the extensor indicis proprius to the EPL as well as address the Mannerfelt lesion by resecting the osteophyte

and doing a local flap transfer of capsular tissue. This helps prevent rupture of adjacent profundus tendons. For an isolated EDM rupture, one should do an end-to-side transfer into the EDC of the small finger. When EDM and EDC of the ring and small finger tendons are ruptured, one should do an end-to-side transfer of the EDC of the ring to the middle finger and EIP transfer to the EDM. When multiple tendons are ruptured, one may also consider transferring one of the FDS tendons or the ECRL.

Flexor tenosynovitis is less common than extensor. Patients have better passive than active motion early on. The tenosynovitis can cause carpal tunnel syndrome and trigger fingers. These conditions should be treated with early tenosynovectomy rather than pulley or transverse carpal ligament release because the releases can lead to bowstringing and increased ulnar and radial deviation deformities. FPL rupture is the most common; and for this, one should debride the osteophyte at the STT joint and do a localized capsular flap to help cover the bones in this region. The tendon should be reconstructed with a small segmental graft or an FDS transfer. Ruptures of the individual digital flexors do quite poorly. Attempts at grafting and transfer of the FDS may provide some function, but it is very difficult to restore good range of motion. One may want to consider fusions of the involved joints.

In addressing the specific problems in rheumatoid arthritis that occur at the joints, we will start at the DRUJ. This frequently develops synovitis, leading to ligamentous attenuation as well as bone and cartilage destruction. The ECU tendon subluxates volarly and ulnarly, and the ulnar head becomes dorsally subluxated. This can lead to the Vaughn-Jackson lesion described earlier. The Darrach procedure, a resection of the ulnar head, is the most widely used procedure for rheumatoid DRUJ disease. When performing it, one should be careful to maintain an adequate periosteal sleeve for later re-suturing or supplement the procedure with an ECU or other tendon-stabilization procedure (Fig. 21–61). This avoids instability of the remaining distal ulna. The Sauve-Kapandji procedure involves fusion of the DRUJ and proximal pseudarthrosis through the ulna. This procedure preserves the TFCC and provides a buttress to ulnar migration of the carpus; however, one can still have proximal stump instability. The procedure is best used for younger patients who have limited disease. The Bowers hemi-resection interposition arthroplasty has little use in rheumatoid patients.

Radiocarpal changes that typically occur in rheumatoid arthritis start with synovitis, resulting in capsular distention and attenuation of the radiocarpal and ulnocarpal ligaments. This leads to intercarpal supination, radial deviation, and ulnar and volar drift deformities. Progression of the disease can lead to volar dislocation of the carpus or eventually a complete destruction of the cartilaginous surfaces of the wrist. Early treatment options include synovectomy, which has generally poor long-term results. When a patient has significant radial deviation deformity, one can consider an ECRL to ECU transfer; it helps balance the wrist and can also help prevent ulnar drift of the MP joints. With extensive radiocarpal but limited midcarpal disease, a radiocarpal arthrodesis is indicated. This helps prevent ulnar drift and continues to allow reasonably good flexion/extension. This procedure should not be used in rapidly progressive disease. In later stages of disease the options include arthroplasty and wrist fusion. Silicon implant arthroplasty was developed by Swanson. It can allow a pain-free arc of motion of 70 to 80 degrees of total combined flexion and extension. Problems with this have included implant failure as well as subsidence into the bone. This procedure should be limited to patients who have very low demand, reasonably good bone stock, and minimal tendon imbalance. Metal and polyethylene total wrist arthroplasties are available, but they have had high rates of loosening and progressive imbalance in several series. Total wrist arthrodesis combined with a Darrach procedure has been a very reliable option for relief of pain and restoration of hand balance in patients with rheumatoid arthritis. The methods for performing an arthrodesis include intermedullary Steinmann pin fixation as described by Nalebuff or new low-profile wrist fusion plates. The position of fusion is widely debated. When a unilateral wrist is fused, neutral to 5 degrees of wrist extension works well. The wrist should also be fused in approximately 10 degrees of ulnar deviation. It is important to avoid fusion in radial deviation. In bilateral fusions it is recommended that one wrist be fused in approximately 20 degrees of flexion to allow for perineal toilet care.

MP joint disease is one of the differentiating hallmarks between rheumatoid arthritis and osteoarthritis. Rheumatoid patients tend to develop a synovitis at the MP joint that attenuates the radial extensor hood sagittal fibers, making them weaker than the ulnar side. This, combined with the radial deviation of the wrist, leads to a moment arm that causes subluxation ulnarly of the extensor tendon. There is a stretch of the radial collateral ligament, and the MP joints tend to drift into ulnar deviation. The joints are further destabilized by the inflammatory destruction of the cartilaginous surfaces, which tends to start on the volar aspect. The ulnar intrinsics contract, creating a volar force, and this leads to ulnar and volar dislocation of the proximal phalangeal bases in late stages. Treatment in early situations is rest, splinting, and corticosteroid injections. Synovectomy can be attempted. This has mixed results but can temporize further problems when combined with ulnar intrinsic release and extensor tendon centralization. In later stages, MP arthroplasty provides an excellent option. Silastic implants as designed by Swanson and modified by others provide very good results with excellent pain relief, much improved arc of motion, improvement of the cosmetic deformity, as well as delay of disease progression. Patients rarely get an increase in strength, but because the arc of motion is in the more functional range they are able to do more functional activities with their hand. Some of the complications of MP arthroplasty in rheumatoid arthritis include recurrent ulnar drift, fracture of the prosthesis,

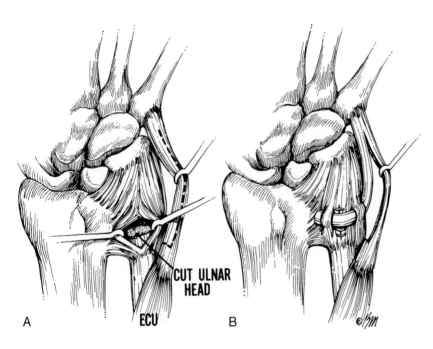

A   **CUT ULNAR HEAD**   **ECU**   B

Figure 21–61. Reconstruction of the distal radioulnar joint after synovectomy and distal ulna excision. *A*, The dorsal capsule of the distal radioulnar joint is opened longitudinally, a synovectomy is performed, and the distal ulna is excised. (The slip of tendon to be stripped from the extensor carpi ulnaris [ECU] is shown by the *dotted line*.) *B*, A strip of ECU is mobilized, passed through the ulnar aspect of the joint capsule and across the dorsal aspect of the joint, and sutured to the dorsal capsule over the radius to correct the supination deformity. The radioulnar joint capsule is imbricated to correct the dorsal subluxation of the distal ulna. The dorsal retinaculum can be used to further reinforce the radioulnar joint capsule. (From Green DP, Hotchkiss RN, Pederson WC [eds]: Operative Hand Surgery, 4th ed. New York, Churchill Livingstone, 1999, p 1689.)

and infection. Infection has very low rates and can be treated reasonably well by resection arthroplasty.

PIP joint involvement in rheumatoid arthritis usually leads to a boutonniére deformity but in some situations can cause a swan-neck deformity. The typical boutonniére deformity is caused by PIP synovitis and attenuation of the extensor tendon central slip. This creates a flexion deformity at the PIP joint, and the lateral bands sublux volarly. Contracture of the lateral bands in this subluxed position leads to a DIP joint hyperextension deformity. Early treatment in situations in which the deformity is passively correctable include PIP joint synovectomy and lateral band reconstruction; and in some cases it can be supplemented by distal Fowler's tenotomy, in which the extensor tendon insertion into the distal phalanx is recessed and the terminal tendon is allowed to drift proximally to create an extensor moment at the PIP joint. In late situations in which is there significant joint destruction and fixed deformity, arthroplasty or fusion is a treatment option.

The typical swan-neck deformity involves DIP flexion and PIP hyperextension deformities. The underlying cause can be one of many, including mallet finger, which leads to excessive extensor force over the PIP joint; PIP volar plate insufficiency, causing a hyperextension deformity at the PIP joint; FDS rupture; or an MP flexion deformity with subluxation causing excessive intrinsic tightness. The treatment is based on the underlying source and the rigidity of the deformity. Treatment options range from extension block splinting, tenotomy of the central slip, proximal Fowler's tenotomy, volar plate advancement, lateral band release or tenodesis volar to the axis of rotation of the PIP joint, spiral oblique retinacular ligament reconstruction, or arthrodesis of the PIP joint in 30 to 50 degrees of flexion. The arthrodesis should only be performed if MP joint is in an acceptable condition or about to undergo an arthroplasty.

Rheumatoid arthritis often involves the thumb. It tends to create characteristic patterns of deformity that fall into one of five classes. Type I is a boutonniére deformity with MP flexion and IP hyperextension. The underlying cause is EPB attenuation secondary to synovitis at the MP joint. This leads to an extensor lag and eventually a flexion contracture at the MP joint. The IP joint drifts secondarily into hyperextension with overpull of the EPL. Early treatment again involves a synovectomy and occasionally an EPL re-route to the base of the proximal phalanx. Unfortunately, this does have high rates of recurrence at the 6-year follow-up. In more advanced states with fixed deformity, an MP joint fusion can produce excellent results, especially if the IP and CMC joints are in good condition. Other options include IP joint fusion and MP joint arthroplasty, or fusion of both the MP and IP joint in advanced disease. Type II rheumatoid thumb is the least common. It involves a subluxated CMC joint with a boutonniére deformity distally. Treatment is to perform a trapeziometacarpal arthroplasty as per the surgeon's choice and then treat the MP and IP joints as described earlier for the boutonniére-type deformity. The type III rheumatoid thumb has a swan-neck deformity with an adducted metacarpal secondary to dorsoradial subluxation of the CMC joint. The treatment is a CMC arthroplasty of choice, fusion of the MP joint in neutral or slight flexion, and release of the first web space as needed. The type IV or "gamekeeper's" thumb has ulnar collateral ligament disruption at the MP joint secondary to synovitis, causing an instability at the MP joint. Early treatment involves synovectomy and ulnar collateral ligament reconstruction and adductor fascial release as needed. In later stages, one can perform an MP arthroplasty with an ulnar collateral ligament reconstruction or an MP joint fusion. Type V thumb has a swan-neck deformity secondary to MP joint disease with an intact trapeziometacarpal joint. Here the rheumatoid synovitis causes volar plate attenuation and a resultant MP hyperextension deformity. The IP joint drifts into a secondary flexion deformity. Unlike type II, the CMC joint has no disease and therefore this can be treated with MP volar plate advancement or MP joint fusion alone.

Other Arthritides

Psoriatic arthritis is an uncommon arthritis present in 5 to 10% of patients with generalized psoriasis. Hand involvement can be severe. Synovial disease here leads to either osteolysis or ankylosis and autofusion. Osteolysis most commonly involves the DIP joint with erosion of the middle phalangeal condyles into a spike, creating "pencil in cup" deformities. This can occur at all finger joints and cause severe deformity in a situation called arthritis mutilans. In this there is telescoping of the fingers, giving an appearance that has been called "opera glass hand" (Fig. 21–62). Spontaneous fusion can occur mainly at the DIP joints and occasionally at the PIP joints. This almost never occurs at the MP joints. Periarterial soft tissue thickening can give the fingers a "sausage" digit appearance. It is rare to have tendon involvement or rupture. Wrist involvement is fairly common, and one is most likely to see an ankylosis and then spontaneous fusion.

There is no role for synovectomy or tendon surgery in this disease. When the wrist is involved, arthrodesis and Darrach's resection are indicated. In the thumb, CMC arthroplasty and MP and IP joint fusions are indicated. In the other digits, osteotomy or arthroplasty can be performed for PIP ankylosis in poor position. Bone graft and fusion is often required to restore length and halt disease when osteolysis occurs at the DIP or PIP joints.

Gouty arthritis is a disease of monosodium urate crystal deposition. Hand surgeons are often consulted to help make the diagnosis and differentiate from infection or to treat the hand manifestations. Diagnosis is made by aspirating or obtaining tissue samples of the involved tissues or joints. Under polarized microscopy, one sees negatively birefringent, needle-like crystals. Treatment for acute flares involves use of indomethacin, colchicine, and other medications. Corticosteroid injections are warranted for patients who do not respond to oral medications. Patients who are also hyperuricemic should be maintained after their initial flare-up with anti-uricemic medications such as probenecid. Surgical interventions can consist of debridement of crystalline deposits when there is a large ulcerated tophus or tenosynovectomy for carpal tunnel syndrome refractory to medical treatment. In rare instances, tendon transfers for ruptures are indicated. A severe joint involvement can warrant debridement or arthrodesis.

Calcium pyrophosphate deposition disease or pseudogout is similarly a crystalline deposition disease. Here,

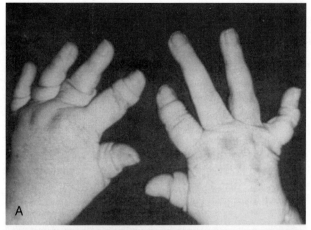

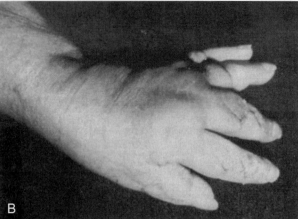

Figure 21–62. *A,* Arthritis mutilans with typical "opera-glass" hand deformities. *B,* Fusions of the interphalangeal joints of the index and middle fingers and of the interphalangeal and metacarpophalangeal joints of the thumb using iliac crest bone grafts to restore pinch function. (From Green DP, Hotchkiss RN, Pederson WC [eds]: Operative Hand Surgery, 4th ed. New York, Churchill Livingstone, 1999, p 1656.)

calcium pyrophosphate dihydrate crystals, which are positively birefringent and rhomboid-shaped, become deposited in joints or soft tissues. Frequently, on x-rays one sees chondrocalcinosis. This disease can affect the wrist in particular and presents as an acute arthritis with diffuse dorsal edema. It is often difficult to distinguish from a septic arthritis. A patient's major symptoms can be those of carpal tunnel syndrome; if these symptoms are chronic or severe, carpal tunnel release may be needed.

Systemic lupus erythematosus (SLE) is an autoimmune disease with multisystemic involvement. Approximately 90% of patients have arthritic manifestations. The hand often has rheumatoid-like joint deformity and tenosynovitis. The joint deformity is not accompanied by the articular destruction present in rheumatoid arthritis. Patients can get volar MP joint subluxation and ulnar subluxation of the extensor tendons. However, initial treatment is usually medical. Splinting does little to help, and soft tissue reconstructions hold up poorly in this disease. MP arthroplasty can be helpful in chronic situations, and shortening osteotomies can also help correct some deformities.

Scleroderma, also known as progressive systemic sclerosis, is a disease in which the hand is nearly always involved to some degree. The most common hand manifestation is Raynaud's phenomenon, which is present in 90% of patients. Unlike the reversible Raynaud's disease that strikes young females, this tends to be a progressive problem that leads to skin ulcerations and eventual irreversible ischemia. Many patients go on to necrosis of digits that either autoamputate or require formal amputation. Digital artery sympathectomy or, in some cases, superficial arch reconstructions can be very useful for preventing spasm and improving flow. Other problems resulting from scleroderma include PIP joint flexion contractures; in severe cases, one can consider an osteotomy for better functional position, especially if the contracture is causing a skin ulceration.

HAND STIFFNESS

Stiffness in the hand can be due to a number of different causes. It leads to decreased function and sometimes chronic pain in the hand. A logical approach to the evaluation of hand stiffness includes making a diagnosis. The history should address the onset of symptoms, their progression, and the presence or absence of any history of trauma (even minor). Physical examination should start with careful inspection. Is there any visible deformity? Are there any skin color changes? Is there still swelling of the digits? Active and passive range of motion should be carefully recorded. Specific tests for contracture include Bunnell's intrinsic tightness test (Fig. 21–63). This involves passive extension of the MP joint and then an attempted passive flexion of the PIP joint. If PIP joint flexion in this position is restricted, one should flex the MP joint to relax the intrinsics and again passively flex the PIP joint. If more PIP flexion is present with the MP joint flexed, then the intrinsic muscles are tight. In a reverse situation in which flexion of the PIP joint is greater with MP joint extension, one may have an extrinsic contracture. If the PIP joint motion is equally tight in both MP joint flexion and extension the underlying problem is most likely contracture of the joint capsule itself.

Flexion contractures of a joint should initially be treated with conservative management involving static splinting and range of motion exercises in an organized occupational therapy program. If this fails, and the patient has a functional deficit secondary to the contractures, surgery should be performed with resection of all tight structures volar to the axis of rotation. Particular attention should be paid to the volar plate and its proximal attachments. The lateral edges of this can thicken greatly and become pathologic "check-rein ligaments," which need to be released. Extension contractures rarely involve the joint capsule alone. Again, conservative management should be initiated first with splinting and active and passive range of motion exercises. Operative treatment involves dorsal capsulectomy, release of collateral ligaments, and freeing of volar plate adhesions. Then active and passive range of motion should be checked; if the patient still has no flexion, a flexor tendon adhesion that needs to be released is often present as well.

MP joint stiffness is usually an extension contracture

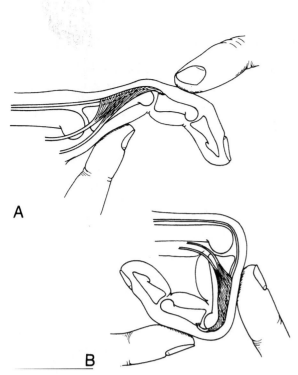

Figure 21–63. Intrinsic tightness test. In most cases of intrinsic tightness, there is less flexion of the proximal interphalangeal joint when the metaphalangeal joint is held extended *(A)* than when the metaphalangeal joint is flexed *(B)*. (From Smith RJ: Intrinsic muscles of the fingers: Function, dysfunction, and surgical reconstruction. AAOS Instructional Course Lecture V24. St. Louis, CV Mosby, 1975.)

from poor positioning in immobilization. Treatment should start with static splinting first, but long-standing contracture often needs operative release. This should be started with dorsal capsulectomy, and the collateral ligament should be released at the metacarpal head if necessary. Again, volar plate adhesions need to be freed up.

Intrinsic contractures should be treated based on the origin and nature of the contraction. If it is secondary to a mallet finger, then one may need to release the central slip to help re-balance the digits or reconstruct the terminal tendon insertion. Otherwise the intrinsic tendons can be released through a dorsal approach.

Reflex Sympathetic Dystrophy

Reflex sympathetic dystrophy is a complex disorder involving an excessive response to injury from the sympathetic nervous system. It can be the result of trauma or surgery. In many cases no causative factor is known. It is most commonly seen in the upper extremity after treatment of a distal radius and ulna fracture. Also it can be frequently seen after injury to the superficial radial nerve, for example with de Quervain's release or after open fasciectomy for Dupuytren's release in patients with diathesis or when an associated carpal tunnel release is performed.

The hallmark of this condition is pain that is constant and is made worse with motion. The patient's pain is frequently out of proportion to stimulus and can occur even with light touch. It usually starts out well localized and then spreads broadly over the extremity. Swelling is almost

always present initially. It can complicate efforts for rehabilitation. Stiffness becomes widespread in later stages. The diagnosis is made with a combination of clinical examination and the aid of some "objective" test such as plain x-rays, which can show osteopenia (Fig. 21–64); bone scans, which can be hot in the initial stages (Fig. 21–65); and diagnostic stellate ganglion blocks, which can provide relief. However, no test is definitively diagnostic for this disease.

The initial treatment goal is to break the vicious cycle with aggressive physical therapy and medical management with antidepressants, anticonvulsants, adrenergic agents, calcium channnel blockers, and/or corticosteroids. Some

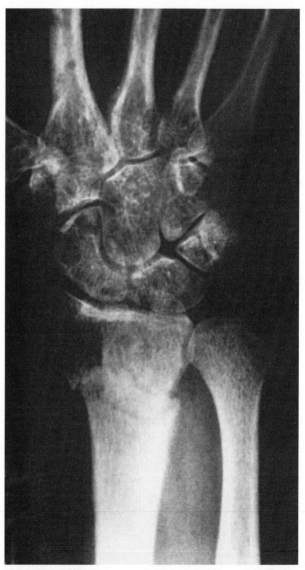

Figure 21–64. Plain x-rays of a patient with type 1 complex regional pain syndrome after fracture of the distal ends of the radius and ulna. The fracture line is visible. There is diffuse osteopenia in addition to juxtacortical demineralization and subchondral erosions and cysts. (From Koman LA, Nunley JA, Goldner JL, et al: Isolated cold stress testing in the assessment of symptoms in the upper extremity: Preliminary communication. J Hand Surg 9A:305–313, 1984.)

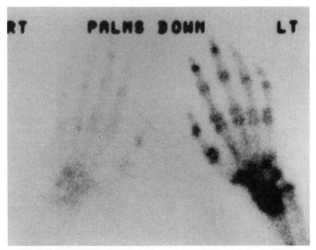

Figure 21–65. An abnormal (phase III) bone scan demonstrating increased periarticular uptake throughout the hand. This is a scan of the patient whose x-ray is seen in Figure 21–64. Notice the increased radiolucency at the fracture site. (From Koman LA, Nunley JA, Goldner JL, et al: Isolated cold stress testing in the assessment of symptoms in the upper extremity: Preliminary communication. J Hand Surg 9A:305–313, 1984.)

more invasive options include nerve blocks, sympathectomy, and peripheral nerve or dorsal column stimulators. One should work in a team-type approach and enlist the help of a pain management specialist and be very aggressive early.

Dupuytren's Disease

Dupuytren's disease is a condition that primarily affects older men of Celtic or Scandinavian heritage. It is characterized by nodule and cord formation in the previously normal fascial tissues of the hand with progressive flexion contractures of the MP and/or PIP joints.

The pathophysiology involves myofibroblastic changes in the fascial bands. The underlying cause is unknown, but decreased oxygen delivery, abnormal genes associated with collagen formation, injury from oxygen free radical formation, and growth factors such as platelet-derived growth factor have all been proposed as stimuli for transformation of the fibroblasts into myofibroblasts. Myofibroblasts contain actin and non-muscle myosin and can contract. Other involved cells include mobile fibroblasts and macrophages. Three stages have been described. The first is a proliferative stage in which large myofibroblasts with minimal extracellular matrix are present and there is increased vascularity in the region. The second stage is an involutional stage in which dense myofibroblasts are found. They tend to align themselves along the stress lines of the fascia in this situation. The final stage is the residual stage, in which myofibroblasts disappear and become replaced by a smaller population of fibroblasts. Patients often present early with nodule formation over the ring and small rays. Initially they are not tender. If tenderness is present, one needs to consider the diagnosis of fibrosarcoma. From the nodular stage the patients tend to progress to a more widespread

involvement and flexion contractures of the MP and PIP joints.

Although work has been done on the development of pharmacologic agents to help slow or reverse the process, there is currently no role for pharmacologic treatment. Stretching and therapy may help with residual hand function, but they have not been proven to retard the formation of the contracture. For contractures at the MP joint most authors believe that a flexion contracture of 30 degrees or greater requires surgical intervention. The disease at the PIP joint is more debated. Some say that any contracture at this joint is an indication for surgery because progressive deformity at the PIP joint is much harder to treat.

The fascial tissues involved include the pretendinous band, the vertical septa around the neurovacular bundles called the ligaments of Legueu and Juvara, the spiral band, the natatory ligament, the lateral digital sheath, and Grayson's ligament. Cleland's ligaments do not develop the disease (Fig. 21–66). When the bands become thickened and contracted, they are called cords. Some of the more common labeled cords include the central cord, the spiral cord, the retrovascular cord, the abductor digiti minimi cord, the isolated cord, and the natatory cord (Fig. 21–67).

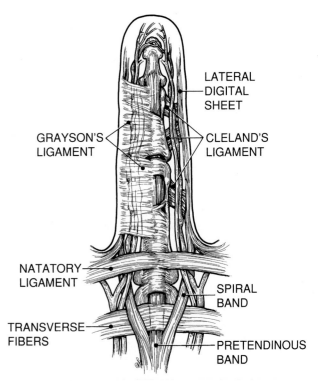

Figure 21–66. Parts of the normal digital fascia that become diseased. Grayson's ligament is shown on the left. It is an almost continuous sheet of thin fascia and is in the same plane as the natatory ligament. Cleland's ligaments are shown on the right. They do not become diseased. The lateral digital sheet receives fibers from the natatory ligament as well as the spiral band. The spiral bands pass on either side of the metaphalangeal joint, deep to the neurovascular bundles, to reach the side of the finger. (From McFarlane RM: Patterns of the diseased fascia in the fingers in Dupuytren's contracture. Plast Reconstr Surg 54:31–44, 1977.)

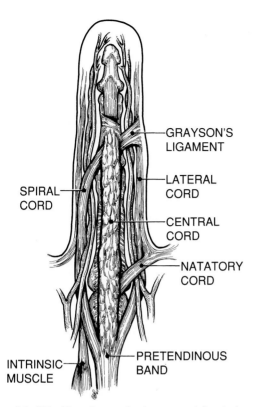

Figure 21–67. The change in the normal fascia bands to diseased cords. The pre-tendinous cord causes metaphalangeal joint contracture, and the others cause proximal interphalangeal joint contracture. When the natatory cord is diseased, it becomes adherent to the pre-tendinous cord. As it is drawn proximally, it appears to bifurcate from the pre-tendinous cord. Grayson's ligament is diseased in two ways. On the right it is shown simply thickened. On the left it has contributed to the attachment of the spinal cord onto the flexor tendon sheath. (Courtesy of Dr. R. M. McFarlane.) (From Green DP, Hotchkiss RN, Pederson WC [eds]: Operative Hand Surgery, 4th ed. New York, Churchill Livingstone, 1999, p 568.)

The spiral and the abductor digiti minimi cords wrap around the neurovascular bundles and push them superficially. One must perform very meticulous dissection around them to avoid injury. By and large, the surgical treatment of this disease involves open excision of the contracted fascial tissues. There are multiple different surgical approaches to perform this. We recommend a volar zig-zag incision with Y-V extensions to allow for skin closure. Overall, the result of first-time release of cords causing MP joint contracture is approximately 80% recovery of full motion. Poorer results are reported for PIP joint contractures and recurrent cases.

Stenosing Tenosynovitis and Tendinitis

Stenosing tenosynovitis is a common condition about the hand and wrist. The tendons are restrained from displacing forces about the hand by the extensor retinaculum and septa, the flexor retinaculum, and the digital fibro-osseous sheaths. If there is thickening of these restraints or of their contents, the tendons become compressed. The tenosyno-

vium becomes inflamed. Its compliance and gliding properties diminish; edema, adhesions, and eventually fibrosis can develop. Normal motion of the tendon is altered, and a vicious cycle of worsening pain and decreased range of motion results unless treatment is initiated.

Causes of these problems have been attributed to repetitive motion, stress, and systemic disease, including diabetes, gout, and hypothyroidism. Some of the more common stenosing tenosynovitides and their treatments are discussed here.

Trigger fingers and thumbs are the most common type of stenosing tenosynovitis that I have encountered. Patients present with pain in the region of the A-1 pulley with finger flexion and extension, and in later stages with difficulty actively extending or flexing the finger. In advanced stages, the PIP joint can lock down in flexion, and forceful popping or triggering is required to gain full extension, hence the name "trigger finger." The thumb is the most commonly involved digit, followed by the ring and middle fingers.

This disease usually originates at the A-1 pulley. The flexor tendon sheath can hypertrophy minimally and start to cause stenosis. The tendon segment just proximal to this constriction develops mechanical alterations and forms a nodular region, further compromising the tendon glide under the sheath. Treatment is initially conservative with nonsteroidal anti-inflammatory medications or local corticosteroid injections and occasionally with splinting of the digit (Fig. 21–68). One should be careful about corticosteroid injections in the tendons in a patient with rheumatoid arthritis, who may already have attenuation of the flexors. The overall results of injection are very good, with up to 70% cured; however, the long-term good results drop below 40% in patients with symptoms of more than 4 months or with multiple digit involvement.

If conservative treatment fails, surgery is recommended. For patients who do not have rheumatoid arthritis, the surgical treatment involves release of the A-1 pulley. When this is performed, one must be very careful to avoid injury to the digital nerve (Fig. 21–69). For patients with rheumatoid arthritis, one should do a flexor tenosynovectomy; the A-1 pulley release is relatively contraindicated because it can lead to bowstringing and further exaggeration of the patient's ulnar deviation deformities. Recent trials of percutaneous releases have shown good results. The most common problems seem to involve incomplete release. There is also significant potential risk of injury to the digital nerves, the blood vessels, and the tendon itself. Because of the superficial and more midline positioning of the digital nerves in the thumb, this technique should probably be avoided in that digit.

De Quervain's disease is a tenosynovitis of the first dorsal compartment of the wrist. It tends to occur most often in middle-aged patients, with women having higher incidence than men. It presents as radial-sided wrist pain worsened by thumb use and ulnar deviation of the thumb and wrist. It can have several underlying causes, including overuse, multiple APL slips, and even a very distal EPB muscle belly. The main differential diagnoses include trapeziometacarpal arthritis and Wartenberg's syndrome. Findings on physical examination include an occasional bogginess of the first dorsal compartment just distal to the radial

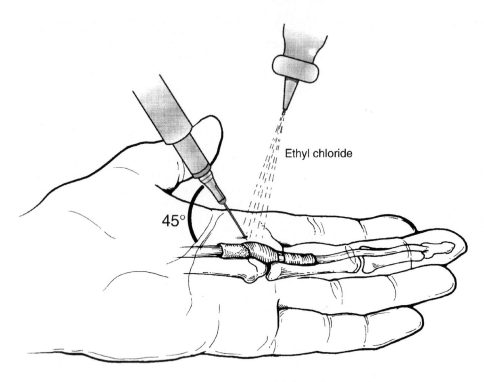

Ethyl chloride

45°

Figure 21–68. Technique of trigger finger injection. (From Green DP, Hotchkiss RN, Pederson WC [eds]: Operative Hand Surgery, 4th ed. New York, Churchill Livingstone, 1999, p 2030.)

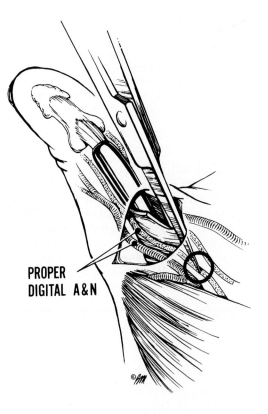

PROPER DIGITAL A&N

Figure 21–69. The digital nerves are vulnerable to injury if the skin incision is deepened too quickly or if scissors are inserted too far proximal without visualizing the nerves *(circle)*. (From Green DP, Hotchkiss RN, Pederson WC [eds]: Operative Hand Surgery, 4th ed. New York, Churchill Livingstone, 1999, p 2031.)

styloid, a positive Finkelstein test, which involves severe pain with forced ulnar deviation of the wrist after passively flexing the thumb, and a negative CMC grind test. When the CMC grind test is positive, one should look more closely and get x-rays for potential CMC arthrosis.

Initial treatment can be with oral NSAIDs or corticosteroid injection followed by thumb spica splinting. This will often allow for a decrease of the inflammation and cure the problem. If conservative treatment fails, surgical release should be done. One should be very careful to avoid injury to the superficial radial nerve branches, because this can lead to reflex sympathetic dystrophy (RSD). One should also carefully protect the radial artery in the approach. Other technical points include being sure to release all of the septa in the first dorsal compartment and to make the initial compartment incision very dorsal to avoid volar subluxation of the tendons (Fig. 21–70).

Intersection syndrome is a condition that involves pain and swelling of the muscle bellies of the APL and EPB proximal to the region of the first dorsal compartment. It is caused by tenosynovitis of the second dorsal compartment and has been associated with repetitive motion and chronic overuse (Fig. 21–71). Initial treatment can involve corticosteroid injection in the region of the second dorsal compartment and wrist extension splinting. However, if these attempts fail, one should consider release of the extensor tendons.

Other instances of stenosing tenosynovitis that have been described around the hand and wrist affect the FCR, FCU, ECU and EPL. The key to treating these conditions is proper diagnosis, and the initial treatment is almost always anti-inflammatory therapy and rest. If these conservative management options fail, then surgical release of the underlying structures nearly always produces reasonably good relief of symptoms.

HAND INFECTIONS

Because of its excellent blood supply the hand has an inherent relative resistance to infection. However, because

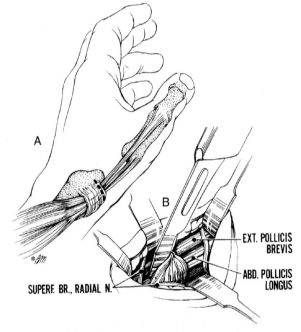

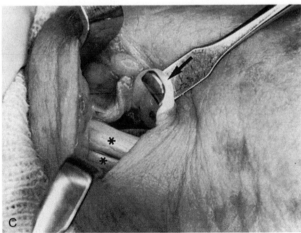

Figure 21–70. Tenovaginotomy for de Quervain's disease. *A,* The first dorsal compartment is approached by a short transverse skin incision. *B,* The annular ligament is incised with scalpel from the snuff-box to the musculotendinous junctions. *C,* Surgical demonstration of a separate compartment for the extensor pollicis brevis *(arrow)* after release of the abductor pollicis longus *(asterisks).* (From Green DP, Hotchkiss RN, Pederson WC [eds]: Operative Hand Surgery, 4th ed. New York, Churchill Livingstone, 1999, p 2037.)

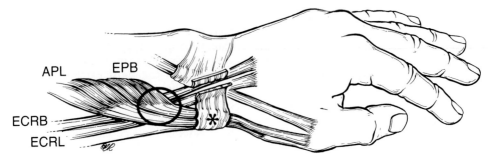

Figure 21–71. The circled area shows where the extensor pollicis brevis (EPB) and abductor pollicis longus (APL) cross the common radial wrist extensors. The location of the first dorsal compartment where de Quervain's disease occurs is indicated with an asterisk. The second dorsal compartment has been released in the manner recommended for treatment of intersection syndrome. (From Green DP, Hotchkiss RN, Pederson WC [eds]: Operative Hand Surgery, 4th ed. New York, Churchill Livingstone, 1999, p 2039.)

of its constant exposure to both minor and major trauma, many hand infections do occur. This is especially true in compromised patients such as diabetics and patients with human immunodeficiency virus (HIV) infection. With improper or delayed treatment the results of an infection in the hand can be devastating to function. For this reason physicians who have any association with hand injuries or emergencies should be familiar with common infectious processes in the hand.

The bacteria most commonly involved in hand infections are *Staphylococcus aureus* and streptococcal species. Infections caused by routine sharp trauma around the hand usually involve one of these two types of gram-positive organisms. More extensive crush wounds, bite wounds, or injuries in intravenous drug abusers or immunocompromised patients such as diabetics and HIV-positive patients are more likely to have polymicrobial infection, with species including gram-negative organisms. Specific injuries such as human and animal bite wounds should point toward additional infection, with organisms such as *Eikenella carotenes* or *Pasteurella multocida*, respectively. The basic principles of treatment include appropriate debridement of all wounds, culture of any abscesses that are present, and appropriate antibiotic therapy, which may have to be empirical if no organism is obtained. Whenever there is an abscess or purulence under pressure one should perform an incision and debridement of the local region. If there is only cellulitis or an infection is caught very early, splinting and appropriate antibiotic therapy will usually effect a cure.

Cellulitis is a spreading subcutaneous tissue infection that does not involve any loculated area of purulence. It usually presents as a painful area of induration and erythema, which can sometimes spread rapidly. One needs to be very careful that there is no underlying abscess or joint space infection. The most common causative organism is group A *Streptococcus*, but other organisms can also cause cellulitis. Attempts at isolating an organism are frequently futile unless there is another source of infection. We recommend empirical therapy with oral antibiotics if the infection is caught within the first 48 hours. If a more severe case is present or if the patient has a delayed diagnosis, then we recommend intravenous antibiotics. Surgical treatment is rarely indicated.

The most common purulent infections of the hand are in the fingertips, particularly in the region of the fingernail. An infection that results in pus underneath the eponychial fold around the nail is called paronychia. It usually occurs after some type of disruption between the seal between the nail and the surrounding nail fold, allowing bacteria to become entrapped underneath the fold. It occurs frequently after manicures, removal of a hang nail, or biting of nails. The organism that causes the paronychia is usually *S. aureus*. If caught in a very early stage, this infection can be treated with warm water soaks and oral antibiotics. When the infection is more involved, decompression of the involved segment of nail fold should be performed under digital block anesthesia (Fig. 21–72). This can be done through various techniques, including removal of the entire nail, removal of a segment of the nail, an incision of the paronychia fold adjacent to the nail, or elevation of the entire nail fold for removal of the base of the nail. Any

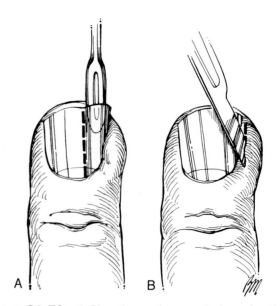

Figure 21–72. *A,* Elevation and removal of one fourth of the nail to decompress the paronychium. *B,* Incision of the paronychial fold with the blade directed away from the nail bed and matrix. (From Green DP, Hotchkiss RN, Pederson WC [eds]: Operative Hand Surgery, 4th ed. New York, Churchill Livingstone, 1999, p 1034.)

time that a segment of nail is removed from the fold in the region of the germinal matrix, the fold should be stented open with gauze. This allows for continued drainage while preventing closure of that segment of nail fold. When the paronychia is chronic, it is much more difficult to eradicate the infection. Marsupialization is one good option for treatment (Fig. 21–73). This involves removal of a crescent-shaped segment of the skin and soft tissue overlying the germinal matrix. This decompresses the infected matrix zone and allows for healing and regrowth of the nail, which can take up to a year.

The other significant infection that often occurs in the tip is called a felon. A felon is an abscess of the pulp space overlying the distal phalanx. These infections can be extremely painful. They, too, can occur after a relatively minor trauma to the region and are most commonly caused by *S. aureus*. Treatment of these infections is complicated by the fact that the pulp space in this region is separated into multiple compartments by fibrous tissue septa that anchor the skin to the bone. All compartments that are involved must be released to get adequate decompression and allow for appropriate treatment of the infection. Surgical decompression is usually performed under digital block with finger tourniquet. Many different incisions have been described; one should be chosen that avoids injury to the digital nerves and vessels and allows for adequate release of all the compartments and continued drainage. Decompression and oral antibiotics are usually adequate to allow for full treatment of this infection.

Another infection that can commonly occur in the fingertip region but also anywhere else around the hand is the herpetic whitlow. This infection presents as a single or group of painful vesicles over the fingertips or other regions of the hand. These frequently appear to be abscesses. The causative organism is a herpes simplex virus, either type 1 or type 2. These infections can be transmitted occupationally to workers who have to deal with secretions, but they can also be caused by exposure to one's own oral or genital lesions. The disease process is usually self-limited with a 7- to 14-day course during which the vesicles coalesce, unroof, and then form ulcers. They then undergo

epithelialization and completely resolve. It is very important to make the diagnosis of herpetic whitlow and avoid any surgical incision or drainage, because this can lead to disseminated infection and/or superinfection. The diagnosis is usually made by history and characteristic clinical findings. Many patients also note symptoms of tingling and paresthesias in the region just before eruption of the vesicles. A definitive diagnosis is made by culture of the vesicles, which can take several days. One can also perform a Tzanck smear on the fluid and find characteristic multinucleated giant cells. This infection is more worrisome in patients with immunocompromise, and one can consider treatment with acyclovir in addition to rest and observation.

Suppurative flexor tenosynovitis is one of the most feared infectious processes in the hand. It involves a purulent infection of the flexor tendon sheath; and if it is not treated adequately and immediately, there is a high risk of severe loss of function secondary to scarring of the tendon sheath or eventual tendon necrosis due to ischemia. The diagnosis is usually made when several of Kanavel's signs are present. These include severe pain to passive extension of the digit, fusiform swelling of the digit, tenderness along the flexor tendon sheath, and maintenance of a semiflexed posture. One can sometimes help confirm the diagnosis and obtain organisms for culture by aspirating the flexor tendon sheath. When these symptoms are caught within the first 24 to 48 hours of their evolution, and one does not suspect a loculated, purulent abscess in the sheath, they can be treated by elevation, splinting, and intravenously administered antibiotics. For all other situations, irrigation and debridement of the sheath is indicated. This can be performed easily with an open incision and drainage through a mid axial approach. Another option that has become extremely popular is closed irrigation as described by Neviaser. The flexor tendon sheath is opened proximally in the region of the A-1 pulley, and a catheter is threaded into the sheath. A secondary incision is made into the sheath distally, and intermittent or continuous lavage of the tendon sheath is performed (Fig. 21–74).

When treatment is either inadequate or delayed, results can be devastating, as noted earlier. One can also develop infection of adjacent structures including the spread to other tendon sheaths or spread to the ulna and radial bursa as well as an infection of the surrounding joints and soft tissues. The ulna bursa is an extension of the flexor tendon synovial sheath, and it surrounds the synovial sheets around all of the flexor tendons in the region of the carpal tunnel. Infections can rapidly spread down the flexor tendon sheath into this region. The radial bursa is an extension of the FPL synovial sheath, and in some situations this can connect with the ulnar bursa; infections can cause a so-called horseshoe abscess (Fig. 21–75). It is important to recognize these variations of simple flexor tenosynovitis and treat them with appropriate widespread decompression.

There are many different contained spaces of the hand in which abscesses can occur. These include the subcutaneous space, the dorsal subaponeurotic space, the thenar and hypothenar spaces, the midpalmar space, and the interdigital web spaces (Fig. 21–76).

Subcutaneous abscesses can occur nearly anywhere in the hand. They present as areas with cellulitis and increased

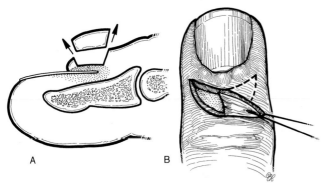

Figure 21–73. Eponychial marsupialization for chronic paronychia. *A*, Lateral view showing the area of wedge-shaped excision. Undisturbed matrix is stippled. *B*, Dorsal view of the crescent-shaped area of excision extending to the margins of the nail folds on each side. (From Green DP, Hotchkiss RN, Pederson WC [eds]: Operative Hand Surgery, 4th ed. New York, Churchill Livingstone, 1999, p 1036.)

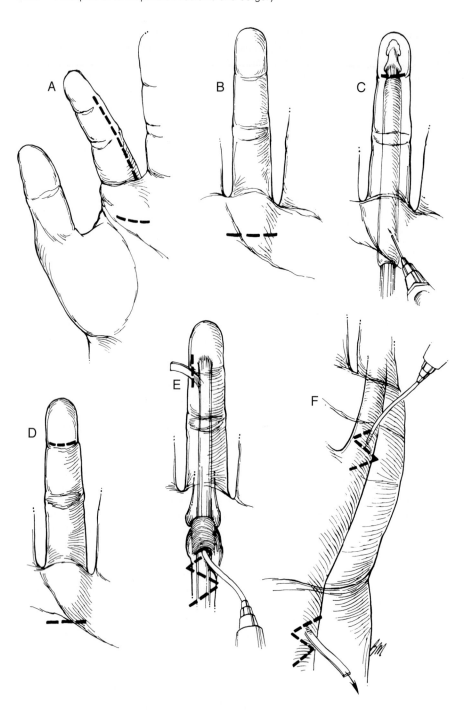

Figure 21–74. Incisions for drainage of tendon sheath infections. *A*, Open drainage incisions. *B*, Single incision for instillation treatment of tendon sheath infections. *C*, Sheath irrigated by means of a needle proximally and a single distal incision. *D*, Incisions for through-and-through intermittent irrigation. *E*, Closed tendon sheath irrigation technique. *F*, Closed irrigation of the ulnar bursa. (From Green DP, Hotchkiss RN, Pederson WC [eds]: Operative Hand Surgery, 4th ed. New York, Churchill Livingstone, 1999, p 1043.)

warmth with localized areas of fluctuants. Aspiration of the area will usually reveal a purulent fluid, and culture of this fluid can aid with diagnosing the involved organism. The most common bacterium causing this is *S. aureus*. Treatment involves incision of the fluctuant regions, adequate drainage, irrigation, packing, and immobilization. After approximately 2 days the packing is removed and soaks should be initiated. The wound should be allowed to heal by secondary intent. During this entire time appropriate antibiotic therapy should be maintained.

The dorsal subaponeurotic space is the region bounded by the fascia and the extensor tendons of the palm dorsally and by the interosseous muscles and the metacarpals volarly. Patients present with impressive dorsal hand swelling,

pain, and a deep area of fluctuance. Treatment involves irrigation and debridement through two longitudinal incisions, with routine postoperative management and healing by secondary intent. Early motion is very important, and use of the extensor tendon should be avoided, to prevent injury or desiccation of the tendons.

Web space abscesses present as pain and swelling in the affected web space and are characterized by abduction of the involved digits. When decompressing these abscesses one must be very careful to explore both volarly and dorsally to avoid missing a "collar button abscess." In this situation, an abscess that starts either volarly or dorsally tracks over the deep transverse metacarpal ligament or through a space in the palmar fascia to create a dumbbell-

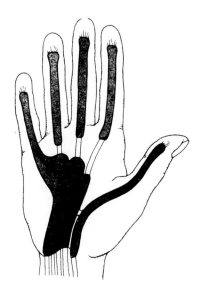

Figure 21–75. Tendon sheaths of the flexor tendon. Note communication of small finger sheath with ulna bursa. (From The Hand, 2nd ed. Aurora, CO, American Society for Surgery of the Hand, 1983, p 96.)

shaped abscess with two large areas of fluctuance connected by a thin bridge.

The thenar space is a potential space bounded on the radial side by the thumb metacarpal. It is bounded volarly by the flexor tendons to the index, ulnarly by the fascia overlying the middle finger metacarpal, and dorsally by the adductor pollicis muscle (see Fig. 21–76). Infections in this region need to be carefully explored, and frequently both volar and dorsal incisions are required because the infection can track over the adductor tendon into the potential space between the adductor and the first dorsal interosseous muscle. These incisions should be made with great care to avoid causing a web space contracture.

The midpalmar space is bounded by the fascial membrane overlying the third metacarpal on the radial side (see Fig. 21–76). Overlying it volarly are the middle and ring finger flexor tendons and neurovascular bundles. Ulnarly,

the hypothenar musculature restricts it, and, dorsally, the metacarpals and interossei provide a roof. Infections in this region can lead to significant dorsal swelling, and one must be careful to recognize that the infection is on the volar aspect of the hand rather than on the dorsal aspect when approaching this for surgery.

Septic arthritis of joints can also occur in the hand and wrist. They are usually due to either direct penetration of the joint through trauma or seeding from a distant source of bacteremia. Pain and swelling accompanied by a lack of range of motion are the hallmarks of this disease. Aspiration of the joint is important in helping make the diagnosis. Early treatment is required because the inflammatory process that the body provides to help eliminate the bacteria in the joint can cause rapid destruction of the cartilage. This type of infection is usually treated with formal incision and drainage followed by intravenous antibiotic therapy and dressing changes to allow for healing by secondary intention. Early motion is recommended as well. Some have advocated serial aspiration to decrease the bacterial load and remove the inflammatory factors in the pus from the joint; however, results from this treatment are variable.

Bite wounds to the hand are the source of many infections and will often require debridement and antibiotics. Animal bites (particularly cat and dog bites) tend to have mixed flora, with both aerobic and anaerobic organisms present. *P. multocida* is a frequently found organism but *Streptococcus*, *Staphylococcus*, and anaerobic species are also frequently present. Most of these injuries should be treated with extension of the wounds, irrigation, and intravenous or oral antibiotic therapy. Human bite wounds can occur through two methods. One is through a direct and intentional bite to the hand, which usually leaves a near circumferential volar and dorsal area of crush and laceration. The more common bite wound is one in which a clenched fist strikes a mouth and involves a bite wound only on the dorsum of the hand, usually in the region of the MP joints. These so-called fight bites can involve laceration of the extensor tendon, penetration of the MP joint capsule, fractures, or even retained tooth fragments within the joint. These injuries can present early with a

Figure 21–76. Cross-sectional anatomy of the hand demonstrating the thenar, midpalmar, hypothenar, interdigital (web), and dorsal subaponeurotic spaces. (From Jebson PJ: Deep subfascial space infections. Hand Clin 14:558, 1998.)

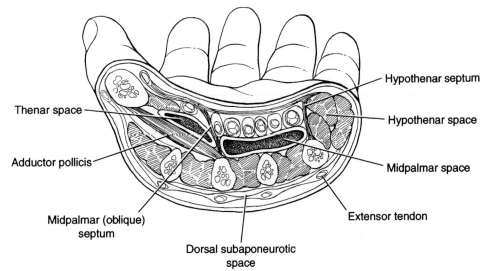

Thenar space

Adductor pollicis

Midpalmar (oblique) septum

Dorsal subaponeurotic space

Hypothenar septum

Hypothenar space

Midpalmar space

Extensor tendon

relatively benign-appearing superficial skin wound. Because of the positioning of the hand in a clenched fist, the level of injury of the tendon sheath or the joint is very different from that of the skin when examined with the MP and IP joints fully extended. Treatment of this includes extending the wounds and performing a meticulous exploration to ensure that all injuries are appropriately treated. Copious irrigation and repair of the lacerated tendon are important. The initial wound should be left open, but the extension can be closed and the patient should be started on early range of motion exercises. Appropriate choice of antibiotics is very important. α-Hemolytic streptococci and *S. aureus* are the most common pathogens from the human bite type infection. *E. corrodens* is cultured from between 7 to 30% of these infections. Ampicillin or penicillin should be included in the treatment of human bite wounds for this reason.

Osteomyelitis in the hand is most commonly caused either by contiguous spread of an abscess or secondary to an open fracture. Hematogenous spread is quite rare in the hand. Infection rates for open fractures of the hand range from 1 to 11%. Patients often present with pain, erythema and swelling. Recurrent presumed soft tissue infection after initial antibiotic treatment should alert one to the possibility of this process. When caught very early, osteomyelitis in the hand can often be treated with intravenous antibiotics in the short term followed by oral antibiotics. However, many surgeons prefer to use open debridement and curettage of the affected bone even in the early setting.

Necrotizing fasciitis is an infection that is most often caused by group A β-hemolytic streptococci. In some situations, particularly in diabetics, it can be caused by polymicrobial infection. This potentially life-threatening disease involves infection along the fascial planes and can present initially with relatively benign findings on physical examination. It tends to progress very rapidly, and mortality rates of 10 to 30% have been reported. Patients tend to present with an extremely painful, clearly demarcated cellulitis that is often accompanied by induration and swelling. There is rapid spread of the disease along the extremity. An elevated white blood cell count is almost always present. MRI can be extremely helpful in confirming this diagnosis; edema and swelling of the fascial planes is a strong indicator that this disease may be present. Early and aggressive surgical debridement is indicated. At surgery, a brown watery fluid is found along the involved fascial planes and multiple debridements are usually required. Frequently, if the limb can be completely preserved, further tissue coverage procedures are required. Antibiotic coverage should be started empirically with inclusion of penicillin, an aminoglycoside, and either clindamycin or metronidazole to cover any infection with anaerobic organisms. Careful hemodynamic monitoring is also very important.

One must keep in mind atypical hand infections such as mycobacterial and fungal infections, particularly when patients have unusual presentation or immunocompromise or chronic infections unresponsive to standard antibiotics. Mycobacterial infections can include standard tuberculosis or other pathogens, including *M. marinum*, the most common atypical mycobacterial infection. *M. avium-intracellulare* is very common in patients with the acquired immunodeficiency syndrome. Other offending agents include *M.*

kansasii and *M. terrae*. These infections present as a very indolent onset usually after a puncture wound or some other exposure or arising in an immunocompromised host. These cases are often initially missed, and they have a delay in treatment. Diagnosis requires a biopsy for histopathology that shows granuloma formation. Acid-fast bacilli seen on special stainings help make the diagnosis. Cultures should be performed in Löwenstein-Jensen medium at 30 degrees for up to 8 weeks. Abscesses, tenosynovitis, and joint or bone involvement require aggressive debridement and several months of antibiotic therapy.

Fungal infections of the hand can be broken down into four major categories: cutaneous, subcutaneous, deep, and systemic. Cutaneous infections are mainly found around the nail folds or the inner digital areas and the palms. They can often be treated with topical therapy; however, nail removal, marsupialization, and, occasionally, systemic therapy can be required.

Subcutaneous infections are often caused by sporotrichosis after puncture wound with a thorn, a scratch, or a splinter. The treatment is oral potassium iodide therapy. Deeper fungal infections can either affect the tenosynovium of the flexor extensor compartments, or present as separate arthritis or osteomyelitis. Specific fungal culture is required to make the diagnosis. Treatment requires debridement and systemic antifungal therapy. In some cases the fungi are so resistant to therapy that amputations are required.

CONGENITAL HAND DISORDERS

Congenital upper extremity anomalies present at birth are relatively rare problems, but the general orthopaedist does occasionally perform the initial evaluation. Frequently, upper extremity anomalies are not detected before birth. The parents are expecting a completely "normal baby," and families are often angry, frustrated, or guilt ridden. By being able to discuss the basic causes, treatment, and prognosis in a caring and informative way a surgeon can help families gain positive outlook, develop realistic reconstructive goals, and even better accept the child. Definitive treatment for most of these differences is, however, usually referred to a hand surgeon.

Embryology

Limb differentiation takes place in a very specific sequence (Fig. 21–77). The upper limb bud first appears as bulges of the mesenchymal tissue alongside somites C5 to T1 on day 26 after fertilization. Growth is controlled by a rim of tissue at the tip of the bud apical ectodermal ridge and proceeds proximally to distally. By day 33 the shoulders, arms, forearms, and hand paddles have formed, and at the end of the sixth week of gestation the limb buds have a clear resemblance to mature limbs. Soon after, chondrification of all the bones occurs, with the distal phalanges being the last to start. Finger rays become visible as longitudinal thickenings of the digital plates. Programmed cell death (apoptosis) occurs to separate the individual fingers, first at the central three digit, and then later for the pre-axial (thumb) and post-axial (small finger) digits. The fingers are completely separated by 8 weeks' gestation.

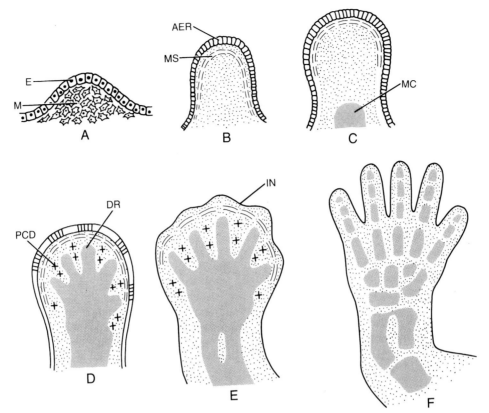

Figure 21–77. Normal limb development after fertilization. *A*, 28 days. *B*, 34 days. *C*, 36 days. *D*, 40 days programmed cell death of mesenchymal tissue between digital ray mesenchymal condensations. *E*, 42 days. *F*, 50 days; individual digits and web spaces are well defined. E, ectoderm; M, mesoderm; AER, apical ectodermal ridge; MS, marginal sinus; MC, mesenchymal condensation; PCD, physiologic cell death; DR, digital ray; IN, interdigital notch. (From Jebson PJ: Deep subfascial space infections. Hand Clin 1998;14:558.)

Muscles differentiate in situ by day 50. Joints form in the upper limb by formation of "mini clefts" in the inner zones between bones. Cavitation of the wrist and finger joints starts around 48 days. It then requires muscle activity to progress. The hands begin to move at 9 weeks. Skin creases develop soon after. Dermal ridges form in the third and fourth months. Nail formation begins in the fifth month. At birth, all systems in the hand show fully developed patterns except the nervous system. Myelinization is not complete until 2 years of age.

Incidence and Etiology

The overall incidence of congenital anomalies throughout the body is 6 to 7%, or 1 in 13, of all live births. Multiple anomalies secondary to chromosomal abnormalities are present in 0.5%. Upper extremity anomalies are present in 1 of 626 live births, but only about 10% of these patients have any significant cosmetic or functional deficit.

The cause for 40 to 50% of congenital hand anomalies is unknown. The rest are due to environmental or genetic causes. Flatt describes three sequences that lead to anomalies:

1. A malformation sequence, which is the result of poor tissue formation. These problems are intrinsic to the fetus and are caused by a wide variety of factors such as skeletal dysplasias, inborn errors of metabolism, and genetic abnormalities.

2. A deformation sequence; here the fetus is initially normal but the environment places an abnormal stress on it. Examples include constriction ring syndrome and packaging disorders secondary to bicornuate uterus.

3. A disruption sequence; in this situation a normal fetus develops tissue breakdown after being subjected to injury caused by infectious, vascular, or metabolic factors. One of the best examples of this is the thalidomide tragedy of the 1960s in Europe.

Genetic abnormalities can be of single gene, multiple gene, or chromosomal origin. Hand anomalies are frequently associated with autosomal dominant single-gene defects with sporadic penetrance. Prime examples of this are syndactyly and polydactyly.

Classification

A comprehensive classification scheme for hand differences was developed by Swanson and associates. It has seven major categories:

    I. Failure of formation of parts (arrest of development): includes amputations and club hands

    II. Failure of differentiation (separation of parts): includes syndactyly, camptodactyly, clinodactyly, and trigger and clasp thumb

    III. Duplication: includes polydactyly

IV. Undergrowth
V. Overgrowth
VI. Congenital constriction ring syndrome
VII. Generalized skeletal abnormalities

This classification scheme helps group different hand anomalies by the pathologic process involved. A more detailed description of the specific anomalies is provided next.

Goals and Timing of Treatment

The main goal of treatment for congenital hand differences is to maximize function and appearance. Function can be further broken down into three major aspects: (1) the ability to control the placing of the hand in space, (2) full skin coverage with good sensation, and (3) satisfactory grasp and precision handling. One cannot always supply all three aspects to both hands: most of these children have normal sensibility, but they frequently lack the correct anatomical parts for normal prehension.

Although one can never make these hands totally normal, so much can be done that families and physicians should be cautiously optimistic that real improvements can be effected. The process, however, may be a long and dynamic one.

The timing of any surgical intervention is important but quite variable. The hand becomes an integrated tool by 1 year of age; grasp and pinch are well developed and accurately controlled. Fine tuning of coordination and increase in strength continue to age 3, and emotional control and ability to cooperate start at about this age.

The overriding factor should be the generalized well-being of the child, and the surgeon needs to work closely with the pediatrician to ensure this. One should nearly always wait until cardiac and other anomalies are stabilized. For constriction bands causing vascular compromise, one may need to operate in the first days of life. Rapidly progressing deformities need to be corrected early, in the 3- to 6-month time period. Most other problems can be treated in the 6- to 18-month time frame; but when phalangeal osteotomies are required, one should consider waiting until after 18 months of age to allow for involution of the endosteal artery. For microsurgical reconstructions one may want to wait until age 4 to allow vessels to reach adequate caliber. It is best to complete the treatment course before the child starts school.

Failure of Formation—Transverse

These anomalies present as congenital amputations, and they are classified by naming the bony level at which the limb ends. They can occur at any level, with the most common being the proximal forearm, which occurs in one in 20,000 live births. The cause is usually unknown, but autosomal recessive inheritance may be involved. The treatment is usually conservative. Passive mittens are made between 3 to 6 months ("sit to fit"). This accustoms a child to a prosthesis and encourages the use of the arm instead of ignoring it completely. At 12 to 18 months, this is switched to an actively open split hook. A Krukenberg procedure, which turns the residual forearm into a volun-

tary hook, is now recommended only for blind bilateral patients.

Most finger-level amputations are well tolerated. For multiple finger absences, complex reconstructions including ulnar post reconstruction, phalangeal transfer, and microvascular toe-to-hand transfers are available but seldom necessary.

Failure of Formation—Longitudinal

This subgroup is defined as all failures of formation not including congenital amputations. One of the most dramatic examples is phocomelia. It is usually rare, but in the 1960s there were a large number of children born with it in Europe as a result of the use of thalidomide. There are three types: complete, with the hand attached to the shoulder with no intervening segment; proximal, in which the hand is attached to an abnormal humerus and often deformed forearm; and distal, in which the hand is attached to the humerus with no intervening forearm. Treatment is almost always non-operative, with surgery only indicated for shoulder instability, minor lengthenings, and thumb opposition. Some patients benefit from prosthesis use and limb training (Fig. 21–78).

Radial Club Hand

This is a preaxial deformity with complete or partial absence of the radius. It occurs in 1 in 100,000 newborns with 50% bilateral involvement. It is commonly associated with thumb aplasia and visceral anomalies, some of which may make surgery life threatening. A few of the associated syndromes include Holt-Oram (cardiac anomalies), Fanconi's anemia (aplastic anemia and genital urinary abnormalities), TAR (thrombocytopenia and absent radius) syndrome, and VATER (vertebral anomalies, imperforate anus, tracheoesophageal aplasia, and renal anomalies) syndrome.

The forearm is short, the wrist is radially deviated, and the ulna is short and bowed. There are many muscular and neurovascular deficiencies. The muscles from the lateral epicondyle are frequently absent, worsening the problem of poor wrist and finger extension. The superficial radial nerve is usually absent. The ulnar and median nerves and ulnar artery are usually unaffected. The most widely used classification scheme was developed by Bayne. Type I involves a short distal radius with a delayed appearance of the distal epiphysis. Type II has a hypoplastic radius with defective proximal and distal epiphyseal growth. Type III patients have partial absence of the middle and distal thirds of the radius. Type IV, the most common category, involves complete absence of the radius (Fig. 21–79).

Treatment is controversial, but most would agree that absence of elbow motion is a contraindication for surgery. For type I and mild type II disorders, the treatment is serial casting and stretching and occasional release of tight bands. Patients with severe type II and types III and IV disorders benefit from serial casting and stretching, followed by surgical realignment of the carpus with the forearm. The options for realignment are fusion, centralization, or radialization; and there is considerable debate as to the procedure of choice. Centralization involves releasing the tight radial-sided tendons and ligaments, creating a notch in the

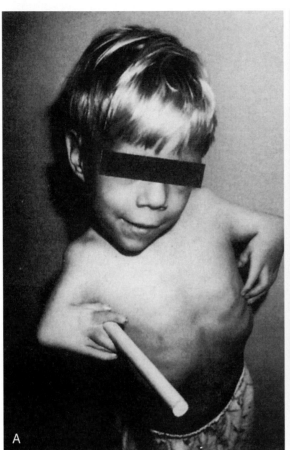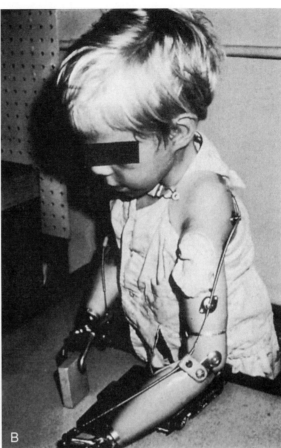

Figure 21–78. *A,* The clinical appearance of a boy with bilateral phocomelia that includes digital deformities, but the digits are partly functional. *B,* The same patient fitted with bilateral upper limb phocomelic prostheses partly controlled by the functional digits. (From Green DP, Hotchkiss RN, Pederson WC [eds]: Operative Hand Surgery, 4th ed. New York, Churchill Livingstone, 1999, p 340.)

carpus by excising central carpal bones, placing the ulnar head into the newly formed carpal notch, and pinning it through the intermedullary canal of the third metacarpal all the way down into the ulnar shaft. The procedure is supplemented by ulnar osteotomy and advancement of the ulnar-sided tendons to further reduce deformity and minimized recurrence (Fig. 21–80). Buck-Gramcko recommended radialization in an effort to further enhance stability while maintaining length. It involves pinning the carpus on the radius in an ulnarly deviated position, transfer of the radial tendons to the ECU, and an ulnar osteotomy as needed to correct severe bowing (Fig. 21–81). Any thumb hypoplasia present should be treated after the correction of the club hand.

Ulnar Club Hand

This is an ulnar deviation and bowing deformity due to complete or partial absence of the ulna. It is about four times less common than radial club hand. It tends to be associated with skeletal abnormalities only, the most common being proximal focal femoral deficit, clubfoot, and spina bifida. About half of the patients have abnormalities of the contralateral upper extremity. Often there is some process other than ulnar deficiency. Fifty percent of patients

have an ipsilateral radial head dislocation. Bayne has classified this deformity into four general groupings. Type I involves only hypoplasia of the ulna. Type II, the most common variety, shows partial absence of the ulna. Type III shows complete ulnar absence, and type IV has associated radiohumeral synostosis.

Despite sometimes severe deformity, the function of these patients is usually quite good. The wrist has a stable base on the radius, and the elbow often functions well if there is no radioulnar synostosis. The rare situation when surgery is indicated includes severe anterior bowing that directs the hand posteriorly and can be corrected with closing wedge osteotomy; fixed pronation deformity, which can be corrected with rotational osteotomy; pain and excessive prominence of a dislocated radial head treatable by radial head resection; and the rare situation of an unstable ulna that can be fixed with radioulnar synostosis.

Central Ray Deficiency

This condition involves a failure of formation of the central rays of the hand, resulting in a splint, cleft, or lobster-claw hand. It represents about 4% of all congenital hand anomalies. There are two main types: (1) typical, in which there is a central V-shaped cleft due to absence of the

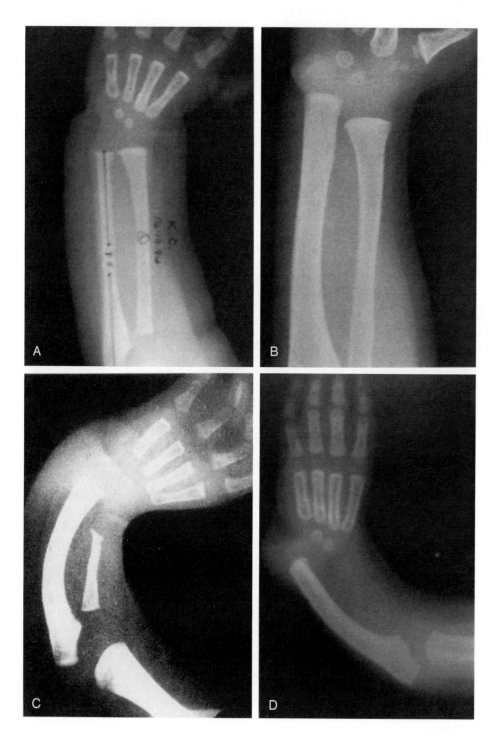

Figure 21–79. Types 1 *(A)*, 2 *(B)*, 3 *(C)*, and 4 *(D)* radial deficiency. (From Green DP, Hotchkiss RN, Pederson WC [eds]: Operative Hand Surgery, 4th ed. New York, Churchill Livingstone, 1999, p 340.)

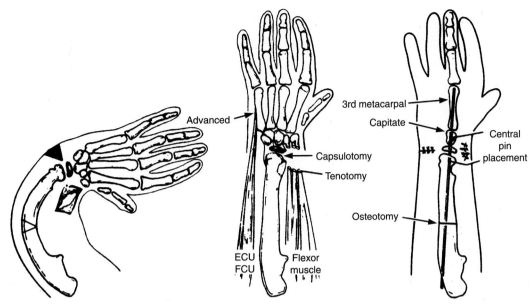

Figure 21–80. Principles of centralization. (From Lourie GM, Lins RE: Radial longitudinal deficiency: A review and update. Hand Clin 14:91, 1998.)

middle ray only and which may include syndactyly between the ulnar or radial digits; and (2) atypical, in which only a thumb and small finger are present. For many patients, function is acceptable and no treatment is required. For severe deformities, closure of the cleft is recommended. The associated syndactyly also must be addressed and the thumb function re-established with creation of a web space.

Failures of Differentiation

SYNDACTYLY

Failure of separation of the digits is one of the most common congenital hand anomalies. It occurs in 1 in 2000

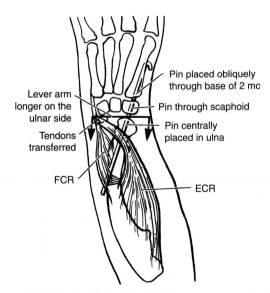

Figure 21–81. Radialization. ECR, extensor carpi radialis; FCR, flexor carpi radialis. (From Bayne LG, Costas BL, Lourie GM: The upper limb. *In* Morrissy RT, Weinsten SL [eds]: Lovell and Winter's Pediatric Orthopaedics, 4th ed, vol 2. Philadelphia, Lippincott-Raven, 1996, p 792.)

newborns, is bilateral in 50% of cases, and is most frequently found in white male infants. Syndactylies are classified as complete if the digits are joined all the way to the tip and as incomplete if they are not. Simple syndactylies have only soft tissue involvement, whereas complex ones have bony fusion as well. Dobyns suggested a further category called "complicated" to include such variances as multiple adjacent digit involvement, associated symphalangism, associated clinodactyly, and other complicating deformities. The most frequently encountered digits are middle/ring (50%), then ring/small (30%), followed by the less common index/middle (15%) and thumb/index (5%) combinations (Fig. 21–82).

Surgical separation is usually recommended between the ages of 6 to 18 months, with occasional earlier releases for rapidly progressive deformity, especially when the size is mismatched, ring/small fingers are involved, or in cases of acrosyndactyly. Careful attention to detail is very important in planning and executing this surgery. The incisions should be planned to allow proper reconstruction of the web space and the tip. Full-thickness skin grafts are always needed, because the total skin available is not enough to cover two independent digits. The bifurcation of the digital nerves is nearly always distal to its normal position in complete syndactyly, and meticulous dissection is required to separate these nerves. Anomalous interconnections between the tendons and the vessels may be present. One should never separate both sides of a digit at the same setting, because vascular compromise may result.

CAMPTODACTYLY

Camptodactyly is an isolated congenital flexion deformity of the PIP joint. The contractured or deformed structures include the skin, the fascia, the tendon sheath, the FDS tendon, intrinsic tendons, the neck of the proximal phalanx, and the central slip insertion. The treatment consists of stretching for mild cases and surgical release for contractures greater than 90 degrees. FDS transfers to the

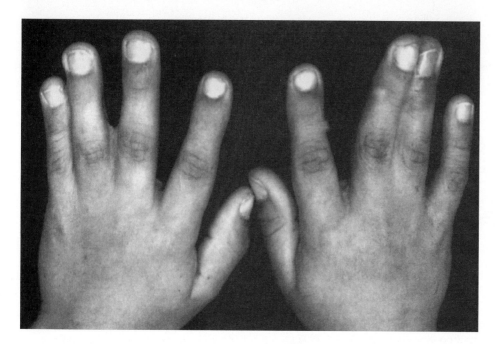

Figure 21–82. Simple, incomplete syndactyly of the left long-ring web space, simple complete syndactyly of the left ring-small web, and complete complex syndactyly of the right long-ring web. (From Green DP, Hotchkiss RN, Pederson WC [eds]: Operative Hand Surgery, 4th ed. New York, Churchill Livingstone, 1999, p 417.)

extensor mechanism and osteotomies of the proximal phalanx have been reported with mixed results.

CLINODACTYLY

Clinodactyly is a congenital lateral deviation of a digit. It is more common in the small finger than in triphalangeal thumbs. Usually the finger curves toward the midline of the hand secondary to a middle phalanx deformity in which the distal articular surface is not parallel to the proximal surface. There are three forms of clinodactyly: (1) minor angulation with normal length, which is very common; (2) minor angulation with short length, which occurs in over 25% of Down syndrome patients but is otherwise rare; and (3) marked angulation, which is usually the result of a delta phalanx.

Delta phalanges are triangular or trapezoidally shaped bones, usually at the level of the middle or proximal phalanx. The proximal phalanx is oriented along the lateral aspect of the phalanx in a C shape rather than the normal flat transversely oriented physis. The epiphysis grows around this physis and spans one entire side of the bone as well as the proximal and distal aspects, leading to the concept of a longitudinally bracketed physis. This orientation leads to progressive angular deformity of the digit as the phalanx continues to grow.

Treatment is rarely indicated in types I and II. Stretching and splinting are almost never effective. One can consider a closing wedge osteotomy if parents insist on correction of the cosmetic deformity (Fig. 21–83). For delta phalanges, surgery is indicated for progressive deformity. Early excision alone can be done for triphalangeal thumbs. Opening or closing wedge osteotomies combined with a partial disruption of the abnormal segment of the physis should be done for more advanced stages or other digits, and this produces reasonably good results (Fig. 21–84).

TRIGGER THUMB

Trigger thumb is due to constriction of the flexor pollicis longus by the A-1 pulley. The thumb is usually held in fixed IP joint flexion and rarely does it trigger like a classic adult stenosing tenosynovitis. Attempts to extend the joint cause pain. One can sometimes feel a prominence in the tendon by the pulley called Notta's node. Only 25% of cases are actually noted at birth. Dirham and associates state that 30% resolve spontaneously by 1 year. Others do well with surgical release of the A-1 pulley. This must be done with great care because the digital nerves are very superficial in this region and can be cut easily.

CONGENITAL CLASPED THUMB

Congenital clasped thumb is characterized by extreme MP flexion and palmar adduction of the thumb that persists beyond the age of 3 months. Mih recently synthesized a

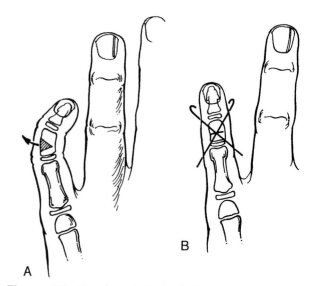

Figure 21–83. *A* and *B*, A closing wedge osteotomy through the abnormal middle phalanx can be best accomplished on the convex side of the digit. (Adapted from Flatt AE: The Care of Congenital Hand Anomalies, 2nd ed. St. Louis, Quality Medical Publishing, 1994, pp 207–217.)

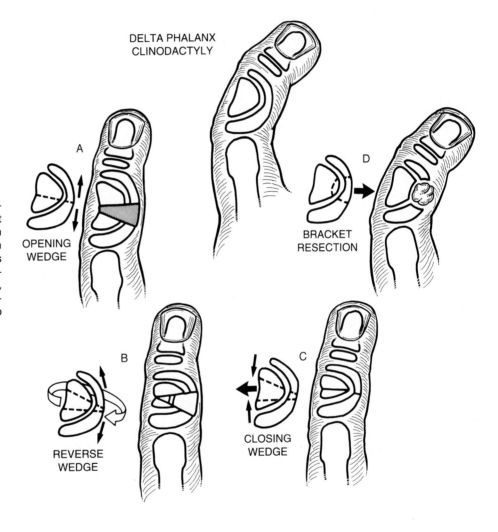

Figure 21–84. The four surgical options for the treatment of clinodactyly caused by a delta phalanx. (Adapted from Upton J: Congenital anomalies of the hand and forearm. *In* McCarthy JG [ed]: Plastic Surgery, vol 8: The Hand [pt 2]. Philadelphia, WB Saunders, 1990, pp 5337–5340.)

new classification scheme for these thumbs: type I—supple, with only an abnormal extensor abnormality; type II—complex, with associated joint contracture, collateral ligament abnormalities, first web space contracture, and thenar muscle hypoplasia; and type III—associated with arthrogryposis or windblown hand syndrome.

Initial treatment consists of serial casting in extension and abduction for 3 to 6 months. If this conservative approach fails, there is a probable absence or insufficiency of the extensor pollicis brevis. One should transfer the EIP (frequently absent) or FDS of the ring finger to the base of the thumb proximal phalanx. In complex cases, one may also need to release the first dorsal interosseous muscle, the adductor pollicis, and both heads of the FPB. The FPL may need lengthening, and the web space may need to be reconstructed. Type III deformity is probably due more to contracture of the web space and volar structures, and the extensor tendons may not be absent. One may need to perform capsulodesis or chondrodesis of the MP joint to maintain proper extension, supplementing with opponensplasty as needed. For the windblown hand, web space reconstruction, MP fusion, and opponensplasty may be required.

DUPLICATION

Polydactyly vies with syndactyly for the most common congenital hand difference. Reported incidences vary from 1 in 300 in African-Americans to 1 in 3000 for whites. The classification was detailed by Stelling and Turek: type I is an extra soft tissue mass without bone; type II is a normal-appearing digit that articulates with the phalanx or metacarpal; and type III is an extra digit with its own metacarpal. This scheme is useful for thinking of the duplicate digits in broad terms, but treatment is guided by separate classifications based on the site of the duplication: preaxial, central, or postaxial.

PREAXIAL

Duplication of the thumb can occur at any level. It almost always interferes with normal function and therefore benefits from surgical correction. The old concept that simple ablation of one duplicate would solve all problems has largely been discarded. These problems are not simple; there is a re-operation rate of over 25% for late deformity. Ezaki has stated that thumb function can never be made completely normal, and the goal should be reconstructing the best thumb possible from the available tissue. Wassel's classification aids in planning the surgery (Fig. 21–85). For types I and II, a Bilhaut-Clouquet type of combination procedure can be performed, but it is difficult to get consistently good results. The best option for all types seems to be ablation of the more hypoplastic duplicate with reconstruction of the remaining one in a fashion that minimizes later deformity and maximizes stability and function (Figs. 21–86 and 21–87). The most common type is the Wassel IV, with duplication of the entire proximal and distal phalanx. It often requires excision of the excess metacarpal head, reorientation of the articular surface, and reconstruction of the collateral ligaments (Fig. 21–88). These procedures can be quite difficult, and the Wassel IV duplication is a risk factor for requiring later operations for deformity.

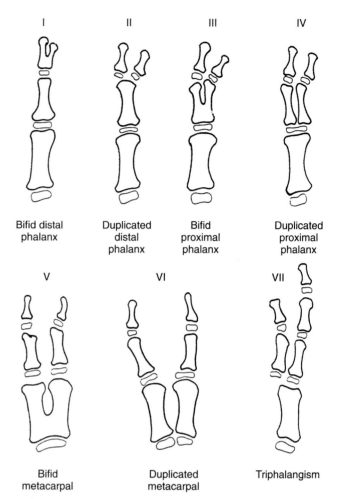

Figure 21–85. Classification of thumb duplication proposed by Wassel in 1969. (From Wassel HD: The results of surgery for polydactyly of the thumb: a review. Clin Orthop 64:175, 1969.)

Other risk factors include a preoperative zigzag deformity and radial deviation of both duplicates.

CENTRAL POLYDACTYLY

Central polydactyly can be further separated into index polydactyly and long/ring polydactyly, with the latter being more of a true central polydactyly and the former an independent entity. Index polydactylies are rare. When present, they impinge on the first web space and limit thumb access to the other digits. Normal pinch function is virtually impossible. The treatment for this involves whatever surgery is required to obtain good hand function, either through ablation of the duplicate or even ray amputation.

Duplication of long and ring fingers is a more common problem, often complicated by having incompletely formed digits linked by syndactyly. The treatment can be retention of the better duplicate if it is at least three fourths of normal size, has stability, is not excessively deviated, and has motor function. In other situations, the best option may be ray resection to achieve appropriate function.

POSTAXIAL (ULNAR) POLYDACTYLY

Temtamy and McKusick categorized this quite common condition into two types: type A is a well-developed super-

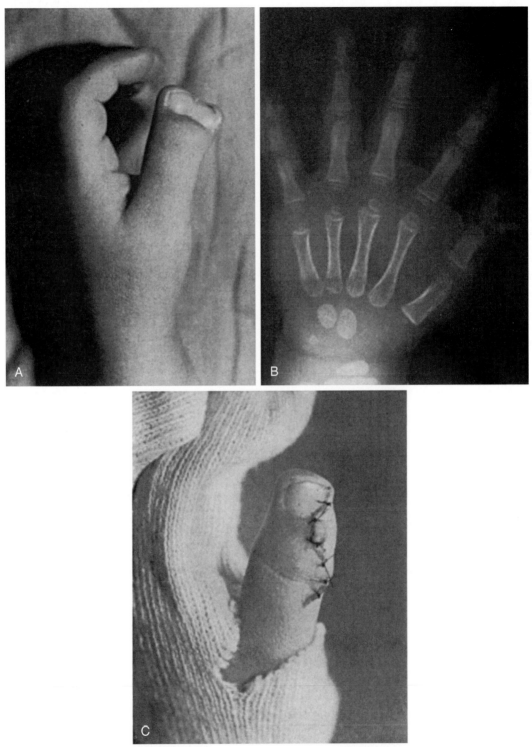

Figure 21–86. Clinical photograph *(A)*, radiograph *(B)*, and postoperative result *(C)*, of a Wassel type II duplication treated with ablation of the radial accessory digit and reconstruction of the radial perionychium utilizing a radial soft tissue flap from the deleted part. (From Simmons BP: Polydactyly. Hand Clin 1:545–565, 1985.)

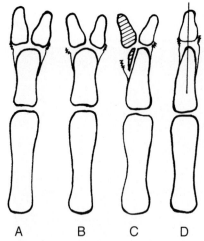

Figure 21–87. Depiction of surgical correction of a Wassel type II thumb with ablation of the radial digit and narrowing of the articular head of the proximal phalanx. Note the preservation of the radial collateral ligament that is reattached to the centralized ulnar distal phalanx. A Kirschner wire is utilized to maintain the reduction during the healing phase postoperatively. (From Manske PR: Treatment of duplicate thumb using a ligamentous/periosteal flap. J Hand Surg [Am] 14:728, 1989.)

numary digit with articulation on the fifth metacarpal, and type B is a common skin tag with no bone, tendon, or nail element. Type B can be suture ligated in the nursery if the pedicle is very narrow. One should do this with caution: reports of exsanguination and retention of the digit for

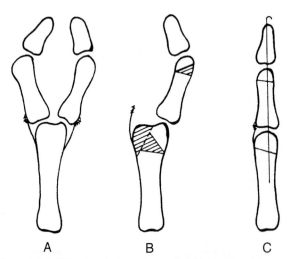

Figure 21–88. Depiction of surgical correction of a Wassel type IV duplication. The radial digit is ablated with preservation of the radial collateral ligament with a proximally based periosteal flap. The metacarpal head articular surface is thinned removing the radial facet, and a closing wedge osteotomy is used to realign the metacarpophalangeal joint. A proximal phalanx osteotomy is added to align the thumb axis, and the collateral ligament is reattached restoring radial stability. A Kirschner wire maintains the reduction postoperatively during bone and soft tissue healing. (From Manske PR: Treatment of duplicate thumb using a ligamentous/periosteal flap. J Hand Surg [Am] 14:728, 1989.)

more than a month have been made. All other patients should have formal surgical removal of the duplicate digit and reconstruction of the retained digit as needed.

THUMB HYPOPLASIA

Normal thumbs extend approximately to the level of the PIP joint. In opposition they reach the base of the small of finger but do not extend beyond the ulnar border of the hand. Thumb hypoplasia involves a congenitally small or absent thumb. The condition is frequently associated with other anomalies and syndromes such as radial clubbing, Holt-Oram syndrome, and Fanconi's anemia, or it can occur as an isolated abnormality. The Blauth classification is very helpful in understanding the spectrum of deformities and directing treatment (Fig. 21–89):

  I. Minor hypoplasia: the thumb is slightly short, but all elements are present.
 II. Adduction contracture of the first web space, laxity of the MP joint ulnar collateral ligament, hypoplasia of the thenar muscles, and normal skeletal articulations.
III. All of the features of II plus
    A. Extrinsic tendon abnormality, hypoplastic metacarpal, and stable CMC joint.
    B. Partial metacarpal aplasia, unstable CMC joint.
IV. Pouce flottant: this digital thumb joined only by neurovascular bundle and skin
 V. The absent thumb

Type I thumbs rarely have any functional deficit, and surgical treatment is almost never necessary. Types II and III require exploration of the flexor and extensor tendons and reconstruction of anomalies, release of the first web space, opponensplasty, and MP stabilization. Types IIIB, IV, and V have almost no prospect for functional reconstruction; the hypoplastic digit should be removed, and an index pollicization should be performed.

CONSTRICTION RING SYNDROME

This group of anomalies involves circumferential bands in an extremity, and in some cases can be limb threatening. There are many theories regarding its origin, including an intrinsic defect of the germ plasm causing soft tissue slough and healing to form a band, abnormal skin creases, and decreased uterine volume. It occurs in 1 in 150,000 live births and is sporadic rather than inherited. There is a 20 to 56% rate of associated anomalies, mainly clubfeet, cleft lip and palate, meningoceles, and cranial defects. There is a greater frequency in the central digits. Patterson has classified the syndrome into four groups: (1) simple constriction ring, (2) constriction rings with distal deformity with or without lymphedema, (3) constrictions rings with soft tissue fusion of the distal parts "acrosyndactyly," and (4) intrauterine amputation. The treatments for types 1 and 2 involve excision of the ring and multiple Z-plasties (Fig. 21–90). Patients with type 3 require surgery between 6 to 12 months of age to halt the rapidly progressive deformity. The surgery involves separation of the digits to provide the best possible function. The principles of syndactyly surgery should be followed as closely as possible. For patients with type 4 who have good function, no treatment may be necessary. Otherwise, a variety of procedures are available,

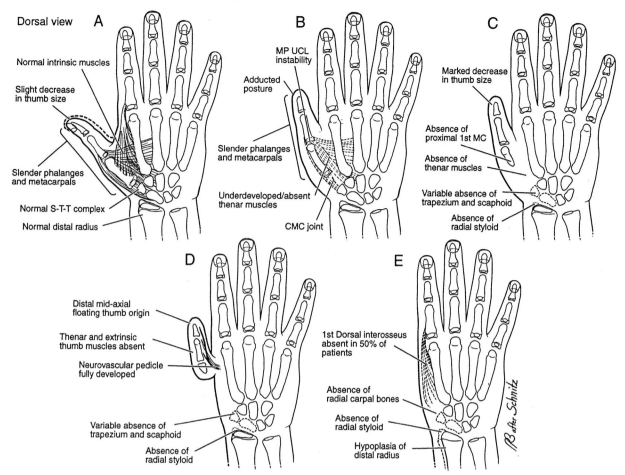

Figure 21–89. Classification of congenital thumb hypoplasia. *A*, Grade I. *B*, Grade II. *C*, Grade III. *D*, Grade IV. *E*, Grade V. (Copyright, Kevin D. Plancher, M.D., Stamford, CT.)

Figure 21–90. The depth and configuration of each constriction ring vary tremendously. Distal edema is more common with deeper grooves. *A* and *B*, Surgical correction includes excision of all skin in the side walls and debulking of dorsal excess adipose tissue. *C*, Subcutaneous advancement flaps are mobilized as needed to correct the contour deformity. *D*, Skin and subcutaneous closures are preferably staggered and Z-plasties are positioned along the side of the digit with a straight line closure dorsally. (From Upton J, Tan C: Correction of constriction rings. J Hand Surg [Am] 16:947, 1991.)

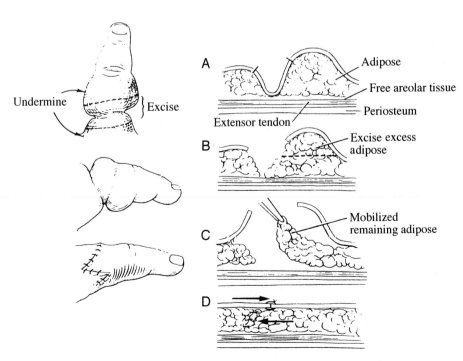

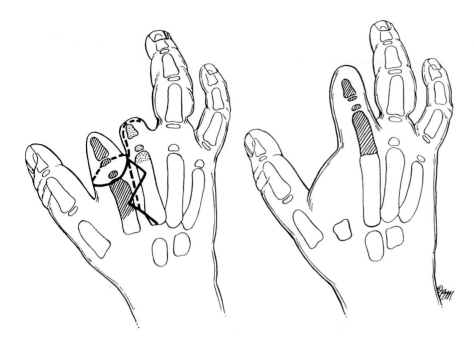

Figure 21–91. It is sometimes possible to deepen the thumb web and lengthen the long finger at the same time by adding the deleted index finger to the distal end of the long finger. (From Dobyns JH: Congenital ring syndrome. *In* Green DP, Hotchkiss RN, Pederson WC [eds]: Operative Hand Surgery, 2nd ed, New York, Churchill Livingstone, 1988, p 515; with permission.)

including on-top plasties (Fig. 21–91), distraction lengthening, and microvascular toe-to-hand transfers.

Selected Readings

Flatt AE (ed): The Care of Congenital Hand Anomalies, 2nd ed. St. Louis, Quality Medical Publishing, 1994.

Green DP, Hotchkiss RN, Pederson WC (eds): Operative Hand Surgery, 4th ed. New York, Churchill Livingstone, 1999.

Jebson PJL, Louis DS (eds): Hand Infections. Hand Clin 14(1), 1998.

Lichtman DM, Alexander AH (eds): The Wrist and its Disorders, 2nd ed. Philadelphia, WB Saunders, 1997.

Manske PR (ed): Hand Surgery Update. American Academy of Orthopaedic Surgeons, 1996.

Mih AD (ed): Congenital Hand Disorders. Hand Clin 14(1), 1998.

Osterman AL (ed): Basic Wrist Arthroscopy and Endoscopy. Hand Clin 10(4), 1994.

Chapter 22

The Hip and Femur

Brian G. Evans, M.D.

The primary function of the lower extremities is locomotion. Any alteration of the function of the lower extremities will affect that individual's ability to walk and run. The hip is the most proximal joint in the lower extremity. Alteration in the hip due to disease will significantly affect the biomechanics of gait and place abnormal stress on the joints above and below the hip.

This chapter will briefly review the anatomy of the hip and its relationship to normal and pathologic gait. The important history and physical examination findings of hip pathology will be discussed. Diseases affecting the hip will be reviewed and treatment outlined. The options for surgical management of end stage disease of the hip will be reviewed. The indications and outcome for each treatment option will also be presented. In addition, trauma to the pelvis, acetabulum, and proximal femur will be summarized and treatment alternatives outlined.

ANATOMY

Development of the Hip

The hip joint is a ball-and-socket joint with the round femoral head articulating within the round acetabular socket. The acetabulum is formed from three structures: the ischium, the ilium, and the pubis. In skeletally immature patients these three bones are joined in the medial acetabulum by the triradiate cartilage, which is a growth plate for the medial acetabulum. Also, appositional growth from the edges of the acetabulum result in increased depth of the acetabulum. Normal development of the acetabulum requires the femoral head to articulate with the acetabular cartilage. If the femoral head is chronically dislocated or subluxed within the acetabular fossa the acetabular socket will not develop fully. This will result in developmental dysplasia of the hip (DDH). The severity of this condition is determined by the degree of subluxation of the femoral head. If DDH is identified at birth or soon thereafter, the hip can be reduced either with casting or surgery. This correction can allow the hip to grow and develop almost normally. If the hip is left subluxed or dislocated, the acetabulum will be shallow and predispose the patient to develop osteoarthritis as an adult. This condition is reviewed in greater detail in Chapter 15 on pediatric orthopaedic conditions.

Osteology and Musculature of the Hip

The innominate bone consists of the ilium, ischium, and pubis, which are joined in the area of the acetabulum (Fig. 22–1). The ilium is a large flat bone providing broad surfaces for muscular attachment. The ischium extends posteriorly and forms the posterior aspect of the acetabulum. The ischium joins the ilium superiorly and the pubis inferiorly through the inferior pubic ramus. The ischium also serves as the origin of the hamstring and short external rotator muscles of the hip. The pubis consists of the superior pubic ramus, inferior pubic ramus, and the pubic symphysis. The superior pubic ramus joins the pubic symphysis with the ilium, and the inferior pubic ramus connects the pubic symphysis with the ischium. The pubis serves as the site of insertion of the musculature of the abdominal wall as well as the site of origin for the adductor muscles of the thigh.

The acetabulum is formed at the junction of the ilium, ischium, and pubis. The ilium forms the superior dome of the acetabulum. The ischium forms the posterior acetabulum and the pubis the anterior acetabulum. The lateral opening of the acetabulum forms a horseshoe with the open end directed inferiorly. The medial base of the acetabulum contains a depression called the acetabular fovea, which is filled with a fatty tissue called the pulvinar and the ligamentum teres. The ligamentum teres extends from the acetabular fovea (to) the fovea of the femoral head. The artery of the ligamentum teres is a branch of the obturator artery and supplies approximately 10 to 20% of the bone of the femoral head. The fovea of the femur, which is a depression on the femoral head, serves as the site of attachment of the ligamentum teres. Attached to the rim of the horseshoe is a fibrocartilaginous labrum, which is similar to the meniscus in the knee. This structure serves to improve stability and to cushion the femoral neck when the femur is rotated and impinges upon the acetabular rim at the extremes of motion. The hip joint capsule is a dense fibrous structure extending from the base of the intertrochanteric region of the femur to the acetabular rim. Within the capsule are the iliofemoral and pubofemoral ligaments anteriorly and the ischiofemoral ligament posteriorly. These ligaments, along with the ligamentum teres and the labrum, augment the stability of the hip joint.

The femoral head is essentially spherical in geometry (Figs. 22–2 and 22–3). The spherical portion of the femoral head is covered by articular cartilage. The sphere is altered in two areas: laterally, where the femoral neck begins, and medially at the fovea of the femoral head. The femoral neck joins the femur at an angle of approximately 125 degrees. The neck is also rotated anteriorly 12 to 14 degrees relative to the axis represented by the posterior femoral condyles (Fig. 22–4). The femoral neck flares laterally

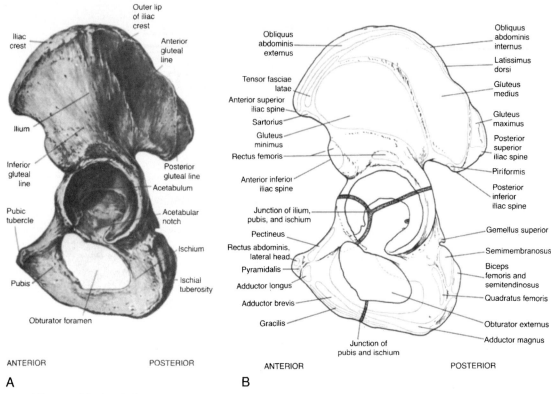

Figure 22–1. *A*, Lateral aspect of left hip bone. *B*, Attachments and epiphyseal lines are shown. (From Williams PL, Warwick R: Gray's Anatomy, 36th ed. New York, Churchill Livingstone, 1980, pp 378–379.)

to join the proximal femur in between the greater and lesser trochanters. The greater trochanter, which is a large osseous prominence at the proximal lateral aspect of the femur, serves as the site of attachment of the abductor musculature. Between the greater and lesser trochanters is an osseous ridge, which serves as the site of attachment of the short external rotators. The lesser trochanter is the site of attachment of the iliopsoas tendon. The iliopsoas tendon leaves the pelvis over the anterior column and superior pubic ramus and then travels over the anterior femoral

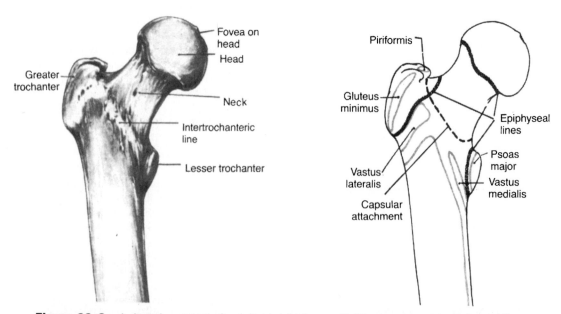

Figure 22–2. *A*, Anterior aspect of proximal right femur. *B*, Attachments and epiphyseal lines (From Williams PL, Warwick R: Gray's Anatomy, 36th ed. New York, Churchill Livingstone, 1980, pp 392–393.)

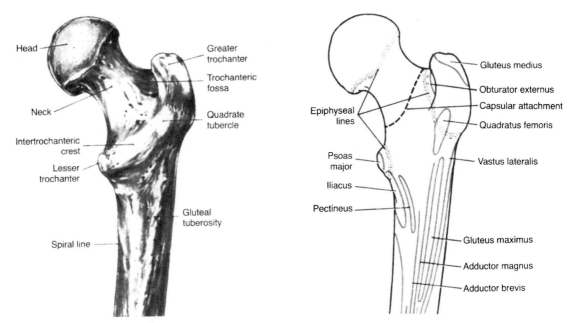

Figure 22-3. *A,* Posterior aspect of proximal right femur. *B,* Attachments and epiphyseal lines. (From Williams PL, Warwick R: Gray's Anatomy, 36th ed. New York, Churchill Livingstone, 1980, p 394.)

neck to insert on the lesser trochanter, which lies on the posterior inferior aspect of the intertrochanteric ridge.

The muscles of the hip form several distinct groups. The anterior muscles are the hip flexors, which consist of the iliopsoas and rectus femoris and sartorius muscles. The femoral nerve innervates the rectus femoris and sartorius muscles. Motor branches from spinal roots L2, L3, and L4 innervate the iliopsoas. The lateral muscle group consists of the abductors, the gluteus medius, gluteus minimus, and tensor fascia lata. These muscles are essential for normal gait. They stabilize the pelvis in single limb stance phase of normal gait. The anterior third of the gluteus medius muscle is also the principal internal rotator of the hip. The superior gluteal nerve innervates the gluteus medius, gluteus minimus, and tensor fasciae latae. Surgical dissection that extends greater than 5 cm proximal to the greater

trochanter can disrupt the nerve and will result in a limp. The posterior muscles form two layers (Fig. 22–5). The superficial layer consists of the gluteus maximus, the primary extensor of the hip, which is innervated by the inferior gluteal nerve. The deep layer consists of the short external rotators of the hip, the piriformis, superior gemellus, obturator internus, inferior gemellus, obturator ex-

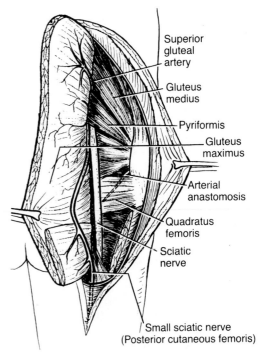

Figure 22-5. Major anatomic features exposed by reflection of right gluteus maximus. (From Steinberg M [ed]: The Hip and Its Disorders. Philadelphia, WB Saunders, 1991.)

Figure 22-4. Average rotary, or torsion, angle of the femur. It may be anteverted (A) or retroverted (R). (From Steinberg M [ed]: The Hip and Its Disorders. Philadelphia, WB Saunders, 1991.)

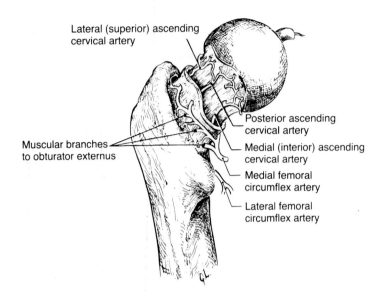

Lateral (superior) ascending cervical artery

Posterior ascending cervical artery

Medial (interior) ascending cervical artery

Muscular branches to obturator externus

Medial femoral circumflex artery

Lateral femoral circumflex artery

Figure 22–6. Arterial supply to the head and neck of the posterior aspect of the left proximal femur. Note the extracapsular arterial ring on the surface of the capsule, the ascending cervical arteries on the neck of the femur, and the intra-articular subsynovial arterial ring at the articular cartilage margin. (From Steinberg M [ed]: The Hip and Its Disorders. Philadelphia, WB Saunders, 1991.)

ternus, the quadratus femoris, and the gluteus minimus and medius. These muscles externally rotate the femur and provide abduction. Small branches from the sacral plexus innervate the short external rotators. The medial muscle group consists of the pectineus; adductor brevis, longus, and magnus; and the gracilis. The adductors and gracilis are supplied by the obturator nerve, with the posterior portion of the adductor magnus also receiving innervation from the tibial division of the sciatic nerve. The femoral nerve innervates the pectineus.

The sciatic nerve crosses the hip joint posteriorly (See Fig. 22–5). It exits the pelvis through the superior sciatic notch, under the piriformis muscle, and lies superficial to the short external rotators. The nerve has two distinct divisions within the single nerve sheath—the tibial and peroneal divisions. The peroneal division is more susceptible to injury at all levels along the course of the sciatic nerve. The increased susceptibility is due to the more lateral location and a more tenuous blood supply of the peroneal division within the sciatic nerve sheath. Therefore, a partial injury to the sciatic nerve will commonly result in a foot drop, clinically similar to the deficits seen in an isolated injury to the common peroneal nerve injury at the level of the fibular neck. One anatomic point with important clinical relevance is that the peroneal division of the sciatic nerve has only one motor branch in the posterior thigh supplying the short head of the biceps femoris. Determining if the short head of the biceps is normally innervated can assist in determining the level of peroneal nerve injury clinically (i.e., the hip or knee).

Vascular Anatomy of the Proximal Femur and Femoral Head

The medial and lateral femoral circumflex vessels in conjunction with the artery of the ligamentum teres provide the vascular supply to proximal femur and femoral head (Fig. 22–6). The medial femoral circumflex artery extends posteriorly and ascends proximally deep to the quadratus femoris muscle. At the level of the hip it joins an arterial ring at the base of the femoral neck. The lateral femoral

circumflex artery extends anteriorly and gives off an ascending branch, which also joins the arterial ring at the base of the femoral neck. This vascular ring gives rise to a group of vessels, which run in the retinacular tissue inside the capsule to enter the femoral head at the base of the articular surface (Fig. 22–7). These vessels provide 80 to 90% of the blood supply to the femoral head. The artery of the ligamentum teres, a branch of the obturator artery, travels within the ligamentum teres and supplies only 10 to 20% of the blood supply to the femoral head.

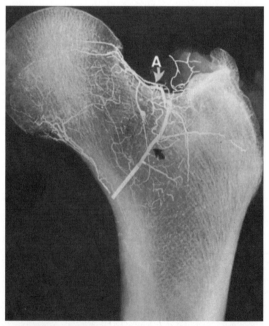

Figure 22–7. Mercury injection of the posterior ascending basal branch joining the superior gluteal to form the trochanteric anastomosis. The lateral ascending rami (A) contribute to the epiphysis, to the descending metaphyseal vessels, and to the subcapital anastomosis. (From Harty M, Joyce JJ: Surgical approaches to hip and femur. J Bone Joint Surg 1963; 45:1.)

BIOMECHANICS

The joint reaction force is the sum of all forces that cross a joint. These forces include components from gravity, body weight, and muscle forces acting upon the joint. In two-legged stance with both feet on the ground and static conditions a joint reaction force of approximately 1.3 to 1.5 times body weight will cross each hip joint. However, in single-limb stance this force will increase to 2.5 to 3 times body weight across the hip joint. The primary contribution to the increase is the force generated by the abductor muscles to maintain balance and to keep the pelvis level. If the system is in motion, such as during walking, the joint reaction forces can be as high as 4 times body weight.

Several studies have measured the actual joint reaction forces during rehabilitation using an implanted-instrumented prosthesis. The greatest joint reaction force was noted when the patients arose from a low chair or during stair climbing. However, even non–weight-bearing activities such as getting onto a bedpan were found to have a joint reaction force of 1.5 to 1.8 times body weight. The lowest joint reaction forces with ambulation were recorded when patients used touch-down weight bearing. Touch-down weight bearing allows the patient to rest the foot on the ground to balance the weight of the leg but not to step down or bear weight on the involved lower extremity.

GAIT

As mentioned previously, the principal function of the lower extremities is ambulation. In gait analysis a gait cycle examines one leg, beginning with heel strike, and continues until the next heel strike of the same leg (Fig. 22–8). Gait can be divided into two principal phases: stance and swing. The stance phase is defined as that portion of the gait cycle when the foot is in contact with the ground. The swing phase is the portion of each step when the foot is not in contact with the ground. The stance phase makes up 60% of each step, and the remainder is made up by the swing phase. Therefore, for 20% of the gait cycle both feet are in contact with the ground. Normal gait requires a stable pelvis, which is provided by the hip abductor muscles. Normal gait also requires 40 degrees of hip flexion and 10 degrees of internal rotation and external rotation.

PATIENT EVALUATION

History

The evaluation of a patient with hip pain requires careful attention to the history, physical examination, and radiographic studies. The character, nature, and duration of the patient's pain should be documented. Acute or recent onset pain will be associated more commonly with trauma or infection. Chronic and gradually progressive pain is associated with arthritic conditions. Intra-articular pain is usually described as a deep aching pain. Pain from the hip joint will commonly be noted anteriorly in the groin or in the region of the greater trochanter. Hip pain can radiate down the inner and anterior thigh to the knee with little or no pain in the area of the hip. Only rarely will hip pain radiate distal to the knee. In adolescent patients it is not uncommon for hip pathology to present as knee pain. Therefore, a thorough physical and radiographic evaluation of the hips is necessary to identify the pathology in these patients. Posterior pain and buttock pain is more commonly associated with lumbar spine pathology. Spine pain also will more commonly radiate down the posterior thigh and below the knee. The insidious onset of a deep boring pain and pain that awakens the patient at night suggest either infection or neoplastic disease.

Hip pain is commonly aggravated by activity and relieved by rest. Patients will report difficulty donning and doffing their shoes and socks and difficulty with toenail care on the involved extremity. As the pain progresses, patients will begin to have pain with prolonged sitting and at night as they try to sleep. Patients with hip arthritis will report that if they have been sitting for a prolonged period of time, then when they get up to walk, the hip will feel out of place or painful for the first few steps. This feeling usually will resolve quickly after a few minutes of walking.

The use of a cane, walking stick or crutch should be documented. The patient may also have begun to take over-the-counter anti-inflammatory medication or pain relievers. The medication and the amount the patient is taking as well as the level of relief this provided needs to be recorded. The patient's walking tolerance can be measured in terms of blocks the patient can walk or in terms of how many minutes the patient can be ambulatory doing activities such as grocery shopping or walking in a mall. Documentation of this data will give a detailed picture of the degree of pain and the patient's functional limitations.

Patients should also be questioned about past problems with the hip such as hip dislocation at birth, delays in ambulation as an infant, and any bracing needed as a child. If previous surgery or trauma to the hips has occurred, this

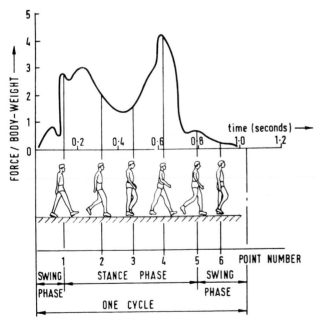

Figure 22–8. Magnitude of the resultant hip joint reaction force during walking. (Modified from Paul JP: Proc Instit Mech Engrs 1967; 181:8.)

should be explored in detail. The past medical history and any medications the patient is taking should be noted. This information can have implications for the patient's hip problems and may have an impact upon what treatment may be instituted.

Physical Examination

The most important aspect of the physical examination in patients with hip disease is evaluation of their gait pattern. The gait will reveal important information about the patient's ambulatory status and the pain. Patients with significant hip pain will manifest a coxalgic gait. This gait pattern is represented by a reduced stance phase on the painful leg, and the shoulders lurch laterally over the affected hip. Patients with mild pain or weakness in the abductor muscles may have a stance phase equal to the opposite leg, but the shoulders will continue to lurch over the affected leg. This lurch results in moving the center of gravity closer to the center of rotation of the hip. This in turn reduces the force necessary to stabilize the pelvis in stance phase. This gait is referred to as a Trendelenburg gait (equal stance phase and the shoulders lurching over the affected hip).

The hip should be inspected for previous scars, swelling, bruises, or abrasions. The region then should be palpated to identify areas of focal tenderness such as over the greater trochanter, sciatic nerve, or anterior hip capsule. The range of motion of the hip should then be determined. Normal range of motion of the hip is flexion to 130 degrees, extension to 20 degrees, adduction to 30 degrees, abduction to 40 degrees, internal rotation to 30 degrees, and external rotation to 70 degrees. When assessing the range of motion of the hip it is important to stabilize the lumbar spine. Motion in the lumbar spine may be attributed to the hip if the examiner is not careful. The Thomas test will stabilize the lumbar spine to measure for a flexion contracture of the hip (Fig. 22–9). Movement of the pelvis with abduction and adduction can be accurately assessed by placing a hand on the opposite anterior superior iliac spine and recording the patient's motion as the amount of motion prior to pelvic abduction.

To assess the function of the hip abductor muscles, the examiner has the patient standing while the involved leg is lifted off the floor. The patient should now be standing on the uninvolved leg and the pelvis should remain level.

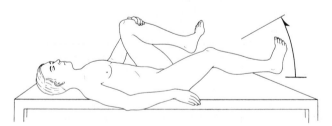

Figure 22–9. Thomas' test. After simultaneous flexion of both hips, each hip may be extended separately to record the arc from the horizontal to the femoral shaft. This indicates the degree of passive flexion contracture of the hip. (From Steinberg M [ed]: The Hip and Its Disorders. Philadelphia, WB Saunders, 1991.)

The patient then stands on the involved leg and lifts the uninvolved leg off the floor. If the pelvis is level, then the patient has normal strength of the abductor muscles. If the pelvis becomes lower on the elevated leg, then the abductor muscles are weak or the hip that is weight bearing is painful. This is referred to as the Trendelenburg sign.

A careful neurologic examination and lumbar spine examination are essential to assessing the possibility of spine pathology producing pain radiating to the hip. Patients with significant arthritic disease in the hip will also commonly have spine pathology as well. Hip arthritis and restriction in hip range of motion can exacerbate spine pathology. The limited range of motion of the hip will result in increased motion at the lumbosacral junction. This motion can aggravate degenerative facet arthropathy and lumbar stenosis. Replacement of the hip and improvement in the range of motion in the hip, however, can relieve stress from the lumbosacral junction and subsequently relieve the patient's pain.

In addition, the pulses should be palpated in the foot and ankle. Significant reduction may indicate vascular insufficiency and may require further evaluation. Vascular compromise may impair wound healing or may lead to acute vascular crisis in the early postoperative period if this is not recognized and treated prior to any elective hip procedure. In addition, if any significant vascular reconstruction has been done in the area of the involved hip, care needs to be taken at the time of surgery to avoid damage to the previous reconstruction.

Radiographic Evaluation

Routine radiography of the pelvis and hips is the most useful study in evaluating hip disease. Standard AP (anteroposterior) radiography of the pelvis will reveal the lower lumbar spine, sacroiliac joints, innominate bone, pubic symphysis, hip joint, and proximal femurs (Fig. 22–10). Frequently in unilateral disease the normal side can be used for comparison (Fig. 22–11). Lateral views of the proximal femurs can also be helpful in defining disease and in determining the size and location of a pathologic lesion. Four pelvic oblique views can be obtained to further evaluate the pelvis and acetabulum, particularly in cases of trauma. These are the inlet, outlet, and Judet's views. Judet's views are 45-degrees pelvic oblique views. They are useful for examination of the acetabulum. The obturator oblique is a 45-degrees internally rotated view of the pelvis (Fig. 22–12). The obturator foramen is roughly perpendicular to the beam, and the iliac crest is in line with the beam. This view will clearly demonstrate the anterior column and posterior rim of the acetabulum. The iliac oblique view is a 45-degrees externally rotated view of the pelvis and acetabulum (Fig. 22–13). The iliac wing is perpendicular to the beam, and the superior and inferior pubic rami are parallel to the beam. This view will clearly demonstrate the anterior rim and the posterior column of the acetabulum.

The inlet and outlet views are useful for patients with pelvic trauma to demonstrate translation of the involved hemipelvis (Fig. 22–14). The inlet view is taken with the beam oriented cephalad to caudad at 45-degrees to demonstrate the anterior or posterior translation of the involved hemipelvis. The outlet view is taken with the

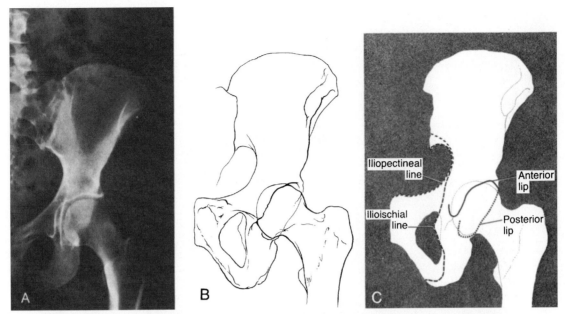

Figure 22–10. *A*, AP radiograph of the left hemipelvis. *B*, Diagram demonstrating the anatomic landmarks seen on the AP radiograph. *C*, The major landmarks identified by various lines, as follows: diagonal dashes, the iliopectineal line (anterior column); straight dashes, the ilioischial line (posterior column); solid line, the anterior lip of the acetabulum; dotted line, the posterior lip of the acetabulum. The same identifying lines are used in Figures 22–12 and 22–13. (From Tile M: Fractures of the Pelvis and Acetabulum. Baltimore: Williams & Wilkins Co, 1984.)

beam oriented 45-degrees from caudad to cephalad. This provides a true AP view of the sacrum. Also, this view can clearly demonstrate any superior or inferior translation of the hemipelvis.

Computed tomography (CT) of the pelvis is most helpful in evaluating trauma. In some centers this has replaced and certainly augments the use of oblique pelvic radiography (Fig. 22–15). CT imaging is particularly helpful in demonstrating fractures in the posterior pelvis and sacrum, which may be poorly visualized in routine radiography. Fractures to the acetabulum are well visualized on CT scan images. CT images can clearly delineate the extent of the

fracture as well as demonstrate any intra-articular fragments, which may be present. The CT can also be converted into a three-dimensional image to more clearly demonstrate the fracture pattern. CT imaging can also be utilized to demonstrate other nontraumatic pathology. For example, anterior osteoarthritis, which may be subtle on the plain radiographs, can readily be appreciated on CT images. Avascular necrosis may also be evaluated with this technique. CT images can augment plain radiography in demonstrating early collapse of the femoral head, which may affect the treatment options available to the patient.

Magnetic resonance imaging (MRI) of the hips is indi-

Figure 22–11. A 75-year-old patient had severe right hip pain. The radiograph reveals a normal left hip and advanced arthritic changes in the right hip. The right hip demonstrates a lateral femoral neck osteophyte, subchondral sclerosis of the subchondral bone, and a subchondral cyst in the femoral head.

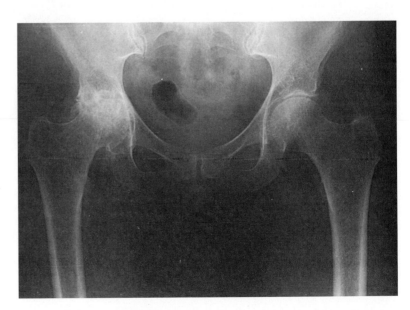

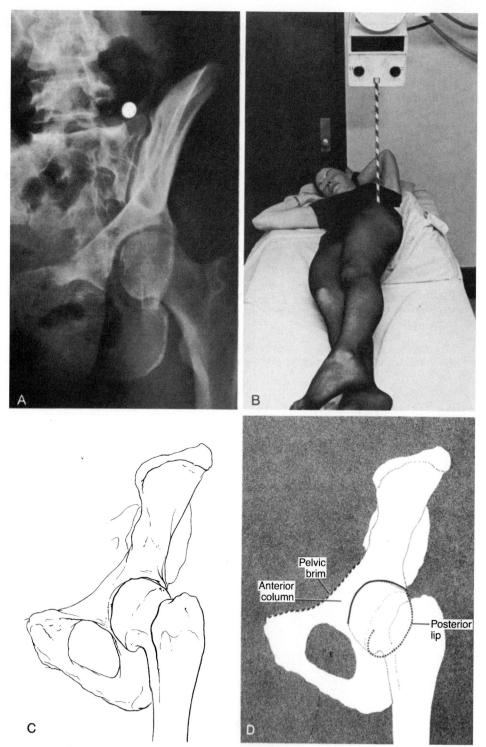

Figure 22–12. *A*, Obturator oblique radiographic view of the left hemipelvis. *B*, This view is taken by elevating the affected hip 45 degrees to the horizontal by means of a wedge and directing the beam through the hip joint with a 15-degree upward tilt. *C*, Diagram demonstrating the anatomy of the pelvis on the obturator oblique view. *D*, Diagram demonstrating the important anatomic landmarks by various lines (described in Figure 22–10 *C*). In this view, note particularly the pelvic brim, indicating the border of the anterior column and the posterior lip of the acetabulum. (From Tile M: Fractures of the Pelvis and Acetabulum. Baltimore: Williams & Wilkins Co, 1984.)

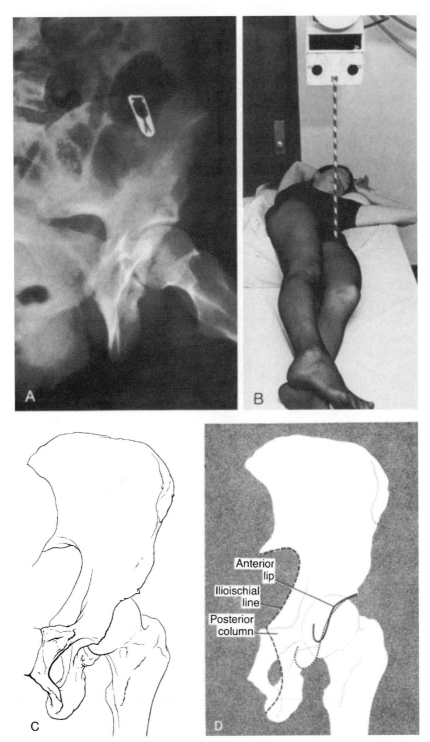

Figure 22–13. *A,* Iliac oblique radiographic view of the left hemipelvis. This view is taken placing the patient in 45 degrees of external rotation by elevating the uninjured side on a wedge, as shown in *B. C,* Diagram demonstrating the anatomic landmarks of the left hemipelvis on the iliac oblique view, further clarified in *D* by the various lines described for Figure 22–10. This view best demonstrates the posterior column of the acetabulum, outlined by the ilioischial line, the iliac crest, and the anterior lip of the acetabulum. (From Tile M: Fractures of the Pelvis and Acetabulum. Baltimore: Williams & Wilkins Co, 1984.)

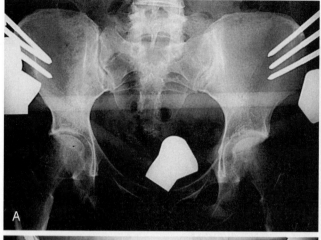

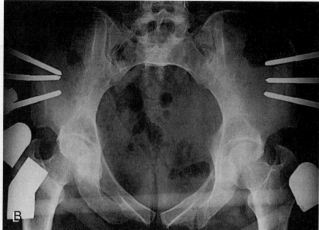

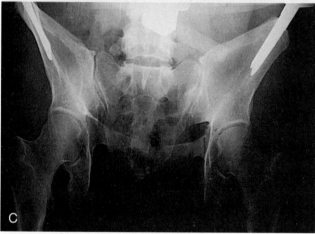

Figure 22–14. These radiographs show a 36-year-old female who sustained a pelvic fracture as a result of a motor vehicle accident. She has had a pelvic external fixation frame applied as treatment. *A,* An AP radiograph. *B,* An inlet view clearly demonstrates the pelvic ring and any anterior or posterior translation. *C,* An outlet view clearly demonstrates an AP view of the sacrum and reveals any superior translation of the involved hemipelvis.

cated in patients in whom a periarticular lesion is suspected or to evaluate for the presence of avascular necrosis (AVN) of the femoral heads (Fig. 22–16). MRI is a very sensitive and specific tool for the evaluation of AVN. It can readily demonstrate the avascular segment prior to changes on the plain radiographs. MRI can also be helpful in demonstrating a tear in the acetabular labrum. This is best demonstrated by the use of MRI arthrography. MRI contrast material is injected intra-articularly, and an MRI of the hip is obtained. The contrast will outline the labrum so that any defect in labrum can be identified.

The technetium 99 pyrophosphate dimethylphosphate (MDP) bone scan can be helpful in evaluating the pelvis. The bone scan can be used as a sensitive indicator of osseous disease in the pelvis. Metastatic disease, occult fractures, infection, or osteomyelitis can be identified (Fig. 22–17). The bone scan is most helpful as a general skeletal screening tool for metastatic disease. The bone scan is very sensitive but is not specific. Therefore, other studies such as MRI or CT may be necessary to fully evaluate the nature and extent of any identified pathology.

Hip aspiration and arthrography can be helpful in the evaluation of pathology. Aspiration can be used to evaluate hip sepsis in both a native hip as well as after hip arthroplasty. Aspiration is best performed under fluoroscopic guidance. An arthrogram can then be utilized to confirm the intra-articular position of the needle. Arthrography can also be utilized to assess loosening of a hip

prosthesis. The contrast material can be noted flowing around the loosened implant demonstrating the separation of the implant, cement, and bone. Not infrequently, patients will present with a history of both hip and spine pathology. Injection of local anesthetic with or without a corticosteroid medication into the hip under fluoroscopic guidance can be helpful in differentiating the pain coming from the hip with that coming from the spine. If the intra-articular local anesthetic results in significant relief of pain, the pain is most likely intra-articular in origin. If the local anesthetic agent does not alter the pain, extra-articular or spine disease should be investigated. Aspiration of the hip should be performed under fluoroscopic guidance.

The patient's history and physical examination direct the use of these radiographic techniques. The appropriate use of these diagnostic tests can result in cost-effective and accurate diagnosis and properly directed treatment.

HIP PATHOLOGY

A variety of soft tissue conditions can affect the hip. These conditions are not uniformly associated with trauma or injury; however, an injury can be the inciting event. Trochanteric bursitis is a common condition of the hip. The pain results from inflammation within the trochanteric bursa, which is located over the lateral aspect of the greater trochanter under the fasciae latae. It is associated with pain

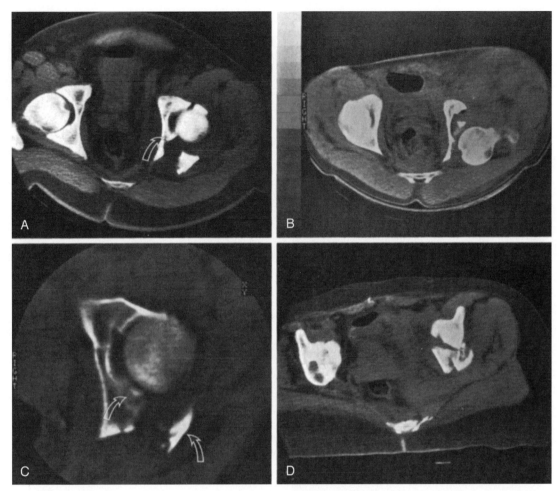

Figure 22–15. *A,* CT scan demonstrating a transverse fracture of the acetabulum; both the anterior column fracture and the large posterior wall fracture are clearly seen. The arrow points to a comminuted rotated bony fragment. *B,* CT scan through the central portion of the acetabulum, showing a posterior dislocation of the hip with two large posterior wall fragments trapped within the joint, preventing reduction. The CT scan is most helpful in determining the presence and size of retained bony fragments in the joint. *C,* CT scan through the central portion of the acetabulum. Note the large displaced posterior wall fracture on the lower right. The other arrow on the left points to an impacted fracture of the articular surface. These depressed articular fractures are best seen on CT scanning. *D,* CT scan through the acetabular dome of a patient with a severely comminuted acetabular fracture. Note the comminuted fragments and the degree of displacement of the posterior column. (From Tile M: Fractures of the Pelvis and Acetabulum. Baltimore: Williams & Wilkins Co, 1984.)

over the lateral aspect of the hip in the region of the greater trochanter. The pain is a deep ache centered over the greater trochanter with radiation both proximally to the pelvic brim and distally, extending all the way to the knee occasionally. The pain is exacerbated by adduction of the hip with the knee extended. No pathologic changes are noted on either plain radiographs or MRI. The treatment consists of stretching the fasciae latae and the iliotibial band, and nonsteroidal anti-inflammatory medications. If these conservative measures are unsuccessful, the patient may benefit from physical therapy with the use of local modalities such as ultrasound and iontophoresis. These modalities can be augmented with a corticosteroid injection into the bursa. If these nonoperative modalities fail to relieve the pain, the bursa can be surgically excised. However, this option is rarely required.

The iliotibial band and the trochanteric bursa can also be involved in the snapping hip. The iliotibial band snapping over the trochanteric bursa and the greater trochanter causes this condition, which is not always painful. The treatment is similar to that for trochanteric bursitis. Snapping in the hip can also occur anteriorly. The iliopsoas tendon can snap over the anterior aspect of the hip where the tendon exits the pelvis over the anterior pelvic brim. This results in an anterior snap with flexion and extension. The amount of pain associated with the snap is variable. The treatment is directed toward alleviation of the pain. Nonsteroidal anti-inflammatory medications can be helpful at alleviating the pain. Stretching of the iliopsoas with hip extension can also help to reduce the symptoms.

Another cause of a snapping hip is a tear in the acetabular labrum. The acetabular labrum is a dense fibrocartilag-

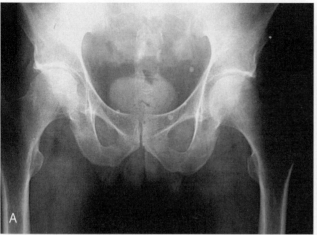
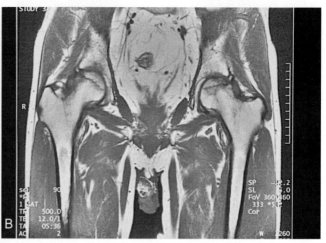
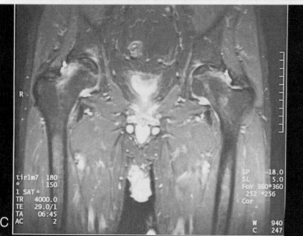

Figure 22–16. A 34-year-old male had a history of 4 months of increasing bilateral hip pain. *A,* His AP pelvic radiograph is essentially normal. *B,* A T$_1$-weighted MRI of the pelvis and hips demonstrates a line of decreased signal intensity across the superior third of the femoral head. This line represents the new bone laid down at the periphery of the lesion that serves to wall off the lesion. *C,* A T$_2$-weighted image demonstrates the same line of decreased signal intensity across the femoral head. However, this image also demonstrates a zone of increased signal intensity consistent with the fibrovascular response to the necrotic bone.

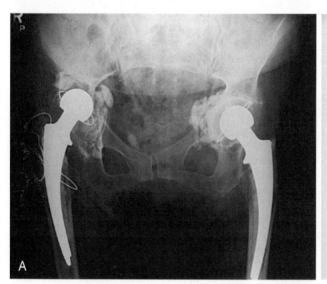
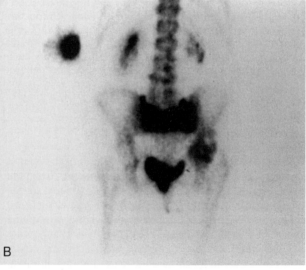

Figure 22–17. An 84-year-old female presented with severe hip pain after a car ride. The patient had bilateral hip replacements done approximately 15 years prior to presentation. *A,* An AP pelvic radiograph demonstrates significant diffuse osteopenia and two hip replacements. Both appear to have some loosening of the acetabular components but demonstrate no acute changes. *B,* A delayed image from a ^{99}Tc-MDP bone scan demonstrates significant uptake in the left acetabulum. However, there is diffuse marked increased uptake throughout the sacrum. This pattern of uptake is consistent with a sacral insufficiency fracture.

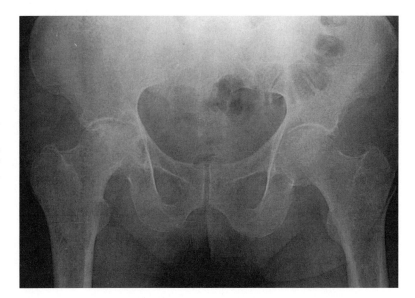

Figure 22–18. A 60-year-old male experienced 6 months of increasing right hip pain. He has a history of corticosteroid administration for treatment of a malignancy. The AP radiograph demonstrates collapse of the superior aspect of the femoral head.

inous structure that is attached to the acetabular rim. This structure can be injured much like the meniscus in the knee. The labrum is more prone to injury in patients with acetabular dysplasia. In this condition the acetabulum is shallow and the labrum hypertrophies and becomes weightbearing. A tear in the acetabular labrum presents clinically with pain in the hip anteriorly, particularly with internal rotation. This injury is also commonly associated with a click noted when the hip is flexed and extended. The diagnosis can be confirmed with an MRI obtained after the injection of intra-articular contrast dye. The accuracy of this assessment is approximately 85%; without the intra-articular contrast material the accuracy is only 50 to 60%. When a tear is identified but the pain is mild, no treatment is necessary. If, however, the injury is painful or the click limits activity, then the tear should be excised or repaired. This can be done either arthroscopically or with an open hip arthrotomy.

Intra-articular loose bodies can occur either as a result of trauma or as a result of synovial chondromatosis. In synovial chondromatosis the synovium will develop osteochondral loose bodies that will be free in the articular space. In the knee these loose bodies will cause a great deal of mechanical symptoms, such as locking. In the hip there is not enough free space for the loose body to cause locking. However, these loose bodies can restrict motion and cause pain. Synovial chondromatosis can be difficult to diagnose. The plain radiographs are usually normal or will demonstrate the very subtle stippled calcifications of the osteochondral fragments. The MRI or CT scan can be helpful in demonstrating the loose bodies and the expansion of the synovial space and effusion. The treatment is surgical. An arthrotomy is performed and the fragments are removed. Synovectomy can be performed, although care should be taken to preserve the vascularity of the femoral head.

Avascular necrosis (AVN) is a condition that most commonly affects the femoral head. However, this condition can also affect the proximal humerus, knee, and talus. The specific mechanism causing AVN is unclear. Several factors have been associated with increased risk of developing this condition. The most common factors are trauma to the femoral head or neck, systemic corticosteroid administration, and excessive alcohol intake (Fig. 22–18). In addition to these factors, many other less common factors such as hemoglobinopathies, metabolic conditions, and inflammatory conditions can cause AVN. However, in as many as one third of patients with nontraumatic AVN no specific etiology can be identified, and those cases are considered to be idiopathic AVN.

In all cases of AVN there is compromise of the blood supply of the femoral head. This most commonly occurs in the antero superior portion of the femoral head, leading to necrosis of a portion of the subchondral bone. If the avascular segment is large and in a weight-bearing area, the stability of the subchondral bone will be compromised as the necrotic trabeculae weaken. This process occurs over 6 to 24 months. Although MRI or ⁹⁹Tc-MDP bone scan can demonstrate the lesion early, the plain radiographs are frequently normal after the segment becomes avascular. Over time the round femoral head will weaken and then develop an area of collapse. At this point the joint is no longer round and congruent and without intervention frequently will progress to degenerative arthritis.

The lesion of AVN has a very typical pathologic and radiographic pattern. The lesion is most commonly in the anterior and superior subchondral bone of the femoral head. There are several distinct zones to the lesion (Fig. 22–19). The outer zone is an area of increased vascularity and inflammation that is in response to the necrotic segment. The next layer is a dense area of sclerotic bone, which is laid down around the necrotic segment in an attempt to heal the lesion. However, this simply serves to wall off the lesion and prevents vascular invasion and healing of the lesion. Inside the sclerotic bone is the necrotic bone with the trabecular structure that is relatively intact. Histologically the necrosis of the bone is demonstrated by trabecular bone with empty lacunae. Closer to the subchondral bone is the area of collapse of the trabecular bone. The outer layer is composed of the subchondral bone and articular cartilage. Radiographically a subchondral radiolucent line referred to as a crescent sign demonstrates this region (Fig.

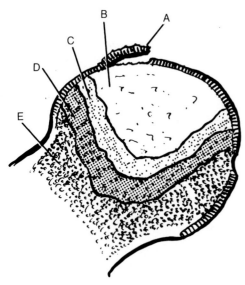

Figure 22–19. Schematic drawing of a femoral head with avascular necrosis. A = Articular cartilage; B = necrotic bone and marrow elements; C = reactive fibrous tissue; D = hypertrophic bone, composed of living and dead trabeculae; E = normal trabeculae of femoral neck. (From Steinberg M [ed]: The Hip and Its Disorders. Philadelphia, WB Saunders, 1991.)

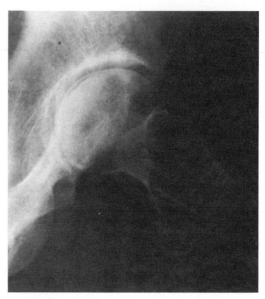

Figure 22–20. Crescent sign seen in lateral radiograph (stage III). (From Steinberg M [ed]: The Hip and Its Disorders. Philadelphia, WB Saunders, 1991.)

22–20). Frequently, after collapse of the subchondral bone, a defect through the cartilage and the subchondral bone will allow articular fluid to enter the necrotic area. This will further impair healing of the lesion.

In early cases prior to collapse of the femoral head attempts can be made to save the femoral head and restore viability to the necrotic bone. These techniques are surgical. There are several variations; however, all involve drilling a core tract into the avascular portion of the femoral head in an attempt to restore vascularity to the necrotic bone and possibly heal the lesion (Fig. 22–21). Several techniques have been described to augment this procedure. These include the use of autologous cancellous bone grafting, bone graft substitutes, allograft cortical or cancellous bone, and using one of the patient's fibulas on a vascular pedicle to place vascularized bone into the lesion.

Of patients who have documented AVN that is untreated, 70% will require a total hip replacement within 5 years. Patients who have had a core decompression type procedure will require a total hip replacement in 30 to 35% of cases by 5 years. The results are improved compared to the natural history; however, the success rate is lower than we would prefer. Vascularized fibular grafting has demonstrated an improvement in the survivorship of the involved hip. However, there can be significant weakness in foot and ankle function on the involved side after harvesting the fibula.

For patients with small lesions that have already undergone subchondral collapse an osteotomy may be done to rotate the necrotic collapsed segment out from under the weight-bearing area of the hip. However, commonly the lesion is extensive, and not enough viable bone remains to allow the necrotic segment to be rotated out of the weight-bearing area of the hip. As the AVN progresses and the hip becomes severely degenerated, hip replacement offers

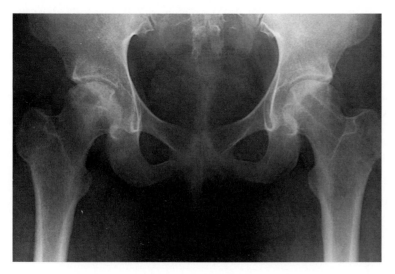

Figure 22–21. A 20-year-old female with systemic lupus erythematosus had been treated with corticosteroids. She presented with bilateral hip pain. The patient was noted to have bilateral avascular necrosis of the femoral heads. Core decompression and grafting was done on the left hip. The core tract is noted in the femoral neck and extending into the femoral head.

Table 22–1. Categories of Hip Arthritis

Category	Examples	Etiology
Osteoarthritis	Primary osteoarthritis Secondary osteoarthritis	Idiopathic Congenital Developmental Avascular necrosis Posttraumatic
Inflammatory arthritis	Rheumatoid arthritis Ankylosing spondylitis Psoriatic arthritis Systemic lupus erythematosus	Immunogenic
Infectious	Pyogenic Lyme disease Nonpyogenic	*Staphylococcus aureus, S. epidermidis,* gonococcal infection *Borrelia* *Mycobacterium*
Other	Crystals Hemophilia	Gout, pseudogout Hemosiderin deposition

the most reliable means of restoring function and relieving pain. Many of the patients are relatively young to receive a total hip replacement. The average age of patients with AVN is approximately 35 to 45 years. The results of cemented arthroplasty in this population have not been as successful as in patients with osteoarthritis. Noncemented fixation does appear to have less loosening compared to cemented fixation in this population. However, the rate of other complications such as dislocation, infection, and hematoma are increased in this population, regardless of the method of fixation of the components.

HIP ARTHRITIS

A wide variety of arthritic conditions can affect the hip joint. Although the medical therapy can vary on the basis of the specific diagnosis, the operative treatments fall into several broad categories and will be discussed as such. Arthritis is defined as any condition that results in articular cartilage damage with resulting pain and limitation of the motion of a joint. Hip arthritis can be divided into several broad categories (Table 22–1).

The clinical presentation of hip arthritis is a gradual increase in pain and limitation of motion. Frequently patients will complain of a reduction in their ability to walk for distances. Patients will also notice a marked stiffness in the joint when they have been sitting for a period of time and then stand. The joint will feel out of place or stiff. This symptom will resolve usually after a few steps. As the arthritis progresses and the joint begins to lose motion, patients will also notice a reduction in their ability to care for their own toe nails and difficulty with activities such as putting on socks or stockings and tying their shoes. A limp will also commonly occur in patients with hip arthritis, particularly after long walks or at the end of the day.

Radiographic and etiologic criteria can assist in dividing the patients into two broad categories—osteoarthritis and inflammatory arthritis—based upon the history and the radiographic appearance of the hip joints. Osteoarthritis has four classic features on plain radiography: localized joint space narrowing, subchondral sclerosis, osteophyte

formation, and subchondral cysts. In rheumatoid arthritis, which is a classic example of an inflammatory arthritis, the radiographic features are periarticular osteopenia, diffuse or global joint space narrowing, and occasionally subchondral cysts. In inflammatory arthritis of the hip, protrusio deformity of the femoral head beyond the ilioischial line can be noted as well. In most cases of arthritic disease in the hip no additional studies, other than plain radiography, are necessary for the evaluation.

The nonoperative treatment will vary on the basis of the specific diagnosis. Osteoarthritis, whether primary or secondary, is treated in a similar fashion. The treatment for the majority of patients with osteoarthritis is nonoperative. There are five primary interventions in the nonoperative management of the patient with osteoarthritis (Table 22–2). These five interventions can be used in isolation or in combination based upon the specific clinical situation in which the patient presents. Nonsteroidal anti-inflammatory agents (NSAIDS) can be very effective in reducing the pain and improving function. However, there is a large individual variation in the efficacy and side effects with each of these agents. Therefore, patients should be tried on several NSAIDs from different chemical classes prior to abandoning this limb of therapy. The principal side effect of NSAID is GI intolerance with the possibility of ulcer formation. NSAIDs can also affect renal and hepatic function, and in the long-term use of these agents renal and hepatic function tests should be followed. In addition, these medications can affect platelet function and may have an adverse effect on bleeding times. These medicines should not be used in patients requiring anticoagulation therapy or within 5 to 7 days prior to any surgical intervention.

Table 22–2. Five Primary Interventions in the Nonoperative Management of Osteoarthritis

Nonsteroidal anti-inflammatory medications
Physical therapy
Intra-articular injection of corticosteroids
Assistive devices
Modification of activities

The new cyclooxygenase-2 (COX-2) inhibitors may offer lower side effects compared to the nonspecific cyclooxygenase inhibitors that represent the majority of the NSAIDs on the market; however, this concept needs to be demonstrated in large clinical trials. The COX-2 inhibitors will also have less effect on platelet function and may be safe to use for patients on anticoagulation therapy. The efficacy of these medicines for pain relief will probably be similar to that noted with traditional NSAIDs.

Intra-articular corticosteroid injections are helpful for the treatment of an acute exacerbation in pain. Intra-articular injections are more beneficial in the treatment of shoulder and knee pathology compared to the hip. They have not been as widely utilized for arthritis of the hip, in part due to the difficulty in ensuring the injection is in fact intra-articular. Fluoroscopy is helpful in ensuring proper placement of the needle. Injection of the hip with local anesthetic can be helpful in differentiating referred back pain from intra-articular hip pathology. Also, there are patients who will have a strong referred pain from the hip to the knee. In these patients an intra-articular hip injection will relieve the knee pain and confirm the site of origin of the knee pain. However, injections are limited in their ability to provide long-term relief of symptoms. Corticosteroid injection for arthritis should not be done more than three times per year. If the patient requires more frequent injections for pain control, other therapeutic measures or surgery should be considered. Repeated injection of the joint is not indicated and will result in acceleration of the articular cartilage degeneration, increasing the risks of complications such as infection.

Physical therapy can be beneficial in reducing pain and improving range of motion for osteoarthritis involving the knee or shoulder, but limited benefit has been found for the treatment of osteoarthritis involving the hip. If physical therapy is utilized, it should be done early in the course. As the arthritis progresses, physical therapy will serve only to exacerbate an already painful joint. However, all patients should be encouraged in aerobic fitness to maintain their joint function as well as their general health. Activities such as swimming and cycling have minimal repetitive impact and are excellent for aerobic fitness. Impact activities such as running and racquet sports can further damage an arthritic joint and should be discouraged in a patient with hip arthritis. As the arthritis progresses, the patient will be able to do less and less and may become more sedentary. If this occurs, the symptoms will also increase in severity.

Assistive devices including crutches, cane, and a walker can be quite effective in the relief of stress across the joint surface with ambulation in patients with osteoarthritis involving the lower extremities. A cane used in the contralateral hand of a patient with isolated hip arthritis can reduce the joint reaction force by as much as 30%. However, the use of these devices is associated with a significant change in a patient's perception of themselves and their global health status. Although this modality can be helpful in relieving symptoms and maintaining mobility, it will commonly meet resistance from the patient.

Modification of activities is one of the most significant aspects in the nonoperative management of arthritis. This approach includes modification in a patient's activities of daily living and self-care. Obtaining a handicapped parking permit and devices to assist in putting on shoes and socks can be very helpful for patients with limitations due to hip arthritis. The reduction in certain activities such as running or racquet sports can improve the joint symptoms. However, this change may result in a gradual progressive decrease in the patient's quality of life. The level of social interaction and activities in which the patient can comfortably participate can become markedly reduced. Modification of activities should also address patients who are overweight. Reduction in weight can significantly improve a patient's symptoms, increase their mobility and improve their global health status. In addition, reduction in weight will reduce the stress placed upon the joint replacement if they require surgery.

The nonoperative management of a patient with osteoarthritis involves all the above therapies. However, as the arthritis progresses, pain and limitation of activities will continue to increase. When the patient fails to achieve acceptable symptomatic relief with the nonoperative regimen, joint replacement should be discussed. No significant change in the complexity of the surgery or outcome will be noted in patients with hip arthritis who delay operative intervention with nonoperative treatment. Therefore the timing of the surgical intervention is based entirely upon the patient, the level of pain, and limitations.

SURGICAL MANAGEMENT

Most hip pathology can be managed with one of several options: arthroscopy, arthrotomy, osteotomy, arthrodesis, or arthroplasty (hemiarthroplasty or total hip arthroplasty). Each option has specific indications and contraindications, which will be discussed in the next few sections.

Arthroscopy

Hip arthroscopy is in its infancy compared to this technique in the knee. The indications for hip arthroscopy are the removal of loose bodies from the hip joint, to address acetabular labral pathology, and to identify articular cartilage defects. The technique requires the use of special equipment because of the more extensive soft tissue envelope around the hip compared to the knee. The soft tissue envelope also limits the mobility of the arthroscope within the hip. In addition, the hip capsule is quite thick and the articular space is quite small. Frequently traction is required to gain visualization of the hip joint. The portals must be opened with care to avoid injury to the neurovascular structures surrounding the hip. These issues have significantly slowed the widespread use of this technique in practice today.

Arthrotomy

Arthrotomy involves surgical opening of the hip joint. Many of the indications for hip arthroscopy are also indications for hip arthrotomy, including removal of loose bodies and to address acetabular labral lesions. However, hip arthrotomy can also address the drainage of hip sepsis and hip synovectomy. The hip joint can be exposed and opened

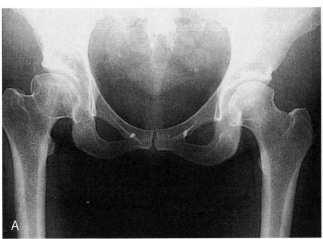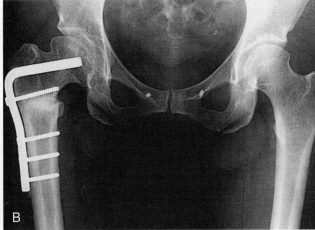

Figure 22–22. A 37-year-old female had 1 year of increasing right hip pain. The initial AP radiograph *(A)* demonstrates a large femoral head with a shortened femoral neck. This most likely is the late result of Perthes' disease of the hip. The patient underwent an osteotomy of the proximal femur to address her hip pain *(B)*.

either from the anterior aspect or the posterior aspect. Anterior approaches are more commonly utilized because this approach is less likely to injure the blood supply to the femoral head, which arises from the medial femoral circumflex vessels along the posterior intertrochanteric line.

The hip joint is then opened, usually from the acetabular edge, with care taken to preserve the acetabular labrum. If the labrum is torn, it can be either excised or repaired, depending on the condition and nature of the tear. A threaded pin can be inserted into the greater trochanter and up into the femoral neck to assist in distraction of the femoral head from the acetabulum and to allow inspection of the hip joint. Any loose bodies or fragments can be removed. If the indication for arthrotomy is synovectomy, it may be necessary to open the hip from the posterior as well as the anterior aspect. This approach does increase the risk of postoperative avascular necrosis, but the synovium of the hip cannot be removed from a single approach.

Osteotomy

Osteotomy involves redirecting the articular surface to move damaged cartilage from the weight-bearing areas of the joint and place a less damaged area of the articular surface in the weight-bearing area of the hip joint (Fig. 22–22). Osteotomy can also reduce joint forces by re-aligning the bone of the pelvis or proximal femur to yield a larger area of contact to distribute the force of weight bearing. During osteotomy the bone of the pelvis or femur is transected, redirected and then fixed rigidly. If the arthritis is localized to only one region of a joint, by performing an osteotomy, the damaged cartilage can be moved away from the weight-bearing area and undamaged articular surfaces are transferred into the high stress area. This will result in reduced pain and prolong the functional life of the patient's native joint. Prerequisites for an osteotomy are that the patient has an adequate range of motion of the joint, that the joint is stable, and that the articular damage involves only a limited area of the joint. If extensive arthritis or an inflammatory arthritis is present, an osteotomy will not be successful.

In properly selected patients hip osteotomies can have a success of greater than 80% at follow-up 8 to 10 years later. For young patients with focal articular damage osteotomy can provide an acceptable result and allow them to retain their own hip joint. This can delay or possibly eliminate the need for replacement with artificial materials, which can wear or become loose. Acetabular osteotomy for developmental dysplasia of the hip can make subsequent total hip arthroplasty easier by redirecting the acetabular bone stock and providing better coverage for an acetabular component (Fig. 22–23). However, osteotomy of the proximal femur can make a future hip replacement more difficult by altering the anatomy of the proximal femur (Fig. 22–24). This may require an additional osteotomy to reconstruct the femur at the time of total hip replacement.

Arthrodesis

Arthrodesis involves the fusion of the proximal femur to the pelvis. This can provide a strong stable painless lower

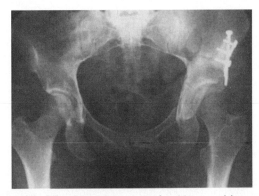

Figure 22–23. AP radiograph of a 26-year-old woman 6 months after a left pelvic osteotomy was performed to deepen her acetabulum and improve coverage of the femoral head. Her primary diagnosis was developmental dysplasia of the hip, which left her with a shallow left acetabulum. (From Wiesel S, Delahay JN [eds]: Essentials of Orthopaedic Surgery, 2nd ed. Philadelphia, WB Saunders, 1997.)

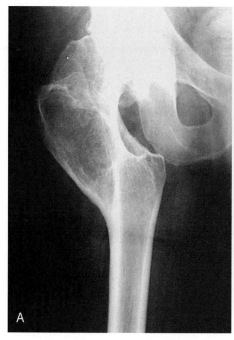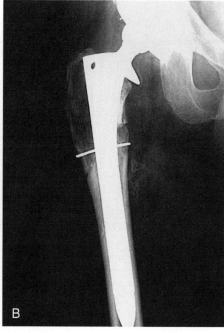

A

B

Figure 22–24. A 56-year-old male had a proximal femoral osteotomy performed for the treatment of slipped capital femoral epiphysis. The patient now had extensive arthritis and required a total hip replacement. *A,* The preoperative radiograph shows the extensive deformity of the femur. *B,* The postoperative radiograph. A proximal femoral osteotomy was required to reconstruct the femur to the total hip replacement. This was fixed with one cerclage cable.

extremity. The patient can return to even heavy labor without the risk of loosening or damage to the arthrodesis. Arthrodesis is indicated in patients who are young with unilateral hip disease with no symptoms or disease involving the lumbar spine, contralateral hip, or the ipsilateral knee. In patients with an inflammatory arthritis or nontraumatic AVN, arthrodesis is relatively contraindicated because these diseases are frequently bilateral. Several studies looking at the long-term results of arthrodesis have found good results lasting greater than 20 years.

However, the hip is stiff and over 15 to 20 years the arthrodesis can result in low back pain and pain in the ipsilateral knee. Several reports have noted between 50 to 60% of patients complaining of pain in the back or knee 25 to 50 years afterward. If the pain is severe, the fusion can be taken down surgically and a total hip replacement performed. The outcome of this surgery depends upon the functional status of the hip abductor muscles. If the surgical arthrodesis involved the removal of the insertion or origin of the hip abductors the patient will have an increased rate of dislocation, pain, and limp after conversion to total hip replacement. These complications can be minimized if the technique used for the arthrodesis spares the hip abductor muscles. The return to a mobile hip can relieve the patient's low back pain; however, the patient may experience pain in the hip that was not present with the arthrodesis.

Hip Replacement Surgery

Total hip replacement (THR) is a common operation today. Approximately 200,000 hip replacements are performed each year. The primary goal of hip replacement is to relieve pain. This can be accomplished in over 95% of patients. The results of THR can last approximately 15 years or more. In fact, one study found that more than 80% of THRs survived a minimum of 20 years. In total hip replacement both the socket and the ball are replaced with metal

and plastic parts. The socket is replaced with either a plastic cup cemented onto the bone or by a metal shell impacted into the prepared acetabular space with a removable plastic liner (Fig. 22–25). The ball is replaced by a metal ball attached to a stem that goes inside the canal of the femur. Two principal types of implants are used today. Those inserted with bone cement and those inserted without cement and designed to allow bone to grow onto or into a porous metal surface (Fig. 22–26). Both techniques have excellent long-term follow-up data supporting their effectiveness.

The principal advantage of utilizing bone cement is that immediate rigid fixation is obtained. The bone does not

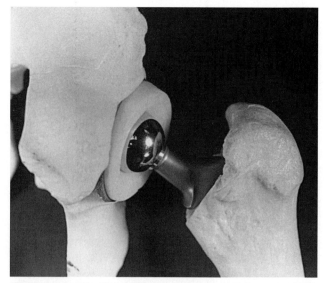

Figure 22–25. Total hip arthroplasty with the acetabular component press fitted onto the pelvis, the femoral component inserted into the femoral canal, and the femoral head articulating with the acetabular polyethylene liner.

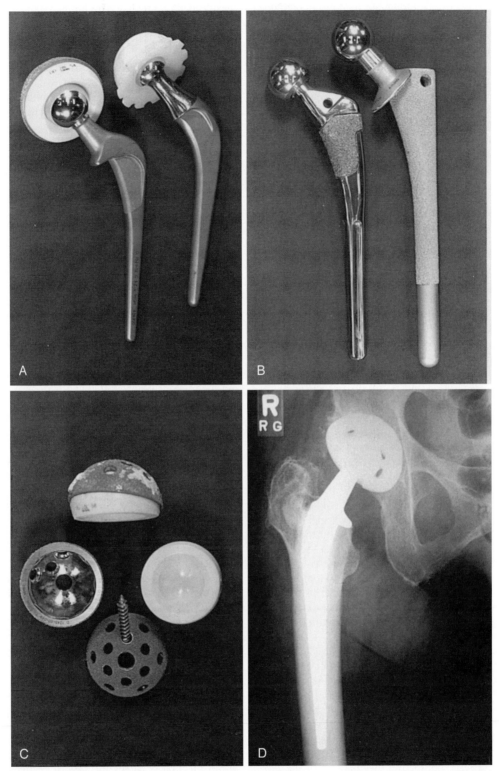

Figure 22–26. *A,* A photograph of two femoral stems and acetabular components. At left is a modular cemented femoral stem with a modular noncemented acetabular component. The right stem is a nonmodular (one-piece) femoral component with an all-polyethylene acetabular component designed for use with cement. *B,* Two modular noncemented femoral stems. The stem on the right has a surface of metal mesh and the stem on the left has metal beads for the bone to grow into. *C,* A modular noncemented acetabular component from several views demonstrating the position of screws, which may be used for ancillary fixation of the metal shell. *D,* A postoperative radiograph of a hybrid hip replacement, with a noncemented acetabular component and a cemented femoral component.

need to respond to the implant to obtain fixation. In patients with an average age of 65 years, excellent survival times of 20 years or greater have been noted. The patients can fully bear weight immediately after the surgery, which facilitates their rehabilitation. In addition the implants are simpler to manufacture and are correspondingly less expensive. Noncemented fixation requires the bone to respond to the implant to provide rigid long-term fixation. The implant has a surface that allows the bone to grow into or onto it in order to stabilize the implant. Many surgeons will keep the patient on restricted weight bearing for the first 6 weeks postoperatively to allow for the bone in-growth. If the bone does stabilize the implant as the bone remodels over time, rigid fixation should be maintained over the long term.

Noncemented fixation is compromised by the presence of thigh pain. This mechanical pain occurs over the anterior thigh. It is mechanical in nature, increasing with weight bearing, and usually relieved by rest. Usually thigh pain can be controlled with NSAIDs or mild narcotic analgesics. In a small number of patients, 1 to 2%, the pain can be severe. In these cases stem revision is indicated. Thigh pain is present in 5 to 15% of patients. Thigh pain is not uniformly associated with loosening of the stem. Thigh pain usually peaks by 6 months postoperatively, but it can persist for up to 18 to 24 months. In a small number of patients it can persist indefinitely. Thigh pain is seen only rarely in cemented fixation and is usually associated with loosening.

Total hip arthroplasty is performed from either an anterior, posterior, or transtrochanteric approach. The transtrochanteric approach utilizes an osteotomy of the greater trochanter to mobilize the abductors to gain access to the hip joint. This has the advantage of providing excellent exposure by lifting the abductors superiorly, allowing visualization of both the anterior and posterior column of the acetabulum. In addition, advancing the trochanter distally to tighten the abductors and reduce the risk of postoperative dislocation can increase the stability of the total hip. However, historically there has been a trochanteric osteotomy nonunion rate of 5 to 15%. Trochanteric nonunion will result in a persistent limp and an increased rate of dislocation postoperatively. The transtrochanteric approach currently is used primarily for revision procedures for which additional exposure is required.

The posterior approaches are the most commonly used for total hip replacement. The dissection is carried posterior to the trochanter. The short external rotators are divided, and a posterior capsule is opened. This creates a defect in the posterior capsule. The hip is dislocated posteriorly by flexion, adduction, and internal rotation. The posterior approach provides an excellent extensile exposure to the pelvis, hip, and femur. In addition, the gluteus medius and minimus are preserved, optimizing the function of the hip abductors postoperatively. However, postoperatively the patients are most at risk for a posterior dislocation with flexion, adduction, and internal rotation. The rate of instability after a posterior approach is 2 to 5% in primary total hip replacement.

Anterior approaches to the hip are also commonly employed for total hip replacement. These approaches enter the hip from in front of the greater trochanter by detaching a portion of the gluteus medius and minimus. The anterior capsule is then opened. The hip is extended, adducted, and externally rotated to dislocate the femoral head, and the arthroplasty is completed. This approach can yield extensile exposure proximally and distally. This approach leaves the posterior capsule intact, protecting the patient from a posterior dislocation. The rate of instability is 1 to 2% in most series. Thus, the rate of instability is less with the anterior approach compared to the posterior approach. However, by detaching a portion of the gluteus medius from the trochanter, the muscle is weakened, which can lead to a greater incidence of limp and pain in the postoperative period. Furthermore, if the repair of the detached gluteus medius pulls off of the trochanter, the patient may be left with a persistent Trendelenburg limp.

All approaches can provide good exposure and a successful arthroplasty. However, there is a trade-off in terms of stability and function. The posterior approach does not violate the abductors and has a low incidence of limp postoperatively. However, the posterior capsule is opened and the rate of instability is increased. Although the anterior approaches leave the posterior capsule intact with a correspondingly lower rate of instability, the abductor mechanism is partially detached, and this may leave the abductors weak and yield an increased rate of limp postoperatively.

The patient is mobilized to a chair the day of surgery and then begins physical therapy. If the femoral component is cemented, the patient may fully bear weight on the operative leg immediately. If porous in-growth fixation is utilized, some surgeons will allow only restricted weight bearing for 6 weeks to allow for bone in-growth. The best exercise in the postoperative period is walking. Hip abduction exercises may be done as well with a posterior approach. However, if an anterior approach was utilized the active abduction exercises may be delayed to allow the gluteus medius repair to heal.

Patients need to be careful not to flex the hip beyond 90 degrees and to keep their legs abducted and neutrally rotated for the first 6 weeks to prevent the femoral head from dislocating out of the acetabular component. The rate of instability and the position of greatest instability vary with the approach used for the arthroplasty, as outlined earlier. With anterior approaches the greatest instability is with extension and external rotation. The patients usually report a dislocation occurring while they are standing and pivoting or while they are supine in bed with the legs adducted and the feet externally rotated. In contrast posterior instability occurs when the hip is in a flexed, adducted, and internally rotated position. Patients report instability when they are getting up from a chair, off the toilet, or out of an automobile. The rate of dislocation is greatest in the first 6 weeks postoperatively. If a dislocation does occur within the first 6 weeks the rate of recurrent instability is approximately 30% with the majority having a single event. However, if the first dislocation occurs after the first 6 months, the rate of recurrent instability increases to 60% with the majority of patients having recurrent instability, often requiring revision surgery to address the problem.

The treatment of a dislocated hip is to first reduce the hip, usually with conscious sedation. Occasionally a general anesthetic may be required for reduction. The patient is placed into a brace for a period of 6 weeks. The patients can bear weight as tolerated. If the patient does have recurrent instability, revision may be necessary. Prior to revision it is helpful to determine the precise position of the components. Plain radiography can accurately determine the vertical inclination of the component, however, it is the degree of anterior rotation of the component that is a greater factor in instability after total hip replacement. Accurate assessment of the anterior rotation of the component can be best assessed by the use of CT imaging. If CT scan imaging cuts are also taken through the femoral condyles, the rotation of both the femoral and acetabular components can be determined. This information is important to aid in identifying the cause of the recurrent instability and to plan appropriate reconstructive surgery to correct the problem.

Aseptic loosening of the implant from bone occurs at a low rate with modern techniques. A recent study reviewed the minimum 20-year follow-up of patients after cemented THR revealed approximately 90% of patients had retained their original implant until they had died or their minimum 20-year follow-up evaluation. Revision surgery had been performed on 15% of the surviving patients. Eleven percent of the revisions were for aseptic loosening. The rates of loosening of the femoral component and acetabular component were 3 and 10%, respectively, in surviving patients. Eighty-five percent of the patients who survived a minimum of 20 years had retained their initial implants. Another study demonstrated the rate of femoral loosening is greater in the first five years and the rate decreases after five years. Acetabular loosening, however, was noted to increase over time when cemented components were used. A rate of cemented acetabular revision or radiographic loosening was noted to be approximately 50% at greater than 10 years. The use of modern cementing techniques has decreased the rate of early failure of cemented stems. Modern techniques, however, have not resulted in any significant change in the rate of acetabular loosening.

The survival of cemented implants in patients under 50 years of age is less than that noted in older patients. This is most likely related to the higher demands and higher activity level in younger patients. In an attempt to reduce the rate of aseptic loosening after THR surgeons have tried to achieve implant fixation directly to bone. This can be achieved through the use of porous surfaces made of small beads or wires sintered onto the base stem. If this surface is closely approximated to bone and essentially no motion occurs at the interface with bone, trabeculae will interdigitate into the porous surface and secure the implant. Little long-term data exist to support the use of porous ingrowth devices. However, the early and intermediate data are encouraging. The rate of early loosening of the porous in-growth femoral implants is comparable in most series to cemented stems. The rate of loosening appears to vary with the stem design for the porous in-growth devices. Therefore, data should be analyzed individually for each implant. Porous in-growth hemispheric acetabular components, however, appear to have a lower rate of loosening compared to cemented acetabular components. Although fixation of the metal shell to bone would be maintained, some early designs developed problems with the interface between the polyethylene liner and the metal shell. Motion and wear would occur at this interface as well as the articulating interface, leading to the development of wear debris and failure of the metal or the polyethylene liner and the need for revision surgery. In addition, the importance of high-quality, thick polyethylene liners for the noncemented acetabular components was not appreciated early. This resulted in a number of patients having early failure due to wearing down or fragmentation of the polyethylene liners (Fig. 22–27). The current recommendations are for a polyethylene thickness of at least 8 mm.

Modern liner shell interfaces should be conforming, with the polyethylene liner supported by the metal shell across the entire nonarticulating surface. The liner should not bear stress on the rim only but be uniformly supported. Most designs limit the holes in the metal shell. The holes in the shell can provide a direct conduit for wear debris to the implant bone interface. This debris can lead to an osteolytic reaction and subsequent loosening of the acetabular shell. Early designs had many holes in the metal shell for the use of ancillary fixation screws to fix the shell to bone prior to bone in-growth. Currently most surgeons press fit the metal shell on the bone by underreaming the acetabular bed and then inserting a slightly larger metal shell into the acetabular bed. This can provide an excellent initial stability and eliminate the need for screws and screw holes in many cases.

At the present time a "hybrid" total hip arthroplasty is recommended for the majority of patients receiving THR. This includes the use of a cemented femoral stem and a porous in-growth acetabular component. This arthroplasty takes advantage of the excellent long-term fixation of the cemented femoral stems and the improved fixation with modern cementing as well as the very encouraging results with the use of porous in-growth acetabular components.

Complications

The most frequent complication after THR is thromboembolic disease. This includes deep venous thrombosis and pulmonary embolism. Early in the history of THR the rate of fatal pulmonary embolism was 1 to 2%. However, at that time patients were kept on bed rest for as long as 2 to 3 weeks and kept up to 6 weeks in the hospital. Early mobilization of patients has undoubtedly contributed to the significant reduction in the rate of fatal pulmonary embolism. However, significant reduction has also occurred through the use of anticoagulant prophylaxis, regional anesthesia, shorter operating times, and lower blood loss. In the United States THR is considered a significant risk factor for thromboembolic disease (TED), and therefore the routine use of medical or mechanical prophylaxis has been recommended. At present the rate of TED ranges between 5 and 20%. The rate of fatal pulmonary embolism is low, approximately 0.01%. The principal methods of prophylaxis are low-dose warfarin (Coumadin), aspirin, low-molecular-weight heparin, and pneumatic compression stockings. Warfarin has the greatest volume of data supporting its use. Warfarin is started the evening prior to surgery or on the day of surgery. It is recommended that the therapy be continued for 6 weeks postoperatively. The medication needs to be monitored closely to keep the level within a safe range. The prothrombin time (PT) is held between 16 and 18 sec and the INR (international normalized ratio) is

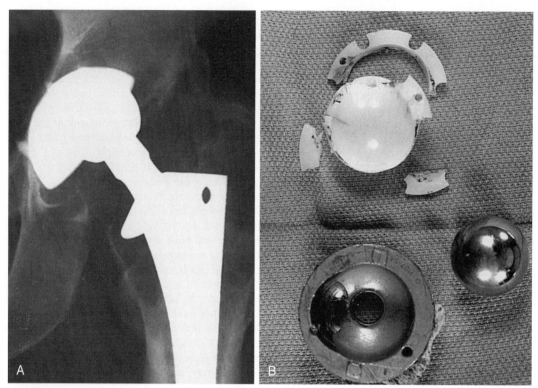

Figure 22–27. *A*, An AP radiograph of the left hip of a 52-year-old male 5 years after a noncemented total hip arthroplasty demonstrates a markedly eccentric position of the femoral head within the acetabular component. *B*, The same patient's retrieved acetabular component and femoral head. The polyethylene is fragmented and was found displaced within the shell, allowing the femoral head to articulate with the metal acetabular shell.

1.25 to 1.5. This drug has been shown in many studies to be a safe and effective method of prophylaxis. The monitoring of warfarin is of particular concern. Occasionally patients will have a dramatic elevation of their PT and INR with the first dose. This will lead to a risk of postoperative bleeding and hematoma at the operative site. As the length of stay in the hospital has decreased to 3 or 4 days or less, this has made the use of warfarin increasingly difficult. It frequently will take 5 to 7 days to get a patient equilibrated on a steady dose of warfarin. This adjustment is more difficult to accomplish in the outpatient setting. Currently this is managed with the use of home nursing services and frequent monitoring.

Low-molecular-weight heparin formulations were developed in part to provide safe and effective prophylaxis against thromboembolic disease. Subcutaneous unfractionated heparin has been used historically in the general surgical population. It has not been found to be effective in the orthopaedic population. Intravenous unfractionated heparin offers effective prophylaxis and treatment of thromboembolic disease. However, heparin requires even greater monitoring when used intravenously because it fully anticoagulates the patient immediately. If this occurs within the first 3 days postoperatively, the incidence of wound hematoma is greater than 50%; thus, this drug is infrequently used in the postoperative orthopaedic patient. Low-molecular-weight heparin is more selective in the interruption of the coagulation cascade. This results in a more controlled effect and patients do not require monitoring. The current

protocols are for 2 weeks of therapy. Most studies demonstrate efficacy comparable with warfarin for total hip replacement.

Aspirin has been used for deep venous thrombosis (DVT) prophylaxis historically. Aspirin irreversibly inhibits platelet function and theoretically will reduce the rate of formation of DVT. Little data directly support its routine use in THR; however, several studies demonstrate acceptable prophylaxis with the use of aspirin and hypotensive epidural anesthesia (HEA). HEA is an excellent anesthesia technique for THR; however, it requires careful patient monitoring and a dedicated anesthesia team. This form of anesthesia results in reduced blood loss while maintaining blood flow in the lower extremities. This reduces the need for transfusion postoperatively, which has been shown to increase the risk of DVT. In addition, the reduction in blood loss results in less activation of the coagulation cascade, again minimizing the risk of DVT. Although this technique has been shown to be very effective, it has not been widely applied because of concerns about the reduction of mean arterial blood pressure in elderly patients, which may result in stroke, renal failure, or myocardial infarction.

Dislocation of the prosthetic femoral head from the acetabular component occurs in 2 to 5% of patients after THR. As discussed previously the incidence and direction vary with the operative approach. Postoperatively patients are instructed to not bend their replaced hip beyond 90 degrees and to keep their legs abducted and in neutral rotation. These restrictions should be followed closely for the first 6 to 8 weeks following surgery. After this time the patient should have formed a sufficient pseudocapsule to protect against dislocation. However, a replaced hip is always at greater risk for dislocation compared to a native hip joint. The majority of patients who dislocate their hip in the early postoperative period can be reduced without additional surgery and protected with a hip abduction brace for 6 weeks to allow healing of the pseudocapsule. The risk of recurrent instability after an early dislocation is approximately 30%. In addition to lack of patient compliance, the other causes of dislocation are component malposition, excessive soft tissue laxity, and impingement of the prosthetic or osseous structures, resulting in levering of the femoral head out of the acetabulum. If a patient recurrently dislocates, revision surgery may be indicated.

The most devastating complication after THR is deep sepsis. Early postoperative infection occurs in approximately 0.3 to 0.5% of cases after primary THR. Late infection resulting from hematogenous spread can occur in 1 to 2% of patients. If detected within the first 2 weeks postoperatively, aggressive open débridement and synovectomy combined with intravenous antibiotics may be successful. However, if the infection recurs after débridement or is detected beyond 2 weeks, treatment must include removal of the prosthetic components and all cement. The prosthesis is left out for at least 6 weeks. An antibiotic impregnated spacer may be placed at the time of débridement. This will provide a local depot of antibiotic at the site of the infection. Recent work has demonstrated the effectiveness of a prosthesis covered in antibiotic-impregnated cement inserted at the time of the débridement to maintain the articular space and soft tissue tension and to provide stability to the soft tissues to promote healing. The success of this technique also raises the question of the role of one-stage reconstruction for an infected total hip replacement. Early data from Europe had demonstrated a success rate of 80% with this technique. However, more study is required to define the role of these techniques in the management of the infected arthroplasty. If the pathologic organisms are highly virulent and resistant to antibiotic therapy, reimplantation should be delayed for more

than 12 months. Serum bactericidal titers (SBTs) should be determined and a titer of at least 1:8 is maintained during the 6-week course of therapy. During the antibiotic therapy, patients may be mobilized as tolerated with the use of a walker. Reimplantation can proceed when the wound is sterile if sufficient bone stock and soft tissue integrity remain. The use of antibiotic-impregnated cement for the femoral component is recommended at the time of reimplantation. If the SBT was maintained at greater than 1:8 for 6 weeks, reimplantation of a new prosthesis will be successful in more than 90% of cases. Recent data have demonstrated a higher rate of recurrence for patients reimplanted without cement.

Heterotopic ossification (HO) can form around a THR in 5 to 25% of cases (Fig. 22–28). Heterotopic bone is histologically bone tissue. It forms within the muscle around the hip after arthroplasty. There is a metaplasia that occurs, forming a bone matrix that becomes calcified over the first 6 to 12 months after the surgery. Most commonly, the presence of HO will not compromise the clinical result. Associated risk factors are patients with hypertrophic osteoarthritis, males over the age of 65, HO formation after previous surgery, and ankylosing spondylitis.

HO is graded according to Brooker. Grade 1 consists of isolated islands of bone within the soft tissue between the femur and pelvis. Grade 2 is bone protruding from the proximal femur or pelvis with more than 1 cm of separation. Grade 3 consists of bone protruding from the femur or pelvis with less than 1 cm between the bones. Grade 4 is radiographic ankylosis, with no visible space between the bone protruding from the femur and pelvis. Grades 1 and 2 are rarely symptomatic. Grade 3 patients usually have stiffness and mild pain. Patients with grade 4 usually have marked stiffness and can be very symptomatic.

Patients who are at high risk for this complication can receive prophylaxis using indomethacin for 6 weeks or low-dose radiation therapy. Once HO forms, the patient should be encouraged to maintain range of motion and activity but passive stretching and passive range of motion should be avoided. Surgical intervention is indicated in patients with significant restriction of motion and pain. These problems occur most commonly in patients with

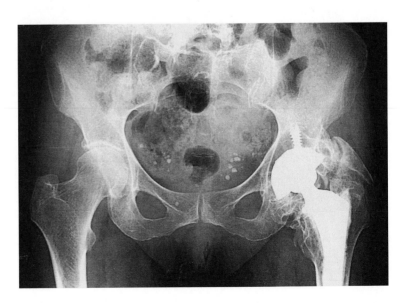

Figure 22–28. An AP radiograph of the pelvis of a 75-year-old male after a left total hip arthroplasty demonstrates Brooker stage III heterotopic ossification about the left hip.

grade 3 and 4 HO. Surgery should be delayed until the HO is mature. This usually takes 12 to 24 months and is indicated by mature appearance on plain radiography, uptake similar to the uninvolved bone of the pelvis on a ^{99}Tc-MDP bone scan, and normal serum alkaline phosphatase level. When the bone is mature it can be surgically excised. Attempts to remove the bone prior to maturity are associated with an increased rate of recurrence. After the bone is excised the patient should receive prophylaxis to prevent recurrence. The prophylaxis is as noted earlier with either indomethacin or radiation therapy. Radiation therapy is preferred in most patients because it is usually a one-dose regimen of 700 to 800 cGy and can be administered either immediately preoperatively of within the first 2 or 3 days postoperatively. In this way the entire treatment regimen is delivered in a controlled setting compared to indomethacin, which is administered for 6 weeks. The rate of recurrence after excision and prophylaxis is approximately 5 to 20%.

The limitations for the long-term fixation of a total hip arthroplasty are loosening and wear. The primary articulation in total hip arthroplasty is a metal ball in a polyethylene socket. The rate of wear is variable, ranging between 0.01 and 0.1 mm each year. The rate of wear is affected by the surface roughness of the femoral head, the quality of the polyethylene, the thickness of the polyethylene, the method of sterilization of the polyethylene, and stress applied to the articulation by the patient. As the implant, particularly the polyethylene liner, wears, the debris that is produced is released into the local tissues. The body has no mechanism to digest or eliminate the polyethylene debris. However, the local macrophages in the area recognize the material as a foreign substance and try to eliminate the debris. The macrophages ingest the material and try to digest it with catabolic enzymes and superoxides. This fails to alter the material. As the debris accumulates within the cell, it breaks down releasing the polyethylene, enzymes, and oxides into the local environment, resulting in a local bone lysis. This process creates cysts in the bone and dissects along the fixation of the implant or cement and bone (see Fig. 22–29). If allowed to continue, the lysis leads to loosening. In addition, failure can occur if the polyethylene is thin at the time of implantation. Thin polyethylene results in increased stress within the polyethylene with weight bearing and a significantly increased rate of wear. This in turn will lead to failure of the polyethylene liner and the need for revision of the implant.

Loosening can also result from mechanical failure of the implant bone interface. The cement mantle can fragment or fracture, leaving the implant loose. In noncemented fixation the implant can also loosen. This can occur when the implant never actually bonds to the bone with bone ingrowth. A fibrous tissue will form instead. This fibrous tissue may not be sufficient to maintain stable fixation of the implant. The implant will then migrate slowly, best appreciated on serial radiographs, and eventually will require revision to provide a stable implant.

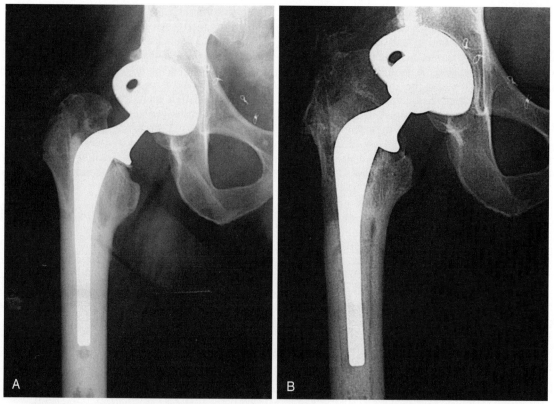

Figure 22–29. *A,* The AP view of the right hip 1 month after a hybrid total hip replacement. *B,* A follow-up radiograph taken 3 years postoperatively demonstrates marked bone loss along the lateral aspect of the femur and a new radiolucent line along the medial border of the implant. These osteolytic changes are in response to polyethylene debris in the periprosthetic tissues.

Similar to the indications for primary arthroplasty, these are elective surgeries. However, in the revision setting it is important to follow the patient closely with plain radiographs. If an accelerated pattern of bone loss is noted, revision surgery should be performed prior to the loss of an extensive amount of bone. The greater the loss of bone at the time of revision the greater the difficulty in obtaining stable fixation for the revision components. This may also lead to a higher rate of repeated revision for aseptic loosening.

TRAUMA

Trauma to the pelvis and femur occur usually as a result of blunt trauma such as a motor vehicle accident or fall. These patients are at high risk for multiple injuries apart from the pelvis and femur, such as significant injuries to the chest, abdomen, and spine in addition to other injuries in the extremities. A careful and thorough approach is required for the evaluation of the trauma patient to ensure optimal care. Injuries to the pelvic ring can damage any of the visceral structures contained within the pelvis. There may be injury to major neurovascular structures as well. Pelvic trauma is one of the true life-threatening injuries in orthopaedics. Proper and prompt initial trauma management and resuscitation are essential for the optimal management and survival of these patients.

Pelvic Trauma

The pelvis is a ring consisting of the two innominate bones joined by the symphysis pubis anteriorly and each attached to the sacrum posteriorly. These three bones are strongly held together by several ligamentous structures. The most important of these are the posterior ligamentous structures reinforcing the sacroiliac joints (Fig. 22–30). The posterior sacroiliac ligaments are much stronger than the anterior structures. The anterior aspect of the innominate bones are joined by the symphysis pubis, which comprises two hyaline cartilage surfaces covered and joined by a dense band of fibrous tissue. The combination of the bones, joints, and reinforcing ligaments creates a stable pelvic ring. This ring structure adds to the strength required for the transfer of weight-bearing forces from the lower extremities to the spine.

Trauma to the pelvis results in disruption in the ring structure. The degree of disruption determines the nature and stability of the pelvis. These injuries can be classified as stable, unstable, and complex injuries (Fig. 22–31). Stable injuries involve only one break in the ring or two areas of injury with minimal displacement. Unstable injuries involve two or more disruptions in the ring of the pelvis with significant displacement. Usually these injuries are only unstable to compression, distraction, or rotation. Complex injuries are severe disruptions to the pelvic ring that are unstable to compression, distraction, rotation, and vertical displacement.

Stable injuries are common in the elderly. They can be seen also in younger patients after trauma. These injuries do not require operative fixation. They are treated symptomatically. Patients remain in bed, progressing to chair until the symptoms subside. Then they are allowed to slowly progress in weight bearing until the fracture heals. Healing usually requires approximately 8 weeks. They can then return to full activities.

Unstable and complex injuries require operative fixation. These injuries, if not fixed, will result in significant alteration of the ability of the pelvis to bear weight. These fractures can also lead to significant alteration in the patient's limb length. The goal of operative fixation is to restore the stability to the pelvis. In unstable fractures the posterior sacroiliac ligaments are usually intact. Therefore, the ring is reconstructed by restoring integrity to the anterior ring with the use of a plate and screws or by the use of external fixation to bridge between the two iliac wings (Fig 22–32). Weight bearing is restricted for the first 6 weeks and then may progress as tolerated. In complex fractures there is no stability to the hemipelvis. The anterior and posterior structures are disrupted and need to be reduced and secured with some form of fixation. The anterior structures can be splinted with either a plate or external fixation, as in the unstable injuries. The posterior structures are reconstructed with either a plate between the two posterior iliac crests or with interfragmentary fixation across the sacroiliac joint or with two threaded bars between the two posterior iliac spines. Weight bearing needs to be restricted for the first 6 weeks and then can be progressed. Patients with pelvic fractures can have significant intrapelvic soft tissue injury as well. These injuries can result in significant urologic dysfunction, difficulty with conception and delivery in women, and chronic pelvic pain. Injuries involving the sacroiliac joints frequently will be associated with posterior pelvic pain with weight bearing. This is diagnosed by the use of an intra-articular injection of a local anesthetic agent under fluoroscopic guidance. If the pain is temporarily relieved, sacroiliac arthrodesis may be indicated.

Acetabular Fractures

Fractures to the acetabulum are usually the result of significant blunt trauma, but they can also occur in the elderly with minimal trauma. Acetabular fractures result in disruption of the articular surface and may result in fracture or contusion of the cartilage of the femoral head, predisposing these patients to posttraumatic osteoarthritis (Fig. 22–33). The risk of degenerative arthritic change is directly related to the degree of disruption of the articular cartilage. Similar to pelvic fractures, these injuries can be associated with significant intrapelvic soft tissue injury. Prior to addressing the acetabular fracture, the trauma team needs to carefully evaluate the patient to be sure that the patient is stabilized and resuscitated. Effective treatment of these injuries is optimized by the use of detailed radiographic evaluation to determine the extent and location of the fractures.

The first study obtained is the AP view of the pelvis (Fig. 22–34). This study can be augmented by the use of 45-degree pelvic oblique radiographs and Judet's views. These views can assist in demonstrating the location of the fractures and the degree of displacement. Further detail can be obtained from pelvic CT scanning to demonstrate the nature of the fracture and the degree of displacement and comminution. Effective management of these injuries requires a detailed understanding of normal pelvic and ace-

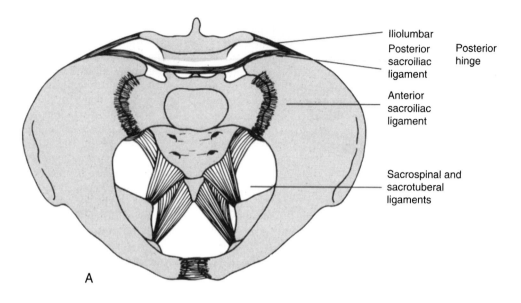

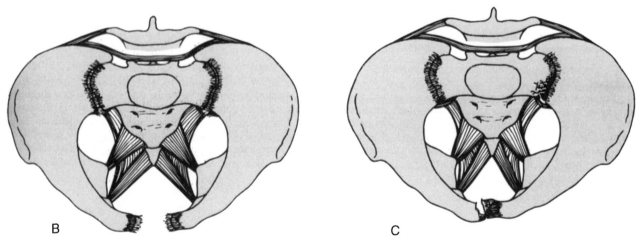

Figure 22–30. Pelvic stability. *A,* The intact ligamentous bony structures of the pelvis maintain its integrity with regard to stability. The posterior hinge, consisting of the posterior sacroiliac ligaments and the iliolumbar ligaments, is imperative to maintain vertical stability. The sacrospinous ligament prevents rotation, and the sacrotuberous ligament prevents vertical migration. As long as these, the anterior sacroiliac, and symphysis are intact, the pelvis will remain stable. If, however, the anterior symphysis is separated or the sacrum is crushed posteriorly, as seen in *B* and *C,* the posterior hinge remains intact and the pelvis is usually stable vertically. The sacrospinous ligaments are intact, and rotatory abnormalities are thus prevented. (From Browner BD [ed]: Fractures in Adults. Philadelphia, WB Saunders, 1998.)

tabular anatomy and a detailed understanding of the individual fracture.

The options for the management of these fractures are either nonoperative treatment with skeletal traction or operative reduction and internal fixation of the fracture. All these patients should be treated with traction initially to allow time to medically stabilize them prior to any operative intervention. The surgery to reduce and fix these fractures can be long and associated with extensive blood loss; therefore, it is essential to ensure that these patients are appropriately stabilized prior to any surgical intervention.

Usually surgical fixation is delayed 3 to 5 days to allow medical stabilization.

Nondisplaced acetabular fractures can be treated nonoperatively with traction. Displaced acetabular fractures should all be treated with operative fixation. However, in addition to nondisplaced fractures, fractures with extensive comminution or extremely poor bone quality, as in the elderly, may be best treated nonoperatively. Attempts at operative intervention in these patients may result in inability to obtain anatomic reduction and poor fixation, while exposing the patient to all the risks of operative interven-

Figure 22–31. Pelvic ring injuries may be classified as stable or unstable depending on the posterior arch integrity. Stable lesions have an intact posterior arch *(A)*, whereas unstable lesions can be divided into incompletely or rotationally unstable injuries with partial integrity of the arch or floor *(B1, B2)* or completely unstable injuries with no part of the floor or posterior arch intact *(C)*. (A–C, Redrawn from Comprehensive Classification of Pelvis Fractures. Bern, Switz., Maurice E. Müller Foundation, 1995.)

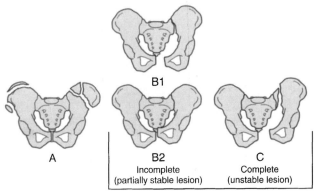

B1

A

B2
Incomplete
(partially stable lesion)

C
Complete
(unstable lesion)

Posterior arch intact   Posterior arch disruption

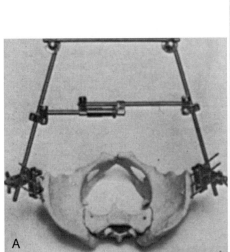

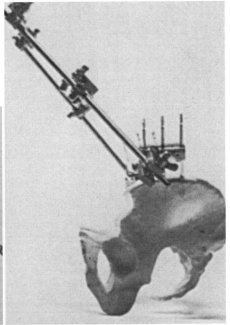

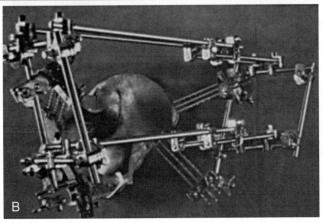

Figure 22–32. Types of external frames. *A,* Trapezoidal (Slatis) frame, which was proposed to be able to control posterior instability. This is a good frame for stabilization of the pelvis because it allows the arms to be moved in an outward direction away from the abdomen for work on the abdomen. *B,* Double-cluster frame of Mears. (From Browner BD [ed]: Fractures in Adults. Philadelphia, WB Saunders, 1998.)

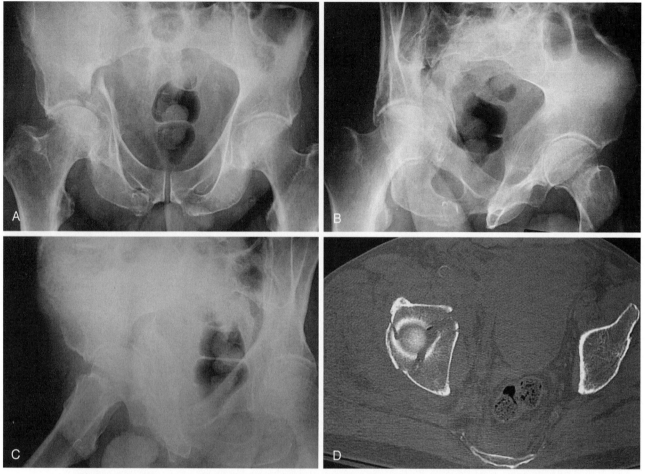

Figure 22–33. *A*, An AP radiograph of the pelvis of a 70-year-old man who fell sustaining an acetabular fracture demonstrates a significant degree of displacement of the posterior column. *B*, The obturator oblique view shows minimal displacement in the anterior column. *C*, The iliac oblique view clearly demonstrates the marked displacement of the posterior column. *D*, A view from the CT scan of the pelvis in the same patient demonstrates the comminution of the acetabular dome.

tion. These fractures can be quite complex to treat operatively and should be managed by surgeons with extensive experience in the operative treatment of acetabular fractures to ensure optimal patient management.

The operative approach to acetabular fractures is determined by the location of the fracture and the maximum displacement. Fractures can be treated by anterior, posterior, or combined approaches. Extensive exposure of the pelvis and acetabulum is frequently required to anatomically reduce these fractures. The goals of operative fixation are anatomic reduction and rigid internal fixation to allow early range of motion. Weight bearing is delayed for 12 weeks to allow for healing (Fig. 22–34).

The degree of trauma to the bone and the soft tissues caused by the injury, in addition to the extensive exposure required for operative fixation, results in an increased risk of heterotopic ossification, neurovascular injury, muscle weakness, avascular necrosis of the fracture fragments, and avascular necrosis of the femoral head. The use of radiation therapy for the reduction of heterotopic ossification should be avoided. If the fracture site is inadvertently exposed in the field of radiation therapy, delayed union or nonunion

may result. Nonsteroidal anti-inflammatory agents, such as indomethacin, can be used for prophylaxis of heterotopic ossification. Neurovascular injury may occur at the time of the injury or as a result of the surgical exposure. The sciatic nerve is injured in up to 13% of patients treated operatively. Injury can also occur to the superior gluteal nerve, which is injured in up to 20% of patients treated operatively. This damage will result in a Trendelenburg limp postoperatively owing to weakness in the gluteus medius and minimus muscles. The superior gluteal artery can be injured in posterior column fractures and with posterior approaches to the pelvis. The femoral nerve, artery, and vein are at risk in ilioinguinal and anterior approaches to the pelvis.

Avascular necrosis of the fracture fragments can be avoided by maintaining soft-tissue attachments to the fracture fragments. Avascular necrosis of the femoral head can be associated with posterior fracture dislocation of the femoral head. A fracture dislocation should be reduced as soon as possible to minimize the risk of avascular necrosis. Posterior approaches to the acetabulum may also result in avascular necrosis of the femoral head because of disrup-

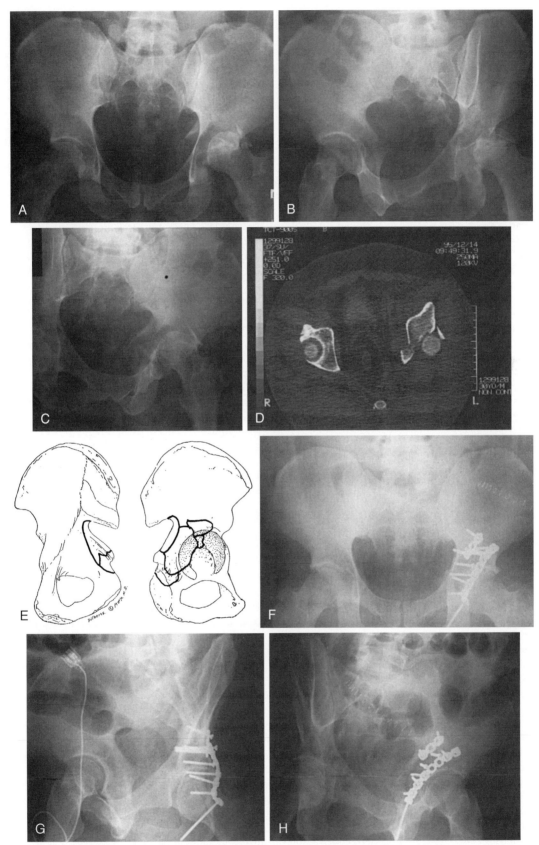

Figure 22–34.   The AP *(A)*, obturator oblique *(B)*, and iliac oblique *(C)* radiographs of a patient with an extended posterior wall acetabular fracture. *D*, CT scan demonstrates that the fracture includes the border of the greater sciatic notch. *E*, The fracture pattern is shown. Postoperative AP *(F)*, obturator oblique *(G)*, and iliac oblique *(H)* radiographs. (From Browner BD [ed]: Fractures in Adults. Philadelphia, WB Saunders, 1998.)

tion of the medial femoral circumflex artery as it ascends in the quadratus femoris muscle to supply the majority of the flow to a vascular ring at the base of the femoral neck, which in turn supplies the femoral head.

Extensive knowledge and experience with acetabular fractures is required to accurately reduce the fractures and to provide rigid fixation without the hardware entering the joint inadvertently. The injury itself places the patient at great risk for posttraumatic arthritis of the hip. Postoperatively these patients should be kept on restricted weight bearing for 12 weeks; however, range of motion should be encouraged early. After 12 weeks the patients can be advanced to unrestricted weight bearing. The patients need to be followed for the development of avascular necrosis or posttraumatic arthritis.

Patients managed nonoperatively are kept in traction for 8 weeks and then on restricted weight bearing for an additional 4 weeks. As for those treated operatively, the patients are allowed to bear weight at 12 weeks. If posttraumatic arthritis or avascular necrosis develops early after operative or nonoperative treatment of these injuries, additional surgery should be delayed for 6 months. This will allow complete healing and remodeling of the fractures and will minimize the risk of heterotopic ossification. If operative intervention is undertaken prior to complete healing of these fractures, nonunion of the acetabular fragments will compromise fixation of the implants in total hip replacement and may compromise healing and fixation in an arthrodesis.

Hip Dislocations

Hip dislocations are usually the result of major trauma. The hip can dislocate anteriorly, posteriorly, inferiorly, or centrally. The hip most commonly dislocates posteriorly. This can occur, for example, when a patient is involved in a motor vehicle accident and the leg is driven posteriorly by impact with the dashboard. If the hip is abducted and externally rotated, it may dislocate anteriorly. A hip dislocation may be associated with a fracture of the acetabulum, femoral head, or both. Dislocation of the hip is a relative surgical emergency. The longer the femoral head is out of the acetabulum, the greater the incidence of posttraumatic avascular necrosis of the femoral head. The blood supply to the femoral head can be stretched or occluded by the dislocation. These injuries can also be associated with injuries to either the femoral or more commonly the sciatic nerve. Frequently, these injuries will not recover or recover only partially.

Dislocation of the hip requires careful radiographic evaluation both before and after reduction. Prior to reduction careful radiographic assessment of the femoral neck is required to determine if a femoral neck fracture is present. If this fracture is present, then careful open reduction may be necessary. After reduction it is essential to determine if there are osseous fragments that were pulled back into the hip at the time of the reduction. If so, operative intervention would be required to remove such fragments.

If the femoral neck is intact, a gentle closed reduction can be undertaken. This can be accomplished with either conscious sedation or a general anesthetic. General anesthesia is preferred when it can be done in a timely fashion to allow for the least traumatic reduction to be performed with complete muscle relaxation. After reduction, the hip should be tested for stability. In the absence of a significant acetabular fracture, the hip is usually very stable after reduction. If the acetabulum is fractured, the hip may be unstable after reduction, and therefore should be splinted in a stable, reduced position or in skeletal traction. Radiographic evaluation should then be obtained to evaluate the fracture pattern and to plan for surgical intervention. These fractures are treated surgically as indicated by the nature of the acetabular fracture to restore stability to the hip.

Central fractures are usually found in elderly osteopenic patients. They can occur from a simple fall onto the lateral aspect of the hip. The femoral head is driven into the acetabulum. These fractures are commonly associated with extensive comminution of the medial wall of the acetabulum. These fracture dislocations are usually best treated with traction. Attempts to operatively repair the medial wall are at best frustrating because of the comminution, poor quality of the bone, and the location of the fracture deep within the pelvis.

All hip dislocations require a detailed CT scan after the hip is reduced to demonstrate that a concentric reduction has been obtained and that there are no intra-articular fragments. If fragments are present, then the patient will require an arthrotomy and débridement of the fragments within the joint. If the fragments are left intra-articularly, significant arthritis will result. If no fracture is present, these injuries can be treated with 6 weeks of restricted weight bearing followed by weight bearing as tolerated. If a fracture is present and the hip is unstable after attempts at reduction, the acetabular fracture should be treated surgically.

Femoral head fractures may also be present and are classified according to the position of the fracture in relation to the fovea of the femoral head. Fractures inferior to the fovea, if nondisplaced, can be treated nonoperatively. If displaced, they can be treated either by excision of the fragment if the hip is stable or with internal fixation if the hip is unstable without the fragment. If the fracture is above the femoral fovea, it must be treated with internal fixation to restore the weight-bearing articular surface. If the fragment is treated with internal fixation, weight bearing should be restricted for 12 weeks.

Femoral Neck Fractures

Fractures of the femoral neck are quite common in the elderly population. They are usually the result of a low-energy injury, such as a simple fall. Femoral neck fracture in a younger patient is a far more significant injury because of the greater force required to cause it. The leg is commonly noted to be shortened and externally rotated, particularly if the fracture is displaced. Femoral neck fractures are graded by the Garden classification (Fig. 22–35), which divides these injuries into four grades. Grade 1 is an impacted or incomplete fracture. Grade 2 is a complete nondisplaced fracture. Grade 3 is a displaced fracture with the trabecular pattern of the femoral head not lining up with the corresponding pattern on the acetabular side. This form implies that there is some remaining tissue intact between the two fragments. In grade 4 injuries the trabecular pattern

Figure 22–35. Garden's classification: *A,* Stage I is an incomplete fracture commonly known as an abduction, or implicated, fracture. The medial trabeculae at the junction of the head and neck sometimes appear to be bent, rather than broken, in the manner of a greenstick fracture. *B,* Stage II is a complete fracture without displacement. The alignment of the medial trabeculae in the two fragments is undisturbed. *C,* Stage III is a displaced fracture in which the direction of medial trabeculae shows that the fracture has rotated in medially. *D,* Stage IV is a completely displaced fracture with loss of intimate contact between the fragments: The head fragment is free to return to its normal position in the acetabulum, as shown by the parallel direction of its medial trabeculae, which now line up with their counterparts in the pelvis. (From Garden RS: J Bone Joint Surg (Br) 1964;46: 630.)

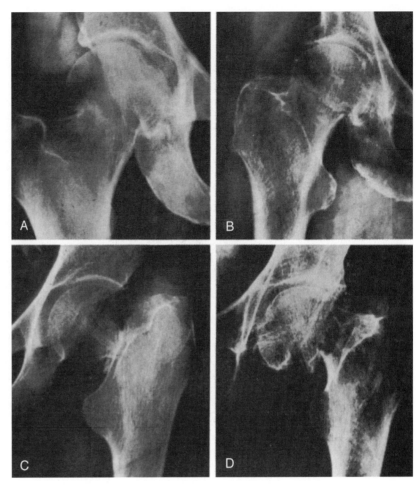

of the femoral head lines up with the acetabular pattern, implying complete displacement, and no tissue is intact between the two fragments. Many surgeons simplify this classification into two categories, combining the Garden 1 and 2 injuries into impacted or nondisplaced fractures and combining Garden 3 and 4 injuries into displaced fractures. This approach offers a more practical grouping that is simple to grade and has importance in prediction of outcome and in the selection of treatment alternatives.

The displacement of the fracture has significant implications for the viability of the femoral head. The blood supply of the femoral head, as indicated earlier, is provided in a series of fine blood vessels that travel within the synovial retinaculum and enter the head at the base of the articular cartilage. These vessels can be tethered, stretched, or occluded by a femoral neck fracture, particularly if the fracture is displaced. Such distortion or disruptions can lead to posttraumatic avascular necrosis. In nondisplaced fractures and impacted fractures, the rate of avascular necrosis is 13 to 20%. In displaced fractures the rate of avascular necrosis can be as high as 25 to 40% if the fracture is reduced and fixed within the first 24 hours. If a longer delay is noted in the fixation of the fracture, the rate of avascular necrosis can increase to almost 100% at 1 week after the fracture. For these reasons, if a displaced fracture is to be fixed, this procedure should be done as soon as possible to reduce the risk of posttraumatic avascular necrosis.

The treatment alternatives for these fractures vary with the displacement and with the age of the patient. The majority of these injuries are in the elderly. A fracture, which is impacted in a valgus position, can be stable. In fact, occasionally patients will present with this fracture several weeks after the injury fully weight bearing with persistent hip pain. These fractures are stable with a low risk of displacement. However, if displacement occurs, the difference in the treatment and the implications for avascular necrosis are significant. Therefore, many surgeons will recommend fixation of these fractures. In this population, if the fracture is nondisplaced or impacted, it should be treated with multiple screws. One study determined that three screws in a triangular or square parallel pattern gave optimal fixation. An alternative method is to use a sliding compression hip screw with an additional parallel screw or pin to prevent rotation of the femoral head on the neck. Fixation of the fracture is appropriate for all nondisplaced or impacted fractures, regardless of the patient's age (Fig. 22–36).

Displaced fractures are treated differently, depending upon the patient's age. In the elderly these fractures are probably best treated by replacement of the femoral head with a hip hemiarthroplasty (Fig. 22–37). This procedure uses a femoral stem similar to that used for a total hip replacement. However, instead of the small femoral head used for a total hip replacement, a larger head is placed to fill the entire native acetabulum. The acetabulum is left

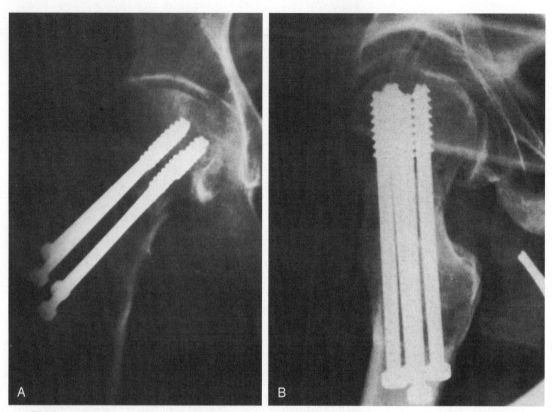

Figure 22–36. A slightly displaced varus fracture that needed only a little improvement in the AP plane *(A)*. Note how well it is fixed in the lateral plane *(B)*. (From Steinberg M [ed]: The Hip and Its Disorders. Philadelphia, WB Saunders, 1991.)

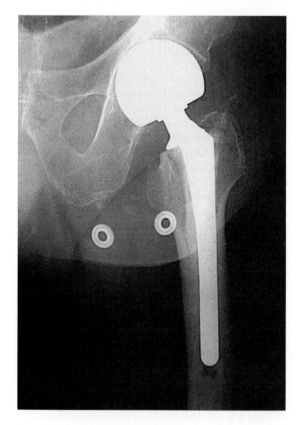

Figure 22–37. A postoperative radiograph of an 85-year-old woman who had sustained a displaced femoral neck fracture. She had a hemiarthroplasty performed with a cemented femoral stem.

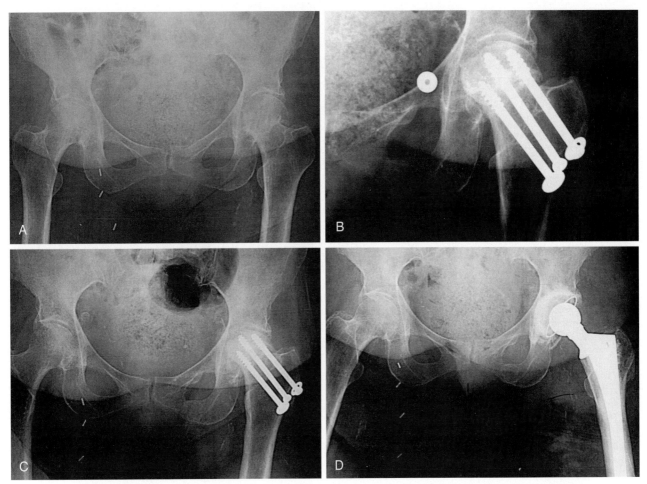

Figure 22–38.   *A,* An AP radiograph of the pelvis of an 81-year-old woman who had sustained a severely impacted left femoral neck fracture. This injury was treated with three cannulated screws *(B).* The fracture did not heal and collapsed further. The screws were noted to extend beyond the articular surface *(C).* She then had a cemented total hip replacement for definitive management *(D).*

unresurfaced. Replacement is used instead of operative fixation because of the high rate of avascular necrosis and nonunion of these fractures. If the fracture were fixed and avascular necrosis or a nonunion were to occur, additional surgery would be required to replace the hip (Fig. 22–38). Also, hemiarthroplasty gives the patient a construct on which they can immediately bear weight, facilitating rehabilitation.

In younger patients all attempts should be made to save the patient's native femoral head. Therefore, the majority of these patients should have the fracture reduced and fixed. It is essential to try to fix the fracture anatomically. Malreduction will increase the risk for nonunion and avascular necrosis. The reduction should also be relatively atraumatic to minimize the risk of additional damage to the blood supply of the femoral head. The fixation should also be as rigid as possible because any motion at the fracture site will impair healing.

Postoperatively the patients who have been treated with internal fixation should be restricted from full weight bearing on the leg for a period of 8 to 12 weeks. This is particularly true of the displaced fractures that have been reduced and fixed. Serial radiographs should be taken to look for migration of the fracture fragments or the hardware. Avascular necrosis of the femoral head may not become evident clinically or radiographically for as long as 2 to 5 years after the fracture.

If a nonunion or migration of the hardware is noted and the femoral head is viable, attempts can be made to create a valgus osteotomy, revise the fixation, and bone graft the fracture. This approach will convert the shear at the fracture site to compressive loading to promote healing. If avascular necrosis develops or the hardware damages the articular cartilage, a total hip replacement is the only remaining alternative.

Intertrochanteric Hip Fractures

The intertrochanteric region of the femur extends from the base of the femoral neck including the greater trochanter and ending at the lesser trochanter. The intertrochanteric line runs from the greater trochanter to the lesser trochanter and is the junction between the diaphyseal and metaphyseal regions of the proximal femur. The femoral neck joins the femur at an angle of approximately 125 degrees. This

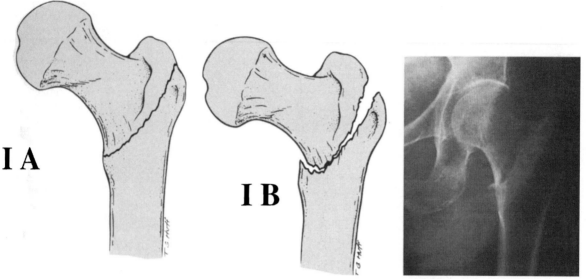

Figure 22–39. Diagrams and radiographic examples of the Evans-Jensen classification of intertrochanteric fractures. Type I fractures are two-part fractures, either nondisplaced (type IA) or displaced (type IB).

puts a significant angular force on the upper femur with a fracture.

Fractures in this region of the femur are far more common in the elderly. In fact, on average, intertrochanteric femoral fractures occur in patients 10 to 12 years older than the patients with a fracture of the femoral neck, and they also have a significant female predominance. These fractures usually present after a simple fall. The leg is shortened and externally rotated. Rarely are femoral neck or intertrochanteric femur fractures associated with a neurovascular injury. However, if this fracture is seen in a younger patient without some form of metabolic bone disease, the energy absorbed by the fracture is far greater, and the risk of other injuries is far greater.

These injuries are best classified by the Evans-Jensen classification (Fig. 22–39), which divides them into stable and unstable varieties based upon the direction of the fracture line and the integrity of the lesser trochanter and the posteromedial cortex of the femur. The stability of the fracture is based on the ability to achieve a stable reduction and the risk of subsequent displacement after fixation. In most intertrochanteric fractures, the major fracture line is parallel to the intertrochanteric line from the greater to the lesser trochanter. If the medial cortex of the distal fragment is intact, then a stable reduction can usually be obtained and maintained. If, however, the posteromedial cortex of the proximal fragment is fractured, the fracture is prone to displacement even if it is anatomically reduced. A variant of the intertrochanteric femur fracture is the reverse obliquity fracture. In this injury the fracture line runs from the base of the femoral neck transversely across the femur, exiting laterally at the level of the lesser trochanter on the lateral cortex. This injury is less stable because the fracture, when reduced and loaded, will tend to shear; the more common intertrochanteric fracture will be loaded in compression. The type of fixation used for these injuries will also vary to accommodate for the fracture configuration.

Nonoperative management of these injuries requires 8

to 12 weeks of traction followed by 4 to 8 weeks of non–weightbearing. These fractures will heal because they have excellent vascularity of the metaphyseal bone. Frequently, when these fractures are treated nonoperatively, significant shortening and an external rotation deformity will result. Thus, although these fractures will heal when treated nonoperatively, the risks of this course of treatment are significant. The patients will suffer decubiti, pneumonia, atelectasis, urinary tract infections, and generalized muscle atrophy. These complications are not tolerated well in the elderly and can result in a mortality rate of up to 55% in those treated nonoperatively. The nonoperative management is to be reserved for patients who have severe medical complications precluding anesthesia and patients with severe contractures. In these select few patients, they can be managed with an alternative nonoperative protocol, which keeps the patients comfortable at bed rest for a few days then mobilizes the patients from bed to chair. This protocol accepts a malunion, but minimizes the risks of protracted bed rest required by traction.

The vast majority of these fractures should be treated operatively. Most intertrochanteric femur fractures can and should be anatomically reduced and fixed. The most common method of fixation at this time is the sliding hip compression screw (Fig. 22–40). This device allows for the fracture to compress with impaction of the fracture while maintaining fixation of the fragments. If the fracture has a large posterior fragment, this should be reduced and fixed with either an interfragmentary screw or a cerclage wire. Fixation of this fragment will substantially increase the rigidity of the construct. However, occasionally fixation cannot be accomplished because of marked comminution. In that setting a shorter barrel side plate may be necessary to allow the greater degree of impaction, which will occur at the fracture site.

The reverse obliquity fracture requires a different form of fixation. Because of orientation of the fracture, if a standard sliding hip screw is used compression will not

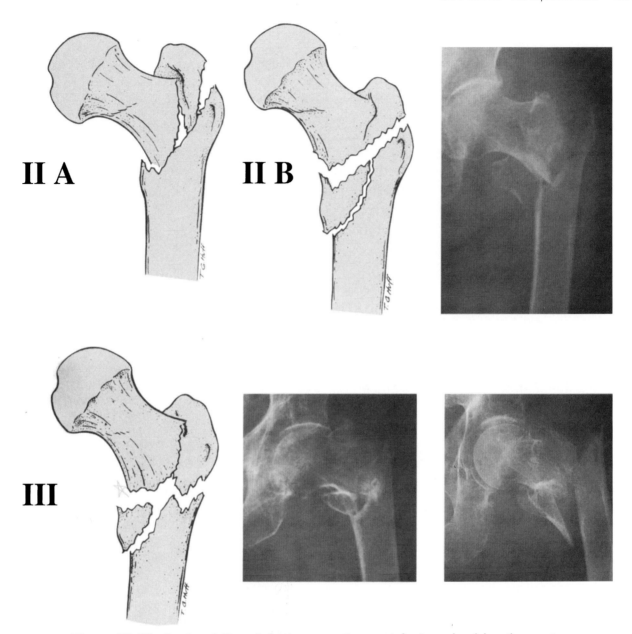

Figure 22–39 *Continued.* Type II fractures are three-part fractures involving the greater trochanter (type IIA) or the lesser trochanter (type IIB). Type III fractures involve both trochanters. Difficulty with reduction and fracture instability increase with fracture type. (From Browner BD [ed]: Fractures in Adults. Philadelphia, WB Saunders, 1998.)

occur at the fracture site (Fig. 22–41). The proximal fragment will slide along the fracture line, and the femur will move medially. The reverse obliquity fracture is best treated with a 95-degree blade plate or a 95-degree dynamic compression screw (Fig. 22–42). Although this construct will not allow for dynamic compression at the fracture, it will provide rigid fixation and maintain alignment of the fragments.

Other methods of treatment are available. An intramedullary hip screw is available. This can provide good fixation, however, there is a significant learning curve to its use. The use of a hemiarthroplasty for the fixation of an intertrochanteric femur fracture is rarely indicated. This method of addressing the intertrochanteric femur fracture has been found to have a greater incidence of complications

postoperatively. After the fixation of an intertrochanteric hip fracture the patient should be on limited weight bearing for 8 weeks. In patients with a reverse oblique fracture, touchdown weightbearing only should continue for 12 weeks. Loss of fixation after treatment of an intertrochanteric femur fracture occurs in approximately 13% of cases. If the proximal fragment is viable and the hardware has not penetrated the articular surface to damage the hip joint, attempts can be made to revise the fixation. If the joint has been damaged or the femoral head is no longer viable, joint replacement is the only option.

Subtrochanteric Femur Fractures

The region of the femur from the level of the lesser trochanter extending 5 cm distally is the subtrochanteric zone

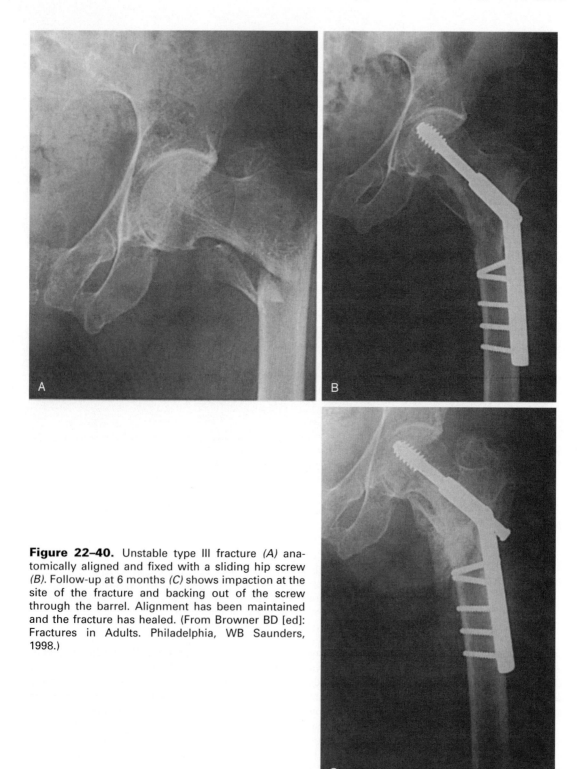

Figure 22–40. Unstable type III fracture *(A)* anatomically aligned and fixed with a sliding hip screw *(B)*. Follow-up at 6 months *(C)* shows impaction at the site of the fracture and backing out of the screw through the barrel. Alignment has been maintained and the fracture has healed. (From Browner BD [ed]: Fractures in Adults. Philadelphia, WB Saunders, 1998.)

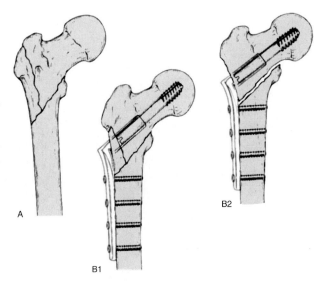

Figure 22–41. *A,* Reverse oblique intertrochanteric fracture. Lateral comminution is common. *B1* and *B2,* Telescoping of the sliding hip screw does not promote interfragmentary compression because of the orientation of the fracture plane. Stability requires secure impaction of the fracture, with either osteotomy of the distal piece to provide mechanical engagement or an implant that resists progressive medial displacement of the shaft. (From Browner BD [ed]: Fractures in Adults. Philadelphia, WB Saunders, 1998.)

of the femur. This region is unique because of the extreme stress applied to the bone at this level. The lateral femur is subjected to an extreme tensile stress while the medial cortex is subjected to high compressive stress. These dramatic forces result in difficulty in maintaining the reduction and fixation of a fracture. Historically there have been many types of fixation utilized to manage this difficult fracture (Fig. 22–43). Currently the intramedullary devices appear to be optimal for fixation of a subtrochanteric fracture without intertrochanteric extension.

These fractures occur in two populations. One is the elderly; usually these fractures are low energy and are long spiral fractures. Occasionally they are comminuted; however, usually they are in two or three major fragments. The other population is the younger patient with major blunt trauma. These are higher energy injuries and are frequently comminuted. The challenge in the management of these fractures is obtaining a reduction and healing the medial cortex in order to restore the compressive side of the construct.

Subtrochanteric fractures can be treated nonoperatively

by the use of traction and followed by the use of a cast or brace. This method of treatment requires 8 to 12 weeks of traction and bed rest. The muscle forces on the proximal femur place the proximal fragment in flexion and abduction (Fig. 22–44). In traction the distal fragment should be therefore flexed and abducted to align the distal fragment with the proximal fragment. The significant muscle forces acting upon this fracture also increase the rate of nonunion or malunion of this fracture.

In most patients these injuries are the result of major trauma. In that setting and also to avoid the complications of prolonged bed rest required by traction, subtrochanteric femur fractures are best treated by surgery. The goals of surgery are the anatomic reconstruction of the femur and rigid internal fixation. This approach allows for rapid mobilization of the patient, although weight bearing should be restricted for the first 6 to 8 weeks. The rapid mobilization will minimize the risks and complications of bed rest. Operative fixation of subtrochanteric fractures is a significant physiologic challenge to the trauma patient. There can be significant operative time and blood loss. Care must be

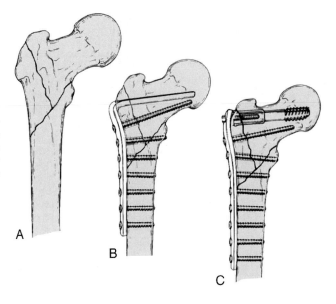

Figure 22–42. *A,* Reverse oblique intertrochanteric fracture, illustrating typical lateral comminution. *B,* Anatomic reduction and fixation with a blade plate angled at 95 degrees. *C,* Anatomic reduction and fixation with a condylar compression screw angled at 95 degrees. (From Browner BD [ed]: Fractures in Adults. Philadelphia, WB Saunders, 1998.)

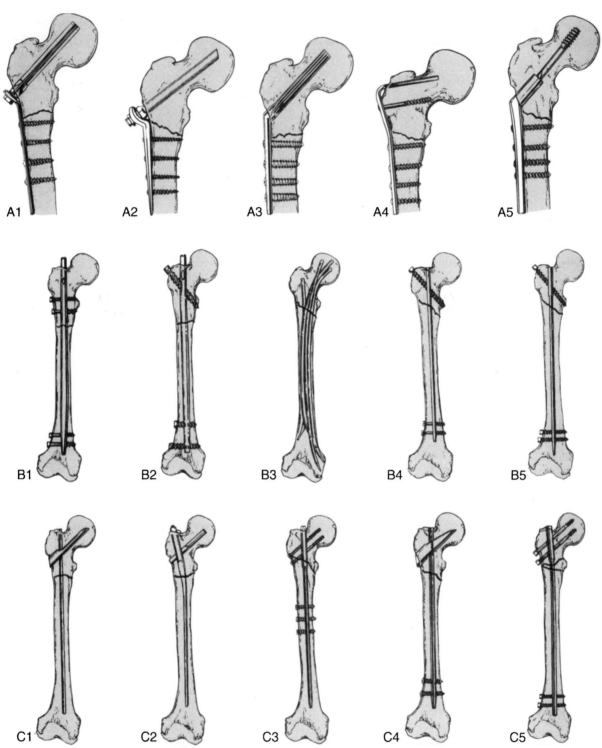

Figure 22–43. *A*, Evolution of plate design. (1) Thornton device. (2) McLaughlin nail plate. (3) Jewett nail plate. (4) AO blade plate. (5) Richards hip compression screw. *B*, Centromedullary and condylocephalic devices. (1) Küntscher interlocking screws and detensor. (2) Klemm-Schellmann device with diagonal proximal locking screw. (3) Ender condylocephalic devices. (4) Grosse-Kempf interlocking device. (5) Russell-Taylor closed-section interlocking femoral nail. *C*, Cephalomedullary implants with proximal fragment stabilization by internal fixation into the femoral head and neck. (1) Küntscher Y nail. (2) Zickel device. (3) Huckstep nail. (4) Williams Y nail. (5) Russell-Taylor reconstruction interlocking nail. *(A–C* redrawn from Calandruccio RA, Chairman, AAOS Committee on the History of Orthopaedic Surgery. Internal fixation devices for fractures of the proximal femur. Exhibit at the 55th Annual Meeting, Atlanta, February 4–9, 1988.) (From Browner BD [ed]: Fractures in Adults. Philadelphia, WB Saunders, 1998.)

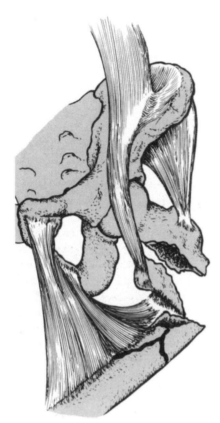

Figure 22–44. Pathologic anatomy: additional deforming forces on a subtrochanteric fracture. (Modified from Froimson AL: Treatment of comminuted subtrochanteric fractures of the femur. Surg Gynecol Obstet 1970; 131:465, by permission of Surgery, Gynecology, & Obstetrics.)

taken intraoperatively and postoperatively to ensure that appropriate fluid and blood replacement are provided to the patient. The patient may require ICU monitoring postoperatively to ensure a safe outcome.

Multiple classifications of these injuries are available. The most functional is the Russell-Taylor classification (Fig. 22–45), which looks primarily at the intertrochanteric area and the piriformis fossa. This helps to determine the method of fixation to be recommended. If the fracture extends into the piriformis fossa, it is a combination of both an intertrochanteric fracture and a subtrochanteric fracture. This fracture pattern can be best treated with a sliding hip screw device. If, however, the fracture does not involve the piriformis fossa, the sliding hip screw device is not optimal. In this setting the sliding device will not be effective at allowing fracture compression because the sliding mechanism will not cross the fracture site. Better fixation can be obtained with the use of a 95-degree blade plate or an intramedullary rod. The rod used in this circumstance must have the capacity to provide proximal fixation into the femoral head and neck by the use of screws, nails, or a blade device, which are inserted through the rod. In addition, distal screws passing through both the bone and the rod will control rotation at the fracture site.

If the fracture is comminuted with large fragments, these should be reconstructed with interfragmentary screw fixation or with the use of cerclage wire or cable fixation

(Fig. 22–46). It is particularly important to reconstruct the medial weight-bearing cortical bone to optimize the potential for healing and minimize the risk of hardware failure. In addition, comminuted fractures should be bone grafted with either cancellous iliac crest bone or with bone reamed from the femoral canal during rod placement. Bone graft will augment fracture healing and will reduce the rate of nonunion and hardware failure.

Postoperatively the patient should be placed on restricted weight bearing until fracture callus is noted on plain radiography. In the treatment of all fractures the internal fixation placed surgically is not sufficient to maintain fixation indefinitely. There is a requirement for the fracture to heal to maintain long-term stability and to restore the full load-carrying capacity of the bone. The internal fixation is an internal splint that stabilizes the bone to allow healing. If the bone does not heal, either the metal implants will break or they will come loose from the bone. Early weight bearing may result in loss of fixation of the hardware, which may lead to a malunion or a nonunion of the fracture. Delay in fracture healing can also lead to failure of fixation. The factors associated with delayed healing are poor nutritional state, infection at the fracture site, motion at the fracture site, and extensive injury to the soft tissues around the fracture (either at the time of the injury or at the time of surgical fixation).

The time to fracture healing is approximately 8 to 12 weeks. Weight bearing should be delayed until fracture callus is noted on plain radiographs. When mature callus is noted then the patient can be returned to full activities. In young patients (under 40 years of age) the hardware should be removed 18 to 24 months postoperatively. This allows time for remodeling of the fracture callus and for the bone to gain adequate strength to maintain stability after the internal fixation is removed.

Femur Fractures

Femur fractures are usually the result of blunt trauma such as a motor vehicle accident. As with many of the previous fractures, femur fractures are commonly associated with injury to other major organ systems. Therefore, these patients must be evaluated by an experienced trauma surgeon to ensure that they have been adequately stabilized and fluid resuscitated. These fractures are generally classified by the fracture pattern and according to the degree of comminution present (Fig. 22–47). Grade 1 injuries are transverse or short oblique fractures with no significant comminution. Grade 2 fractures have a butterfly fragment or a comminuted segment that is less than 50% of the width of the bone. Grade 3 fractures have comminution of greater than 50% of the bone but have enough bone intact on both the proximal and distal fragments to asses the true length of the femur. Grade 4 fractures have such extensive comminution that the length of the bone cannot be assessed without a radiograph of the uninjured femur.

These fractures are best treated within the early postinjury period. Frequently these patients will develop significant pulmonary compromise after the trauma. If the surgery is delayed, the patient may not be able to undergo surgery until the pulmonary compromise resolves. If the surgery is done as soon after the trauma as possible after initial

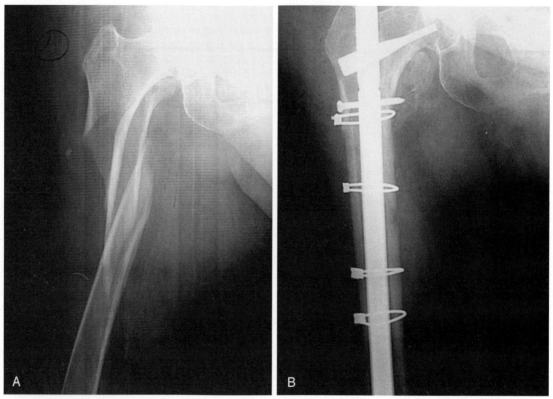

Figure 22–45. *A,* This 79-year-old woman sustained a fall, resulting in a subtrochanteric femur fracture with a large oblique segmental fragment. *B,* The patient was treated by reduction of the fracture with cerclage cables, and then an intramedullary rod was placed and fixed proximally and distally to allow an anatomic reduction of the subtrochanteric region of the femur. (From Browner BD [ed]: Fractures in Adults. Philadelphia, WB Saunders, 1998.)

fluid resuscitation, the patient's postoperative care can be optimized even if pulmonary complications develop because the patient can be mobilized to facilitate pulmonary function. This has resulted in a lower mortality rate for femoral fractures treated within the first 24 hours after injury.

Femoral fracture can be treated either operatively or nonoperatively in skeletal traction. As noted earlier, these fractures are best managed operatively to facilitate the patient's management. If traction is utilized, the protocol is similar to that for the subtrochanteric femur fractures. The patient is in traction for 8 weeks, then managed with restricted weight bearing for an additional 4 weeks. Care must be taken to ensure that the femur is held in proper alignment in traction. The hip is usually flexed 20 degrees and the leg is held in the neutral rotation, with no abduction or adduction.

The majority of femur fractures should be managed operatively. The optimal treatment for most femur fractures is the use of an intramedullary rod. This rod is then fixed proximally and distally with screws that traverse the bone through the rod and then enter the bone on the other side. These screws control the rotation and length of the fracture while the fracture is healing. Care must be taken to ensure that the femur is reconstructed with the appropriate length and rotation. If the femur is lengthened and the bone ends are not in contact, then a nonunion may develop. Bone grafting is rarely necessary as the fracture is bone grafted

by material from the femoral canal that is pushed out at the fracture site during surgical preparation of the canal prior to rod placement.

Postoperatively these patients can be mobilized with restricted weight bearing on the involved leg. Weight bearing is restricted until fracture callus is noted. This usually occurs at 6 to 8 weeks postoperatively. At that point weight bearing can be progressed as tolerated. Complete fracture healing has usually occurred by 8 to 12 weeks. Patients can then progress to full activities. The rod should be removed in patients under the age of 40 not but until 18 to 24 months after fracture healing. When the rod has been removed the patient should be placed on crutches for an additional 6 weeks to allow the bone to remodel and accommodate the removal of the rod to minimize the risk of refracture.

If fracture callus is not noted by 8 to 12 weeks postoperatively, healing can be stimulated by several options. The interlocking screws can be removed from one or both ends of the rod to allow impaction of the fracture site. The fracture can be operatively bone grafted with autogenous graft from the iliac crest, or the rod can be revised and the intramedullary canal reamed to generate bone graft and hopefully stimulate healing. In addition, the surgeon should suspect the possibility of deep infection as the cause for the delayed union. The results of an erythrocyte sedimentation rate and C-reactive protein analysis may be helpful in determining the presence of infection. If infection is sus-

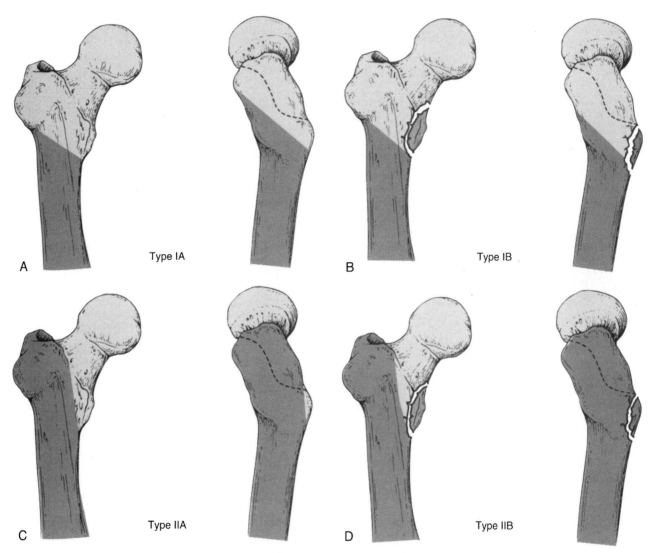

Figure 22–46. Russell-Taylor classification of subtrochanteric fractures. *A,* Type IA: Fracture extension with any degree of comminution from below the level of the lesser trochanter to the isthmus with no extension into the piriformis fossa. *B,* Type IB: Fracture extension involving the lesser trochanter to the isthmus with no extension into the piriformis fossa. *C,* Type IIA: Fracture extension into the piriformis fossa. Stable medial construct. *D,* Type IIB: Fracture extension into the piriformis fossa in the lesser trochanteric area with no stability of the medial femoral cortex. (*A–D,* modified from Tencer AF, et al: Orthop Biomech Lab Report #002. Mcmphis, Richards Medical Co., 1985.)

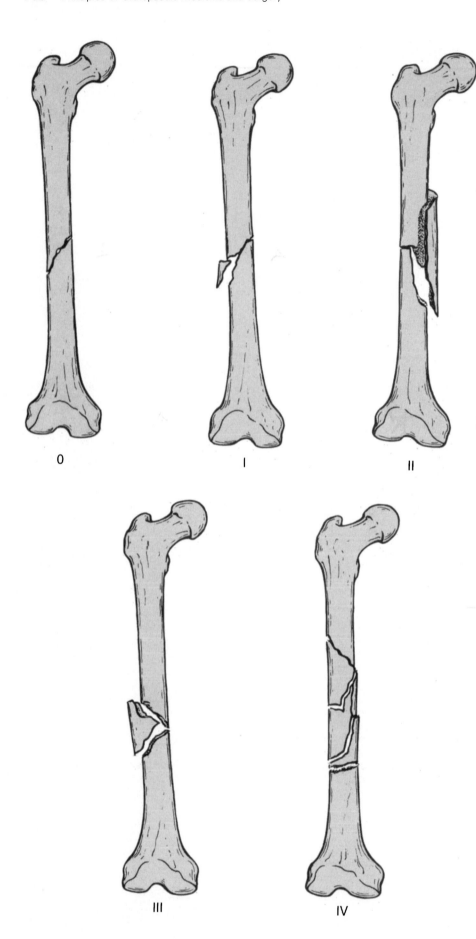

0

I

II

III

IV

Figure 22–47. Winquist and Hansen's classification of comminution. 0, No comminution. I, Insignificant butterfly fragment. II, Large butterfly fragment of less than 50% of the width of the bone. This leaves approximately 50% of the cortex from the proximal fragment in contact with the distal fragment. III, Large butterfly fragment of more than 50% of the width of the bone. This leaves less than 50% cortical contact between the proximal and the distal fragments. IV, Segmental comminution. (From Browner BD [ed]: Fractures in Adults. Philadelphia, WB Saunders, 1998.)

pected, then an operative biopsy and culture may be indicated. If the rod and femur are found to be infected, the treatment is to remove the rod, ream the canal, and replace the rod. The patient is then placed on a 6 week course of appropriate intravenous antibiotics. If the fracture is not healed and the infection is due to a particularly virulent organism, the patient should be managed in skeletal traction after the removal of the intramedullary rod.

SUMMARY

As noted initially, disorders involving the hip and femur are manifested by alteration in the patient's ability to ambulate. Diagnosis and treatment require a careful history, thorough physical examination, and the appropriate use of radiographic studies. When the proper diagnosis is made, for most nontraumatic disorders it is usually best to begin with a nonoperative approach. If the nonoperative treatment alternatives are not successful, then operative intervention is indicated and will result in an excellent outcome in the majority of patients.

Bibliography

Brooker AF, Bowerman JW, Robinson RA, Riley LH: Ectopic osification following total hip replacement: Incidence and a method of classification. J Bone Joint Surg 1973;55(A):1629–1632.

Collier JP, Sutula LC, Currier BH, et al; Overview of polyethylene as a bearing material: comparison of sterilization methods. Clin Orthop Rel Res 1996;333:76–86.

Evans BG, Salvati EA: Total Hip Arthroplasty in the Elderly: Cost Effective Alternatives. Instructional Course Lectures, AAOS, Vol. 43, 1994.

Evans BG, Salvati EA: The rationale for cemented total hip arthroplasty. Orthop Clin North Am 1993; 24(4):599–610.

Evans BG: Late complications and their management. *In* Callaghan JJ, Rosenberg AG, Rubash HE (eds): The Adult Hip. 1998, pp 1149–1161.

Garvin K Evans BG, Salvati EA, Brause B: Palacos gentamicin for the treatment of deep periprosthetic hip infections. Clin Orthop Rel Res 1994;298:97–105.

Gruen TA, McNiece GM, Amstutz HC: "Modes of failure" of cemented stem-type femoral components. A radiologic analysis of loosening. Clin Orthop Rel Res 1979;141:17–27.

Healy WL, Lo TCM, DeSimone AA, et al: Single-dose irradiation for the prevention of heterotopic ossification after total hip arthroplasty: A comparison of doses of five hundred and fifty and seven hundred centigray. J Bone Joint Surg 1995;77A:590–595.

Jasty M, Anderson MJ, Harris WH: Total hip replacement for developmental dysplasia of the hip. Clin Orthop Rel Res 1995;311:40–45.

Schulte KR, Callaghan JJ, Kelley SS, Johnston RC: The outcome of Charnley total hip arthroplasty with cement after a minimum twenty year followup: The results of one surgeon. J Bone Joint Surg 1993;75A:961–971.

Steinberg ME: Early Diagnosis, Evaluation and Staging of Osteonecrosis. Instructional Course Lectures, Vol. 43, 1994, pp 513–518.

Trousdale RT, Ekkernkamp A, Ganz R, Wallrichs SL: Periacetabular and intertrochanteric osteotomy for the treatment of osteoarthrosis in dysplastic hips. J Bone Joint Surg 1995;77A:73–85.

Wedge JH, Cummiskey DJ: Primary arthroplasty of the hip in patients who are less than twenty-one years old. J Bone Joint Surg 1994;76A:1732–1742.

Wiklund I, Romanus B: A Comparison of quality of life before and after arthroplasty in patients who had arthrosis of the hip joint. J Bone Joint Surg 1991;73A:765–769.

Willert HG, Bertram H, Buchhorn GH: Osteolysis in alloarthroplasty of the hip. The role of ultra-high molecular weight polyethylene wear particles. Clin Orthop 1990;258:95–107.

Woo RYG, Morrey BF: Dislocation after total hip arthroplasty. J Bone Joint Surg 1982;64A(9):1295–1306.

Chapter 23

The Knee and Leg

Benjamin Shaffer, M.D.

Whether impacting the career of the elite athlete or threatening the independent function of a geriatric patient, knee problems are one of the most common orthopaedic complaints. Rather than focusing on how frequent the knee is subjected to trauma and disease, it is with wonder that we should marvel at this joint's ability to withstand the rigors and stresses to which it is normally subjected in the course of a lifetime. Recent advances in both technologic imaging and surgical intervention have improved our diagnostic acumen and rendered possible the increase in longevity of this important joint. The purpose of this chapter is to review the knee and leg's functional anatomy, and describe techniques for evaluation, imaging, and treatment of common problems of the knee and leg.

FUNCTIONAL ANATOMY

The knee is actually composed of three separate articulations: the tibiofemoral, patellofemoral, and proximal tibiofibular joints. The joint most commonly referred to when describing the "knee joint" is the *tibiofemoral joint*, in which the distal femoral condyles articulate with the proximal tibial plateaus (Fig. 23–1). The distal femur is composed of the medial and lateral femoral condyles with the slightly larger medial side accounting for the valgus orientation of the normal knee joint. In the anterior portion of the distal femur is a shallow sulcus, known as the trochlear groove, in which the patella tracks (Fig. 23–2). Inspection of the distal femur end-on shows an intercondylar notch in between the medial and lateral femoral condyles. The cruciate ligaments of the knee are found within this intercondylar notch (Fig. 23–2). Other important bony landmarks include the medial epicondyle on the medial aspect of the femoral condyle, to which the adductor magnus attaches proximally, and the medial collateral ligament slightly more distally. The lateral epicondyle marks the proximal attachment site of the lateral collateral ligament.

The tibiofemoral joint is essentially a modified hinge joint, with the greatest motion in the sagittal plane. However, some motion is also present in the coronal (varus and valgus) and axial plane (internal and external rotation). The femoral condyles articulate with the chondral surfaces of the proximal tibia known as the plateau. Both medial and lateral plateaus are relatively flat in shape when viewed in the coronal plane (see Fig. 23–1). However, when viewed sagitally (from the side), the contour of the compartments is somewhat different, with the medial side demonstrating a gentle concavity into which the medial condyle fits, and the lateral side actually has a convexity, somewhat

incongruous with the mating lateral femoral condyle. If left to its bony architectural design, the inherent stability afforded the tibiofemoral joint would be limited. However, fortuitously nature has provided a rather dynamic structural solution to permit freedom of movement while simultaneously ensuring joint congruity. This solution is in the form of the menisci, fibrocartilage structures that interface between the adjacent articular surfaces and provide joint congruence (Figs. 23–3 and 23–4).

The medial meniscus is somewhat semicircular in shape and the lateral more circular in design (Fig. 23–5). They are firmly connected to the tibial plateaus, attached through ligament fibers to the tibia (meniscotibial ligaments, also known as "coronary" ligaments and meniscofemoral ligaments). Although they are attached, some movement is permitted both menisci. This mobility, normally greater on the lateral side than the medial side, allows the menisci to conform to the dynamically moving joint surfaces and

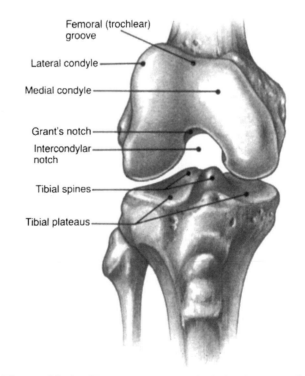

Figure 23–1. Observe the bony articulation between the convex medial femoral condyles and the somewhat flatter and sometimes actually convex tibial plateaus. (From Wiesel SW, Delahay JN: Essentials of Orthopaedic Surgery, 2nd ed. Philadelphia, WB Saunders, 1997.)

711

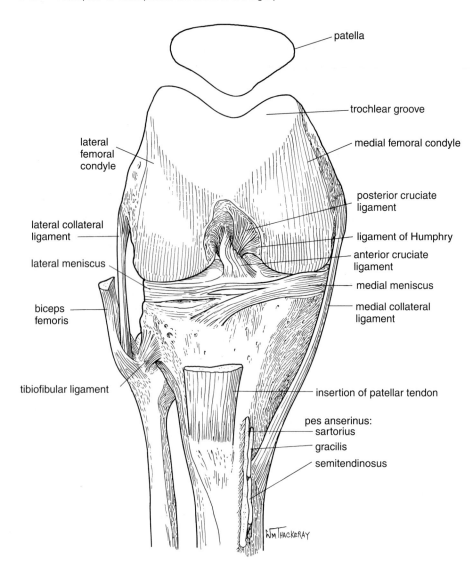

Figure 23–2. Anterior view of the distal femur demonstrates the trochlear groove with which the patella articulates (the patellofemoral joint). (From Insall JN, et al: Surgery of the Knee, 2nd ed. New York, Churchill Livingstone, 1993.)

Figure 23–3. This anteroposterior view demonstrates the congruity rendered the tibiofemoral articulation between the otherwise somewhat incongruous surfaces of the femoral condyles and the tibial plateaus. (From Wiesel SW, Delahay JN: Essentials of Orthopaedic Surgery, 2nd ed. Philadelphia, WB Saunders, 1997.)

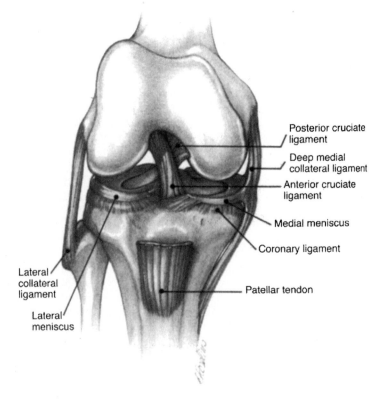

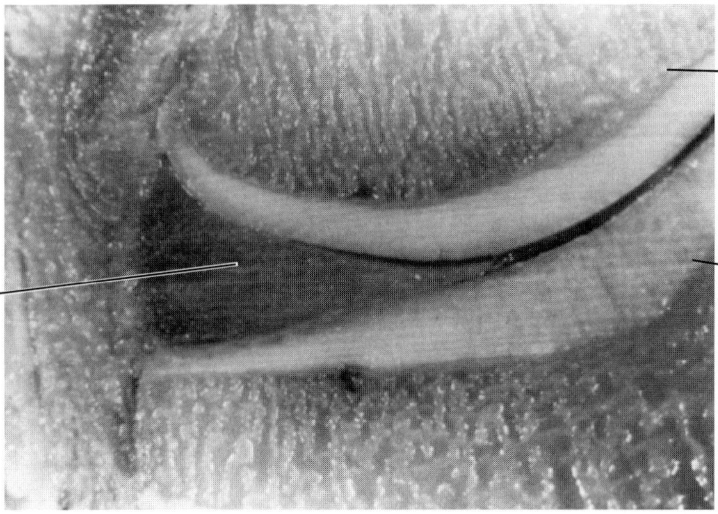

Figure 23–4. In this close-up sagittal view, observe the relative incongruity of the articular surfaces between the femur and tibia. The meniscus compensates for this relative lack of joint congruity. (From Insall JN, et al: Surgery of the Knee, 2nd ed. New York, Churchill Livingstone, 1993.)

avoid the sheer stresses otherwise imposed if anatomically constrained. The lateral side's greater mobility, estimated at an anterior-posterior movement of approximately 1 cm (compared with the medial's 0.5 cm), is a consequence of its nonattachment along the posterolateral aspect of the knee, at the "popliteal hiatus" (Fig. 23–6).

The menisci provide several important functions, of which the most significant, transmission of joint stresses, derives from its conforming anatomic design. The menisci distribute the normal forces across the joint surfaces, decreasing peak contact stresses and better distributing joint loads. This is thought to directly preserve articular cartilage; conversely, absence of the meniscus risks injury to articular cartilage, which has a dramatically increased joint reaction force in areas where the meniscus is no longer present. Several biomechanical studies have demonstrated an approximate 300% increase in contact pressures following meniscus removal. The medial meniscus is thought to transmit up to 50% of joint forces across its compartment, in comparison with up to 70% on the lateral side. Additional functions of the meniscus include improved joint stability, impact absorption, and articular nourishment.

The bone of the distal femur and proximal tibia is covered by a highly organized structure of hyaline or articular cartilage. Varying in thickness according to location, it is thickest over the patella, where it is 6 to 7 mm, or more than a quarter of an inch thick. This is some of the thickest articular cartilage in the human body. The cartilage biochemically is composed of type II collagen, whose unique structure accounts for the ability of this dynamic structure to absorb impact and accommodate the variable forces of compression, tension, and sheer seen in this joint.

Although joint congruence through bone and meniscal anatomy provides some inherent stability, most joint security is conferred by the surrounding soft tissue structures, including the joint capsule and the ligaments. The capsule of the knee joint is a variably thick structure lined by synovium. This layer is responsible for fluid generation that accounts for the knee's low coefficient of friction. Perhaps the most important macromolecule synthesized by the synovium is hyaluronic acid, which serves to lubricate the joint surfaces. External to the synovium is the fibrous capsular envelope of the knee, which varies in thickness according to the region investigated. Somewhat thin in the

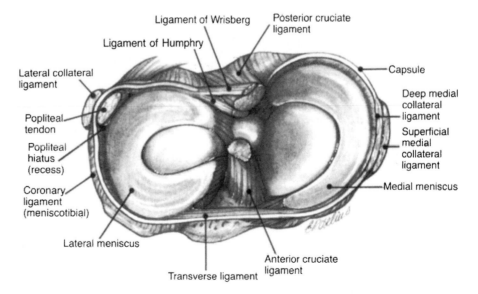

Figure 23–5. In this axial (overhead) view, note the relatively more circular shape of the lateral meniscus in comparison with the semicircular design of the medial meniscus. (From Wiesel SW, Delahay JN: Essentials of Orthopaedic Surgery, 2nd ed. Philadelphia, WB Saunders, 1997.)

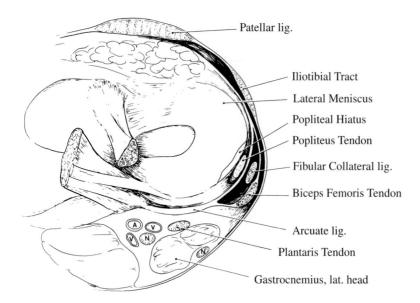

Patellar lig.

Iliotibial Tract

Lateral Meniscus

Popliteal Hiatus

Popliteus Tendon

Fibular Collateral lig.

Biceps Femoris Tendon

Arcuate lig.

Plantaris Tendon

Gastrocnemius, lat. head

Figure 23–6. In this axial image, note that the circular lateral meniscus is circumferentially attached except along its posterolateral corner, where the presence of the popliteal tendon precludes normal attachment. This "hiatus" through which the popliteal tendon traverses toward attachment on the lateral femur allows for the increased mobility seen in the lateral meniscus compared with that seen on the medial side. (From Arnoczky SP, et al: Basic science of the knee. *In* Operative Arthroscopy, 2nd ed. Philadelphia, Lippincott-Raven, 1996.)

anterior portion of the knee, it is thicker and reinforced by numerous discrete fibrous ligament complexes posteriorly, laterally termed the arcuate ligament and medially the posteriomedial oblique ligament.

The ligaments of the knee are responsible for most joint stability and include the collateral ligaments and the cruciate ligaments. These ligaments are discrete collagen bundles that connect one bone to another. The cruciate ligaments work together to "guide" the articular surfaces during knee motion. They are critical in maintaining this normal relationship. The anterior cruciate ligament (ACL) originates from a broad footprint on the anteromedial tibia, passes through the intercondylar notch, and attaches to the posterior lateral aspect of the notch on the lateral femoral condyle. The ACL is the primary restraint to anterior tibial translation (Fig. 23–7).

The posterior cruciate ligament (PCL) criss-crosses the ACL within the intercondylar notch, arising on the posterior aspect of the tibial plateau and inserting anteromedially in the notch along the medial femoral condyle. The PCL is thought to be crucial to normal knee mechanics as well, and is the primary restraint to posterior tibial translation (Fig. 23–8).

The collateral ligaments provide stability in the coronal plane to varus and/or valgus stresses. The medial collateral ligament (MCL) is composed of two discrete parts: a superficial and a deeper component. The superficial MCL arises from the medial epicondyle of the femur and travels inferi-

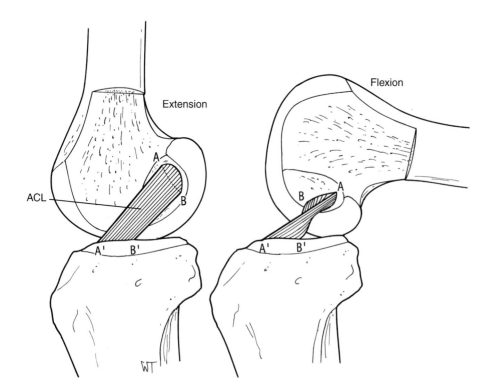

Extension

Flexion

ACL

Figure 23–7. This side view of the knee shows the anterior cruciate ligament (ACL) arising from the anteromedial tibia and inserting on the posterior aspect of the lateral femoral condyle. Rather than simply straight fibers, the ACL demonstrates a somewhat spiral course along its path. The ACL maintains normal rotational stability of the knee and prevents anterior tibial translation. (From Insall JN, et al: Surgery of the Knee, 2nd ed. New York, Churchill Livingstone, 1993.)

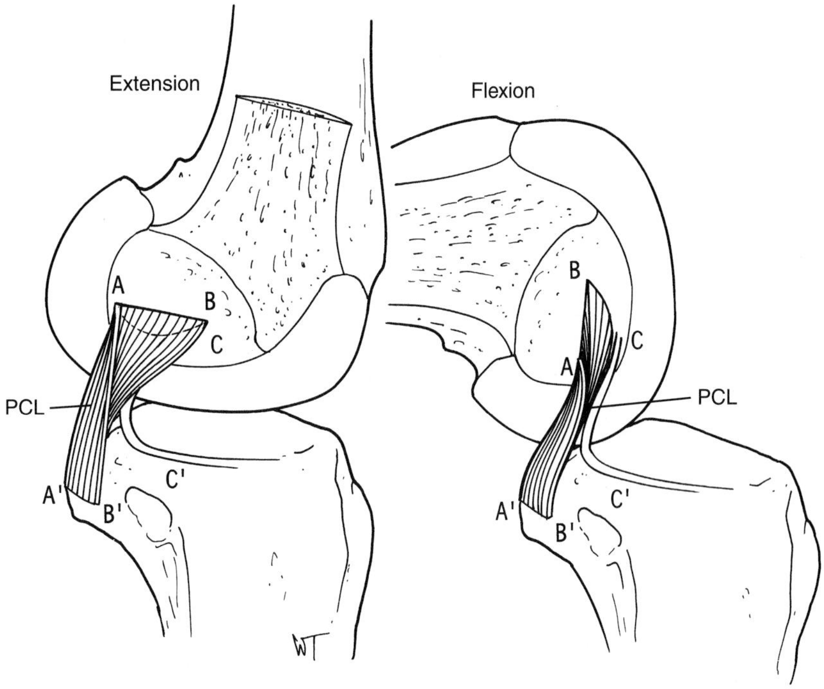

Figure 23–8. The posterior cruciate ligament (PCL) can be seen to arise from the anterior and medial aspect of the medial femoral condyle and to insert on the posterior aspect of the tibia. It is responsible for preventing posterior tibial translation. (From Insall JN, et al: Surgery of the Knee, 2nd ed. New York, Churchill Livingstone, 1993.)

orly to its broad proximal medial tibial attachment approximately 8 cm inferior to the medial joint line. The deep MCL is composed of the capsule of the medial knee joint (Fig. 23–9). The lateral collateral ligament travels from the lateral femoral epicondyle to the fibula head. It can be palpated when the knee is placed in the "figure of four" position (Fig. 23–10). A number of other important fibrous structures contribute to normal knee stability. These include the arcuate complex posterolaterally and the posterior oblique ligament posteromedially.

The second "joint" in the knee is the patellofemoral joint, in which the patella articulates with the femoral condyles. The patella is a sesamoid bone encased within the quadriceps mechanism. By elevating the quads mechanism anterior to the center of the joint, the patella effectively increases the muscle's moment arm. The patella is thought to decrease the force necessary to achieve extension through this mechanical advantage. Clinical data support the patella's value in noting the approximately 30% weakness in quadriceps function among patients in whom it has been removed.

The patella articulates with the distal femur in its trochlear groove. The posterior surface of the patella contains medial and lateral facets that congruently track within the trochlear groove in a very specific manner (Fig. 23–11). The patella is loosely held in place by this anatomic convex-concave arrangement, as well as by the medial and lateral retinacular ligaments. The patellofemoral joint carries large loads, particularly during activities in which the knee is flexed. For example, stair climbing and jumping are calculated to result in patellofemoral forces that are between three and eight times body weight, respectively.

The third and final joint of the knee complex is the proximal tibiofibular joint. The neglected "step-child" of the knee, it is easily overlooked and an occasionally unrecognized source of knee or leg pain. A diarthrodial joint, the articular surfaces are surrounded by a synovial-lined capsule with strong reinforcing anterior and posterior ligaments. This joint is at risk of developing the same pathology as that seen in other joints, including arthritis, trauma, and synovial disease.

The most important muscles around the knee include the quadriceps mechanism anteriorly, the hamstrings posteriorly, the pes tendons medially, and the iliotibial band laterally. The quadriceps are composed of four muscles (therein lies the name), including the rectus femoris, vastus intermedius, vastus lateralis, and vastus medialis. These muscles all arise from the femur and collectively insert along the patella, which through the patellar tendon attaches to the tibial tubercle (Fig. 23–12). All four are innervated by branches of the femoral nerve.

Posteriorly, the hamstrings arise from the ischial tuberosity and travel distally to attach to the posterior tibia and fibula. Medially, the semimembranosis and semitendinosis attach to the proximal tibia and posteromedial capsule. The biceps femoris inserts along the fibular head laterally. Branches of the sciatic nerve are responsible for their innervation. The hamstrings function to flex the knee.

The tendons of the gracilis, semitendinosus, and sartorius are found medially. These tendons, arising from the pubis, ischial tuberosity, and anterior superior iliac spine, respectively, insert over the anteromedial aspect of the proximal tibia superficial to the MCL. The appearance of these three structures led Greek observers to describe the structure as a "pes anserine" in deference to its resemblance to a duck's webbed foot. Clinically, this structure is responsible for symptoms when its underlying bursa becomes irritated (pes bursitis) and is a popular source of autograft tissue during reconstructive surgery.

Laterally, the iliotibial band (ITB) is a strong sinewy broad flat band that arises from the iliac crest, receives insertions of the gluteus maximus and tensor fascia lata, and travels inferiorly to attach to Gerty's tubercle on the proximal anterolateral tibia. From 0 to 30 degrees, the ITB contributes to knee extension. Beyond 30 degrees, the ITB is thought to flex the knee. The ITB is clinically relevant in causing a friction syndrome over the lateral aspect of the knee known as runner's or cyclist's knee. The ITB is also thought mechanically responsible for the "pivot shift" maneuver seen in ACL insufficiency.

Posteriorly, there are several other muscle groups of importance, including the medial and lateral gastrocnemii, which arise from their respective posterior femoral condyles, along with an indirect slip from the posterior knee capsule. The gastrocnemii combine with the soleus to form the triceps surae muscle, whose tendonous portion inserting on the calcaneus is known as the achilles tendon. Deep to the gastrocnemii, arising from the midpoint of the posterior proximal tibia, is the popliteus muscle, which travels superolaterally, enters the joint directly behind the lateral meniscus and exits again to attach just inferior to the lateral epicondyle (Fig. 23–13). This structure is important in

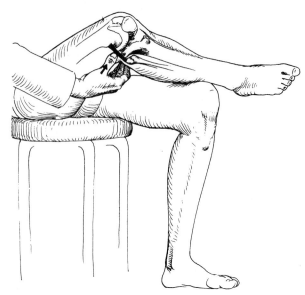

Figure 23–10. The lateral collateral ligament (LCL) is a distinct structure arising from the lateral epicondyle of the femur and inserting onto the fibular head, providing stability to varus stress. It is best appreciated by placement of the leg in the "figure-of-four" position, in which the LCL is felt as a discrete cord along the lateral aspect of the knee. (From Hoppenfield S: Physical examination of the knee. *In Physical Examination of the Spine and Extremities*. New York, Appleton-Century-Crofts, 1976, p 182.)

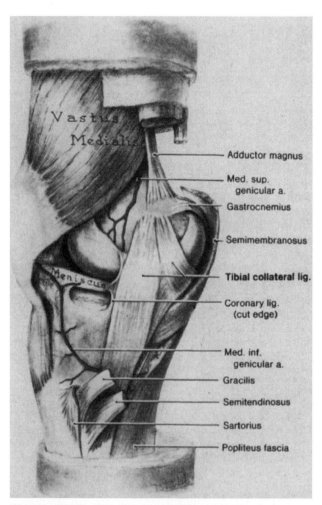

Vastus Medialis

Meniscus

- Adductor magnus
- Med. sup. genicular a.
- Gastrocnemius
- Semimembranosus
- **Tibial collateral lig.**
- Coronary lig. (cut edge)
- Med. inf. genicular a.
- Gracilis
- Semitendinosus
- Sartorius
- Popliteus fascia

Figure 23–9. The medial collateral ligament (MCL) is composed of two portions—an extra-articular superficial band and an intra-articular component, consisting of the deep capsule of the knee. The MCL provides restraint against valgus stresses. (From Fu FH, Harner C, Vince KG, Miller MD: Basic Science in Knee Surgery, Vol 1. Baltimore, Williams and Wilkins, 1994.)

contributing to normal knee function by "unlocking" the tibial plateau and internally rotating it at the beginning of knee flexion.

There are a number of bursae in the knee, including the prepatellar, pes, iliotibial, and semimembranosus bursae (Fig. 23–14). Each of these bursae are synovial-lined "potential" sacs that serve as lubricated interfaces between adjacent moving surfaces. The prepatellar bursa is detected only when it becomes symptomatic and "inflates" in response to trauma or irritation, most commonly seen in patients with trauma to the front of the knee. Repetitive or direct trauma leads to inflammation, occasional thickening, and swelling. The pes bursa lies between the pes tendons and the underlying anteromedial tibia. Inflammation here often leads to anteromedial knee pain. Laterally, inflammation and irritation of the ITB over the lateral epicondyle is a common problem in running athletes and cyclists, leading to ITB friction syndrome. And finally, a bursa in the posteromedial aspect of the knee between the posteromedial capsule and the semimembranosis can become swollen and historically has been called a Baker cyst. More recently, clinicians have come to recognize that this structure in fact is a prominent semimembranosus bursa.

Important neurovascular structures about the knee include the posterior femoral artery becoming the popliteal artery at the adductor hiatus. Distal to the joint, the popliteal artery divides into an anterior branch, which penetrates the interosseous membrane, and the posterior branch, which continues inferiorly. A lateral or peroneal branch trifurcates from this point in the proximal posterior leg as well. This trifurcation is of clinical significance because of its vulnerability during leg trauma (Fig. 23–15). In addition

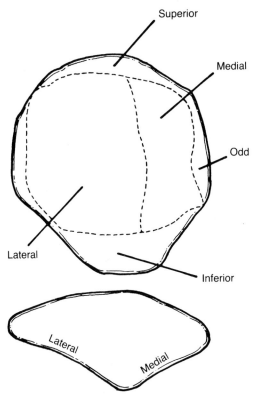

Figure 23–11. The facets of the patella are seen here on this view of the articular cartilage of the patella, including the larger lateral, the smaller medial facet, and the "odd" facet with which the patella articulates against the femur only when the knee is flexed beyond about 135 degrees. (From Scott WN [ed]: Arthroscopy of the Knee. Diagnosis and Treatment. Philadelphia, WB Saunders, 1990.)

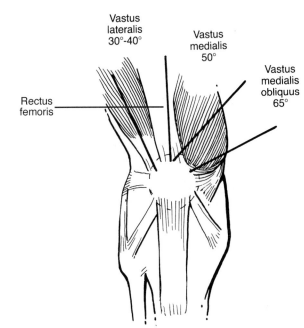

Figure 23–12. The quadriceps mechanism includes the four (quad) muscles in the anterior aspect of the knee, including the rectus femoris, vastus medialis, vastus lateralis, and vastus intermedius. Collectively, these muscles blend together and through the patellar tendon attach to the tibial tubercle. (From DeLee JC, Drez D Jr: Orthopaedic Sports Medicine: Principles and Practice, Vol 2. Philadelphia, WB Saunders, 1994.)

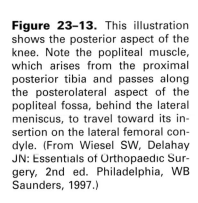

Figure 23–13. This illustration shows the posterior aspect of the knee. Note the popliteal muscle, which arises from the proximal posterior tibia and passes along the posterolateral aspect of the popliteal fossa, behind the lateral meniscus, to travel toward its insertion on the lateral femoral condyle. (From Wiesel SW, Delahay JN: Essentials of Orthopaedic Surgery, 2nd ed. Philadelphia, WB Saunders, 1997.)

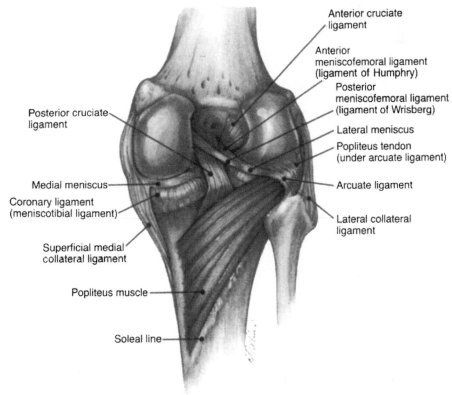

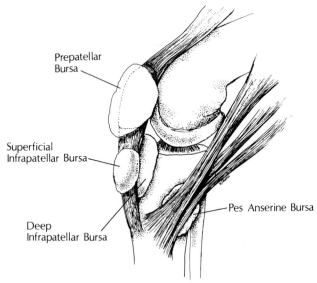

Figure 23–14. Common bursae of the knee include the prepatellar, infrapatellar, and pes anserine bursae. (From Insall JN, et al: Surgery of the Knee, 2nd ed. New York, Churchill Livingstone, 1993.)

to the tibial and peroneal divisions of the sciatic nerve contributing to motor and sensory function, there are several smaller nerves of some clinical significance. The infrapatellar branch of the saphenous nerve travels along the medial aspect of the knee and provides sensation to the

anteromedial and lateral sensory dermatomes (Fig. 23–16). This nerve's proximity to common surgical incisions puts it at risk of neuroma and risk of sensory loss in affected dermatomes. The obturator nerve to the distal medial thigh is of little usual significance in the adult population, but in the skeletally immature age group may be a source of referred pain. Hip pathology presenting as "knee pain" is a tribute to this particular nerve referral pattern. The peroneal nerve trunk providing motor and sensation to the anterior and lateral compartment of the leg and foot is vulnerable in its course traveling anterior around the fibula neck, where the superficial branch continues distally and the deep branch dives into the anterior compartment (Fig. 23–17). The nerve is at considerable risk in its vulnerable location with both traumatic and iatrogenic injury from surgical exploration or reconstruction on the lateral side of the knee. The superficial peroneal nerve is at risk during surgery of the lateral compartment of the leg.

In the leg, there are four muscular compartments, including anterior, lateral, superficial posterior, and deep posterior (Fig. 23–18). Each has specific muscle groups and neurovascular supply surrounded by a fascial envelope. The risk of increased pressure within this envelope due to trauma, disease, or overuse makes recognition and understanding of the anatomy of each of these compartments clinically important. The anterior compartment is composed of the tibialis anterior, extensor hallicus longus, and extensor digitorum longus. The deep peroneal nerve and anterior tibial artery provide neurovascular supply. The

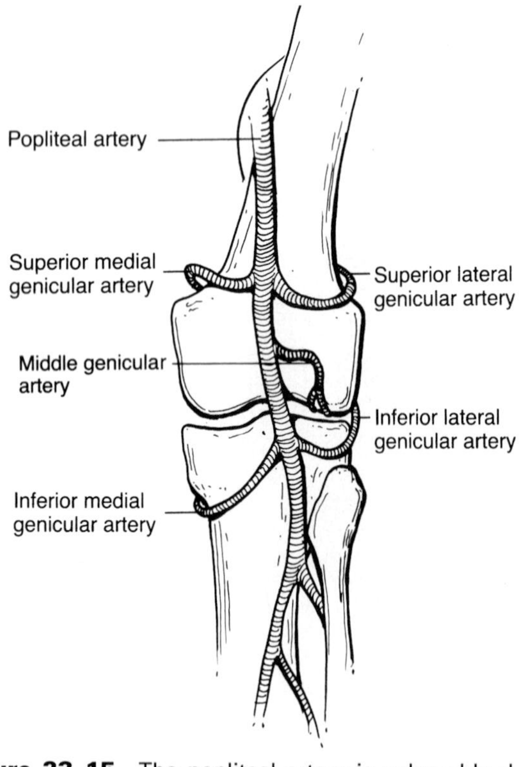

Figure 23–15. The popliteal artery is vulnerable during knee dislocations because of its tethered position between the relatively fixed adductor hiatus proximally and the passage through the interosseous membrane distally. (From DeLee JC, Drez D Jr: Orthopaedic Sports Medicine: Principles and Practice, Vol 2. Philadelphia, WB Saunders, 1994.)

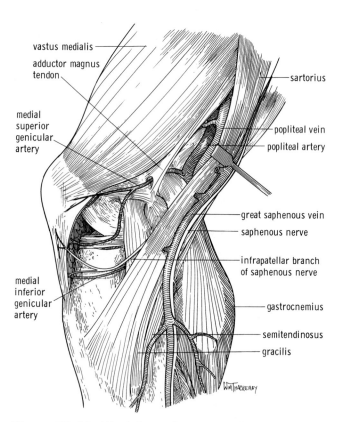

Figure 23–16. The infrapatellar branch of the saphenous nerve travels along the posteromedial aspect of the knee joint and is vulnerable to blunt trauma and iatrogenic injury during surgical repair. (From Insall JN, et al: Surgery of the Knee, 2nd ed. New York, Churchill Livingstone, 1993.)

lateral compartment is composed of the peroneus longus and brevis, with the tertius contributing in the inferior fourth. The superficial peroneal nerve contributes motor supply to this compartment, which is divided from the anterior compartment by the lateral intermuscular septum. Posteriorly, there are two separate compartments: the deep and the superficial. The deep is composed of the flexor digitorum, flexor hallicus longus, and posterior tibialis. The superficial compartment is composed of the soleus, the gastrocnemii, and the plantaris tendon. All posterior compartment muscles are supplied by the posterior tibial nerve.

EVALUATION OF KNEE AND LEG PROBLEMS

The evaluation of knee and leg problems depends upon understanding normal knee anatomy, techniques of physical

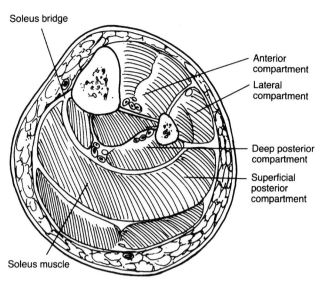

Figure 23–18. This cross-section of the leg through its midportion demonstrates the four compartments, including the anterior, lateral, superficial posterior, and deep posterior. (From DeLee JC, Drez D Jr: Orthopaedic Sports Medicine: Principles and Practice, Vol 2. Philadelphia, WB Saunders, 1994.)

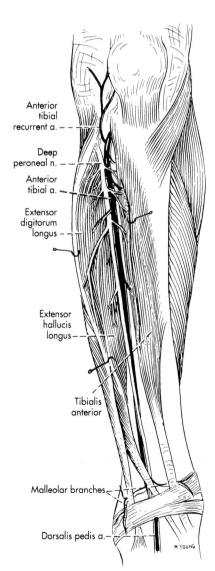

Figure 23–17. The peroneal nerve travels around the neck of the fibula, where it is vulnerable to direct trauma and injury during knee dislocations. (From Jenkins DB: Hollinshead's Functional Anatomy of the Limbs and Back, 6th ed. Philadelphia, WB Saunders, 1991, p 296.)

examination, and familiarity with common knee conditions. A history and physical examination, complemented as necessary by x-ray, can diagnose most problems. Special tests are not commonly required, although sophisticated imaging tests are sometimes helpful.

Although familiarity with how to perform a systematic knee examination approach is important, a comprehensive examination is not usually required in every patient. Instead, the examination should be tailored to the patient's presentation. For example, examination of a 72-year-old with progressive knee pain should be different than the evaluation of an 18-year-old football player following a traumatic injury. Understanding *how* to perform a basic overall examination is an important skill, but knowing *when* to perform the various specific examination techniques is a learned art. A thorough history usually alerts the examiner to the most likely diagnostic conditions and facilitates a tailored examination in the context of this diagnostic differential.

Advantage should be taken of the body's symmetry. The opposite knee and leg serves as an excellent "control" that by comparison helps distinguish normal from abnormal with respect to atrophy, swelling, motion, strength, and stability. Because of normal variability within the population, use of the patient's opposite limb makes diagnostic evaluation more accurate.

Finally, remember that knee symptoms can be caused by pathology elsewhere. Common sources of referral in adults are the spine and hip, and in children, knee pain is considered due to hip pathology until proven otherwise.

History

Obtaining a careful history is as important as the actual physical examination. The most common presenting symptoms include pain, swelling, giving way, clicking, catching, and locking. Determine the chief complaint. The most common complaint is that of knee pain. How did it begin? Was it acute or insidious in onset? Was it related to a traumatic event, and if so, how specifically did it occur? Clues to the type of injury are ascertained by the pattern of trauma. For example, the patient sustaining a blow to the anterior knee following a fall would likely have a fracture or injury to the posterior cruciate ligament. Acute pain, pop, and swelling in an athlete following planting of the foot and pivoting suggest tear of the ACL. Understanding the specific mechanism of injury, enhanced by soliciting observations from witnesses, may help better elucidate the nature of the injury.

What is the nature of the pain? A dull, aching discomfort that is poorly localized and occurs in the front of the knee is typical of patellar disorders. Conversely, sharp, catching pain that occurs with twisting, turning, or squatting may reflect a meniscus tear. A boring, aching pain that is constant and feels like a toothache may suggest osteonecrosis.

Where is the pain localized? Discomfort around the front of the knee that is poorly localized often reflects patellofemoral disorders. In contrast, more localized pain over the medial or lateral joint line may suggest a structural origin for the pain, such as chondral or meniscal pathology. Pain over the posterolateral aspect of the knee that radiates into the leg may be due to problems of the proximal tibiofibular joint.

Does the pain radiate anywhere? In children, hip pathology may present as knee pain, and asking about pain in the thigh or hip may be rewarded by directing inquiry to the true source of symptoms. In adults, ask about hip and back problems that can occasionally masquerade as knee problems or radiate into the knee. Problems of the proximal tibiofibular joint typically radiate into the anterolateral leg.

When does the pain occur, and what activities exacerbate symptoms? Most knee problems that are mechanical in origin (i.e., torn menisci, damaged articular cartilage) are worsened with activity and improved with rest. For example, meniscus tears are typically painful with protracted activity in which there is loading of the joint, such as in walking, twisting, turning, squatting, and of course more vigorous activities such as running or jumping. Cycling and rowing may cause pain over the lateral aspect of the knee in patients with ITB friction syndrome. Basketball and volleyball, with their repetitive jumping demands, may lead to anterior knee pain in patients with patellar tendonitis.

Likewise, degenerative arthritis is typically exacerbated by increased activity. Conversely, some symptoms are seemingly improved with activity, such as patellofemoral pain syndrome, which commonly causes discomfort with protracted sitting, with aching and stiffness that often feels better a few moments after arising. Pain that is constant, even at rest, suggests osteonecrosis, tumor, or infection.

What improves the symptoms? Rest and activity modification almost always improve symptoms. Exceptions include more serious problems such as osteonecrosis, tumor, infection, and thrombophlebitis. Have anti-inflammatory medications been helpful? What other treatments has the patient received, and what was the response? Ask about activity modifications, medications, injections, physical therapy, and surgery.

What other symptoms does the patient have? Does the patient experience clicking? Many patients note clicking in their knee, which may be asymptomatic. Generally, clicking is caused by mechanical "twanging" of inelastic synovial bands within the patellofemoral joint. These bands are usually vestigial remnants of synovial development. Their postnatal persistence is variable, usually of little clinical consequence, and arthroscopically appear as cobweb-like structures within the patellofemoral joint, referred to as "plicae synovialis" (Fig. 23–19). Be sure to ask if clicking is painful. Usually it is painless and unrelated to presentation. This is not to say that all clicking is harmless. Sometimes, the clicking is distinctly painful, and the most likely conditions to consider in such cases are a meniscal tear, a symptomatic plica, and degenerative chondral pathology.

Does the knee swell? Swelling is a nonspecific finding. Determine the frequency of the swelling, relationship to activities, and whether the knee has been aspirated. Effusions (fluid within the knee) can occur for several reasons, including synovial disorders such as inflammatory arthritis, gout, pseudogout, infection, and traumatic injury (hemarthrosis or bleeding into the joint). In addition to swelling, does the patient notice any masses? Vague fullness in the popliteal region is usually due to Baker's cyst, a semimembranosus bursa containing synovial fluid. In distinction is the typical discrete grape-size mass directly over the joint line indicative of a meniscal cyst associated with meniscal degeneration and tearing. Swelling directly over the patella following direct trauma or repetitive pressure on the front of the knee may be due to prepatellar bursitis (housemaid's knee). Has the mass changed in size or shape? A mass that is synovial-based often will wax and wane in dimension. A solid mass will not fluctuate in size.

Does the patient complain of the knee "giving way"? This generally reflects *functional* weakness, in which the quadriceps suddenly stops contracting, allowing the knee to involuntarily bend or "give way." This process is often due to "reflex inhibition of pain," in which sudden impending joint overload or pain stimuli through a reflex arc cause the quads to stop firing. Giving way is a nonspecific symptom that can occur in patellofemoral pain syndrome, patellar instability, meniscal tears, ligament injuries, and chondral problems. A second reason for giving way is actually quad weakness.

Instability is a common complaint, although not necessarily specific. Patients should be specifically questioned as to what they mean by "unstable." Are they describing "giving way," or is it true instability, in which they have felt or observed their knee to be unstable? The most common instability occurs at the patellofemoral joint, with lateral patellar dislocation from the trochlear groove. ACL-injured patients may describe their knee as "going out" and feel the subluxation during twisting, pivoting, or cutting activities.

Has the knee locked? Locking is a very specific phenomenon, and almost always reflects meniscal pathology. Locking implies a transient inability to flex or straighten the knee, lasting from minutes to days. Generally the knee is fixed in 10 to 20 degrees of flexion and cannot be straightened. Episodes may occur spontaneously or follow a twist or squat. In locked knees, the meniscus is usually torn and is subluxed within the joint in the configuration

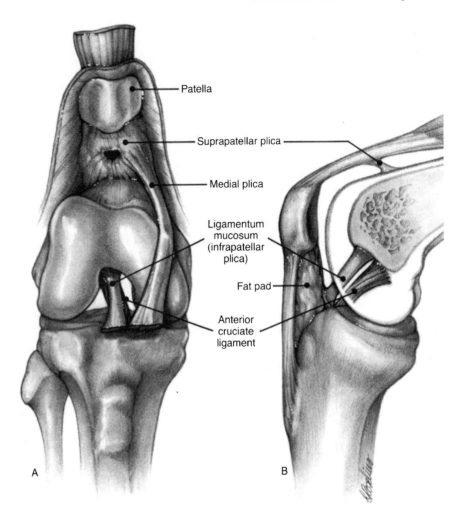

Figure 23–19. Plicae are normal variants, vestigial remnants of development. The most common are the suprapatellar, medial, and ligamentum mucosum. Occasionally, traumatized plicae may become symptomatic and lead to painful clicking in the knee. (From Scott WN [ed]: Arthroscopy of the Knee: Diagnosis and Treatment. Philadelphia, WB Saunders, 1990.)

Patella

Suprapatellar plica

Medial plica

Ligamentum mucosum (infrapatellar plica)

Fat pad

Anterior cruciate ligament

A

B

of a bucket handle (Fig. 23–20). Some patients complain or admit to locking episodes in which their knee seems to get "stuck" for a few seconds. This can occur for a variety of reasons. Instead of smooth gliding and rotation, the knee joint surfaces "jam" together, creating a momentary pause in motion. Chondral injury, loose bodies, patellofemoral pain syndrome, and synovial irritation can all lead to this transient "pseudo-locking."

Is there associated numbness or tingling? Neurologic complaints are uncommon and may be from referred sources such as spinal stenosis. Localized nerve problems can occur as a result of direct compression on the tibial nerve within the popliteal space (i.e., Baker's cyst), compression of the deep peroneal nerve at the fibular neck, or irritation of the infrapatellar branch of the saphenous nerve with burning dysesthesias over the medial aspect of the proximal tibia.

Ask about previous treatment and response to medications, corticosteroid injections, physical therapy, and surgery. Obtaining copies of previous operative reports and arthroscopic photos is instrumental in understanding the patient's diagnosis and previous treatment and establishing a treatment strategy. Discussion of the patient's response to treatment with the trainer, previous physician, and/or physical therapist can be enlightening.

Leg problems usually present with localized complaints such as pain, swelling, numbness, or weakness. The relationship of symptoms to activities, and response to treat-

ment, must be determined. In the patient with "shin splints," pain is usually related to running and is usually relieved with rest. In distinction, stress fractures usually occur with activity but often persist after cessation of exercise, at rest, and occasionally at night. Leg discomfort localized to the soft tissue that worsens dramatically with activity and requires cessation as a result of the discomfort may suggest exertional compartment syndrome. Pain and swelling in the posterior calf that is abrupt in onset and following "pushing off" when running for a tennis ball may reflect a tear of the gastrocnemius, commonly known as tennis leg.

How do the symptoms interfere with activity? This information will influence diagnostic and therapeutic decision making. Understanding the patient's motivation and goals strongly influences treatment strategy. A younger or middle-aged patient with stress reaction or fracture, whose goal is to complete a marathon, will require a different type and level of management when compared with the older patient with osteoarthritis, whose goal is to ambulate with a little less pain. Only by understanding the patient's personal and professional circumstances can the care provider best serve the patient's needs.

Physical Examination

A thorough systematic examination technique is important to master, even though all elements are rarely invoked

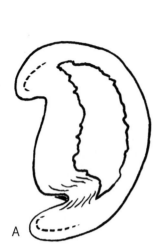
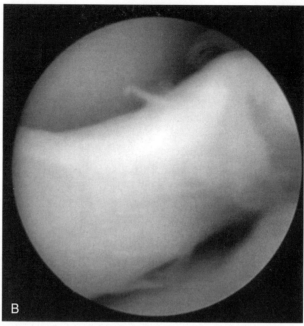

Figure 23–20. A "bucket-handle" tear of the medial meniscus results when a longitudinal tear of the meniscus allows displacement of the inner body of the meniscus, like the handle of a bucket. Such pathology is the most common reason for a "locked" knee. *A,* Diagram of typical bucket handle tear. *B,* Arthroscopic view of displaced bucket-handle fragment. (From McGinty JB, Caspari RB, Jackson RW, Poehling GG [eds]: Arthroscopic Meniscectomy in Operative Arthroscopy, 2nd ed. Philadelphia, Lippincott—Raven, 1996.)

on any one single patient. Physical examination includes inspection, palpation, and assessment of motion, laxity, strength, neurovascular status, and the patellofemoral joint. The examination begins with ensuring that the patient is properly attired to permit visualization of both lower extremities, including the feet.

INSPECTION

Examination begins with inspection. Observe the patient's gait. This requires having the patient walk down a hallway at his or her normal cadence. Observe for evidence of pain, which causes an antalgic gait. In this gait, more time is spent on the unaffected leg during the stance phase of walking. Also note the presence of abnormal motion, either in the form of stiffness (a "stiff knee" gait) or abnormal varus, valgus, or hyperextension exaggeration (thrust) (Fig. 23–21). Such observations may be appreciated only through this dynamic gait inspection. Observing the patient's feet for normal heel-toe gait is also useful. Look specifically for evidence of pronation, in which the medial arch dynamically "collapses" during the stance (weight-bearing) phase. Such a pattern may have treatment implications in patients with patellofemoral disorders and shin splints.

Observe the patient's alignment when standing. Usually in 5 to 7 degrees of valgus, malalignment may not be obvious with the patient supine. Valgus malalignment is more common in patients with inflammatory arthritis. Static inspection involves examination for skin integrity, looking for ecchymoses, abrasions, open wounds, and swelling. Trauma patients must be inspected carefully, including the popliteal fossa to ensure that an occult laceration or abra-

sion (and possible underlying open fracture) does not escape detection. Moderate to significant swelling can usually be detected simply by observing the soft tissue contour in comparison with the opposite knee.

PALPATION

Palpate the extremity for tissue swelling, turgor, integrity, tenderness, and crepitus. Moderate swelling can usually be readily detected upon inspection. However, the location of fluid is not always obvious. This can be ascertained with careful examination techniques. Joint effusion can be detected by the ballottement test or the fluid wave test. In the ballottement test, fluid is milked from the suprapatellar pouch inferiorly into the knee joint. With fluid confined to the space beneath the knee cap, direct pressure by a finger on the anterior aspect of the patella leads it to be temporarily depressed toward the femur and bounce back, floating on a bed of fluid (Fig. 23–22). When swelling is present over the anterior patella and seems circumscribed but is not ballottable, a prepatellar effusion may be present.

A smaller amount of intra-articular fluid can be detected by the "fluid wave" test. In this technique, one hand is used to try to circumscribe the patella on the medial side, with the other hand positioned over the lateral aspect of the knee. As one hand applies gentle pressure, the other is used to try to sense the transmission of a "fluid wave" on the other side (Fig. 23–23). Such detection is subtle and requires practice.

All fluid within the knee may not be intra-articular or within a confined bursa, and may in fact be within the soft tissues itself. In such cases, the prominent soft tissues about the knee may feel "swollen" or "boggy," and may reflect synovial edema.

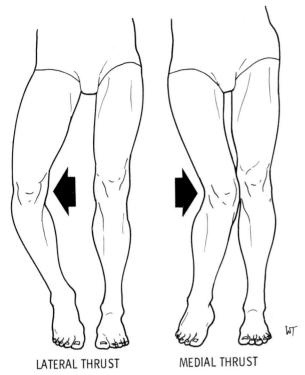

LATERAL THRUST   MEDIAL THRUST

Figure 23–21. Dynamic inspection of gait sometimes demonstrates an otherwise undetectable "thrust" during the stance phase of gait. Such a thrust may occur either in the anterior-posterior plane (recurvatum or hyperextension thrust) or in the coronal plane as shown here, in either varus or valgus direction. (From Insall JN, et al: Surgery of the Knee, 2nd ed. New York, Churchill Livingstone, 1993.)

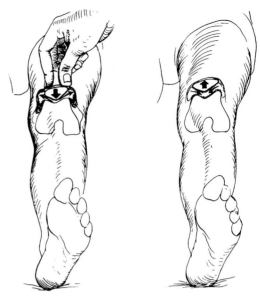

Figure 23–22. The ballottement test is performed by circumscribing the patella, milking fluid out of the suprapatellar pouch, and applying pressure on the patella. Ballottement occurs when there is sufficient fluid present under the patella, which "bounces back," confirming an effusion within the knee. (From Fu FH, Harner C, Vince KG, Miller MD: Basic Science in Knee Surgery, Vol 1. Baltimore, Williams and Wilkins, 1994.)

Next, palpate for tissue integrity. Palpate the soft tissue structures about the knee and leg for any structural defects. Examples include loss of integrity between the quadriceps tendon and the superior pole of the patella in a patient with a quadriceps tendon rupture, and the inferior pole of the patella and patellar tendon in a patient with a patellar tendon rupture. Although the medial collateral ligament and intra-articular cruciate ligaments cannot be distinctly palpated, the lateral collateral ligament (LCL) can be appreciated by placing the knee into the "figure-of-four" position (see Fig. 23–10). Failure to palpate its discrete

structure from the femoral epicondyle to the fibular head indicates compromise of the LCL.

Palpation for tenderness is the most familiar aspect of the knee examination and requires attention to detail. The knee should be palpated from proximally to distally in a systematic manner to ensure completeness. Diagnostic accuracy and patient comfort can be improved by examining less symptomatic areas first for reassurance and demonstration of the intended gentleness of the examination. Particularly in traumatized (physically and sometimes emotionally) patients, care and gentleness will often be rewarded by improved diagnostic accuracy. Examination of the patient's countenance during the examination sometimes adds to examination reliability.

Anteriorly, palpate over the quadriceps mechanism, including the rectus femoris, vastus lateralis and vastus medi-

Figure 23–23. A fluid wave may be elicited in patients with a small effusion. The patella is circumscribed by both hands, and application of force on one side yields a palpable "thrill" by the opposite hand. (From Insall JN, et al: Surgery of the Knee, 2nd ed. New York, Churchill Livingstone, 1993.)

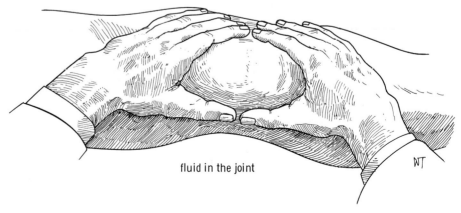

fluid in the joint

alis, the retinaculum, patella, patellar tendon, and tibial tubercle insertion. Medially, palpate over the medial epicondyle, the medial joint line, the course of the superficial medial collateral ligament (MCL), the tibial MCL insertion, the pes tendons and their insertion, and the medial joint line. Palpate for tenderness over the anteromedial knee between the joint line and the medial epicondyle, the most common site of a pathologic plica. Laterally, palpate the lateral epicondyle, the fibular collateral ligament, fibular head, Gerty's tubercle, and lateral joint line. Palpate both joint lines from anterior (on either side of the patellar tendon) to posterior. Joint line tenderness is one of the most reliable findings of a torn meniscus. Posteriorly, palpate the popliteal fossa for tenderness or a mass.

Crepitus refers to a grating sensation and is felt by placing one's hand over the patellofemoral joint while the patient actively extends the knee. Although grating does not necessarily reflect underlying degenerative pathology, its presence should be determined and compared with the opposite side.

MOTION

Next, assess the patient's active and passive range of motion. Inability to *actively* extend the knee may be present for a number of reasons (pain, swelling, effusion, mechanical block). In some cases, inability to extend the knee reflects structural compromise to the extensor mechanism such as with a quadriceps tendon tear, a patellar fracture

with retinacular injury, or a patellar tendon disruption. Alternatively, loss of active motion may reflect nerve injury.

With the patient lying supine, determine the degree of restriction, if any, in extension and flexion. Lack of full extension passively may be due to an effusion, MCL sprain, or a "locked" knee with a meniscus tear. Loss of extension can be accurately measured by comparing heel height difference with the patient prone. Each centimeter of difference roughly approximates 1 degree of extension loss (Fig. 23–24). Loss of flexion is a nonspecific finding and can occur as a result of trauma, the presence of an effusion, ligament injury, painful patellofemoral disorders, or meniscal injury/tear.

LIGAMENT ASSESSMENT

Assessment for ligament integrity is perhaps the most difficult portion of the knee examination. Examining both knees will allow comparison with a normal "control" knee in most cases, and help determine whether the ligament tested is abnormal for that particular patient. Ligaments should be tested by stressing the joint in the direction usually protected by the specific ligament in question. This can be done discretely for each of the four major knee ligaments—the MCL, ACL, PCL, and LCL.

The MCL is the most commonly injured ligament of the knee. Although its course can be traced from the femur's medial epicondyle to the proximal medial tibia, it

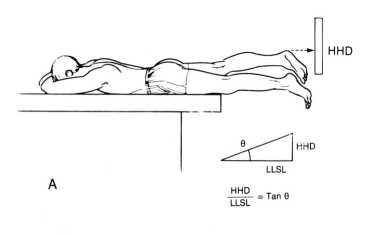

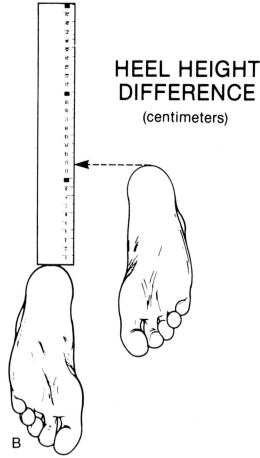

Figure 23–24. Loss of normal extension can be more accurately determined by placing the patient prone and measuring the difference in heel height, with each centimeter roughly approximating 1 degree of extension loss. (From DeLee JC, Drez D Jr: Orthopaedic Sports Medicine: Principles and Practice, Vol 2. Philadelphia, WB Saunders, 1994.)

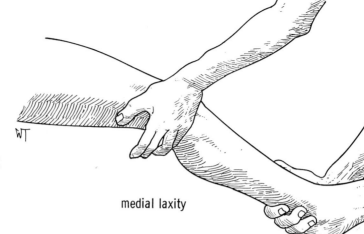

Figure 23–25. Medial collateral ligament (MCL) laxity is determined by applying a valgus stress to the slightly (15 to 30 degree) flexed knee. The degree of opening, the quality of the end point, and the reproduction of symptoms during this maneuver help ascertain the presence and degree of MCL injury. (From Insall JN, et al: Surgery of the Knee, 2nd ed. New York, Churchill Livingstone, 1993.)

medial laxity

cannot be palpated as a distinct structure. Tenderness to palpation, however, does correspond to the site of the tear. Integrity of the MCL is tested by applying a valgus stress to the slightly (15 to 30 degree) flexed knee. The easiest way to apply such a stress is with the patient supine and the knee slightly flexed off the side of the table, with the patient's foot and ankle securely seated in the examiner's axilla. The examiner's hands are then free to apply the valgus stress to the proximal tibia and better sense the degree of medial joint line opening and the nature of the end point (Fig. 23–25). Ligament injuries are generally graded according to a I to III (mild, moderate, severe) classification scheme, or by actually estimating the number of millimeters of joint opening (i.e., <5 mm, 5 to 10 mm, >10 mm). Injury is suggested by the presence of (1) abnormal amount of "opening" compared with the opposite side; (2) the abnormal quality of the end point, with a "soft" feel upon application of stress rather than a firm or discrete end point; (3) the reproduction of symptoms (usually pain); or (4) a combination of these findings. Injury to the MCL usually leads to both pain and slight opening when valgus stress is applied.

The anterior cruciate ligament (ACL) is the next most common injury and is particularly frequent among athletes involved in pivoting and cutting sports. Physical examination of this structure is more difficult than that of the MCL and requires practice. A number of examinations have been described, including the Lachman, the anterior drawer, and the pivot shift test. The most reliable is the Lachman test, named for the Temple University professor who popularized this particular technique of examining for ACL insufficiency. With the patient supine, the knee is gently flexed between 15 and 30 degrees. With the femur held securely, the tibia is firmly grasped and an effort made to translate the tibia anteriorly. The test is positive if the tibia translates anteriorly to a degree greater than the opposite side, or shows an abnormal end point (Fig. 23–26).

Placement of a pillow behind the patient's knee may aid in relaxation and facilitate a more accurate examination. This test is positive even in the face of swelling and pain, although apprehension on the part of some patients will make detection of ACL injury difficult. The test should be graded according to the amount of translation, using a 1 to 3 + scale, or by actually estimating the amount of translation in millimeters. This latter is perhaps more accurate, particularly with experience. By placing the thumb of the examining hand (the hand on the proximal tibia) over the medial joint line while performing the anterior translation maneuver, the depth to which the thumb "falls into" the anterior tibial crest helps more specifically gauge the amount of translation, and may be a helpful way of better estimating the degree of translation.

The anterior drawer test has been used more frequently historically but is less reliable than the Lachman examination in detecting instability, particularly in acute injury. In this test, the knee is flexed to approximately 70 to 90 degrees with the patient supine. While the foot is fixed

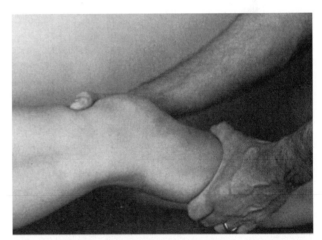

Figure 23–26. The Lachman test is the most sensitive and reliable physical examination to determine injury to the anterior cruciate ligament (ACL). The test is performed with the knee in 15 to 30 degrees of flexion and, while holding the thigh (femur), attempting to anteriorly translate the tibia. The degree of translation and quality of the end point, in comparison with the opposite side, help determine the presence of ACL injury. (From Garrick JE, Webb DA: Sports Injuries: Diagnosis and Management. Philadelphia, WB Saunders, 1990.)

(usually by the examiner seated upon it), both hands encircle the proximal tibia and attempt to translate it anteriorly, again noting both the translation amount and the proprioceptive nature of the end point (Fig. 23–27). Some clinicians have further recommended positioning of the foot in various degrees of rotation to more specifically elicit different laxity patterns. However, interpretation of these modifications in the acutely injured knee is of little practical value. Swelling, pain, and hamstring muscle spasm usually preclude reliably performing the anterior drawer test, and for this reason, it is much less useful than the Lachman.

The pivot shift test involves the simultaneous application of valgus and rotational stress to the knee to elicit anterolateral instability. The ACL is thought to provide not only anterior stability, but also rotational stability, preventing anterior and lateral subluxation of the tibial plateau. When the knee subluxes, it usually does so anterolaterally. The pivot shift test is designed to reproduce this functional instability pattern and is specific to the ACL-injured knee. In the traditional description of this test, the patient is placed supine. The foot of the affected limb is grasped and an internal rotation force applied to the leg by holding the foot in internal rotation. Using the heel of the other hand, a valgus stress is applied to the proximal tibia as the knee is flexed from the extended position. Because the ACL-deficient knee is subluxed anterolaterally in the extended position, it "reduces" with a palpable and visible "clunk" at about 30 degrees of knee flexion (Fig. 23–28). By extending the knee from the flexed position, this same shift can be elicited, this time anterolaterally subluxing the tibia from the reduced position. An alternative technique for eliciting the pivot shift involves placing the foot of the injured extremity in the examiner's axilla, and gently grasping the proximal tibia. By applying a valgus and rotational stress directly below the joint line, the shift is more easily detected and controlled. Subtle instability can be better detected in this manner. The value of the pivot shift is in demonstrating functional laxity, rather than just the static laxity seen with the Lachman examination. A patient with a positive pivot shift is at risk of instability during pivoting or cutting activities. Patients will often remark during the examination that the maneuver reproduces the feeling they experience when their knee "goes out." This test is rarely helpful in evaluating the acutely injured knee because of pain, swelling, and guarding.

The posterior cruciate ligament is injured much less frequently than the ACL and occurs most commonly from athletic injury and motor vehicle accidents in which a direct posterior force is applied to the proximal anterior tibia. There is no "reverse Lachman" examination; testing for PCL laxity requires placing the knee of the supine patient at approximately 70 to 90 degrees and inspecting for evidence of a "sag sign" of the proximal posterior tibia relative to the opposite knee (Fig. 23–29). Note the amount of sag by directly observing the anterior proximal tibial contour from the side. The opposite knee can be viewed for comparison at the same time in profile. The posterior drawer test involves the application of a posterior force to the 70 to 90 degree flexed knee to determine the amount of posterior laxity present (Fig. 23–30). Because the tibia may already be resting slightly posteriorly, it should first be "reduced" by anteriorly translating the proximal tibia; then, from this "neutral" position, posterior force is applied to the proximal tibia and the amount of translation and the nature of the end point are observed and compared with the opposite side.

The quadriceps active test is yet a third examination technique helpful for detecting PCL injury. In this test, the

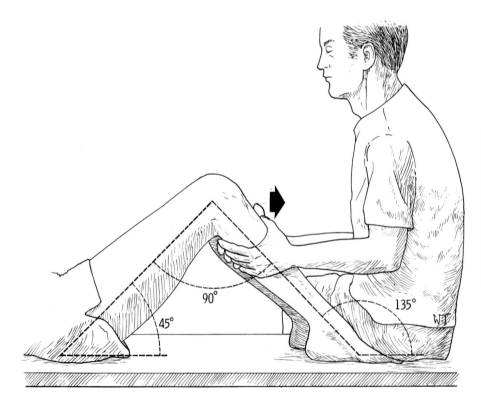

Figure 23–27. The anterior drawer test is performed with the knee flexed approximately 70 to 90 degrees and an attempt is made to anteriorly translate the tibia relative to the femur, observing both the amount of translation and the nature of the end point, compared with the opposite side. (From Insall JN, et al: Surgery of the Knee, 2nd ed. New York, Churchill Livingstone, 1993.)

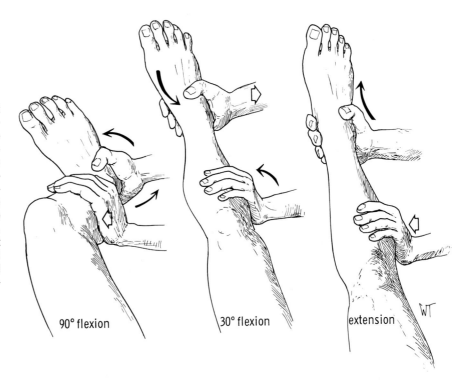

Figure 23–28. The pivot shift test is positive in patients with ACL insufficiency and is a passive maneuver that demonstrates transient tibiofemoral subluxation. While one applies a valgus stress to the internally rotated foot, the knee is extended from a flexed position. If the ACL is deficient, with flexion, the tibia reduces back into position. This phenomenon is seen at about 30 degrees of flexion. (From Insall JN, et al: Surgery of the Knee, 2nd ed. New York, Churchill Livingstone, 1993.)

90° flexion   30° flexion   extension

knee is again positioned at 70 to 90 degrees of flexion with the patient supine. With the foot of the affected limb immobilized (by either the examiner's hand or by the examiner seated upon the foot), the patient is asked to "straighten out" his or her leg. In so doing, the quadriceps contracts. In the normal knee, the force generated results in an isometric quads contraction and no visible effect on knee motion. In the PCL-deficient knee, however, the posteriorly subluxed tibia translates forward under active contraction of the quads as a result of the anteriorly oriented vector of the patellar tendon (Fig. 23–31).

The lateral collateral ligament (LCL) is the least commonly injured knee ligament. The ligament can be palpated for tenderness along its course from the lateral epicondyle to the fibular head and can be brought into relief in the "figure-of-four" position. Testing for ligament integrity is performed by placing a varus stress on the slightly (15 to 30 degree) flexed knee and noting the amount of opening, the nature of the end point, and the degree to which this stress reproduces symptoms (Fig. 23–32). Grading is similar to that in other knee ligament injuries, using a 0 to 3 + scale, or assessing opening in either degrees or, more commonly, millimeters. As in testing other knee ligaments, comparison with the opposite side is crucial to determine the significance of any observed laxity.

STRENGTH

Strength assessment should be carried out to determine muscle or nerve injury. Ask the patient to perform a straight leg raise, lifting the leg off the examining table. He or she

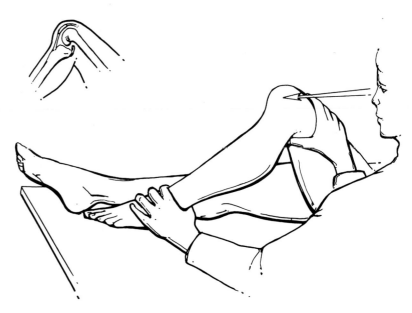

Figure 23–29. Posterior cruciate ligament (PCL) injury is best demonstrated on physical examination through inspection of the anterior tibial contour from the side, looking for the "sag sign," owing to posterior subluxation of the tibia on the femur. (From DeLee JC, Drez D Jr: Orthopaedic Sports Medicine: Principles and Practice, Vol 2. Philadelphia, WB Saunders, 1994.)

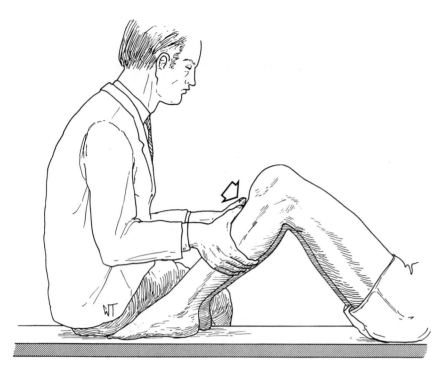

Figure 23–30. The posterior drawer test is performed with the knee flexed 70 to 90 degrees and demonstrates PCL laxity. (From Insall JN, et al: Surgery of the Knee, 2nd ed. New York, Churchill Livingstone, 1993.)

may not be able to do this owing to pain, swelling, and apprehension, but the ability to do so confirms function of the femoral nerve and the extensor mechanism.

PATELLOFEMORAL JOINT ASSESSMENT

Examination of the patellofemoral joint begins with inspection, noting the dynamic gait, including the feet for pronation. The presence of pronation is a common accompaniment of patellofemoral pain syndrome.

Inspect for atrophy, and in particular note the quadriceps development. The vastus medialis obliquis (VMO) at the superomedial border of the patella strongly influences patellar tracking. Having the patient "push down" with the legs while lying supine allows observation of VMO development. Next, inspect for malalignment. Patellofemoral pain due to malalignment and patellar instability are two frequent clinical problems in which abnormal patella positioning or tracking is thought to play a part. Observe the "Q angle," normally up to 15 degrees, and slightly higher in women than men. This angle is made by a line from the

anterior superior iliac spine to the mid-patella intersecting with a line from the mid-patella to the patellar tendon's tibial tubercle insertion (Fig. 23–33). Angles greater than 15 degrees are thought to contribute to malalignment.

Palpate the extensor mechanism for tenderness, integrity, and crepitus. Palpation should include the medial and lateral retinaculum. Identifying the area of tenderness is crucial during planning for surgical repair when indicated. Palpate the quadriceps muscles and the patella itself. Patients with symptomatic bipartite patellas may have tenderness localized to the non-united fragment (Fig. 23–34). Alternatively, some patients with radiographically evident abnormal ossification centers will have no localized tenderness whatsoever. Palpate over the proximal and distal pole of the patella for tenderness, and palpate the patellar tendon and tubercle itself for tenderness and masses. Irregular ossification or scar tissue formation may lead to nodularity within the tendon itself. Prominence of the tibial tubercle at the site of the patellar tendon insertion, with or without tenderness, may be present due to Osgood-Schlatter syn-

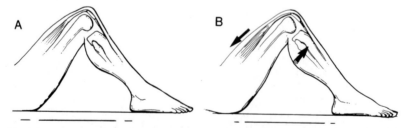

Figure 23–31. The quadriceps active test demonstrates PCL injury. With the patient supine and the knee flexed 70 to 90 degrees and the foot held by the examiner, the patient is asked to extend the knee. Doing so in a normal knee causes no change, but in the PCL-deficient knee, the tibia actively shifts forward from its subluxed position as a result of quads contraction. (From Stanitski CL, et al: Pediatric and Adolescent Sports Medicine, Vol 3. Philadelphia, WB Saunders, 1994.)

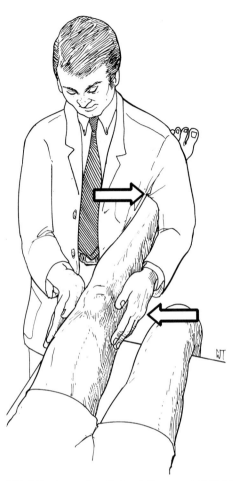

Figure 23–32. Lateral collateral ligament (LCL) laxity is assessed by applying a varus stress to the slightly (15 to 30 degree) flexed knee, noting the reproduction of symptoms, the amount of opening, and the nature of the end point, in comparison with the opposite side. (From Insall JN, et al: Surgery of the Knee, 2nd ed. New York, Churchill Livingstone, 1993.)

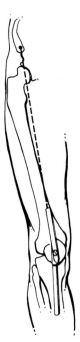

Figure 23–33. The "Q" or quadriceps angle is determined by measuring the angle made by a line drawn from the anterior superior iliac spine to the mid-patella, bisecting a line drawn from the mid-patella to the tibial tubercle. Normal should be less than 15 degrees. (From DeLee JC, Drez D Jr: Orthopaedic Sports Medicine: Principles and Practice, Vol 2. Philadelphia, WB Saunders, 1994.)

drome. Palpate the medial and lateral patellar facets for tenderness by displacing the patella medially and laterally, respectively. The presence of medial facet tenderness is the most common location of pain in patients with patellofemoral pain syndrome. Some examiners have described the patellofemoral compression test as a useful indicator of patellofemoral pathology. The test involves the gentle application of a compressive force to the patella into the trochlear groove, attempting to elicit pain that reproduces the symptoms. The problem with this test is its nonspecificity, as discomfort is frequently elicited as a result of painful impingement of the highly innervated synovial lining.

Palpate the extensor mechanism for integrity. This can be done by using your fingers to palpate for a defect along the course of the quadriceps to their patellar insertion, and along the patellar tendon from patella to tibial tubercle.

Palpate for patellofemoral crepitus. This is best performed with the patient seated. Place your hand directly over the anterior patella and note the amount of crepitus or grating in the patellofemoral joint. Remember to palpate

the opposite knee, as crepitus may be asymptomatic and not directly responsible for patient symptoms.

Next, inspect and palpate for patella alignment. Can the patella be easily translated side to side? Can the patella be everted (lifted up on its lateral side)? Normally the patella can be slightly translated both medially and laterally. Re-

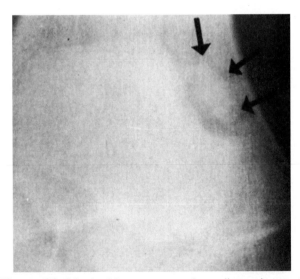

Figure 23–34. In this anteroposterior radiograph, a typical bipartite configuration to the patella can be seen. Note the smooth margins along the easily misdiagnosed "fracture" line. (From Stanitski CL, et al: Pediatric and Adolescent Sports Medicine, Vol 3. Philadelphia, WB Saunders, 1994.)

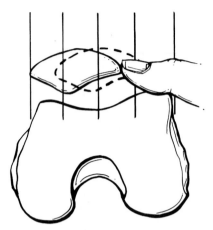

Figure 23–35. Peripatellar soft tissue laxity is determined by attempting to translate the patella medially, observing the amount of translation. When the patella translates more than 50% of its diameter, the amount of soft tissue laxity is thought to be potentially abnormal, a positive "medial glide" sign. (From DeLee JC, Drez D Jr: Orthopaedic Sports Medicine: Principles and Practice, Vol 2. Philadelphia, WB Saunders, 1994.)

striction may be normal for that patient, so it must be compared with the opposite side. Failure to translate the patella medially during the patellar glide test may suggest lateral patella retinacular tightness. Translation of more than 50% of the patella's width laterally suggests medial retinacular laxity (Fig. 23–35). Increased laxity in both medial and lateral translation suggests the possibility of generalized ligamentous laxity.

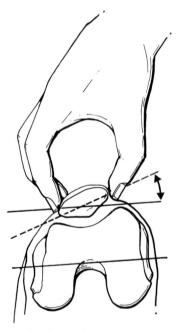

Figure 23–36. With the knee extended, an attempt is made to passively evert the patella. Failure to do so beyond 15 to 20 degrees suggests relative tightness of the lateral retinaculum. (From DeLee JC, Drez D Jr: Orthopaedic Sports Medicine: Principles and Practice, Vol 2. Philadelphia, WB Saunders, 1994.)

Next, perform the patellar tilt test by trying to evert the patella by lifting up its lateral side (Fig. 23–36). Normally the patella is evertable at least to neutral. Failure to elevate it to about 15 degrees of eversion suggests a tight lateral retinaculum, the most common physical finding in patients with patellofemoral pain syndrome. Again, remember to compare the degree of tightness with the opposite knee.

Examine for maltracking by inspection. Seated, the patellas should sit within their groove. Occasionally, they will display lateral orientation suggestive of "grasshopper eyes," associated with patellar instability (Fig. 23–37). Have the patient actively extend the knee. In the seated position, observe the course the patella tracks from flexion to terminal extension. Normal excursion of the patella involves tracking in multiple planes, and its course is not simply direct superior translation. Slight side-to-side movement and subtle rotational movement may accompany normal patella tracking. Observe for any differences between the symptomatic and asymptomatic knee. The "J" or "jump" sign can sometimes be observed in patients with patellofemoral instability, in which the patella actually is seen to "jump" at about 20 degrees as it reduces into the trochlear groove from its laterally subluxed position (Fig. 23–38). Slight lateral excursion during terminal extension may be normal, especially if present on both sides.

Patellar instability assessment should also include examining for apprehension. The apprehension test is performed

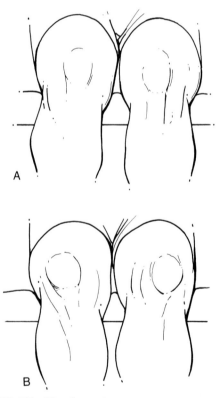

Figure 23–37. The "grasshopper eyes" sign is observed by inspection of the patella's position when viewed from the front of the knee. Note the normal appearance in *A*, in comparison to the abnormal posture seen in the "grasshopper eyes" appearance shown in *B*. (From DeLee JC, Drez D Jr: Orthopaedic Sports Medicine: Principles and Practice, Vol 2. Philadelphia, WB Saunders, 1994.)

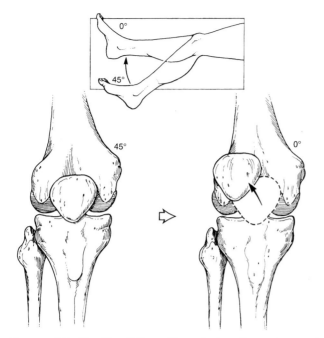

Figure 23–38. The "J" or "jump" describes abnormal patella tracking, seen when the patient is asked to actively extend the knee. The patella often follows a lateral subluxing course, but in near full extension will often dramatically relocate (jump) into the trochlear groove. (From Scuderi G: Physical examination of the patellofemoral joint. *In*: The Patella. New York, Springer-Verlag, 1995.)

with the patient supine and by applying gentle pressure to laterally translate the patella while observing the patient's countenance (Fig. 23–39). The patient may become anxious and/or actually implore the examiner to discontinue the manipulation because of the feeling of impending instability.

NEUROVASCULAR ASSESSMENT

Neurovascular assessment completes the knee examination and includes examination of neurovascular function both around the knee and distally at the foot and ankle. At the knee, several nerves can be involved in clinical problems, the most common of which is the vulnerable peroneal nerve as it courses along the fibular neck. Another im-

portant cutaneous nerve is the infrapatellar branch of the saphenous nerve, traveling along the inferomedial aspect of the knee. Reproduction of pain, dysesthesias, or paresthesias on palpating over these nerves may suggest their clinical involvement. Palpate the posterior tibial pulse over the posteromedial aspect of the ankle, and the dorsalis pedis pulse over the foot's dorsum.

EXAMINATION OF THE LEG

Examination of the leg includes many of the same components incorporated in a careful knee examination, including inspection, palpation, strength, and neurovascular assessment. Many of these will not be reviewed, but some of the more salient and relevant clinical highlights will be emphasized. Inspect for ecchymoses, swelling, deformity, and abrasions or lacerations. Open fractures may occur with only a slight puncture of the skin, but even this "minimal" compromise may have clinical importance. Palpate for tenderness and swelling. In the patient with "shin splints," tenderness is often palpable along the mid to distal thirds of the anteromedial tibias bilaterally. In the patient with a tibial stress fracture, tenderness is usually more localized and may be accompanied by palpable callus in the vicinity of the fracture site.

Palpate the leg for tenderness and swelling. In the patient with acute injury to the medial gastrocnemius head (tennis leg), there may be tenderness over the posteromedial calf. Patients with a deep venous thrombosis may also have localized tenderness, accompanied at times by a painful "cord" representing a thrombosed vessel. Palpation of the leg for swelling and tissue tenseness is important in patients with suspected compartment syndrome. Tissue tenseness, in which the compartment pressure may be elevated sufficiently to render the compartment ischemic, is an important early objective finding in patients with compartment syndrome. Pain on passive toe extension or flexion may further corroborate clinical suspicion of this entity. Palpation of distal pulses is an important component of the workup of compartment syndrome and for any patient with trauma, but it must be remembered that the presence of a pulse does not ensure vascular patency.

EXAMINATION FOR SOURCES OF REFERRED PAIN

Because pain in the knee or leg may represent referral from a more proximal source, one should always consider

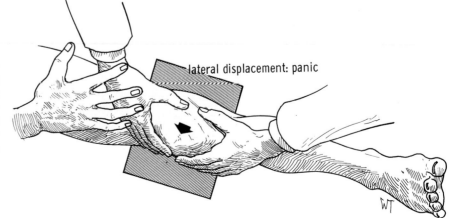

Figure 23–39. Attempts to translate the patella laterally will yield apprehension in some patients with patellar instability who are intolerant of the impending subluxation feeling. (From Insall JN, et al: Surgery of the Knee, 2nd ed. New York, Churchill Livingstone, 1993.)

lateral displacement: panic

additional physical examination techniques depending upon clinical suspicion. Specifically, examination of the hips or back may yield findings in the older patient with hip osteoarthritis or stenosis of the lumbar spine. In children, knee symptoms should be considered owing to hip pathology until proven otherwise, and warrants hip examination.

X-RAY EXAMINATION

Radiographs are a helpful adjunct to knee and leg evaluation, particularly in the traumatized patient. In the absence of trauma, patients do not always require radiographic evaluation, particularly when the diagnosis is clinically apparent. Patients with persistent symptoms unresponsive to initial treatment, those with a history of acute or traumatic onset, and those with physical examination findings suggestive of mechanical or structural pathology (malalignment, crepitus, restricted motion, loss of integrity) deserve x-ray evaluation.

The x-rays obtained depend upon the patient's presentation. The basic workup should include an AP, lateral, and patellofemoral view. The AP view should be taken during weight bearing (unless the patient is unable to do so) to facilitate detection of malalignment or joint space narrowing, sometimes undetectable on non–weight-bearing views (Fig. 23–40). Both knees should be imaged for comparison purposes. Inspect for soft tissue abnormalities, bone density, and joint height. The patellofemoral view (also known as the "sunrise," Merchant, or Laurin view, depending upon the imaging technique) demonstrates the relationship between the patella and the femur's trochlear groove, and can demonstrate joint space narrowing and osteophytes, as well as osteochondral fragments following patellar instability events (Fig. 23–41).

A number of other views have been described to evaluate the knee, including the tunnel view, the PA flexion weight-bearing view, oblique joint views, and views to evaluate the tibial plateau. The "tunnel" view is obtained by directing the x-ray beam into the intercondylar notch or tunnel with the knee flexed about 30 degrees (Fig. 23–42). The knee flexion angle allows visualization of the intercondylar notch contents and also the posterior aspect of the femoral condyles. Lesions located more posteriorly on the femoral condyles, such as osteochondritis dissecans or osteonecrosis, may be seen only on this view. Likewise, osteochondral fragments within the knee may be better appreciated on this view than the routine AP. Joint space narrowing may also be more readily detected with the knee flexed. A specific view has been described in which a weight-bearing PA view is obtained with the knee flexed approximately 30 degrees, demonstrating joint line narrowing earlier than when relying on the conventional AP weight-bearing images (Fig. 23–43).

Radiographic evaluation of the leg involves AP and lateral views and should include the knee and the ankle

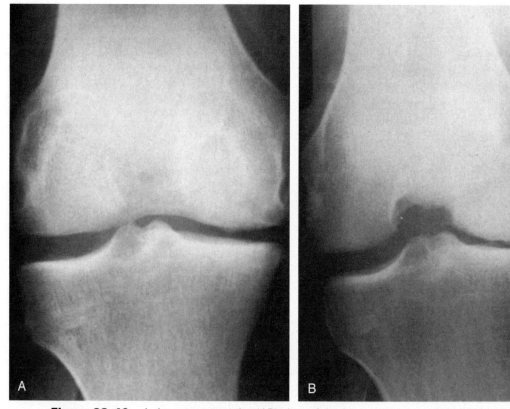

Figure 23–40. *A,* An anteroposterior (AP) view of the knee, which reveals mild degenerative changes and minimal apparent narrowing. Note the importance of obtaining weight-bearing AP films, which in this case *(B)* reveal the marked narrowing and more advanced "bone on bone" changes underestimated by the conventional AP view. (From DeLee JC, Drez D Jr: Orthopaedic Sports Medicine: Principles and Practice, Vol 2. Philadelphia, WB Saunders, 1994.)

joint. Oblique views are sometimes helpful in better demonstrating subtle callus formation or evaluation of bony lesions.

MAGNETIC RESONANCE IMAGING (MRI)

MRI is unnecessary in the evaluation of most knee problems. However, when indicated, it remains the definitive investigative tool for diagnosing a number of disorders with a high degree of sensitivity and accuracy unparalleled by any other noninvasive technique. With the exception of arthroscopy, MRI is the gold standard for diagnostic imaging of the knee. It is particularly helpful in demonstrating meniscus pathology, with an approximately 95% accuracy for detecting meniscus tears (Fig. 23–44). It is similarly good in identifying developmental meniscal abnormalities such as discoid menisci, and nearly 100% sensitive in identifying ligamentous pathology. It is equally good in detecting injuries to the ACL, PCL, MCL, and LCL and has been found effective in more complex instability patterns, including injury to the posterolateral corner of the knee.

MRI reveals the presence of fluid, which on T2-weighted images demonstrates a high-intensity (bright) signal. Effusions, hematoma, soft tissue and bone edema, Baker's cysts, meniscal cysts, synovial pathology, osteochondral lesions, and musculoskeletal neoplasms can all be

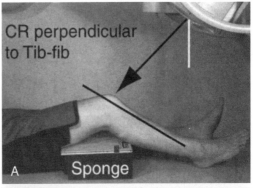

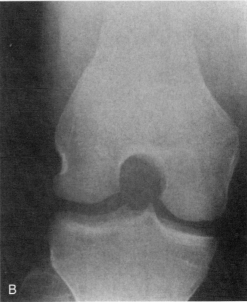

Figure 23–42. *A*, Technique for generating the *(B)* "notch" view of the knee. (From Pavlov H, Burke M, Giesa M, Seager KR: Knee. Orthopaedist's Guide to Plain Film Imaging. New York, Thieme, 1999.)

seen with great resolution using MRI (Fig. 23–45). MRI can also detect non-displaced and stress fractures not visible on plain x-rays. Newer scan sequences can demonstrate even chondral pathology.

Limitations of MRI include its cost and its demonstration of abnormalities that may in fact be incidental and not the source of the patient's symptoms. Age-related degenerative changes, particularly within the menisci, make clinical correlation with any MRI findings imperative.

BONE SCAN

Some conditions are not visible using conventional plain films. Bone scan is a physiologic test in which a dye labeled with radioisotope (technetium pyrophosphate) is injected intravenously to enhance the detection of bone pathology. Following injection, the skeletal area of interest is scanned to detect focal areas of increased dye. Increased uptake reflects increased blood flow to the affected area. This flow is nonspecific and does not necessarily identify the exact pathologic process responsible. For example, increased tracer uptake or a "hot spot" in a patient with leg pain may represent osteomyelitis, bone tumor, or a stress

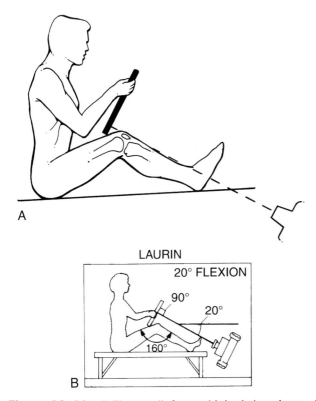

Figure 23–41. *A*, The patellofemoral joint is best imaged through a tangential film, obtained here by the method of Laurin. (From DeLee JC, Drez D Jr: Orthopaedic Sports Medicine: Principles and Practice, Vol 2. Philadelphia, WB Saunders, 1994.) Note the relationship of the patella to the trochlear groove in *B*. (From Scuderi G: Physical examination of the patellofemoral joint. *In* The Patella. New York, Springer-Verlag, 1995.)

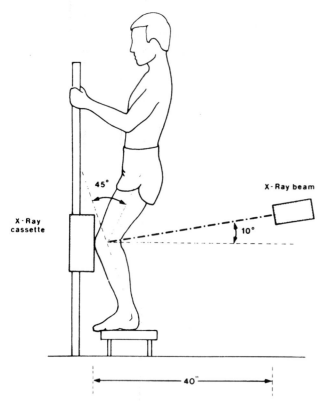

Figure 23–43. Thirty-degree flexion posteroanterior weight-bearing view permits better appreciation of joint space narrowing than seen with standard anteroposterior weight-bearing views. (From DeLee JC, Drez D Jr: Orthopaedic Sports Medicine: Principles and Practice, Vol 2. Philadelphia, WB Saunders, 1994.)

fracture. More accurate interpretation of scan results is assisted by knowing the "phase" in which uptake occurs (early soft tissue phase, intermediate bone flow phase, or late pooling phase). Because of the nonspecificity of this test, results must be interpreted in the context of the patient's presentation and other findings. One of the most

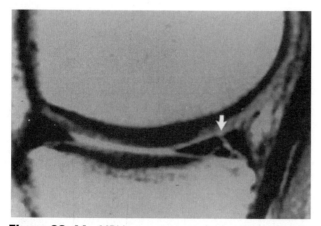

Figure 23–44. MRI is very accurate in demonstrating meniscus tears. Note the abnormal linear signal *(white arrow)* in the posterior horn of the medial meniscus, indicative of a tear. (From Browner BD, Jupiter JB, Levine AM, Trafton PG: Skeletal Trauma, Vol 1. Philadelphia, WB Saunders, 1998.)

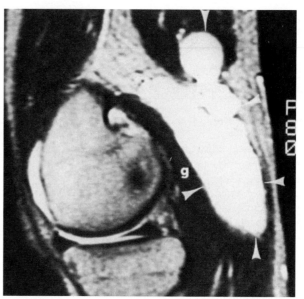

Figure 23–45. Recurrent knee swelling accompanied by a prominence within the popliteal fossa led this patient to have an MRI, which on sagittal T2-weighted images demonstrates the clear-cut appearance of a Baker cyst. Note the similar high signal intensity *(white appearance)* of the joint effusion and the popliteal cyst. (From DeLee JC, Drez D Jr: Orthopaedic Sports Medicine: Principles and Practice, Vol 2. Philadelphia, WB Saunders, 1994.)

common indications for use of a bone scan is in the runner with persistent leg pain, in whom "shin splints" have not yielded to treatment. Increased focal uptake on the bone scan confirms the suspected "stress fracture" common to this athletic population (Fig. 23–46). Conversely, the patient with shin splints (medial tibial stress syndrome) will demonstrate more diffuse uptake along the midshaft tibia (Fig. 23–47).

ARTHROGRAM

Arthrography involves the injection of radiopaque contrast dye into the knee joint. Historically an important imaging tool in facilitating meniscal, osteochondral, and ligament injury diagnosis, it has been replaced by the noninvasive and much more accurate MRI. Rarely, contrast material may be injected intra-articularly prior to MRI sequencing to enhance diagnostic yield (known as MR arthrography).

ARTHROSCOPY

The gold standard for intra-articular imaging is the arthroscope. Introduced for clinical applications in the late 1970s, this extraordinarily useful tool allows for both diagnostic evaluation and definitive treatment. Minimally invasive, the small camera is manipulated throughout the knee to view the entire intra-articular domain, including the medial and lateral compartments, the patellofemoral joint, and the intercondylar notch. In addition to decreased morbidity compared with open joint surgery (complications like pain, stiffness, infection, nerve injury), arthroscopy provides visualization that is superior to that of conventional open techniques because of the magnification afforded by the fiberoptic and lens technology. In addition, arthroscopic images in situ reflect the true intra-articular anatomy unlike the disturbed anatomic relationships seen when the knee is opened. Diagnostic arthroscopy, however, is an expensive and invasive resource and should be utilized only when other evaluative methods have not successfully afforded the diagnosis.

ELECTRODIAGNOSTIC TESTS

Electrodiagnostic testing is useful in evaluating nerve function. Electromyography (EMG) involves the insertion of electrodes within specific muscles and recording the electrical signal generated at rest and with activity. Abnormal patterns of activity can reflect various pathologic states, such as denervation (loss of normal nerve input, such as may occur when a nerve is injured), or disease (neuropathy such as may occur with diabetes or neurologic disorder). The second electrodiagnostic test commonly used assesses nerve conduction velocity (NCV). Analysis of the exact pattern of electrical activity and nerve speed facilitates diagnosis of the etiology and site of nerve involvement.

COMPARTMENT PRESSURE MEASUREMENTS

Compartment syndrome, in which intra-compartmental pressure exceeds the gradient necessary for normal arterial flow, can lead to limb ischemia and necrosis and is one of the most devastating complications of lower extremity trauma. Exertional compartment syndrome can also occur

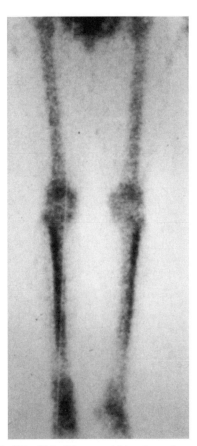

Figure 23–47. This 18-year-old hockey player complaining of chronic "shin splints" demonstrated diffuse uptake of technetium dye on bone scan, consistent with a "stress reaction." (From Stanitski CL, DeLee JC, Drez D Jr: Pediatric and Adolescent Sports Medicine, Vol 3. Philadelphia, WB Saunders, 1994.)

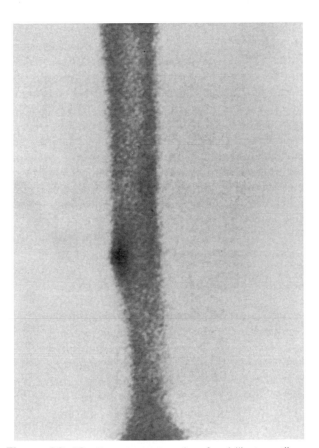

Figure 23–46. Bone scan reveals a focal "hot spot" consistent with a stress fracture in this tibia. Note the surrounding increased diffuse uptake as well, more consistent with stress "reaction."

as a consequence of exercise. Both conditions require compartment pressure testing for diagnostic confirmation. This test involves insertion of a catheter or needle into the suspected compartment(s) for direct pressure measurement (Fig. 23–48). This is most commonly performed in the compartments of the leg, including the anterior, lateral, superficial posterior, and deep posterior. Variable criteria exist for both acute posttraumatic compartment syndrome and exertional compartment syndrome. In traumatic compartment syndrome, pressures should probably be below 30 mmHg. In exertional compartment syndrome, pressures at rest should be no higher than 15 mmHg and should return below this level upon cessation of exercise. Commonly, pressures are interpreted in the context of the patients' diastolic blood pressure or their opposite extremity.

TREATMENT OF KNEE AND LEG PROBLEMS

Knee and leg problems can be treated algorithmically. Consider whether the problem is traumatic or atraumatic. Initial treatment of trauma to the knee or leg relies on the mnemonic "RICE," which refers to rest, ice, compression, and elevation. Minimizing hemorrhage and edema is critical. Patients should be placed in a knee immobilizer or

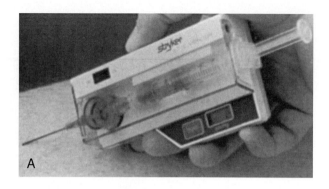

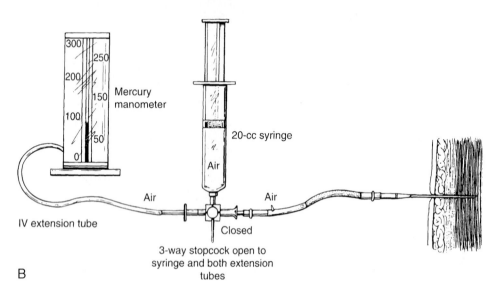

Figure 23–48. Compartment pressure measurements can be obtained by several techniques. In *A*, a Stryker measurement tool is used with disposable needles. In *B*, a needle manometer has been set up using equipment available within hospitals and operating room facilities. Both techniques permit accurate direct intra-compartmental pressure. (From Browner BD, Jupiter JB, Levine AM, Trafton PG: Skeletal Trauma, Vol 1. Philadelphia, WB Saunders, 1998.)

leg splint and made non–weight bearing until definitive diagnostic evaluation has been rendered. Neurovascular assessment is a high priority, particularly in tibia fractures. Open injuries must be treated promptly with inspection for and sterile coverage of any open wounds.

Definitive treatment usually depends upon the exact diagnosis. Some knee injuries will be treatable empirically based on a presumed diagnosis. The aggressiveness of diagnostic evaluation obviously depends upon many variables, including the severity of the injury, risk to the neurovascular structures and the limb, the patient's activity level, and goals.

Common nonoperative treatment for knee and leg problems includes activity modification (rest), tincture of time, anti-inflammatory medications, physical therapy modalities (ice, heat, ultrasound, electrical stimulation), and exercise (stretching, manipulation, strengthening). Operative options for knee disorders include surgical intervention via arthroscopic or open (arthrotomy) techniques. Leg fractures may be treated with casting and external or internal fixation, and compartment syndromes are managed with fascial release.

Initial treatment of atraumatic conditions of the knee and leg may also involve activity modification, use of anti-inflammatory medications, physical therapy modalities, and exercises. Definitive treatment depends upon many variables, including the diagnosis, degree to which symptoms interfere with activity, patient activity level, and goals. The

aggressiveness of diagnostic workup may vary based on patient considerations. For example, the weekend recreational athlete with occasional mild patellar tendonitis symptoms and nondiscrete physical examination findings may be treated empirically without requiring further diagnostic studies. Conversely, the scholarship basketball player with recurrent anterior knee pain, focal tenderness, and patellar tendon nodularity may well require an MRI for definitive evaluation of patellar tendon injury. Definitive treatment for atraumatic conditions can include nonoperative and operative strategies. Nonoperative alternatives are similar to those afforded traumatized patients, such as activity modification, use of casting or bracing, anti-inflammatory medications, physical therapy, and occasionally the judicious use of cortisone injections. Operative alternatives include arthroscopic and open techniques.

COMMON KNEE AND LEG PROBLEMS: EVALUATION AND TREATMENT

Treatment of lower extremity knee and leg problems requires understanding basic anatomy, knowledge of physical and diagnostic examination techniques, and familiarity with common conditions. The following section reviews the most common traumatic and atraumatic conditions of the knee and leg.

Traumatic Conditions of the Knee

DISTAL FEMUR FRACTURES

Fractures of the distal femur may occur in either the supracondylar or the intracondylar region and are often intra-articular. Their management is sometimes difficult, owing to fracture displacement and associated soft tissue injury.

Presentation. Most fractures occur as a consequence of direct trauma. In younger patients, this often occurs due to a motor vehicle accident or a fall from a height. Older patients with osteoporotic bone may suffer a fracture from a fall onto the flexed knee. Patients present with pain, swelling, and deformity in the supracondylar area of the distal femur.

Relevant Anatomy. The gastrocnemius muscles attach to the most distal portion of the condyles, accounting for the usual posterior displacement and angulation. The pull of the quadriceps and hamstrings causes fracture shortening.

Classification. Several classification schemes exist, of which perhaps the most used is the AO/ASIF classification, which divides the fractures according to whether they are intra- or extra-articular. Type A is extra-articular, B is unicondylar, and C is intra-articular (Fig. 23–49).

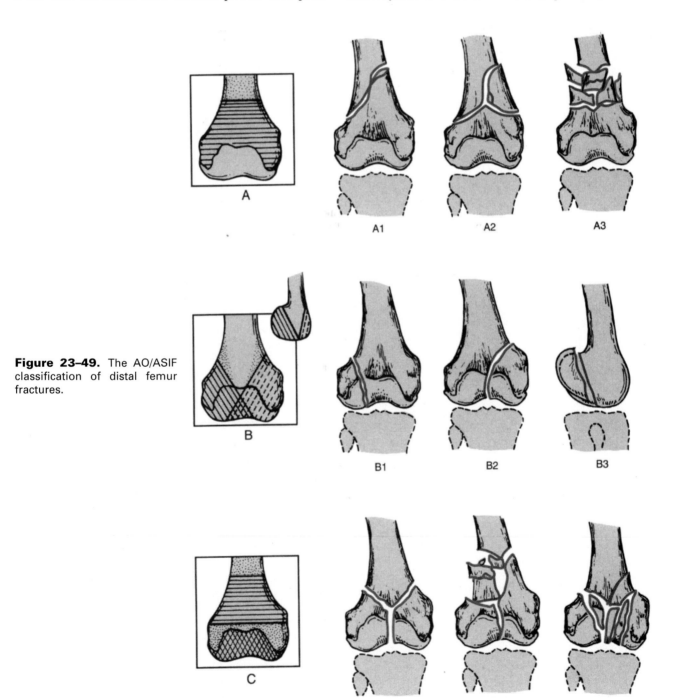

Figure 23–49. The AO/ASIF classification of distal femur fractures.

Physical Examination. Painful swelling and deformity are present over the distal femur, often accompanied by false motion at the fracture site. The proximity of neurovascular structures to the fracture site mandates prompt assessment. Fullness or swelling in the popliteal area, particularly when accompanied by weak distal pulse or other signs of ischemia (pallor, cool skin), suggests vascular injury.

X-Ray Evaluation. X-rays should include a minimum AP, lateral, and two oblique projections. Evaluation for intra-articular displacement is the key to treatment.

Special Tests. CT scans may help in surgical planning by identifying the location and relationship of the various fragments, particularly when intra-articular.

Definitive Treatment. Nonoperative treatment is possible in extra-articular and non-displaced intra-articular fractures, and generally consists of fracture reduction (when necessary) by traction, followed by early application of a cast-brace. Reduction usually requires placement of two pins—one through the supracondylar fragment and the other through the proximal tibia. Difficulty in controlling fracture fragments, particularly when intra-articular, makes nonoperative management difficult. Common complications include prolonged bed rest with its attendant problems and knee stiffness. Surgical intervention involves open reduction and internal fixation, usually indicated when the fracture is intra-articular, poorly reduced or maintained by closed means, open, associated with multiple trauma, or due to pathologic conditions (tumor).

PATELLA FRACTURES

Fractures of the patella are relatively common, accounting for approximately 1% of all skeletal injuries. They are more common in men and occur in all age groups.

Presentation. Acute anterior knee pain follows a fall or direct trauma.

Mechanism of Injury. Injury is due to direct or indirect force. Direct force from a fall or direct trauma to the front of the knee (dashboard injury) often leads to a stellate or comminuted fracture pattern. Indirect injury due to quads contraction (while attempting to suddenly decelerate) usually causes a transverse fracture pattern, sometimes extending laterally into the retinaculum.

Relevant Anatomy. The patella is the largest sesamoid bone in the body, encased within the extensor mechanism of the quadriceps. The patella increases the mechanical advantage of the quadriceps mechanism as well as protects the femoral condyles from direct trauma. Medial and lateral retinacular expansions may be compromised during fracture. Disruption may prevent active knee extension.

Classification. Classification is divided into nondisplaced or displaced patterns. Nondisplaced can be described as stellate, transverse, vertical, or osteochondral. Displaced can be transverse, polar (apical or basal), stellate, or osteochondral (Fig. 23–50).

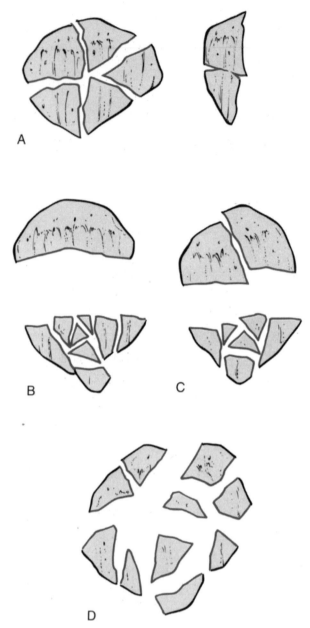

Figure 23–50. Patella fractures can be classified based on the degree of displacement or fracture pattern. *A*, Fragments are displaced no more than 3 mm from one another and thus are considered nondisplaced. *B*, Displaced transverse patellar fracture, with comminution of the distal pole. *C*, Longitudinal fracture in the proximal fragment. *D*, Significant comminution of the entire patella. (From Browner BD, Jupiter JB, Levine AM, Trafton PG: Skeletal Trauma, Vol 1. Philadelphia, WB Saunders, 1998.)

Physical Examination. Painful swelling, ecchymoses, and tenderness to palpation are all present. Evaluate for ability to actively extend the knee or perform a straight leg raise, which suggests integrity of the retinaculum.

X-Ray Evaluation. AP, lateral, and sunrise (tangential) views of the patella should be obtained. The tangential view provides the best opportunity to gauge the presence of an osteochondral fracture.

Differential Diagnosis. A bipartite patella, in which an ossification center persists, is occasionally mistaken for a fracture (see Fig. 23–34). It is almost always superolateral and has smooth margins. Up to 50% are bilateral.

Special Tests. Special tests are not usually necessary.

Definitive Treatment. Nonoperative treatment in either a cylinder cast or occasionally a knee immobilizer is sufficient for non- or minimally displaced fractures in which the retinaculum is intact (the patient is able to do a straight leg raise). Operative treatment is reserved for displaced fractures or open injuries. Surgery involves either internal fixation using wires and retinacular suture repair, partial patellectomy, or, in severely comminuted cases, total patellectomy.

TIBIAL PLATEAU FRACTURES
Tibial plateau fractures constitute approximately 1% of all fractures.

Presentation/Mechanism of Injury. Knee pain following major trauma due to motor vehicle, industrial, or athletic accident accounts for most presentations. The most common scenario is that of a pedestrian with pain and/or deformity following a "bumper" injury. The degree of displacement and extent of comminution are influenced by many factors, including the force of the trauma, the quality of the bone, and the age of the patient.

Relevant Anatomy. The tibial plateau is composed of medial and lateral condyles. The medial is larger and concave from anterior to posterior and medial to lateral. The lateral plateau is smaller in size and convex in shape. The two plateaus are separated by an intercondylar eminence that serves as attachment for the anterior cruciate ligament. Because the medial articular surface and its associated condyle is stronger than the lateral plateau, and because of the normal valgus angle of the knee, fractures involving the lateral compartment are more common. Adjacent soft tissue and neurovascular structures are at risk in these injuries, particularly those that involve extensive comminution and larger amounts of the plateaus. The popliteal vessel trifurcates just below the knee and is at risk of proximal tibial fractures. Laterally, the peroneal nerve is at risk as it winds around the neck of the fibula.

Classification. There are several classification schemes, the most useful of which is that by Schatzker, in which the plateau fracture types are divided according to their pattern and location. In Type I, there is a split fracture of the lateral tibial plateau. Type II involves a split with associated depression of the lateral plateau. In a Type III, the lateral plateau is depressed. Type IV fractures involve the medial plateau. In Type V injury, the fracture is bicondylar, involving both medial and lateral plateaus. Finally, in the Type VI fracture, the fracture extends into the proximal tibial metaphysis.

Physical Examination. Swelling and ecchymoses are frequently present. Neurovascular assessment is critical, particularly in cases of high-energy trauma. Remember to evaluate the leg for compartment syndrome. Evaluation for stability is an important component of determining treatment. This involves the application of gentle stresses to the knee to determine the degree of stability. With the knee in extension, a varus or valgus force is applied depending upon the compartment involved, and the tendency to open up is determined. Similarly an anterior and/or posterior force may be gently applied to determine the presence of associated ligamentous injury. Pain often precludes a satisfactory evaluation, which requires intra-articular local anesthetic injection or general anesthesia.

X-Ray Evaluation. AP, lateral, and oblique projections are helpful in evaluation of proximal tibial fractures.

Special Tests. Stress tests are sometimes helpful to establish the stability of the injury and assess associated ligamentous damage. This sometimes requires anesthesia and can be performed under fluoroscopy. CT scans are helpful in determining the degree of intra-articular displacement. Because management often hinges on the amount of fracture displacement, CT scans are commonly indicated in the workup of tibial plateau fractures.

Differential Diagnosis. Because knee dislocations may be accompanied by a tibial plateau fracture, one must consider this possibility when evaluating any patient with distal femoral or proximal tibial trauma. The relatively high percentage of vascular injuries mandates their consideration in any patient with knee trauma. There are a number of commonly associated injuries accompanying fractures of the tibial plateau. These include meniscal tears in up to 50% and ligament disruptions in up to 30%. Young patients with strong bone are at highest risk of associated ligament disruptions.

Definitive Treatment. Nonoperative treatment may be sufficient for non- or minimally displaced fractures and those that are "stable." Treatment most commonly involves non–weight bearing in a fracture brace for up to 3 months (until metaphyseal bone has healed). Operative intervention is reserved for displaced (usually greater than 5 mm articular incongruity), unstable, or open fractures. Surgical treatment most commonly involves open reduction and internal fixation using plates and screws, but associated open or soft tissue injuries may alternatively lead to use of an external fixator (Fig. 23–51). Vascular injuries usually require repair. Nerve injuries are usually neuropraxias. When treating an open injury or performing an open reduction and internal fixation, nerve exploration may be warranted. A high index of suspicion for the development of compartment syndrome must be maintained. Complications of tibial plateau fractures include stiffness, malunion, nonunion, infection, wound problems, compartment syndrome, nerve injury, and posttraumatic arthritis.

KNEE DISLOCATION
Dislocation of the knee is an uncommon but serious orthopaedic injury involving complete separation of the tibiofemoral joint. It is limb-threatening and should be considered an orthopaedic emergency.

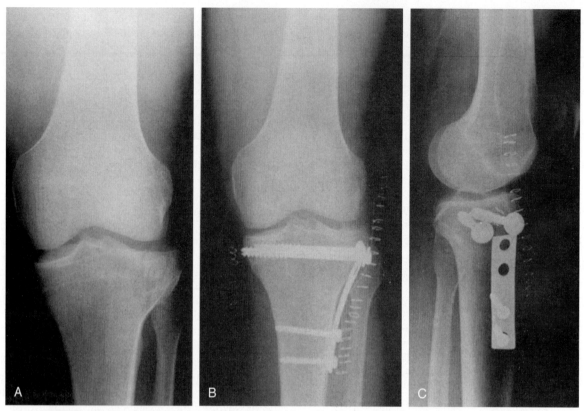

Figure 23–51. *A,* This type II tibial plateau fracture shows both a split and a compression component. *B and C,* Treatment involved open reduction and internal fixation (ORIF) using plate, screws, and bone grafting. (From Browner BD, Jupiter JB, Levine AM, Trafton PG: Skeletal Trauma, Vol 1. Philadelphia, WB Saunders, 1998.)

Presentation. The severity of trauma involved often means this may be but one of the orthopaedic problems with which the patient is presenting. Patients may have an isolated injury to their leg following a traumatic injury from a fall, an athletic event, or collision. The patient or the EMT may describe an awkward position of the limb at the scene of the accident, which with intended manipulation or unintentional movement reduced into more normal alignment. The patient notes a great deal of pain and swelling and is unable to bear weight. Sometimes the patient presents weeks or even months after an injury, and only in retrospect is it apparent that the patient had suffered an unrecognized knee dislocation.

Mechanism of Injury. Substantial trauma is necessary to disrupt the knee joint. High-energy injury usually occurs as a result of motor vehicle accidents, with lower energy injury occurring during athletic events or falls.

Relevant Anatomy. The tibiofemoral joint stability is afforded predominantly by soft tissue, particularly the cruciate and collateral ligaments. Both cruciates and at least one collateral are usually torn for a knee to dislocate. The vascular structures within the immediate vicinity, including the popliteal artery and vein and tibial nerve, are at substantial risk owing to their tethering proximally at the adductor hiatus and distally at the trifurcation (Fig. 23–52). The neurologic structures including the tibial nerve and pero-

neal nerve are at risk posteriorly in the popliteal fossa and laterally at the fibular neck, respectively.

Classification. Dislocations are classified according to the displacement of the tibia relative to the femur. The most common dislocation is anterior due to knee hyperextension, accounting for 30 to 50% of all dislocations. Posterior is the next most common and occurs from a posteriorly directed force against the anterior proximal tibia, a so-called dashboard injury. Medial, lateral, and rotational dislocations are less common and usually due to varus, valgus, and combination mechanism injuries, respectively.

Physical Examination. The examination findings vary with the type of dislocation and the timing of evaluation. At the scene of the injury, the knee will have an abnormal appearance, with obvious deformity accompanied by swelling. Following reduction (spontaneously or preceding the evaluation), the knee may be relatively normal to inspection, but has swelling and marked tenderness and the patient is usually very apprehensive to any but the most gentle manipulation. Examination of the unconscious patient usually reveals gross abnormal motion on laxity testing. Because of the frequency of associated neurovascular injuries, examination of the neurovascular structures is a priority with this injury. Vascular injury with either intimal damage or rupture of the popliteal artery occurs in 20 to 60% of knee dislocations, owing to a bow stringing of the

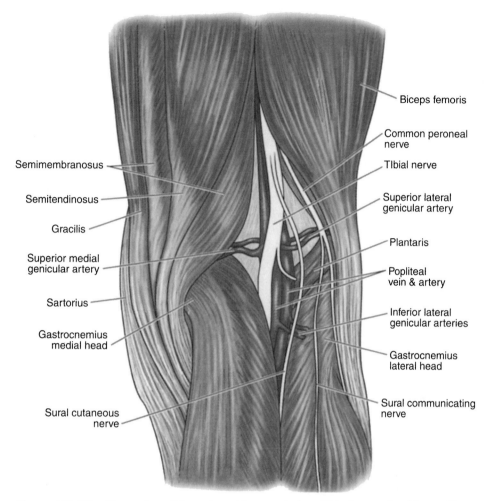

Semimembranosus

Semitendinosus

Gracilis

Superior medial
genicular artery

Sartorius

Gastrocnemius
medial head

Sural cutaneous
nerve

Biceps femoris

Common peroneal
nerve

Tibial nerve

Superior lateral
genicular artery

Plantaris

Popliteal
vein & artery

Inferior lateral
genicular arteries

Gastrocnemius
lateral head

Sural communicating
nerve

Figure 23-52. Illustration of the vulnerable vascularity within the popliteal fossa. (From Insall JN, Scott WB [eds]: Surgery of the Knee, 3rd ed. Philadelphia, Churchill Livingstone, 2001, p 62.)

vessel across the popliteal fossa. Remember to check the distal pulses. Collateral circulation is usually inadequate to provide sufficient circulation to the leg. Capillary refill and pulses may both be intact despite significant vascular compromise. Neurologic injury, most commonly to the peroneal nerve, can occur in up to 35% of cases and requires careful neurologic evaluation to detect.

X Ray Evaluation. AP, lateral, and oblique radiographs of the knee joint are the minimum necessary for proper evaluation. Equally important are post-reduction x-rays to evaluate for congruency of reduction, presence of intra-articular or avulsion fragments, and associated fractures. Joint space widening may indicate inadequate or incomplete reduction.

Differential Diagnosis. Fractures of the distal femur, proximal tibia, or patella can all present with an acutely painful swollen knee. Radiographs usually help make the diagnosis. However, remember to consider dislocation in the differential diagnosis of other, less severe appearing knee injuries, in which reduction of the dislocation prior to the examination leads to underrecognition of a more serious injury.

Special Tests. The high incidence of vascular injury usually mandates arteriography in every knee dislocation (Fig. 23–53). In the circumstance of a clearly compromised limb in which operative intervention is intended, this sometimes time-consuming step may be unnecessary. MRI helps assess the extent of injury for treatment purposes, particularly when elective reconstruction is being considered following nonoperative management.

Definitive Treatment. Prompt reduction following neurovascular assessment, followed by a careful repeat neurovas-

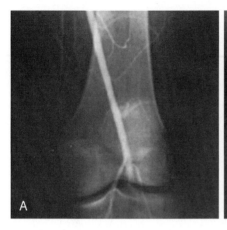 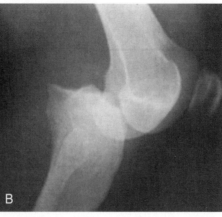

Figure 23–53. Note the occlusion of the popliteal artery demonstrated by arteriography *(A)* following reduction of a posterior knee dislocation *(B)*. (From Browner BD, Jupiter JB, Levine AM, Trafton PG: Skeletal Trauma, Vol 1. Philadelphia, WB Saunders, 1998.)

cular check and post-reduction films is mandatory. Ischemic threat to the limb obligates expeditious reduction. Splinting of the extremity should follow reduction, along with elevation and ice to further decrease swelling. Reduction maneuvers vary according to the type of dislocation but usually require longitudinal traction and some gentle manipulation. Closed reduction is usually achievable, although some dislocations are irreducible as a result of buttonholing of the bone through soft tissue. Indications for open treatment include an open injury, inability to achieve closed reduction, associated residual soft tissue interposition, and vascular injury.

In the absence of these specific indications for surgery, definitive treatment is controversial, with some recommending closed management with initial splinting and elevation followed by definitive casting and brace application. Complications of this approach include stiffness and, in some cases, residual instability. Open treatment involves direct repair of the soft tissues and/or associated ligament avulsions. Proponents of surgical intervention claim more predictable stability and opportunity to rehabilitate the knee more aggressively, and decreased risk of stiffness. Complications of open repair include stiffness, infection, and risks of anesthesia.

QUADRICEPS TENDON RUPTURE

Rupture of the quadriceps tendon is relatively common in the middle-aged individual, usually with complete tearing of the attachment near the superior pole of the patella.

Presentation. The patient experiences acute pain in the knee following a stumble or trip, in which the forceful contraction of the quadriceps mechanism exceeds its inherent strength.

Mechanism of Injury. The reflex contraction of the quads to decelerate the body overpowers the inherent strength of the tissue, usually leading to a complete rupture of the quadriceps tendon within 1 cm of the superior pole of the patella. Histologic studies have demonstrated degenerative pathology within the substance of the quads tendon, predisposing to injury in this vicinity.

Relevant Anatomy. The quadriceps mechanism consists of the rectus femoris and the vastus intermedius, lateralis, and

medialis. The four muscles become tendinous in their distal portion and coalesce to attach and envelop the patella. Extensions of the distal tendinous portions of the muscles account for the medial and lateral retinaculum.

Classification. Although tendon injuries, known as "strains," can be classified according to the severity of injury as grade I, II, and III, most tendon injuries of the quads are grade III tears, with complete disruption of the extensor mechanism and loss of normal continuity.

Physical Examination. The patient has a swollen and painful knee, often with ecchymoses. He or she is unable to walk normally, and there is a palpable defect above the patella in the quadriceps tendon. The patient is unable to extend the knee or do a straight leg raise. In rare cases of partial rupture, a straight leg raise may be possible.

X-Ray Evaluation. AP and lateral x-rays usually demonstrate soft tissue swelling and patella baja as a result of inferior patella displacement (Fig. 23–54).

Differential Diagnosis. Rupture of the patellar tendon can also lead to knee pain, but the defect and tenderness lie over the inferior pole, patellar tendon, or tibial tubercle. On x-ray, patella tendon ruptures demonstrate patella alta, with a high-riding patella (Fig. 23–55).

Special Tests. MRI confirms the tear but is unnecessary in most cases.

Definitive Treatment. Quadriceps (and patellar tendon) ruptures are treated surgically with direct reapproximation of tendon to the superior border of the patella, followed by immobilization and rehabilitation. Complications include knee stiffness and weakness.

PATELLA DISLOCATION

Dislocation of the patella is a relatively common occurrence and accounts for most patients claiming an episode of "knee dislocation." Dislocation is almost always lateral.

Presentation. Acute pain following an incident in which the knee "went out of place" is the most common description of a patella dislocation. Occasionally the patient will

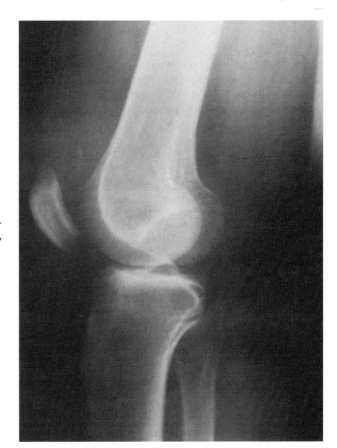

Figure 23–54. X-ray of patella baja following quads rupture. (From Fu FH, et al: Knee Surgery, Vol 1. Baltimore, Williams & Wilkins, 1994.)

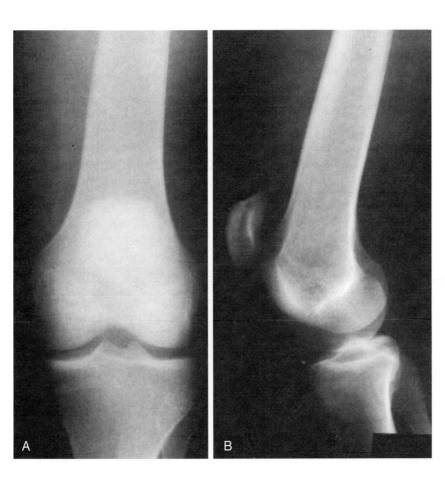

Figure 23–55. *A* and *B*, These AP and lateral radiographs demonstrate the typical appearance of patellar tendon rupture with associated patella alta. Note that this finding is best appreciated on the lateral *(B)* view. (From DeLee JC, Drez D Jr: Orthopaedic Sports Medicine: Principles and Practice, Vol 2. Philadelphia, WB Saunders, 1994.)

not only observe the laterally displaced patella, but will also assist in its reduction.

Mechanism of Injury. Patella dislocations usually occur during a maneuver in which the knee is flexed and rotated. In such a position, the patella may be poorly engaged in its groove and vulnerable to lateral subluxation or dislocation. Contributing factors include a high "Q angle" (greater than 15 degrees), tight lateral retinaculum, and loose medial restraints. Generalized ligamentous laxity (thumb-to-the-forearm sign, knee, elbow, and metacarpophalangeal joint hyperextension) is a risk factor for patellar instability.

Relevant Anatomy. The patella lies superior to the trochlear groove into which it engages with knee flexion. Some patients are at risk of instability as a result of anatomic risk factors including poor VMO development, high Q angle, and retinacular soft tissue imbalance.

Classification. Patellar instability can occur in the form of dislocations, in which the patella completely displaces out of the groove, or subluxation, in which there remains some articular contact. Sometimes, differentiating the two is not possible by history.

Physical Examination. When the patella is dislocated, the contour of the knee is abnormal and displays a prominence laterally and a void anteriorly where the patella is usually located. Most patellar dislocations, however, are seen after either spontaneous or manipulated reduction, in which case findings are nonspecific and include swelling, tenderness, and ecchymoses. Tenderness is often present over the lateral aspect of the knee, specifically over the lateral femoral condyle, and medially over the facet and the site of retinacular injury.

X-Ray Evaluation. AP, lateral, and tangential (sunrise) views are necessary to evaluate the suspected or observed patellar dislocation. One should inspect for evidence of an osteochondral fragment, best seen on the lateral or sunrise view (Fig. 23–56).

Special Tests. Special tests are not usually necessary. Occasionally, the diagnosis is in doubt; in such cases, MRI is helpful.

Differential Diagnosis. Patellar dislocation can be differentiated from the knee (tibiofemoral) dislocation by the degree of associated soft tissue injury. Tenderness over the patellar facets and retinaculum, absence of tenderness elsewhere, and normal anterior-posterior and medial-lateral stability indicate a patella dislocation. The more difficult differential is in the young patient with a seemingly trivial injury in which "something felt like it went out of place." The list of diagnostic possibilities in this scenario includes reflex inhibition of pain in patellofemoral pain syndrome, patella subluxation, medial meniscus tear, medial collateral ligament sprain, and ACL injury. Each of these can be best differentiated using standard examination techniques, occasionally requiring more sophisticated imaging such as MRI.

Definitive Treatment. Prompt reduction, evaluation to rule out associated displaced osteochondral fractures, occasional aspiration of the hemarthrosis for comfort, and immobilization in either a knee immobilizer or cylinder cast for 3 to 4 weeks represent the treatment of choice. Operative treatment is reserved for the presence of displaced osteochondral fragments or recurrent instability despite an adequate program of activity modification and physical therapy strengthening.

MEDIAL COLLATERAL LIGAMENT SPRAIN

Sprain of the medial collateral ligament (MCL) is the most common knee ligament.

Presentation/Mechanism of Injury. The most common presentation is that of acute medial knee pain following trauma. This often involves an acute valgus stress such as in football, soccer, or skiing. Patients may have gotten "clipped" over the lateral aspect of the knee or leg, or their ski tip may have caught an edge in the snow.

Relevant Anatomy. The MCL is composed of two distinct structures—a deep and a superficial ligament. The deep portion is actually the medial capsule of the knee joint. The superficial MCL is a discrete structure arising from the medial epicondyle and traveling distally to span out and attach over the proximal tibia anteromedially.

Classification. MCL sprains are graded from I to III depending on the severity of injury. In a grade I sprain, there

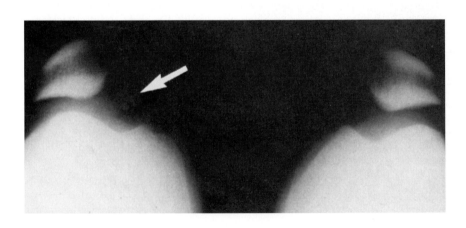

Figure 23–56. Note the presence of the rather large osteochondral fragment (arrow) following acute patellar dislocation in this patient. (From DeLee JC, Drez D Jr: Orthopaedic Sports Medicine: Principles and Practice, Vol 2. Philadelphia, WB Saunders, 1994.)

is a small amount of injury and no detectable laxity. Grade II (moderate) sprains involve stretching and disruption of part of the ligament, with accompanying greater degrees of pain, swelling, and joint laxity. In Grade III injuries, the ligament is completely disrupted, with concomitant pain, tenderness, laxity, and disability.

Physical Examination. Findings vary with the degree of injury (see Fig. 23–25). In a grade I mild sprain, there may be little in the way of ecchymoses or swelling, some localized tenderness and pain, but no opening on valgus stress with the knee in slight flexion. Grade II sprains are more severe and will usually be accompanied by a more substantial amount of tenderness, pain on stress testing, and a discernible opening on valgus stress that is different from the opposite side. The tenderness can often be localized to the femoral or tibial attachment. In a grade III sprain, the knee "opens up" to valgus stress and is often quite painful. There is usually little swelling because of extravasation of blood into the surrounding soft tissues. Opening of the knee in full extension indicates additional ligamentous injuries to the ACL or PCL.

X-Ray Evaluation. AP and lateral x-rays are usually negative.

Special Tests. MRI is rarely necessary but may be helpful in evaluating the painful patient in whom physical examination is difficult and/or additional ligament injury is suspected. Occasionally patients with MCL sprains present with "locked" knees in which extension is impossible. An MRI helps by ruling out the presence of a bucket handle meniscus tear blocking extension and will incidentally confirm the suspected diagnosis of MCL sprain, clearly visible on MR examination (Fig. 23–57). In the skeletally imma-

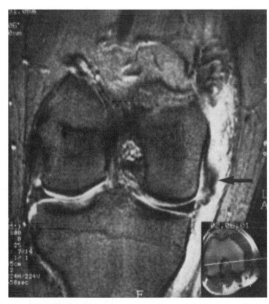

Figure 23–57. MRI demonstrates disruption of the medial collateral ligament, normally attached distally, and here "wrinkled" in appearance *(arrow).* (From DeLee JC, Drez D Jr: Orthopaedic Sports Medicine: Principles and Practice, Vol 2. Philadelphia, WB Saunders, 1994.)

ture patient, a stress radiograph may be useful to rule out fracture through the distal femoral physis (growth plate) rather than the medial collateral ligament (Fig. 23–58).

Differential Diagnosis. The most important differential is that of distal femoral physeal injury in the skeletally immature population. Other diagnoses that can present similarly to MCL sprains include meniscus tears, ACL injuries, patellar subluxations, pes tendonitis, and acute chondral or osteochondral injuries of the knee. Medial meniscus injuries can be distinguished from MCL tears by the lack of pain or opening on valgus stress in the knee with a meniscus tear. Also, MCL tears are often tender above and/or below the joint line along the course of the MCL, whereas meniscal tears are usually tender only over the joint.

Definitive Treatment. Treatment is nonoperative and involves a period of immobilization whose duration depends upon the degree of injury and the presence of associated injury. Grade I sprains are usually treatable with early range of motion exercises and early return to activity. Grade II injuries may require a period of immobilization followed by return to activity with a protective knee brace. Grade III injuries are sometimes casted or immobilized for 2 to 4 weeks, followed by rehabilitation to return normal motion and strength, with full return to activity taking from 6 to 8 weeks or longer. When associated with other injuries, the MCL is still usually treated nonoperatively. In cases of knee dislocation, primary repair of the MCL is sometimes performed.

ANTERIOR CRUCIATE LIGAMENT SPRAIN (ACL TEAR)
Arguably the most common career-threatening injury to the athlete's knee, anterior cruciate ligament (ACL) injury occurs in an estimated 250,000 people annually.

Presentation. The classic presentation is the acute onset of pain and swelling accompanied by a "pop" when coming down from a rebound, landing awkwardly, or twisting the knee. Most injuries involve contact or collision sports but do not involve actual contact during the injury. The athlete is rarely able to continue activity. Occasionally the person has a much less traumatic history, with a simple twist or turn precipitating knee symptoms. Usually through a careful history, the patient may admit to a previous injury that was undiagnosed or unrecognized as an ACL tear.

Mechanism of Injury. Virtually all ACL sprains are a consequence of a singular traumatic event and are not due to overuse. The exact mechanism varies according to the sport involved, but most injuries occur when the athlete plants his or her foot and cuts or pivots. Alternatively, the person may come down from a rebound and hyperextend the knee. In skiing, the ski tip may get caught in the snow when turning and the binding fail to release. At the moment of injury, a force, which exceeds the strength of the normal ACL, results in some fiber failure, stretching, and if sufficiently strong, complete ligament tearing.

Relevant Anatomy. The ACL is one of two cruciate ligaments (the other being the posterior cruciate ligament [PCL]) of the knee, named for their "crucial" role in

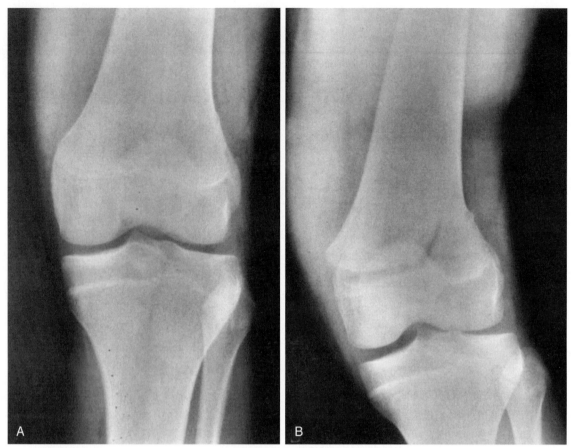

Figure 23–58. *A,* Anteroposterior radiograph of a 14-year-old boy after sustaining a valgus injury to his knee in a football game. Physical examination suggested MCL injury with opening on valgus stress, but tenderness was over the distal femur. Initial x-rays show only subtle findings suggestive of fracture. Stress views, however, clearly demonstrate the Salter-Harris Type II distal femoral physeal injury in *B.* (From Stanitski CL, DeLee JC, Drez D Jr: Pediatric and Adolescent Sports Medicine, Vol 3. Philadelphia, WB Saunders, 1994.)

maintaining normal femorotibial alignment. Arising from the anteromedial tibia, the ACL is a thick bundle of collagenous tissue that traverses through the intercondylar notch of the knee to insert posterolaterally on the lateral femoral condyle (see Fig. 23–7). The ACL is normally covered by a thin synovial membrane. Nutrition and vascularity are provided by vessels entering the ACL at its origin and insertion, and through the fat pad directly anteriorly. The function of the ACL is to maintain normal alignment between the femoral condyles and the tibial plateau, particularly during rotatory (twisting, pivoting, cutting) activity. In the absence of the normal ACL, abnormal stresses are imparted to the articular cartilage and the menisci during twisting or cutting activities, during which the knee may sublux (partially dislocate). Recurrent such episodes are thought to lead to cumulative meniscal and chondral damage and eventually degenerative arthritis.

Classification. Like any ligament injuries, the ACL may be partially (grade I), significantly (grade II), or completely (grade III) torn. Although it is not always possible to distinguish a grade I from a II, it is recognition of the patient with a grade III complete ACL tear that is most important for prognostic and therapeutic reasons.

Physical Examination. If seen within the first week or so of injury, the athlete may still be on crutches and will have obvious swelling of the knee. The amount of effusion may preclude patients from completely straightening their knee on the examining table. On the other hand, if they are being seen after a recent "reinjury," the knee may look remarkably benign, with normal gait and little swelling. The hallmark of all tests for ACL integrity relies on assessing the amount of translation between the tibia and the femur, and the quality of the end point of that translation, best detected by the Lachman examination. With the patient supine and the knee gently flexed between 15 and 30 degrees, and the thigh firmly held by one hand of the examiner, the other hand grasps the proximal tibia just distal to the knee and attempts to gently translate it anteriorly (see Fig. 23–26). Comparison to the opposite side helps distinguish normal from abnormal. Timing of the examination influences the findings. When examined acutely at the time of injury, for example, swelling is minimal and a positive examination is relatively easy to detect when present. After several hours, the degree of swelling (from bleeding within the knee joint known as a *hemarthrosis*) and guarding (due to pain) makes this examination more difficult. Because meniscal and associate

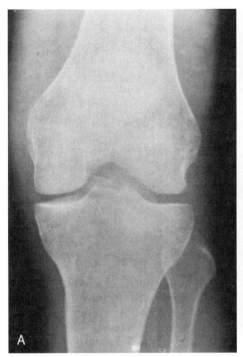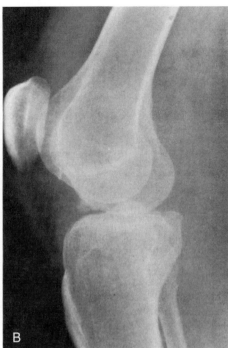

Figure 23–59. Intercondylar eminence fracture representing an avulsion fracture of the ACL origin, seen on the anteroposterior *(A)* and lateral *(B)* views. (From Rockwood C Jr, Green DP, Bucholz R, Heckman JD: Fractures in Adults, 4th ed. Philadelphia, Lippincott-Raven, 1996.)

ligament (most commonly the medial collateral ligament) injuries are common with ACL injury, examine for joint line tenderness and evidence of abnormal laxity to valgus and varus stress.

X-Ray. X-rays are usually normal. When chronic, there may be peaking of the intercondylar eminences. Occasionally the ACL tears by avulsion from its tibial insertion rather than the usual mid-substance tear, visible on x-ray as a fracture of the intercondylar eminence (Fig. 23–59).

Differential Diagnosis. An acute patellar dislocation will lead to pain, swelling, guarding, and a similar clinical picture. However, tenderness is along the medial retinaculum, and the Lachman will be negative. Meniscal injuries commonly accompany ACL tears, so inability to completely extend the knee or significant joint line tenderness on palpation may be due to a meniscus tear. If the Lachman examination is easy to perform and feels negative, you are probably dealing with a meniscal injury and no more than a grade II ACL. Conversely, inability to adequately perform a Lachman, or an equivocal Lachman, precludes you from ruling out an ACL injury, and you may not be able to definitively establish the diagnosis at the time of your initial examination.

Special Tests. Several tests have been described as attempts to facilitate the diagnosis of ACL tears. In the *pivot shift* test, the tibial and femoral articular surfaces actually shift during a provocative physical examination maneuver. With the patient supine and the knee extended, a valgus stress is applied to the knee, the foot is internally rotated, and the knee is slowly flexed. At approximately 30 degrees of knee flexion, the tibia will often shift or "jump," confirming instability due to ACL injury. Such a pivot shift is negative if the ACL is intact and not stretched out. This test is not

very reliable in the acute setting because of guarding and pain, but under anesthesia is a helpful confirmatory test.

A recently developed test that is useful in clinical assessment of ACL injury is the KT-1000, a ligament laxity testing machine (Fig. 23–60). Studies have shown that a side-to-side difference of 3 mm or more reflects ACL injury. Patients with less than 5 mm have been shown to be better able to "cope" with chronic ACL insufficiency than those with more than this amount of instability.

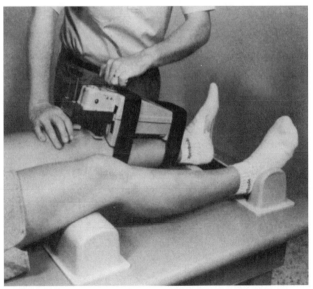

Figure 23–60. The KT-1000 arthrometer is a device that permits objective measurement of the amount of anterior tibial translation, and is the equivalent of an "instrumented Lachman" test. (From Andrews JR, Harrelsen GL: Physical Rehabilitation of the Injured Athlete. Philadelphia, WB Saunders, 1991.)

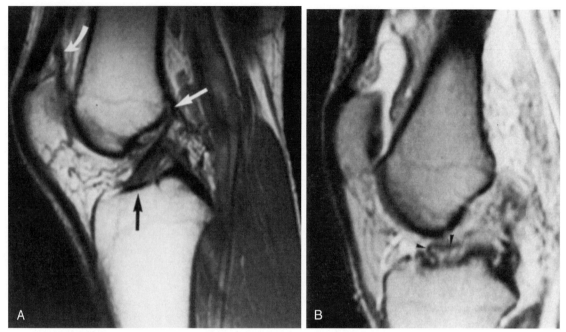

Figure 23–61. MRI is very sensitive and accurate in defining ACL tears. In *A*, observe the distinct normal-appearing striated fibers of the ACL along its normal course. (From Insall JN, et al: Surgery of the Knee, 2nd ed. New York, Churchill Livingstone, 1993.) In *B*, observe in this T2-weighted sagittal image the absence of distinct striated fibers running in the direction of the normal ACL. This absence is diagnostic of an ACL disruption. (From DeLee JC, Drez D Jr: Orthopaedic Sports Medicine: Principles and Practice, Vol 2. Philadelphia, WB Saunders, 1994.)

The most definitive noninvasive diagnostic test is an MRI, which is virtually 100% sensitive to ACL injury (Fig. 23–61). Unfortunately, the test is so sensitive that even a partial tear appears abnormal. In the patient with a typical history and obvious physical examination findings, MRI adds little to the diagnosis and does not usually influence treatment decision making. Occasionally, diagnostic confirmation requires examination under anesthesia and arthroscopic evaluation.

Definitive Treatment. Historically, treatment of ACL injuries has been nonoperative, relying on strengthening exercises, brace wear, and activity modification. The natural history of the ACL-deficient knee and technical refinements in surgical technique have changed this perspective. The ACL has poor healing potential because of its intra-articular location, where synovial fluid interferes with normal fibrin clot formation and organization. Recurrent instability follows, with progressive injury to the menisci and chondral surfaces. Such cumulative wear and tear changes lead to sports disability and, eventually, arthritis.

Nonoperative treatment means emphasis on physical therapy to restore motion and strength, and return to activity with a functional brace designed to decrease the risk of recurrent instability. Activity modification includes the elimination of more aggressive pivoting and cutting sports (football, rugby, downhill skiing, volleyball, singles tennis) and substituting less demanding straight-line activities (cycling, swimming, running, cross-country skiing, rollerblading).

Operative treatment involves surgical reconstruction in which autograft (tissue from the patient) is arthroscopically implanted as a substitute. The most common grafts are the central third patellar tendon and hamstrings autograft (Fig. 23–62). Less commonly used are allografts, tissues harvested from cadavers. With a slightly higher failure rate, slower incorporation, and risk of disease transmission, they remain a good backup when autograft tissue is unavailable or contraindicated. Approximately 90% of patients undergoing ACL reconstruction can expect to return to activity following a postoperative rehabilitation program.

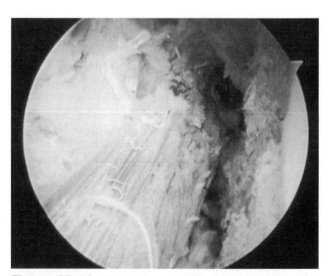

Figure 23–62. Illustration of ACL reconstruction using mid-third patellar tendon graft. (From McGinty JB, Caspari RB, Jackson RW, Poehling GG: Operative Arthroscopy, 2nd ed. Philadelphia, Lippincott-Raven, 1996.)

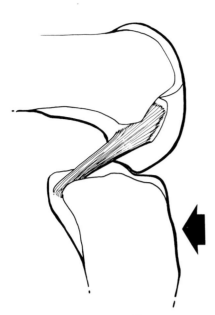

Figure 23–63. PCL injury usually occurs as a result of a fall or dashboard injury against the flexed knee, with consequent strain and tearing of the PCL fibers. (From DeLee JC, Drez D Jr: Orthopaedic Sports Medicine: Principles and Practice, Vol 2. Philadelphia, WB Saunders, 1994.)

POSTERIOR CRUCIATE LIGAMENT INJURY

Injury to the PCL occurs about 20 times less commonly than to the ACL. This relative infrequency leads to a poorer understanding of its natural history and treatment strategies compared with the more common ACL and MCL injuries. It is most commonly injured during knee dislocations.

Presentation/Mechanism of Injury. The mechanism of injury varies, but the most common involves a direct blow to the anterior aspect of the knee with the ankle plantarflexed (Fig. 23–63). In this position, the brunt of the posterior load is absorbed by the PCL (rather than the patella), which is disrupted usually in its mid-portion. Other mechanisms include dashboard-type injuries and severe hyperextension. The patient presents with an obviously injured and painful knee. Associated injuries are common, including additional ligament injuries such as the MCL, ACL, LCL, and the posterolateral corner.

Relevant Anatomy. The PCL provides approximately 95% of the primary restraint to posterior tibial translation. It arises from the posterior tibia just below the articular surfaces and travels anteriorly to insert on the medial femoral condyle along the anterior intercondylar notch (see Fig. 23–8). Its fibers are stout and in fact stronger than the ACL. Directly anterior and posterior to the femoral origin lie the meniscofemoral ligaments of Humphry and Wrisberg, respectively, which serve as attachments from just in front of and behind, respectively, the PCL femoral attachment to the posterior horn of the lateral meniscus (Fig. 23–64). Their contribution to normal knee stability and mechanics is not well understood at this time.

Classification. PCL injuries are graded from I to III like other ligaments. Grade III injuries represent complete tears. Associated ligament injury to the posterolateral corner may cause greater degrees of laxity and may account for some purportedly "isolated" PCL injuries with substantial laxity.

Physical Examination. Physical findings depend upon injury severity. A grade I injury may have mild swelling, anterior tenderness, and only slight posterior laxity. The patient with an isolated grade III tear will have a posterior sag sign in which when viewed from the side, the anterior contour of the tibia is subluxed posteriorly on the femoral condyle (see Fig. 23–29). Normally, there should be an approximately 1 cm step-off of the tibia anteriorly relative to the femur. Absence of this normal step-off is an indication of probable PCL disruption. Other tests that confirm PCL insufficiency include the posterior drawer test, the quadriceps active test, and knee hyperextension. Patients with chronic PCL insufficiency often complain of patellofemoral and medial joint symptoms as a consequence of increased stresses to these compartments.

X-Ray Evaluation. AP and lateral views are usually normal. Patients with chronic PCL insufficiency may have degener-

Figure 23–64. From this posterior view of the knee with the capsule removed, one can appreciate the two meniscofemoral ligaments that contribute to posterior stability as secondary restraints to the PCL. The anterior meniscofemoral ligament is termed the ligament of Humphry, and the posterior the ligament of Wrisberg. Each arises from along the intercondylar notch near the PCL femoral insertion and attaches to the posterior horn of the lateral meniscus. (From DeLee JC, Drez D Jr: Orthopaedic Sports Medicine: Principles and Practice, Vol 2. Philadelphia, WB Saunders, 1994.)

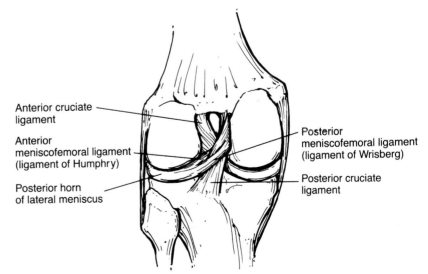

Anterior cruciate ligament

Anterior meniscofemoral ligament (ligament of Humphry)

Posterior horn of lateral meniscus

Posterior meniscofemoral ligament (ligament of Wrisberg)

Posterior cruciate ligament

ative changes in the patellofemoral and/or medial compartments.

Special Tests. Special tests are usually unnecessary. When indicated, MRI is nearly 100% accurate (Fig. 23–65). Bone scan may be useful in evaluating the medial and patellofemoral compartments in patients with chronic PCL insufficiency.

Differential Diagnosis. Additional ligament injuries must be ruled out, either by physical examination, MRI, or examination under anesthesia. The PCL must be considered injured until proven otherwise following a knee dislocation. The most important differential is to distinguish the "isolated" PCL from that associated with injury to the posterolateral structures. The latter involves injury to a number of nearby structures that can lead to a chronic and difficult to treat knee instability pattern. Physical examination techniques, which facilitate identification of posterolateral injury, include the posterolateral drawer test and the external rotation test. These tests take advantage of the fact that the posterolateral structures are responsible for preventing posterolateral translation or external rotation of the tibial plateau relative to the femur. When these structures are compromised, external rotation at 30 degrees of knee flexion will be increased when compared with the opposite normal knee. Similarly, the tibia will drop posterolaterally on the affected side more than the unaffected side. At 90 degrees, if the PCL is intact, the increased translation and rotation will decrease compared with that seen at 30 degrees. If the PCL and posterolateral corner are both compromised, external rotation and posterolateral subluxation will both be present at both 30 and 90 degrees. This differential is very important because failure to recognize contributory posterolateral instability will lead to underrecognition and undertreatment of this severe injury pattern.

Definitive Treatment. Treatment initially involves RICE and immobilization or hinge-brace type of casting or bracing until swelling and pain subside, followed by rehabilitation. The majority of PCL injuries are treated nonoperatively. The natural history of the isolated PCL-deficient knee is variable, with some patients functioning well and others developing insidious progressive disability. Surgical reconstruction is reserved for patients with chronic symptoms refractory to medical management or patients with grade III "isolated" PCL injuries in which posterior translation is greater than 10 mm. Reconstruction involves arthroscopic implantation of auto- or allograft substitutes.

Long-term results have not approached the surgical success seen following ACL reconstruction.

LATERAL COLLATERAL LIGAMENT

Injuries to the lateral collateral ligament (LCL) are very uncommon, and when they do occur, it is usually in association with other ligament injuries such as knee dislocations or posterolateral corner injuries.

Presentation. The presentation is that of a significantly traumatized knee with pain, swelling, and inability to bear weight.

Mechanism of Injury. An acute varus stress is responsible for injury to the LCL, which is the primary restraint to this motion.

Relevant Anatomy. The LCL is a distinct collagenous structure traveling from the lateral epicondyle of the femur to attach to the fibular head (see Fig. 23–10). Other structures of importance on the lateral side include the arcuate complex composed of thickening of the posterolateral capsule, the biceps tendon, the iliotibial band, and the popliteus tendon. The peroneal nerve courses around the fibular neck and dives deep into the anterior compartment as the deep peroneal nerve and sends a branch into the lateral compartment as the superficial peroneal nerve. The nerve is vulnerable during injury to the lateral side of the knee.

Classification. Grades I, II, and III reflect mild, moderate, and complete ligament tears.

Physical Examination. Pain, swelling, ecchymoses, and tenderness over the lateral side of the knee are common. Examine for associated nerve injury due to the peroneal nerve's proximity. Ligament integrity can be palpated with the knee in the figure-of-four position, and tested by applying a varus stress with the knee in slight flexion (see

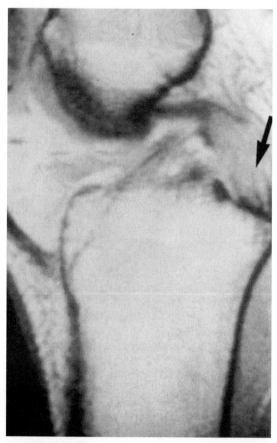

Figure 23–65. This sagittal MRI demonstrates tearing of the PCL in its distal portion, just proximal to its tibial insertion. (From DeLee JC, Drez D Jr: Orthopaedic Sports Medicine: Principles and Practice, Vol 2. Philadelphia, WB Saunders, 1994.)

Fig. 23–32). Associated injury to the posterolateral corner is suggested if there is increased external rotation or posterior translation of the tibia at 30 degrees of knee flexion. Lateral opening in full extension suggests additional injury to the ACL and/or PCL.

X-Ray Evaluation. AP and lateral x-rays should be obtained to identify any avulsion components or suggestions of other injury.

Special Tests. MRI confirms the injury and excludes other diagnostic possibilities.

Differential Diagnosis. Associated injuries to other ligaments, most commonly the posterolateral corner, and the possibility of knee dislocation must be considered.

Definitive Treatment. Treatment of isolated LCL injuries is usually nonoperative, with cast immobilization for a 6-week period followed by rehabilitation. For patients with associated posterolateral corner pathology, or those with varus alignment (in which the ligament is prognostically doomed as a result of varus stresses during weight bearing), primary surgical repair is considered.

Atraumatic Conditions of the Knee

MENISCAL TEAR

Meniscal tears are one of the most common problems seen in the knee and account for the most common indication for arthroscopy.

Presentation. Acute or insidious onset of pain or aching may herald tear of the medial or lateral meniscus. Occasionally, in addition to pain, there may be a history of having heard a pop at the time of injury, usually when the patient twisted, squatted, or came down on the leg in an awkward manner. In older patients, symptom onset is usually related to something innocuous, such as stepping off a curb or getting out of the car. There may or may not be a history of swelling associated with the pain. Occasionally there may be a history of actual mechanical locking, in which the knee has been temporarily "stuck" in a certain position.

Mechanism of Injury. Trauma can be responsible for meniscal tearing, although with age the fibrocartilaginous disks stiffen, degenerate, and tear with little trauma. Simple sheer or rotational stresses are sufficient to cause a tear.

Relevant Anatomy. The menisci are the fibrocartilaginous semilunar-shaped disks that occupy the medial and lateral compartments of each knee, providing the congruency between the convex femoral condyles and somewhat flat tibial plateau (see Figs. 23–4 and 23–5). Their predominant function is that of load distribution with secondary contribution to stability, shock absorption, and cartilage nutrition. The medial meniscus is circumferentially attached to the capsule and has little mobility. In contrast, the lateral meniscus has no capsular attachment posterolaterally at the popliteal hiatus, accounting for its significantly greater mo-

bility. This differential in mobility probably contributes to the fact that symptomatic medial meniscus tears outnumber lateral meniscus tears by an average of 4 to 1.

Classification. Tears are classified by their configuration and location (Fig. 23–66). Common examples are longitudinal (parallel to the circumference), radial (perpendicular to the circumference), cleavage (in the plane of the meniscus, parallel to the superior and inferior surfaces), and complex (in which there is a combination of more than one specific pattern). Tears can also be described based on their proximity to the blood supply, which influences likelihood of healing when tears are repaired. Tears can be described as occurring at the red-red zone (at peripheral meniscosynovial junction with vascularity present on both sides of the tear), the red-white zone (vascularity on the peripheral side of the tear only), and the white-white zone (neither side of the tear is vascular) (Fig. 23–67).

Physical Examination. Look for evidence of atrophy of the thigh muscles, effusion (joint swelling), and restricted motion. The most common finding is joint line tenderness that reproduces the patient's pain. Pain with forced flexion is another good sign. The McMurray test, in which internal and external rotation of the knee from full flexion to 90 degrees of flexion causes pain and occasional clicking and is reasonably specific (Fig. 23–68). Occasionally, the McMurray test will yield a palpable click over the joint line, reflecting the intermittently entrapped and freed meniscal fragment.

X-Ray. X-rays are usually negative. X-rays in which the meniscus has been removed show classic Fairbanks changes including squaring of the femoral condyle, sclerosis, joint space narrowing, and osteophyte formation (i.e., degenerative post-meniscectomy changes) (Fig. 23–69).

Differential Diagnosis. The differential includes injury to the articular cartilage (chondral or osteochondral fracture[s]), synovial disorders, and ligament injuries.

Special Tests. MRI has proven extremely reliable in the confirmation of meniscal tears, with an accuracy rate of better than 95% (see Fig. 23–44). Because of the frequency with which MRI detects asymptomatic degenerative tears with age, close clinical correlation is important.

Definitive Treatment. Meniscus tears are often successfully treated nonoperatively with activity modification, anti-inflammatory medication, and time. A number of proven meniscal tears will improve symptomatically if given enough time and relative rest. Indications for surgical intervention include persistent symptoms unresponsive to nonoperative treatment, a "locked" knee in which the meniscus is mechanically blocking knee extension, and meniscus pathology identified during ligament surgery.

Historically, surgical treatment involved opening up the joint (arthrotomy) and removing the entire meniscus, which predictably led to arthritis in the involved compartment. Since the advent of arthroscopy, efforts are made to remove only the damaged portion and to leave as much normal meniscus as possible in hopes of avoiding degenerative

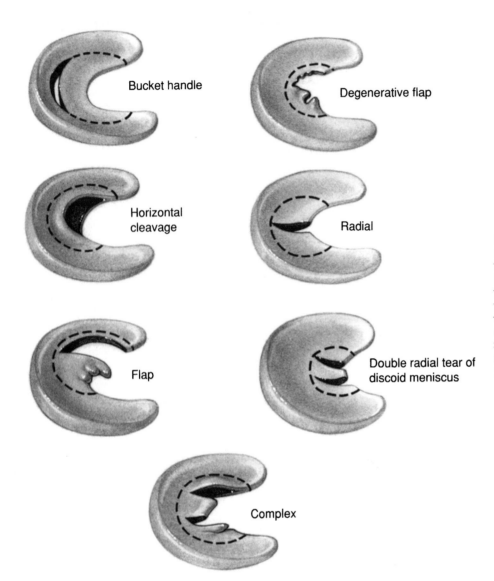

Figure 23–66. Meniscus tears may be classified according to the tear pattern, as well as their location and repairability. Illustrated are the most common variations in tear patterns with their associated descriptive names. (From Insall JN, et al: Surgery of the Knee, 2nd ed. New York, Churchill Livingstone, 1993.)

Figure 23–67. This schematic drawing shows the "zones" of the meniscus based on the degree of vascularity. The periphery, where the vascularity is excellent, is termed the "red" zone, with healing potential due to vascular proximity excellent. Next to this is the "red-white" zone, in which there is good vascularity on the peripheral side of the tear, but not necessarily the central (or white) side. Healing here is not quite as predictable. Finally, the most central type of tears, away from the vascular periphery, are known as "white-white" zone tears, with neither the periphery nor the central portion in proximity to good vascularity. These tears have poor healing prognosis. (From Andrews JR, Timmerman LA: Diagnostic and Operative Arthroscopy. Philadelphia, WB Saunders, 1997.)

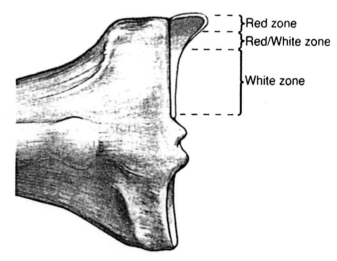

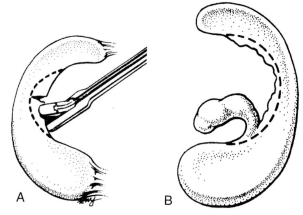

Figure 23–70. Meniscectomy involves removal of the portion of damaged meniscus thought responsible for the symptoms. Note the partial meniscectomy performed for a radial type in *A*, in comparison with a degenerative flap tear in *B*. (From Miller MD, et al: Arthroscopy: Correlative Atlas. Philadelphia, WB Saunders, 1997.)

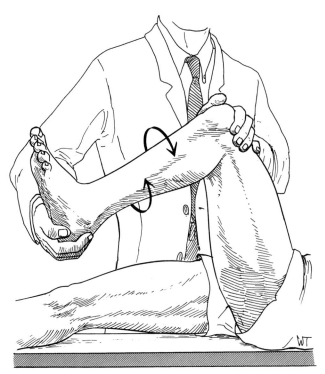

Figure 23–68. With the patient supine, the McMurray sign is elicited by flexing the knee completely and then alternately internally and externally rotating the foot. The reproduction of symptoms of pain, along with a click over the affected joint line, suggests meniscal pathology.

arthritic changes (Fig. 23–70). Unfortunately, despite such efforts, many studies show that even partial meniscectomies lead to degenerative changes with time (see Fig. 23–69). Under some circumstances, meniscus tears can be repaired rather than excised. Repairable tears are longitudinal in configuration and within the peripheral third of the meniscus where vascularity makes healing possible (Fig.

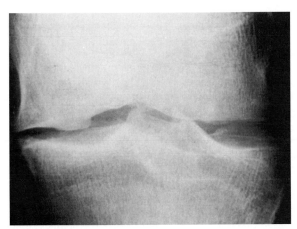

Figure 23–69. In this anteroposterior view of the knee of a 20-year-old man following a complete medial meniscectomy at age 10, the typical post-meniscectomy changes described by Fairbanks can be seen, including flattening of the joint surfaces, joint space narrowing, and sclerosis of the affected compartment. (From Insall JN, et al: Surgery of the Knee, 2nd ed. New York, Churchill Livingstone, 1993.)

23–71). Only about 5% of meniscus tears are repairable. Research into meniscal replacement through cadaveric substitute, biologic scaffold, or synthetic implant is an area of intense current interest.

PATELLOFEMORAL PAIN SYNDROME (ANTERIOR KNEE PAIN)

Patellofemoral pain syndrome is one of the most common causes of knee pain. Historically termed *chondromalacia* (literally, softening of the articular cartilage), the pain is usually due to patellar malalignment rather than chondral breakdown.

Presentation. Patients present with vague pain in the front of the knee, often bilaterally, and usually with no history of specific injury. Pain is exacerbated by activities in which the knee is flexed, such as stair climbing or squatting. Stiffness and aching are often present with prolonged sitting and first arising. This is referred to as the "movie sign." Unlike other mechanical knee problems, activity such as walking usually makes the symptoms better rather than worse.

Mechanism of Injury. Most patients with patellofemoral symptoms have underlying patellar malalignment. Abnormal patella tracking leads to abnormal pressure on the articular cartilage. Although the articular cartilage is without sensory nerve endings, the underlying subchondral bone is not, and the abnormal forces from asymmetrical loading are perceived as pain. Rarely is there actual structural injury to the patella articular surface, whose thickness of 7 mm is the thickest hyaline cartilage in the body. When such softening does occur, it is known as chondromalacia. The terms chondromalacia and patellofemoral pain syndrome are not synonymous. Chondromalacia specifically refers to the condition in which there is pathologic softening of the cartilage surface.

Relevant Anatomy. The patella functions to effectively lengthen the lever arm of the quadriceps muscle. In full

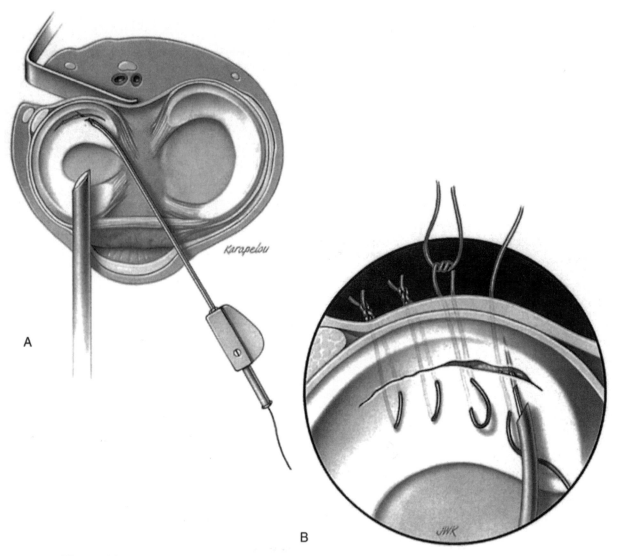

Figure 23–71. In this arthroscopic "inside-out" meniscal repair, sutures are arthroscopically passed across the longitudinal tear in the posterior aspect of the lateral meniscus. Note the retractor posterolaterally, positioned to capture the passed sutures to protect against iatrogenic neurovascular injury. (From Miller MD, et al: Arthroscopy: Correlative Atlas. Philadelphia, WB Saunders, 1997.)

extension (standing or supine), the patella lies superior to the trochlear groove. As the knee is flexed, the patella begins articulating with the trochlear groove, with progressively increasing contact with knee flexion.

Classification. Although there is no specific classification system for patellofemoral pain syndrome, there are three different types of patients presenting with this complaint. The most common are those with patellar malalignment. The second group are patients with patellar hypermobility. Third are those with no identifiable malalignment.

Physical Examination. Look at the patient's overall alignment. As the patient stands and walks, inspection for possible pronation may indicate one of the predisposing causes of patellofemoral strain. With the patient seated, observe the position of the patellas, which in some appears as "grasshopper eyes" with lateral tilt (see Fig. 23–37). In-

spect for active malalignment by having the patient actively extend the knee while seated. The "J" sign occurs if the patella jumps back into its groove near terminal extension after tracking laterally.

Inspect the quadriceps for overall development and specifically the VMO. Atrophy or hypoplasia contributes to maltracking. Inspect for passive malalignment by noting the Q angle (see Fig. 23–33). Slightly higher in females than males, the normal Q angle is approximately 10 degrees and should not exceed 15 degrees. With the patient supine, look for patella mobility. Inability to elevate the lateral aspect of the patella to a neutral position indicates tightness of the lateral retinaculum and is known as a positive "patellar tilt" sign (see Fig. 23–36). Ability to laterally displace the patella more than 50% of its width suggests lax medial retinacular restraints, another finding in malalignment as well as instability (see Fig. 23–35). If the patient displays apprehension when attempting lateral patellar displacement, there may be actual instability contributing to or responsible for the patient's symptoms (see Fig. 23–39).

In the seated position, palpate over the patellofemoral joint while the patient actively extends the knee, noting any crepitus. Palpate for crepitus in the opposite knee also, since crepitus may be normal in that patient. Crepitus may reflect articular pathology or may be due to intermittently entrapped and bowstringed synovial bands within the patellofemoral joint. Palpation of the medial and lateral patellar facets is often tender.

X-Ray. X-ray evaluation should include the usual AP and lateral views of the knee, but in addition, a view tangential to the patellofemoral joint is necessary. A tangential view (sunrise, Merchant, Laurin) helps evaluate patellofemoral congruency and arthritis.

Differential Diagnosis. In children, anterior knee pain is presumed hip pathology until proven otherwise. When localized to tender tibial tubercle, the condition may be Osgood-Schlatter syndrome, a consequence of repetitive traction stresses to the vulnerable tibial tubercle apophysis. Local tenderness and radiographic changes with fragmentation and enlargement of the tibial tubercle apophysis confirm the diagnosis. In older adolescents and adults, anterior knee pain may occur more over the patellar tendon rather than the patella itself, known as patellar tendinitis (or jumper's knee). Another cause of anterior knee pain is bipartite patella, in which a separate ossification center persists, most commonly at the superolateral aspect of the patella. These are usually incidental and rarely account for patient symptoms. The presence of tenderness directly over the fragment may indicate this as the source of symptoms. Occasionally, the fragment requires removal.

Special Tests. There are no special tests necessary to confirm the diagnosis of patellofemoral pain syndrome. Some clinicians have found tangential x-rays at different angles of knee flexion helpful in better evaluating the relationship of the patella to the trochlear groove. However, such tests are static and do not take into account dynamic forces of muscle pull during activity. This limits the usefulness not only of x-rays, but also of CT and MRI.

Definitive Treatment. Remember that most patients with patellofemoral pain syndrome have no actual articular cartilage damage. The mainstay of treatment is to identify and correct any malalignment or tracking disorder. Physical therapy emphasizes VMO development through "short arc" quadriceps exercises. Some patients benefit from McConnell taping of the patella into a corrected tracking position (Fig. 23–72). Arthroscopy is reserved for patients with persistent symptoms. Occasionally, arthroscopic release of the tight lateral retinaculum improves symptoms.

ILIOTIBIAL BAND FRICTION SYNDROME

Also known as cyclist's or runner's knee, this syndrome is a common overuse injury seen about the knee.

Presentation. Pain is over the lateral side of the knee, usually related to running. Symptoms are often preceded by a change in training regimen, such as an increase in mileage, intensity, terrain surface, or shoe wear. Conversely, cyclists may admit to increased mileage or change in terrain.

Mechanism of Injury. Repetitive motion of the tense iliotibial band over the lateral epicondyle is thought to set up a bursitis between the epicondyle and tendon. Patients in whom one leg is longer than the other may be predisposed.

Relevant Anatomy. The iliotibial band is a sinewy structure whose origin is in the gluteus maximus and the insertion of the tensor fascia lata. Traveling distally along the lateral thigh, it travels over the femur's lateral epicondyle and inserts on Gerty's tubercle.

Physical Examination. Examination reveals focal tenderness over the lateral epicondyle. Occasionally, the Ober test will be positive. In this test, the patient is placed laterally on the unaffected side. Starting with the hip abducted and the knee flexed 90 degrees, the hip is gently extended, adducted, and then flexed in an adducted position. Tightness and irritation over the iliotibial band will be rewarded by discomfort indicative of a positive test.

X-Ray Evaluation. X-rays are negative in this entity.

Differential Diagnosis. Pain on the lateral side may reflect lateral meniscus pathology or a proximal tibular fibular joint problem.

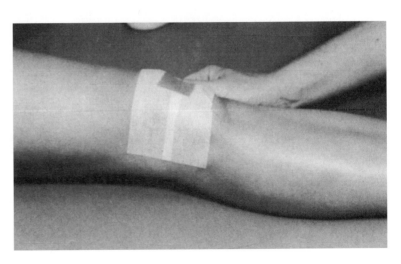

Figure 23–72. Specific taping techniques have been shown to influence patellar tracking and alignment and therefore improve symptoms in some patients with patellofemoral disorders. This technique is best known for the physical therapist who developed and popularized this technique, known as the McConnell method. (From Andrews JR, Harrelsen GL: Physical Rehabilitation of the Injured Athlete. Philadelphia, WB Saunders, 1991.)

Special Tests. There are no special tests for diagnosing this condition.

Definitive Treatment. Treatment is nonoperative and includes activity modification, anti-inflammatory medications, and a thorough stretching program of the iliotibial band, hamstrings, and glutei. Most patients are able to return to their previous level of activity. Rarely are corticosteroid injections or surgical intervention warranted.

BAKER'S CYST

Described by Baker in the late 1800s, this condition is a well-known accompaniment of several knee disorders. Rather than a discrete entity, it is actually a normal anatomic structure that becomes prominent in response to knee pathology.

Presentation. Most Baker's cysts come to the physician's attention when discovered by MRI. Occasionally the patient will note a prominence in the popliteal area. Less commonly, patients may present with acute pain and swelling in their proximal calf as a consequence of cyst rupture, with spilling of the synovial contents into the calf.

Relevant Anatomy. This structure is a normal bursa of the semimembranosis and is present in an estimated 35 to 50% of patients. Synovial fluid generated within the knee in response to meniscal, chondral, or synovial pathology can lead to bursal distention due to direct communication with the joint.

Physical Examination. Baker's cysts are almost always located posteromedially. Usually there is an indistinct fullness in the popliteal fossa.

X-Ray Evaluation. X-rays are unhelpful in evaluation of Baker's cysts, although occasionally osteochondral fragments can be seen posteromedially.

Differential Diagnosis. The presence of a neoplasm must be considered in the patient presenting with fullness or a palpable mass in the popliteal fossa. Imaging is almost always carried out to rule out this possibility. In the patient with acute pain and swelling of the proximal calf, consideration must be given to a deep venous thrombosis. Meniscal cysts are differentiated in their size and location. They are very discrete grapelike structures that occur directly along the joint line and are most commonly associated with meniscus tears (Fig. 23–73).

Special Tests. Special tests are unnecessary in patients with a typical history. Imaging by MRI demonstrates the cyst and other intra-articular problems and is the diagnostic test of choice. Aspiration of the mass yields golden-yellow viscous synovial fluid. Its viscosity mandates use of a large-bore needle, such as an 18 gauge, to ensure successful aspiration.

Definitive Treatment. Baker's cysts are often brought to the fore by an MRI performed for other knee symptoms. Most cysts will resolve upon definitive treatment of the intra-articular problem—i.e., debridement of the meniscal tear or chondral fragmentation. Occasionally the cyst itself produces symptoms due to its size. Aspiration, followed by corticosteroid injection, is an alternative but if unsuccessful may require surgical excision.

OSTEOCHONDRITIS DISSECANS

Although chondral or osteochondral problems can be caused by acute trauma, a more common cause is osteo-

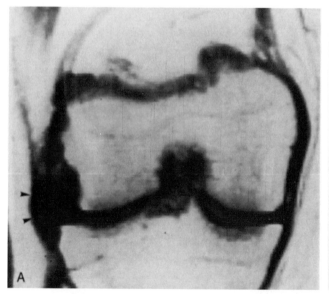 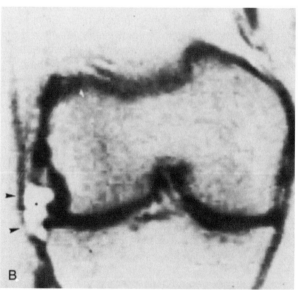

Figure 23–73. These coronal images demonstrate the typical appearance of a meniscal cyst, seen as a prominence on the T1-weighted image *(A)* and as a bright-intensity discrete signal on the T2-weighted sequence *(B)*. Discrete and about the size of a grape, these cysts form in relation to associated meniscal pathology, usually with degeneration and cleavage tearing. Treatment involves debridement and cyst decompression, usually achievable arthroscopically. (From DeLee JC, Drez D Jr: Orthopaedic Sports Medicine: Principles and Practice, Vol 2. Philadelphia, WB Saunders, 1994.)

chondritis dissecans. In this condition, a portion of the normal articular surface is "dissected" away from its underlying subchondral bed.

Pathophysiology. This condition has been attributed to a vascular insult to the growing epiphysis of skeletally immature patients. The condition is most frequently seen in the medial femoral condyle of the knee (Fig. 23–74), but has been described in other joints as well, including most commonly the elbow (capitellum) and ankle (talus).

Presentation. The most common presentation is that of an adolescent or young adult with joint symptoms. Intermittent pain, swelling, or catching related to activities is present.

Physical Examination. Physical findings are usually nonspecific, and the diagnosis is afforded by x-rays or diagnostic imaging studies.

X-Rays. X-rays show a localized area of radiolucency (decreased density) in the area of the OCD (Fig. 23–74). Often the osteochondral fragment is sclerotic (increasingly dense) and may be partially or completely detached from its underlying bed.

Special Tests. Special tests are rarely necessary, although MRI may help in further localization and treatment planning (Fig. 23–75).

Classification. Osteochondral injuries have been classified based on the fragment's relationship to the bone from which it arises (Fig. 23–76). In a grade I, the lesion is

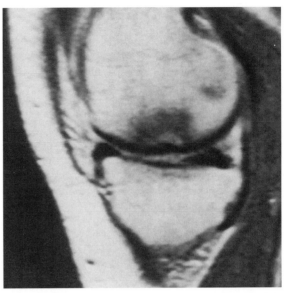

Figure 23–75. In comparison with x-ray, MRI better delineates the extent of the lesion, here involving a substantial portion of the weight-bearing surface of the medial femoral condyle. (From Insall JN, et al: Surgery of the Knee, 2nd ed. New York, Churchill Livingstone, 1993.)

incomplete, without actual complete fracture from the underlying subchondral bed into the joint. In a grade II, there is a fracture line extending from the subchondral bone to the joint, but the fragment is still within the bed. In a grade III lesion, the fragment is loose, with a fracture plane around the lesion, which loosely lies in its bed. In grade IV injury, the fragment has become detached and is free within the joint. This scheme helps determine treatment.

Treatment. Treatment varies according to the lesion's size, location, stage, and age of the patient. In skeletally imma-

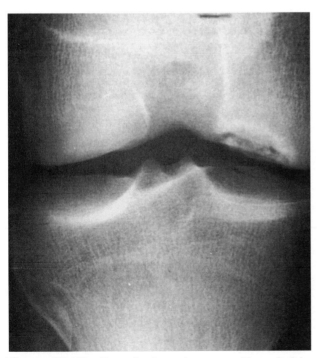

Figure 23–74. Note the irregular area with underlying radiolucency over the femoral condyle, typical of osteochondritis dissecans. (From Insall JN, et al: Surgery of the Knee, 2nd ed. New York, Churchill Livingstone, 1993.)

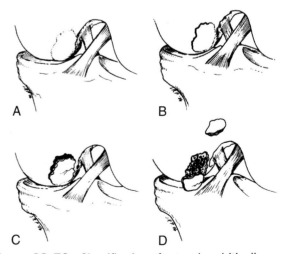

Figure 23–76. Classification of osteochondritis dissecans (OCD). *A* shows an in situ lesion. In *B*, there is early separation but the lesion is still within its base. In *C*, the lesion has partially detached, and in *D*, there is complete detachment of the osteochondritic fragment. (From Miller MD, et al: Arthroscopy: Correlative Atlas. Philadelphia, WB Saunders, 1997.)

ture patients, non-displaced osteochondral fragments are thought to have healing potential with immobilization. Conversely, in older adolescents or young adults, particularly when there is evidence of fragment displacement, definitive treatment involves debridement and sometimes attempted fixation (Fig. 23–77). A number of strategies have been devised for treating the defect left behind following debridement of an osteochondral defect. These include (1) abrasion and/or drilling to stimulate and enhance biologic repair with fibrocartilage tissue, (2) transplantation of small (6 to 10 mm diameter) osteochondral "plugs" from healthy non–weight-bearing areas of the knee to the damaged weight-bearing areas, and (3) harvesting of cartilage to be grown and later implanted.

DEGENERATIVE ARTHRITIS

Degenerative arthritis is the most common cause of knee pain in the older adult. The knee is the most common site of degenerative osteoarthritis in the body.

Presentation. Patients with arthritis can present in a variety of ways, but most commonly complain of pain that is insidious and slowly progressive, associated with stiffness and occasionally swelling, worse with activity, and relieved by rest. Symptoms are usually more significant in one knee, although both may be affected.

Pathophysiology. The pathophysiology of osteoarthritis is poorly understood but involves damage to the highly organized articular cartilage and supporting subchondral bone. Despite numerous biochemical, histologic, and clinical observations, the etiology remains unknown. Primary (degenerative) osteoarthritis or secondary (posttraumatic) osteoarthritis both lead to the chondral damage, increased subchondral bone stress, and eventually exposed subchondral bone.

Relevant Anatomy. The weight-bearing chondral surfaces are the most commonly affected areas of disease, with progressive loss of cartilage thickness in areas of greatest stress concentration.

Physical Examination. An antalgic gait is often present. Most patients with degenerative osteoarthritis have a tendency toward varus malalignment. Swelling is often present during periods of exacerbation. Motion is frequently mildly restricted, with flexion contracture (inability to passively extend the knee fully) common. Flexion is often limited as well. Tenderness is nonspecific, although medial joint line pain is most common. Crepitus of the patellofemoral joint is a frequent finding.

X-Ray Evaluation. Weight-bearing AP films demonstrate loss of normal joint height, along with the other findings typical of osteoarthritis, including sclerosis, osteophyte formation, and juxta-articular cysts (Fig. 23–78). Observe for evidence of malalignment, either varus or valgus, by comparing the knees on a weight-bearing film (see Fig. 23–40). Occasionally very early arthritis will fail to show obvious findings. Because the true AP view normally reveals only the anterior to mid weight-bearing portions of the joint in profile, having the patient flex during the x-ray may better demonstrate the more typically present wear seen on the more posterior aspect of the condyles. Thus, in trying to accurately assess the true extent of arthritis, particularly in patients in whom standard AP weight-bearing views are underwhelming, an additional film of 30 to 45 degrees of knee flexion in a PA direction is taken. This view often reveals more substantial arthritis that may not have been recognized on the more standard image (see Fig. 23–43). A lateral film demonstrates the tibiofemoral and patellofemoral joints. A sunrise view reveals the patellofemoral articulation.

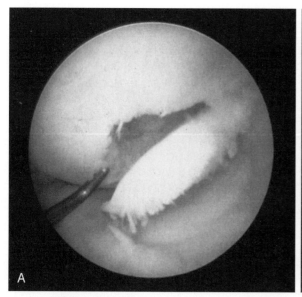
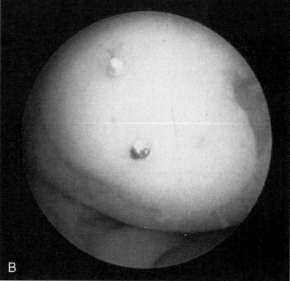

Figure 23–77. In *A*, note the arthroscopic appearance of osteochondritis dissecans that has not been completely displaced from its bed. In *B*, observe the appearance after debriding the base of the lesion and performing arthroscopic pin fixation. (From Scott WN: Arthroscopy of the Knee: Diagnosis and Treatment. Philadelphia, WB Saunders, 1990.)

Special Tests. Special tests are usually unnecessary. MRI is rarely necessary in the evaluation or management of osteoarthritis. Full-length-standing films are helpful to better assess overall alignment. Bone scans are sensitive to detection of osteoarthritis when not visible radiographically, but this test is not very specific.

Differential Diagnosis. The differential diagnosis for osteoarthritis includes all other conditions that can lead to knee pain and swelling. This includes inflammatory types of arthritis, of which the best known is rheumatoid arthritis. Inflammatory arthritides often present with bilateral knee symptoms and other joint involvement as well. Soft tissue bogginess of the surrounding synovium is more likely than true effusions. Systems review may be positive for associated conditions involving the eyes, skin, or gastrointestinal tract, and a family history may be positive for inflammatory arthritis. Physical examination often shows a tendency toward neutral or valgus alignment. X-ray changes suggest more of an osteopenic picture (decreased bone density) rather than a sclerotic appearance (Fig. 23–79). Peri-articular erosions may be present as well.

Metabolic arthritis such as gout or pseudogout may present with pain and/or swelling. Effusions are common. A history of gout elsewhere or great toe symptoms (the most common musculoskeletal site for gout) combined with an elevated serum uric acid level suggests the presence of gout. Synovial fluid analysis demonstrating the typical appearance of sodium urate crystals confirms the

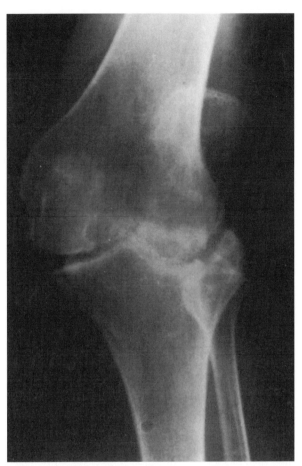

Figure 23–79. This anteroposterior radiograph shows end stage findings of fixed valgus deformity in a patient with long-standing rheumatoid arthritis. (From Insall JN, et al: Surgery of the Knee, 2nd ed. New York, Churchill Livingstone, 1993.)

diagnosis. Pseudogout or calcium pyrophosphate crystal disease often demonstrates faintly visible calcifications within the menisci seen on x-ray (Fig. 23–80). Joint aspiration analysis yields rhomboid-shaped crystals.

Osteonecrosis is a distinct entity that presents with knee pain with or without swelling. However, the onset is usually acute, with pain more localized to the medial compartment and persistent even at rest. X-rays may demonstrate an area of radiolucency, although this condition is sometimes radiographically undetectable in its early stages and may require more sensitive imaging such as MRI or bone scanning (Fig. 23–81).

Septic arthritis must be considered in the adult with acute onset of pain and swelling. However, these patients usually have significant pain with any knee motion and have hot, swollen, painful knees. Knee joint aspiration with synovial fluid analysis confirms the diagnosis, with a high number of white cells (usually >100,000 cells/mm³), elevated proportion of segmented white cells, and a Gram stain that demonstrates bacteria.

Natural History. The natural history of osteoarthritis is variable. In some patients, symptoms will be mild and easily controlled by activity modification and analgesics. In others, the pain and disability will be progressive and inexora-

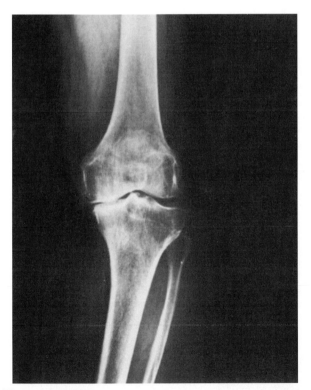

Figure 23–78. In this weight-bearing anteroposterior view, observe the typical radiographic changes of degenerative osteoarthritis, including joint space narrowing with varus alignment and sclerosis. (From Insall JN, et al: Surgery of the Knee, 2nd ed. New York, Churchill Livingstone, 1993.)

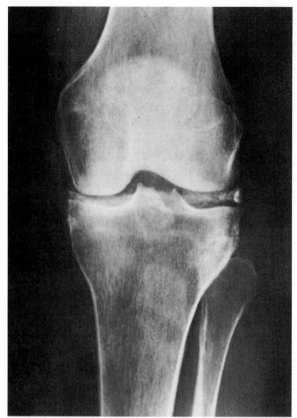

Figure 23–80. Typical findings indicative of chondrocalcinosis, or pseudogout, are seen in the lateral compartment of this patient's knee, with rather typical-appearing calcifications distributed along the lateral joint line. (From Insall JN, et al: Surgery of the Knee, 2nd ed. New York, Churchill Livingstone, 1993.)

transmission to the medial compartment during weight bearing. This alignment pattern prevents them from "unloading" this medial compartment, and as stress to this area increases, the joint wear worsens, further leading to increased compartment stress and further deformity.

Definitive Treatment. Treatment ranges from simple reassurance to joint replacement. In general, treatment is symptomatic. There are no techniques that will "reverse" the condition. With the exception of treating focal cartilage defects in patients with isolated articular cartilage lesions, there is no medical or surgical method for cartilage regeneration in osteoarthritis. Current emphasis, therefore, is on palliative relief of symptoms. Fortunately, there are a wide variety of satisfactory options. The specific type of treatment depends upon the patient, severity of arthritis, the level of disability, patient goals, and medical condition. Treatment strategy must be individualized, particularly since x-ray appearance and function are not always related. Many patients with rather significant appearing disease by x-ray function quite well, whereas others with minimal evidence of degenerative change by radiographs require operative intervention.

Treatment options usually begin with activity modification and analgesics. Activity modification may mean having to eliminate certain activities that overload the joint, such as running or tennis, and substituting less demanding activities, such as walking, swimming, or cycling. Exercise in general has been found very helpful in patients with mild to moderate arthritis. An aquatics therapy program, in which gravity is somewhat reduced by exercising in a pool, may further improve symptoms.

Anti-inflammatory medications are a mainstay of current treatment, with many patients able to manage symptoms with long-term use. However, potential renal or hepatic toxicity warrants blood testing approximately every 4 months in cases of chronic use. Recent interest in the use of over-the-counter supplements such as the cartilage precursors chondroitin and glucosamine sulfate supplements has led to their increased use as adjuncts for treating

ble. Generally, the condition is slowly progressive with symptoms related to activity. Patients with considerable malalignment (i.e., varus deformity) are at risk of progression because of the biomechanical predisposition to stress

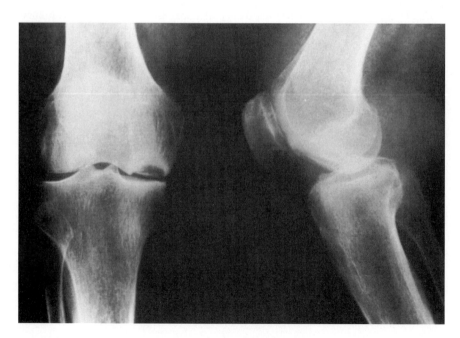

Figure 23–81. Note the significant focal area of radiolucency over the medial femoral condyle in this patient with relatively late-stage osteonecrosis. The calcification within the center of the lesion is indicative of calcified cartilage. (From Insall JN, et al: Surgery of the Knee, 2nd ed. New York, Churchill Livingstone, 1993.)

symptomatic mild to moderate osteoarthritis. Although there is no evidence that they contribute to actual regeneration of new cartilage, many studies have demonstrated their efficacy in some patients.

Judicious use of intra-articular cortisone injections is particularly helpful in controlling exacerbations. When overutilized, however, cortisone has been shown to actually accelerate degeneration of articular cartilage. Limiting injections to no more than three over the course of a year is probably acceptable. Interest in the recently FDA-approved hyaluronic acid derivatives to enhance the normal lubricating mechanism of the knee has led to their use in the form of serial injections. However, proof of their clinical efficacy is pending.

Ambulatory aides such as a cane or walker are effective in decreasing pain but are not well tolerated for long-term use by most patients. Special "unloading" knee braces may decrease stress in the affected compartment and are rarely effective for long-term use.

Surgical options are available for patients with symptoms unresponsive to nonoperative management. These include arthroscopic debridement, high tibial osteotomy (HTO), knee replacement, and arthrodesis. Arthroscopy is useful for patients with mild or moderate osteoarthritis, particularly when mechanical symptoms such as catching, clicking, or locking are present. In these circumstances, a minimally invasive arthroscopic "clean-out" with removal of loose bodies, meniscal flap tears, chondral irregularities, and osteophytes can improve symptoms and functioning. Generally thought to be palliative, arthroscopic debridements are effective in about 75% of patients. However, the results often deteriorate with time and often require further intervention.

HTO can be a very effective treatment for patients with relatively localized medial compartment arthritis and mild to moderate varus deformity. In this procedure, a triangular wedge of bone is removed from the proximal tibia to change the alignment and redistribute loading toward the lateral compartment (Fig. 23–82). This is effective in about 90% of patients for up to 10 years but often is a precursor to definitive joint replacement surgery. The procedure is most effective in patients who are relatively younger (under the age of 60) and have "isolated" medial compartment disease. The presence of significant patellofemoral and/or lateral compartment disease is a contraindication.

Joint replacement is the mainstay of surgical intervention for osteoarthritis and posttraumatic arthritis of the knee. In this procedure, the joint surfaces are replaced with metal and plastic articulating components whose low-friction interface provides remarkably pain-free and effective functioning in the majority of patients in whom they are implanted. Total knee replacements include resurfacing of the tibial, femoral, and patellar articular surfaces (Fig. 23–83). Hemi-arthroplasty, in which only the femoral and tibial surfaces of the affected compartment are replaced, is a far less common alternative for patients with isolated compartment pathology. Complications of joint replacement include persistent pain (<10%), bleeding (usually treated by auto-transfusing patients with their own pre-donated blood), infection (<1%), and component wear. Current implants are thought to have relative longevity depending upon the patient's age, demands, and weight,

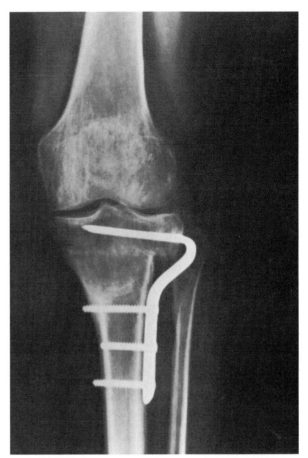

Figure 23–82. This anteroposterior radiograph demonstrates the neutral alignment achieved following high tibial osteotomy (HTO) for varus malalignment and medial compartment osteoarthritis. A blade plate device has been used to achieve fixation. (From Insall JN, et al: Surgery of the Knee, 2nd ed. New York, Churchill Livingstone, 1993.)

with an estimated 10- to 15-year life expectancy. Results of revision surgery are good but not quite as favorable as those following initial implantation.

A final alternative of mostly historical interest in the treatment of end stage arthritis is that of arthrodesis, or knee fusion. This procedure is very effective for pain relief, but because it does so by completely eliminating all knee motion and renders the patient permanently stiff, it is an unappealing option to most patients. It is reserved for patients in whom knee replacement is not an alternative, including those with failed and unsalvageable knees following previous joint replacement, those with chronic infection, and those with a compromised and dysfunctional extensor mechanism.

OSTEONECROSIS

Osteonecrosis is a relatively uncommon but distinct entity in which part of the subchondral bone undergoes necrosis or death. Known as a "heart attack" of the knee, this condition most commonly affects the medial femoral condyle and frequently leads to collapsed degenerative arthritis.

Presentation. The typical presentation is that of acute onset of pain unrelated to any particular activity. The onset is so

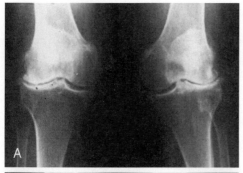
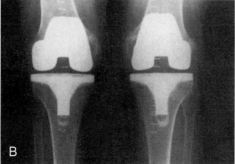

Figure 23–83. In *A*, note the significant lateral joint compartment narrowing in this 70-year-old female with progressive bilateral knee pain unresponsive to non-operative measures. *B* shows the anteroposterior radiograph following bilateral knee replacements, performed as a one-stage procedure in this patient. (From Wiesel SW, Delahay JN: Essentials of Orthopaedic Surgery, 2nd ed. Philadelphia, WB Saunders, 1997.)

abrupt that patients can usually describe the specific time of onset even months later. Patients are commonly over age 60 (4:1) and are more frequently female (3:1).

Pathophysiology. The pathophysiology is unknown, although a vascular insult is thought to initiate the cascade of subsequent changes in the bone, including focal necrosis, surrounding edema, attempted repair and sclerosis and frequent subchondral bone weakening, collapse, and degenerative joint changes. Some have also speculated on the role of trauma, but this remains unproven.

Relevant Anatomy. Most commonly, the medial femoral condyle is affected. The disease has also been reported to occur in the tibial plateau and the lateral femoral condyle as well.

Classification. Classification is radiographic, with five stages describing progression of the process (Fig. 23–84). In stage 1, x-rays are completely normal. Bone scan and MRI may detect lesions early in their course before obvious on plain films, but changes may be subtle even using these imaging modalities. In stage 2, there may be very early changes such as focal radiolucency with some flattening of the associated joint surface, indicative of impending subchondral fracture. Stage 3 shows the typical x-ray appearance of osteonecrosis, including the focal area of radiolucency accompanied by distal sclerosis. In stage 4, the distal fragment is more calcified in appearance with an

obvious radiolucency surrounded by a sclerotic halo. Stage 5 shows degenerative changes, with joint space narrowing, sclerosis, osteophyte formation, and perhaps the formation of juxta-articular cysts—findings indicative of osteoarthritis.

Physical Examination. Examination findings are usually those of the painful knee. The patient may have an antalgic gait. Malalignment due to angulatory deformity is uncommon early but may develop with disease progression. Mild swelling and tenderness to palpation over the (usually medial) affected compartment are common. Motion may be restricted, and manipulation during the examination will often be uncomfortable.

X-Ray Evaluation. Radiographs vary depending upon the stage of the disease. Plain films are commonly normal early on. Classic findings include an area of focal radiolucency, surrounded by a sclerotic reactive border.

Special Tests. MRI is probably the most sensitive and specific test to detect abnormal marrow signal in the associated subchondral bone. Bone scans are also effective in early detection, although not as accurate as MRI.

Differential Diagnosis. The differential diagnosis is fairly broad and includes all causes of knee pain. However, the presentation is so classic that the nature of the symptoms (localized pain, constant, at rest, accompanied by nocturnal awakening), rapidity of onset, and the presence of typical radiolucency is very specific. Other causes of acute knee pain should be considered, including acute chondral, synovial, or meniscal injury or exacerbation; metabolic arthritis; septic arthritis; and tumor. Radiographically, osteochondritis dissecans (OCD) can look similar, but most patients with OCD are relatively young (under age 40), have mechanical symptoms (catching, clicking, and locking), and have relatively little pain.

Natural History. The natural history of this process is poorly understood, with most patients progressing toward degenerative joint disease. The most important prognostic factors are probably the size and stage of the lesion. Large lesions and those in which a subchondral fracture line is already seen have a generally poor prognosis. A smaller lesion in which bone edema alone is seen may respond more favorably and reconstitute itself.

Definitive Treatment. Treatment is intended to relieve pain and minimize progression. Unfortunately, many patients presenting with this condition already have evidence of substantial subchondral involvement. In these patients, knee replacement has been the most predictable and successful form of management. When detected at an earlier stage and when smaller in size, nonoperative treatment may be effective such as use of anti-inflammatory medication, activity modification, and ambulatory aids. Arthroscopic efforts to stimulating healing through drilling, lavage, or debridement have met with limited success. Current efforts at core drilling and bone grafting of the lesion or arthroscopic autograft transplantation using osteoarticular plugs may provide relief in some patients.

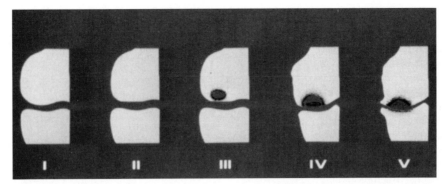

Figure 23–84. Osteonecrosis is classified radiographically into five stages according to x-ray appearance. In I, films are entirely normal. In II, there may be a subtle but detectable area of slight flattening of the femoral condyle. Stage III shows typical findings indicative of the early stage of the disease, including local radiolucency and a possible halo of surrounding bony reaction. Stage IV shows progression with calcification of the cartilage lesion within the process; in Stage V, there is degenerative progress, with joint space narrowing, subchondral sclerosis, and osteophyte formation typical of osteoarthritis. (From Insall JN, et al: Surgery of the Knee, 2nd ed. New York, Churchill Livingstone, 1993.)

Common Traumatic Conditions of the Leg

FRACTURES OF THE TIBIA/FIBULA

Fractures of the tibial and fibular shaft are the most common long bone fractures.

Presentation. Patients present with acute leg pain accompanied by deformity and swelling following a traumatic injury.

Mechanism of Injury. There are three common mechanisms of injury. Direct trauma can be from high-energy injury, such as that experienced when a pedestrian is struck by a car bumper, or a low-energy injury from a direct blow from an athletic event. Indirect trauma can occur when the foot is fixed and the leg is torqued, as may occur during athletic events or from a fall from a small height. Finally, fractures can occur as a result of penetrating injury such as seen with gunshot wounds.

Relevant Anatomy. The tibia and fibula are long bones, with the tibia demonstrating a rather triangular cross section. Its anterior border is rather sharp, subcutaneous, and quite vulnerable to trauma. The fibula is connected proximally to the posterolateral proximal tibia at the proximal tibiofibular joint. Distally, the fibula articulates with the distal tibia laterally at the ankle mortise. Four distinct compartments contain the soft tissue and neurovascular components of the leg and include the anterior, lateral, superficial posterior, and deep posterior compartments. The blood supply is nearly entirely from the popliteal artery, which in the proximal third of the leg sends branches anteriorly through the interosseous membrane to provide blood supply to the anterior and lateral compartments through the anterior tibial and peroneal vessels. The origin of this vasculature, at the trifurcation in the proximal leg, is a site of vulnerability, with potential vascular compromise, ischemia, and limb loss following trauma to this area. Nerve supply is via the common peroneal nerve and the posterior tibial nerve.

Classification. The simplest classification is descriptive, in which the fracture pattern, location (proximal, middle, distal), type and degree of displacement and angulation (20% anterior, 50% posterior, 10 degrees varus angulation, etc.), and presence of associated soft tissue injury (open with small puncture wound, open with 12-cm laceration and protruding bone) are characterized.

Physical Examination. Physical examination should focus on close inspection to rule out an open fracture.

X-Ray Evaluation. X-rays include an AP and lateral view including the knee and ankle.

Special Tests. Further films are obtained depending on clinical suspicion of associated joints and/or other injuries in these often multiply injured patients. Doppler evaluation of vascular status is necessary if there is any question about vascular integrity, and an arteriogram is the definitive test for demonstrating vascular integrity or compromise.

Differential Diagnosis. There is very little in the differential diagnosis of this injury, but the most important accompanying clinical problem is that of associated neurovascular compromise and compartment syndrome. Ischemia due to vascular compromise from fracture displacement and malalignment, soft tissue swelling, and vascular injury jeopardizes the leg's vulnerable soft tissue compartments. A high index of suspicion for the development of compartment syndrome must be maintained.

Definitive Treatment. Treatment depends upon the type of fracture. For closed fractures, nonoperative treatment is often acceptable, with closed reduction and cast application. General guidelines for acceptable reduction include less than 5 degrees of varus or valgus angulation, less than 10 degrees of anterior or posterior angulation, less than 10 degrees of rotational deformity, less than 1 cm of shortening, less than 5 mm of distraction, and more than 50% cortical contact. When treated nonoperatively, a long leg cast is employed, with initial non–weight-bearing transitioning to progressive weight bearing as the fracture begins to heal. Healing averages 16 weeks, and risk of displacement warrants frequent follow-up evaluation to ensure maintenance of reduction. Closed treatment is most effective for low-energy fractures with little displacement, with healing rates as high as 97%.

Unstable fractures, those in which reduction cannot be achieved or maintained, are usually candidates for internal fixation. Although plates and screws have been historically popular, current treatment methods emphasize placement of intramedullary rods for fracture fixation (Fig. 23–85). Immediate weight bearing, decreased functional disability, and more predictable fracture union occur with this method of treatment.

Open fractures must be treated with attention to wound management and fracture stability. Antibiotics should be instituted as soon as the open fracture is identified. Tetanus prophylaxis should be administered in patients with inadequate immunizations.

Open wounds must be sterilely covered, splinted, and treated as a surgical emergency, with prompt irrigation and debridement of the wound and fracture site. Repeat surgical debridements are usually necessary to ensure adequate removal of all potentially necrotic and infectious material, some of which may not be evident at the time of first surgical exploration. Definitive soft tissue and wound management may be required, including recurrent debride-

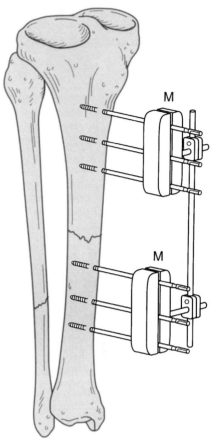

Figure 23–86. A common treatment option for stabilizing an open tibia fracture is application of an external fixator, which both stabilizes the fracture and permits access to the often-injured soft tissue structures. (From Browner BD, Jupiter JB, Levine AM, Trafton PG: Skeletal Trauma, Vol 1. Philadelphia, WB Saunders, 1998.)

ments, use of split-thickness skin grafts, local muscle flap coverage, and transfer of a "free flap." Definitive fracture management depends upon the nature of the injury, associated soft tissue problems, presence of compartment syndrome, and degree of bone comminution. The most common treatment is use of an external fixator, a device in which the bones are definitively stabilized using a frame whose minimal profile permits both fracture stabilization and soft tissue wound management (Fig. 23–86). Recently, emphasis on using internal fixation with unreamed intramedullary rods has led to their common use in grade I and grade II injuries.

Complications of tibia fractures are numerous, including delayed union, non-union, malunion, joint stiffness, thromboembolic disease, compartment syndrome, neurovascular injury, skin problems, infection, and limb loss.

COMPARTMENT SYNDROME

Compartment syndrome refers to a condition in which pressure within a soft tissue compartment of an extremity exceeds the pressure necessary for normal blood flow, leading to muscle ischemia, pain, and potential necrosis.

Mechanism of Injury. Most commonly described in the leg, compartment syndrome is usually a sequelae of traumatic

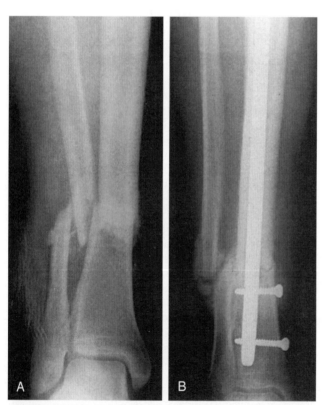

Figure 23–85. This tib-fib fracture was considered unstable and was treated by intramedullary (IM) rod fixation. Note the transfixing screws ("locks") placed in *B*, taken 5 months post-injury. (From Browner BD, Jupiter JB, Levine AM, Trafton PG: Skeletal Trauma, Vol 1. Philadelphia, WB Saunders, 1998.)

injury such as a tibia fracture in which intracompartmental bleeding leads to swelling within an otherwise restricted compartment. Progressive swelling impedes blood flow and necrosis ensues. Any of the four compartments can be affected, including the anterior, lateral, superficial posterior, and deep posterior. Failure to recognize and treat promptly can jeopardize limb viability. This is a limb-threatening emergency!

Presentation. There is severe pain in the leg and foot, often incompletely blunted by narcotic analgesics administered in treating the (usually) associated tibia fracture. The patient may note numbness or tingling of the foot.

Relevant Anatomy. The four compartments of the leg include the anterior, lateral, superficial, and deep posterior compartments surrounded by relatively unyielding fascial envelopes (see Fig. 23–18). Each compartment contains specific musculature and neurovascular structures at risk with progressive swelling.

Classification. There is no classification for compartment syndrome.

Physical Examination. The most reliable finding is that of soft tissue tightness or tenseness in the leg. Other signs include pain on passive extension or flexion of the toes. Sensation may be decreased distally, although this may be a consequence of nerve trauma and is less specific. The presence of a palpable pulse does not rule out compartment syndrome.

X-Ray Evaluation. X-rays are routinely important in evaluation of anyone with suspected compartment syndrome and should include AP and lateral views of the leg.

Special Tests. Compartment pressure measurement is the most important diagnostic test for evaluating patients with suspected compartment syndromes. Compartment pressures should be measured if there is any question regarding the possibility of this syndrome, particularly in the unconscious patient.

Direct measurement of the compartments can be achieved by introducing an 18-gauge needle connected to a pressure transducer (see Fig. 23–48). Disposable measurement kits are also available. Pressures exceeding 30 mmHg may indicate compartment syndrome.

Differential Diagnosis. Pain due to fracture and soft tissue injury is sometimes difficult to differentiate from that due to compartment syndrome. In general, in the conscious patient with a compartment syndrome, pain will often be disproportionate to the injury, narcotic analgesics may be insufficient to control the pain, and physical findings will indicate tenseness of the soft tissue and pain with passive motion of the toes. The key to establishing the diagnosis is to maintain a high index of suspicion for this potentially limb-threatening complication.

Definitive Treatment. Emergency fasciotomies with release of the constricted compartments are the definitive treatment. Release of the soft tissue fascial envelopes should be carried out for all four compartments and is usually performed through separate medial and lateral incisions. Sometimes, prominent muscle herniation through the open wounds will prevent skin closure and require delayed closure or split-thickness skin grafting.

Common Atraumatic Conditions of the Leg

OVERUSE: "SHIN SPLINTS" (MEDIAL TIBIAL STRESS SYNDROME)

One of the most common problems seen among runners is "shin splints," also known as medial tibial stress syndrome.

Presentation. The presentation is indicative of its name. Pain over the shins or posteromedial tibias occurs, usually as a consequence of running, often on hard, flat terrain. Discomfort is usually during the activity, but with continued running can lead to pain even with walking.

Pathophysiology. The pathophysiology of this condition is not well understood. Historically, this condition was thought a consequence of one of several entities, including periostitis, posterior tibial tendonitis, soleus tendonitis, or early stress reaction in the bone. There is no absolute consensus on the etiology of this condition, although there is wide agreement that it is related to soft tissue response to overuse. Periostitis of the soft tissue muscular attachment along the posteromedial tibia is thought to be the most likely cause of this syndrome.

Relevant Anatomy. Medial tibial stress syndrome occurs over the posterior mid to distal third of the tibia.

Classification. There is no clinical classification for medial tibial stress syndrome.

Physical Examination. Diffuse tenderness to palpation is usually present over the posteromedial mid to distal third of the tibia. Active plantarflexion and inversion of the hindfoot against resistance may be painful.

X-Ray Evaluation. X-rays are usually negative but are important to rule out the presence of a stress fracture.

Special Tests. A number of tests have been described, including injection into adjacent soft tissue with local anesthetic. However, relief does not completely confirm the diagnosis or definitively exclude the possibility of a stress fracture. Bone scans demonstrate diffuse uptake of the tracer along the distal third of the tibia (see Fig. 23–47).

Differential Diagnosis. The main differential to consider is that of a stress fracture, which is well demonstrated on bone scan as a focal "hot spot," in comparison to the more diffuse dye uptake in tibial stress syndrome.

Definitive Treatment. Definitive treatment is rest. Usually activity modification results in near-immediate improvement. When an athlete can return to his or her running depends upon the severity, intensity, duration, and goals of the individual patient. Ice massage several times a day over the painful area combined with use of anti-inflammatory medications helps. Some studies have suggested that the use of arch supports may help those with marked pronation. Heel cord stretching may also be useful in some patients. Cross-training to maintain conditioning through swimming, cycling, and even running with a weighted-vest in a pool are encouraged while the condition resolves. Importantly, prevention of this condition is possible through correcting any identified training errors such as excessive mileage, hard surfaces, and inadequate shoewear.

EXERTIONAL COMPARTMENT SYNDROME

Compartment syndrome, in which elevated compartment pressure can lead to muscle ischemia, pain, and potential necrosis, most commonly occurs in the traumatized extremity. However, this condition can also occur in the absence of discrete trauma. Among athletes, a more common presentation is referred to as exertional compartment syndrome.

Pathophysiology. This entity occurs as a consequence of progressive increased compartmental pressure due to activity, most commonly occurring in the leg while running. Progressive muscle hypertrophy and swelling during activity compromise the normal blood supply, leading to potential ischemia and pain.

Presentation. Unlike stress reactions or shin splints, where pain is usually bearable and can often be "run through," pain with exertional compartment syndrome usually is severe enough to force the athlete to stop. Unlike stress reactions or fractures, the symptoms promptly vanish after cessation of activity. The distinct presentation is highly suggestive of exertional compartment syndrome.

Physical Examination. Physical examination is unremarkable. There is no particular focal tenderness or neurologic abnormality.

X-Rays. X-rays are negative.

Special Tests. The diagnosis of exertional compartment syndrome is established by compartment pressure measurements, at rest and following activity. Using a small (16- or 18-gauge) needle attached to a pressure manometer set-up, each of the four compartments are measured in both legs and recorded (see Fig. 23–48). The athlete runs on a treadmill until symptomatic. Measurements are then repeated and compared to pre-exercise measurements. The exact criteria necessary for diagnosing compartment syndrome are somewhat variable, but in general pressure measurements in excess of 15 mmHg at rest, or greater than 20 mmHg 5 to 15 minutes post-exercise, are suggestive of exertional compartment pressure syndrome. X-rays, bone scans, and MRIs are all negative.

Differential Diagnosis. In the patient with equivocal intracompartmental pressure readings and the presence of bone tenderness, medial tibial stress syndrome is a more likely diagnosis.

Treatment. Treatment is simple. The athlete can either modify his or her activity (i.e., give up running) or have the affected compartment(s) surgically decompressed. This surgical procedure involves a small incision over the affected compartment followed by incision of the surrounding constricting fascial envelope. The outcome is predictably good.

SUMMARY AND CONCLUSIONS

Evaluation and management of problems of the knee and leg require familiarity with anatomy, examination techniques, and common conditions. An algorithmic approach facilitates diagnostic workup and definitive treatment in most cases. Problems of the knee can be divided into traumatic and atraumatic conditions for ease of diagnostic consideration. The most common problems involve overuse injury to the soft tissue structures about the knee, including the extensor mechanism (patellofemoral pain syndrome, patellar tendonitis, and Osgood-Schlatter syndrome) and iliotibial band, and degenerative conditions (osteoarthritis). Common traumatic conditions include ligament injuries and fractures. In the leg, traumatic injuries to the tibia and compartment syndrome constitute the most common and serious problems facing the practitioner. Atraumatic injuries to the leg including "shin splints" and exertional compartment syndrome can be differentiated and treated based on appropriate evaluation techniques. Nonoperative treatment is effective in managing most atraumatic conditions, whereas surgical intervention is often required to treat fractures and traumatic soft tissue injuries.

Bibliography

Fu F, Harner C, Vince KG: Knee Surgery, Vols 1 and 2. Baltimore, Williams & Wilkins, 1994.

McGinty JB: Operative Arthroscopy, 2nd ed. Philadelphia, Lippincott–Raven, 1996.

Chapter 24

The Foot and Ankle

Paul S. Cooper, M.D.

ANATOMY

The management of disorders involving the foot and ankle requires thorough knowledge of both the anatomy and the pathomechanics of these structures. The bony anatomy of the foot and ankle consists of the tibia and fibula in the leg and the 26 major bones that compose the foot. The *tibia* is a triangular bone with an anterior crest that starts at the proximal border as the tibial tubercle. This bone expands to become the tibial plateau at the level of the knee joint proximally, whereas distally the diaphysis terminates into the metaphyseal plafond, creating the medial malleolus. The lateral surface has a sulcus to accommodate the adjacent fibula, forming the *distal tibiofibular* joint. The geometry of the distal end of the tibial plafond is quadrilateral in shape and articulates with the talar dome to form the tibiotalar, or ankle, joint. The *fibula* is a triangular bone that lies lateral and slightly posterior to the tibia. It is held adjacent to the tibia by a thick interosseous membrane and is held distally by the inferior tibiofibular ligaments. The fibula contributes to the tibiotalar joint by forming the lateral malleolus of the ankle joint. The relationship of the fibula to the tibia is not static. With ankle dorsiflexion, the fibula translates laterally, migrates proximally, and rotates externally. This allows for the accommodation of the trapezoid-like talar dome.

The osseous structure of the foot is composed of 7 tarsals, 5 metatarsals, and 14 phalanges. The hindfoot consists of the talus and calcaneus bones. The *talus*, or astragalus, consists of a body, neck, and head. Approximately 60% of this structure is covered by articular cartilage. The unique trapezoidal geometry of the superior surface of the body, which is wider anteriorly, allows for stability in the mortise during dorsiflexion. The lateral and medial surfaces of the body articulate with corresponding articular surfaces of both the lateral and the medial malleoli. Posteriorly, a sulcus is formed between the posterolateral and posteromedial tubercles to accommodate the flexor hallucis longus tendon. On occasion, an accessory bone, the *os trigonum*, is attached to the posterolateral process. This accessory bone is often bilateral and is found in approximately half of all feet. The inferior surface of the talus articulates with the corresponding facet of the os calcis to create the *subtalar joint*. The talar neck is directed inferomedially and in a plantar direction, with the undersurface contributing to the sinus tarsi and tarsal canal to accommodate the artery of the tarsal sinus. The talar head is supported through an articulation with the navicular and anterior processes of the calcaneus. Medially, the calcaneonavicular ligament, or

spring ligament, provides support for the talar head in a fashion similar to that of a hammock or sling. The blood supply to the talar body is composed of branches from the posterior and anterior tibial arteries with additional contribution from the peroneal artery. The artery of the tarsal canal is formed by the anastomosis between the posterior tibial artery medially and the dorsalis pedis and peroneal arteries laterally. The tarsal canal artery supplies the middle one half to two thirds of the talar body. The sinus tarsi artery supplies the lateral 25% of the body; the head and neck are supplied by superior neck vessels from the anterior tibial artery branches of the tarsal sinus artery. This variation in extra-osseous and intra-osseous anastomoses leads to the high incidence of osteonecrosis associated with displaced fractures and dislocations.

The *calcaneus*, or os calcis, is the largest bone in the foot; the longitudinal axis is directed dorsally and laterally. The bone has been likened to an irregular cube with six surfaces. The inferior surface articulates with the talus in three facets: anterior, middle, and posterior, creating the *subtalar joint*. The largest, the posterior facet, articulates with the corresponding posterior calcaneal articular facet of the talus. The calcaneal groove is located between the middle and posterior articular surfaces and, with the adjacent talar sulcus, creates the *sinus tarsi*. The sinus tarsi, with the tarsal canal, contains the interosseous subtalar ligaments, the primary stabilizers for eversion of the subtalar joint. The subtalar joint is composed of three articular facets. The middle articular facet overlies the sustentaculum talus and is often confluent with the anterior articular facet. These two facets articulate with the adjacent undersurface of the talar head. The subtalar axis projects anteromedially to posterolaterally on the horizontal plane and mediocephalad to laterocaudad on the coronal plane, with a mean angle of 82 degrees plus or minus 4 degrees off the vertical axis. Distally, the calcaneus articulates with the cuboid in a concavo-convex arrangement, or saddle joint. The sustentaculum tali are medial projections that create a groove to accommodate the tendon sheath of the flexor hallucis longus. The sustentaculum also serves as the insertion site of the tibial calcaneal branches of the deltoid ligament and of the superior-medial attachment of the spring ligament. The inferior surface of the calcaneus is triangular, with two tubercles at the posterior aspect of the base. The medial tubercle is the main weight-bearing area and the origin of the plantar fascia and flexor digitorum brevis muscle. The lateral tubercle is the origin of the long plantar ligaments and the short plantar calcaneal cuboid ligaments. The lateral wall is flat and contains the trochlear process, which forms a groove for the peroneus longus tendon. The cortical bone of the calcaneus is weak in the central body, with tension trabeculae from the inferior cortex and compression trabeculae converging to support the anterior and posterior facets of the subtalar joint. Condensation of the supportive compact bone under the facets is referred to as the *thalamic* portion. The calcaneus functions as a lever arm for transmission of force from the Achilles tendon complex and provides subtalar mobility with inversion and eversion during the stance phase of gait.

The midfoot consists of the navicular and cuboid bones and three cuneiform bones. The convex surface of the *tarsal navicular* bone articulates with the distal convex aspect of the talar head and lies medial to the cuboid bone. It functions as a keystone for the medial longitudinal arch of the foot. The distal surface is composed of three facets that articulate with the medial, middle, and lateral cuneiform bones, respectively. Medially, the navicular bone extends to form the insertion site for the posterior tibial tendon. In up to 10% of cases, this medial extension may develop as an unfused accessory navicular bone, or *os tibiale externum*. The *cuboid* bone forms the lateral column through an articulation between the calcaneus proximally and the fourth and fifth metatarsals distally. There are additional articulations with the lateral cuneiform and navicular bones. Laterally, a groove accommodates the peroneus longus tendon as it courses plantarly in the deep layer of the foot. The three cuneiform bones are geometrically wedge-shaped, tapering plantarly to contribute to formation of the transverse arch of the foot. Distal articulations with the first, second, and third metatarsals, respectively, contribute to formation of part of the tarsometatarsal, or *Lisfranc's joint*. The middle cuneiform bone is shorter axially than the medial or lateral cuneiform bone, adding greater stability to the second tarsometatarsal joint. This is considered architecturally to be a mortise-and-tenon configuration, or a "keystone" (Fig. 24–1).

The forefoot consists of the metatarsal and phalangeal bones. Five metatarsals terminate distally with articulations to the proximal phalanges, creating the *metatarsophalangeal (MTP) joints*. The normal parabola in most humans consists of a curve, with the second metatarsal being longest and the first metatarsal being shortest and widest. Successive metatarsals, from the third to the fifth, are successively shorter, creating a tapered effect at the outer border of the foot. The fifth metatarsal has a prominent styloid process proximally, to which the peroneus brevis tendon attaches. Each of the lesser toes (two through five) has three phalanges—a proximal, a middle, and a distal (terminal) phalanx. The hallux has only two phalanges—proximal and distal. In the lesser toes, articulation between the proximal and middle phalanges is trochlea-shaped. Each distal phalanx terminates in a tuft of bone and serves as an anchor for the toe pad. Underlying the first MTP joint are the two *sesamoid* bones, which articulate with the plantar aspect of the metatarsal head. The tibial and fibular sesamoid bones are encased by the flexor hallucis brevis (FHB) tendon, which proceeds to insert at the base of the proximal phalanx, adding a mechanical advantage to the tendon pull. On occasion, the lesser metatarsals may have sesamoid bones underlying the MTP joints in similar positions.

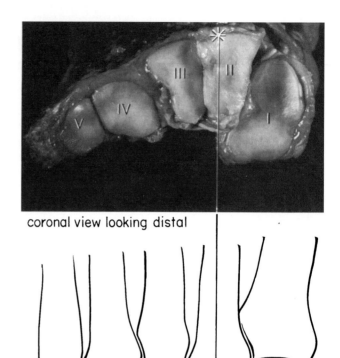

coronal view looking distal

Figure 24–1. The relationship of the bases of the five metatarsal joints. (From Jahss M [ed]: Disorders of the Foot and Ankle: Medical and Surgical Management, 2nd ed, Vol I. Philadelphia, WB Saunders, 1991, p 18.)

The ankle is a diarthrodial joint. It consists of the articulation between the talus and the confluence of the tibia and fibula, or *mortise*. The ankle joint is modeled as a single axis joint with an axis of 88 degrees at approximately the distal ends of the medial and lateral malleoli. Dorsiflexion of the ankle joint is therefore coupled with eversion of the foot, whereas plantarflexion is combined with inversion. Unloaded dorsiflexion is coupled with internal rotation of the tibia, whereas plantarflexion is accompanied by external rotation. The distal fibula has a dual function. It provides a static buttress for the talus laterally. During movement, it translates laterally, with migration of an average of 2.4 mm distally, in addition to rotating externally during the stance phase of gait. The dynamic ability of the fibula to alter its relationship through the tibiotalar joint is related to the wedge-shaped, trapezoidal nature of the talar trochlea. The fibula bears one sixth of transmitted weight during the stance phase of gait.

Ligamentous structures of the ankle joint include the medial deltoid ligament complex and the lateral ankle ligament complex. The *deltoid* ligament, or medial collateral ligament, is fan-shaped and has both superficial and deep components. The superficial components attach from the medial malleolus to the navicular and calcaneus bones and the posterior talus. The deep portion of the deltoid ligament is the primary contributor to the medial stability of the ankle joint and has two components, which attach to the medial talus. The lateral ligament complex consists of three major ligaments, including the *anterior talofibular (ATFL)*, the *calcaneofibular (CFL)*, and the *posterior talofibular (PTFL) ligaments* (Fig. 24–2). The ATFL is a thickening of the anterior portion of the joint capsule and originates from the anterior-distal fibula to insert onto the lateral neck of the talus. It is considered to be the primary restraint against anteriorly directed forces when the ankle is in the neutral position. The ATFL acts as a restraint against inversion stresses in the plantarflexed foot. The CFL is a distinct structure originating from the fibular tip and inserting on the lateral calcaneus. It is a primary restraint against varus talar tilt when the ankle is in a neutral or dorsiflexed position. Biomechanical studies suggest that the combination of the ATFL, CFL, and PTFL contributes to anterior restraint. The deep deltoid ligament is considered to be only a secondary restraint. The angle created between the ATFL and CFL averages 105 degrees in the sagittal plane. It is thought that individuals in whom greater angles separate the two ligaments may be more susceptible to recurrent sprains. Studies indicate that the ATFL is significantly more vulnerable to failure than are the other lateral ligaments. This correlates clinically, as the ATFL is the most common of the three ligaments to be injured in plantarflexion and inversion injuries.

Ligaments of the ankle syndesmosis include the anterior, posterior tibiofibular, and interosseous ligaments. With ankle dorsiflexion, the intermalleolar distance is widened and the distal fibula rotates externally. Injuries to these ligaments may occur with hyperdorsiflexion and the external rotation mechanism, creating a "high" ankle sprain, which is seen especially in athletes.

Subtalar joint motion occurs between the talus and the calcaneus in a single oblique axis plantarlateral from the talar neck through the sinus tarsi to the lateral wall of the calcaneus. The axis averages 23 degrees in the horizontal plane from the longitudinal axis of the foot and 42 degrees in the sagittal plane (Fig. 24–3). The subtalar joints' range of motion varies from 10 to 60 degrees, depending on the type of foot pattern; a cavus foot has less range of motion than does a planovalgus foot. This joint has been likened to an Archimedes right-handed screw, in which forward translation of the talus is linked with inversion, or a varus heel. Using the mitered hinge model, inversion of the subtalar joint is associated with tibial external rotation, whereas eversion is associated with tibial internal rotation. Ligamentous resistance to subtalar joint inversion is provided primarily by the inferior extensor retinaculum when the joint is in neutral and dorsiflexed positions. The CFL, the ligament of the anterior capsule, the posterior subtalar joint, the interosseous talocalcaneal ligaments, and the ligament of the tarsal canal contribute to subtalar joint stability at various joint positions.

The transverse tarsal, or *Chopart's joint*, is the sum of the saddle-shaped calcaneocuboid and the cup-shaped talonavicular joints. With the calcaneus in the valgus position, or eversion, the joints have parallel axes of rotation, resulting in a flexible transverse tarsal articulation. In the varus position (inversion), the axes of rotation diverge, resulting in a rigid midfoot. At heel strike, it is important for the transverse tarsal joint to be unlocked so as to dissipate the shock forces. However, during the later stages of the stance phase of gait, the locking of the transverse tarsal joint provides optimal stability for the push-off phase.

The midfoot joints are stabilized by multiple ligaments and by the intrinsic bony architecture of the wedge-shaped cuneiform bones. This section of the foot is primarily a stable segment designed to handle the stresses of the stance

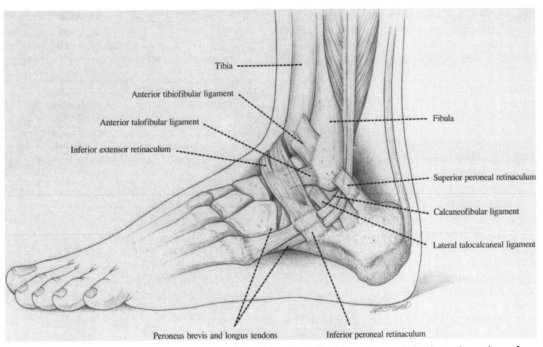

Figure 24–2. The normal anatomy of the lateral ankle ligaments and the lateral portion of the extensor retinaculum. (From Hamilton WG: The modified Brostrom procedure for acute and chronic ankle instability. Oper Tech Orthop 1992;2:143.)

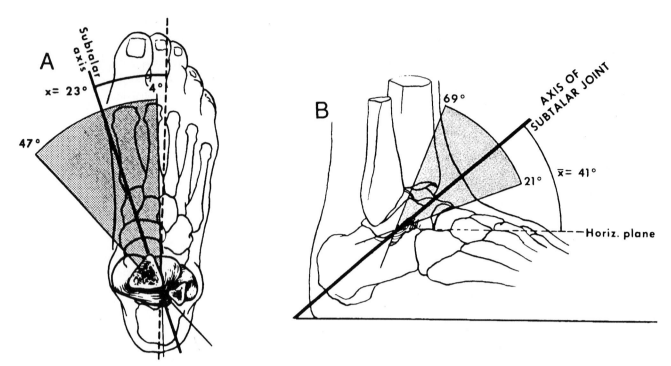

Figure 24–3. Subtalar joint axis and variations. *A*, Anteroposterior plane. *B*, Lateral plane. (From Drez D, DeLee J: Biomechanics and orthotics of the foot in athletes. Oper Tech Sports Med 1994;2[1].)

phase of gait; little motion occurs at any of the joints. Stabilizing ligaments include Chopart's ligament, which is a V-shaped structure composed of the lateral calcaneonavicular and the medial calcaneocuboid ligaments. They originate in the anterior process of the calcaneus and the navicular and cuboid bones, respectively. Long (superficial) and short (deep) plantar ligaments span from the os calcis to the cuboid bone and metatarsals (Fig. 24–4). The short ligaments also connect the calcaneus plantarly to the cuboid, navicular, and cuneiform bones. These ligaments serve as static stabilizers of the longitudinal arch. The tarsometatarsal ligaments include dorsal, plantar, and interosseous components; each of the metatarsal bases is stabilized by adjacent interosseous ligaments between the respective metatarsal bases. There is, however, no true transverse interosseous ligament between the first and second metatarsal bases. Instead, there is an oblique ligament that connects the first cuneiform bone to the second metatarsal ligament; it is known as *Lisfranc's ligament.* In addition to dorsiflexion and plantarflexion, the first metatarsal–medial cuneiform articulation has rotatory motion predominantly in supination that has been demonstrated with ground reaction forces.

The MTP joints of the lesser toes are stabilized by fibrocartilaginous plantar plates originating from the metatarsal heads and inserting on the bases of the proximal phalanges. The plates are supported by a deep transverse metatarsal ligament, which serves as an insertion point for the flexor tendon sheath and the plantar aponeurosis. Medial and lateral collateral ligaments also stabilize the MTP joints. Vertical fibers extending from the plantar plate connect to the plantar aponeurosis, skin, and transverse ligaments by way of the extensor expansion (Fig. 24–5). The

combination of plantar plates and collateral ligaments resists the dorsal instability created by ground reaction forces through the MTP joint during the later stance phases of gait. Attenuation of these structures, secondary to synovitic processes, results clinically in dorsal subluxation or dislocation. The hallux MTP joint has an excursion range of a 70-degree arc dorsally to accommodate the toe-off phase of gait. The metatarsal head articulates with two plantar sesamoid bones, which are centered through a midline crista; the sesamoid bones are stabilized in relation to each other by the intersesamoidal ligament complex. They are further stabilized by the pull of the flexor digitorum brevis tendon proximally, the abductor hallucis medially, and the adductor hallucis laterally (Fig. 24–6).

The muscles of the foot and ankle are divided into extrinsic and intrinsic muscles. The extrinsic muscles are encased in four leg compartments: the superficial and deep posterior compartments, the lateral compartment, and the anterior compartment. These muscles originate proximal to the ankle joint and insert within the foot. The majority of these muscle-tendon units cross more than one joint and thus have complex functions. The superficial posterior compartment includes the *gastrocnemius, plantaris,* and *soleus* muscles. The gastrocnemius muscle originates in the medial and lateral femoral condyles and crosses the knee joint to join with the soleus muscle, which arises from the posterior aspect of the proximal tibia and fibula. The tendon fibers of the soleus merge with gastrocnemius tendon fibers to form the *tendocalcaneus,* or *Achilles tendon.* The Achilles tendon rotates 90 degrees to insert on the posterosuperior tuberosity of the os calcis (Fig. 24–7). The plantaris originates in the lateral femoral condyle and soon becomes tendinous at the proximal ⅙ junction as it courses between

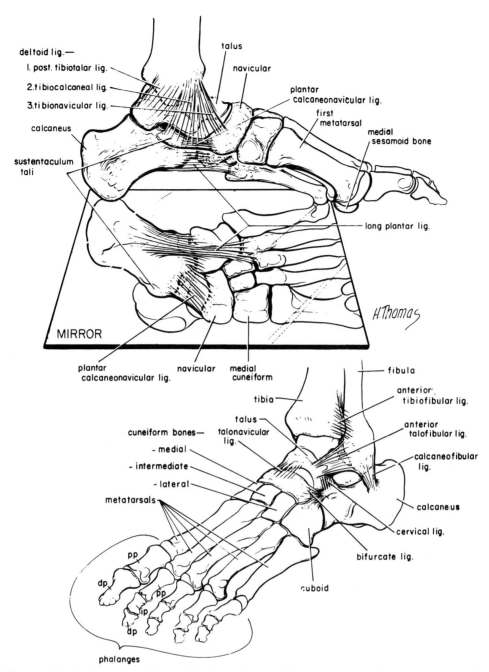

Figure 24–4. Skeleton of the adult foot showing ligamentous attachments. pp, proximal phalanx: ip, intermediate phalanx; dp, distal phalanx. (From Jahss M [ed]: Disorders of the Foot and Ankle: Medical and Surgical Management, 2nd ed, Vol I. Philadelphia, WB Saunders, 1991, p 15.)

the soleus and the gastrocnemius muscles to attach medial to the Achilles tendon on the os calcis. This muscle is variable in presentation, being absent up to 7% of the time. The muscles of the superficial posterior compartment are innervated by the tibial nerve and function as the primary plantarflexors of the ankle and foot. These muscles assist secondarily in inversion of the hindfoot.

The deep posterior compartment contains three muscles, which serve as invertors of the foot and as secondary plantarflexors (Fig. 24–8). The *tibialis posterior* muscle originates in the interosseous membrane and posterior tibia

to course behind the medial malleolus and insert on the navicular tuberosity. The tendon then courses underneath the talus to contribute static support for the longitudinal arch through fibers into the calcaneonavicular ligament, cuneiform ligaments, and plantar capsules of the middle and lateral cuneiform bones, cuboid bones, and lesser metatarsal bones. The primary function of the tibialis posterior muscle is inversion and abduction of the foot; it is also a secondary plantarflexor of the ankle. The dynamic function of the tendon is to support the longitudinal arch of the foot by stabilizing the talonavicular joint. The *flexor digitorum*

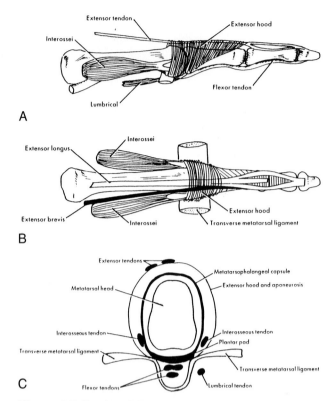

Figure 24–5. *A* to *C*, The anatomy of the lesser toe. (From Mizel M: Correction of hammertoe and mallet toe deformity. Oper Tech Orthop 1992;2:[3].)

longus (FDL) muscle originates in the interosseous membrane and passes between the posterior talar processes and then courses under the flexor retinaculum along with the posterior tibial tendon and the *flexor hallucis longus* (FHL) muscle. The FDL crosses medially and plantarly under the medial longitudinal arch at the knot of Henry along with the FHL. Distally in the foot, the FDL divides into four slips and receives insertions of the quadratus muscle. The FDL terminates by inserting on the base of the proximal phalanx of the lesser toes. The FDL serves as a weak ankle plantarflexor as well as a toe flexor, which is especially important during the final stages of gait. The FHL originates in the interosseous membrane and posterior tibia and is the most lateral muscle in the posterior deep compartment. It courses between the medial and lateral posterior talar process to travel in a fibro-osseous tunnel beneath the sustentaculum talus and then travels through the flexor tunnel between the sesamoid bones to insert on the plantar aspect of the distal phalanx. It functions as a weak plantarflexor of the ankle and a primary flexor of the hallux.

The lateral compartment contains the peroneal muscles. The *peroneus longus* muscle originates in the upper two thirds of the lateral fibula and intermuscular septum and fascia. This muscle courses posterolateral to the peroneus brevis muscle at the level of the lateral malleolus. Distally, it courses underneath the cuboid base of the fifth metatarsal to insert on the base of the first metatarsal and the medial cuneiform bone. The function of the peroneus longus is plantarflexion of the first ray and weak ankle plantarflexion and foot abduction. The *peroneus brevis* muscle originates from the distal two thirds of the fibular intermuscular septum and passes distally behind the lateral malleolus. It lies superficial to the calcaneofibular ligaments to insert on

the styloid process of the fifth metatarsal (Fig. 24–9). This muscle functions as a weak ankle plantarflexor and as a primary evertor of the foot.

The anterior leg compartment contains the *tibialis anterior*, the *extensor hallucis longus (EHL)*, and the *extensor digitorum longus (EDL)* muscles (Fig. 24–10). These muscles serve as primary dorsiflexors of the ankle and foot and

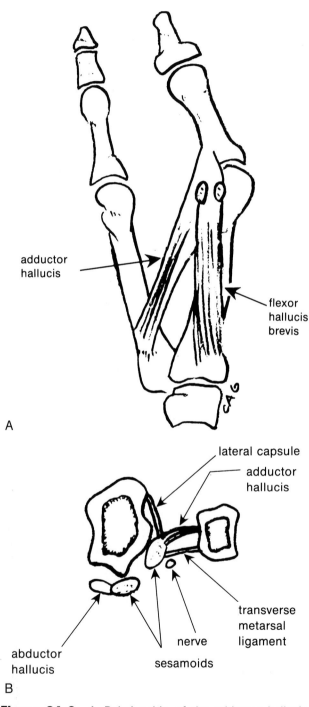

Figure 24–6. *A*, Relationship of the adductor hallucis, flexor hallucis brevis, and sesamoid bones to the first metatarsal. *B*, Coronal section of structures at the level of the sesamoid bones. (From Guanche CA, Rudicel SA: The Mann hallux valgus repair of bunion deformities. Oper Tech Orthop 1992;2:168.)

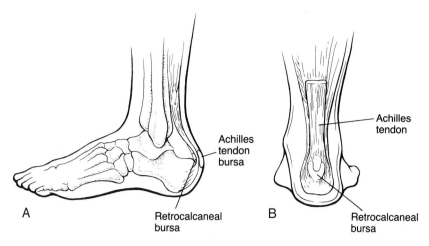

Figure 24–7. *A,* The bursa and tendon sheath that are associated with the Achilles tendon. The Achilles tendon bursa lies between the skin and the tendon, and the retrocalcaneal bursa lies between the tendon and the os calcis. *B,* An end-down, or Harris, view of the heel demonstrating that the Achilles tendon inserts medially and laterally but not in the central area where the retrocalcaneal bursa is. (From Gould J [ed]: Operative Foot Surgery. Philadelphia, WB Saunders, 1994, p 977.)

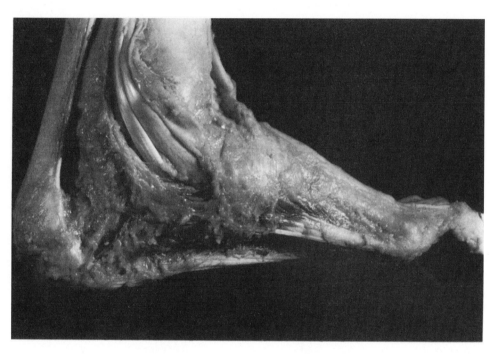

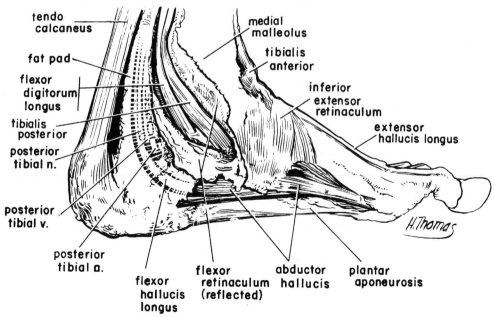

Figure 24–8. Medial view of the adult foot. (From Jahss M [ed]: Disorders of the Foot and Ankle: Medical and Surgical Management, 2nd ed, Vol I. Philadelphia, WB Saunders, 1991, p 23.)

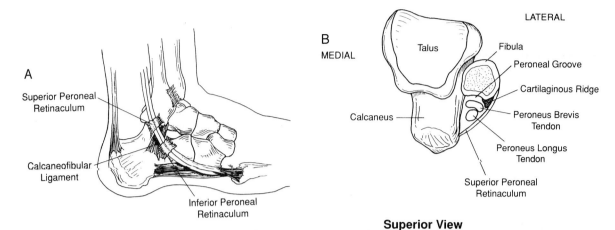

Superior View

Figure 24–9. Anatomic relationships of the ankle with the peroneal tendons held in position by the superior and inferior peroneal retinacula and the fibrous rim on the posterolateral aspect of the fibula. The calcaneofibular ligament lies below the peroneal tendons. *A*, Lateral view. *B*, Superior view. (From Clanton TO, Schon LS: Athletic injuries to the soft tissues of the foot and ankle. *In* Mann RA, Coughlin MJ [eds]: Surgery of the Foot and Ankle, 6th ed. St. Louis, Mosby-Year Book, 1993, p 1169.)

are innervated by the deep peroneal nerve. The tibialis anterior muscle originates from the lateral tibial condyle and the interosseous membrane and septum. It courses beneath the superior and inferior extensor retinaculum to insert on the medial border of the medial cuneiform bone and the base of the first metatarsal. The primary functions of the tibialis anterior are dorsiflexion of the ankle and

inversion of the subtalar joint. The EHL muscle originates in the middle two thirds of the anterior fibula and interosseous membrane and courses medially to the neurovascular bundle (the dorsalis pedis and deep peroneal nerve) to insert on the distal phalanx of the hallux. It functions as the primary extensor of the hallux, a weak dorsiflexor of the ankle, and an invertor of the foot. The EDL originates

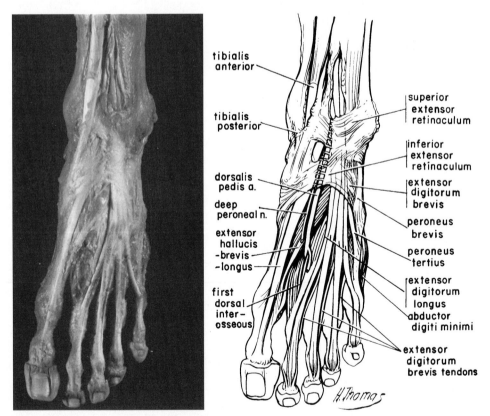

Figure 24–10. Dorsal view of the adult foot. (From Jahss M [ed]: Disorders of the Foot and Ankle: Medical and Surgical Management, 2nd ed, Vol I. Philadelphia, WB Saunders, 1991, p 19.)

in the lateral tibial condyle, interosseous membrane, and intermuscular septa. This muscle runs lateral to the neurovascular bundle to insert on the dorsal aspect of the extensor hood of the lesser MTP joints. The extensor tendon divides at the insertion into one central and two lateral slips. The central slip inserts onto the base of the middle phalanx, and the lateral slips terminate in the extensor hood of the distal phalanx. The EDL extends the MTP joints and, secondarily, through the extensor hood, extends the proximal interphalangeal (PIP) and distal interphalangeal (DIP) joints.

The intrinsic muscles of the foot are arranged in four plantar layers, and there is a single dorsal muscle, the *extensor digitorum brevis (EDB)*. The EDB originates in the superolateral calcaneus and sinus tarsi to lie along the dorsolateral aspect of the second, third, and fourth tendons of the EDL. It inserts onto the lateral capsule of the MTP joints of the toes. The lateral terminal branch of the deep peroneal nerve innervates the muscle. The medial part of the EDB muscle is termed the *extensor hallucis brevis (EHB)*, which inserts onto the base of the hallux.

The first, or superficial, layer of the intrinsic plantar muscles originates in the medial border of the os calcis and includes the *flexor digitorum brevis (FDB), abductor hallucis, and abductor digiti minimi (ADM)* muscles. These muscles lie deep to the plantar fascia in distinct compartments. The ABD originates in the medial aspect of the calcaneus to insert on the medial base of the proximal phalanx with the tendon of the medial head of the FHB. The tendon blends with the capsule of the first MTP joint. The FDB lies deep to the plantar fascia on the plantar aspect of the os calcis intermuscular septum and forms four tendons that attach to the PIP joints of the second through fifth toes. During its course, each tendon divides to allow the FDL tendons to pass through. The ADM originates from the lateral calcaneus to insert on the plantar plate and lateral phalanx of the fifth toe. This muscle functions to abduct and flex the small toe.

The second layer contains the muscles for toe motion control and includes the quadratus plantae and lumbrical muscles as well as the tendons of the FHL and FDL. The quadratus plantae muscle originates from the calcaneal tuberosity and plantar ligament (Fig. 24–11). The two heads coalesce to insert into each FDL tendon. This muscle assists the FDL in toe flexion. The lumbrical muscles originate along the medial side of the FDL tendons to pass plantar to the deep transverse metatarsal ligament, with insertions on the dorsal extensor expansions of the proximal phalanges. These muscles serve to maintain an intrinsic balance of extension of the PIP joint and flexion at the MTP joint.

The third layer is composed of intrinsic muscles assisting in first and fifth toe function. The FHB originates in the posterior tibial tendon and divides into two heads, each containing a sesamoid bone, which insert on the base of the first metatarsal. The medial head runs with the abductor hallucis tendon, and the lateral head joins with the adductor hallucis (ADH) tendon. The action of this muscle is to flex the MTP joint and stabilize it during the toe-off stance phase of gait. The adductor hallucis muscle has an oblique and transverse head; the oblique head originates in the base of the cuboid bone and second, third, and

fourth metatarsals. The transverse head originates in the plantar plates and transverse metatarsal ligaments of the third, fourth, and fifth metatarsals. The adductor hallucis inserts via a conjoined tendon onto the lateral aspect of the fibular sesamoid bone and plantar lateral plate at the base of the proximal phalanx. The action of the adductor hallucis is adduction of the hallux, and contractures contribute to hallux valgus deformities.

The fourth and deepest layer contains the seven interosseous muscles and the insertions of the peroneus longus and anterior and posterior tibial tendons. The interossei muscles are divided into two groups, with four dorsal interossei and three plantar interossei. The dorsal interossei move the toes toward the longitudinal axis of the second metatarsal (adduction), and the plantar interossei move them away from the axis (abduction). Together, the interossei muscles help to flex the MTP joints while extending the interphalangeal joints of the toes via the extensor hood and, in conjunction with the lumbricals, to maintain an intrinsically balanced foot.

The neurovascular structures of the foot and ankle include five major nerve branches and three arteries. The tibial and common peroneal nerves are the terminal branches of the sciatic nerve, which arises from the lumbosacral plexus. The common peroneal nerve (L5) is the smaller of the two branches of the sciatic nerve and courses lateral to the biceps femoris tendon and lateral head of the gastrocnemius, curving to meet the head of the fibula, where it is susceptible to trauma and compression. The nerve courses through the anterior compartment of the leg, where it divides into superficial and deep branches. The superficial peroneal nerve courses through the lateral compartment between the peroneus longus muscle and the neck of the fibula. Following muscular branches to the peroneus longus and brevis, the nerve terminates approximately 10 to 15 cm above the lateral malleolus through a fascial defect, continuing subcutaneously to provide sensory innervation to the dorsal aspect of the foot and toes. The remaining branch, the deep peroneal nerve (the anterior tibial nerve), supplies the extrinsic anterior compartment muscles and courses into the foot deep to the EDL muscle along with the anterior tibial artery. The nerve in the foot continues with the dorsalis pedis artery to provide innervation to the intrinsic foot muscles, including the EDB and EHB muscles, and terminates as a cutaneous nerve to the first web space. The sural nerve, a sensory branch of the tibial nerve, divides at the popliteal fossa to pierce the posterior fascia in the center of the calf. It provides sensation to the posterolateral hindfoot and the lateral border of the foot (Fig. 24–12).

The tibial nerve (S1) travels through the popliteal fossa superficial to the artery and vein to enter the deep posterior compartment of the calf and pass under the soleus muscle with the posterior tibial artery. As it courses medial to the Achilles tendon, it gives off branches to the FHL muscle. Proximal to coursing under the flexor retinaculum at the medial malleolus, a sensory branch, the medial calcaneal nerve, is given off and runs superficial to the flexor retinaculum to supply sensation over the medial heel. As the tibial nerve courses through the tarsal tunnel, it divides into the medial and lateral plantar nerves. The medial plantar nerve runs deep to the abductor hallucis muscle to supply intrin-

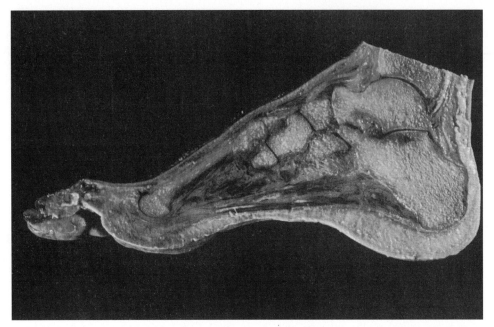

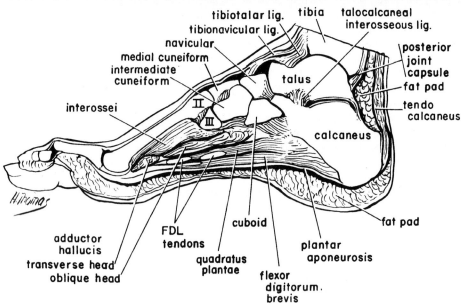

Figure 24–11. Midsagittal section of the adult foot. FDL, flexor digitorum longus. (From Jahss M [ed]: Disorders of the Foot and Ankle: Medical and Surgical Management, 2nd ed, Vol I. Philadelphia, WB Saunders, 1991, p 13.)

sic foot muscles, including the abductor hallucis FDB, FHB, and first lumbrical muscles. Distally, the nerve terminates as the proper digital nerve to the hallux and the first, second, and third web spaces, providing sensation to the medial aspect of the great toe, sole, and ball of the foot. The lateral plantar nerve courses beneath the calcaneus to innervate the abductor digiti quinti and quadratus plantae muscles and then divides into superficial and deep branches. The superficial branch contains the sensory fibers that supply the outer sole area, and a motor branch extends to the short flexor of the fifth toe. The deep branch follows the lateral plantar artery to pass between the adductor hallucis and the interosseous muscles and give small motor branches to the three lateral lumbrical muscles, the interos-

seous muscles; to the second, third, and fourth spaces; and to the transverse head of the adductor hallucis. An anatomic crossover of the lateral and medial plantar nerves is often seen in the third web space and is thought to be the cause of interdigital (Morton's) neuroma in the third plantar web space (Fig. 24–13).

The saphenous nerve is a terminal branch of the femoral nerve, originating in L2 through L4. The nerve courses along the anteromedial aspect of the lower limb posterior to the greater saphenous vein and terminates in two distal branches to provide sensation on the medial side of the ankle and foot.

Vascular supply to the foot and ankle is derived from the anterior, posterior, and peroneal arteries. The anterior

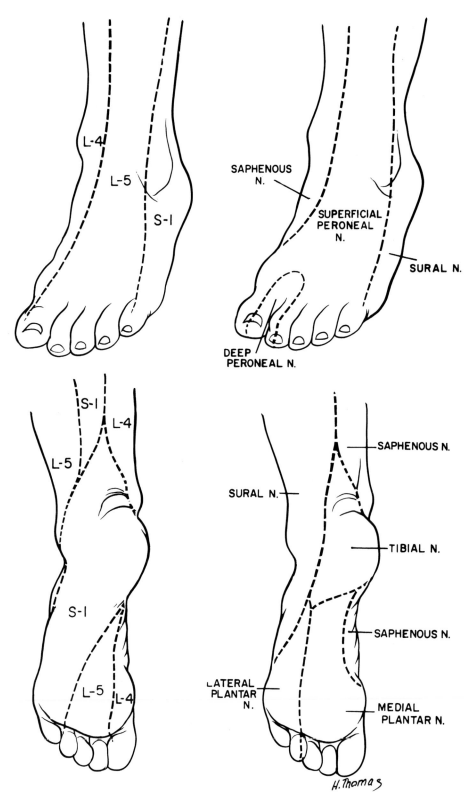

Figure 24–12. Sensory innervation of the foot. (From Jahss M [ed]: Disorders of the Foot and Ankle: Medical and Surgical Management, 2nd ed, Vol I. Philadelphia, WB Saunders, 1991, p 28.)

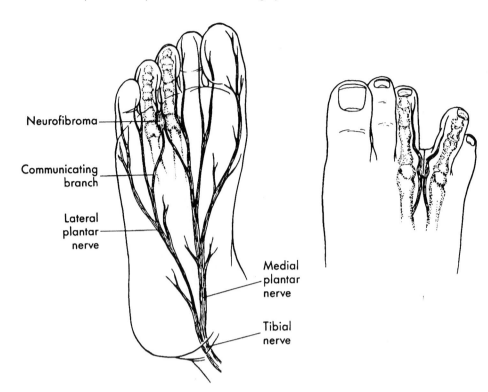

Neurofibroma

Communicating branch

Lateral plantar nerve

Medial plantar nerve

Tibial nerve

Figure 24–13. Most common location of interdigital neuroma: plantar and dorsal views. (From McElvenny RY: Morton's neuroma: The etiology and surgical treatment of intractable pain about the fourth metatarsophalangeal joint [Morton's toe]. J Bone Joint Surg [Br] 1943; 25: 675–679.)

tibial artery branches distal to the popliteus muscle in the popliteal fossa from the popliteal artery. The tibial artery passes under the popliteus muscle and runs over the superior end of the interosseous membranes to travel anterior and medial to the deep peroneal nerve. It courses below the superior and inferior extensor retinaculum to become the dorsalis pedis artery in the foot. At the level of the ankle, the anteromedial and lateral malleolar branches anastomose with the medial and lateral tarsal branches. The artery becomes the dorsalis pedis in the foot and gives off a lateral branch to the sinus tarsi. It then continues as the first dorsal metatarsal artery into the base of the first web space, where another branch, the arcuate artery, contributes to the deep plantar arterial arch. This forms the first plantar metatarsal artery. The posterior tibial artery is the continuation of the popliteal artery, which runs deep to the soleus muscle with the posterior tibial nerve to form the neurovascular bundle known as the tarsal tunnel. Distally in the foot, the vessel divides: the medial plantar artery runs medial to the plantar nerve deep to the abductor hallucis muscle to anastomose with the first plantar metatarsal artery and supply the first, second, and third web spaces of the medial three and a half toes: the lateral plantar artery is larger and passes lateral to the lateral plantar nerve in the middle compartment of the foot, runs to the fifth digit, and then curves under the oblique head of the adductor hallucis muscle to form the deep plantar arch with the perforating branch of the dorsalis pedis and provide four metatarsal arteries to the lateral portion of the four toes. The peroneal artery branch from the posterior tibial artery travels down posterior to the interosseous membrane and deep to the FHL muscle. It terminates at the distal tibiofibular joint to give off branches anteriorly that anastomose with the lateral malleolar artery of the anterior tibial artery.

The venous system of the leg is composed of the super-ficial and deep systems. The superficial system lies in the subcutaneous space and composes most of the venous return through the greater and lesser saphenous veins. These veins drain the dorsum of the foot and ankle and converge at the ankle to merge with the deep venous system. The greater saphenous vein is the largest vein to drain the dorsum of the foot. It courses anterior to the medial malleolus along the medial calf to end in the femoral vein. The lesser saphenous vein runs posterior to the fibula and drains the lateral foot and arch. The deep venous system consists of the venae comitantes of the dorsalis pedis artery. This system receives communication with the saphenous veins through perforating malleolar and metatarsal vessels.

GAIT CYCLE

The gait cycle consists of events occurring from one heel strike to the next heel strike of the same foot. Each cycle averages 120 steps per minute and is traditionally divided into a stance phase that makes up 62% of the cycle and a swing phase that makes up the remaining 38% of the cycle. The initial heel strike (0%) of the gait cycle occurs with the lower extremity in internal rotation, the ankle joint plantarflexed and the subtalar joint everted. The transverse tarsal joint is unlocked to allow for attenuation of the shock force. Pretibial or anterior compartment muscles are active in helping to decelerate the limb. At approximately 15% of the gait cycle, the lower extremity externally rotates with the ankle joint, initiating dorsiflexion, and the subtalar joint inverts (Fig. 24–14). These conditions increase stability through the midfoot to allow it to become a stable platform for push-off. The pretibial muscles are now inactive. The intrinsic muscles are increasingly becoming active

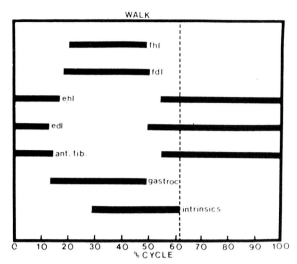

Figure 24–14. Electromyelogram of the extrinsic and intrinsic muscles about the foot and ankle. (From Mankey MG, Mann RA: Biomechanics of the first metatarsophalangeal joint. Sem Arthroplast 1992;3:3.)

and the posterior compartment calf muscles are now firing as toe-off approaches. The stance phase is divided into floor contact reaction, midstance, terminal stance, and pre-swing. At pre-swing, the ankle joint is in plantarflexion. Lift-off is defined as 60% of the gait cycle as the swing phase begins. This is divided into the initial swing and terminal swing phases. Again, the lower extremity is in internal rotation, with dorsiflexion of the ankle and eversion of the subtalar joint. This creates the unlocking of the transverse tarsal joint, and an unstable foot pattern prepares for the initial floor contact event. The pretibial muscles are again active, and the intrinsic and calf muscles are inactive.

CLINICAL EVALUATION OF THE FOOT AND ANKLE

Successful treatment of foot and ankle disorders requires taking a meticulous history and making a careful physical examination so as to achieve an accurate diagnosis. Thorough knowledge of the bony and soft tissue anatomy is integrated into the examination to confirm the diagnosis. Additionally, the kinematics of the foot and ankle do not exist in isolation but are related to the lower extremity as a whole. An ankle disorder may be the initial presentation of a systemic disorder and must therefore be taken in the context of assessing the patient as a whole.

History and Physical Examination

The objective of the history is to narrow the focus and direct attention toward the physical examination and ultimately to formulate the differential diagnosis. It is important to use a questionnaire or to personally record the responses so as to have accurate and complete documentation. Occupation, level of education, socioeconomic status, and level of activity assist in determining the degree to which patients will participate in their care. A medical and surgical history, the mechanism of injury, and the duration

of the symptoms should be elicited. The location and quality of the pain and its relationship throughout the day with activities and activity limitations should be documented. Other symptoms to be documented include timing and duration of swelling, sensation of the ankle giving way, and any noticeable changes in foot alignment. Existing systemic disorders—including inflammatory, infectious, neoplastic, metabolic, and congenital conditions—should be ruled out, placing an emphasis on diabetes and gout. A musculoskeletal history focused on associated conditions involving the spine and lower extremities is helpful in determining their relationship with the current complaints. Family history is helpful because many of the foot and ankle disorders arise from a hereditary predisposition, including congenital abnormalities and inflammatory and metabolic disorders.

General Examination Principles

Disorders of the lower extremities should be evaluated when both stockings and shoes have been removed, so that the legs are fully visible and can be accurately assessed. Gait pattern should be determined with the patient walking both toward and away from the examiner. The style and pattern of gait, foot position (including rotation), and arch configuration should be noted. Similarly, components of gait (including antalgic gait), pelvic tilt, and alterations in cadence, arm swing, and foot and leg positions in both stance and swing phases are evaluated. In the stance phase, emphasis is placed on the relationship of the hindfoot and forefoot positions, as well as on the position of the medial longitudinal arch. Examination on the frontal plane in both single and double stance toe rise and heel rise can provide valuable information.

The examiner should inspect shoes both inside and out for abnormal wear patterns and the supplemental use of orthoses. Asymmetrical shoe wear typified by lateral sole wear is associated with a cavovarus foot; medial wear is typically associated with a planovalgus foot pattern (Fig. 24–15). Orthotic devices should be evaluated for both durability and alignment when the patient is standing.

Once inspection has been completed, localized examination of the bony and soft tissue structures follows. It is helpful to have the patient first indicate specific symptomatic sites. Overall, the areas should be examined for the presence of edema, induration, effusion, skin temperature changes, skin status, and previous sites of surgery or trauma. Systematic examination is divided into subgroups, including the ankle, hindfoot, midfoot, and forefoot.

The Ankle

The ankle joint should first be assessed for evidence of effusion versus local soft tissue swelling. Effusion can best be assessed through ballottement along the anterior ankle joint, either medial to the tibialis anterior tendon or lateral to the EDL tendon. The range of motion of the ankle, which functions as a hinge joint, is normally 20 degrees of dorsiflexion and 50 degrees of plantarflexion. Range of motion should be documented for both active and passive arcs, with the knee in full extension and flexed 90 degrees. Ankle motion is gender-dependent: with increased age,

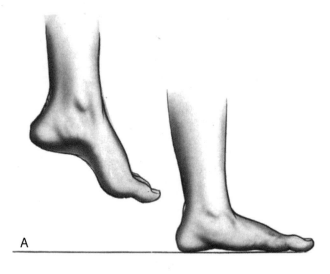

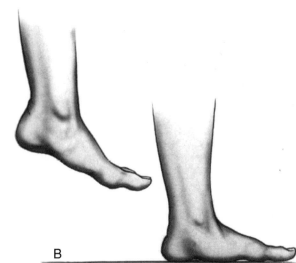

Figure 24–15. *A,* Supple pes planus. *B,* Rigid pes planus. (From Jahss M [ed]: Disorders of the Foot and Ankle: Medical and Surgical Management, 2nd ed, Vol I. Philadelphia, WB Saunders, 1991, p 58.)

men tend to have an increased arc of plantarflexion, whereas older women lose dorsiflexion. Restricted dorsiflexion resulting from an *equinus contracture* creates significant mechanical and functional disability. The ankle restricts the forward progression of the tibia over the foot during the midstance phase of gait. Loss of ankle dorsiflexion may be associated with a tight heel cord, posterior capsular contracture, or anterior bony impingement. Limitation of dorsiflexion with the knee in full extension that improves passively with the knee flexed to 90 degrees indicates a contracture of the gastrocnemius muscle.

Conditions affecting the posterior ankle and hindfoot include those involving the Achilles tendon and the posterior calcaneal tuberosity. Rupture of the Achilles tendon often presents with a palpable gap and swelling, approximately 2 to 4 cm above the site of insertion into the os calcis. The Thompson test is a reliable indicator of the competency of the Achilles tendon unit. With the patient prone and the leg hanging over the edge of the table, the clinician squeezes the patient's calves proximally. An

absence of passive plantarflexion during the squeeze is compatible with a tendon rupture. Another reliable indicator is to observe the resting tension of the foot, which normally ranges from 15 to 25 degrees of plantarflexion in an intact Achilles tendon complex. Achilles tendinosis is defined as an intact Achilles tendon with either fusiform or localized thickening in the tendon or paratenon that is painful to palpation. If the mass moves with passive dorsiflexion or plantarflexion of the ankle, the mass is localized to the tendon proper. However, with ankle range of motion, a nonmobile mass is consistent with paratenon involvement. The retrocalcaneal bursa may become inflamed and may present as a thickening proximal and anterior to the insertion site of the Achilles tendon. Normally, the soft tissues in this area are hollow medially and laterally, but they swell and lose definition in the presence of an inflamed bursa. Tenderness is elicited by squeezing the sides of the bursa. Insertional calcific tendinitis is noted by extreme hypersensitivity to palpation and localized swelling at the insertion site of the Achilles tendon. A posterior ankle impingement, or os trigonum syndrome, may be associated with swelling in the posterior ankle joint. Pain during palpation deep to the retrocalcaneal region, posterolaterally behind the peroneal tendons, in association with pain elicited with passive extreme end-range plantarflexion of the ankle joint is characteristic of this condition.

The lateral ankle joint is one of the most common sites of pathology, which is frequently associated with an ankle sprain. Because of the condensed anatomy in this region, an orderly and specific approach is essential for confirming a diagnosis. Tenderness overlying the ATFL, with or without associated pain along the CFL, is characteristic of a lateral ankle sprain. Stability testing includes the anterior drawer and inversion stress tests. To test the competency of the ATFL, an anterior drawer test is performed with the patient relaxed and the knee bent over the side of the table. One of the examiner's hands is cupped around the posterior heel while the opposite hand stabilizes the anterior tibia. An anteriorly directed force is applied to the heel, with the ankle in approximately 10 degrees of plantarflexion (Fig. 24–16). The degree of laxity is determined by the presence of a firm or soft end point. With the patient in a similar position, inversion stress is applied to the lateral aspect of the heel while stabilizing the medial tibia. Inversion stress tests should be applied in both the dorsiflexion and plantarflexion positions so as to stress the competency of both the CFL and the ATFL, respectively. All ligamentous laxity should be evaluated in comparsion with the contralateral ankle joint and the presence of generalized body ligamentous laxity. Posterolaterally, the peroneus brevis tendon may be palpated for the presence of fusiform swelling posterior and proximal to the tip of the fibula. Additionally, with provocative dorsiflexion and eversion, palpation of the tendons should be performed to denote evidence of subluxation or dislocation. Pain and weakness associated with resisted foot eversion with the ankle plantarflexed can be associated with tendon pathology. Examination of the subtalar joint should quantify the degree of the joint's range of motion in both inversion and eversion. Subtalar synovitis may result from a variety of causes, including arthrosis and inflammatory conditions. Palpating the sinus tarsi region

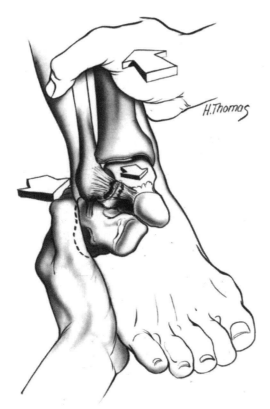

Figure 24–16. The anterior drawer sign, a test for ankle instability. (From Jahss M [ed]: Disorders of the Foot and Ankle: Medical and Surgical Management, 2nd ed, Vol I. Philadelphia, WB Saunders, 1991, p 56.)

and noting fullness or pain may isolate this condition (Fig. 24–17). Additionally, painful or restricted range of motion of the subtalar joint during inversion or eversion is characteristic of this condition. Quantitation of subtalar range of motion should be performed with the ankle positioned in neutral or in several degrees of dorsiflexion so as to control for any adjacent tibiotalar joint contribution. Inversion motion is, on average, greater than eversion by a ratio of 2:1; an individual with a cavovarus foot will have a decreased arc of motion, whereas one with a hypermobile planovalgus foot will be noted to have an increased arc of motion on the sagittal plane.

A *peroneal spastic flatfoot* is a pes planus condition associated with a rigid subtalar joint, pain in the sinus tarsi region, and spasms associated with the peroneal tendons posterior to the fibula and radiating up the lateral aspect of the leg. Disorders involving the peroneus longus tendon include tenderness and swelling distal to the tip of the fibula and beneath the cuboid sulcus. Painful os peroneus syndrome involves an accessory bone within the peroneus longus tendon as it courses under the cuboid bone. Resisted plantarflexion of the first ray during palpation of the tendon in the cuboid sulcus may help to confirm the diagnosis.

Ankle joint symptoms may be related to sprains of the distal tibiofibular joint, anterior impingement syndrome, arthrosis of the ankle joint, entrapment neuropathies, or tendon injuries. The *distal tibiofibular sprain*, or "high ankle sprain," presents as pain on palpation above the level of the ankle joint at the distal tibiofibular joint. Unlike

ankle sprains, swelling is not associated with this injury. Symptoms may be reproduced by the compression test, in which the fibula is squeezed against the tibia at the midlevel, or by the external rotation test, in which the knee is flexed 90 degrees over the table, and an external rotatory force is applied to the foot while the proximal tibia is stabilized.

The *anterior impingement syndrome* presents as a thickening or swelling in a band-like fashion across the anterolateral ankle joint, with tenderness elicited over the anteromedial region. Restricted degrees of dorsiflexion are often associated with this condition. Pain is elicited with passive dorsiflexion of the ankle joint and is relieved with plantarflexion.

Degenerative arthrosis presents with diffuse bandlike swelling and pain across the ankle joint and may have an associated ballotable ankle effusion and crepitus during passive range of motion of the joint.

Entrapment and injuries to either the superficial or the deep peroneal nerve may be associated with scars or traction involved in plantarflexion or inversion injuries. Tinel's sign, or the percussion test, will be positive overlying the nerve on either the anterolateral ankle joint (for the superficial peroneal nerve) or in the midcentral area lateral to the EHL (for the deep peroneal nerve). Anteromedial pain with maximal plantarflexion or, later, pain on palpation of the talar dome may signify either articular injury or an osteochondral talar lesion. Pain in the posteromedial ankle and hindfoot may indicate nerve entrapment and tendon pathology.

A *tarsal tunnel syndrome* consists of entrapment of either the posterior tibial nerve or one of its branches under the flexor retinaculum. A positive percussion test along the course of the neurovascular bundle with hyperesthesia in

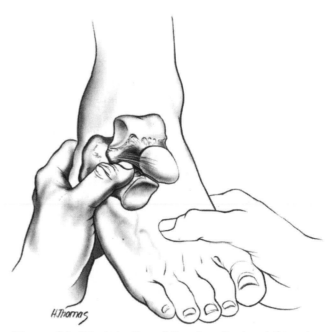

Figure 24–17. Palpation of the sinus tarsi and the anterior talofibular ligament. (From Jahss M [ed]: Disorders of the Foot and Ankle: Medical and Surgical Management, 2nd ed, Vol I. Philadelphia, WB Saunders, 1991, p 55.)

the distribution of either the medial or the lateral plantar nerves in the forefoot is associated with entrapment. The medial calcaneal nerve, which branches proximal to the tarsal tunnel and courses subcutaneously, supplies sensation to the medial aspect of the heel. Trauma to this nerve is often a source of medial heel pain.

A *deltoid sprain* may occur in conjunction with lateral ankle injuries and present as pain with palpation inferior and anterior to the medial malleolus. Rarely do these sprains occur in isolation.

Synovitis and *degeneration* of the posterior tibial tendon are common sources of medial ankle and proximal arch pain. Pain is elicited on palpation of the posterior tibial tendon along the posterior border of the medial malleolus and distally into the longitudinal arch and may be associated with swelling and thickening of the tendon.

Attritional tears, which are seen mainly in middle-aged women, are characterized by progressive loss of a medial longitudinal arch, in association with arch pain. With weight bearing, a marked asymmetry and progressive planovarus foot deformity is noted, as is excessive hindfoot valgus when viewed from behind. The medial longitudinal arch is depressed and the forefoot drifts into abduction; this creates the "too many toes" sign that is seen from behind. The pathognomonic heel-rise test demonstrates the patient's inability to correct the hindfoot valgus. The patient will be unable to perform a single-stance heel rise on the affected limb.

Injuries to the FHL tendon are often seen in dancers and may be associated with a *posterior impingement syndrome*. Pain and inflammation are noted in the tendon along the posterior margin of the ankle, proximal to the medial malleolus. The pain is aggravated by passive motion of the hallux when the ankle is brought from dorsiflexion to plantarflexion. Tears in the tendon and fusiform thickening occur, creating a triggering effect associated with stenosing tenosynovitis. This results in complete loss of passive extension of the hallux when the ankle is in dorsiflexion.

The Heel

Heel pain may have a variety of causes, including nerve entrapment, local stress fracture, and inflammation and trauma to the plantar fascia. Plantar heel pain localized to the central weight-bearing area and elicited on direct palpation can be associated with either atrophy of the heel pad or a subcalcaneal bursitis. *Calcaneal stress fractures* occur as a result of repetitive high-impact loading; diffuse swelling is associated with tenderness elicited by medial and lateral heel compression. *Plantar fasciitis* and traumatic rupture produce tenderness along the central band of the plantar aponeurosis, distal from the origin and along the medial calcaneal tubercle. When passive dorsiflexion occurs, it puts the plantar fascia on stretch, and tenderness with palpation of the plantar fascia is characteristic (Fig. 24–18). In acute cases, a palpable gap and localized swelling may be associated in the midarch region. *Plantar fibromatosis*, like plantar fasciitis, is a painful nodular thickening adherent to the plantar fascia, often in isolation or in satellite in the midsubstance of the plantar fascia. Entrapment of the first branch of the lateral plantar nerve (Baxter's nerve) produces heel pain that is manifested on palpa-

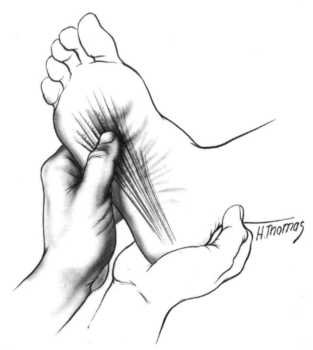

Figure 24–18. Palpation of the plantar fascia. (From Jahss M [ed]: Disorders of the Foot and Ankle: Medical and Surgical Management, 2nd ed, Vol I. Philadelphia, WB Saunders, 1991, p 58.)

tion above the abductor hallucis muscle medially. Direct palpation or percussion may create a bony sensation on the plantar heel that extends over to the lateral border. *Heel pain syndrome*, or heel spurs, is classic heel pain localized to the origin of the plantar fascia on the plantar medial calcaneal tuberosity. Pain is elicited with direct palpation and is often diagnosed through a process of exclusion of the other local diagnostic conditions.

The Midfoot

Injuries involving the midfoot generally involve sprains of the various plantar ligaments of the midtarsus and degenerative conditions secondary to traumatic and inflammatory processes. Selective palpation correlated with the bony anatomy is essential to isolating the specific joint or joints involved. The accessory navicular bone can be a painful symptomatic accessory bone along the medial aspect of the navicular tuberosity, where a component of the posterior tibial tendon inserts. Pain may be elicited with resisted plantarflexion and inversion while palpating the prominence. Sprains of the tarsometatarsal joints may be associated with swelling throughout the midfoot. Pain may be elicited with re-creation of the traumatic event, using a pronation abduction force applied through the forefoot while stabilizing the hindfoot. Any instability through these joints should be recorded. Pain on palpation of the anterolateral process of the calcaneus would be associated with an avulsion injury of the EDB, as a differential diagnosis from a plantarflexion or inversion type of injury.

The Forefoot

Most common disorders of the foot and ankle occur at the forefoot and involve the hallux and lesser toes. Disorders of the hallux include hallux valgus, hallus rigidus, sesamoiditis, and fracture. *Hallux valgus* is a lateral deviation of the great toe at the MTP joint, which may have a number of causes. On inspection, the toe demonstrates lateral drift with associated external rotation or pronation and subluxation in a lateral direction. This creates the painful prominence along the dorsomedial MTP joint commonly referred to as a bunion. The torsion position of the toe creates overloading under the medial base of the proximal phalange, leading to a hyperkeratotic junctional "pinch" callus. Similarly, because of the altered biomechanics, a transfer lesion may occur, with overloading of the second MTP joint, as demonstrated by a painful callus under the second metatarsal head. Compression of the dorsomedial cutaneous nerve of the hallux as it runs over a prominent medial exostosis may cause a burning dysesthetic pain, and a positive percussion test radiates into the hallux.

Sesamoiditis is secondary to inflammation, overload, or fracture under the first metatarsal head that is localized to either the medial or the lateral sesamoid bone. Symptoms may be elicited with passive dorsiflexion of the first MTP joint while palpating the sesamoid complex. *Hallux rigidus* and *hallux limitus* are degrees of arthrosis involving the first MTP joint. The pain is initially localized to the dorsum of the MTP joint. Palpable osteophytes may be noted. A more involved condition associated with advanced hallux rigidus is diffuse *arthrosis*, which is manifested by swelling, thickening of the capsule, and crepitus with axial grind (Fig. 24–19). Motion of the MTP joint is restricted in comparison with that of the opposite foot. First, MTP joint motion is measured with a starting reference position of zero. The hallux is placed in a functional neutral position by aligning the great toe with the plantar surface of the foot. The surface plane is defined as a line connecting the calcaneus tuberosity to the head of the first metatarsal. Sagittal functional motion is noted with plantarflexion and dorsiflexion. Similarly, mobility and subluxation in the coronal plane are recorded.

Disorders of the lesser toes involve deformities of the toes, both fixed and flexible, and include metatarsalgia and

nerve entrapment. A *hammer toe* is characterized by a flexion contracture at the PIP joint with an associated mild extension contracture of the MTP joint. A *claw toe* is an extension of a hammer toe that is typified by hyperextension of the MTP joint and flexion contractures at both the PIP and DIP joints. Mallet toe deformity is an isolated flexion contracture at the DIP joint secondary to an FDL tendon. When examining deformities of the lesser toes, it is necessary to assess the flexibility and stability of the joints, ranging from located to subluxated to frankly dislocated. Additionally, identification of callosities on the dorsum of the PIP joint or at the terminal digit is necessary. A *corn*, or a hyperkeratotic thickening of the skin in response to mechanical pressure against the dorsum of the toe box, caused by shoe wear, is seen commonly and may be painful. A soft corn, or clavus, is typically seen in the fourth web space and is caused by abutment of the proximal phalanx of one toe against the metatarsal head or base of the proximal phalanx of the adjacent fifth toe. A clavus, unlike a hard corn, is soft and macerated, and secondary infection may be present. It is re-created by compressing the two toes and the web space together.

Synovitis is noted to occur in the lesser MTP joints and presents as diffuse swelling and thickening of the joint. Assessment of the degree of extrinsic tightness and reducibility of the MTP joint is performed by the push-up test. The test assesses the reduction of the joint when the clinician pushes dorsally under the corresponding metatarsal head (Fig. 24–20). Palpation by squeezing in a dorsoplantar direction across the MTP joint assesses the fusion and re-creates the pain. *Instability* of the MTP joint is a sequela that results from unremitting synovitis with associated disruption or attenuation of the collateral ligaments and plantar plate. This may best be documented by stabilizing the metatarsal shaft with one hand and grasping the base of the proximal phalanx with the other in an attempt to dorsally translocate the toe (Fig. 24–21). A *crossover toe* deformity is typically localized to the second MTP joint and may be associated with a hallux valgus deformity. If mobile lesser toe MTP joints are involved with dorsal dislocation, underlying inflammatory arthropathy such as rheumatoid arthritis may be responsible.

Metatarsalgia is pain under the metatarsal heads that may result from a variety of causes. Atrophy of the fat pad and inflammatory conditions should be noted, as should the existence of hyperkeratotic lesions. Localized thickening of the plantar skin in reaction to excessive pressure on bony prominences must be distinguished from plantar warts. Calluses are painful when undergoing direct pressure by palpation, and they lack satellite lesions (Fig. 24–22). Plantar warts may have satellite lesions and are most painful with side squeezing. When pared, a callus may have a central seed corn without bleeding, whereas a viral wart typically has punctate, hemorrhagic edges.

A *Morton neuroma* commonly occurs in the third or, less commonly, second web space as a result of traumatized overuse injuries. Plain pressure in the web space elicits tenderness and may re-create the symptoms. Percussion in the plantar web space over the neuroma, with the toes extended, may re-create paresthesia that extends into the digits. A provocative test elicits a click known as a Mulder click when the foot is squeezed during palpation of the

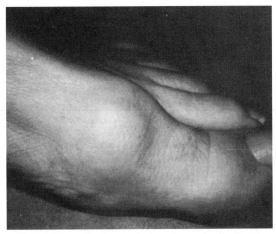

Figure 24–19. Dorsal osteophytes and swelling can be observed in this patient with hallux rigidus. (From Gould J [ed]: Operative Foot Surgery. Philadelphia, WB Saunders, 1994, p 23.)

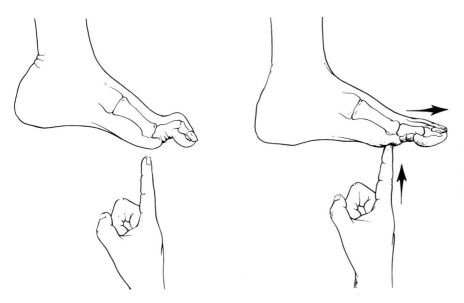

Figure 24–20. The push-up test. When the toes are easily flexible, pushing up on the metatarsal heads resolves the hammer toe deformity. (From Johnson KA: Surgery of the Foot and Ankle. New York, Raven Press, 1989, p 110.)

plantar web space distal to the intermetatarsal ligament (Fig. 24–23). Swelling in both the plantar and dorsal metatarsal regions, proximal to the metatarsal head, may be associated with a stress fracture, which is usually caused by repetitive activities such as marching. An individual with a relatively long, stiff second ray and a cavus foot is particularly at risk for repetitive stress overload and fracture.

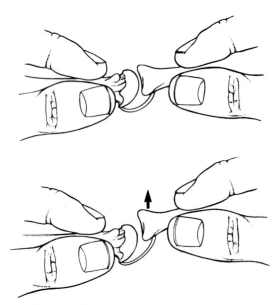

Figure 24–21. The vertical stress test for MTP subluxation. Note that this is *not* a test of dorsiflexion around the joint. The metatarsal head must be stabilized with one hand as the other hand exerts a straight vertical push while grasping the proximal phalanx. No vertical upward movement is a negative test result and indicates a normal volar plate *(top)*. Upward vertical movement is a positive test result and indicates volar plate instability *(bottom)*. (From Gould J [ed]: Operative Foot Surgery. Philadelphia, WB Saunders, 1994, p 38.)

Gait

Gait should be noted, as it commonly deviates in the presence of deformities of the lower extremity. Typical gait is a reciprocal heel-toe pattern. Arthritic conditions of the hindfoot result in a vaulting or circumduction type of gait combined with external rotation to make up for the loss of motion in the involved joints. Equinus contractures result in a delay in heel strike and may be compensated for through a recurvation deformity of the ipsilateral knee. In the valgus foot, posterior tibial tendon insufficiency can be demonstrated as a delay in the rising of the midfoot during the second and third phases of stance.

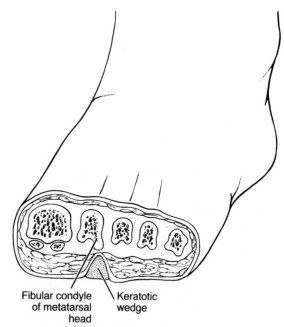

Fibular condyle of metatarsal head   Keratotic wedge

Figure 24–22. A prominent fibular condyle leading to a callus. (From Gould J [ed]: Operative Foot Surgery. Philadelphia, WB Saunders, 1994, p 71.)

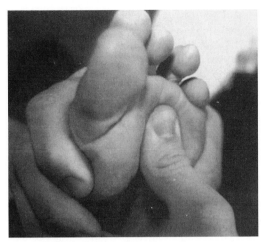

Figure 24–23. Eliciting Mulder's sign. (From Guten G [ed]: Running Injuries. Philadelphia, WB Saunders, 1997, p 166.)

Figure 24–24. Tangential view of normal sesamoids bones. The bony architecture is normal, and the sesamoid bones fit accurately into the groove on the plantar surface of the metatarsal head. (From Jahss M [ed]: Disorders of the Foot and Ankle: Medical and Surgical Management, 2nd ed, Vol I. Philadelphia, WB Saunders, 1991, p 74.)

RADIOLOGY OF THE FOOT AND ANKLE

Radiographic studies of the foot and ankle require a weight-bearing stance when possible. Key views of the foot involve anteroposterior (AP), lateral, and oblique views; those for the ankle involve AP, lateral, and mortise views. The AP view of the foot offers adequate assessment of forefoot and midfoot pathology. The beam is directed 15 degrees from the vertical toward the hindfoot, with the beam centered at the level of the talonavicular and calcaneocuboid joints. To avoid distortion secondary to parallax, each foot should be exposed on a separate flat plate. A lateral view is obtained in a lateral-to-medial projection. The cassette is placed parallel to the medial side of the foot. This allows assessment of the relationship of the talus and calcaneus to that of the midfoot, forefoot, and ankle joint. Oblique views are obtained, including a medial or internal oblique view and additional lateral or external oblique views. A medial oblique view is used to

evaluate the relationship of the lateral tarsometatarsal joints in the midfoot. It is obtained with the knee flexed and the side of the foot angled at 30 degrees to the surface of the cassette; the beam is directed vertically. A reverse oblique view is helpful for visualizing accessory navicula.

Ancillary studies include radiographs to assess sesamoid bones, the os calcis, and the subtalar joint. Visualization of sesamoid bones is difficult because of the overlapping first metatarsal on AP projections and lateral metatarsals on lateral views. The sesamoid view assesses the status of the sesamoid bones axially; a beam is directed tangential to the plantar surface of the sesamoid region while the patient's toes are held in hyperextension (Fig. 24–24). The Harris axial view is used to assess the status of the calcaneal tuberosity associated with calcaneus fractures or in delineating a talocalcaneal coalition (Fig. 24–25). This view is obtained by directing a beam approximately 40

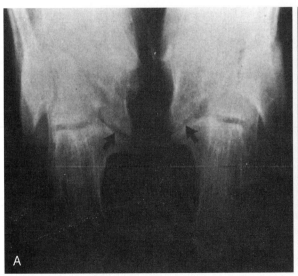

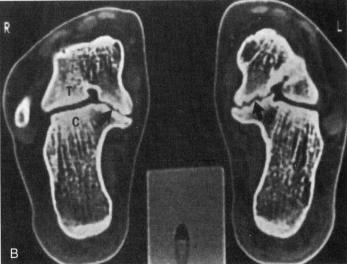

Figure 24–25. Bilateral subtalar coalition. Os calcis view demonstrates bilateral tarsal coalitions *(arrows)*. (From Jahss M [ed]: Disorders of the Foot and Ankle: Medical and Surgical Management, 2nd ed, Vol I. Philadelphia, WB Saunders, 1991, p 124.)

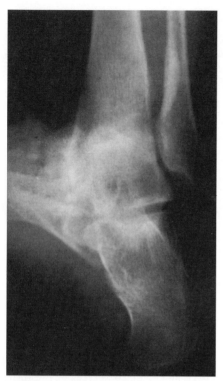

Figure 24–26. A Broden view shows the posterior facet of the subtalar joint and provides an excellent view of the talofibular and tibiofibular joints. (From Jahss M [ed]: Disorders of the Foot and Ankle: Medical and Surgical Management, 2nd ed, Vol I. Philadelphia, WB Saunders, 1991, p 75.)

degrees cephalad to the long axis of the foot with the foot in maximal dorsiflexion. The status of the subtalar joint can best be assessed by using the Broden series of radiographs (Fig. 24–26). They are obtained with the foot positioned so that the ankle is in neutral dorsiflexion and plantarflexion and is internally rotated 45 degrees. Four views are obtained: the beam is angled cephalad at 10, 20, 30, and 40 degrees while it is centered 2 cm anterior and distal to the tip of the lateral malleolus. The 10-degree view demonstrates the posterior portion of the posterior facet; the 20- and 30-degree views demonstrate the medial facet; and the 40-degree angulation demonstrates the anterior portion of the posterior facet. These views are helpful for assessing the status of the posterior facet necessary in cases of intra-articular calcaneus fractures and to delineate subtalar arthrosis.

An AP radiography of the tibiotalar joint allows evaluation of the status of the joint, the relationship of the distal tibia and fibula, the talar dome surface, and the integrity of the tibiofibular syndesmosis. This view is obtained in a weight-bearing mode, with the ankle in neutral dorsiflexion and plantarflexion. The lateral view is also obtained while the patient is standing, and it might be obtained in conjunction with a lateral view of the foot. It is obtained by placing the cassette, which may be propped using a sandbag, parallel to the medial side of the ankle. Evaluation includes the relationship of the tibiotalar joint to the talocalcaneal alignment and the presence of soft tissue swelling or ankle effusion. The mortise view is obtained with the ankle in neutral dorsiflexion and plantarflexion and the leg inter-

nally rotated 20 degrees to create parallelism of the malleoli. This is helpful for assessing the joint space equally on all three sides of the talar dome.

Other views of the ankle include stress radiographs to demonstrate ankle instability and the modified Coby view to assess the mechanical alignment of the tibiocalcaneal relationship. Stress radiographs include the varus, or inverted, stress view; the anterior drawer stress view; and the Broden stress view. In acute situations, an ankle block of 1% lidocaine is recommended. It is also recommended that comparable views be obtained of the contralateral (uninjured) ankle to rule out ligamentous laxity. The varus stress view assesses the anterior talofibular ligament when it is taken with the ankle in plantarflexion (Fig. 24–27). The status of the calcaneofibular ligament is assessed when the ankle is in dorsiflexion. The AP radiograph of the ankle is taken as varus stress is applied to the calcaneus while the tibia is stabilized. It is believed that a difference in talar tilt of more than 10 degrees between the right and left sides is consistent with instability (Fig. 24–28). Anterior drawer stress radiographs are considerably more reliable indicators of instability and have greater specificity for the

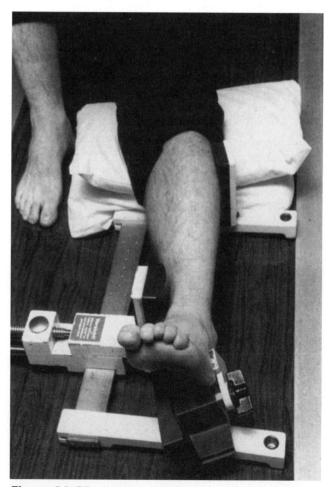

Figure 24–27. Patient positioned for inversion stress examination. The calcaneal attachment is positioned at 18 degrees in order to approximate a mortise view. (From Jahss M [ed]: Disorders of the Foot and Ankle: Medical and Surgical Management, 2nd ed, Vol I. Philadelphia, WB Saunders, 1991, p 82.)

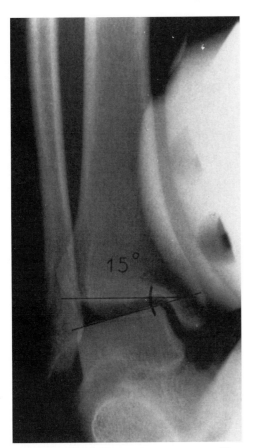

Figure 24-28. Positive inversion stress test. (From Jahss M [ed]: Disorders of the Foot and Ankle: Medical and Surgical Management, 2nd ed, Vol I. Philadelphia, WB Saunders, 1991, p 85.)

status of the anterior talofibular ligament. The patient is positioned supine and a rigid board is placed under the heel; a standard lateral radiograph is then obtained while posterior stress is applied to the distal tibia. A change of 4 mm or more in anterior displacement is considered significant. It has been advocated that a stress radiograph that indicates a difference of 2 mm between the ankles also be viewed as abnormal. A modified Coby view is taken from posterior to anterior, with the beam angled 20 degrees caudad from the horizontal. This allows for assessment of the tibiocalcaneal axis to determine the degree of varus or valgus positioning during weight-bearing.

Ancillary radiographic studies include computed tomography (CT), magnetic resonance imaging (MRI), radionuclide studies, tomography, and dye-injection studies involving tomography and ankle arthrography. CT consists of thin-section images in sagittal, coronal, and axial planes that may detect occult lesions and delineate interarticular pathology better than plain radiographs. Other applications include assessing fractures, such as those of the pilon, talus, and calcaneus, and evaluating osteochondral lesions of the talus and congenital abnormalities in addition to tarsal coalitions. This involves 3- to 5-mm bony and soft tissue windows. Multiplanar reconstructions can yield coronal and axial images. Viewing subtalar joint pathology requires that sections be taken perpendicular to the posterior facet at 30 degrees cephalad. Axial images use cuts

parallel to the sole of the foot. MRI is used to assess soft tissue structures, such as soft tissue tumors, osteomyelitis, avascular necrosis, bone tumors, chondral lesions, and tendon abnormalities, including distinguishing between tenosynovitis and tears. MRI has the advantage of showing structures in more than one plane, thus eliminating the need for reconstructions. T1-weighted images reveal greater anatomic detail. In these images, fat has a high signal intensity and tendons and ligaments have low signal intensities. T2-weighted images have better contrast—tendons and ligaments are dark and fluid is bright—which facilitates assessment of effusions and tenosynovitis. T1 inversion recovery (STIR) allows for visualization of the anatomy and simultaneous assessment of pathology involving the various soft tissue structures.

TRAUMA

Bony traumatic injuries of the ankle mortise include pilon, ankle, and syndesmosis injuries. Pilon fractures are high-energy injuries involving intra-articular fractures of the tibial metaphysis extending into the plafond. The mechanism of injury is primarily axial compression, but there may be a rotatory component. Pilon fractures are classified on the basis of intra-articular incongruity and degree of comminution. Type I fractures are intra-articular fractures without significant articular displacement. Type II fractures have a greater degree of incongruity of the articular surface without comminution. Type III fractures have incongruity in addition to high comminution of the metaphyseal region. Although these fracture patterns may exist in isolation from the distal tibia, distal fibular fracture is commonly involved.

Pilon Fractures

Management of pilon fractures is technically challenging because of their high-energy nature and the potential of extensive soft tissue involvement and comminution in the metaphyseal area of the tibia (Fig. 24-29). Nondisplaced pilon fractures may be treated nonoperatively with immobilization in a cast. Type II and type III fractures involving significant comminution or displacement of the joint or both require open reduction and internal fixation when possible. Surgical approach and type of fixation are dependent on the degree of soft tissue injury and the level of comminution. For lower energy injuries with less comminution, internal fixation using screws and a plate is recommended. A posterolateral incision is made initially to stabilize the fibula with a plate and screws so as to restore fibular length. The pilon fracture is then approached using an anteromedial incision overlying the anterior tibial tendon, maintaining a 7-cm skin bridge. Fragments are reduced and stabilized with K-wires or screw fixation followed by bone grafting of the cancellous defect in the metaphysis. A medial buttress plate is added for stability of the medial column and to prevent a sequela of varus angulation. Newer techniques, especially in high-energy injuries with soft tissue compromise, include the use of combined circular fine wire fixation with limited internal fixation. Reports indicate that outcomes are similar to those

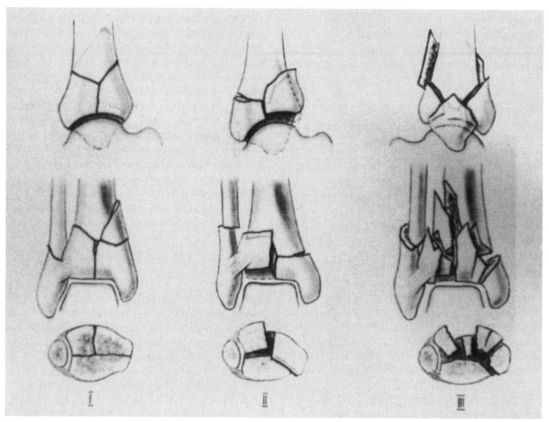

Figure 24–29. The Ruedi and Allgower classification of fractures of the tibial plafond. (From Ruedi TP, Allgower M: The operative treatment of intra-articular fractures of the lower end of the tibia. Clin Orthop 1979;138:105–110.)

involving more extensile approaches in which greater soft tissue stripping is required for plating. When pilon fractures involve skin loss, loss of fixation and infection occur in more than 50% of cases. Typical treatments of type II and type III fractures may yield a 70 to 80% rate of satisfactory outcomes. Outcome is related to the adequacy of reduction, the energy of injury, the degree of comminution, and the extent of articular damage.

Ankle Fractures

Ankle fractures are among the most common fractures treated by orthopaedic surgeons. With an aging population, the incidence and severity of ankle fractures have increased. Focal presentation is a twisting injury of the ankle with immediate pain and inability to bear weight on the ankle. Ecchymosis, deformity, and crepitus may be associated. Radiographic evaluation consists of non–weight-bearing AP, lateral, and mortise views of the ankle joint. Indications for radiography include gross deformity, instability of the ankle, crepitus, localized bone tenderness, swelling, tenderness, and inability to bear weight. Neurologic evaluation of the ankle is based on two major classification systems (Fig. 24–30).

1. The Weber-AO system classifies ankle fractures based on the anatomic level of the fibular fracture. Type A fractures are at or below the level of the ankle mortise. Type B fractures extend obliquely,

proximal to the joint level. Type C fractures are high fibular fractures that start above the tibial plafond, and they are commonly associated with syndesmotic injuries.

2. The Lauge-Hansen classification system (see Fig. 24–30) is based on cadaveric studies of mechanism and severity of injury. This system accounts for both bony and ligamentous injuries to the ankle but suffers from a high degree of interobserver variability in classification. This system uses two terms: The first relates to the position of the foot at the time of the injury, and the second relates to the direction of force applied. The position of supination composes approximately 75% of all cases; this category is divided into adduction and eversion subtypes. Supination-adduction injuries are further classified into two stages: Stage I is a transverse fracture of the lateral malleolus or a tear of the lateral collateral ligaments; stage II is an extension of stage I, with fracture of the medial malleolus. Supination-external rotation fractures are divided into four stages: Stage I is a tear of the anterior capsule and ATFL; stage II is an oblique or spiral fibular fracture, a pattern similar to that of the Weber-AO type B fracture; stage III is a stage II injury plus the fracture of the posterior lip of the tibia; stage IV encompasses the injuries of the first three stages plus a fracture of the medial malleolus or a tear of the deltoid ligament. Alteration of the

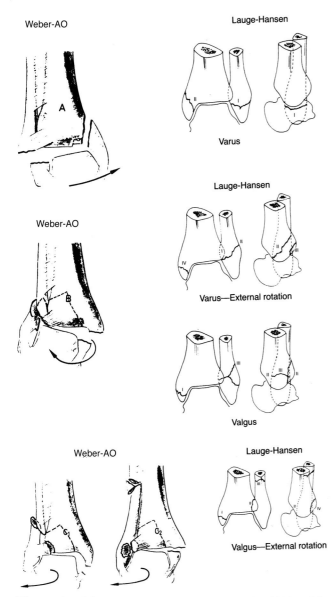

Weber-AO

Lauge-Hansen

Varus

Lauge-Hansen

Varus—External rotation

Valgus

Weber-AO

Lauge-Hansen

Valgus—External rotation

Weber-AO

Figure 24–30. The relationship between the Weber-AO and the Lauge-Hansen classification systems for ankle fractures. The most confusing area is the Weber-AO type B fracture, which corresponds to two different fracture types and mechanisms of injury in the Lauge-Hansen system. (From Gould J [ed]: Operative Foot Surgery. Philadelphia, WB Saunders, 1994, p 330.)

initial foot position from supination to pronation alters the initiation of the injury and thus the fracture pattern. Pronation-related injuries are initiated on the medial side of the ankle as a result of the initial deltoid ligament tension created by a pronated foot position. The pronation-abduction fracture is made up of three stages: Stage I involves a fracture of the medial malleolus or a tear of the deltoid ligament; state II includes stage I plus rupture of the inferior tibiofibular ligament and fracture of the posterior lip or posterior malleolus; stage III is an extension of stage II plus an oblique supramalleolar fracture of the fibula. This correlates

with a Weber-AO type C fracture. Here the fracture pattern extends through the anterior and posterior tibiofibular ligaments but preserves the interosseus ligament. The pronation-eversion fracture is made up of four stages. The first stage is a fracture of the medial malleolus or a tear of the deltoid ligament similar to that of the pronation-abduction stage I injury; stage II consists of a stage I injury plus a tear of the anteroinferior tibiofibular ligament and interosseus ligament; stage III extends the fracture pattern to involve a spiral fracture of the fibula, 7 to 8 cm proximal to the tip of the lateral malleolus; stage IV includes the addition of a fracture of the posterior lip of the tibia resulting from avulsion of the posterorinferior and inferior transverse tibiofibular ligaments. With the increased complexity of the Lauge-Hansen classification system, interobserver agreement is less than 50%, whereas the reliability rate of the Weber-AO system is higher, at approximately 58%.

Management of ankle fractures is related to the degree of lateral fibular displacement and, more specifically, the degree of lateral talar translation. The acceptable range of fibular displacement is between 0 and 5 mm in any direction, whereas less than 2 mm of talar shaft displacement is considered acceptable on plain radiographs (Fig. 24–31). Overlap of the tibia and fibula is measured in the syndesmotic space 1 cm proximal to the tibial plafond. The criterion for a normal relationship is more than 1 mm of overlap on any view or a clear space between the medial border of the fibula and the border of the tibia that measures less than 6 mm on the plain studies.

Simple lateral malleolus fractures (Weber-AO type A) are often reducible and do well with a closed treatment regimen. Good to excellent results have been noted in 95 to 98% of patients in follow-up studies ranging from 3 to 30 years. A non–weight-bearing, short leg cast is applied immediately, and protected weight bearing is instituted in 10 days to 2 weeks for approximately 6 weeks until there is early radiographic evidence of healing. The patient may then receive an ankle brace for an additional month. In bimalleolar ankle fractures and fractures involving deltoid disruption, the medial and lateral supporting structures have been compromised. These fractures are considered unstable and generally require surgical intervention to restore the alignment of the ankle joint. The goal of surgical treatment is to restore normal anatomic relationships and to allow for early range of motion so as to minimize stiffness after injury.

Anatomic reduction yields an 85 to 90% rate of good to excellent results. The surgical approach involves a lateral-longitudinal incision over the fibula and application of a one-third semitubular plate. One screw may be placed from anterior to posterior, perpendicular to the fracture site, to secure reduction. The plate is contoured posterolaterally and stabilized with 3.5-mm cortical screws proximally and 4-mm cancellous screws distally into the metaphyseal bone. In the presence of deltoid tears, the medial joint requires exploration and fibular reduction for restoration of the tibiotalar relationship in most cases. On the rare occasions when reduction cannot be achieved, the deltoid may have flipped into the medial joint space; a medial arthrotomy is

SYNDESMOSIS RADIOGRAPHIC CRITERIA
Mortise View

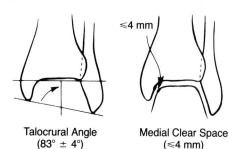

Talocrural Angle
(83° ± 4°)

Medial Clear Space
(≤4 mm)

Talar Tilt
(≤2 mm)

Anteroposterior View

A = Lateral border of
    posterior malleolus
B = Medial border of fibula
C = Lateral border of
    anterior tibial
    tubercle

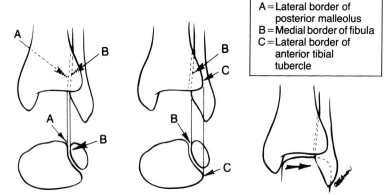

Syndesmosis A
(<5 mm)

Syndesmosis B
(≥10 mm)

Talar Subluxation

Figure 24–31. Radiographic criteria for abnormalities in ankle joint spaces, as suggested by Stiehl. (From Stiehl JB: Ankle fractures with diastasis. Instruct Course Lect 1990;39:95.)

required to remove the interposed soft tissue. If there is an associated medial malleolar fracture, it is stabilized after the lateral malleolus is fixed. In a similar anterior ankle arthrotomy, the medial malleolus is reduced and stabilized under direct visualization of the joint. Grade II 4-mm, cannulated, partially threaded screws approximately 40 mm in length are sufficient. In a smaller fracture or avulsion injury, either a single screw with a K-wire or tension band fixation with K-wires to control rotation is sufficient. Other issues involving ankle fractures include managing the posterior malleolus (in a trimalleolar fracture) and addressing syndesmotic injuries and open ankle fractures. The posterior malleolus involves less than one third to one quarter of the total AP diameter of the tibial joint surface, and no fixation is required. Indirect reduction is achieved with dorsiflexion of the ankle joint in a cast. When the posterior articular surface fragment comprises 25% or less of the total sagittal area, nonoperative treatment has been as successful as surgical fixation. When displacement is greater than 25% or more than 2 mm, reduction by means of percutaneous clamps and fixation from anterior to posterior using a 4-mm cannulated cancellous screw may be required.

Injury of the Syndesmosis

Syndesmotic injuries, with resultant disruption of the syndesmosis and diastasis of the distal tibia and fibula, are associated with higher Weber-AO grades of ankle fractures. Medial stability is often maintained with reduction of medial malleolus fractures. When a deltoid tear occurs and the syndesmotic injury extends 3 to 4.5 cm above the plafond, stabilization of the syndesmosis is recommended in the absence of fibular displacement (see Fig. 24–31). Once the fibula and medial malleolus are reduced, syndesmotic stability is determined on the operating table by stressing and visualizing under fluoroscopy. Reduction and stabilization of the syndesmosis are achieved by using a single 3- to 4.5-mm screw that engages three cortices, including the two fibular cortices and the lateral tibial cortex. The screw should be fully threaded and placed parallel to the plafond without using a lag technique. Overcompression of the fibula against the tibia will result in reduction of ankle dorsiflexion. This is avoided by placing the screw so that the ankle is maintained at 10 to 15 degrees of dorsiflexion. It is recommended that the screw remain in place for a minimum of 10 to 12 weeks; there is debate concerning resumption of weight-bearing status prior to screw removal because of the potential problem of hardware failure. Several studies have demonstrated a minimal rate of screw breakage with early weight bearing. It is believed that engaging three, rather than four, cortices allows for greater motion of the syndesmotic screw, thereby reducing the risk of hardware failure. It has been noted that on removal of the screw at 12 weeks, arthroscopic examination should ascertain the maintaining of reduction of the distal tibiofibular joint; loss of reduction is handled by means of an extended period of screw fixation or by open reduction and internal fixation of the joint. Ankle fractures are treated according to standard trauma principles in cases in which there are open injuries associated with the orthopaedic injury. Cultures should be obtained in the emergency department after the wounds have been irrigated. Broad-spectrum antibiotics, including a second-generation cephalosporin and aminoglycoside, are given. Formal debridement and reduction of the fracture should be performed within 6 hours of injury. In general, grade I, grade II, and grade III open fractures may be treated with immediate open reduction and internal fixation without appreciable increases in infection rates. Wounds in general should be left open, with a delayed closure performed within 5 days. Grade III injuries with excessive contamination or soft tissue damage are managed with external fixation because of associated high-energy injury of soft tissue and the articular surface and because of comminution.

Complications involving ankle fractures include infection, nonunion, malunion, and arthrosis. They are generally related to the amount of energy absorbed by the extremity, the amount of articular damage, and joint displacement. Nonunion of an ankle fracture involves rotatory deformity of the lateral malleolus or proximal migration of the fibula. Patients with insulin-dependent diabetes require an extended period of protected weight bearing to prevent the potential manifestation of Charcot's neuroarthropathy postoperatively. Unlike nondiabetics, who require a limited period of protected immobilization of 6 to 10 weeks, diabetic patients may experience Charcot's neuroarthropathy up to a year after injury. It is therefore recommended that frequent examinations be performed and that patients be warned to notify the surgeon if an unexplained increase in swelling occurs more than 4 months after injury.

Injury of the Hindfoot

Fractures of the hindfoot involve the calcaneus, talus, and tarsal navicular bones. Although they are less common, these fractures have higher complication rates and cause significant alterations in the joint kinematics of the foot. Anatomic reduction and stabilization sufficient to allow early commencement of motion are the goals of treatment.

The talus is covered by articular cartilage on 60% of its surface and articulates with the ankle (tibiotalar joint), calcaneus (subtalar joint), and navicula (talonavicular joint). The joints account for the majority of dorsiflexion, plantarflexion, inversion, and eversion of the foot. The blood supply to the talus is tenuous in the presence of fractures. It comprises an extra-osseous anastomotic sling around the neck of the talus that is formed by the artery of the tarsal canal and the artery of the sinus tarsi (from the posterior tibial, anterior tibial, and peroneal arteries). Blood supply to the talar head arises from the anastomotic sling and from distinct branches of the anterior tibial artery and talonavicular capsule. The talar body receives its blood supply from the posterior capsule of the ankle and the subtalar joints, from branches of the posterior tibial artery that course through the deltoid ligament, and from muscles and tendons attached to the talus proper. Fractures of the

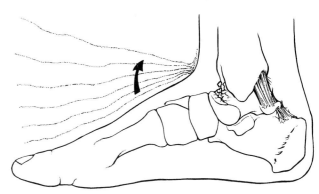

Figure 24–32. The mechanism of injury of most talar neck fractures is hyperdorsiflexion with an axial load. After impingement of the trochlea (the talar neck) on the tibia, the posterior capsule is put under stretch and supination occurs, thus stabilizing the subtalar joint. (From Gould J [ed]: Operative Foot Surgery. Philadelphia, WB Saunders, 1994, p 381.)

talus can involve the head, neck, and body, and associated intra-articular osteochondral lesions can occur. The mechanism of injury in talar neck fractures is hyperdorsiflexion of the foot, which is usually caused by motor vehicle accidents and falls from heights (Fig. 24–32). With dorsiflexion, the neck of the talus impacts along the anterior distal tibia, creating a fracture. If this force is continued, it may move the body of the talus posteromedially to lie behind the medial malleolus, rotating on the deltoid ligament (Fig. 24–33; see Fig. 24–32).

Hawkins' classification categorizes fractures of the talar neck into three patterns (see Fig. 24–33). Type I is a nondisplaced fracture of the neck. Type II is the displacement of the fracture, with subluxation or dislocation of the talar body from the subtalar joint. Type III is a displacement fracture, with subluxation or dislocation of the body from both the ankle and the subtalar joints. Canale added a fourth pattern (type IV), which is a rare variant involving a displaced neck fracture and including dislocation at the talonavicular joint. The Hawkins system is now widely accepted; the prognosis is correlated with the likelihood of osteonecrosis. The incidence of avascular necrosis increases with escalating type. The incidence of injuries involving talus fractures may be as high as 64%, according to one study. Approximately 15 to 20% of talar neck fractures are located at the anterolateral ankle joint. Vascular injury may be associated with the higher grades of Hawkins fractures because the talar body may compress the neurovascular bundle posteromedially. In 25% of talar neck fractures, an associated medial malleolar fracture may be present.

Radiographic assessment of this kind of fracture includes standard AP, mortise, and lateral views of the ankle in addition to AP and lateral views of the foot. A radiographic technique for assessing the alignment of the talar neck on the AP projection requires positioning the ankle in maximal plantarflexion and placing the foot, which is pronated 15 degrees, on a film cassette. The x-ray tube is directed cephalad at 75 degrees from the horizontal (Fig. 24–34). Treatment objectives in cases of talar fracture are to maintain an anatomic union of the fracture site and

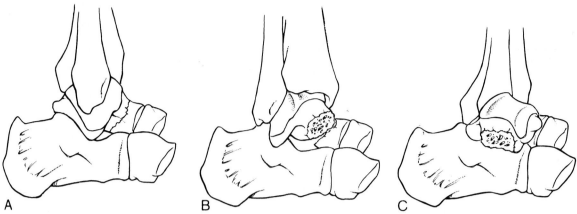

Figure 24–33. Hawkins-type classification of talar neck injuries. *A*, Class I. *B*, Class II. *C*, Class III (From Gould J [ed]: Operative Foot Surgery. Philadelphia, WB Saunders, 1994, p 381.)

minimize post-traumatic arthrosis, osteonecrosis, and varus malalignment. Immediate reduction protects overlying soft tissues and preserves any remaining blood supply to the talar body.

Type I fractures are considered to be nondisplaced. They are rare and may be best treated by immobilization in a cast for 8 to 12 weeks, with the first 4 to 6 weeks in non–weight-bearing status and the ankle in a slight equinus position. There is a potential for late displacement or prolonged joint stiffness because of the immobilization period. Therefore, treatment involving internal fixation and early motion has been advocated for type I fractures, which is similar in management to the higher grade injuries. Type II and more severe fractures are considered to be orthopaedic emergencies requiring initial closed reduction and then open reduction to maintain alignment and fixation. Steps should be taken to minimize varus malalignment because a displacement of more than 5 mm or a malalignment of more than 5 degrees will have an adverse effect on the kinematics of the hindfoot. Open reduction with rigid inter-

nal fixation may be achieved by using one of three surgical approaches to displaced talar neck fractures: anteromedial, anterolateral, or posterolateral. The anteromedial approach is used most widely. It extends between the interval of the tibialis anterior tendon and tibialis posterior tendon. It affords exposure of the talar neck medially and has the potential to allow extension of the exposure so medial malleolar osteotomy can be performed if necessary. The disadvantage of this exposure is the possibility of damaging the deltoid artery, which is the only preserved blood supply. The mediolateral approach affords exposure of the lateral talar neck and subtalar joint. The artery of the tarsal sinus is at risk in this exposure. Often, a combined medial and lateral approach is recommended. Fixation is dependent on the fracture's location, the degree of comminution, the bone quality, and the approach used. In general, either cortical or cancellous screws are preferable to K-wire fixation. Two screws positioned on the anteromedial and anterolateral talar neck to the dome are a popular option (Fig. 24–35). The potential disadvantage is screw head prominence in an

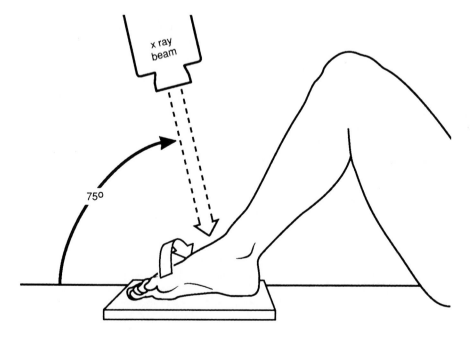

Figure 24–34. Canale view for looking at the neck of the talus. This can also be obtained in the operating room with an image intensifier. The foot is rotated medially 15 to 20 degrees. (From Baumhauer JF, Alvarez RG: Controversies in treating talus fractures. Orthop Clin North Am 1995;26[2]:335–351.)

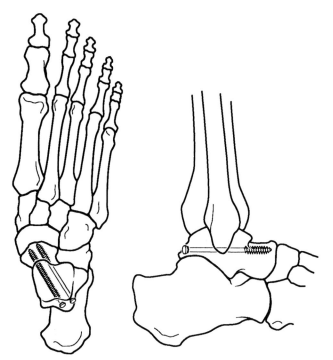

Figure 24–35. AP and lateral views of the foot with screws inserted. The AP shows two parallel screws, one fully threaded and one partially threaded. Screws or threaded pins can be parallel or divergent. (From Baumhauer JF, Alvarez RG: Controversies in treating talus fractures. Orthop Clin North Am 1995;26[2]:335–351.)

articular area of the talus. A posterolateral approach extends from the interval between the Achilles tendon and the peroneal tendons and is useful for posterior-to-anterior screw fixation. Advantages of posterior-to-anterior fixation are improved screw purchase and potential preservation of the blood supply to the talar body. Potential disadvantages are injury to the sural nerve and posterior ankle symptoms resulting from impingement of the prominent screw head.

Postoperatively, the patient is placed in a short leg cast in a neutral position or slight plantarflexion. A removable walker boot worn during a period of non–weight bearing allows for the patient to start early range-of-motion exercises to prevent stiffness. Weight bearing is allowed after 6 weeks, depending on the progress of union as seen radiographically in addition to evidence of vascularity to the talar body. This may be manifested at 8 to 10 weeks by a crescent sign (Hawkins' sign) seen on the AP and mortise views of the talar dome.

Complications involving talar neck fractures include malunion, delayed union, and post-traumatic arthritis. A common complication related to the Hawkins type of fracture is avascular necrosis. The risk ranges from 0 to 10% for Hawkins type I to up to 90 to 100% for types III and IV. Avascular necrosis is monitored by confirming the absence of the Hawkins sign and by taking MRI scans of the talar body. During MRI, there is a potential for scatter caused by stainless steel screws, so titanium screws, which are more MRI compatible, are recommended if such studies are planned for follow-up evaluation. General complications include skin necrosis, infection, delayed union, and

nonunion and may occur in approximately 10% of cases. Additionally, varus malunion, which has a locking effect on the midfoot, may occur in up to 50% of type II and more severe fractures. Arthritis of both the ankle and the subtalar joint may be secondary to arterial compromise, the initial articular cartilage damage from the fracture dislocation, malunion, and prolonged immobilization.

Nondisplaced talar head fractures may be treated with the conservative approach of a short leg, non–weight-bearing cast. Small displaced fractures may be excised or rigidly fixed with headless screws countersunk below the articular surface in a medial approach.

Fractures of the talar body (Fig. 24–36) may occur in the vertical, sagittal, or horizontal plane. Fractures most commonly occur in the lateral talar process and the posterior talar process; osteochondral lesions of the talus are also common. Fractures of the lateral talar process are the second most common fractures of the body of the talus. Fractures frequently remain unrecognized for a prolonged

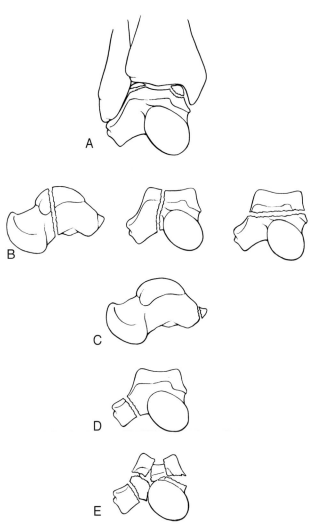

Figure 24–36. Classification of talar body fractures. *A,* Osteochondral fracture (group I). *B,* Sagittal, vertical, and horizontal talar body injuries (group II). *C,* Posterior process fracture (group III). *D,* Lateral tubercle fracture (group IV). *E,* Crush injury (group V). (From Gould J [ed]: Operative Foot Surgery. Philadelphia, WB Saunders, 1994, p 392.)

period after ankle inversion injuries. Displaced fractures are treated with cast immobilization, whereas displaced or comminuted fractures are handled using a sinus tarsi approach and are treated with open reduction and internal fixation or excision. Posterior talar process fractures are distinguished from those of the common accessory ossicle of the os trigonum by evidence of irregular borders at the fracture site. This fracture was initially described by Shepard (1882); two mechanisms are described. The first is excessive ankle dorsiflexion, with or without inversion, that creates tension through the posterior talofibular ligament, which causes an avulsion fracture of the lateral tubercle. The second mechanism involves a hyperplantarflexion injury, which compresses the lateral tubercle between the posterior tibia and calcaneus. Swelling may be present with this injury. Pain is typically aggravated when the foot is in a hyperequinus position, and there is tenderness on palpation anterior to the Achilles tendon. This may be associated with symptoms related to muscle testing of the adjacent FHL. Treatment of an acute fracture includes the use of a non–weight-bearing cast for 4 weeks, followed by the use of a walking cast for an additional 2 weeks or until the patient is asymptomatic. Excision of the symptomatic fragment is recommended in chronic conditions. This is performed through a posterolateral approach in the interval between the peroneal tendons and the FHL. Early weight bearing and active range of motion are encouraged to minimize scarring of the posterior capsule.

Lesions to the talar dome may occur in 6.5% of all ankle sprains and they occur in 1% of all talar fractures. These lesions, initially felt to be congenital-vascular in origin, are currently believed to be related to trauma. With the ankle in dorsiflexion and inversion, an anterolateral fracture may be produced by impaction of the talus. With plantarflexion and inversion, the articular surface of the tibia impacts the superior medial ridge of the talus. Medial lesions are slightly more common (55%) than lateral lesions. The medial lesions are described as cup-shaped; the lateral lesions, described as wafer-like. The Burt and Hardy classification, based on the appearance of the fracture on plain radiographs, has four stages. In stage I there is an area of compressed subchondral bone; in stage II there is

a partially detached fragment; in stage III there is a completely detached, nondisplaced fragment; in stage IV there is a completely detached, displaced fragment (loose body). MRI scans help to determine the stage of the lesion. Both complete and nondisplaced fractures can be treated by cast immobilization—a non–weight-bearing cast for 6 weeks and a weight-bearing cast for an additional 6 weeks until healing is complete. Stages III and IV lesions (and stages I and II lesions that continue to be symptomatic 4 to 6 months after injury) are treated surgically. Small displaced fragments can be removed and the bed of the lesion drilled to restore blood supply and create a fibrocartilaginous replacement (Fig. 24–37). Medial fragments with a significant subchondral bony component may be reduced and stabilized with absorbable pins or screw fixation. Anterolateral lesions may be fixed arthroscopically; often a medial malleolar osteotomy and arthrotomy are required for the posteromedial lesions. Articular defects larger than 1 cm require osteochondral harvesting from the knee joint to replace the defect.

The calcaneus is the most commonly fractured tarsal bone. Fractures are classified as intra-articular or extra-articular (Fig. 24–38). Intra-articular fractures are sustained in the presence of axial loads resulting from falls or motor vehicle accidents (Fig. 24–39). The mechanism of injury is that the lateral talar process is driven into the superior calcaneal surface, creating a primary fracture line that runs from the posterior facet in a lateral to posteromedial direction. A secondary fracture line may occur and extend through the calcaneocuboid joint and lateral calcaneal wall. There may be one or more sagittal fracture lines through the posterior facet. Typically, the anteromedial fragment contains the sustentaculum tali, which is usually nondisplaced because of its attachments to the talus through the interosseous ligament. The calcaneal tuberosity is frequently shortened and misangulated. Diagnosis is made on the basis of history and plain radiographs. Radiographs for this area should include AP, lateral, and Broden's views (Fig. 24–40). Examination and radiographs of the pelvis and thoracolumbar spine may be required because of the axial nature of the injury. Bohler's angle—the angle formed by the most posterosuperior aspect of the calcaneal tuberos-

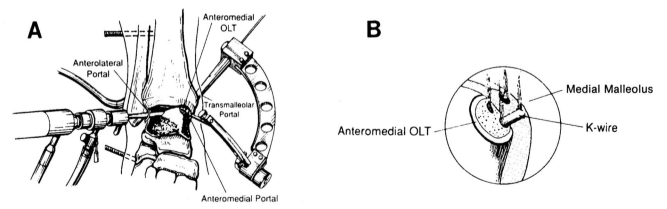

Figure 24–37. *A,* Transmalleolar drilling of an osteochondral lesion of the medial talar dome using a guide. The scope is in the anterolateral portal, and inflow is through the posterolateral portal. *B,* Drill holes are made through the medial malleolus into the talus down to areas of bleeding bone. OLT, osteochondral lesion of talus. (From Philips B: Oper Tech Sports Med 1994;2[1].)

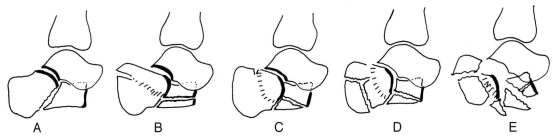

Figure 24–38. Classification of intra-articular fractures of the calcaneus. *A,* Shear. *B,* Tongue type. *C,* Central depression type. *D,* Tongue or central depression with comminution. *E,* Comminuted. (From Paley D, Hall H: Calcaneal fracture controversies: Can we put Humpty Dumpty together again? Orthop Clin North Am 1989;20:667.)

ity, the posterior facet, and the anterior process—is normally in the range of 20 to 40 degrees. In posterior facet intra-articular injuries, this angle may be appreciably reduced to zero degrees or to a negative angle. A Broden view may assess the status of the posterior facet and the degree of comminution and incongruity. CT is a good method of definitively imaging the os calcis. Views are taken in both axial and semicoronal planes, which are positioned 30 degrees of the horizontal to assess the degree of articular displacement and the number, location, and size of the fracture fragments. A classification system for calcaneus fractures has been proposed by Sanders. Determined by CT, the classifications are based on the amount of comminution of the posterior facet, and there is a direct correlation with prognosis. The type I fracture is nondisplaced and has an articular step-off of 2 mm or less.

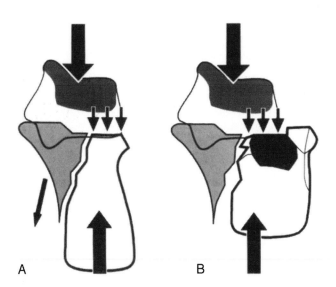

Figure 24–39. *A,* Axial loading forces applied to the calcaneus during fracture. Note the position of the tuberosity relative to the talus. *B,* Resultant deformation of the calcaneus after the fracture. Note that the sustentacular, or constant, fragment stays with the talus, whereas the tuberosity fragment shifts laterally, shortening and widening the heel. Also note the depressed intra-articular fragment that tends to blow out the lateral wall. (Drawings courtesy of Professor Christopher Colton. From Sanders R: Intra-articular fractures of the calcaneus: Present state of the art. J Orthop Trauma 1992;6:252–265.)

Type II and type III fractures have two or three displaced interarticular fragments, respectively, and type IV has four or more fragments (severe comminution). Treatment options include closed treatment with initial casting and early motion, open reduction and internal fixation, and primary arthrodesis. Closed treatment is reserved for patients with minimal deformity and 2 mm or less of articular displacement and for fractures that are so comminuted that bony stabilization cannot be obtained surgically. Poor surgical candidates include those with suboptimal viability, soft tissue compromise, or a complicated medical condition. Closed treatment is acceptable for most Sanders type I fractures. The more severe fractures (type II and type III) have better outcomes with surgical intervention. Disabilities associated with non-reduced calcaneus fractures include overall shortening of the height, a decrease in the talar declination angle, and potential tibiotalar impingement symptoms. Additionally, the blowing out of the lateral wall of the calcaneus may create calcaneofibular abutment symptoms and peroneal entrapment symptoms with tenosynovitis. Heel varus may disturb the ankle and hindfoot kinematics, so a patient may walk on the outer border of the foot because of a locked forefoot. Additionally, because of secondary Achilles tendon shortening and the loss of height, overall plantarflexion strength is diminished.

Open reduction and internal fixation of a calcaneus fractures is indicated predominantly for Sanders type II and type III fractures. Technically, they are two of the most challenging fracture types to address with internal fixation, and they are associated with potentially high complication rates. Because of the traumatized and compromised soft tissues and excessive swelling, surgical intervention should not commence until there is wrinkling of the lateral hindfoot soft tissues. Complications of surgical intervention include residual deformity and the potential for increased range of motion through the subtalar joint. The approach is composed of an L-type incision, as advocated by Benoshca, using both the subtalar and calcaneocuboid joints, with a full-thickness subperiosteal flap involving the peroneal tendons, sural nerve, and calcaneofibular ligament. Fixation involves initially reducing and stabilizing the posterior facet and then attaching the laminate portion of the calcaneus to the main tuberosity and anterior process. The fixation is typically stabilized by using a low-profile steel plate designed for the lateral wall of the calcaneus. Careful handling of soft tissues during exposure is advocated, as is a careful, tensionless skin closure.

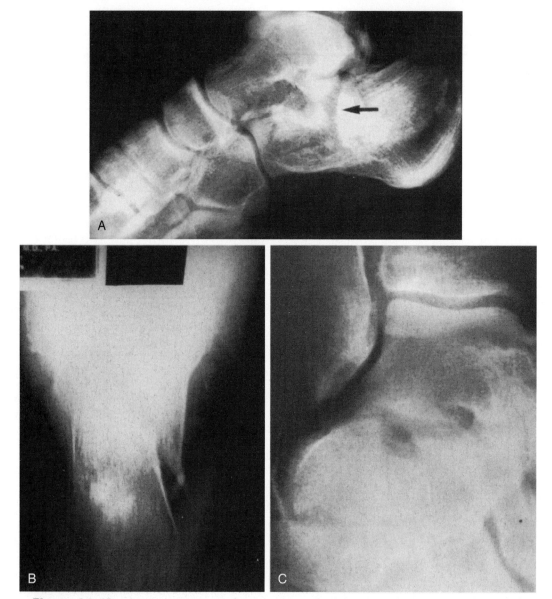

Figure 24–40. *A,* Lateral view of the calcaneus. *B,* Axial view. *C,* Broden's view. (From Sanders R, Gregory P: Operative treatment of intra-articular fractures of the calcaneus. Orthop Clin North Am 1995;26[2]:203–214.)

Non–weight bearing should last for a minimum of 8 weeks, whereas early motion is emphasized once the wound is considered stable. Patients with significant comminution of the posterior facet or delamination of the articular cartilage are candidates for primary subtalar arthrodesis at the time of open reduction and internal fixation. This avoids potential complications such as subtalar joint arthrosis and may allow for earlier return to work. Complications involved in surgical fixation of calcaneus fractures are wound slough, dehiscence, subtalar arthrosis, and damage to the sural and superficial peroneal cutaneous nerves. Breakdown—which may occur in up to one third of cases of calcaneus fractures treated by open reduction with internal fixation—is a drastic complication given the limited amount of soft tissue on the lateral aspect of the calcaneus available to cover the plate and screw fixation. This situation may require a plastic surgery consultation for an ab-

ductor digiti minimi rotation flap or local rotation of the arm of the existing flap and skin grafting posteriorly. Coverage is to be obtained as quickly as possible so as to prevent deep infection and osteomyelitis of the calcaneus. Arthrosis of the subtalar joint is a potential complication. Often, it is not attributed directly to fixation. Because of the axial nature of the injury, it is common for there to be articular cartilage damage that is not apparent on initial inspection at the time of injury but that manifests itself 1 to 2 years after the initial injury.

Extra-articular fractures are those of the anterior process, tuberosity, sustentaculum talus, medial or lateral calcaneus process, and calcaneal body. Anterior process avulsion fractures occur as a result of tension caused by the bifurcated ligament; they are associated with inversion and the plantarflexion injuries. These fractures are best identified on an oblique radiography of the foot. There is tenderness and pain with palpation of the sinus tarsi region, as well as swelling. Although all nondisplaced fractures may be treated with weight-bearing cast immobilization for 4 to 6 weeks, displaced fractures may be treated acutely with open reduction and internal fixation. Chronic, symptomatic nonunions are excised. Posterior avulsion tuberosity fractures occur at the insertion site of the Achilles tendon, where the tensile strength of the tendon exceeds that of the bone. The bony fragment may extend either intra- or extra-articularly to the posterior facet. Displaced fractures are left closed and treated with immobilization, initially in a plantarflexed cast for 3 weeks and subsequently in a neutral cast for an additional 3 to 6 weeks until healing has occurred. Displaced fractures of the tuberosity are best treated with open reduction and internal fixation using screw fixation and early lack of weight bearing followed by range of motion exercises and a removable cast. A complication of closed initial treatment of large displaced fragments is skin necrosis secondary to the pressure of the fragment against the skin and cast.

Injury of the Midfoot

Injuries involving the midfoot include those of the tarso-navicular, cuboid, cuneiform, and tarsometatarsal joints. Diagnosis of isolated fractures of tarsal bones can be made after midfoot joint complex injuries have been ruled out. Fractures of the tarsal navicular bone have been classified as dorsal lip, tuberosity, or stress fractures. Dorsal lip fractures are the most commonly isolated navicular fractures; they involve cortical avulsion of the dorsal lip resulting from an eversion mechanism in the talonavicular joint capsule and anterior fibers of the deltoid ligament. The fracture fragment is best identified in a lateral radiograph and may vary in size and geometry. Differential diagnosis includes an accessory ossicle of the navicular bone and talus. Treatment is usually determined by the symptoms. The majority of cases are treated with short leg walking casts for 4 to 6 weeks. Persistent displacement of the fragment generates a painful prominence and is treated with excision.

Tuberosity fractures result from an eversion mechanism that causes eccentric contraction of the posterior tibial tendon. Local tenderness is elicited and there is pain on resisted inversion. Displacement is often minimal because of the broad attachment of the posterior tibial tendon. Radiographs, including AP and medial oblique studies, best demonstrate this type of fracture. Bilateral studies are often required to rule out the presence of an accessory navicular bone (which may occur in 12% of the population and is bilateral in up to 64%). Additionally, evaluation of the cuboid bone for crush injury should be carried out on the same radiographs. Treatment for nondisplaced or minimally displaced fractures is immobilization for 4 to 6 weeks in a short leg cast. Fractures displaced 1 cm or more should be opened and fixed acutely to preclude dysfunction of the posterior tibial tendon. Symptomatic nonunions may be treated by excising the fragment and advancing the tendon to the remaining tuberosity, with 4 to 6 weeks of cast immobilization.

Navicular body fractures are commonly associated with other foot injuries but may occur in isolation. Typically,

they involve both the talonavicular and the navicular cuneiform joints. Classification of displaced intra-articular fractures is as follows: type I is a transverse fracture in the coronal plane; type II is an oblique fracture with a larger dorsolateral fragment; and type III is a central or lateral comminution. Treatment consists of open reduction and internal fixation when more than 60% of the joint surface is involved. A chronic stress fracture is a variant that occurs in the avascular central third navicular bone and is typically seen in young male athletes performing repetitive high-intensity activities. Clinically, the pain is localized to the dorsolateral aspect of the midfoot and may be difficult to delineate on a plain radiograph. A low index of suspicion is required and may be confirmed by bone scan, CT, or MRI using coronal cuts. Treatment of incomplete stress fractures requires 6 to 8 weeks of cast immobilization. Displaced fractures and nonunions exhibiting excess sclerosis require bone grafting with open reduction and internal fixation (Fig. 24–41A, B). Chronic untreated conditions may result in debilitating pain caused by talonavicular arthrosis, which ultimately necessitates arthrodesis.

Cuboid fractures rarely occur in isolation and are typically associated with injuries involving the midfoot. Two forms of injury exist. The first is an avulsion-type injury associated with an inversion mechanism that may present as a "fleck" sign on the lateral calcaneocuboid joint. The differential diagnosis involves avulsion injury of the anterior process of the calcaneus from the bifurcated ligament. The second and more significant injury is related to abduction of the forefoot by injury of the Lisfranc joints. Lateral displacement of the forefoot results in compression fracture of the cuboid bone, which is known as a nutcracker fracture. Comminution may result, which causes loss of axial length in the lateral column and creates an asymmetrical flatfoot pattern. The treatment of a nondisplaced fracture is a short leg walking cast worn for 4 to 6 weeks. Crush injuries that are displaced or comminuted are best treated with open reduction and internal fixation. The goal is to restore the length of the lateral column and thus the kinematics of the hindfoot. The length may be restored by a bridging external fixator or a buttress plate and graft to fill defects in the cuboid bone. The foot is immobilized in a short leg, non–weight-bearing cast for up to 12 weeks. Ultimately, arthrosis may develop in the adjacent calcaneocuboid joint; it can be adequately treated with arthrodesis.

Injuries to the Lisfranc (tarsometatarsal) joints include a wide spectrum, from subtle sprains to frank fracture-dislocations resulting in gross deformity and significant disability. The tarsometatarsal joint complex is composed of the three cuneiform bones, the cuboid bone, and five metatarsal bases. The bony architecture is similar to that of a Roman arch in design and stability. The keystone of the arch is the second metatarsal, which has wedge-shaped bases that are recessed between the medial and lateral cuneiform bones. The ligamentous support for the tarsometatarsal joint is provided primarily by the stronger plantar interosseous ligaments, particularly the transverse intermetatarsal ligaments, which occur at every base except the first and second tarsometatarsal joints (Fig. 24–42). At this level, the Lisfranc ligament spans the plantar-lateral aspect of the medial cuneiform bone and the medial base of the second metatarsal and functions to resist lateral translation

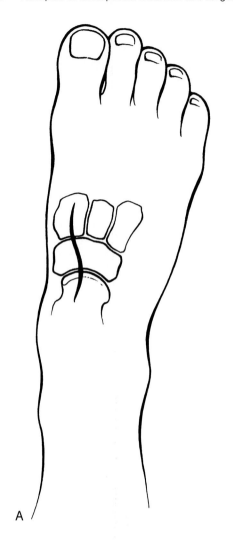

A

Figure 24–41. *A,* The skin incision for open reduction and internal fixation of a displaced navicular stress fracture. *B,* Internal fixation of a displaced navicular stress fracture obtained by inserting two cancellous lag screws. (From Gould J [ed]: Operative Foot Surgery. Philadelphia, WB Saunders, 1994, p 941).

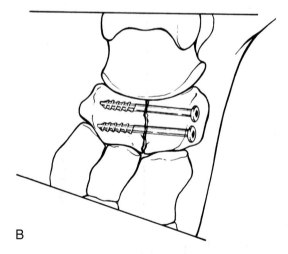

B

of the lesser metatarsals. The first metatarsal-medial cuneiform joint is stabilized by the joint capsule and by insertions of the anterior tibial and peroneus longus tendons.

Both direct and indirect mechanisms of Lisfranc fracture-dislocations have been described. The direct mechanism is a crush injury of the dorsum of the foot, which produces dislocation in the direction of the applied force.

Even trivial trauma can disrupt the weaker dorsal, soft tissue constraints in a plantarflexed foot. High-energy trauma, including heavy crush injuries, produce a spectrum of injuries in addition to the potential for foot compartment syndrome. The second mechanism is indirect; it is a twisting type injury of the forefoot in relation to the midfoot (Fig. 24–43). This pattern is most commonly seen in motor

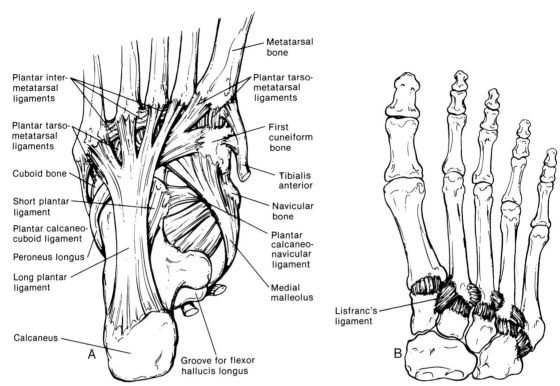

Figure 24–42. *A*, Plantar ligaments involving the tarsometatarsal joints. *B*, Dorsal ligaments of the tarsometatarsal joints. (*A* modified from Rockwood CA Jr, Green DP, Bucholz RW, et al [eds]: Fractures in Adults, 3rd ed. Philadelphia, JB Lippincott, 1992, p 2050; *B* modified from Mann RA: Surgery of the Foot and Ankle, 6th ed. St. Louis, CV Mosby, 1992, p 1677.)

vehicle accidents and equestrian injuries, in which an abduction-directed force may indirectly cause a concurrent lateral column injury (cuboid fracture). Up to 20% of these injuries are missed on initial evaluation because of the broad spectrum of their presentation. Gross deformity of the midfoot is not apparent, and spontaneous reduction (as viewed on non–weight-bearing radiographs) adds to the difficulty of diagnosis. Therefore, a high index of suspicion is necessary if the mechanism of the injury so demands (Fig. 24–44).

Evaluation consists of a history of inability to bear weight and of pain localized in the midfoot. A pronation-abduction test may re-create the symptoms and the pain. Gross incongruity and crepitus of the midfoot is noted on examination of severe, unstable injuries. Findings in the case of a concomitant forefoot compartment syndrome include neurologic and circulatory changes and pain with passive range of motion. Radiographic evaluation includes AP, lateral, and 30-degree-oblique plain radiographs; comparison with the opposite foot is necessary to assess for subtle diastasis. On the AP view, the medial border of the second metatarsal base should line up with the medial aspect of the middle cuneiform bone. An avulsion fracture at the medial base of the second metatarsal extends from the oblique Lisfranc ligament and is diagnostic of the injury. On the oblique view, the medial aspect of the fourth metatarsal base should align with the medial aspect of the cuboid bone. If the patient is able to tolerate weight bearing, standing radiographs are equivalent to stress views and elicit any subtle deviations. Re-creation of the mechanism by means of a pronation-abduction stress radiogaph may

reveal the deformity and document the degree of instability. This is best performed after administering an ankle block. On the lateral view, the dorsal borders of the first and second metatarsals should line up with their respective cuneiform bones without evidence of step-off.

The management of tarsometatarsal joint injuries includes obtaining a stable, painless plantigrade foot by means of anatomic restoration of articular congruency. Treatment options range from closed reduction with cast immobilization for nondisplaced injuries to open reduction and internal fixation for displaced acute fracture dislocations. The management of acute injuries, including closed reduction in a non–weight-bearing cast for 6 to 8 weeks, is limited to grade I and grade II sprains. Evidence of displacement can be demonstrated on weight-bearing or stress radiographs. Loss of reduction resulting from resolution of soft tissue swelling with cast immobilization necessitates open reduction and internal fixation in displaced grade III tarsometatarsal sprains. Fixation methods, including K-wire fixation and rigid screw fixation, have been advocated. K-wire fixation has the potential to result in loss of reduction during the healing process; therefore, screw fixation is currently advocated. Before surgery, the degree of swelling and displacement must be considered. It is preferable to treat closed injuries within 24 hours, but a delay of up to 7 to 10 days will not significantly alter the outcome. Most fracture-dislocations should be reduced and immobilized to minimize the risk of vascular and soft tissue compromise. This may be achieved by manual reduction and longitudinal traction to restore length. Direct pressure over the second metatarsal base, with the patient

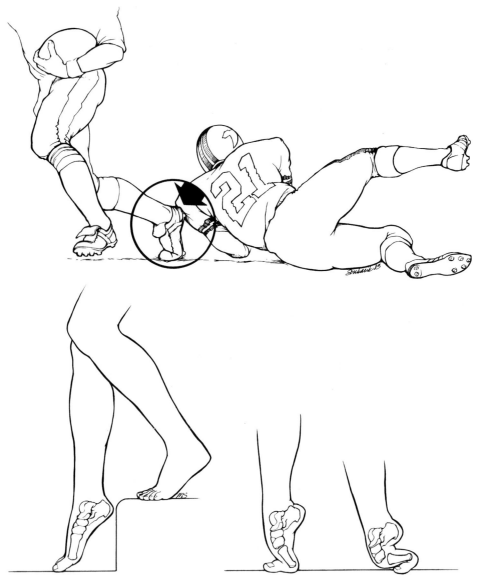

Figure 24–43. Mechanisms of Lisfranc fracture-dislocation. *Top*, Axial load applied to heel with foot fixed in equinus. *Bottom*, Axial load applied by body weight with ankle in extreme plantarflexion. (From Heckman JD: Fractures and dislocations of the foot. *In* Rockwood CA Jr, Green DP, Bucholz RW, et al [eds]: Rockwood and Green's Fracture in Adults, 3rd ed. Philadelphia, Lippincott, 1992, p 2143.)

under anesthesia, is used to reduce the dislocation into the mortise.

The surgical technique involves making two parallel, dorsal, longitudinal incisions over the first and third intermetatarsal spaces. Care should be taken to maintain the soft tissue bridge between the two incisions. Initial reduction consists of stabilization of the medial column involving the first metatarsal–medial cuneiform joint. Any debris in the base of the second tarsometatarsal joint is debrided, the second tarsometatarsal joint is reduced and stabilized, and screw fixation is applied across the third tarsometatarsal joint and, when unstable, through the fifth metatarsal–cuboid joint. Evidence of a lateral cuboid crush injury may require that an external fixator be applied to neutralize the lateral column and maintain length. Postoperatively, the patient is placed in a non–weight-bearing cast for approximately 4 to 6 weeks, followed by a progressive weight-

bearing cast for an additional 4 to 6 weeks. Screws should be removed at approximately 12 to 14 weeks and prior to unrestricted weight bearing.

Complications involving Lisfranc fracture-dislocations include posttraumatic arthrosis, which may be seen in up to 70% of involved injuries. Secondary arthrosis can be adequately treated with arthrodesis of the involved tarsometatarsal joints. The fourth and fifth metatarsal–cuboid joints should be not be included in the fusion mass if at all possible because outcomes are less favorable when global fusion is performed.

Metatarsal fractures are the most common foot fractures, and there are varying degrees of involvement and various patterns. The most common mechanism is a direct blow by a heavy object. Compromise of associated soft tissues is also common. Low-energy injuries result in minimally displaced fractures that are best treated conservatively. High-

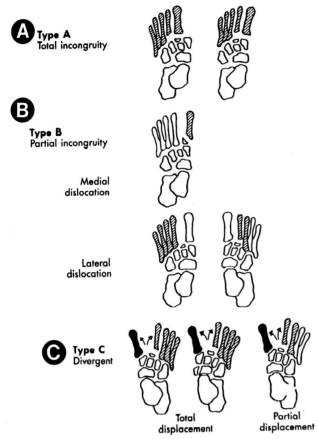

Figure 24–44. Classification of Lisfranc fracture-dislocations. *A,* Type A, total incongruity. *B,* Type B, partial incongruity. *C,* Type C, divergent. (From Whittle A: Fractures of the foot in athletes. Oper Tech Sports Med 1994;2[1].)

energy injuries involving significant deformity may lead to dysfunction, chronic pain, and transfer metatarsalgia and therefore are best treated surgically to achieve anatomic reduction. The mechanism of injury is typically direct pressure applied to the dorsum of the foot by a heavy object. This results in transverse neck fractures in the second, third, or fourth metatarsals or in a combination of these joints. Indirect forces create spiral shaft fractures.

Treatment of nondisplaced fractures involving the lesser metatarsals includes the use of a firm shoe or short leg cast for approximately 3 to 4 weeks, followed by progressive weight bearing as tolerated. Displacement of lesser metatarsal fractures on the sagittal plane can result in intractable plantar keratosis and transfer metatarsalgia with dorsal displacement. A mild angulation on the coronal plane is acceptable. Excessive mediolateral angulation of the central metatarsals may result in mechanical impingement or interdigital nerve compression. The more distal the fracture, the greater the potential for displacement resulting from the lack of soft tissue attachments to provide stability to the distal metatarsal head and neck. Management of displaced fractures includes intermedullary K-wire fixation, plate fixation, or use of the lag screw technique, depending on the pattern of injury. Intra-articular fractures should be treated by attempting to restore articular congruity. The goals of surgery are restoration of length, rotation, and

angulation so as to allow for even weight-bearing distribution. In cases of significant bone loss, restoration of length should be attempted, either initially or as a staged procedure, using bone grafting to achieve the healing of the fracture.

Fractures of the fifth metatarsal bone are classified according to anatomic location and mechanism of injury (Fig. 24–45). Fractures at the base of the fifth metatarsal fall into three anatomic zones.

Zone 1 includes the tuberosity and styloid process, the insertion of the peroneus brevis tendon, and the lateral border of the plantar fascia. Fractures in this location are typically avulsion injuries caused by sudden, reflexive contraction of the peroneus brevis. They occur with plantarflexion-inversion injuries. Treatment is almost always conservative—elastic wrap, a postoperative shoe, or a short leg cast.

Zone 2 is the region distal to zone 1 and comprises the intermetatarsal articulation and the intermetatarsal ligaments. Fractures at the junction of the metaphyseal and diaphyseal regions are termed *Jones fractures* and occur as a result of the nutcracker effect, in which the fifth metatarsal is levered against the stable base of the fourth metatarsal. A vascular watershed zone occurs in this area; distinct, nonoverlapping intermedullary and extra-osseous blood supplies contribute to the high rate of nonunion associated with Jones fractures. A fracture is treated with a non–weight-bearing cast for 6 weeks followed by a progressively weight-bearing cast for an additional 4 to 6 weeks until union has occurred. Closed reduction and percutaneous screw fixation using an intermedullary screw can be performed in special patients such as high-performance athletes.

Zone 3 fractures occur in the metaphyseal-diaphyseal junction distally, from the intermetatarsal ligament into the mid-diaphyseal bone. In this region, presentation is typically secondary to a pre-existing stress fracture or chronic intermedullary sclerosis that is evident on radiographs. Fractures are managed conservatively in a short leg, non–weight-bearing cast for approximately 6 weeks. Surgery is reserved for chronic medullary sclerotic stress fractures,

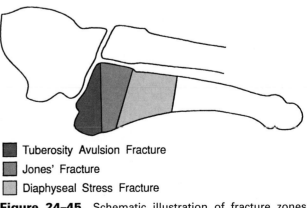

■ Tuberosity Avulsion Fracture
■ Jones' Fracture
□ Diaphyseal Stress Fracture

Figure 24–45. Schematic illustration of fracture zones for proximal fifth metatarsal fractures. (From Lawrence SJ, Botte MJ: Foot Fellow's Review: Jones' fractures and related fractures of the proximal fifth metatarsal. Foot Ankle 1993;14:358–365.)

which may be treated with intermedullary compression screw fixation or onlay bone graft.

Injury of the Forefoot

Fractures of the sesamoid bones occur as a result of direct trauma, frank overuse, or avulsion injuries associated with hyperdorsiflexion injuries ("turf toe"). The sesamoid bones may disrupt the soft tissue that surrounds the sesamoid complex or, alternatively, may dissociate, causing diastasis of the intersesamoid ligament. Radiographic evaluation includes AP, lateral, and axial views (Fig. 24–46). When evaluating sesamoid fractures, it is important to differentiate a bipartite sesamoid bone from a fracture. Bipartite sesamoid bones occur in approximately 25% of individuals, with 80% involving the tibial sesamoid bones. A fracture has irregular edges, as opposed to a bipartite sesamoid bone, which has smooth, relatively sclerotic edges. A bone scan may be helpful in confirming the diagnosis. Initial management of acute fractures involves 3 to 6 weeks of immobilization in a short leg cast with an extended toe plate to minimize the motion of the hallux. Alternatively, a stiff-soled shoe with relief under the sesamoid bones has been recommended. Pain associated with the nonunion of a sesamoid fracture may require either partial or total excision of the affected sesamoid bone. Complications resulting from the excision of a sesamoid bone may include hallux valgus caused by removal of the tibial sesamoid bone, and hallux varus caused by excision of the fibular

sesamoid bone. The potential for transfer sesamoiditis of the remaining sesamoid bones is common. Alternatively, bone grafts have been successfully performed in cases of persistently painful nonunion, and they are recommended, especially for high-performance athletes.

Fracture dislocations of the hallux occur as a result of stubbing or impact by a falling object. Nondisplaced fractures may be treated by the wearing of a shoe postoperatively for approximately 3 to 4 weeks. Fractures may be reduced under regional anesthetic block. Displaced intra-articular fractures involving the MTP and interphalangeal joints may be reduced anatomically and fixed with small or minifragmentation screws. Management of the interphalangeal joint surgically is controversial because sequelae resulting from incongruous joints and fractures involving ankylosis or arthrosis pose a threat of disability. A dislocation of the first MTP joint should be reduced, splinted to the adjacent second toe (with a spacer between the toes), and taped. Occasionally, the buttonholing of the metatarsal head into the short flexor complex creates an irreducible condition that requires open reduction.

Injuries of the lesser toes caused by stubbing or axial loads on the toes may result in joint dislocations or phalangeal fractures. The fifth toe is the most commonly injured; the proximal phalanx is involved more often than the distal or middle phalanx. Phalangeal fractures may be either displaced or nondisplaced but are typically angulated. Reduction of phalangeal fractures includes closed manipulation using the "pencil technique," preceded by a digital block. It is then "buddy-taped" to the adjacent toe, and a stiff-soled shoe or sandal is worn. A fracture that extends intra-articularly involves a displaced condylar fragment at the base of the proximal phalanx. Fractures may require open reduction and K-wire stabilization to prevent significant step-off or diastasis. Sequelae of injuries of the lesser toes include joint instability, incongruence, and arthrosis. These conditions may be treated with resection arthroplasty to address both the deformity and the symptomatic arthrosis.

Dislocations may occur at the MTP joints of the lesser toes as a result of stubbing the toe. The digit displaces dorsally and laterally because of the exertion of a hyperextension force. Treatment involves closed reduction and buddy-taping for 1 to 2 weeks after assessment of the stability of the MTP joint. In complex, irreducible dislocations, the plantar capsule and transverse metatarsal ligament may be displaced dorsally, with buttonholing of the metatarsal head. The metatarsal head may become entrapped between the flexor tendons and lumbricals, creating an irreducible condition. Open reduction and division of the transverse metatarsal ligament and plantar plate may be required.

ACQUIRED DEFORMITIES OF THE FOOT AND ANKLE

Deformities of the Forefoot

DEFORMITIES OF THE FIRST RAY

Disorders of the first ray include hallux valgus (bunion deformities), hallux varus, hallux rigidus, claw hallux deformities, and deformities of the sesamoid complex.

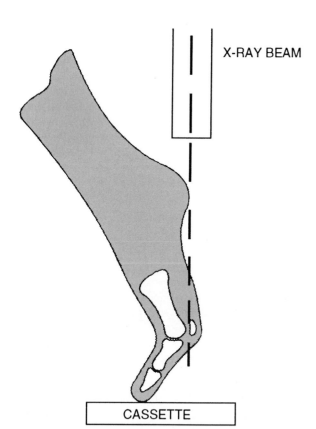

Figure 24–46. Tibial sesamoid view. (From Richardson EG: Injuries to the hallucal sesamoid in the athlete. Foot Ankle 1987;7:229–244.)

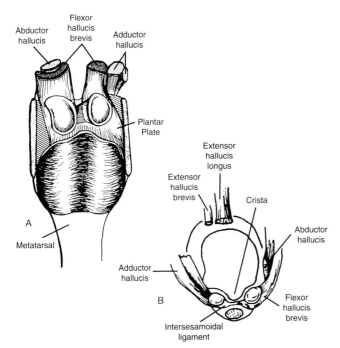

Figure 24–47. *A,* First MTP joint complex, plantar view. The sesamoid bones are embedded in the plantar plane and flexor brevis tendons. The sesamoid complex is flipped over distally. *B,* Axial view through the metatarsal head. The bony landmarks surrounding the ligaments and tendons are labeled. (From Coughlin MJ: Hallus valgus. *In* Springfield DS [ed]: Instructional Course Lecture 46. Rosemont, IL, American Academy of Orthopaedic Surgeons, 1997, pp 357–391.)

Hallux Valgus. Hallux valgus is a condition of the medial prominence of the first MTP joint that involves lateral drifting of the big toe. Predisposing anatomic and genetic factors, including planovalgus foot deformity and ligamentous laxity, increase the risk for development of a hallux valgus deformity. However, it is almost exclusively related to shoe wear. Because of this, 9 of 10 people with bunions are women. Anatomic variances associated with hallux valgus deformity include a rounded first metatarsal head and an increased obliquity or curvature of the first metatarsal medial cuneiform joint. Radiographically, a hallux valgus deformity is defined as an MTP joint angle of more than 15 degrees and an angle between the first and second metatarsals that is more than 9 degrees.

The pathophysiology of the hallux valgus deformity involves derangement of the intrinsic musculature of the foot. Lateral deviation of the base of the proximal phalanx also contributes to pushing the first metatarsal head into increased varus. The medial capsule becomes attenuated, and the lateral structures simultaneously shorten. The balance between the adductor hallucis and abductor hallucis is set and, with the pull of the abductor hallucis in a plantar direction and the pull of the EHL in a dorsal direction, additional adduction forces are present. Also, the abductor hallucis tendon, by migrating in a plantar direction, relinquishes any remaining abductor power as it becomes a flexor tendon. Initially, the FHL tendon, while remaining with the sesamoid complex, migrates laterally and acts as an additional valgus deforming force (Fig. 24–47). Hallux

valgus is thus described as mechanical derangement of the first MTP joint, including a prominent medial eminence, lateral subluxation of the proximal phalanx, and dissociation of the first metatarsal sesamoid complex, with pronation of the hallux and medial drifting of the first metatarsal (metatarsus primus varus).

Symptoms associated with hallux valgus deformity include pain, swelling, and inflammation over the medial eminence caused by shoe wear as well as secondary hypertrophy of the overlying bursa. Patients often complain of the difficulty of finding comfortable shoes yet may ambulate barefoot without difficulty. Pain that accompanies ambulating barefoot may be caused by an arthritic condition of the first MTP joint. Assessment includes a neurovascular examination, especially in the geriatric group, as well as evaluation for associated pes planovalgus deformity of the foot, Achilles tendon contracture, ligamentous laxity, neuromuscular disorders, and underlying systemic disease, including rheumatologic conditions. Initially, assessment should include evaluation for associated lesser toe deformities, including subluxation or dislocation of the lesser MTP joints, transfer callosities under the metatarsal heads, bunionette deformities, corns, and hammer toes. Range of motion of the first MTP joint should be assessed because the normal dorsiflexion required for gait is 70 degrees. Anteroposterior and lateral radiographs determine the degree of hallux valgus deformity, associated metatarsus primus varus, joint congruity, degenerative changes in the first MTP joint, and evidence of sesamoid subluxation. The obliquity and degree of curvature of the first metatarsal medial cuneiform joint relate to the metatarsus primus varus (Fig. 24–48). The angle of the hallux valgus is determined by a line bisecting the first metatarsal and the proximal phalanx. The intermetatarsal angle of the first and second metatarsals is determined by bisecting the longitudinal axis of the first and second metatarsals. Hallux interphalangeus is the angle defined by lines bisecting the proximal

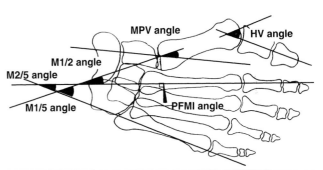

Figure 24–48. The metatarsus primus varus (MPV) angle measures the relationship of the axis of the first metatarsal shaft to the axis of the medial cuneiform. Higher numbers are associated with oblique medial cuneiform articular facets or a high degree of subluxation in an unstable joint. The proximal first metatarsal inclination (PFMI) is the angle that is formed between the proximal articular surface of the first metatarsal and the axis of the second metatarsal. Researchers have determined that the articular surface of the base of the first metatarsal is more reliably measured than the distal articular facet of the medial cuneiform. (From Tanaka Y, Takakura Y, Kumai T, et al: Radiographic analysis of hallux valgus. J Bone Joint Surg 1995;77A:197–204.)

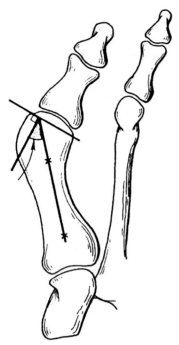

Figure 24–49. The distal metatarsal articular angle is the angle formed between the distal articular surface of the first metatarsal and its shaft. (From Coughlin MJ: Hallux valgus. *In* Springfield DS [ed]: Instructional Course Lecture 46. Rosemont, IL, American Academy of Orthopaedic Surgeons, 1997, pp 357–391.)

and distal phalanges. The distal metatarsal articular angulation is defined as the angle created between a line transversely connecting the proximal edge of the articular surfaces and a line bisecting the longitudinal axis of the first metatarsal (Fig. 24–49). Assessments include the relative length of the first and second metatarsals, the angulation of the first metatarsal medial cuneiform joint, the presence of arthritis in the first MTP joint, and evidence of generalized metatarsus adductus. Initially, the position of the sesamoid bones in relation to the metatarsal head should be assessed.

Based on clinical and radiographic evaluation, a hallux valgus deformity is considered mild when the angle of the hallux valgus is 20 degrees, the medial eminence is painful, and there is minimal metatarsus primus varus, a relatively congruous joint, and anatomic alignment of the sesamoid bones. Moderate hallux valgus deformity involves a hallux valgus angle of 20 to 40 degrees, moderate metatarsus primus varus, and possible loss of congruency and displacement of the sesamoid bones laterally from under the metatarsal head. Severe hallux valgus deformity involves a hallux valgus angle greater than 40 degrees, lateral deviation and significant metatarsus primus varus, incongruity of the first joint (usually), significant pronation of the hallux, and complete subluxation of the sesamoid complex laterally.

Treatment of a hallux valgus deformity in the early stage is conservative and includes selection of appropriate shoes that have a high, wide toe box and a soft leather upper. If associated planovalgus foot deformity exists, orthotic devices may be helpful. Surgical intervention is indicated when conservative measures fail and there is progression of deformity, increasing difficulty with shoe wear, and involvement of the second MTP joint as manifested by a crossover toe deformity or claw toe with instability. Types of surgery include correction of the valgus deformity and pronation of the hallux, resection of the prominent medial eminence of the first metatarsal head, relocation of the sesamoid subluxation, and reduction of the metatarsus primus varus, when present. Factors in the decision-making process concerning the type of surgical procedure to perform include the age and activity level of the patient, the presence of arthrosis, generalized ligamentous laxity, hypomobility of the first ray, congruency of the joint, physical shape of the metatarsal head, and degree of the hallux valgus, intermetatarsal, and distal metatarsal articular angles. It is important to identify the apex of the deformity; it may be at the first metatarsal–medial cuneiform joint, at the first MTP joint, or within the proximal phalanx (hallux interphalangeus). Contraindications to bunion surgery include spasticity, ligamentous laxity as seen in the Marfan and Ehlers-Danlos syndromes, and vascular or skin insufficiency.

Surgical procedures include exostectomy, soft tissue repair, proximal metatarsal osteotomy, distal metatarsal osteotomy, resection arthroplasty, proximal phalangeal osteotomy, and arthrodesis (Fig. 24–50). Exostectomy involves excision of the prominent medial eminence. It is indicated in cases of enlargement of the eminence without significant hallux valgus deformity or metatarsus primus varus. This procedure is performed in conjunction with soft tissue repair. Indications for soft tissue repair include mild to moderate hallux valgus deformity (less than 40 degrees and with a metatarsus primus varus of less than 15 degrees). This may be performed in isolation or in conjunction with a distal metatarsal osteotomy.

The modified McBride procedure corrects all soft tissue components of the MTP joint deformity. Complications that may result from isolated soft tissue repair include recurrence of the deformity and hallux varus. They may be caused by overcorrection at surgery or by removal of the fibular sesamoid bone or division of the lateral tendon of the FHB during exposure.

Distal metatarsal osteotomies include the Mitchell procedure and the chevron (Austin) osteotomy. The Mitchell procedure is indicated for moderate hallux valgus deformities that have an intermetatarsal angle of less than 18 degrees and in patients younger than 50 years of age. Complications involve excessive shortening, avascular necrosis of the metatarsal head, malunion, and nonunion. The chevron osteotomy is indicated in both adolescents and adults when the hallux valgus deformity is 30 degrees and the angle between the first and second metatarsals is 15 degrees or less. The nature of the cut means that it is more stable and has a higher rate of union than that provided by the Mitchell osteotomy. There is increased stability, rapid healing, and minimal shortening. It is indicated in cases of hallux valgus with metatarsus primus varus of mild to moderate deformity in middle-aged patients less than 60 years of age. Contraindications include the presence of arthrosis in the first MTP joint or severe metatarsus primus varus and an age older than 60 years.

A proximal (basilar) metatarsal osteotomy is used in a

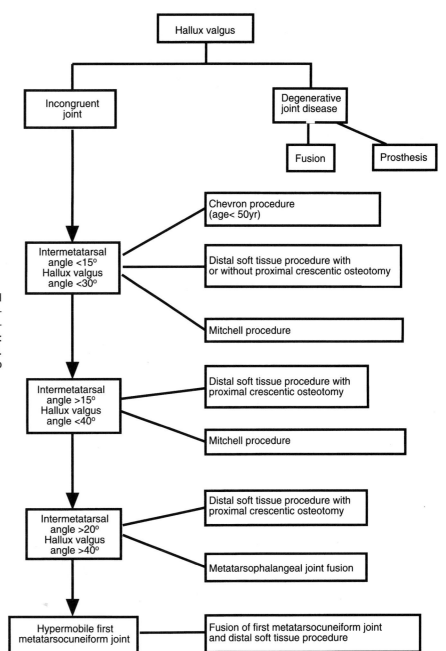

Figure 24–50. Algorithm for surgical decision making in hallux valgus surgery as proposed by Mann and Coughlin. (From Mann RA, Coughlin JA [eds]: Surgery of the Foot and Ankle, 6th ed. St. Louis, Mosby-Year Book, 1993, pp 167–197.)

case in which there is a high degree of hallux valgus deformity associated with metatarsus primus varus greater than 15 degrees and in the presence of an incongruous joint. Techniques include the crescentic and opening and closing wedge osteotomies, as well as the proximal chevron osteotomy. The procedure is performed in conjunction with a distal soft tissue release. Complications include delayed union, nonunion, and malunion including dorsal displacement of the first metatarsal, which may result in transfer metatarsalgia to the second or lesser metatarsal heads. An Akin osteotomy is a closing wedge osteotomy of the proximal phalanx and is the procedure of choice for hallux valgus interphalangeus. It may also be used in conjunction with an osteotomy involving the first metatarsal and for mild pain when hallux valgus deformity is associated with overriding second toe deformity. Contraindications include

stiffness of the adjacent IP joint, potential laceration of the FHL tendon, and nonunion, because this procedure is performed in the middiaphyseal region of the proximal phalanx.

Arthrosis of the first MTP joint in conjunction with hallux valgus may be aggravated or potentiated with surgery. The procedures available for handling arthritic bunion deformities include resection arthroplasty and arthrodesis of the first MTP joint. Resection arthroplasty that involves a section of the base of the proximal phalanx and removal of the medial eminence is known as the Keller procedure. It decompresses the MTP joint section of the proximal phalanx and causes resultant relaxation of contracted lateral structures. Although it was a popular procedure in the past, current primary indications for its performance include impending medial skin breakdown and limited ambulation in patients of advanced age. Occasionally it is used as a salvage procedure in failed bunion surgeries. Complications of resection arthroplasty include lateral-transfer metatarsalgia, excessive shortening of the hallux, loss of purchase of the toe with gait, and cock-up toe deformity. Arthrodesis of the first MTP joint has been a reliable and durable procedure that is indicated for management of severe deformities associated with degenerative joint disease, neuromuscular conditions, and salvaging failed surgeries and in cases of previous infection. It is particularly effective in stabilizing the medial column in a patient with rheumatoid arthritis. Toe position ranges from 10 to 15 degrees of dorsiflexion and 15 to 20 degrees of valgus. Complications include nonunion, malunion, and degenerative arthrosis of the adjacent interphalangeal joint. An alternative, although less popular, option for managing bunion deformity associated with arthrosis is the use of an implant. Previous double-stem polymeric silicone (Silastic) implants met with high failure rates, triggering acute inflammatory reactions and local bone resorption. Patients developed synovitis, bone invasion, and lymphatic involvement with fracture of the implant. Other total toe implants made of polyethylene and hybrids have been described, although to date no long-term follow-up has been done. Implants are not indicated for an active individual who places significant demands on the forefoot.

Hallux Varus. Hallux varus is a medial deviation of the great toe at the MTP joint. Causes include complications related to hallux valgus surgery in which an overcorrection was made and involvement of the capsular structures or rupture of the conjoined tendon, as seen in rheumatic conditions. The deformity has been described in excision of the fibular sesamoid bone as originally described by McBride for a soft tissue bunion procedure. Imbalances created by corrective bunion procedures include overplication of the medial capsule, overpull of the abductor hallucis tendon, medial displacement of the tibial sesamoid bone, excessive resection of the medial eminence, and overcorrection of the first metatarsal in cases of metatarsus primus varus when a proximal first metatarsal osteotomy leads to a negative first intermetatarsal angle. Surgery for a supple deformity and preserved MTP joint involves the use of an EHL tendon transfer under the intermetatarsal ligament and medial capsule lengthening. Invariably, in fixed deformities, the recommendation is for a primary arthrodesis of the MTP joint.

Hallux Rigidus. Hallux rigidus is painful loss of motion of the first MTP joint. Although it may occur bilaterally, often one side is predominantly worse. It generally occurs in middle-aged and older persons but may also occur in active younger people. The causes of hallux rigidus include congenital and juvenile conditions secondary to osteochondritis dissecans of the first metatarsal head. Other causes are improper shoes, occupational stress, a long first metatarsal, and underlying arthritides, including gout, psoriasis, and rheumatoid arthritis. The patient presents with an enlarged first MTP joint, which is warm and swollen and has decreased range of motion, predominantly in dorsiflexion. Symptoms are usually worse in the morning and are aggravated by prolonged walking and standing. Shoes with elevated heels tend to increase the pain. Radiographic examinations appear normal but show enlarging dorsal exostosis on the metatarsal head and the base of the proximal phalanx. With time and severity, a mediolateral exostosis may develop. Radiographs show a decrease in joint space, sclerotic joint margins, flattening of the first metatarsal head without chondral defects, and subchondral cyst formation consistent with progressive arthrosis.

Initial treatment consists of conservative management with orthotic devices and shoe modifications. The goal is reduction of stress across the first MTP joint during gait. Modifications include a stiff sole, a steel shank, or a rocker-bottom attachment to minimize stress during the toe-off phase of stance and gait. A rocker bar may be used to prevent motion. Ancillary treatments include nonsteroidal anti-inflammatory drugs and occasional use of intra-articular steroid injections.

Surgical intervention may be indicated in the event of pain that is unresponsive to conservative measures. Possible treatments include resection arthroplasty, heel cheilectomy, metatarsal or phalangeal osteotomy, implant arthroplasty, and arthrodesis (Fig. 24–51). In an adolescent, removal of a loose body may serve to increase range of motion and reduce pain. Alternatively, if mild involvement is present, a closing dorsal wedge osteotomy of the proximal phalanx will provide a better functioning range of motion and pain reduction. Resection of the dorsal osteophytes has been recommended for most forms of hallux rigidus. This procedure involves removal of the proliferative periarticular bone to alleviate pain associated with

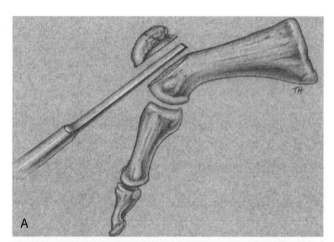

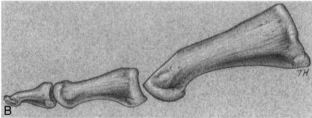

Figure 24–51. *A,* One quarter to one third of the dorsal portion of the metatarsal head is removed with a straight osteotome. This is the critical step in the procedure that allows restoration of dorsiflexion of the great toe. *B,* Appearance of the metatarsal head after removal of dorsal osteophytes. (From Clanton TO, Dorham-Smith: Cheilectomy for the treatment of hallux rigidus. Oper Tech Orthop 1992;2[3].)

dorsiflexion, but it may not improve range of motion. Current studies indicate that in the majority of patients, little or no progression of the degenerative process occurs. It is therefore recommended for cases of mild to moderate degenerative conditions of the first MTP joint. For more severe extensive global arthrosis of the first MTP joint or when cheilectomy has failed, the recommendation for an adult is a Keller procedure or arthrodesis of the first MTP joint. In cases of hallux valgus deformities, the Keller procedure, although yielding satisfactory results, weakens push-off and may create transfer metatarsalgia. It is now recommended that it be used only as a salvage procedure and for elderly sedentary patients. Arthrodesis remains the mainstay salvage procedure for persistent pain in an active patient who demands stability and durability of the first ray.

DISORDERS OF THE SESAMOID COMPLEX

Fractures involving the sesamoid bones may be acute injuries associated with hyperdorsiflexion, such as football injuries, falls from a height, or repetitive stress injuries, as seen in miners and dancers. Physical examination often reveals diminished range of motion at the MTP joint, pain on palpation of the sesamoid bones, and decreased strength of plantarflexion. Pain is often present with weight bearing and ambulation. Other causes of pain include inflammation of the sesamoid bones (sesamoiditis), chondromalacia of the sesamoid bones, osteochondritis dissecans, acute fractures, and chronic stress fractures. Radiographs should include weight-bearing AP and lateral views of the foot in addition to axial and medial sesamoid views to assess alignment of the sesamoids in relation to the first metatarsal head. A common variant seen in approximately 25% of individuals is a bipartite sesamoid bone, with 80% involving the tibial sesamoid bone. Differentiation between a bipartite sesamoid bone and an acute fracture may be difficult. Generally, the sum of the sesamoid fragments should be equal in amount to the adjacent uninvolved sesamoid bone. When the sum is greater than the adjacent sesamoid, a bipartite sesamoid bone exists. Sesamoid views in dorsiflexion should be compared with nonstress views if there is concern that diastasis may occur in either an acute fracture or a bipartite sesamoid bone. Differential diagnosis should also include vascular necrosis, which is typified by a dense sclerotic white sesamoid bone on radiographic examination. Conservative management of acute sesamoiditis includes a dancer pad to unload the symptomatic sesamoid bone, reduction in heel height to a negative-heel shoe, anti-inflammatory medications, and consideration of local steroid injections. Occasionally, casting is necessary in refractory cases. Chronic sesamoiditis of 6 months' to a year's duration that is refractory to conservative measures may be excised with satisfactory results. This should be performed, however, only if just one of the sesamoids is involved. Otherwise, there is potential for transfer and increased symptoms involving the adjacent sesamoid bone, which aggravate the condition. If a sesamoid bone is excised through an inferior medial incision, the lateral sesamoid bone is approached through a dorsal incision in the first web space or through a plantar incision in the same area. If the bone is excised, it is essential to restore the tendinous balance of the FHB or subsequent varus or valgus deformity may develop. Sesamoid bones should

never be excised simultaneously because of the potential for development of a claw toe deformity. Complications involving sesamoid bone excision include diminished range of motion, continued pain, and progressive varus or valgus deformity.

DEFORMITIES OF THE LESSER TOES

Lesser toe deformities include bunionette deformities of the fifth MTP joint; claw, hammer, and mallet toe deformities of all lesser toes; instability with crossover toe deformity; and Freiberg's infraction, which is unique to the second MTP joint.

The bunionette, or Taylor's bunion, is a deformity similar to that of the hallux valgus deformity, but it occurs in the fifth MTP joint and is characterized by the presence of a prominence over the lateral aspect of the fifth metatarsal head. When compressed by shoe wear, the prominence creates pain in the bursa over the fifth metatarsal head and a plantar lateral callosity. When associated with hallux valgus, the forefoot deformity is considered a splay foot. In the majority of cases, a bunionette deformity is associated with a pronated foot. Bunionette deformities are the result of several anatomic variances, as classified by Coughlin, including enlargement of the metatarsal head, bowing or curving laterally of the metatarsal shaft, displacement of the metatarsal head into a more prominent position, or divergence between the fourth and fifth metatarsal rays (Fig. 24–52). Physical examination reveals a prominent, tender lateral eminence. Treatment is uniformly conservative and includes a shoe with a wide toe box and a soft leather upper to reduce extrinsic pressure against the outer border of the foot. If conservative measures fail, surgery may be indicated to excise the prominent lateral eminence in the absence of any additional deformities. If there is lateral bowing of the fifth metatarsal ray or divergence of the fourth and fifth metatarsals, or if the proximal base of the fifth metatarsal has a dysvascular area, proximal metaphyseal-diaphyseal osteotomies are discouraged because of the potential for slow healing and nonunion. Deformities associated with a laterally curved metatarsal may be addressed by performing a distal osteotomy. Given the narrowness of the distal fifth metatarsal, stability of these osteotomies is difficult, limiting the magnitude of correction. Other osteotomies include a distal chevron osteotomy and a closing wedge osteotomy. A deformity associated with divergence between the fourth and fifth metatarsals commonly requires an osteotomy at the mid-diaphyseal region. This permits controlled medial rotation of the distal fragment. The metatarsal is osteotomized obliquely from dorsal-proximal to plantar-distal, and the distal fragment is rotated medially and fixed in position.

Deformities of the lesser toes are classified as either fixed or flexible. Deformities that occur in the sagittal plane include mallet, hammer, and claw toe deformities. Mallet toe is a flexion deformity at the DIP joint. The PIP and MTP joints are not involved. Hammer toe is a flexion deformity that occurs at the PIP joint; the middle and distal phalanges are plantarflexed in relation to the proximal phalanx. Claw toe is a hammer toe deformity with the addition of hyperextension or dorsiflexion at the MTP joint, creating an intrinsic minus position of the lesser toes (Fig.

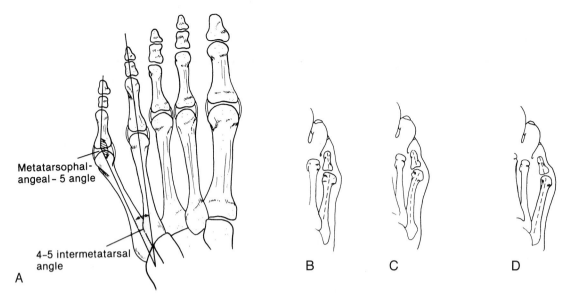

Figure 24–52. *A,* The fifth MTP joint angle; the 4–5 intermetatarsal angle. *B,* Bunionette caused by a prominent fifth metatarsal condyle. *C,* Angulation at the distal fifth metatarsal, causing prominence. *D,* Splayed or increased 4–5 metatarsal angulation, resulting in the bunionette deformity. (*A* and *C* from Mann RA, Coughlin MJ: The Video Textbook of Foot and Ankle Surgery. St. Louis, Medical Video Production, 1991. *B* and *D* from Mann RA, Coughlin MJ: Surgery of the Foot and Ankle, 6th ed. St. Louis, Mosby-Year Book, 1993, pp 442–443.)

24–53). This deformity is commonly seen in neuromuscular conditions, including cerebral palsy.

The causes of mallet and hammer toes include ill-fitting or poorly designed shoes and therefore are more common in women than in men. A restricted toe box creates a buckling effect on the end of the toe, plantarflexing the PIP and DIP joints and contributing to an imbalance in which the extrinsic muscles exert greater pull on the foot than do the intrinsic muscles. The long extensors act on the extensor sling and hood at the proximal phalanx, forcing the MTP joint to dorsiflex, and the long and short flexors curl the toe under. The dorsiflexion force at the

MTP joint is opposed by the underpowered lumbricals and interossei. This dorsiflexed position of the MTP joint secondarily exerts tension on the short flexor, creating a PIP joint flexion contracture. Toe deformities, especially when presenting globally and symmetrically, are associated with the cavus foot deformities seen in neuromuscular conditions such as peripheral neuropathies (e.g., diabetes and Charcot-Marie-Tooth syndrome) and lower motor neuron disorders (e.g., myelodysplasia, poliomyelitis, and multiple sclerosis). Claw toe anatomy, as defined by Myerson in 1989, includes contracture of the dorsal capsular and extensor tendons, dorsal shifting of the intrinsic muscles with volar plate insufficiency, and subsequent joint dislocation.

Symptoms include painful corns over the dorsal bony prominences of the PIP joint and difficulty with shoe wear. Physical examination reveals tender, hyperkeratotic lesions over the dorsal PIP joint and painful terminal corns. With advanced deformities, including claw toe deformities, there may be pain under the metatarsal head, or metatarsalgia. Although the initial deformities are flexible, later soft tissue contractures result in fixed deformities.

Initial management is nonsurgical; the goal is to alleviate the painful callosities and accommodate the deformity. Painful terminal corns of the toes, as seen in mallet toe and hammer toe, can be relieved by using crest pads that elevate the toe tips, thus eliminating the pressure exerted by the sole of the shoe. Shoes with soft leather uppers and wide toe boxes provide the increased volume required by the presence of sagittal plane deformities. Orthotics with metatarsal pads or bars may help to relieve pressure under the metatarsal heads. Strapping flexible deformities with tape or commercially available loop pads can help to rebalance the toe. Conservative measures are relegated to accommodation only (Fig. 24–54).

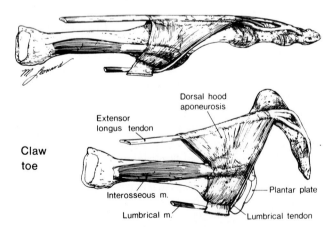

Figure 24–53. Claw toe. The normal and pathologic anatomy of the MTP joint. Note the dorsal subluxation of the interosseous tendon, the tethering of the lumbrical tendon, and the dorsal bowstringing of the extensor hood. (From Meyerson MS: Arthroplasty of the second toe. Sem Arthroplast 1992;3:32.)

Surgery is indicated when conservative measures fail to stabilize the deformity. It is necessary to differentiate between fixed and flexible deformities. The passive pushup test can reveal whether a flexible deformity exists when dorsal displaced pressure is applied under the metatarsal (see Fig. 24–20). In a mallet toe deformity, a tenotomy of the flexor digitorum longus (FDL) at the DIP joint is all that is required if it is flexible. If it is fixed, PIP resection arthroplasty or fusion in conjunction with a tenotomy of the FDL and plantar capsule is necessary. Flexible hammer toe deformities are effectively managed by transferring the FDL to the extensor aponeuroses, which provides dynamic correction (the Girdlestone-Taylor procedure). Alternatively, in fixed PIP flexion deformities, resection arthroplasty or fusion of the PIP joint is indicated. In the presence of metatarsalgia and extension into a hyperdorsiflexion deformity of the MTP joint (a claw toe deformity), dorsal capsulotomy is performed, along with collateral ligament release, plantar plate mobilization, and extenson tendon lengthening at the MTP. This can be performed in conjunction with a flexor-to-extensor tendon transfer in a flexible deformity. In advanced fixed deformities with either subluxation or dislocation of the MTP joint, skeletal shortening (by dorsiflexion or shortening osteotomy or both) at a metatarsal shaft or neck may be required in order to relocate the MTP joint. This procedure is indicated not only in cases of long-standing fixed deformity but also in cases of arthrosis and to minimize vascular embarrassment while attempting reduction.

The fifth toe is predisposed to unique deformities. In addition to the cock-up toe deformity, contractures at the IP joint may present as an overlapping or underlapping of the fifth toe, which creates pressure on the lateral margin of the digit. This often results in dystrophic changes of the lateral nail fold and callosities along the dorsolateral aspect of the interphalangeal joint. These deformities may be addressed by performing soft tissue releases, including the release of the EDL and dorsomedial capsular tissues in conjunction with a resection arthroplasty of the PIP joint. A soft tissue contracture can also be managed by performing a Y-V plasty. A severe deformity requires a transfer of the EDL tendon to the abductor digiti quinti tendon, as described by Lapidus, to derotate the toe and correct the sagittal plane cock-up toe deformity. Mild to moderate cock-up deformities can be addressed by using surgical techniques similar to those used for the central toes. In the case of a severe fixed deformity, however, salvage treatment, including a total proximal phalangectomy and plantar dermadesis (the Ruiz-Mora procedure), is required. This procedure appreciably shortens the digit and relieves the deformity but may result in a secondary bunionette deformity of the toe because of the loss of MTP stability, and it may also create digital corn deformities or a floppy toe.

Conditions unique to the second MTP joint include the crossover toe deformity associated with hallux valgus deformities and avascular necrosis of the second metatarsal head, or Freiberg's infraction. Dorsomedial deviation of the second toe occurs as a result of loss of static stabilizers, including the lateral collateral ligament. Local synovitis creates attenuation of the stabilizers. It is often brought on by progressive hallux valgus deformity, which alters the normal pressure distribution under the first ray and creates overload at the second MTP joint. Synovitis of the second

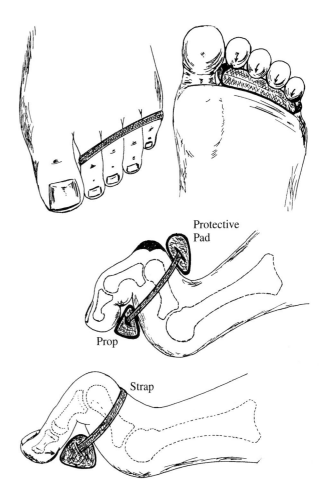

Figure 24–54. The dorsal subluxation test for instability of the MTP joint is performed by grasping the base of the proximal phalanx and attempting to subluxate or dislocate the joint with a dorsally directed force. (From Brahms M: Corns and deformities of the small toes. *In* Jahss D [ed]: Disorders of the Foot and Ankle: Medical and Surgical Management, Vol I. Philadelphia, WB Saunders, 1991, pp 1175–1197.)

MTP joint has been reported in isolation in athletes, particularly in the presence of a Morton foot pattern or a relatively long second metatarsal in relation to the first and third metatarsals. Examination of a symptomatic second MTP joint with synovitis includes a Hamilton-Thompson test, which is a provocative Lockman test that investigates the stability of the collateral ligaments when restraining a dorsally directed force (see Figs. 24–21 and 24–54). Differential diagnosis includes inter-digital neuroma of the second web space, which, although rare, occurs as a secondary phenomenon because of traction from the medially drifting second toe. Deterioration of the MTP joint and static restraints ultimately result in dislocation of this joint.

The treatment of synovitis includes stabilizing the joint by taping and strapping it, making appropriate shoe modifications, using metatarsal pads, placing cushioning under the metatarsal head region, and attaching rocker soles to the outsides of the shoes (Fig. 24–55). Administering anti-inflammatory medications and local corticosteroid injections may help to break the synovitic pattern. Once a deformity has become evident and is reducible by performing the passive push-up test, synovectomy of the second MTP joint in conjunction with flexor-extensor tendon

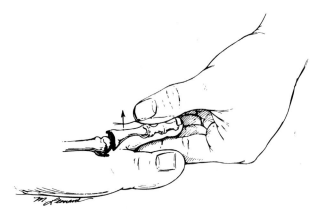

Figure 24–55. Pads and straps designed to alleviate pain caused by hammer toe deformity. (From Kelikian H: Hallux Valgus, Allied Deformities of the Forefoot, and Metatarsalgia. Philadelphia, WB Saunders, 1965, pp 282–334.)

transfer (the Girdlestone-Taylor procedure) helps to reduce and stabilize the joint. In frank dislocations of the second MTP joint, osteotomy of the second metatarsal head allows reduction of the MTP joint while decompressing the forces across the joint. Additionally, if there is arthrosis or a fixed deformity that cannot be reduced, resection arthroplasty of the metatarsal head (the DuVries procedure) may be required. A skeletal shortening procedure may be performed in isolation or in conjunction with flexor-extensor tendon transfer, depending on the severity and instability of the joint. In a crossover toe deformity, additional stabilization may be derived from a flexor-extensor tendon transfer with asymmetrical lateral pull to reduce the drift of the proximal phalanx or from a reconstruction of the lateral collateral ligament using the EDB as a tendon transfer. This may be performed again in conjunction with a metatarsal head osteotomy to reduce the MTP joint. Involvement of both the second and third joints with extensive instability and dislocation may be addressed by performing a partial proximal phalangectomy and partial syndactylization of the second and third toes.

Freiberg's infraction is considered to be a result of both vascular and traumatic insult to the second metatarsal head. It occurs in the early teenage years and manifests as pain and swelling. Radiographic findings include osteochondrosis with central collapse and, over a variable length of time, dorsal osteophyte formation and flattening of the metatarsal head, which create restriction of motion in dorsiflexion as well as pain. End-stage deformity includes arthrosis. Treatment during the early period is non–weight bearing and restricted weight bearing until the acute event has resolved. It may include a metatarsal pad, a rocker-bottom sole, shoes with low heels, and restricted activity. Once the flattening of the head by dorsal osteophytes has caused the blocking of motion, complete excision of the osteophytes by means of synovectomy may be indicated. In cases of focal central degeneration, a dorsiflexion osteotomy that presents healthy plantar articular cartilage to the articulating MTP joint may be indicated. End-stage involvement with global arthrosis may require a distal DuVries resection arthroplasty with interposition of the extensor and flexor tendons to create a soft tissue spacer.

Injuries of the Tendons of the Foot and Ankle

Injuries of the tendons of the foot and ankle may be caused by subacute or chronic inflammatory conditions that result in tendinitis or rupture. *Tendinitis* is a nonspecific term for a variety of pathologic conditions of tendons. Peritendinitis is an inflammatory process of the vascularized connective tissue structures surrounding the tendon and may include the peritenons and tenosynovium. The term *tendinosis* is reserved for a degenerative intratendinous process. Management of most tendinous conditions of the foot and ankle is the same: rest and immobilization combined with anti-inflammatory medication. Various modalities of physical therapy may be used to reduce swelling and inflammation, and there may be a secondary emphasis on strengthening and on expanding range of motion until the inflammation is under control. Disorders of the tendons of the foot and ankle are commonly associated with underlying rheumatic or metabolic conditions and are often the initial presenting symptoms. It is essential, therefore, to rule out systemic and metabolic conditions as the underlying causes, especially in the case of a bilateral presentation. Common disorders of the tendons are those involving the peroneal tendon complex, the anterior tibial tendon, the Achilles tendon, the posterior tibial tendon, and the FHL tendon.

INJURIES RESULTING FROM OVERUSE OF THE PERONEAL TENDON

The peroneal tendon complex consists of the peroneus brevis and longus, which course behind the lateral malleolus. At the level of the ankle joint, the brevis lies behind the fibula, and the longus is slightly posterolateral. They become tendinous prior to reaching the ankle joint in a common sheath. The brevis and longus travel in an anterior fibro-osseous tunnel and have distinct sheaths distal to the fibula. The brevis is separated from the longus by the peroneal tubercle. The peroneus longus inserts on the first metatarsal base and the brevis inserts on the base of the fifth metatarsal. The primary lateral restraint, providing stability against subluxation, is the superior peroneal retinaculum. Secondary stability is afforded by the posterior aspect of the lateral malleolus, which creates a peroneal groove with variable sulcus depth. This is increased by a fibrocartilaginous rim on the lateral border.

Peroneal tendon disorders include injury and degeneration of the peroneus brevis or longus and instability of the peroneal tendon complex.

Injuries of the peroneus brevis tendon occur at the level of the fibular groove, proximal to the ankle joint. There is direct contact with the sharp ridge as the tendon changes course by 45 degrees. Extrinsic pressure is added by the overlying peroneus longus tendon. Injuries of the peroneus longus occur at the cuboid tunnel, where the peroneus longus is in direct contact with the lateral calcaneal wall and undergoes a 45-degree-angle change at the cuboid facet to enter the deep soft tissues of the foot. Overall, injuries of the peroneus brevis tendon are much more common than those of the longus and may be identified at the time of lateral ankle ligament reconstruction (Fig. 24–56).

Diagnosis may occur as long as 8 years or more after the time of injury. Peroneus brevis tendon injuries may manifest as tenosynovitis, a longitudinal split, or subluxa-

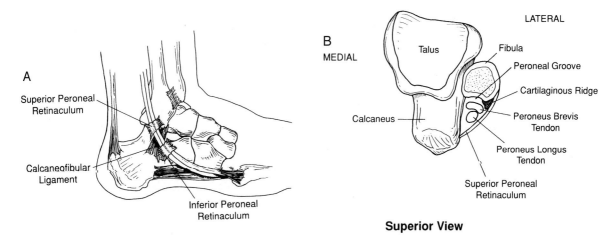

Figure 24–56. Anatomic relationships of the ankle. The peroneal tendons are held in position by the superior and inferior peroneal retinacula and the fibrous rim on the posterolateral aspect of the fibula. The calcaneofibular ligament lies below the peroneal tendons. *A,* Lateral view. *B,* Superior view. (From Clanton TO, Schol LS: Athletic injuries to the soft tissues of the foot and ankle. *In* Mann RA, Coughlin MJ [eds]: Surgery of the Foot and Ankle, 6th ed. St. Louis, Mosby-Year Book, 1993, p 1169.)

tion or frank dislocation of the tendon. The patient has a history of an inversion-supination sprain or of repetitive injury and lateral instability. Injury may also occur secondary to forced dorsiflexion during push-off. There is often painful swelling in the retromalleolar area and lateral ankle discomfort without any antecedent trauma. Differential diagnosis should include an inflammatory condition. Physical examination often finds fullness along the tendon and diffuse tenderness, pain with resisted eversion or passive stretch, increased localized tenderness at the posterior ridge of the fibula (associated with longitudinal splits), and weakness in eversion. There is little pain associated with frank rupture. Examination should also include assessment of stability of the ankle ligaments, both the ATFL and the CFL. Subluxation and dislocation may be determined by the presence of a snapping, popping sensation with resisted eversion while the posterior fibular border is palpated. A fixed dislocation may present with vague lateral ankle findings, including chronic swelling and fullness over the distal lateral fibula. Radiographic studies are often normal. Occasionally, a fleck sign signifying evulsion of the posterior distal fibula at the level of the superior peroneal retinaculum may correlate with a peroneal dislocation. Stress radiographs of the ankle may be required to rule out associated ankle instability. Other studies that are helpful in assessing peroneal pathology include MRI and ultrasonography. Tenography is no longer commonly used as a diagnostic test.

Medical management of peroneal tendon pathology includes cast immobilization for 2 to 3 weeks, peroneal strengthening exercises, physical therapy, anti-inflammatory medication, and the use of a lateral heel wedge to minimize excursion of the peroneal tendons. If there is evidence of acute rupture, with subluxation or dislocation of the peroneal tendon, cast immobilization is required for as long as 4 to 6 weeks and is followed by an ankle brace.

Indications for operative treatment are persistent pain and failure of conservative treatment. The goals of surgery are to reconstruct the superior peroneal retinaculum where

it has become attenuated, to perform a tenosynovectomy with decompression of the peroneal tendons, to debride the flattened and attritted peroneus brevis, and to perform tubularization and repair using nonabsorbable sutures. Frank rupture of the tendon may require end-to-end repair. If there is a significant gap, tenodesis to the adjacent peroneal tendon is recommended. Chronic subluxation or instability of the tendon with range of motion on the operating table may mean that repair of a patulous superior peroneal retinaculum is necessary. Additionally, if there is a low-lying peroneus brevis muscle–tendon junction or if an anomalous muscle of the peroneus cortis is present, a volume reduction of the contents of the peroneal complex is required. The retinaculum is advanced and secured to bone, or pants-over-vest repair is performed. Associated lateral ligament instability may require a modified Brostrom procedure for stabilization. Severe dislocations of peroneal tendons require reduction of the tendons and repair of the superior peroneal retinaculum in acute injuries; alternatively, if the superior peroneal retinaculum is associated with bony evulsion, open reduction and internal fixation with miniscrews or sutures are indicated. In cases of chronic dislocation, the fibular-groove–deepening procedure is performed by creating a trough in the posterior aspect of the fibula, or the lateral bone block technique may be performed to deepen the groove. If attenuated, the superior peroneal retinaculum may have to be reconstructed using local soft tissues.

Complications of peroneal tendon surgery include sural neuritis, superficial peroneal nerve neuritis and neuroma, recurrent pain, propagation of tendinosis or tear, possible recurrent instability, and excessive stiffening and arthrofibrosis.

Peroneus longus tendon tears, like brevis injuries, may manifest as tenosynovitis, tendinosis, or rupture. A unique condition not seen in the peroneus brevis tendon is the painful os peroneal syndrome, which consists of a stenosing peroneus longus tenosynovitis caused by an enlarged peroneal tubercle, chronic os peroneum pathology, or exostosis after ankle calcaneal fracture. Clinical presentation includes plantar lateral foot pain that is nonspecific. The injury is associated with a supination-inversion mechanism and may be aggravated by weight bearing or heel rise. Physical examination reveals localized tenderness in the region of the cuboid tunnel or peroneal tubercle. There may or may not be associated swelling, pain that increases with heel rise, resisted plantarflexion of the first metatarsal, or forced inversion, supination, and adduction of the foot. There is mild weakness to resisted eversion, and these patients may have associated lateral ankle ligament instability. Radiographic studies may demonstrate a fracture or diastasis of the os perineum with proximal migration that is best seen on an oblique view. Additionally, Harris axial views may demonstrate an enlarged peroneal tubercle, and weight-bearing tibial calcaneal views may demonstrate lateral calcaneal impingement. MRI may be helpful in assessing tenosynovitis, tendinosis, and rupture. CT may be helpful in assessing stenosing tenosynovitis caused by an enlarged peroneal tubercle (giant peroneal tubercle syndrome).

Nonoperative treatment is similar to that for other tendon injuries, including cast immobilization, anti-inflammatory medications, physical therapy, and orthotic modifications that provide arch support and stabilization of the first metatarsal; later, a heel wedge or flare may be used. Indications for surgery are similar to those in peroneus brevis tendon injuries. The approach is distal to the fibula at the level of the calcaneal-cuboid joint. Surgery involves decompression of the peroneus longus sheath and debridement and repair of any associated tendinosis. If chronic rupture is present, it is recommended that tenodesis to the adjacent peroneus brevis be performed. With evidence of os peroneal pathology, excision followed by primary end-to-end repair of the peroneus longus is recommended. Peroneal tendinitis related to lateral calcaneal-fibular abutment may require lateral wall decompression or resection of an enlarged peroneal tubercle. Complications of surgery include sural neuritis or neuroma and persistent, recurrent pain. Development of varus foot deformity has not been described.

INJURIES RESULTING FROM OVERUSE OF THE ANTERIOR TIBIAL TENDON

Injuries of the anterior tibial tendon are relatively rare. Tenosynovitis may result from irritation by footwear or ski boots, but it is often attributed to an underlying rheumatic condition. When this type of injury does occur, it is associated with a generalized inflammatory condition or it appears in the elderly. Tenosynovitis is often related to overuse; discomfort and stiffness at the start of exercise improve with continued activity. Acute rupture may be secondary to open fracture or laceration and presents as acute foot drop and fatigue, with pain and swelling anteriorly. A chronic rupture may occur because of hypervascularity and attrition under the superior extensor retinaculum or because of extrinsic pressure from a dorsal exostosis. Generally, men 45 years old or older are at risk, and a high incidence is associated with diabetes and inflammatory conditions. These injuries involve minimal trauma, and there is usually an appreciable delay in diagnosis. A patient may present with an appreciable foot slap, weakness, or

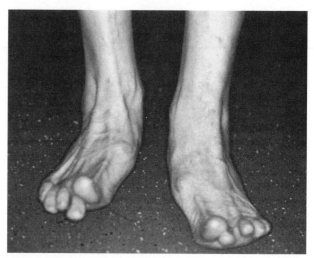

Figure 24–57. This elderly patient has loss of the normal contour of the tibialis anterior tendon in the left ankle. (From Mankey MG: Anterior tibial tendon ruptures. Foot Ankle Clin 1996;1:316.)

fatigue with ambulation. Physical examination may show diffuse swelling over the anterior ankle and a mass proximal to the ankle joint, which is considered a pseudotumor. The patient demonstrates a steppage gait, with foot drop and an inability to walk on the heels. A palpable gap may be present in acute injury that is not demonstrated in a chronic condition (Fig. 24–57). Manual muscle testing reveals weak dorsiflexion against resistance. In chronic conditions, there may also be signs of accessory tendon recruitment, which is manifested by hyperactivity of extrinsic muscles and associated clawing of the lesser toes and hallux. The differential diagnosis includes peroneal nerve injury and herniated disk with radiculopathy, so a neurologic examination is important. Diagnostic studies using plain radiographs are often normal. Ultrasonography and MRI may best delineate a rupture, which is often 3 cm proximal to the insertion site. Management is similar to that of other acute tendon injuries; transition into an ankle-foot orthosis is allowed after cast immobilization for 3 to 4 weeks. In the elderly and in sedentary individuals, rupture may be treated with casting followed by orthosis. Often, an individual regains a normal gait but has decreased ankle motion and strength. Surgery is indicated when a patient is younger or is an active individual with an acute rupture. Primary end-to-end repair may be achieved when the proximal tendon has not retracted appreciably. When avulsion of the tendon's insertion has occurred, the tendon is reinserted at a more proximal location and the retinaculum is released to gain length. In a neglected chronic rupture in which a large gap exists, either a turndown flap or a free tendon graft using the EHL may be required. Complications involving anterior tibial tendon surgery include injury to the deep or superficial peroneal nerve, rerupture, and a tenodesis effect in the adjacent tendons. The goal of repair is improvement in gait, strength, and function.

INJURIES RESULTING FROM OVERUSE OF THE FLEXOR HALLUCIS LONGUS

When overuse takes place, tenosynovitis can develop from mechanical irritation within the fibro-osseous tunnel under the sustentaculum tali, where the FHL courses. It is termed *dancer's tendinitis* because it is most common in ballet dancers and athletes who are involved in repetitive push-off activities. The tendinitis may lead to the formation of a nodule on the tendon and the triggering of the tendon as it passes through the fibro-osseous tunnel (hallux saltans). The clinical presentation is posteromedial ankle pain and occasional snapping deep to the flexor retinaculum. Pain is worse with activity and better with rest. Occasionally, there is difficulty in moving the hallux and locking of the toe. Physical examination shows tenderness over the course of the FHL tunnel and varying degrees of swelling. There may be a catching or triggering effect with passive dorsi-flexion of the ankle joint as the patient actively attempts to flex the toe. This is aggravated by passive and active range of motion against the resistance of the hallux during dorsiflexion and plantarflexion.

Differential diagnosis of posterior medial ankle pain in athletes and dancers includes FHL tendinitis, posterior tibial tendinitis, soleus syndrome, and posterior fibrous tunnel coalition. Additionally, differentiation is made between FHL tendinitis and posterior impingement syndrome, which presents with posterolateral pain rather than postero-medial pain, with tenderness behind the fibula as opposed to tenderness over the FHL tendon, and with pain that is commonly elicited by plantarflexion of the ankle (positive plantarflexion).

As with most tendon injuries, plain radiographs fail to show any significant pathology. An os trigonum may be present and must be considered in the differential diagnosis of posterior hindfoot pain. MRI will show stenosis resulting from hypertrophy of the muscle or tendon swelling and tenosynovitis of the FHL to confirm the diagnosis. Initial management of acute inflammatory symptoms should be conservative, as with other tendon injuries. Chronic symptoms, including triggering, are less likely to respond to conservative measures and may have to be treated by surgical intervention. This involves the release of the fibro-osseous tunnel through a posteromedial approach to eliminate the stenosis. Synovectomy and repair of the associated FHL tear have proved beneficial.

INJURIES RESULTING FROM OVERUSE OF THE ACHILLES TENDON

Disorders of the Achilles tendon include peritendinitis, tendinosis, partial and complete rupture, and insertional tendinitis–retrocalcaneal bursitis. Achilles tendinitis is a painful inflammation of the surrounding peritenon (peritendinitis) or degenerative changes within the tendon (tendinosis) that occur approximately 4 to 6 cm proximal to the insertion site on the os calcis. The region of the Achilles tendon complex is considered vulnerable and prone to overuse because of its poor vascularity. Achilles tendinosis is seen most commonly in runners with a history of altered training or shoe wear. Pain is present along the Achilles tendon, approximately 4 to 6 cm proximal to the insertion site, and may be associated with swelling. The pain is aggravated by activity and relieved by rest. Uphill running or walking is especially painful. Predisposing factors in Achilles tendon injuries include lower extremity malalignment, a tight Achilles tendon with poor flexibility, and errors made during training in running. Physical examination includes evaluation of the alignment and flexibility of the heel cord and palpation of the cord, insertion, and retrocalcaneal area. Symptoms include tenderness at the site of the inflammatory process and pain that is aggravated by dorsiflexion of the ankle. When significant tendinosis exists, a fusiform tender mass within the substance of the tendon occurs 4 to 6 cm proximal to the insertion site. Peritendinitis is distinguished from true tendinosis by the fact that it is a fusiform mass that is mobile, as opposed to being an immobile mass as is found in isolated tendinosis (Fig. 24–58). Peritendinitis is associated with common signs of inflammation, including pain, swelling, warmth, local tenderness, and occasional crepitus with range of motion of the ankle. Tendinosis often lacks the signs of inflammation and commonly has palpable tendon nodules and diffuse thickening of the tendon. The combination of the two, termed *peritenonitis*, shows inflammation, palpable tendon nodules, and tendon thickening. Tendinosis is characterized by a gradual onset of pain, stiffness, and diffuse tenderness and swelling at the tendon complex. When it is associated with peritendinitis, crepitation is occasionally present. Diagnostic studies include MRI in the rare cases in which confirmation by clinical examination is difficult (Fig. 24–59). These studies can distinguish between peritendinitis, which presents as the swelling and thickening of the outer sheath, and the intratendinous degeneration associated with tendinosis. Further studies, including ultrasonography, have been used and have the advantage of allowing a dynamic evaluation of the tendon. On rare occasions, a plain lateral radiograph of the ankle

Figure 24–58. *A*, Generalized swelling seen with Achilles peritendinitis and tendinosis. *B*, Localized swelling often seen with clinical diagnosis of tendinosis. (From Leach RE, James S, Wasilewski S: Achilles tendinitis. Am J Sports Med 1981;9:93–98. With permission of McGraw-Hill, Inc.)

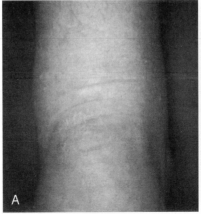
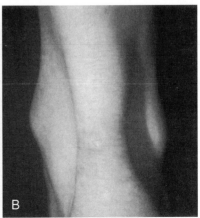

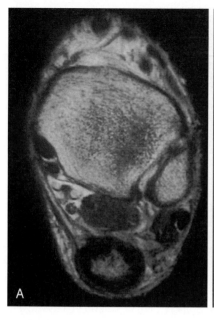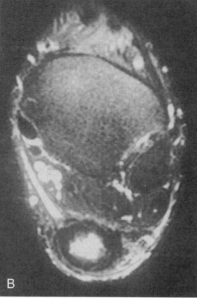

Figure 24–59. Achilles tendinosis with mucoid degeneration. *A*, Axial T2 image. *B*, Axial fat-suppressed turbo spin echo images. Note marked tendon enlargement with central intrasubstance mucoid degeneration. (From Mammone JF: MR imaging of the foot and ankle. Clin Pod Med Surg 1997;14:320.)

demonstrates the calcific deposition associated with Achilles tendinosis.

Treatment of Achilles tendon overuse injuries is primarily conservative. It includes correction of malalignment, application of ice, anti-inflammatory medications, and range-of-motion exercises for the ankle, including stretching and strengthening the plantarflexors and dorsiflexors of the ankle. Physical therapy modalities such as ultrasonography are effective. In the presence of calcific tendinosis, acetic acid iontophoresis, which alters the pH and dissolves calcium deposits, can be effective. Use of local steroid injections is not recommended because of the potential for tendon rupture and subcutaneous atrophy. A heel lift may be helpful in reducing symptoms during daily activities. Conservative management of Achilles tendon overuse injuries may mean that a period of 4 to 6 months is necessary for resolution of symptoms.

Surgery is reserved for patients in whom conservative management (a minimum 6-month course) has failed and for patients with moderate to extensive tendinosis because there is a high rate of rupture.

Surgery for peritendinitis includes excision of the thickened, scarred peritenon. In cases of a partial tear or tendinosis, the tendon is split longitudinally and the pathologic tissue is debrided using side-to-side repair; in cases of severe, extensive tendinosis, augmentation with the adjacent FHL tendon is recommended. Complications include postoperative tendon rupture, difficulty of wound healing, injury to the adjacent sural nerve, and scarring of the tendon to the peritenon.

Posterior heel pain may present as a spectrum of diseases ranging from retrocalcaneal bursitis to insertional Achilles tendinitis. Superficial posterior heel pain may be retrocalcaneal bursitis secondary to irritation caused by shoe wear. The retrocalcaneal burst, located between the posterior angle of the os calcis and the Achilles tendon, may become inflamed and hypertrophied. An enlarged posterosuperior calcaneal process is called a Haglund deformity. Retrocalcaneal bursitis is more commonly present

in middle-aged to elderly women than in men. The tenderness is medial and lateral to the Achilles tendon and adjacent to the bursa. The tendon is often less tender posteriorly. Careful palpation may differentiate a painful bursa anterior and superior to the os calcis and with fullness anterior to the tendon from insertional Achilles tendinitis, which causes pain directly at the point of posterior insertion. Continuity of the Achilles tendon complex is established based on heel rise strength and Thompson's test.

Diagnostic studies for insertional tendinosis and Haglund's deformity include a standing lateral radiograph of the foot to profile the shape and the appearance of the calcaneal prominence. Abnormal calcifications such as insertional Achilles tendon osteophytes are noted. The pitch angle of the calcaneus and the degree of prominence of the posterosuperior tuberosity (as defined by the Fowler and Phillip angle) delineate the degree of involvement (Fig. 24–60). The erosive pattern of insertional Achilles tendinitis may be a systemic condition such as seronegative arthropathy or gout. As in other Achilles tendon pathologic conditions, MRI can identify suspected insertional Achilles tendinopathy.

The treatment for isolated retrocalcaneal bursitis is conservative; it uses heel lifts to move the bursal prominence forward and away from the Achilles tendon and a firm heel counter to minimize excursion of the Achilles tendon. Anti-inflammatory medications and occasional casting or bracing are beneficial. Foot orthoses may correct any hindfoot malalignment. When associated with a Haglund deformity, surgical intervention may be required in order to resolve the symptoms. A Haglund deformity is treated in a similar fashion—modified shoe wear and orthoses to alleviate the pressure. In insertional Achilles tendinitis, a more aggressive form of rest such as casting and pedorthic management may resolve the inflammation and prevent chronic changes in the tendon. In refractory cases of insertional Achilles tendinitis associated with Haglund's deformity and retrocalcaneal bursitis, surgical resection of the bursa and excision of the posterosuperior process of the calcaneus may be

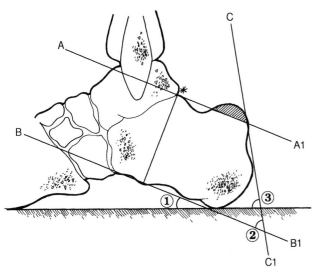

Figure 24–60. A–A1 is the parallel pitch line, drawn parallel to B–B1 starting from the posterior lip of the taloarticular facet (*). The posterosuperior calcaneal tuberosity existing above the A–A1 line *(hatched area)* is considered excessive. The calcaneal pitch angle (1) added to the Fowler and Phillips calcaneal angle (2) equals the number angle (3). Less than 90 degrees is considered normal. (From Gerken AP, McGarvey WC, Baxter DE: Insertional Achilles tendinitis. Foot Ankle Clin 1996;1:240.)

indicated. Attention is also directed toward debridement and repair of the Achilles tendon insertion and resection of any calcific deposition or osteophytes.

Ruptures of the Achilles tendon are classified as acute or neglected (chronic). They commonly occur in middle-aged men who are in moderately poor physical condition, and the location is usually the hypovascular zone approximately 3 to 5 cm proximal to the insertion. Ruptures occur as the result of the forceful eccentric contraction of an elongating triceps sura. An alternative mechanism is uncontrolled dorsiflexion of the ankle; rarely are they the result of direct trauma (Fig. 24–61). Symptoms include severe, sudden pain in the back of the calf that is described as "being hit by a bat" and is often associated with immediate swelling. In some cases, a patient continues to play sports, which contributes to the 25% rate of missed diagnoses. Diagnosis is made by palpating a defect 2 to 6 cm above the insertion of the Achilles tendon. In obese patients and individuals with severe bleeding or swelling, a gap may not be evident. The patient is placed in the prone position; two findings are consistent with full rupture of the tendon. The first is loss of passive resting tension in comparison to the opposite (unaffected) extremity, which causes the foot to be at a right angle to the remainder of the lower extremity. The second finding is based on the reliable Thompson test, which is performed with the patient prone and the foot hanging over the edge of the examination table. The midcalf muscle is squeezed. If the tendon is intact, the ankle should passively plantarflex, but if it has ruptured, no plantarflexion occurs. Radiographic studies reveal blunting of the retrocalcaneal space or, on rare occasions, bony avulsion fractures of the posterior calcaneus. In difficult cases, MRI or ultrasonography serve to confirm the diagnosis.

Treatment of an acute rupture of the Achilles tendon

can be nonoperative or operative. Nonoperative methods include a non–weight-bearing, long leg cast worn with the ankle in plantarflexion for 4 to 6 weeks and followed by the wearing of a short leg walking cast worn with the ankle in a neutral position for an additional 4 to 6 weeks. After a period of immobilization of up to 3 months, a good, stiff, supportive lace-up shoe with a heel lift is worn for an additional 1 to 2 months. The advantages of the nonoperative methods are the avoidance of complications (surgery involves wound slough and the possibility of infection), the lack of hospitalization, and a return to activities in the same amount of time as that possible after open repair. Disadvantages include a higher rerupture rate and the prolonged immobilization.

Operative methods include direct repair of the two ends of the tear. Advantages over nonoperative treatment include a lower rerupture rate (less than 4%) and proper adjustment of tendon tension, which cannot be obtained with casting alone. Disadvantages include wound complications, infection, and adhesions of the tendon in addition to sural nerve injury. To date, no study has clearly defined the best treatment for acute ruptures. Factors to be considered include age, overall medical condition, and level of activity.

Chronic, neglected ruptures are defined as tendons that go untreated for longer than 3 to 6 months. Patients often complain only of weakness and do not recall significant pain at the time of injury. The initial lack of immobilization and unprotected, continued use create a large gap between the ends of the tendon, leading to significant weakness in push-off, which manifests as difficulty in ascending stairs and hills. Treatment options for a neglected rupture include, from a conservative standpoint, bracing with an ankle foot orthosis for the elderly and for poor surgical candidates.

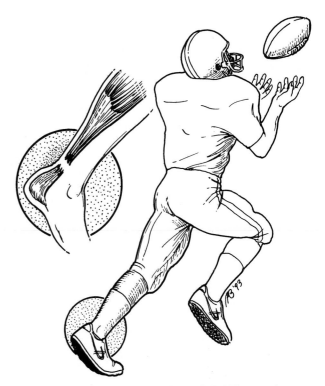

Figure 24–61. The mechanism of Achilles tendon rupture. (From Greenfield J, Stanish WD: Tendinitis and tendon ruptures. Oper Tech Sports Med 1994;2[1]:10.)

For younger, active individuals, reconstruction with a Y-V plasty advancement flap for smaller defects is advocated; intercalary grafts using the plantaris or FHL and connecting to the calcaneal tuberosity are reserved for larger defects.

INJURIES RESULTING FROM OVERUSE OF THE POSTERIOR TIBIAL TENDON

Overuse of the posterior tibial tendon causes conditions that range from mild tendinitis to tenosynovitis to complete rupture and asymmetrical flatfoot deformity. Posterior tibial dysfunction may occur secondary to trauma, inflammatory arthropathies, or attritional degenerative conditions. Causes may include trauma, degeneration secondary to a hypovascular area 0.5 cm distal to the medial malleolus, seropositive and seronegative rheumatic conditions, obesity, and overpronation that causes excessive strain on the tendon. A less common presentation occurs at the insertion onto the navicular bone either as calcific tendinosis or as a symptomatic accessory navicular bone. Predisposing factors include hypertension, obesity, diabetes, steroid exposure, and prior surgery or trauma that compromises blood flow to the tendon in 60% of cases. A lack of traumatic history is seen in more than 50% of patients. Early stages include pain, swelling, and fullness localized to the posterior medial hindfoot. With progressive deterioration of the tendon and resultant incompetent function, a progressive asymmetrical flatfoot deformity develops because of overpull on the peroneal tendons. Late symptoms include progression of deformity, difficulty with shoe wear, and lateral calcaneal-fibular impingement. Clinical examination in the early stages reveals tender, boggy edema at the level of the medial malleolus, a secondary heel cord contracture, and weakness in inversion in a foot that is plantarflexed and abducted in a non–weight-bearing position. Patients are unable to perform a single heel-toe rise on the affected side and often, in a double-stand toe rise, there is no inversion of the heel. With advanced forefoot abduction and collapse, the "too many toes" sign occurs when visualized from behind in a resting stance, as does increased heel valgus (Fig. 24–62). With advanced collapse, there is evidence of loss of the medial longitudinal arch and there are varying degrees of inflexibility. The Jack test consists of passively dorsiflexing the hallux; restoration of the medial longitudinal arch occurs in flexible conditions. Diagnostic studies consist of plain, standing films, including weight-bearing AP and lateral views of the foot. The opposite (uninvolved) extremity is used for comparison. Bilateral, modified Cobey views allow for assessment of the mechanical tibio-calcaneal axis so the extent of valgus deformity can be delineated in both the subtalar area and the ankle joint in cases of advanced collapse. On weight-bearing AP radiographs, the relationship of the talar head to the navicular bone in terms of the percentage uncovered increases in the talar–first metatarsal angle, and talocalcaneal divergence is noted. The lateral view indicates peritalar subluxation, as typified by the talonavicular sagging of a plantarflexed talus and the negative talar–first metatarsal angle (Fig. 24–63). Although it is a clinical diagnosis, MRI can confirm the status of the tendon and the extent of involvement. Findings based on the sagittal cuts of an MRI scan indicate heterogeneous changes in the tendon, tendon swelling that makes it more than twice the size of the

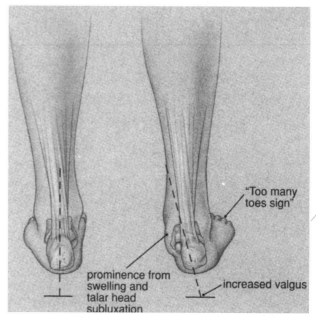

Figure 24–62. A posterior view shows a typical deformity in the right foot with swelling over the degenerated tendon, prominence of the talar head medially, and increased heel valgus. Forefoot abduction and heel valgus cause the "too many toes" sign, which can be noted by making a comparison with the opposite foot. (From Deland J: Posterior tibial tendon insufficiency. Oper Tech Orthop 1992;2:158.)

adjacent FDL tendon, and fluid resulting from tenosynovitis, which is known as the ring sign (Fig. 24–64).

The classification system proposed by Johnson (1986) is dependent on the flexibility of the flatfoot deformity. Stage I describes pain and swelling, mild posterior tibial tendon weakness, and the absence of the flatfoot deformity. Stage II involves posterior tibial tendon disruption and the presence of a flatfoot deformity that is flexible. Stage III is reserved for rigid flatfoot deformity. Treatment options are determined by the stage at presentation. Stage I conditions with minimal deformity may be addressed with orthotics, anti-inflammatory medications, and physical therapy. In fulminant tenosynovitis, cast immobilization or a modified ankle-foot orthosis is used to decrease tendon strain. Resistant tenosynovitis that is refractory to conservative measures requires a tenosynovectomy to halt development of tendinosis. Stage II, defined as a flexible but reducible flatfoot, can be treated conservatively with an ankle-foot orthosis indefinitely or can be surgically reconstructed, repairing the posterior tibial tendon by performing an FDL tendon transfer. For distal pathology involving a symptomatic accessory navicula at the tendon insertion onto the navicula, a modified Kidner procedure can be expected to produce good results. Initial high rates of failure of isolated tendon transfer led to the addition of ancillary bone procedures to increase the durability and longevity of the tendon transfer. Two popular procedures are lateral column lengthening through the os calcis (the Evans procedure) or calcaneocuboid joint in the form of an arthrodesis. The second involves a medial calcaneal heel slide acting as a second tendon transfer so as to augment the transfer of the FDL. In more severe flexible deformities and stage III rigid

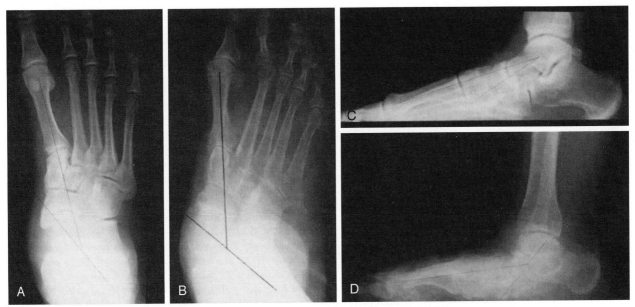

Figure 24–63. Anteroposterior and lateral weight-bearing radiographs. *A*, Moderate talonavicular subluxation. Note the increased talometatarsal angulation. *B*, Severe talonavicular subluxation. *C*, Moderate talometatarsal angulation in a patient with posterior tibial tendon dysfunction. *D*, Severe talometatarsal angulation. Note the plantarflexed talus. (From Slovenkai MP: Clinical and radiographic evaluation. Foot Ankle Clin 1997;2:250–251.)

deformities, arthrodesis is the mainstay of treatment. Isolated arthrodeses that include the subtalar joint, talonavicular joint, and calcaneocuboid joint have been proposed. In severe rigid deformities and those with associated forefoot varus, a triple arthrodesis of all three hindfoot joints is recommended.

Heel Pain

Plantar heel pain is one of the most common and potentially disabling conditions to affect the foot. There are a

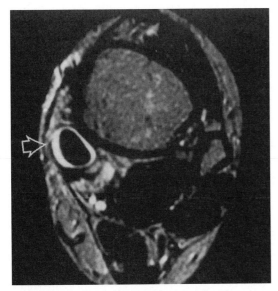

Figure 24–64. T2-weighted MRI scan showing tenosynovitis. Note the edema around the posterior tibial tendon. (From Slovenkai MP: Clinical and radiographic evaluation. Foot Ankle Clin 1997;2:253.)

multitude of potential causes for heel pain, including tumors, infection, stress fractures, inflammatory arthropathies, and compressive or metabolic neuropathies. The history of the patient's pain and a physical examination help to form a differential diagnosis; emphasis should be placed on characterizing the pain, including onset, duration, nature, localization, and relationship to physical activity. Discoloration, wounds, bumps, blisters, and tender areas, including nerve branches, should be documented.

The most common plantar heel pain is associated with a chronic injury–reparative process that leads to microtears, necrosis, and chondroid metaplasia at the origin of the plantar fascia. Heel pain syndrome is synonymous with such lay terms as *heel spur syndrome* and *plantar fasciitis*. It is typically localized in the plantar fascia origin on the plantar medial calcaneal tuberosity. The onset is insidious and is often preceded by overuse. Symptoms include morning stiffness and pain that resolve during the day. Classically, pain is most severe when arising and taking the first step on the floor or after sitting for a protracted period. It may decrease after prolonged walking and may be intolerable when jumping and running. Typically, it is a middle-aged woman, 40 to 65 years of age, who presents after recent weight gain or overuse, for example, vacation or shopping. The patient may have a pronated foot pattern or a history of wearing high-heeled shoes.

Wearing high-heeled shoes typically alleviates symptoms, whereas going barefoot and wearing flat shoes increase symptoms. Physical examination reveals a point of tenderness at the plantar medial origin of the plantar fascia on the os calcis. There is a moderately to severely tight Achilles tendon complex and restricted ankle dorsiflexion. There may be some fullness and warmth in the area of the plantar medial heel and, occasionally, associated fat pad or heel pad atrophy. The patient localizes the pain to the origin of the plantar fascia, but the central band in the midfoot is not tender. The pain typically is not elicited by passive dorsiflexion of the toes, which applies traction to the plantar fascia. Radiographs include lateral weight bearing, which may demonstrate a plantar spur; this in turn is often associated with the FDB origin and signifies chronicity. Rarely does a spur develop at the true origin of the plantar fascia. A bone scan is positive in almost all studies but is nonspecific and therefore is of little diagnostic help. Radiographs rule out other sources of heel pain, including calcaneal stress fractures and tumors. Potential diagnoses of plantar medial heel pain include calcaneal stress fracture, fat pad atrophy, fat pad inflammation, plantar fascial rupture, heel spur fracture, plantar fasciitis, and compression of the first branch of the lateral plantar nerve (Baxter's nerve).

In almost all cases of heel pain syndrome, management is primarily conservative and consists of rest, anti-inflammatory medications, and orthotic devices. Studies have indicated that an inexpensive, over-the-counter heel-cushion pad is as effective as a custom-made orthosis when combined with a stretching regimen. Stretching exercises are the hallmark of conservative treatment of heel pain syndrome. They involve isolating and stretching the plantar fascia, soleus, and gastrocnemius components of the Achilles tendon complex. Management also includes a night

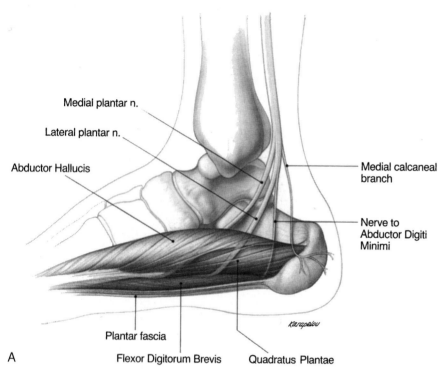

Medial plantar n.

Lateral plantar n.

Abductor Hallucis

Medial calcaneal branch

Nerve to Abductor Digiti Minimi

Plantar fascia

Flexor Digitorum Brevis

Quadratus Plantae

A

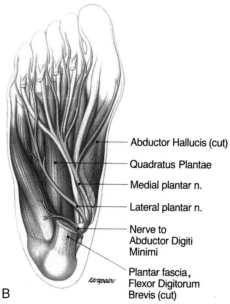

Abductor Hallucis (cut)

Quadratus Plantae

Medial plantar n.

Lateral plantar n.

Nerve to Abductor Digiti Minimi

Plantar fascia, Flexor Digitorum Brevis (cut)

B

Figure 24–65. Tarsal tunnel anatomy. (From Beskin J, Baxter D: Tarsal nerve entrapment. Oper Tech Orthop 1992;2:164.)

splint on the plantar fascia, which helps to keep the posterior calf muscles in a stretched position while the patient sleeps. The healing time is 2 to 6 months. In refractory cases, a single cortisone injection in the plantar fascia, either in isolation or in conjunction with cast immobilization, may be effective. Surgery is relegated to chronic conditions that have lasted more than 6 months or a year, cases that are refractory to conservative measures, and those with associated entrapment of the first branch of the lateral plantar nerve.

True plantar fasciitis is an inflammation of the greater central band of the plantar fascia in the midarch. The pain is often elicited by passive dorsiflexion of toes, and tenderness is elicited by palpation of the midfoot region rather than the heel. An orthosis with a plantar fascial groove to relieve the pressure on the plantar fascia, taping and strapping of the foot, and physical therapy that includes phonophoresis and other modalities are invariably effective. Like heel pain syndrome, plantar fasciitis may take 6 months or longer to resolve.

Plantar fascial rupture is characterized by plantar heel pain and has sudden onset. Ruptures are not common but have been attributed to cortisone injections in the plantar fascia proper. Management of an acute injury requires a radiographic study to rule out associated spur fracture or calcaneus body fracture. Treatment includes rest, anti-inflammatory medications, crutches, and possibly immobilization in a cast for 6 to 10 weeks.

Two lesser conditions, heel pad atrophy and subcalcaneal bursitis, are characterized by pain localized in the central weight-bearing area of the heel, beneath the calcaneal tuberosity. Commonly self-limiting, these disorders may be treated by using viscoelastic heel cups, which have characteristics similar to those of the heel pad. In a persistent case of subcalcaneal bursitis, a cortisone injection could be beneficial. Multiple cortisone injections in the plantar heel pad may create the condition of heel pad atrophy. Fat pad atrophy occurs in the elderly. Clinical examination reveals a soft, flattened heel pad that allows easy palpitation of the calcaneal tubercle. The pain is worst over the central weight-bearing portion of the heel; direct compression duplicates the patient's symptoms. Palpation does not elicit radiation of the pain. The plantar fascia is not tender. There is no role for surgery in this condition.

Entrapment of the first branch of the lateral plantar nerve occurs in approximately 15% of patients with chronic plantar heel pain. Chronic inflammation of the nerve is associated with plantar fasciitis and may occur concurrently. The exact site of entrapment is deep to the fascia of the abductor hallucis, sandwiched between the superomedial margin of the quadratus planti muscle (Fig. 24–65). Findings on examination include maximal tenderness in the area of the abductor hallucis muscle, and the plantar heel pain is re-created on palpation. Management includes conservative care similar to that for proximal plantar fasciitis. Surgical decompression is reserved for cases in which conservative treatment has failed after a course of more than 6 months. This surgery is typically performed in conjunction with a partial plantar fascial release.

Acute and Chronic Ankle Sprains

Soft tissue trauma at the level of the ankle is one of the most common injuries; sprains of the lateral ankle liga-

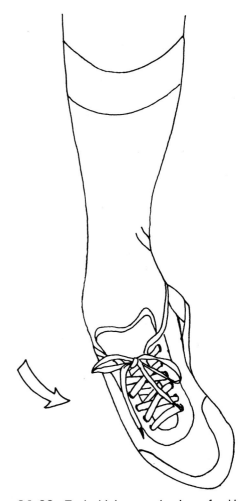

Figure 24–66. Typical injury mechanism of ankle sprain: plantarflexion, inversion, and adduction. (From Drez D, DeLee J: Management of ankle sprains. Oper Tech Sports Med 1994;2:60.)

ments predominate. The incidence of ankle sprains is 1 in 10,000 people per day, adding up to a total of 27,000 injuries. Sprains are most commonly associated with basketball, soccer, and volleyball.

The normal mechanism of injury is plantarflexion-inversion (Fig. 24–66). It is important to specify this because eversion injuries of the ankle are associated with different injury patterns. An ankle in a neutral position or dorsiflexion that undergoes an inversion injury experiences an isolated calcaneofibular ligament injury or subtalar dislocation. An external rotation–eversion injury may cause the sprain of both the deltoid and the syndesmotic ligaments. A plantarflexion-inversion injury pattern most commonly involves the ATFL, the capsule, and, less commonly, the CFL. Injuries of the PTFL rarely occur (Fig. 24–67). In a plantarflexion-inversion sprain, the patient may have noticed a pop when the injury occurred and an immediate inability to bear weight. Often the patient's history is positive for previous sprains.

Physical examination includes palpation of the tender areas in the ligamentous anatomy on the anterolateral aspect of the ankle joint. Because of the condensed anatomy and the acute nature of the injury, it is often difficult initially to define the specific structures involved. The

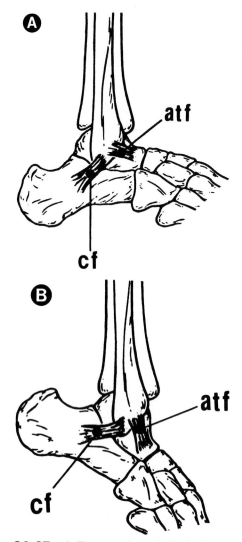

Figure 24–67. *A,* The anterior talofibular ligament runs parallel to the axis of the foot when the foot is in a neutral position. *B,* When the foot is plantarflexed, the ATFL assumes a course parallel to the axis of the tibia and fibula. (From Drez D, DeLee J: Management of ankle sprains. Oper Tech Sports Med 1994; 2:60.)

patient may have to return several weeks later, once the swelling and pain are under control, for further examination. The presence of ecchymoses and swelling in addition to the active and passive ranges of motion of ankle and subtalar joints should be documented. Assessment of the overall alignment of the lower extremity and of the relationship of the heel to the lower limb can help to determine the existence of a pronated or supinated foot pattern. A systematic approach to the anterolateral ankle includes assessment of the skin, nerves, and tendon structures in addition to the ligamentous and bony components to the ankle joint.

Several diagnostic maneuvers can help to specify and differentiate the specific ligaments involved. Each is a provocative test to re-create and assess the degree of laxity of the underlying ligament. The anterior drawer test is performed to determine the integrity of the ATFL. With the ankle in 10 degrees of plantarflexion, the foot is pulled

anteriorly as the examiner attempts to translate the talar dome in relation to the tibial plafond. The amount of translation is recorded in millimeters; there are three grades. A stable grade I injury demonstrates minimal anterior motion and a firm end point; grade II involves moderate laxity and a firm end point; grade III involves severe anterior motion and a soft end point. The talar tilt test evaluates excessive inversion or adduction by means of a varus-directed force that is applied to the lateral hindfoot while the distal medial tibia is stabilized. The results of both tests should be compared with those on the opposite (uninvolved) side. In dorsiflexion-eversion injuries, the status of the syndesmotic ligament and the distal tibiofibular joint should be assessed. A positive fibular squeeze test recreates symptoms above the level of the ankle joint; it is performed by squeezing the fibula and tibia together at the midpoint of the calf. The external rotation stress test, in which the foot is externally rotated while in a neutral position and the knee is flexed to 90 degrees, demonstrates a syndesmotic injury if pain is produced over the interosseous membrane and distal tibiofibular joint.

The differential diagnosis for lateral hindfoot injuries associated with the plantarflexion-inversion mechanism is substantial. Superficially, a neurapraxia may occur that involves either the superficial peroneal or the sural nerve distribution. Numbness in the nerve distribution and a Tinel sign are common findings. Injuries to the peroneal tendon complex may involve an acute tear or a subluxation or dislocation anteriorly. Fractures may occur at the anterior process of the os calcis, the base of the fifth metatarsal, or the lateral talar process. Intra-articular osteochondral lesions of the talus occur as the result of a shearing effect on the joint's surface that is caused by the anterolateral rotatory instability associated with injuries of the ankle ligaments.

The diagnostic study is a three-view series of plain radiographs of the ankle. Stress views may be helpful to document the number of ligaments injured and the extent of injury involved. The anterior drawer stress test, with the ankle in slight plantarflexion and the tibia stabilized, is considered abnormal if there is a difference of more than 4 mm between the translation on the injured and the uninjured sides or if it is more than 5 mm total (Fig. 24–68A). The criteria for declaring abnormal the findings of a stressed AP tilt study are variable; a tilt of more than 9 degrees is considered abnormal by some authors, and a tilt of more than 15 degrees is considered abnormal by others. Some studies indicate that more than 6 degrees of difference between the injured side and the uninvolved side is abnormal (see Fig. 24–68B). Although stress views may be helpful, there are wide variations in the recommendations for load, relaxation, manual versus mechanical stressing, duration of load, use of anesthesia, measurement method, and foot positions. Subtalar instability, which may occur in isolation or in conjunction with ankle instability, can be assessed in stressed Broden's views taken at 40 degrees. It is believed that a loss of parallelism in comparison to the nonstressed Broden view, or more than 3 mm of distal translation of the calcaneus on the talus in the anterior drawer on a lateral view, is abnormal. Syndesmotic injuries may demonstrate abnormalities on the weight-bearing AP and mortise ankle radiographs. The normal syndesmotic

Figure 24–68. *A,* On anterior drawer stress radiographs, anterior talar displacement is determined by measuring the shortest distance between the most posterior articular surface of the tibia and the talar dome. *B,* On talar tilt radiographs, talar tilt is the angle between two lines drawn parallel to the tibial plafond and the talar dome; during stress, the ankle is in a neutral position but is internally rotated 10 to 20 degrees. (From Drez D, DeLee J: Management of ankle sprains. Oper Tech Sports Med 1994;2:58–61.)

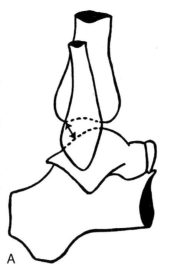
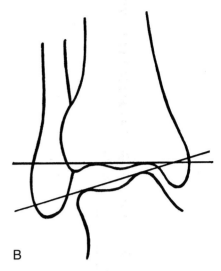

A

B

relationship is measured 1 cm above the tibial plafond. The tibiofibular clear space should be less than 6 mm. The tibiofibular overlap at that level, on the anteroposterior view, should be more than 6 mm, or 42% of the fibular width, and more than 1 mm on the mortise view to be considered normal.

Grade I and grade II ankle sprains are uniformly treated conservatively with rest, ice, elevation, compression, and protective weight bearing for the first 5 to 7 days. Rehabilitation emphasizes proprioception, strengthening, and stretching. This is followed by agility and sport-specific exercises to return the patient to the previous level of athletic activity and prevent recurrent ankle sprain. Management of grade III ankle ligament sprains is somewhat controversial. The majority of the literature supports nonoperative management for grade I and grade II injuries and the addition of a walking cast or a removable walker boot for 4 to 6 weeks for grade III injuries. It is important to immobilize the ankle between neutral to 10 degrees of dorsiflexion so as to approximate the torn ends of the ATFL. After 6 weeks, the approach is similar to that of grade I and grade II injuries. Operative intervention has been advocated for acute grade III ankle sprains in high-performance athletes only. To date, no study has proved that surgery is a superior treatment for ankle sprains. Surgical intervention creates the potential for longer rehabilitation and more complications than does conservative treatment. Furthermore, a patient can undergo surgery at a later date, if necessary; this approach has demonstrated consistently good results. In general, use of an ankle brace does not impede performance; it is easy to apply, improves balance, and does not loosen over time as taping does. The patient may be weaned from the brace as soon as approximately 50% of strength and range of motion has been achieved. Proper choice of shoes has been shown to help prevent recurrent injuries; shoes with high tops are better for resisting inversion. Several studies have demonstrated that the use of a brace or tape plus high-topped shoes is superior. Residual symptoms occur in 20 to 40% of athletes with ankle sprains. The most common cause is incomplete or suboptimal rehabilitation.

Chronic ankle instability and a history of repeated, isolated ankle sprains are secondary to mechanical instability or incompetence of the lateral ankle ligaments. When a patient complains of feeling that the ankle is giving way and he or she lacks confidence with activities, the condition is equivalent to a proprioceptive deficit, which is described as functional instability. Initial management includes conservative treatment with appropriate additional physical therapy, excellent arch support, and proprioceptive and peroneal strengthening. This approach has been reported to be effective in 50% of cases of chronic ankle pain. In refractory cases of mechanical instability, surgery has been recommended to restore stability to the lateral ankle ligaments. Typical procedures fall into two main categories of anatomic and nonanatomic procedures. The most popular anatomic procedure, the Brostrom procedure, uses the original ligaments to retension the ATFL and CFL. Its advantage is that it preserves the peroneals; however, it may be less successful in patients who have generalized hypermobility or a subtalar component in the ankle instability. The nonanatomic procedures have been reported to have an 80 to 90% success rate. They use the peroneus brevis tendon in various degrees to weave together the lateral ankle ligaments (Fig. 24–69). Multiple techniques and procedures have been described, but to date no ideal procedure exists. Nonanatomic ligament reconstruction has the potential for overtightening, which causes excessive stiffness in addition to the loss and weakening of the peroneus brevis tendon.

A common source of chronic ankle symptoms after a sprain is an osteochondral lesion of the talus. This mechanism involves the lateral subluxation and rotation of the talus around the deltoid ligament axis, a circumstance present in true mechanical instability. It may cause either medial or lateral osteochondral lesions of the talus, as the convex talus abuts the anterior edge of the tibia. Studies have independently reported rates of occurrence as high as 7% after ankle sprains. Symptoms are often vague, mild, and intermittent and include stiffness, swelling, catching, clicking, and occasionally giving way. The mechanism of injury remains controversial. The two main pathologies attributed to this disorder are spontaneous osteonecrosis

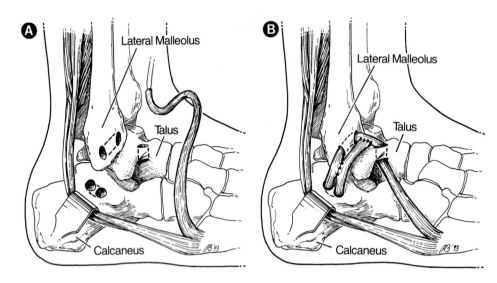

Figure 24–69. *A* and *B,* Modification of Elm technique. Graft is passed through tunnels in the talus, calcaneus, and lateral malleolus deep to the peroneal tendon. (From Drez D, DeLee J: Management of ankle sprains. Oper Tech Sports Med 1994;2[1].)

and trauma. Lateral lesions are produced by strong inversion of a dorsiflexed foot; the tibia is internally rotated. A strong inversion force to a plantarflexed foot produces medial lesions, and the tibia is externally rotated (Fig. 24–70).

The incidence of osteochondral lesions of the talus is 4% of all cases of osteochondritis dissecans. Patients are usually in their second or third decade. Medial dome lesions are more common than lateral lesions, yet lateral lesions are more often associated with trauma. The incidence of bilaterality is 10%. Medial dome lesions are located posteriorly, whereas lateral dome lesions are found anteriorly. Lateral lesions are shallow, wafer-shaped, and commonly displaced; medial lesions are deeper, cup-shaped, and nondisplaced.

Physical examination reveals tenderness medially or laterally, pain on range of motion, overall decreased motion, swelling, weakness, and occasional instability. Lesions are categorized according to the Berndt-Hardy classifications, which are based on plain radiographic studies.

Stage I: a small area of compression
Stage II: a separate, nondisplaced fragment
Stage III: a hinged, detached fragment
Stage IV: a frank, loose body.

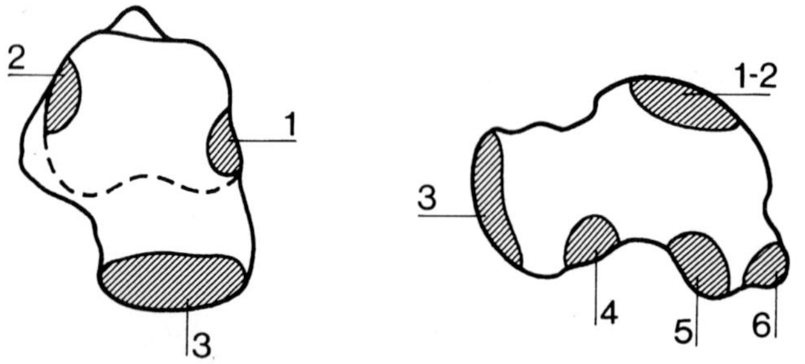

Figure 24–70. Localized necrosis of the talus. 1 and 2, crest of the trochlea; 3, head of the talus; 4 and 5, base of the talus; 6, posterior talar tubercle (os trigonum). (From Jahss M [ed]: Disorders of the Foot and Ankle: Medical and Surgical Management, 2nd ed, Vol I. Philadelphia, WB Saunders, 1991, p 621.)

Further diagnostic workup may include CT and MRI. CT scans have been shown to be particularly helpful preoperatively and for staging.

Acute stage I and stage II lesions are best managed nonoperatively at first, with non–weight-bearing cast immobilization and activity restriction. Treatment depends on lesion size and location and the patient's age, activity level, and symptoms. Chronic stage I and stage II lesions and acute stage III and stage IV lesions are treated surgically. Options in surgical treatment include excision of loose bodies, drilling of intact lesions, debridement and drilling of unstable lesions, or bone grafting with internal fixation (Fig. 24–71). Generally, patients 15 years old or younger have better healing potential following excision of a lesion.

Arthritic Conditions of the Foot and Ankle

Although the ankle joint is more commonly injured than the foot, it less commonly becomes symptomatically degenerative. Causes of ankle joint degeneration include primary osteoarthritis, trauma secondary to avascular necrosis, osteochondritis dissecans, synovial chondromatosis, and rheumatic conditions.

Conservative management of ankle conditions includes taking anti-inflammatory medications, wearing a lace-up style ankle brace and a solid ankle cushioned heel (SACH) rocker-bottom shoe to absorb and minimize ankle excursion, and receiving cortisone injections. Bracing may include an ankle-foot orthosis or a patellar tendon-bearing modification to minimize joint motion and unload axial forces, respectively (Fig. 24–72). Surgical management of early ankle arthrosis is dependent on the extent and location of the arthrosis. It is not uncommon for the anterior ankle joint to develop osteophytes at the talus and tibia; they create a bony or a soft tissue impingement lesion. These impingement syndromes are best treated by arthroscopic or open resection of the osteophytes. Ankle arthrodesis remains the salvage procedure of choice in cases of recalcitrant ankle pain and global involvement of the ankle; a satisfaction rate as high as 90% has been observed. An alternative to ankle arthrodesis is the third-generation total ankle prosthesis. Prior generations met with higher failure

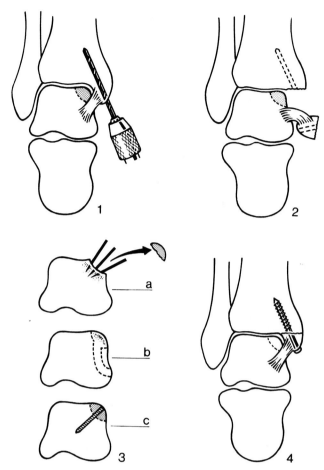

Figure 24–71. Surgical treatment of osteochondritis of the talus. *1,* Transmalleolar approach to the talus. Before the osteotomy, the malleolus is drilled. *2,* The medial malleolus is retracted downward. *3,* One of three possible approaches may be used: *a,* the ossicle is removed and the matrix is drilled; *b,* the necrotic tissue underneath the joint cartilage is removed; or *c,* a free body with normal cartilage is fixed with a pin. *4,* The tibial malleolus is replaced and fixed with an AO screw. (From Jahss M [ed]: Disorders of the Foot and Ankle: Medical and Surgical Management, 2nd ed, Vol I. Philadelphia, WB Saunders, 1991, p 624.)

rates and difficulty in salvage. Total ankle arthroplasty may be indicated in patients who have rheumatoid arthritis and in less active patients who have osteoarthritis. The potential advantages over arthrodesis are minimization of stress on adjacent joints and early mobilization with an improved gait pattern as a result of motion retention. Contraindications include significant ligamentous laxity and varus and valgus deformities of more than 20 degrees.

OSTEOARTHRITIS

The Hindfoot. Osteoarthritis of the hindfoot is most commonly due to trauma leading to abnormal loading stresses and altered biomechanics. Most cases are related to calcaneus fractures, but high-energy injuries of the ankle and midfoot may affect the subtalar joint secondarily and lead to symptomatic arthrosis. Subtalar arthrosis is frequently mistaken for ankle pain; it presents with swelling and pain after exertion. The patient complains of difficulty with

ambulation on uneven surfaces. Physical examination shows pain in the sinus tarsi region laterally and limitation of inversion and eversion. Radiographic studies, including weight-bearing lateral and Broden's views, demonstrate narrowing of the joint space, subchondral sclerosis, and, occasionally, lateral wall osteophytes. Radiographs of the ankle allow evaluation of the lateral recess for evidence of impingement in cases of calcaneus fractures and severe pes planovalgus deformities.

Goals of treatment include, as with other arthritic joints, pain relief, correction and prevention of deformities, and restoration and preservation of function. Nonoperative management includes anti-inflammatory medications, reduced activity, and shoe modification using orthoses. Control of subtalar motion requires a University of California Berkley Laboratory (UCBL) orthosis or an ankle-foot orthosis (Fig. 24–73). Surgery is reserved for refractory cases; it entails primary subtalar arthrodesis and bone grafting. In cases involving significant calcaneal loss of height such as prior calcaneal fracture malunions, restoration of the axial height may be accomplished by means of a distraction bone block arthrodesis of the subtalar joint using a tricortical iliac crest graft.

The Midfoot. Osteoarthritis in the midfoot is most commonly secondary to trauma such as midtarsal intra-articular fracture and Lisfranc fracture-dislocation at a tarsometatarsal joint. It may be localized to involved joints or may be more global in nature. Prominent dorsal osteophytes may cause irritation and nerve compression if lace-up shoes are worn. Physical examination may reveal mild swelling of the midfoot over dorsal prominences or asymmetrical loss of the medial longitudinal arch secondary to collapse resulting from previous fracture. Radiographs should include an AP projection angled 15 degrees cephalad to maximize visualization of the tarsometatarsal joints. An internal oblique radiograph best projects the middle and lateral columns at a 45-degree angle. An external oblique view may similarly delineate the status of the medial column. Lateral radiographs demonstrate the apex of deformity in the presence of longitudinal arch loss. Ancillary studies such as collimated technetium Tc 99m bone scans and CT help to confirm and correlate a patient's complaints with specific symptomatic joints.

Conservative treatment includes shoe modifications, orthoses, and anti-inflammatory medications. Shoes are padded on the uppers to prevent irritation of the dorsal osteophytes, and the outer sole provides plantar support. Surgical management of symptomatic midfoot arthrosis is reserved for cases refractory to conservative measures. Preoperatively, selective lidocaine blocks may help to delineate the specific joints to be addressed. Surgical options include (1) osteophyte excision when the primary complaints are due to dorsal skin or nerve irritation and (2) arthrodesis with bone grafting and rigid internal fixation in the presence of focal and global symptomatic arthrosis involving the midtarsus (Fig. 24–74).

RHEUMATOID ARTHRITIS

Rheumatoid arthritis is a systemic disease that commonly involves the foot, where there are many joints lined with synovium, so active rheumatoid disease may produce wide-

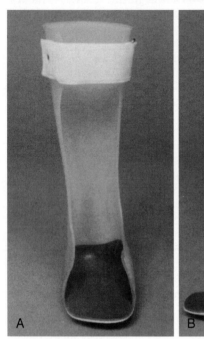
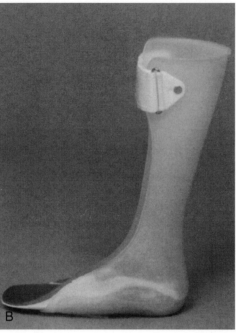

Figure 24–72. Frontal view *(A)* and side view *(B)* of a long, solid, ankle-foot orthosis for a patient with stage III posterior tibialis tendon dysfunction who is symptomatic secondary to lateral fibular abutment. A semirigid orthosis is placed inside to better accommodate the forefoot's deformity. (From Sferra JJ, Rosenberg GA: Nonoperative treatment of posterior tibial tendon pathology. Foot Ankle Clin 1997;2:267.)

Figure 24–73. Frontal view *(A)* and side view *(B)* of a UCBL orthotic made of ⁹⁄₁₆-inch polypropylene. PPT is used to pad any bony prominence of the medial column. (From Sferra JJ, Rosenberg GA: Nonoperative treatment of posterior tibial tendon pathology. Foot Ankle Clin 1997;2:265.)

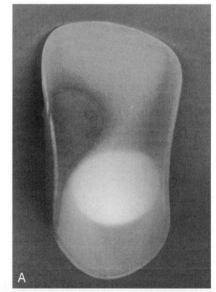
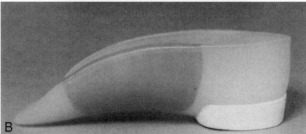

DEGENERATIVE PATTERNS

I. Arthritic or decompensated first metatarsal–medial cuneiform joint

SURGICAL OPTIONS

Fusion of the first metatarsal–cuneiform joint with two-screw fixation and an iliac crest bone graft

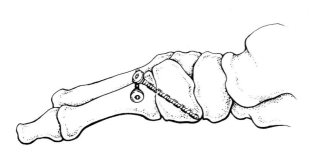

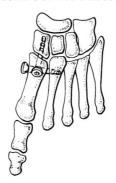

Type I

II. Overload, degenerative joint disease, or both of the second metatarsal with an incompetent first ray; short or hypermobile first ray

III. Diastasis

Fusion of the first and second metatarsal–cuneiform joints with the optional use of a stabilization screw for the first metatarsophalangeal joint and an iliac crest bone graft

Reduction of the Lisfranc ligament region with a lag screw between the first cuneiform and the base of the second metatarsal and an iliac crest bone graft

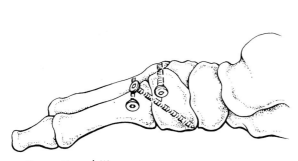

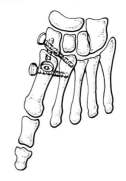

Types II and III

IV. Global involvement

a. Trauma

b. Charcot's foot
c. Rheumatoid arthritis

Reduction of subluxation with an optional small distractor

a. Screws at the bases of the first, second, and third metatarsal–cuneiform joints
b. Optional pin fixation for the fourth and fifth rays
c. Iliac crest bone grafting

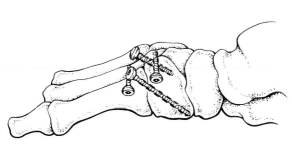

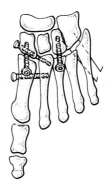

Type IV

Figure 24–74. Surgical options for specific types of midfoot breakdown. (From Gould J [ed]: Operative Foot Surgery. Philadelphia, WB Saunders, 1994, p 174.)

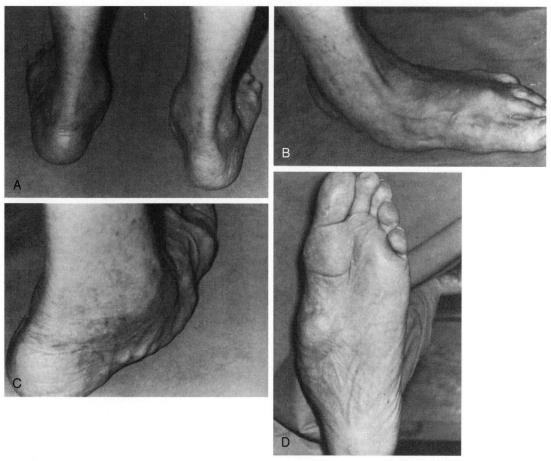

Figure 24–75. *A* and *B*, Posterior and lateral standing views of a patient with rheumatoid arthritis demonstrating loss of posterior tibial tendon function, collapse of the medial longitudinal arch, and increased hindfoot valgus on the left. *C*, Note the prominence of the head of the talus along the medial foot, which is associated with forefoot pronation. *D*, Callosity on the posterior medial aspect of the same foot. (From Gould J [ed]: Operative Foot Surgery. Philadelphia, WB Saunders, 1994, p 293.)

spread foot pain. The disease affects both the synovial lining of the joints and the tendons of the foot and ankle. Rheumatoid involvement of the ankle is found in 9 to 42% of such patients and its extent is related to duration of systemic illness. Physical examination reveals antalgic gait, global swelling, and decreased sagittal plane motion. There is coronal plane malalignment, which manifests as a valgus deformity of the hindfoot; it may originate in the ankle or, more commonly, in the subtalar joint. An increasing valgus deformity, with resultant subtalar joint pain, is related to calcaneofibular abutment and sinus tarsi impingement. Weight-bearing radiographs of the ankle and foot are essential for delineating the apex of the deformity and the presence of valgus angulation at either the ankle or the subtalar joint. Radiographic changes often precede a restricted level of function and profusion of symptoms.

The Ankle. Management of a rheumatoid ankle includes education, activity modification, intermittent corticosteroid injections, optimal medical management, and the use of an ankle or patellar tendon–bearing (PTB) ankle-foot orthosis and shoe modifications. Surgical options include synovectomy, ankle arthrodesis, and total ankle arthroplasty. Syno-

vitis in the ankle can be treated with an open or arthroscopic synovectomy. The washout may decrease the synovitic load on the ankle joint but is a temporizing measure at best. Arthrodesis remains the only reliable and durable procedure to treat a painful rheumatoid ankle. Indications include intractable pain, significant deformity, loss of range of motion, failed prior arthrodesis, and total arthroplasty. Techniques are similar to those described for osteoarthritis of the ankle, but there is the need for additional fixation due to the poor bone quality. In the presence of subtalar joint involvement, as seen in cases of global talar avascular necrosis resulting from steroid use, a tibiotalar calcaneal arthrodesis may be required. It can be performed by internal fixation using cannulated screws or a retrograde intermedullary rod. Total ankle arthroplasty has historically been plagued by dismal long-term results. Preliminary results of third-generation arthroplasties may signify a resurgence in the use of this procedure. Its advantage over arthrodesis in the rheumatoid patient is the minimization of stress transference to adjacent joints, which occurs in an isolated ankle fusion. Additionally, maintaining a mobile segment between the MTP and knee joints avoids a severely stiff gait with bilateral involvement.

The Hindfoot. Rheumatoid involvement of the hindfoot typically presents with pain "around the ankle" and is often associated with edema and synovitis of the subtalar joint that becomes worse with weight bearing (Fig. 24–75). The patient complains of a collapsed hindfoot and lateral impingement pain. Nonoperative treatment of hindfoot arthrosis includes the use of a soft UCBL with a rocker sole, a small heel lift, and medial or lateral flaring of the outer sole to add stability. With early hindfoot collapse an off-the-shelf athletic ankle brace is helpful; an ankle-foot orthosis is necessary for advanced deformities.

Operative treatment of rheumatic disorders of the hindfoot includes arthrodesis of the subtalar joint, the talonavicular joint, or both, and of the calcaneocuboid joint (triple arthrodesis). Hindfoot surgery, in the presence of other major involvement of the lower extremity, requires that the hip or knee be aligned initially so as to determine overall alignment and thus position the hindfoot properly. The goal of hindfoot arthrodesis in a rheumatoid patient is to provide pain relief, improve function and alignment, and provide a stable platform for ambulation.

The Midfoot. Midfoot involvement in rheumatoid arthritis is not seen as commonly as is forefoot and hindfoot involvement. Unremitting synovitis results in capsular weakening, which creates subluxation and a painful, debilitating flatfoot condition. Evaluation reveals hypermobility of the midtarsus joints in both the sagittal and transverse planes and the presence of mild warmth and fullness. Discomfort is elicited with range of motion of the central three tarsometatarsal joints. When a planovalgus foot deformity develops, the fourth and fifth metatarsal cuboid joints are often spared because of the added laxity of the subtalar and midtarsus joints. This results in forefoot abduction relative to the hindfoot and in the shortening of the peroneal tendons and the tightening of the gastrocnemius-soleus complex. This results in the alteration of the gait cycle; excessive midfoot collapse and pronation of the foot occur early in the cycle, and the foot does not return to a neutral, stable platform before terminal stance and toe-off.

Radiographic evaluation of midfoot deformities includes standing AP, lateral, and oblique radiographs to assess the congruency of the tarsometatarsal joints and the evidence of subluxation of the first tarsometatarsal joint. There is a widened space between the medial cuneiform bone and the lateral base of the second metatarsal in the Lisfranc region. As is true in most cases of flat feet acquired in adulthood, an increased talar–first metatarsal angle is consistent with a forefoot abduction deformity. A standing lateral view demonstrates dorsal osteophytes over the first and second tarsometatarsal joints. Management consists of arresting the midfoot synovitis by means of a short leg, weight-bearing cast for 4 weeks followed by orthoses with medial heel wedges or, in advanced cases, ankle-foot orthoses. Stretching the Achilles tendon complex helps to relieve midfoot stresses. Cortisone injection is limited to the first tarsometatarsal joint in conjunction with casting. Surgery is reserved for patients with greater functional demands who refuse treatment by the wearing of braces. The technique involves stabilizing the medical arch by means of arthrodesis so as to restore weight-bearing status and thus minimize the pain in arthritic lateral joints. Typically, the

first, second, and third tarsometatarsal joints are involved in fusion; rarely, the fourth and fifth metatarsal cuboid joints are included.

The Forefoot. Involvement of the forefoot is the initial presentation of patients with rheumatoid arthritis in 17% of cases. Ultimately, the feet are involved in 89% of patients with rheumatoid arthritis. Initially unilateral in presentation, patients eventually develop symmetrical bilateral involvement. The forefoot is by far the most commonly involved area.

The pathophysiology entails synovitis in the MTP joints, which causes articular cartilage destruction and ligamentous and capsular laxity. Intractable synovitis results in the weakening of the stabilizing structures of the MTP joints, so they sublux dorsally as a result of ground reaction forces. The destabilization of the MTP joints pulls the plantar weight-bearing pad and plantar plate distally, uncovering the metatarsal head and creating intractable metatarsalgia. The first ray commonly deforms as a hallux valgus secondary to the laterally directed force of shoe wear and the loss of the second toe buttress (Fig. 24–76). The physical presentation is pain secondary to metatarsalgia caused by exposed plantar metatarsal heads. Associated fixed flexion deformities of the PIP and DIP joints create painful dorsal and terminal callosities, respectively. Conservative management includes splinting and strapping the toes, cortisone injections, and combined soft orthotics and stiff-soled rocker shoes to offload the MTP joints and minimize laxity. Toe spacers, sleeves, and crest pads offload and protect painful callosities by splinting and straightening the toes.

Indications for operative intervention include reduction of pain, improved ambulatory function, improved shoe-wear options, and cosmesis. Surgery involves the stabilization of the first ray, the reduction of the lesser MTP joints,

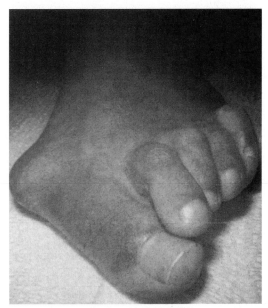

Figure 24–76. Hallux tortus. Severe hallux valgus with an associated pronation deformation. (From Holmes G: Reconstruction of the forefoot in rheumatoid arthritis. Sem Arthroplast 1992;3[1]:11.)

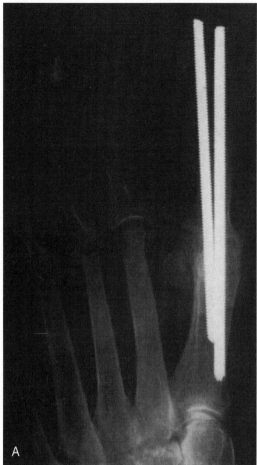

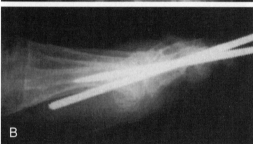

Figure 24–77. Anteroposterior *(A)* and lateral *(B)* views of MTP arthrodesis using threaded Steinmann pins. (From Holmes GH: Reconstruction of the forefoot in rheumatoid arthritis. Sem Arthroplast 1992;3:14.)

and the relocation of the fat pads so as to provide a suitable weight-bearing structure. It usually includes arthrodesis of the first MTP joint to provide permanent stability to the medial column and PIP and metatarsal head resection arthroplasties to relocate the lesser toes (Fig. 24–77). Complications of forefoot surgery in cases of rheumatoid arthritis include problems with wound healing, infection, nonunion, malunion, recurrence of deformities of the lesser toes, and recurrent metatarsalgia.

Neural Conditions of the Foot and Ankle

Nerve entrapment may involve any of the five major nerves that cross the foot and ankle. The most common conditions

are tarsal tunnel syndrome at the level of the ankle and interdigital neuroma in the plantar forefoot. Entrapment of the posterior tibial nerve within the fibro-osseous tunnel posterior and distal to the medial malleolus is referred to as tarsal tunnel syndrome (Fig. 24–78). The cause is identified in only about 50% of cases; it may be extrinsic or intrinsic. Malalignment causes a planovalgus foot deformity that stretches the tibial nerve. Intrinsic conditions include proliferative rheumatoid synovitis and exostosis adjacent to the tarsal tunnel. Extrinsic causes are common and include tumor within the tarsal tunnel, lipoma, ganglion cyst, varicosity, neurilemoma, and anomalous muscles. Tarsal tunnel syndrome is a complex of symptoms characterized by burning pain in the arch, vague numbness in the toes, and pain that is accentuated by ambulation and is also present at night. Motor deficits and intrinsic muscle paresis and paralysis are common late findings. A patient may present with proximal medial radiation of pain to the midcalf. Tarsal tunnel syndrome has been positively correlated with pregnancy; bilaterality is rare.

Physical findings in about half of patients include a positive percussion test over the posterior tibial nerve that re-creates the pain. A Tinel sign may be present along with numbness of the sole and tenderness behind and below the medial malleolus. Electromyographic nerve conduction studies are helpful in ruling out lumbar disk disease as the source of the symptoms. Diagnostic findings for medial plantar nerve involvement include terminal latency in the abductor hallucis of more than 6.2 msec. Similarly, a prolonged latency of more than 7 msec in the abductor digiti quinti is consistent with lateral plantar nerve involvement. Sensory latencies, however, are the most sensitive tests in more than 90% of cases. Bilateral lower extremities should be tested to rule out involvement of the lower lumbar root and proximal neurologic pathology. MRI may be helpful in delineating space-occupying lesions.

Treatment includes anti-inflammatory medications and medial wedges and orthoses to control hindfoot valgus and decrease the tension across the tunnel. Cortisone injection and bracing to rest the nerve may be helpful. Surgery involves decompressing the flexor retinaculum overlying the tarsal tunnel and must be extended to include releasing the superficial calcaneal branch of the tibial nerve and tracing the plantar branches distally through the abductor hallucis muscle. Resection of any space-occupying lesions is included. Internal neurolysis is indicated where nerve fibrosis occurs. Tarsal tunnel release produces improvement in 75% of cases and no change in 25%. When space-occupying lesions are identified, good results can be expected in 95% of cases.

Plantar interdigital nerves are terminal branches of the medial and lateral plantar nerves. Morton's neuroma is believed to be a reaction of the plantar interdigital nerve to compression by the distal transverse metatarsal ligament; tight shoes create traction in the interdigital nerve around the intermetatarsal ligament (Fig. 24–79). The unique anatomy of the third interdigital nerve, which is composed of contributions from both the lateral and the medial plantar nerves, puts the third web space at greatest risk for development of Morton's neuroma (Fig. 24–80). The distribution of idiopathic Morton's neuroma is as follows: 85% of cases occur in the third web space and 15% in the second web

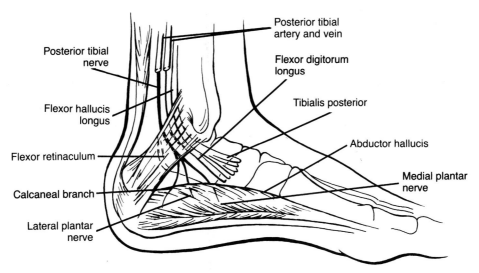

Figure 24–78. Anatomy of the tarsal tunnel and the posterior tibial nerve. (From Gould J [ed]: Operative Foot Surgery. Philadelphia, WB Saunders, 1994, p 188.)

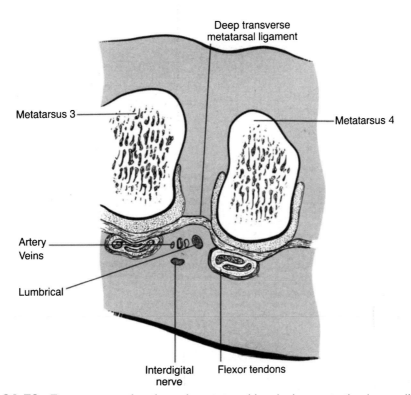

Figure 24–79. Transverse section through metatarsal heads demonstrating bones, ligament, tendons, and nerve. (From Gould J [ed]: Operative Foot Surgery. Philadelphia, WB Saunders, 1994, p 114.)

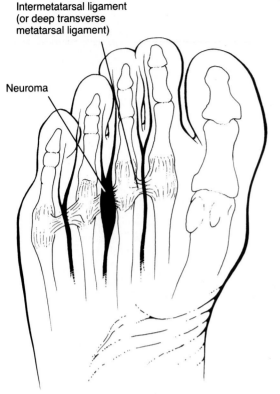

Intermetatarsal ligament
(or deep transverse
metatarsal ligament)

Neuroma

Figure 24–80. Nerve passing over deep metatarsal ligament as seen from the plantar aspect. (From Gould J [ed]: Operative Foot Surgery. Philadelphia, WB Saunders, 1994, p 114.)

ganglion cysts. Symptoms include vague, intermittent pain that increases in intensity and duration with weight bearing. Wearing wide shoes and rubbing the feet typically help. It is usually localized but may radiate into the third and fourth digits. Diagnosis is confirmed in the presence of decreased sensation in the third and fourth toes and a palpable plantar nerve that elicits a Mulder click, in which the neuroma pops out from between the compressed metatarsal heads. Diagnosis may be confirmed by injecting a local anesthetic into the third web space. Treatment consists of modifying shoes and placing metatarsal pads proximal to the third and fourth metatarsal heads to help spread the transverse metatarsal ligament and unload the impingement on the underlying nerve. External shoe modifications, including a metatarsal bar, may help to unload the forefoot. Administering local steroid injections in addition to anti-inflammatory medications has also been advocated.

Operative intervention is reserved for refractory cases. A dorsal approach is used to resect an approximately 3-cm length of the nerve. Surgical resection of the neuroma yields good to excellent results in 75 to 80% of cases. Complications that may arise in neuroma resection include symptomatic end-stump neuroma and recurrence. With recurrence, a plantar approach to the intermetatarsal space may be used when resecting the neuroma to a more proximal level.

Selected Bibliography

Gould J (ed): Operative Foot Surgery. Philadelphia, WB Saunders, 1994.

Guten G (ed): Running Injuries, 1st ed. Philadelphia, WB Saunders, 1997.

Jahss M (ed): Disorders of the Foot and Ankle: Medical and Surgical Management, 2nd ed. Philadelphia, WB Saunders, 1991.

Mann R, Coughlin M (eds): Surgery of the Foot and Ankle, 6th ed. Philadelphia, Mosby, 1993.

Myerson M (ed): Foot and Ankle Clinics. Philadelphia, WB Saunders, 2000.

Sarrafian S (ed): Anatomy of the Foot and Ankle, 2nd ed. New York, JB Lippincott, 1993.

space. Neuromas do not form in the first and fourth web spaces. In assessing a patient with symptomatic interdigital neuroma, it is important to assess for adjacent MTP synovitis, crossover toe deformities that create traction against the adjacent nerve, synovial cysts in the MTP joint, and

Index

Note: Page numbers followed by f refer to figures; page numbers followed by t refer to tables.

A

Abrasive wear, 47, 47f
Abscess(es)
Brodie's, 153
hand, 651–653
spinal infection and, 493, 497, 498f, 499, 500f, 501
Absorptiometry, dual energy x-ray, in assessment of bone density, 94, 202–203, 205f
Abused child(ren), 434–435
characteristic fractures in, 435, 435f
Accretion, following initial calcification, in mineral phase of bone, 31, 31f
Acetabular labrum, 276, 677, 679
Acetabulum, 667, 668f. See also *Hip.*
development of, 667
fractures of, 691–692, 694, 696
computed tomography of, 84f, 673, 677f
radiography of, 691, 694f, 695f
osteotomy of, 683, 683f
position of femoral head in, 351, 353f. See also *Femur, head of.*
Achilles tendon, 770, 773f
injuries resulting from overuse of, 780, 813f, 813–815, 814f
rupture of, 780, 815–816
mechanism of injury in, 815, 815f
Thompson test for, 780, 815
Achondroplasia, 316–317, 317f
Acidosis, renal tubular, 219
Acromegaly, 219
Acromioclavicular joint, 512, 513f, 518–519, 520f. See also *Shoulder.*
arthritis of, 551–553
diagnosis of, 552
lidocaine injection test in, 552, 553f
radiography in, 552, 552f
treatment of, 552–553
corticosteroid injection in, as therapy for arthritis, 552
cross-body adduction testing of, 548, 550f, 552
lidocaine injection in, to test for arthritis, 552, 553f
separation or sprain of, 539–541
classification of, 539f, 539–540
diagnosis of, 266, 267f, 540, 540f
stress x-rays in, 269, 269f, 540, 541f
mechanism of injury in, 539, 539f

Acromioclavicular joint *(Continued)*
"step-off" due to, 540, 540f
treatment of, 540–541
Zanca view of, 529, 531f
in detection of arthritic changes, 552, 552f
Acromion
classification of structure of, 547, 550f
ossification of
axillary radiographic view in detection of, 415f, 547, 549f
risk of impingement associated with, 547
Acute hematogenous osteomyelitis, 148–153. See also *Osteomyelitis.*
Adamantinoma, 179–180
Adduction contracture, of hip, in cerebral palsy, 325
Adduction testing, cross-body, of acromioclavicular joint, 548, 550f, 552
Adenoma, parathyroid, 207
Adhesive capsulitis, 553–554
arthrographic diagnosis of, 529, 553–554
Adhesive wear, 47, 47f
Adolescent(s). See also *Child(ren).*
bunion deformity in, 372–373
idiopathic scoliosis in, 388
treatment of, 388, 390–392
Adson test, 52, 54f
Advancement flaps, 295f, 295–296, 296f
V-Y, 295–296, 296f
for fingertip injuries, 627, 627f
Aggrecan, in articular cartilage, 19, 19f
Aging
and changes in articular cartilage, 21
and changes in electrophysiologic responses, 101
and development of osteoporosis, 211t, 212
Alcoholic(s), Saturday night palsy in, 108
Alendronate, for osteoporosis, 213
Allen test, 526, 603, 604f
Allopurinol, for gout, 255
Aluminum blocks, x-ray absorption by, as referent for bone densitometry, 202, 204f
Alveolar rhabdomyosarcoma, 194
Alveolar soft tissue sarcoma, 191
American Rheumatological Association (ARA) criteria, for characteristics of rheumatoid arthritis, 243t
Amitriptyline, for fibromyalgia, 247
Amputation
congenital, 656
neuroma formation following, 189

Amputation *(Continued)*
osteomyelitis management via, 144
replantation following, in hand and finger surgery, 632–633
tumor resection via, 166
Anatomic snuffbox, palpation over, 60, 60f
Ancient medicine, fracture treatment in, Hippocrates and, 117, 117f
Anesthesia, in Civil War–era medicine, 118f
Aneurysmal bone cyst, 172, 173f
spinal involvement in, 487, 488f
Angiogenesis, in wound healing, 281, 283
Angiolipoma, 186
Angiosarcoma, 181, 188f
Angiosomes, 292f
Angular deformity, of knee, in child with cerebral palsy, 327
Angular limb malalignment, 307
Anisotropic vs. isotropic materials, 36f
Ankle. See also *Foot.*
anatomy of, 767–778
arthritis involving, 822–823, 826
treatment of, 822–823, 824f
Broden view of, 77, 80f, 786, 786f, 796f
calcaneonavicular bar between bones of, 371
coalition of bones of, 371
calcaneonavicular bar in, 371, 371f
talocalcaneal bar in, 371, 371f, 372, 372f
deep peroneal nerve entrapment at, 110, 781
equinus deformity of, in child with cerebral palsy, 327–328
fractures of, 788–790, 789f
in child, 432, 432f, 433f
Harris view of, 77, 80f, 785
hindfoot views of, 77, 80f. See also *Hindfoot/heel.*
instability of, 821
surgery for, 821, 822f
testing for, 69–70, 70f, 268, 269f, 780, 781f
joint spaces of, radiographic criteria for abnormalities in, 790f
ligaments of, 768, 769f
medial malleolar fracture of, in child, 432, 432f
pain in, nonarthritic regional syndromes associated with, 239t
physical examination of, 69–70, 779–782
for instability. See *Ankle, instability of, testing for.*
for subtalar synovitis, 780–781, 781f
posterior tibial nerve entrapment at, 110, 781–782, 828

ISBN 0-7216-8189-1

90038

9 780721 681894